The American Psychiatric Association Publishing

TEXTBOOK of

PSYCHOSOMATIC MEDICINE

and CONSULTATION-LIAISON

PSYCHIATRY

THIRD EDITION

The American Psychiatric Association Publishing

TEXTBOOK of

PSYCHOSOMATIC MEDICINE
and CONSULTATION-LIAISON PSYCHIATRY

THIRD EDITION

EDITED BY

James L. Levenson, M.D.

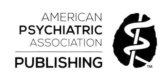

AMERICAN
PSYCHIATRIC
ASSOCIATION
PUBLISHING

If you wish to buy 50 or more copies of the same title, please go to www.appi.org/specialdiscounts for more information.

Copyright © 2019 American Psychiatric Association Publishing
ALL RIGHTS RESERVED

Manufactured in the United States of America on acid-free paper
22 21 20 19 18   5 4 3 2 1
Third Edition

Typeset in Palatino and Helvetica Neue.

American Psychiatric Association Publishing
800 Maine Avenue S.W., Suite 900
Washington, DC 20024
www.appi.org

Library of Congress Cataloging-in-Publication Data
Names: Levenson, James L., editor.
Title: The American Psychiatric Association Publishing textbook of psychosomatic medicine and consultation-liaison psychiatry / edited by James L. Levenson.
Other titles: American Psychiatric Publishing textbook of psychosomatic medicine
Description: Third edition. | Washington, D.C. : American Psychiatric Association Publishing, [2019] | Preceded by American Psychiatric Publishing textbook of psychosomatic medicine : psychiatric care of the medically ill / edited by James L. Levenson. 2nd ed. 2011. | Includes bibliographical references and index.
Identifiers: LCCN 2018023613 (print) | LCCN 2018024419 (ebook) | ISBN 9781615371990 (ebook) | ISBN 9781615371365 (hardcover : alk. paper)
Subjects: | MESH: Psychophysiologic Disorders—therapy | Psychophysiologic Disorders—diagnosis | Psychosomatic Medicine—methods | Referral and Consultation
Classification: LCC RC49 (ebook) | LCC RC49 (print) | NLM WM 90 | DDC 616.08—dc23
LC record available at https://lccn.loc.gov/2018023613

British Library Cataloguing in Publication Data
A CIP record is available from the British Library.

This book is dedicated to all of those from whom I have learned:

To my teachers and supervisors,
my colleagues in and outside of psychiatry and psychosomatic medicine,
from whom I have learned to be a better psychiatrist and physician.

To my students, residents, and fellows,
from whom I have learned to be a better teacher.

To my patients,
from whom I have learned to be a better doctor and therapist.

To my family and friends,
from whom I have learned to be better in love and friendship.

Contents

PART I
General Principles in Evaluation and Management

PART II
Symptoms and Disorders

PART III
Specialties and Subspecialties

PART IV
Treatment

Contributors

Yesne Alici, M.D.
Assistant Attending Psychiatrist, Clinical Director of the Psychiatry Service, Department of Psychiatry and Behavioral Sciences, Memorial Sloan-Kettering Cancer Center, New York, New York

Andrew R. Alkis, M.D.
Consultation-Liaison Psychiatrist, Psychiatry Inpatient Services, Novant Health, Forsyth Medical Center, Winston-Salem, North Carolina

David J. Axelrod, M.D., J.D.
Associate Professor, Department of Internal Medicine, Jefferson Medical College; Director, Sickle Cell Program, Thomas Jefferson University Hospital, Philadelphia, Pennsylvania

Robert Bahnsen, M.D.
Clinical Assistant Professor, Department of Psychiatry and Human Behavior, Thomas Jefferson University, Philadelphia, Pennsylvania

Rosemary Basson, M.D.
Clinical Professor, Department of Psychiatry, University of British Columbia, Vancouver, British Columbia, Canada

Madeleine Becker, M.D., M.A.
Director, Consultation Liaison Psychiatry and Hospital Psychiatry, Thomas Jefferson University Hospital, Department of Psychiatry and Human Behavior, Philadelphia, Pennsylvania

Charles H. Bombardier, Ph.D.
Professor, Department of Rehabilitation Medicine, University of Washington School of Medicine, Seattle, Washington

John Michael Bostwick, M.D.
Professor of Psychiatry, Mayo Clinic College of Medicine, Rochester, Minnesota

William Breitbart, M.D.
Chairman, Jimmie C. Holland Chair in Psychiatric Oncology, Department of Psychiatry and Behavioral Sciences; Attending Psychiatrist, Supportive Care Service, Department of Medicine, Memorial Sloan-Kettering Cancer Center; Professor of Clinical Psychiatry, Department of Psychiatry, Weill Medical College of Cornell University, New York, New York

Rebecca W. Brendel, M.D., J.D.
Director of Law and Ethics, Center for Law, Brain, and Behavior, and Psychiatrist, Massachusetts General Hospital, Boston, Massachusetts; Director, Master of Bioethics Degree Program, and Assistant Professor of Psychiatry, Harvard Medical School, Boston, Massachusetts

E. Sherwood Brown, M.D., Ph.D.
Professor, Aradine S. Ard Chair in Brain Science, and Vice Chairman for Clinical Research, Department of Psychiatry, The University of Texas Southwestern Medical Center, Dallas, Texas

Brenda Bursch, Ph.D.
Professor, Departments of Psychiatry and Biobehavioral Sciences, and Pediatrics, David Geffen School of Medicine at UCLA, Los Angeles, California

Alan J. Carson, M.Phil., M.D., FRCPsych, FRCP
Dr Reader in Neuropsychiatry, Centre for Clinical Brain Sciences, University of Edinburgh, Edinburgh, United Kingdom

Keira Chism, M.D., M.A.
Associate Director, Consultation Liaison and Hospital Psychiatry, Transplant Psychiatry, Thomas Jefferson University Hospital, Department of Psychiatry and Human Behavior, Philadelphia, Pennsylvania

Harvey Max Chochinov, M.D., Ph.D., FRCPC
Distinguished Professor, Department of Psychiatry; Co-Director, Psycho-Social Oncology Research Group; Director, Manitoba Palliative Care Research Unit, Faculty of Medicine University of Manitoba, Winnipeg, Manitoba, Canada

Michael R. Clark, M.D., M.P.H., M.B.A.
Chair, Department of Psychiatry & Behavioral Health, Inova Health System, Falls Church, Virginia

Catherine C. Crone, M.D.
Associate Professor, Department of Psychiatry, George Washington University School of Medicine, Washington, DC; Clinical Professor of Psychiatry, Virginia Commonwealth University, Richmond, Virginia; Vice Chair, Department of Psychiatry, Inova Fairfax Hospital, Falls Church, Virginia

Ericka L. Crouse, Pharm.D., BCPP, BCGP
Associate Professor, Department of Pharmacotherapy and Outcomes Science, Virginia Commonwealth University School of Pharmacy, Richmond, Virginia

Daniel Cukor, Ph.D.
Associate Professor, Department of Psychiatry and Behavioral Sciences, SUNY Downstate Medical Center, Brooklyn, New York

Mary Amanda Dew, Ph.D.
Professor of Psychiatry, Psychology, Epidemiology, Biostatistics, and Clinical and Translational Science; Director, Clinical Epidemiology Program, Western Psychiatric Institute and Clinic; Director, Quality of Life Research, Artificial Heart Program Adult Cardiothoracic Transplantation, University of Pittsburgh School of Medicine and Medical Center, Pittsburgh, Pennsylvania

Andrea F. DiMartini, M.D.
Professor of Psychiatry and Surgery, Western Psychiatric Institute and Clinics, University of Pittsburgh School of Medicine and Medical Center, Starzl Transplant Institute, Pittsburgh, Pennsylvania

Andrew Edelstein, M.D.
Instructor in Clinical Psychiatry, Department of Psychiatry and Behavioral Sciences, Memorial Sloan-Kettering Cancer Center, New York, New York

Natacha D. Emerson, Ph.D.
Postdoctoral Fellow, Department of Psychiatry and Biobehavioral Sciences, David Geffen School of Medicine at UCLA, Los Angeles, California

Steven A. Epstein, M.D.
Professor and Chair, Department of Psychiatry, Georgetown University School of Medicine and Physician Executive Director, MedStar Behavioral Health, Washington, D.C.

Jesse R. Fann, M.D., M.P.H.
Professor, Department of Psychiatry and Behavioral Sciences, and Adjunct Professor, Department of Rehabilitation Medicine, University of Washington School of Medicine; Adjunct Professor, Department of Epidemiology, University of Washington School of Public Health; Director, Psychiatry and Psychology Service, Seattle Cancer Care Alliance; Affiliate Investigator, Clinical Research Division, Fred Hutchinson Cancer Research Center, Seattle, Washington

Charles V. Ford, M.D.
Professor, Department of Psychiatry and Behavioral Neurobiology, University of Alabama at Birmingham, Birmingham, Alabama

Andrew Francis, Ph.D., M.D.
Professor of Psychiatry, Associate Director of Residency Training, and Director of Neuromodulation Services, Penn State Medical School, Hershey Medical Center, Hershey, Pennsylvania

Oliver Freudenreich, M.D.
Co-Director, Schizophrenia Clinical and Research Program, Massachusetts General Hospital; Associate Professor of Psychiatry, Harvard Medical School, Boston, Massachusetts

Gregory L. Fricchione, M.D.
Director, Benson–Henry Institute for Mind–Body Medicine, Massachusetts General Hospital; Professor of Psychiatry, Harvard Medical School, Boston, Massachusetts

Patricia Gracia-Garcia, M.D., Ph.D.
Psychiatrist, Hospital Universitario Miguel Servet, Zaragoza, Spain

Mark S. Groves, M.D.
Assistant Clinical Professor, Departments of Psychiatry and Neurology, Icahn School of Medicine at Mt. Sinai, New York, New York

Angela S. Guarda, M.D.
Associate Professor, Department of Psychiatry and Behavioral Sciences; Director, Eating Disorders Program, Johns Hopkins Medicine, Baltimore, Maryland

Madhulika A. Gupta, M.D., M.Sc., FRCPC
Professor, Department of Psychiatry, Schulich School of Medicine and Dentistry, University of Western Ontario, London, Ontario, Canada

Elspeth Guthrie, M.B., Ch.B., FRCPsych, M.Sc., M.D.
Professor of Psychological Medicine, Institute of Health Sciences, University of Leeds, Leeds, West Yorkshire, United Kingdom

Raed Hawa, M.D.
Associate Professor, Department of Psychiatry, University of Toronto, Centre for Mental Health, University Health Network, Toronto, Ontario

Peter Henningsen, M.D.
Professor and Chair, Department of Psychosomatic Medicine and Psychotherapy, TUM University Hospital, Munich, Germany

J. Greg Hobelmann, M.D., M.P.H.
Chief Medical Officer, Ashley Addiction Treatment, Havre de Grace, Maryland

Michael R. Irwin, M.D.
Distinguished Professor of Psychiatry and Biobehavioral Sciences, UCLA David Geffen School of Medicine; Norman Cousins Chair for Psychoneuroimmunology, UCLA Semel Institute for Neuroscience and Human Behavior; and Director, Cousins Center for Psychoneuroimmunology, Los Angeles, California

Richard Kennedy, M.D.
Assistant Professor, Division of Gerontology, Geriatrics, and Palliative Care, Department of Medicine, University of Alabama at Birmingham, Birmingham, Alabama

Paul L. Kimmel, M.D.
Clinical Professor of Medicine, Division of Renal Diseases and Hypertension, Department of Medicine, George Washington University, Washington, D.C.

Cynthia K. Kirkwood, Pharm.D., BCPP
Executive Associate Dean for Academic Affairs; Professor, Department of Pharmacotherapy and Outcomes Science, Virginia Commonwealth University School of Pharmacy, Richmond, Virginia

Christopher Kogut, M.D.
William and Ruth McDonough Professor in Graduate Psychiatric Education and Director of Residency Education, Virginia Commonwealth University School of Medicine, Richmond, Virginia

Lois E. Krahn, M.D.
Professor of Psychiatry, Mayo Clinic College of Medicine; Center for Sleep Medicine, Mayo Clinic, Scottsdale, Arizona

Juliet Kroll, M.A.
Graduate Research Assistant, Clinical Psychology, Department of Psychology, Southern Methodist University, Dallas, Texas

Alexandra Kulikova, M.S.
Clinical Research Coordinator, Department of Psychiatry, The University of Texas Southwestern Medical Center, Dallas, Texas

Jeanne M. Lackamp, M.D.
Associate Professor, Department of Psychiatry, University Hospitals Cleveland Medical Center, Case Western Reserve University School of Medicine, Cleveland, Ohio

Albert F.G. Leentjens, M.D., Ph.D.
Associate Professor of Psychiatry, Department of Psychiatry, Maastricht University Medical Center, Maastricht, The Netherlands

James L. Levenson, M.D.
Professor of Psychiatry, Medicine, and Surgery, Virginia Commonwealth University School of Medicine, Richmond, Virginia

Madeline Li, M.D., Ph.D., FRCPC
Associate Professor, Department of Psychiatry, University of Toronto; Clinician Scientist, Department of Psychosocial Oncology and Palliative Care, Princess Margaret Hospital, Toronto, Ontario, Canada

Ted S. Liao, M.D.
Assistant Professor of Clinical Psychiatry, Georgetown University School of Medicine; Associate Director of Consultation-Liaison Psychiatry Fellowship and Associate Director of Psychiatry Residency Training Program, MedStar Georgetown University Hospital, Washington, D.C.

Antonio Lobo, M.D., Ph.D.
Emeritus Professor. Department of Medicine and Psychiatry, University of Zaragoza, Aragon Health Research Foundation (IIS Aragón), Zaragoza, Spain

Constantine G. Lyketsos, M.D., M.H.S.
Elizabeth Plank Althouse Professor, Department of Psychiatry and Behavioral Sciences, Johns Hopkins University School of Medicine, and Chair, Department of Psychiatry, Johns Hopkins Bayview Medical Center, Baltimore, Maryland

Mary Jane Massie, M.D.
Professor of Clinical Psychiatry, Weill Medical College of Cornell University; Attending Psychiatrist, Memorial Sloan-Kettering Cancer Center, New York, New York

Cheryl McCullumsmith, M.D., Ph.D.
Associate Professor, Department of Psychiatry and Behavioral Neuroscience, University of Cincinnati, Cincinnati, Ohio

David J. Meagher, M.D., MRCPsych, Ph.D.
Professor of Psychiatry, Graduate Entry Medical School, University of Limerick, Limerick, Ireland

Weronika Micula-Gondek, M.D.
Assistant Professor, Department of Psychiatry and Behavioral Sciences, Johns Hopkins Medicine, Baltimore, Maryland

Kimberley Miller, M.D., FRCPC
Assistant Professor, Department of Psychiatry, University of Toronto; Attending Psychiatrist, Princess Margaret Cancer Centre, Toronto, Ontario, Canada

Philip R. Muskin, M.D., M.A.
Professor of Psychiatry and Senior Consultant in Consultation-Liaison Psychiatry at Columbia University Medical Center; Faculty, Columbia University Psychoanalytic Center for Training and Research, New York, New York

Alyson K. Myers, M.D.
Medical Director, Inpatient Diabetes, North Shore University Hospital, Manhasset, New York; Assistant Professor, Donald and Barbara Zucker School of Medicine at Hofstra/Northwell, East Garden City, New York; and Assistant Professor, Merinoff Center for Patient-Oriented Research at the Feinstein Institute, Northwell Health, Manhasset, New York

Ariana Nesbit, M.D., M.B.E.
Forensic Psychiatry Fellow, Department of Psychiatry, Division of Psychiatry and the Law, University of California, Davis Medical Center, Sacramento, California

Patrick G. O'Malley, M.D., M.P.H., FACP
Professor of Medicine, Uniformed Services University of the Health Sciences, Bethesda, Maryland

Chiadi U. Onyike, M.D., M.H.S.
Associate Professor, Department of Psychiatry and Behavioral Sciences, Division of Geriatric Psychiatry and Neuropsychiatry, Johns Hopkins School of Medicine, Baltimore, Maryland

James A. Owen, Ph.D. (Deceased)
Associate Professor, Department of Psychiatry and Department of Pharmacology and Toxicology, Queen's University; Director, Psychopharmacology Lab, Providence Care Mental Health Services, Kingston, Ontario, Canada

Miguel Ángel Quintanilla, M.D., Ph.D.
Attending Psychiatrist, Hospital Clínico Universitario; Instructor in Psychiatry, Department of Medicine and Psychiatry, University of Zaragoza, Zaragoza, Spain

J. J. Rasimas, M.D., Ph.D.
Associate Professor of Psychiatry & Emergency Medicine, University of Minnesota Medical School; Director of Consultation-Liaison Psychiatry, Hennepin County Medical Center, Minneapolis, Minnesota

Keith G. Rasmussen, M.D.
Professor, Mayo Clinic Department of Psychiatry and Psychology, Rochester, Minnesota

Peter M. Rees, M.D., Ph.D.
Neurologist (retired), formerly at Burnaby Hospital, Burnaby, British Columbia, Canada

Thomas Ritz, Ph.D.
Professor of Psychology and Director, Psychobiology of Stress, Emotion, and Chronic Disease Research Program, Department of Psychology, Southern Methodist University, Dallas, Texas

Gary Rodin, M.D., FRCPC
Professor, Department of Psychiatry, University of Toronto; Head, Department of Supportive Care, Princess Margaret Cancer Centre, Toronto, Ontario, Canada

Joshua Rosenblat, M.D.
Resident in Psychiatry, Clinician Scientist Program, University of Toronto, Toronto, Ontario, Canada

Deborah Rosenthal-Asher, Ph.D.
Memory and Psychological Services, Inc., Brecksville, Ohio

Pedro Saz, M.D., Ph.D.
Professor of Psychiatry, Department of Medicine and Psychiatry, University of Zaragoza, Zaragoza, Spain

Ronald Schouten, M.D., J.D.
Director, Law and Psychiatry Service, Massachusetts General Hospital, and Associate Professor of Psychiatry, Harvard Medical School, Boston, Massachusetts

Peter A. Shapiro, M.D.
Professor of Psychiatry, Columbia University Medical Center; and Director, Consultation-Liaison Psychiatry Service, New York Presbyterian Hospital–Columbia University Medical Center, New York, New York

Michael C. Sharpe, M.A., M.D., FRCP, FRCPsych
Professor of Psychological Medicine, University of Oxford, Oxford, United Kingdom

Akhil Shenoy, M.D., M.P.H.
Assistant Professor of Psychiatry, Columbia University College of Physicians and Surgeons; Liaison to the Center for Liver Disease and Transplantation, New York–Presbyterian Hospital Columbia University Medical Center, New York, New York

Felicia A. Smith, M.D.
Chief, Psychiatric Consultation Service; Director, Division of Psychiatry and Medicine, Massachusetts General Hospital; Assistant Professor of Psychiatry, Harvard Medical School, Boston, Massachusetts

Sanjeev Sockalingam, M.D.
Associate Professor, Department of Psychiatry, University of Toronto, Centre for Mental Health, University Health Network, Toronto, Ontario

Wolfgang Söllner, M.D.
President, European Association for Psychosomatic Medicine; Professor of Psychosomatic Medicine and Psychotherapy, Paracelsus Medical University, General Hospital Nuremberg, Germany

Loretta Sonnier, M.D.
Assistant Professor, Department of Psychiatry and Behavior Sciences, Tulane University, New Orleans, Louisiana

Theodore A. Stern, M.D.
Chief Emeritus, Psychiatric Consultation Service, Massachusetts General Hospital; Ned H. Cassem Professor of Psychiatry, Harvard Medical School, Boston, Massachusetts

Donna E. Stewart, C.M., M.D., FRCPC
University Professor and Professor of Psychiatry, Obstetrics and Gynecology, Anesthesia, Family and Community Medicine, and Surgery, University of Toronto Faculty of Medicine; Senior Scientist, Toronto General Hospital Research Institute; Director of Research, University Health Network Centre for Mental Health, Toronto, Ontario, Canada

Jon Stone, Ph.D., FRCP
Dr Reader in Neurology, Centre for Clinical Brain Sciences, University of Edinburgh, Edinburgh, United Kingdom

Margaret L. Stuber, M.D.
Professor and Associate Chair, Medical Student Education, Department of Psychiatry and Biobehavioral Sciences, David Geffen School of Medicine at UCLA, Los Angeles, California

Simone N. Vigod, M.D., M.Sc., FRCPC
Associate Professor, Department of Psychiatry, University of Toronto; Shirley A. Brown Memorial Chair in Women's Mental Health, Women's College Research Institute, Women's College Hospital, Toronto, Ontario, Canada

Michael Weaver, M.D., DFASAM
Professor and Medical Director, Center for Neurobehavioral Research on Addiction, Department of Psychiatry and Behavioral Sciences, McGovern Medical School, Houston, Texas

Chelsey Werchan, M.A.
Graduate Research Assistant, Clinical Psychology, Department of Psychology, Southern Methodist University, Dallas, Texas

Elizabeth A. Wise, M.D.
Geriatric Psychiatry Fellow, Department of Psychiatry and Behavioral Sciences, Johns Hopkins University School of Medicine, Baltimore, Maryland

Adam Zeman, M.A., D.M., FRCP
Professor of Cognitive and Behavioural Neurology, Cognitive Neurology Research Group, University of Exeter Medical School, St. Luke's Campus, Exeter, United Kingdom

Disclosure of Interests

The following contributors to this textbook have indicated a financial interest in or other affiliation with a commercial supporter, manufacturer of a commercial product, and/or provider of a commercial service as listed below:

E. Sherwood Brown, M.D., Ph.D.   *Research Grant:* Otsuka.

Alan J. Carson, M.Phil., M.D., FRCPsych, FRCP   Neither I nor my immediate family have any links or financial conflicts of interest with pharmaceutical companies or similar entities. I have given lectures on neuropsychiatric topics at drug company symposia on approximately 10 occasions and received fees of less than $250 dollars on each occasion. I never directly promoted a particular agent. I have received fees for giving independent testimony in court on a variety of neuropsychiatric topics (50% pursuer, 50% defender). I am listed at Companies House London as a director of Dr Jon Stone Ltd, which is a personal services company through which any private medical earnings exclusively for medicolegal work I have are collected and taxed (this is a standard UK arrangement for payment). I am a paid editor of the *Journal of Neurology, Neurosurgery, and Psychiatry.*

Oliver Freudenreich, M.D. *Consultant (Advisory Board):* Alkermes, Janssen, and Neurocrine; *Research Grants:* Avanir, Janssen, Otsuka, and Saladax; *Honoraria:* Global Medical Education (CME speaker and content developer), Neurocrine (CME talk), and UpToDate (content developer and editor); *Royalties:* Wolters-Kluwer (content developer), UpToDate (content developer and editor).

Patricia Gracia-Garcia, M.D., Ph.D. I have received honoraria, travel funds, and subscriptions for a scientific meeting from Servier.

Miguel Ángel Quintanilla, M.D., Ph.D. Funding for congress from Lundbeck; grants for survey from Servier.

Jon Stone, Ph.D., FRCP Neither I nor my immediate family have any links or financial conflicts of interest with pharmaceutical companies or similar entities. I have received fees for giving independent testimony in Court on a variety of neuropsychiatric topics (60% pursuer, 40% defender). I am listed at Companies House London as a director of Dr Jon Stone Ltd, which is a personal services company through which any private medical earnings exclusively for medicolegal work I have are collected and taxed (this is a standard UK arrangement for payment). I receive royalties from UpToDate for articles relating to conversion disorder. I run a self-help website (www.neurosymptoms.org) that is free to users and carries no advertising or sponsorship.

Simone N. Vigod, M.D., M.Sc., FRCPC *Research Support:* Canadian Institutes for Health Research, Ontario Ministry of Health and Long-Term Care, University of Toronto, and Women's College Hospital in Toronto; *Royalties:* UpToDate (writing of several chapters on maternal mental health).

Adam Zeman, M.A., D.M., FRCP I received an unrestricted grant of £15,132.53 from UCB in 2018 to fund development of our sleep disorders service though creation of a "Clinical Physiologist Sleep Specialist" role. I undertake occasional medicolegal work, and am sole Director of a company providing this service, Azimuth Medical Consultants Ltd.

The following contributors stated that they had no competing interests during the year preceding manuscript submission:

Andrew R. Alkis, M.D.; David J. Axelrod, M.D., J.D.; Robert Bahnsen, M.D.; Rosemary Basson, M.D.; Madeleine Becker, M.D., M.A.; Charles H. Bombardier, Ph.D.; William Breitbart, M.D.; Rebecca W. Brendel, M.D., J.D.; Brenda Bursch, Ph.D.; Keira Chism, M.D., M.A.; Catherine C. Crone, M.D.; Daniel Cukor, Ph.D.; Mary Amanda Dew, Ph.D.; Andrea F. DiMartini, M.D.; Natacha D. Emerson, Ph.D.; Jesse R. Fann, M.D., M.P.H.; Charles V. Ford, M.D.; Andrew Francis, Ph.D., M.D.; Gregory L. Fricchione, M.D.; Angela S. Guarda, M.D.; Madhulika A. Gupta, M.D., M.Sc., FRCPC; Peter Henningsen, M.D.; Lois E. Krahn, M.D.; Jeanne M. Lackamp, M.D.; Albert F. G. Leentjens, M.D., Ph.D.; James L. Levenson, M.D.; Antonio Lobo, M.D., Ph.D.; Weronika Micula-Gondek, M.D.; Alyson K. Myers, M.D.; Patrick G. O'Malley, M.D., M.P.H., FACP; J. J. Rasimas, M.D., Ph.D.; Keith G. Rasmussen, M.D.; Deborah Rosenthal-Asher, Ph.D.; Pedro Saz, M.D., Ph.D.; Peter A. Shapiro, M.D.; Michael C. Sharpe, M.A., M.D., FRCP, FRCPsych; Akhil Shenoy, M.D., M.P.H.; Sanjeev Sockalingam, M.D.; Loretta Sonnier, M.D.; Margaret L. Stuber, M.D.; Michael Weaver, M.D., DFASAM.

Foreword

Wolfgang Söllner, M.D.

James Levenson's new *Textbook of Psychosomatic Medicine and Consultation-Liaison Psychiatry* continues a distinguished tradition of textbooks on Psychosomatic Medicine that began with Dunbar's *Psychosomatic Diagnosis* (1943), Weiss and English's *Psychosomatic Medicine: The Clinical Application of Psychopathology to General Medical Problems* (1949), and Alexander's *Psychosomatic Medicine—Its Principles and Applications* (1950). On the basis of available knowledge at that time, these authors described, above all, mental syndromes accompanying physical illnesses and theoretical foundations for the interaction between body and mind. For the latter, there was a lack of empirical evidence, and so these theories often remained speculative. Twenty years later, Schwab (1968), Lipowski et al. (1977), and Hackett and Cassem (1978) published the first textbooks for psychiatrists working in the general hospital, reflecting the rapidly growing field of consultation-liaison (C-L) psychiatry. These leaders based their textbooks on the increasing clinical experience of the field and the growing insights of empirical research on the of physical and psychiatric disorders. Another 20 years later, this work was continued with the first and second editions of *The American Psychiatric Publishing Textbook of Consultation-Liaison Psychiatry*, edited by Rundell and Wise (1996) and Wise and Rundell (2002), respectively.

With the establishment of Psychosomatic Medicine (now Consultation-Liaison Psychiatry) as an official subspecialty of psychiatry in the United States, the Academy of Psychosomatic Medicine undertook support for creation of a new comprehensive textbook of psychosomatic medicine for the field, aimed at both trainees and advanced practitioners. Jim Levenson shouldered this task, and in his *Textbook of Psychosomatic Medicine* (2005) and *Textbook of Psychosomatic Medicine: Psychiatric Care of the Medically Ill*, Second Edition (2011), provided up-to-date, evidence-based information on the diagnosis and treatment of three groups of clinical problems: 1) comorbid psychiatric and general medical disorders complicating each other's course and treatment (complex diseases), 2) health anxiety and somatic symptom disorders, and 3) mental disorders that are a consequence of a primary medical condition or its treatment. In all three areas, the body of research has grown rapidly in the past two decades. To keep pace with this growth, it has been necessary to publish updated editions at increasingly shorter intervals. Hence, within a period of only 13 years, this textbook now appears in its third edition. Once again, James Levenson has succeeded in recruiting renowned experts from North America and Europe as authors of the textbook chapters. This group of outstanding clinicians, educators, and researchers offer practical guidance on key clinical issues encountered by psychiatrists working with medically ill patients, as well as an overview of the latest findings from empirical research in the field of C-L psychiatry.

The publication of this third edition of the *Textbook of Psychosomatic Medicine* coincided with the change in the official name of the subspecialty, paralleled by the Academy of Psychosomatic Medicine's change of its name to the Academy of Consultation-Liaison Psychiatry. Thus, the textbook now includes "and Consultation-Liaison Psychiatry" in its title, while retaining the earlier designation "Psychosomatic Medicine" for continuity. The scientific and clinical interrelatedness of these two traditions, psychosomatic medicine and C-L psychiatry, is still high. For many years, the two disciplines had divergent emphases, with C-L psychiatry primarily focused on clinical work and psychosomatic medicine on research. In a 1985 paper tracing the evolving relationship of the two fields, one of the pioneers of C-L psychiatry, John Schwab, wrote: "Consultation-liaison work became the clinical arm of psychosomatic medicine" (Schwab 1985, p. 585); and in a 2001 article on the mutual influence and overlap of the scientific literature of the two fields, Don Lipsitt wrote: "If, in fact, general hospital psychiatry was the soil in which the roots of C-L psychiatry were planted, then it is likely that psychosomatic medicine was the fertilizer that nourished its growth" (Lipsitt 2001, p. 897). Lipsitt opined that basic research examining the interaction of psychological and physiological aspects of medical illness was nourishing the development of health care in this clinical field. However, as the editor of the present textbook previously lamented, C-L psychiatrists have not made sufficient use of the broad research opportunities offered by the clinical field of C-L psychiatry (Levenson 1994). This third edition of the *Textbook of Psychosomatic Medicine and Consultation-Liaison Psychiatry* demonstrates that the historical division of emphases—clinical work in C-L psychiatry versus research in psychosomatic medicine—can no longer be upheld. C-L psychiatry has become increasingly research oriented. In particular, health services research has burgeoned within the past 15 years. The development, implementation, and evaluation of new models of integrative and collaborative care not only are intellectually challenging but also are opening up new opportunities for concrete improvements in clinical care.

Editing a textbook of psychosomatic medicine represents a unique challenge. Psychosocial issues may influence the development, course, and treatment of every disease affecting every organ system (Engel 1977). The relatedness of body and mind and the different biological pathways by which body and mind interact are fascinating topics of ongoing psychosomatic research. Taking all of these issues into account would require a volume that far exceeds the scope of a textbook, encompassing psychopathophysiology, diagnosis, and treatment of all medical diseases, as well as basic psychosomatic science from stress research, psychoneuroendocrinology, psychoneuroimmunology, and epigenetics, among other areas. Jim Levenson's textbook offers a pragmatic solution that reconciles the competing demands of utility and comprehensiveness. In it, he and his co-authors have focused on psychosocial aspects and psychiatric comorbidity—from a health care perspective—associated with the most relevant medical diseases, as well as on the mental disorders that are most prevalent in the general hospital—in short, the clinical issues and situations that most often lead to referrals to C-L psychiatrists.

Although this textbook is primarily written for psychiatrists working in the general hospital, it is also of interest to general practitioners and specialists in other medical disciplines. In particular, in the chapters on the different organ systems and on specific medical treatments (such as organ transplantation and palliative care), readers will find valuable information on psychosocial aspects of illness and the diagnosis and treatment of mental comorbidities in physical disorders.

At the international level, few textbooks have attempted to capture the full range of this scientific and clinical field. With the exception of Lloyd and Guthrie's *Handbook of Liaison Psychiatry* (2007) and the German textbook *Uexküll: Psychosomatic Medicine,* which recently appeared in its eighth edition (Köhle et al. 2017), there is a lack of comprehensive textbooks of Psychosomatic Medicine and C-L Psychiatry. Jim Levenson's *Textbook of Psychosomatic Medicine and Consultation-Liaison Psychiatry* ably fills this gap and will appeal to a wide range of readers in countries around the world.

References

Alexander EJ: Psychosomatic Medicine—Its Principles and Applications. New York, WW Norton, 1950

Dunbar HF: Psychosomatic Diagnosis. New York, PB Hoeber, 1943

Engel GL: The need for a new medical model: a challenge for biomedicine. Science 196(4286):129–136, 1977 847460

Hackett TP, Cassem NH (eds): Massachusetts General Hospital Handbook of General Hospital Psychiatry. St. Louis, MO, CV Mosby, 1978

Köhle K, Herzog W, Joraschky P, Kruse J, Langewitz W, Söllner W (eds): Uexküll, Psychosomatische Medizin: Theoretische Modelle und Klinische Praxis, 8th Edition. Munich, Germany, Urban & Fischer (Elsevier), 2017

Levenson JL: Achieving excellence in consultation-liaison research: barriers and opportunities. Psychosomatics 35(5):492–495, 1994 7972665

Levenson JL (ed): The American Psychiatric Publishing Textbook of Psychosomatic Medicine. Arlington, VA, American Psychiatric Publishing, 2005

Levenson JL (ed): The American Psychiatric Publishing Textbook of Psychosomatic Medicine: Psychiatric Care of the Medically Ill, 2nd Edition. Arlington, VA, American Psychiatric Publishing, 2011

Lipowski ZJ, Lipsitt DR, Whybrow PC (eds): Psychosomatic Medicine: Current Trends and Clinical Applications. New York, Oxford University Press, 1977

Lipsitt DR: Consultation-liaison psychiatry and psychosomatic medicine: the company they keep. Psychosom Med 63(6):896–909, 2001 11719628

Lloyd G, Guthrie E (eds): Handbook of Liaison Psychiatry. Cambridge, UK, Cambridge University Press, 2007

Rundell JR, Wise MG (eds): The American Psychiatric Press Textbook of Consultation-Liaison Psychiatry. Washington, DC, American Psychiatric Press, 1996

Schwab JJ: Handbook of Psychiatric Consultation. New York, Appleton-Century-Crofts, 1968

Schwab JJ: Psychosomatic medicine: its past and present. Psychosomatics 26(7):583–585, 588–589, 592–593, 1985 3895279

Weiss E, English OS: Psychosomatic Medicine: The Clinical Application of Psychopathology to General Medical Problems. Philadelphia, Saunders, 1949

Wise MG, Rundell JR (eds): The American Psychiatric Publishing Textbook of Consultation-Liaison Psychiatry: Psychiatry in the Medically Ill, 2nd Edition. Washington, DC, American Psychiatric Publishing, 2002

Preface

James L. Levenson, M.D.

What is Psychosomatic Medicine? In the past, Psychosomatic Medicine has had ambiguous connotations, alternatively "psychogenic" or "holistic," but it is the latter meaning that has characterized its emergence as a contemporary scientific and clinical discipline (Lipowski 1984). In this book, *Psychosomatic Medicine* refers to a specialized area of psychiatry whose practitioners have particular expertise in the diagnosis and treatment of psychiatric disorders and difficulties in complex medically ill patients (Gitlin et al. 2004). We treat and study three general groups of patients: 1) those with comorbid psychiatric and general medical illnesses complicating each other's management, 2) those with somatoform and functional disorders, and 3) those with psychiatric disorders that are the direct consequence of a primary medical condition or its treatment. Psychosomatic Medicine practitioners work as hospital-based consultation-liaison psychiatrists (Kornfeld 1996), on medical–psychiatric inpatient units (Kathol and Stoudemire 2002), and in settings in which mental health services are integrated into primary care (Unützer et al. 2002). Thus, the field's name reflects the fact that it exists at the interface of psychiatry and medicine.

Historical Background

Psychosomatic Medicine and Consultation-Liaison Psychiatry have a rich history. The term *psychosomatic* was introduced by Johann Heinroth in 1818, and Felix Deutsch introduced the term *psychosomatic medicine* around 1922 (Lipsitt 2001). Psychoanalysts and psychophysiologists pioneered the study of mind–body interactions from very different vantage points, each contributing to the growth of Psychosomatic Medicine as a clinical and scholarly field. The modern history of the field (see Table 1) perhaps starts with the Rockefeller Foundation's funding of psychosomatic medicine units in several U.S. teaching hospitals in 1935. Lipowski described the nascent field of consultation-liaison psychiatry in 1971 (Lipowski 1971). The National Institute of Mental Health made it a priority to foster the growth of consultation-liaison psychiatry through training grants (circa 1975) and a research development program (circa 1985).

TABLE 1.   **Key dates in the modern history of psychosomatic medicine and consultation-liaison psychiatry**

1935	Rockefeller Foundation opens first Consultation-Liaison (C/L)–Psychosomatic Units at Massachusetts General, Duke, and Colorado
1936	American Psychosomatic Society founded
1939	First issue of Psychosomatic Medicine
1953	First issue of Psychosomatics
1954	Academy of Psychosomatic Medicine (APM) founded
1975	National Institute of Mental Health (NIMH) Training Grants for C/L Psychiatry
1985	NIMH Research Development Program for C/L Psychiatry
1991	APM-recognized fellowships number 55
2001	Subspecialty application for Psychosomatic Medicine
2003	Approval as subspecialty by American Board of Medical Specialties
2018	Subspecialty renamed C/L Psychiatry by American Board of Psychiatry and Neurology

This specialized field has had many names, including *medical–surgical psychiatry, psychological medicine,* and *psychiatric care of the complex medically ill.* In 2001, the Academy of Psychosomatic Medicine applied to the American Board of Psychiatry and Neurology (ABPN) for recognition of Psychosomatic Medicine as a subspecialty of psychiatry, choosing to return to the name for the field embedded in our history, our journals, and our national organizations. Psychosomatic Medicine was formally approved as a psychiatric subspecialty by the American Board of Medical Specialties (ABMS) in 2003, with subsequent approvals received from the American Psychiatric Association, the ABPN, and the Residency Review Committee (RRC) of the Accreditation Council for Graduate Medical Education (ACGME). Since the first certifying examination in 2005, 1,544 psychiatrists (as of 2018) have been certified in Psychosomatic Medicine/Consultation-Liaison Psychiatry in the United States.

In the spring of 2017, the Academy of Psychosomatic Medicine once again applied to the ABPN for approval of a name change for the subspecialty, this time to Consultation-Liaison Psychiatry. Approval was granted in October 2017, and on November 28, 2017, the ABPN announced that, effective January 1, 2018, the name of the Psychosomatic Medicine subspecialty certification would become Consultation-Liaison Psychiatry. In its official announcement, the ABPN stated its belief that the new name "better describes the discipline's key focus of treating behavioral conditions in patients with medical and surgical problems" (Faulkner 2017). In a member-wide vote in November 2017, the Academy of Psychosomatic Medicine officially changed its name to the Academy of Consultation-Liaison Psychiatry.

Psychosomatic Medicine is a scholarly discipline, with classic influential texts (Table 2), many devoted journals (Table 3), and both national (Table 4) and international (Table 5) professional/scientific societies. The Academy of Consultation-Liaison Psychiatry (ACLP; formerly the Academy of Psychosomatic Medicine) is the only U.S. national organization primarily dedicated to Consultation-Liaison Psychiatry as a psychiatric subspecialty. The American Psychosomatic Society (APS), an older

TABLE 2. Selected classic texts in psychosomatic medicine and consultation-liaison psychiatry

1935	*Emotions and Body Change* (Dunbar)
1943	*Psychosomatic Medicine* (Weiss and English)
1950	*Psychosomatic Medicine* (Alexander)
1968	*Handbook of Psychiatric Consultation* (Schwab)
1978	*Organic Psychiatry* (Lishman)
1978	*Massachusetts General Hospital Handbook of General Hospital Psychiatry* (Hackett and Cassem)
1993	*Psychiatric Care of the Medical Patient* (Stoudemire and Fogel)

TABLE 3. Selected journals in psychosomatic medicine

Journal name	Date of initial publication
Psychosomatic Medicine	1939
Psychosomatics	1953
Psychotherapy and Psychosomatics	1953
Psychophysiology	1954
Journal of Psychosomatic Research	1956
Advances in Psychosomatic Medicine	1960
International Journal of Psychiatry in Medicine	1970
General Hospital Psychiatry	1979
Journal of Psychosomatic Obstetrics and Gynecology	1982
Journal of Psychosocial Oncology	1983
Stress Medicine	1985
Psycho-Oncology	1986

TABLE 4. National organizations

Academy of Consultation-Liaison Psychiatry (formerly Academy of Psychosomatic Medicine)

Association for Medicine and Psychiatry

American Psychosomatic Society

American Association for General Hospital Psychiatry

Society for Liaison Psychiatry

Association for Academic Psychiatry—Consultation-Liaison Section

American Neuropsychiatric Association

American Psychosocial Oncology Society

North American Society for Psychosomatic Obstetrics and Gynecology

TABLE 5. **International organizations**

European Association for Psychosomatic Medicine

International Organization for Consultation-Liaison Psychiatry

World Psychiatric Association—Section of General Hospital Psychiatry

International College of Psychosomatic Medicine

International Neuropsychiatric Association

International Psycho-Oncology Society

cousin, is primarily devoted to psychosomatic research, and its members come from many disciplines (Wise 1995). While consultation-liaison psychiatry and psychosomatic medicine first flourished in the United States, exciting work now comes from around the world. APM's counterpart in Europe is the European Association for Psychosomatic Medicine (EAPM), which was formed in 2012 by the merger of the European Association of Consultation-Liaison Psychiatry and Psychosomatics (EACLPP) and the European Conference on Psychosomatic Research (ECPR) (Söllner and Schüssler 2012). Associations or special interest groups for psychosomatic medicine and consultation-liaison psychiatry now exist in many countries, including Argentina, Brazil, Germany, Italy, the Netherlands, Portugal, Spain, Canada, and the United Kingdom. The international nature of the field is reflected in the fact that the Foreword and 11 of the textbook's 39 chapters and were authored by psychiatrists from outside the United States, including Canada, the United Kingdom, Germany, Ireland, the Netherlands, and Spain. The first edition of this book has been translated into Chinese and Spanish.

Third Edition of the Textbook

There are 88 contributors to the third edition of this textbook, 30 of them new authors. Twenty-four of the contributors are from countries other than the United States. Four chapters are entirely newly authored. The remaining 35 chapters have all been extensively revised.

This book is organized into four sections. Chapters 1–3 cover general principles in evaluation and management, legal and ethical issues, and psychological reactions to illness. Chapters 4–16 are devoted to psychiatric symptoms and disorders in the medically ill. Chapters 17–35 address issues within each of the medical specialties and subspecialties. The final 4 chapters review psychiatric treatment in the medically ill, including psychopharmacology, psychotherapy, electroconvulsive therapy, and palliative care.

This book has attempted to capture the diversity of our field, whose practitioners vary on the emphasis they give to the syllables of "bio-psycho-social." There is not unanimity among us on some questions, and diverse opinions will be found in this book. Psychosomatic Medicine has evolved, since its start, from a field based on clinical experience, conjecture, and theorizing into a discipline grounded in empirical research that is growing and spreading its findings into many areas of medical care.

Acknowledgments

I owe an enormous debt of gratitude to the many people who made this book possible. First, to the contributors, who were patient under repeated onslaughts of red "track-changes" from me. Laura Roberts and John McDuffie at American Psychiatric Association Publishing (APAP) gave advice and encouragement from start to finish, and I am grateful to all of the APAP staff, including Greg Kuny, Rebecca Richters, Susan Westrate, Judy Castagna, and Teri-Yaé Yarbrough.

Finally, this book would not have been possible without enthusiastic support from my chair, Joel Silverman; the help of my assistant, Pam Copeland; and the patience and tolerance of my wife, Janet Distelman.

References

Faulkner LR: Memorandum, American Board of Psychiatry and Neurology, November 28, 2017. Available at: https://www.abpn.com/wp-content/uploads/2017/11/PSM-Name-Change-Memo.pdf. Accessed March 12, 2018.

Gitlin DF, Levenson JL, Lyketsos CG: Psychosomatic medicine: a new psychiatric subspecialty. Acad Psychiatry 28(4):4–11, 2004 15140802

Kathol RG, Stoudemire A: Strategic integration of inpatient and outpatient medical-psychiatry services, in The American Psychiatric Publishing Textbook of Consultation-Liaison Psychiatry. Edited by Wise MG, Rundell JR. Washington, DC, American Psychiatric Publishing, 2002, pp 871–888

Kornfeld DS: Consultation-liaison psychiatry and the practice of medicine. The Thomas P. Hackett Award lecture given at the 42nd annual meeting of the Academy of Psychosomatic Medicine, 1995. Psychosomatics 37(48):236–248, 1996 8849500

Lipowski ZJ: Consultation-liaison psychiatry in general hospital. Compr Psychiatry 12(5):461–465, 1971 5124938

Lipowski ZJ: What does the word "psychosomatic" really mean? A historical and semantic inquiry. Psychosom Med 46(2):153–171, 1984 6371870

Lipsitt DR: Consultation-liaison psychiatry and psychosomatic medicine: the company they keep. Psychosom Med 63(6):896–909, 2001 11719628

Söllner W, Schüssler G: New `European Association of Psychosomatic Medicine' founded. J Psychosom Res 73(5):343–344, 2012 23062806

Unützer J, Katon W, Callahan CM, et al: Collaborative care management of late-life depression in the primary care setting: a randomized controlled trial. JAMA 288(22):2836–2845, 2002 12472325

Wise TN: A tale of two societies. Psychosom Med 57(4):303–309, 1995 7480559

PART I

General Principles in Evaluation
and Management

CHAPTER 1

Psychiatric Assessment and Consultation

Felicia A. Smith, M.D.
James L. Levenson, M.D.
Theodore A. Stern, M.D.

Psychosomatic medicine is rooted in consultation-liaison psychiatry, having expanded from a handful of general medical wards in the 1930s to specialized medical units throughout various parts of the health care delivery system. Practitioners in this psychiatric subspecialty assist with the care of a variety of patients, especially those with complex conditions such as cancer, organ failure, HIV infection, dementia, delirium, agitation, psychosis, substance use disorder or withdrawal, somatic symptom disorder, personality disorders, and mood and anxiety disorders, as well as suicidal ideation, treatment nonadherence, and aggression and other behavioral problems (Gitlin et al. 2004; Hackett et al. 2010). In addition, ethical and legal considerations are often critical elements of the psychiatric consultation. In the medical setting, prompt recognition and evaluation of psychiatric problems are essential because psychiatric comorbidity commonly exacerbates the course of medical illness, causes significant distress, prolongs hospital length of stay, and increases costs of care.

In this introductory chapter, we present a detailed approach to psychiatric assessment and consultation in medical settings. Successful psychiatric consultants must be flexible when evaluating affective, behavioral, and cognitive disturbances in the medically ill. In the final section of the chapter, we briefly outline the benefits of psychiatric consultation for patients as well as for the greater hospital and medical communities.

Psychiatric Consultation in the General Hospital

Psychiatrists who work in medical settings are charged with providing expert consultation to medical and surgical patients. In many respects, the psychiatric care of such patients is no different from the treatment of patients in a psychiatric clinic or in a private office. However, the constraints of the modern hospital environment demand a high degree of adaptability. Comfort, quiet, and privacy are scarce commodities in medical and surgical units, and the consultant's bedside manner is important in compensating for this. Interruptions by medical or nursing staff, visitors, and roommates erode the privacy that the psychiatrist usually expects (Eshel et al. 2016). Patients who are sick, preoccupied with their physical condition, and in pain are ill-disposed to engage in the exploratory interviews that often typify psychiatric evaluations conducted in other settings. Monitoring devices replace the plants, pictures, and other accoutrements of a typical office. Nightstands and tray tables are littered with medical paraphernalia commingled with personal effects.

The consultant must be adept at gathering the requisite diagnostic information related to a patient's condition and must be able to tolerate the sights, sounds, and smells of the sickroom. Additional visits for more history are often inevitable. In the end, the diagnosis will likely fall into one (or more) of the categories outlined in Lipowski's (1967) timeless classification (Table 1–1).

Although the consultant is summoned by the patient's primary care team, in many cases the visit is unannounced and is not requested by the patient, from whom cooperation is expected. Explicitly acknowledging this reality is often sufficient to gain the patient's cooperation. Cooperation is enhanced if the psychiatrist sits down and operates at eye level with the patient. By offering to help the patient get comfortable (e.g., by adjusting the head of the bed, bringing the patient a drink or a blanket, or adjusting the television) before and after the encounter, the consultant can increase the chances of being welcomed then and for follow-up evaluations.

When psychiatrists are consulted for a patient's unexplained physical symptoms or for pain management, it is useful to empathize with the distress that the patient is experiencing. This avoids conveying any judgment on the etiology of the pain except that the patient's suffering is real. After introductions, if the patient is in pain, the consultant's first questions should address this issue. Failing to do so conveys a lack of appreciation for the patient's distress and may be taken by the patient as disbelief in his or her symptoms. Starting with empathic questions about the patient's suffering establishes rapport and also guides the psychiatrist in setting the proper pace of the interview. Finally, because a psychiatric consultation will cause many patients to fear that their physician thinks they are "crazy," the psychiatrist may first need to address this fear.

Process of the Consultation

Although it is rarely as straightforward as the following primer suggests, the process of psychiatric consultation should, in the end, include all the components explained below and summarized in Table 1–2.

Speak Directly With the Referring Clinician

Requests for psychiatric consultation are notorious for being vague and imprecise (e.g., "rule out depression" or "patient with schizophrenia"). They sometimes signify

---

TABLE 1–1. **Categories of psychiatric differential diagnoses in the general hospital**

Psychiatric presentations of medical conditions

Psychiatric complications of medical conditions or treatments

Psychological reactions to medical conditions or treatments

Medical presentations of psychiatric conditions

Medical complications of psychiatric conditions or treatments

Comorbid medical and psychiatric conditions

Source.　Adapted from Lipowski 1967.

TABLE 1–2. **Procedural approach to psychiatric consultation**

Speak directly with the referring clinician.

Review the current records and pertinent past records.

Review the patient's medications.

Gather collateral data.

Interview and examine the patient.

Formulate diagnostic and therapeutic strategies.

Write a note.

Speak directly with the referring clinician.

Provide periodic follow-up.

---

only that the team recognizes that a problem exists; such problems may range from an untreated psychiatric disorder to the experience of countertransferential feelings. In speaking with a member of the team that has requested the consultation, the consultant employs some of the same techniques that will be used later in examining the patient; that is, he or she listens to the implicit as well as the explicit messages from the other physician (Murray and Kontos 2010). Is the physician angry with the patient? Is the patient not doing what the team wants him or her to do? Is the fact that the patient is young and dying leading to the team's overidentification with him or her? Is the team frustrated by an elusive diagnosis? All of these situations generate emotions that are difficult to reduce to a few words conveyed in a consultation request; moreover, the feelings often remain out of the team's awareness. This brief interaction may give the consultant invaluable information about how the consultation may be useful to the team and to the patient.

Review the Current Records and the Pertinent Past Records

When it is done with the curiosity of a detective on the trail of hidden clues, reading a chart can be an exciting and self-affirming part of the consultation process. Although it does not supplant the consultant's independent history-taking or examination, the chart review provides a general orientation to the case. Moreover, the consultant is in a unique position to focus on details that may have been previously overlooked. For example, nurses often document salient neurobehavioral data (e.g., the level of awareness and the presence of confusion or agitation); physical and occupational therapists estimate functional abilities crucial to the diagnosis of cognitive disorders and to the choice of an appropriate level of care (e.g., nursing home or assisted-living facility); and speech pathologists note alterations in articulation, swallowing, and language, all of which may indicate an organic brain disease. All of them may have written progress notes about adherence to treatment regimens, unusual behavior, interpersonal difficulties, or family issues encountered in their care of the patient. These notes may also provide unique clues to the presence of problems such as domestic violence, factitious illness, or personality disorders.

Review the Patient's Medications

Construction of a medication list at various times (e.g., when at home, on admission, on transfer within the hospital, and at present) is a good, if not essential, practice. Special attention should be paid to medications with psychoactive effects and to those associated with withdrawal syndromes (both obvious ones like benzodiazepines and opiates and less-obvious ones like antidepressants, anticonvulsants, and beta-blockers). Review of orders is not always sufficient, because—for a variety of reasons—patients may not always receive prescribed medications; therefore, medication administration records should also be reviewed. Such records are particularly important for determining the frequency of administration of medicines ordered on an as-needed basis. For example, an order for lorazepam 1–2 mg every 4–6 hours as needed may result in a patient receiving anywhere from 0 mg to 12 mg in a day, which can be critical in cases of withdrawal or oversedation.

Gather Collateral Data

Histories from hospitalized medically ill patients may be especially spotty and unreliable, if not nonexistent (e.g., with a patient who is somnolent, delirious, or comatose). Data from collateral sources (e.g., family members; friends; current and outpatient health care providers; and case managers) may be of critical importance. However, psychiatric consultants must guard against prizing any single party's version of historical events over another's; family members and others may lack objectivity, be in denial, be overinvolved, or have a personal agenda to advance. For example, family members tend to minimize early signs of dementia and to overreport depression in patients with dementia. Confidentiality must be valued when obtaining collateral information. Ideally, one obtains the patient's consent first; however, this may not be possible if the patient lacks capacity or if a dire emergency is in progress (see Chapter 2, "Legal and Ethical Issues"). Moreover, in certain situations there may be contraindications to contacting some sources of information (e.g., the partner of a woman who is experiencing abuse). Like any astute physician, the psychiatrist collates and synthesizes all available data and weighs each bit of information according to the reliability of its source.

Interview and Examine the Patient

Armed with information elicited from other sources, the psychiatric consultant now makes independent observations of the patient. For non-English-speaking patients, a translator should be employed. Although using family members may be expedient, their presence often compromises the questions asked and the translations offered because of embarrassment or other factors. It is therefore important to utilize hospital translators or, for less common languages, services via telephone. This can be difficult, but it is necessary in obtaining a full and accurate history.

The process and content of the psychiatric interview must be adapted to the consultation setting. To establish rapport and to have a therapeutic impact, the psychiatrist should assume an engaging, more spontaneous stance (typically, after explaining the purpose of the visit and inquiring about the patient's physical complaints) and deviate from the principles of anonymity, abstinence, and neutrality that help form the foundation for psychodynamic psychotherapy (see Perry and Viederman 1981). Long silences common in psychoanalytic psychotherapy are rarely appropriate with medical patients, who have not sought out psychiatric assessment and who may lack the stamina for long interviews. Deeply exploring traumatic events may not be ideal; it is often sufficient to acknowledge the patient's past hardships and provide a perspective of what treatment after discharge can offer. Neither a rigidly biological approach (which can impede rapport) nor an exclusively psychoanalytic inquiry should be adopted. It is especially important to elicit patients' beliefs about their illness (what is wrong, what caused it, what treatment can do) so that emotional responses and behaviors can be placed in perspective. Although the psychiatric consultant often works under pressure of time (e.g., conducting the evaluation between medical tests and procedures), an open-ended interview style should be used when possible.

Mental Status Examination

A thorough mental status examination is central to the psychiatric evaluation of the medically ill patient. Because the examination is hierarchical, care must be taken to complete it in a systematic fashion (Hyman and Tesar 1994). The astute consultant will glean invaluable diagnostic clues from a combination of observation and questioning.

Level of consciousness. Level of consciousness depends on normal cerebral arousal by the reticular activating system. A patient whose level of consciousness is impaired will inevitably perform poorly on cognitive testing. The finding of disorientation implies cognitive failure in one or several domains. It is helpful to test the patient's orientation near the start of the mental status examination, as it will provide an immediate clue about cognitive functioning.

Attention. The form of attention most relevant to the clinical mental status examination is the sustained attention that allows one to concentrate on cognitive tasks. Disruption of attention—often by factors that diffusely disturb brain function, such as drugs, infection, or organ failure—is a hallmark of delirium. Sustained attention is best tested with moderately demanding, nonautomatic tasks, such as reciting the months backward or, as in the Mini-Mental State Examination (MMSE; Folstein et al. 1975), spelling *world* backward or subtracting 7 serially from 100. Serial subtraction is intended to be a test of attention, not arithmetic ability, so the task should be adjusted to the patient's native ability and educational level (serial *3*s from 50, serial *1*s from 20). An inattentive patient's performance on other parts of the mental status examination may be affected on any task requiring sustained focus.

Memory.   Working memory is tested by asking the patient first to register specific information (e.g., three words) and then to recall that information after an interval of at least 3 minutes, during which other testing prevents rehearsal. This task can also be considered a test of recent memory. Semantic memory is tapped by asking general knowledge questions (e.g., "Who is the president?") and by naming and visual recognition tasks. The patient's ability to remember aspects of his or her history serves as a test of episodic memory (as well as of remote memory). Because semantic and episodic memories can be articulated, they constitute declarative memory. In contrast, procedural memory is implicit in learned action (e.g., riding a bicycle) and cannot be described in words. Deficits in procedural memory can be observed in a patient's behavior during the clinical evaluation.

Executive function.   Executive function refers to the abilities that allow one to plan, initiate, organize, and monitor thought and behavior. These abilities, which localize broadly to the frontal lobes, are essential for normal social and professional performance but are difficult to test. Frontal lobe disorders often make themselves apparent in social interaction with a patient and are suspected when one observes disinhibition, impulsivity, disorganization, abulia, or amotivation. Tasks that can be used to gain insight into frontal lobe function include verbal fluency, such as listing as many animals as possible in 1 minute; motor sequencing, such as asking the patient to replicate a sequence of three hand positions; the go/no-go task, which requires the patient to tap the desk once if the examiner taps once, but not to tap if the examiner taps twice; and tests of abstraction, including questions like "What do a tree and a fly have in common?"

Language.   Language disorders result from lesions of the dominant hemisphere. In assessing language, one should first note characteristics of the patient's speech (e.g., nonfluency or paraphasic errors) and then assess comprehension. Naming is impaired in both major varieties of aphasia, and anomia can be a clue to mild dysphasia. Reading and writing should also be assessed. Expressive (Broca's or motor) aphasia is characterized by effortful, nonfluent speech with use of phonemic paraphasias (incorrect words that approximate the correct ones in sound), reduced use of function words (e.g., prepositions and articles), and well-preserved comprehension. Receptive (Wernicke's or sensory) aphasia is characterized by fluent speech with both phonemic and semantic paraphasias (incorrect words that approximate the correct ones in meaning) and poor comprehension. The stream of incoherent speech and the lack of insight in patients with Wernicke's aphasia sometimes lead to misdiagnosis of a primary thought disorder and psychiatric referral; the clue to the diagnosis of a language disorder is the severity of the comprehension deficit. Global dysphasia combines features of Broca's and Wernicke's aphasias. Selective impairment of repetition characterizes conduction aphasia. The nondominant hemisphere plays a part in the appreciation and production of the emotional overtones of language.

Praxis.   *Apraxia* refers to an inability to perform skilled actions (e.g., using a screwdriver, brushing one's teeth) despite intact basic motor and sensory abilities. These abilities can be tested by asking a patient to mime such actions or by asking the patient to copy unfamiliar hand positions. Constructional apraxia is usually tested with the Clock Drawing Test. Gait apraxia involves difficulty in initiating and maintaining gait despite intact basic motor function in the legs. Dressing apraxia is difficulty in dressing caused by an inability to coordinate the spatial arrangement of clothing on the body.

Mood and affect.   Mood and affect both refer to the patient's emotional state, mood being the patient's perception and affect being the interviewer's perception. The interviewer must interpret both carefully, taking into account the patient's medical illness. Normal but intense expressions of emotion (e.g., grief, fear, or irritation) are common in patients with serious medical illness but may be misperceived by nonpsychiatric physicians as evidence of psychiatric disturbance. Disturbances in mood and affect may also be the result of brain dysfunction or injury. Irritability may be the first sign of many illnesses, ranging from alcohol withdrawal to rabies. Blunted affective expression may be a sign of Parkinson's disease. Intense affective lability (e.g., pathological crying or laughing) with relatively normal mood occurs with some diseases or injuries of the frontal lobes. In addition, depressed or euphoric affect may be a medication side effect.

Perception.   Perception in the mental status examination is primarily concerned with hallucinations and illusions. However, before beginning any portion of the clinical interview and the mental status examination, the interviewer should establish whether the patient has any impairment in vision or hearing that could interfere with communication. Unrecognized impairments have led to erroneous impressions that patients were demented, delirious, or psychotic. Although hallucinations in any modality may occur in primary psychotic disorders (e.g., schizophrenia or affective psychosis), prominent visual, olfactory, gustatory, or tactile hallucinations suggest a secondary medical etiology. Olfactory and gustatory hallucinations may be manifestations of seizures, and tactile hallucinations are often seen with substance use disorders.

Judgment and insight.   The traditional question for the assessment of judgment—"What would you do if you found a letter on the sidewalk?"—is much less informative than questions tailored to the problems faced by the patient being evaluated; for example, "If you couldn't stop a nosebleed, what would you do?" "If you run out of medicine and you can't reach your doctor, what would you do?" Similarly, questions to assess insight should focus on the patient's understanding of his or her illness, treatment, and life circumstances.

Further guidance on mental status examination.   An outline of the essential elements of a comprehensive mental status examination is presented in Table 1–3. Particular cognitive mental status testing maneuvers are described in more detail in Table 1–4.

Physical Examination

Although the interview and mental status examination as outlined above are generally thought to be the primary diagnostic tools of the psychiatrist, the importance of the physical examination should not be forgotten, especially in the medical setting. Most psychiatrists do not perform physical examinations on their patients. The consultation psychiatrist, however, should be familiar with and comfortable performing neurological examinations and other selected features of the physical examination that may uncover the common comorbidities in psychiatric patients. At an absolute

---

TABLE 1–3. **The mental status examination**

Level of consciousness

Alert, drowsy, somnolent, stuporous, comatose; fluctuations suggest delirium

Appearance and behavior

Overall appearance, grooming, hygiene

Cooperation, eye contact, psychomotor agitation or retardation

Abnormal movements: tics, tremors, chorea, posturing

Attention

Vigilance, concentration, ability to focus, sensory neglect

Orientation and memory

Orientation to person, place, time, situation

Recent, remote, and immediate recall

Language

Speech: rate, volume, fluency, prosody

Comprehension and naming ability

Abnormalities including aphasia, dysarthria, agraphia, alexia, clanging, neologisms, echolalia

Constructional ability

Clock drawing to assess neglect, executive function, and planning

Drawing of a cube or intersecting pentagons to assess parietal function

Mood and affect

Mood: subjective sustained emotion

Affect: observed emotion—quality, range, appropriateness

Form and content of thought

Form: linear, circumstantial, tangential, disorganized, blocked

Content: delusions, paranoia, ideas of reference, suicidal or homicidal ideation

Perception

Auditory, visual, gustatory, tactile, and olfactory hallucinations

Judgment and insight

Understanding of illness and consequences of specific treatments offered

Reasoning

Illogical versus logical; ability to make consistent decisions

---

Source.   Adapted from Hyman and Tesar 1994.

---

minimum, the consultant should review the physical examinations performed by other physicians. However, the psychiatrist's examination of the patient, especially of central nervous system functions relevant to the differential diagnosis, is often essential. A more complete physical examination is appropriate on medical-psychiatric units or whenever the psychiatrist has assumed responsibility for the care of a patient's medical problems. Even with a sedated or comatose patient, simple observation and a few maneuvers that involve a laying on of hands may potentially yield significant findings. Although it is beyond the scope of this chapter to discuss a com-

TABLE 1–4. **Detailed assessment of cognitive domains**

Cognitive domain	Assessment
Level of consciousness and arousal	Inspect the patient.
Orientation to place and time	Ask direct questions about both of these.
Registration (recent memory)	Have the patient repeat three words immediately.
Recall (working memory)	Have the patient recall the same three words after performing another task for at least 3 minutes.
Remote memory	Ask about the patient's age, date of birth, milestones, or significant life or historical events (e.g., names of presidents, dates of wars).
Attention and concentration	Subtract serial 7s (adapt to the patient's level of education; subtract serial 3s if less educated). Spell *world* backward (this may be difficult for non–English speakers). Test digit span forward and backward. Have the patient recite the months of the year (or the days of the week) in reverse order.
Language	(Adapt the degree of difficulty to the patient's educational level.)
Comprehension	Inspect the patient while he or she answers questions.
	Ask the patient to point to different objects.
	Ask yes-or-no questions.
	Ask the patient to write a phrase (paragraph).
Naming	Show a watch, pen, or less familiar objects, if needed.
Fluency	Assess the patient's speech.
	Have the patient name as many animals as he or she can in 1 minute.
Articulation	Listen to the patient's speech.
	Have the patient repeat a phrase.
Reading	Have the patient read a sentence (or a longer paragraph if needed).
Executive function	Determine whether the patient requires constant cueing and prompting.
Commands	Have the patient follow a three-step command.
Construction tasks	Have the patient draw interlocked pentagons.
	Have the patient draw a clock.
Motor programming tasks	Have the patient perform serial hand sequences.
	Have the patient perform reciprocal programs of raising fingers.
Judgment and reasoning	Listen to the patient's account of his or her history and reason for hospitalization. Assess abstraction (similarities: dog/cat; red/green). Test the patient's judgment about simple events or problems: "A construction worker fell to the ground from the seventh floor of the building and broke his two legs; he then ran to the nearby hospital to ask for medical help. Do you have any comment on this?"

prehensive physical examination, Table 1–5 provides an outline of selected findings of the physical examination and their relevance to the psychiatric consultation.

Formulate Diagnostic and Therapeutic Strategies

By the time the consultant arrives on the scene, routine chemical and hematological tests and urinalyses are almost always available and should be reviewed along with any other laboratory, imaging, and electrophysiological tests. The consultant then considers what additional tests are needed to arrive at a diagnosis. Before ordering a test, the consultant must consider the likelihood that the test will contribute to making a diagnosis.

While there is an extensive list of studies that could be relevant to psychiatric presentations, the most common screening tests in clinical practice are listed in Table 1–6. It was once common practice for the psychiatrist to order routine batteries of tests, especially in cognitively impaired patients, in a stereotypical diagnostic approach to the evaluation of dementia or delirium. In modern practice, tests should be ordered selectively, with consideration paid to sensitivity, specificity, and cost-effectiveness. Perhaps most important, careful thought should be given to whether the results of each test will affect the patient's management. Finally, further studies may be beneficial in certain clinical situations as described throughout this book.

Routine Tests

A complete blood cell count may reveal anemia that contributes to depression or infection that causes psychosis. Leukocytosis is seen with infection and other acute inflammatory conditions, lithium therapy, and neuroleptic malignant syndrome, whereas leukopenia and agranulocytosis may be caused by certain psychotropic medications. A serum chemistry panel may point to diagnoses as varied as liver disease, eating disorders, renal disease, and malnutrition—all of which may have psychiatric manifestations (Alpay and Park 2004). Serum and urine toxicological screens are helpful in cases of altered sensorium and obviously whenever substance use, intoxication, or overdose is suspected. Because blood tests for syphilis, thyroid disease, and deficiencies of vitamin B_{12} and folic acid (conditions that are curable) are readily available, they warrant a low threshold for their use. In patients with a history of exposures, HIV infection should not be overlooked. Obtaining a pregnancy test is often wise in women of childbearing age to inform diagnostically as well as to guide treatment options. Urinalysis, chest radiography, and electrocardiography are particularly important screening tools in the geriatric population. Although it is not a first-line test, cerebrospinal fluid analysis should be considered in cases of mental status changes associated with fever, leukocytosis, meningismus, or unknown etiology. Increased intracranial pressure should be ruled out before a lumbar puncture is performed, however. More detailed discussion of specific tests is provided in relevant chapters throughout this text.

TABLE 1–5. **Selected elements of the physical examination and significance of findings**

Elements	Examples of possible diagnoses
General	
General appearance healthier than expected	Somatic symptom disorders
Fever	Infection or NMS
Blood pressure or pulse abnormalities	Withdrawal, thyroid or cardiovascular disease
Body habitus	Eating disorders, polycystic ovaries, or Cushing's syndrome
Skin	
Diaphoresis	Fever, withdrawal, NMS
Piloerection ("gooseflesh")	Opioid withdrawal
Dry, flushed	Anticholinergic toxicity, heatstroke
Pallor	Anemia
Changes in hair, nails, skin	Malnutrition, thyroid or adrenal disease, polycystic ovaries
Jaundice	Liver disease
Characteristic stigmata	Syphilis, cirrhosis, or self-mutilation
Bruises	Physical abuse, ataxia, traumatic brain injury
Eyes	
Mydriasis	Opiate withdrawal, anticholinergic toxicity
Miosis	Opiate intoxication, cholinergic toxicity
Kayser-Fleischer rings	Wilson's disease
Neurological	
Tremors	Delirium, withdrawal syndromes, parkinsonism, lithium toxicity
Primitive reflexes present (e.g., snout, glabellar, grasp)	Dementia, frontal lobe dysfunction
Hyperactive deep tendon reflexes	Withdrawal, hyperthyroidism
Ophthalmoplegia	Wernicke's encephalopathy, brain stem dysfunction, dystonic reaction
Papilledema	Increased intracranial pressure
Hypertonia, rigidity, catatonia, parkinsonism	EPS, NMS
Abnormal movements	Parkinson's disease, Huntington's disease, EPS
Abnormal gait	Normal-pressure hydrocephalus, Parkinson's disease, Wernicke's encephalopathy
Loss of position and vibratory sense	Vitamin B_{12} deficiency

Note. EPS=extrapyramidal symptoms; NMS = neuroleptic malignant syndrome.

TABLE 1–6.   Common tests in psychiatric consultation
Complete blood count
Serum chemistry panel
Thyroid-stimulating hormone (thyrotropin) concentration
Vitamin B_{12} (cyanocobalamin) concentration
Folic acid (folate) concentration
Human chorionic gonadotropin (pregnancy) test
Toxicology
Serum
Urine
Serological tests for syphilis
HIV tests
Urinalysis
Electrocardiogram

Neuroimaging

The psychiatric consultant must also be familiar with neuroimaging. Neuroimaging may aid in the differential diagnosis of neuropsychiatric conditions, although it rarely establishes the diagnosis by itself (Dougherty and Rauch 2004). In most situations, magnetic resonance imaging (MRI) is preferred over computed tomography (CT). MRI provides greater resolution of subcortical structures (e.g., basal ganglia, amygdala, and other limbic structures) of particular interest to psychiatrists. It is also superior for detection of abnormalities of the brain stem and posterior fossa. Furthermore, MRI is better able to distinguish between gray matter and white matter lesions. CT is most useful in cases of suspected acute intracranial hemorrhage (having occurred within the past 72 hours) and when MRI is contraindicated (in patients with metallic implants). Dougherty and Rauch (2004) suggest that the following conditions and situations merit consideration of neuroimaging: new-onset psychosis, new-onset dementia, delirium of unknown cause, prior to an initial course of electroconvulsive therapy, and an acute mental status change with an abnormal neurological examination in a patient with either a history of head trauma or an age of 50 years or older. Regardless of the modality, the consultant should read the radiologist's report, because other physicians tend to dismiss all but acute focal findings and, as a result, misleadingly record the results of the study as normal in the chart. Psychiatrists recognize, however, that even small abnormalities (e.g., periventricular white matter changes) or chronic changes (e.g., cortical atrophy) have diagnostic and therapeutic implications (see Chapter 5, "Dementia," Chapter 7, "Depression," and Chapter 30, "Neurology and Neurosurgery").

Electrophysiological Tests

The electroencephalogram (EEG) is the most widely available test that can assess brain activity. The EEG is most often indicated in patients with paroxysmal or other symptoms suggestive of a seizure disorder, especially complex partial seizures or pseudoseizures (see Chapter 30, "Neurology and Neurosurgery"). An EEG may also be helpful in distinguishing between neurological and psychiatric etiologies for a mute, uncommunicative patient. An EEG may be helpful in documenting the presence of generalized slowing in a delirious patient, but it rarely indicates a specific etiology of delirium and it is not indicated in every delirious patient. However, when the diagnosis of delirium is uncertain, EEG evidence of dysrhythmia may prove useful. For example, when the primary treatment team insists that a patient should be transferred to a psychiatric inpatient service because of a mistaken belief that the symptoms of delirium represent schizophrenia or depression, an EEG can provide concrete data to support the correct diagnosis. EEGs may also facilitate the evaluation of rapidly progressive dementia or profound coma; but because findings are neither sensitive nor specific, they are not often helpful in the evaluation of space-occupying lesions, cerebral infarctions, or head injury (Bostwick and Philbrick 2002). Continuous EEG recordings with video monitoring or ambulatory EEG monitoring may be necessary in order to document abnormal electrical activity in cases of complex partial seizures or when psychogenic seizures are suspected. As with neuroimaging reports, the psychiatric consultant must read the EEG report, because nonpsychiatrists often misinterpret the absence of dramatic focal abnormalities (e.g., spikes) as indicative of normality, even though psychiatrically significant brain dysfunction may be associated with focal or generalized slowing or with sharp waves. Other electrophysiological tests may be helpful in specific situations; for example, sensory evoked potentials to distinguish multiple sclerosis from conversion disorder, or electromyography with nerve conduction velocities to differentiate neuropathy from malingering.

Other Tests

Other diagnostic tools may also prove useful as adjuncts. Neuropsychological testing may be helpful in diagnosis, prognosis, and treatment planning in patients with neuropsychiatric disorders. Psychological testing can help the consultant better understand a patient's emotional functioning and personality style. For example, elevations on the Hypochondriasis and Hysteria scales of the Minnesota Multiphasic Personality Inventory and a normal or minimally elevated result on the Depression scale constitute the so-called conversion V or psychosomatic V pattern, classically regarded as indicative of a significant psychological contribution to the etiology of somatic symptoms but now recognized as confounded by medical illness.

Write a Note

The consultation note should be clear, concise, and free of jargon and should focus on specific diagnostic and therapeutic recommendations. Although an understanding of the patient's psychodynamics may be helpful, the consultant should usually avoid speculations in the chart regarding unconscious motivations. Consultees fundamentally want to know what is going on with the patient and what they should and can do about it; these themes should dominate the note. Mental health care professionals are trained to construct full developmental and psychosocial formulations, but these do not belong in a consultation note (although they may inform key elements of the assessment and recommendations). Finger-pointing and criticism of the primary care team or other providers should be avoided. The consultant should also avoid rigid insistence on a preferred mode of management if there is an equally suitable alternative (Kontos et al. 2003).

The consultation note should include a condensed version of all the elements of a general psychiatric note with a few additions (Querques et al. 2012). The consultant should begin the note with a summary of the patient's medical and psychiatric history, the reason for the current admission, and the reason for the consultation. Next should be a brief summary of the current medical illness with pertinent findings and hospital course; this summary is meant to demonstrate an appreciation for the current medical issues rather than to repeat what has already been documented in the chart. It is often helpful for the consultant to include a description of the patient's typical patterns of response to stress and illness, if known. Relevant physical and neurological examinations, as well as germane laboratory results or imaging studies, should also be summarized rather than pasting in the entirety of test results. The consultant should then list the differential diagnosis in order of decreasing likelihood, making clear which is the working diagnosis or diagnoses. If the patient's symptoms are not likely to be due to a psychiatric disorder, this should be explicitly stated. Finally, the consultant should make recommendations or clearly describe plans in order of decreasing importance. Recommendations include ways to further elucidate the diagnosis as well as therapeutic suggestions. It is especially important to anticipate and address problems that may appear at a later time (e.g., offering a medication recommendation for treatment of agitation in a delirious patient who is currently calm). For medication recommendations, brief notation of side effects and their management is useful. The inclusion of a statement indicating that the consultant will provide follow-up will reassure the consulting team, and the consultant should include contact information in the event that they have further questions.

Speak Directly With the Referring Clinician

The consultation ends in the same way that it began—with a conversation with the referring clinician. Personal contact is especially crucial if diagnostic or therapeutic suggestions are time-sensitive. Some information or recommendations may be especially sensitive, whether for reasons of confidentiality or risk management, and are better conveyed verbally than fully documented in the chart. The medical chart is read by a variety of individuals, including the patient at times, and, thus, discretion is warranted.

Provide Periodic Follow-Up

Many consultations cannot be completed in a single visit. Rather, several encounters may be required before the problems identified by both the consultee and the consultant are resolved. Moreover, new issues commonly arise during the course of the consultative process, and a single consultation request often necessitates frequent visits, disciplined follow-up, and easy accessibility. All follow-up visits should be documented in the chart. Finally, it may be appropriate to sign off of a case when the patient is stabilized or when the consultant's opinion and recommendations are being disregarded.

Role of Other Providers

Although the emphasis of this chapter is on the psychiatrist as consultant, the value of members of other professions, working together as a team, should not be over-

looked. Psychologists play an essential role in performing neuropsychological and psychological assessments and providing psychotherapeutic and behavioral interventions. Psychiatric clinical nurse specialists provide services to the nursing staff that parallel those that the psychiatrist provides to the medical team. They are especially helpful in organizing interdisciplinary care conferences and nursing behavioral treatment plans that include behavioral contracts with patients. Social workers and care coordinators facilitate transfers and set up aftercare. Chaplains address the spiritual needs of patients in distress. Finally, communication with primary care physicians and outpatient psychiatrists remains of utmost importance, since the primary care physician is well positioned to provide and coordinate ongoing care after discharge.

Consultation and Collaborative Care in the Outpatient Setting

Whereas the majority of this chapter has focused on psychiatric consultation in the inpatient setting, it could be argued that the consultation psychiatrist provides an even greater impact by working collaboratively with primary care physicians in the outpatient domain (Stern et al. 2004). Many studies over the past 35 years have established both the high prevalence of mental disorders in outpatient medical settings and the fact that more people with mental disorders present to general medical settings than to psychiatrists (Unützer et al. 2006). In their report for the President's New Freedom Commission on Mental Health, Unützer et al. (2006) described a number of common barriers to effective mental health care at the interface with medicine, including the following: incorrect identification of symptoms by patients or reluctance to seek psychiatric care due to stigma; lack of mental health care training for primary care providers; lack of time to fully address mental health issues in brief clinical encounters in the primary care setting; and restrictions in insurance coverage for mental health care services. The elderly, children and adolescents, ethnic minorities, and uninsured individuals are especially susceptible to having their needs unmet in this regard (Unützer et al. 2006). Given that general medical settings comprise such a significant portion of the mental health care system, what strategies may be used to improve quality and efficacy of care?

Initial studies that focused on the improvement of mental health care in general medical settings stressed diagnosis and screening techniques (Gilbody et al. 2001; Spitzer et al. 1999) (see a detailed description of screening tools for this population later in this chapter). Subsequent inquiries then combined screening with systematic feedback of diagnoses to the primary care providers. These studies revealed that whereas screening and giving feedback to providers often increase the rate of diagnosis of mental disorders, they are not sufficient to improve patient outcomes (Katon and Gonzales 1994; Klinkman and Okkes 1998). Similar results were obtained when researchers looked at the efficacy of employing treatment guidelines for the care of common psychiatric disorders in primary care settings in combination with developing comprehensive training for providers (Hodges et al. 2001; Simon 2002). A simple referral to a psychiatrist is often inadequate for a myriad of reasons, including lack of access to mental health care practitioners (especially for underserved populations), lack of patient follow-through (e.g., the patient never makes it to the appointment), and inability to pay for mental health care services. Although adequate screening, use of practice guidelines, provider training, and referral to specialists are all important components of improving mental health care in general medical settings, research has shown that these alone are inadequate (Unützer et al. 2006). The development of collaborative care models represents a potential solution to this problem.

Collaborative care refers to the joining together of mental health care providers with primary care physicians and their teams to deliver specialized care within the outpatient primary care setting. Consultation psychiatrists are uniquely positioned for this role, given the focus of psychosomatic medicine at the interface of medicine and psychiatry. While specific models of collaborative care vary, effective programs generally share certain key components. The first is systematic care management (often by a trained nurse, social worker, or psychologist). The care manager helps identify patients in need, coordinates an initial treatment plan, educates patients, provides follow-up, monitors progress, and helps change the treatment course as needed. These tasks may be performed in person (e.g., in the primary care clinic) or by telephone (Worth and Stern 2003). The next essential piece is consultation and appropriate sharing of information among the primary care provider, the care manager, and the consulting psychiatrist (Unützer et al. 2006). This does not necessarily mean that the psychiatric specialist provides a consultation for every patient; in fact, research has shown that the most efficient and cost-effective measures often involve a stepwise approach in which progressively more intensive interventions are applied until a successful outcome is achieved (Katon et al. 2005, 2008; Richards et al. 2008). Thus, stepped care for a patient with depression might involve an initial intervention of prescription of an antidepressant by the primary care provider along with care management either by phone or in person, as detailed above. If the patient remains symptomatic, the next step would be referral for brief psychotherapy or other behavioral interventions and/or a switch to another medication. While much of this process takes place under the supervision of a consulting psychiatrist, referral to mental health care specialists is generally reserved for treatment nonresponders. For example, in the IMPACT (Improving Mood—Promoting Access to Collaborative Treatment) randomized trial for depressed elderly patients in primary care, consulting psychiatrists saw only about 10% of patients but served as key members of the collaborative team by providing consultation and education to care managers and primary care providers (Hunkeler et al. 2006; Unützer et al. 2002). Collaborative care models have been shown to improve outcomes and enhance patient function and quality of life as well as to be cost-effective (Rossom et al. 2017). For further discussion of collaborative care, see Chapter 37, "Psychotherapy."

Screening

As mentioned in the previous section, the use of screening tools may be helpful in specific situations. For example, even though a comprehensive assessment of cognitive function is not required for every patient, even a slim suspicion of the possibility of a cognitive deficit should prompt performance of cognitive screening. Although individualized mental status examinations performed as part of a psychiatrist's clinical interview are much preferred to standardized tests, screening tests may be particularly useful in case finding (e.g., in primary care settings as part of a collaborative care approach) and in research. The same has been proposed for a variety of other psychiatric disorders, including depressive, anxiety, and substance use disorders. An important note in this regard, however, is that screening is unlikely to be helpful without a systematic approach to treatment and may even have negative effects (Thombs et al. 2012) (see also the discussion of collaborative care above). This is evidenced by a meta-analysis that showed that when used alone, screening questionnaires for depression did not have an impact on the actual detection and management of depression by clinicians in non–mental health care settings (Gilbody et al. 2008). Such findings underscore the importance of collaboration between psychosomatic medicine specialists and general medical teams (in both the outpatient and inpatient settings), with screening tools as just one aspect of this collaboration. Selected instruments are described below; others are discussed in the relevant chapters in this book.

Tests such as the MMSE and the Montreal Cognitive Assessment (MoCA) are helpful adjuncts to quickly identify potential cognitive disorders. The MMSE is a 19-question test that provides an overview of a patient's cognitive function at a moment in time; it includes assessment of orientation, attention, and memory. It is of limited use without modification, however, in patients who are deaf or blind, who are intubated, or who do not speak English. The MMSE is also particularly insensitive in measuring cognitive decline in very intelligent patients, who may appear less impaired than they really are. The MoCA is a more recently developed and validated bedside test (Nasreddine et al. 2005) that takes approximately 10 minutes to administer. It incorporates some elements of the MMSE (i.e., tests of memory, attention, and orientation) with more complex tests of visuospatial and executive function (i.e., clock drawing and an adaptation of the Trail Making Test part B). Although the MoCA is not specifically validated for delirium, it has been shown to be more sensitive than the MMSE in detecting cognitive impairment from a variety of causes. The MMSE and the MoCA may be supplemented with other tests—including Luria maneuvers and cognitive estimations (e.g., How many slices are there in an average loaf of white bread? How long is the human spinal cord?)—that further assess the functioning of frontal–subcortical networks. A formal neuropsychological battery may be useful if these bedside tests produce abnormal results. In a patient with an altered level of awareness or attention, formal cognitive tests should be deferred until the sensorium clears, because clouding of consciousness will produce uninterpretable results.

Other screening instruments may also help to identify patients in medical settings who could benefit from a comprehensive psychiatric interview. The Patient Health Questionnaire (PHQ), an abbreviated form of the Primary Care Evaluation of Mental Disorders (PRIME-MD), is a three-page questionnaire that can be entirely self-administered by the patient (Spitzer et al. 1999). In addition to the assessment of mood, anxiety, eating, alcohol use, and somatization disorders, the PHQ screens for posttraumatic stress disorder and common psychosocial stressors and also elicits a pregnancy history. The PHQ is valid and reliable and has improved the diagnosis of psychiatric conditions in primary care and other ambulatory medical settings (Spitzer et al. 1999); it may also have a role at the bedside. Subsets of the PHQ's items have been validated for specific screening purposes. For example, the nine-item PHQ-9, a self-administered depression-specific questionnaire that can be completed by the patient in roughly 2 minutes (Gilbody et al. 2007a; Kroenke et al. 2001), has been shown to perform as well (in a range of countries, populations, and clinical settings) as longer clinician-administered instruments that screen for depression in medical settings (Gilbody et al. 2007b); it can also be used to monitor the severity of depression. The PHQ-2 for depression, which includes just the items for mood and anhedonia, is sensitive and specific for both major depressive disorder and other depressive disorders, performing almost as well as the PHQ-9 (Löwe et al. 2005).

The PHQ-15 assesses 15 somatic symptoms and is useful as an index of somatization (Kroenke et al. 2002). The Generalized Anxiety Disorder 7-item (GAD-7) scale is a valid and efficient tool for screening for generalized anxiety disorder and assessing its severity (Spitzer et al. 2006).

The Clinical Outcomes in Routine Evaluation—Outcome Measure (CORE-OM; Barkham et al. 2001) is a 34-item instrument that measures a range of mental health problems as well as functional capacity and risk of harm to self or others that has been validated for assessment of depression in the primary care setting (Gilbody et al. 2007a).

The General Health Questionnaire (GHQ) is another instrument originally developed in the 1970s to screen for psychiatric disorders in medical outpatients (Goldberg and Blackwell 1970). The original 60-item version has been replaced with well-validated 28- and 12-item versions. The GHQ has been translated into numerous languages worldwide and is cross-culturally validated (Tait et al. 2003). Because of its emphasis on identifying new symptoms, the GHQ is most useful for assessing state rather than trait conditions (Tait et al. 2003).

The CAGE questionnaire is a well-known screening device developed by Ewing (1984) to identify alcohol use disorder. Two or more positive responses on the four-question screen correlates with an 89% chance of alcohol use disorder (Mayfield et al. 1974) (see Chapter 16, "Substance-Related Disorders"). Other screening tests are described in the chapters covering specific syndromes (e.g., depression, anxiety, delirium).

Practice Guidelines

Groups from several countries have developed psychosomatic medicine practice guidelines that detail professional standards for psychiatric consultation in nonpsychiatric settings, referencing the appropriate knowledge base as well as delineating integrated clinical approaches, effective methods, and ways to enhance adherence to recommendations made by the consulting psychiatrist (Bronheim et al. 1998; Leentjens et al. 2009; Royal Colleges of Physicians and Psychiatrists 1995). Although a complete review of these guidelines is beyond the scope of this chapter, they may serve as excellent additions to the information provided here. Especially helpful are practice guidelines informing evaluation of specific disorders (e.g., delirium [Leentjens and Diefenbacher 2006]) or specific tasks (e.g., psychosocial evaluation of living unrelated organ donors [Dew et al. 2007]; management of patients who engage in self-harm [Carter et al. 2016]).

Benefits of Psychiatric Services

The benefits of psychiatric services in health care delivery are significant. An extensive body of evidence has demonstrated a link between comorbid psychopathology and increased length of hospital stay and, consequently, increased inpatient costs. Levenson et al. (1990) described a longer median length of hospital stay (a 40% increase) and hospital costs that were 35% higher in medical inpatients with depression, anxiety, cognitive dysfunction, or high levels of pain (independent of severity of medical illness). Depressed elderly patients in another sample had more hospitalizations and longer hospital stays (Koenig and Kuchibhatla 1998). Although it was hoped that psychiatric consultation might decrease lengths of stay and inpatient costs, it has been difficult to prove and is not where its primary value lies. Patients benefit from the reductions in mental suffering and improvements in psychological well-being that result from more accurate diagnosis and more appropriate treatment. The adverse effects of psychopathology on specific medical disorders, and the benefits of treating it, are reviewed in remaining chapters of this textbook. Providers of health care profit from the added diagnostic and therapeutic expertise of the psychiatric consultant as well as from a better understanding of health behaviors. The hospital milieu also benefits from having readily available medically knowledgeable psychiatrists, whose assistance improves the care of the complex patients described in the rest of this textbook, contributing to better risk management and a safer and more pleasant work environment.

Conclusion

Psychiatric assessment and consultation can be crucial to seriously ill medical patients. The psychosomatic medicine psychiatrist is an expert in the diagnosis and care of psychopathology in the medically ill. Psychiatric consultation affords a unique ability to offer a panoramic view of the patient, the illness, and the relationship between the two. The psychiatric consultant will be called on to help diagnose, understand, and manage a wide array of conditions; when effective, the consultant addresses the needs of both the patient and the medical–surgical team. In this manner, psychiatric consultation is essential to the provision of comprehensive care in the medical setting.

References

Alpay M, Park L: Laboratory tests and diagnostic procedures, in Massachusetts General Hospital Psychiatry Update and Board Preparation, 2nd Edition. Edited by Stern TA, Herman JB. New York, McGraw-Hill, 2004, pp 251–265

Barkham M, Margison F, Leach C, et al; Clinical Outcomes in Routine Evaluation-Outcome Measures: Service profiling and outcomes benchmarking using the CORE-OM: toward practice-based evidence in the psychological therapies. J Consult Clin Psychol 69(2):184–196, 2001 11393596

Bostwick JM, Philbrick KL: The use of electroencephalography in psychiatry of the medically ill. Psychiatr Clin North Am 25(1):17–25, 2002 11912938

Bronheim HE, Fulop G, Kunkel EJ, et al; The Academy of Psychosomatic Medicine: The Academy of Psychosomatic Medicine practice guidelines for psychiatric consultation in the general medical setting. Psychosomatics 39(4):S8–S30, 1998 9691717

Carter G, Page A, Large M, et al: Royal Australian and New Zealand College of Psychiatrists clinical practice guideline for the management of deliberate self-harm. Aust N Z J Psychiatry 50(10):939–1000, 2016 27650687

Dew MA, Jacobs CL, Jowsey SG, et al; United Network for Organ Sharing (UNOS); American Society of Transplant Surgeons; American Society of Transplantation: Guidelines for the psychosocial evaluation of living unrelated kidney donors in the United States. Am J Transplant 7(5):1047–1054, 2007 17359510

Dougherty DD, Rauch SL: Neuroimaging in psychiatry, in Massachusetts General Hospital Psychiatry Update and Board Preparation, 2nd Edition. Edited by Stern TA, Herman JB. New York, McGraw-Hill, 2004, pp 227–232

Eshel N, Marcovitz DE, Stern TA: Psychiatric consultations in less-than-private places: challenges and unexpected benefits of hospital roommates. Psychosomatics 57(1):97–101, 2016 26671624

Ewing JA: Detecting alcoholism. The CAGE questionnaire. JAMA 252(14):1905–1907, 1984 6471323

Folstein MF, Folstein SE, McHugh PR: "Mini-mental state": a practical method for grading the cognitive state of patients for the clinician. J Psychiatr Res 12(3):189–198, 1975 1202204

Gilbody SM, House AO, Sheldon TA: Routinely administered questionnaires for depression and anxiety: systematic review. BMJ 322(7283):406–409, 2001 11179161

Gilbody S, Richards D, Barkham M: Diagnosing depression in primary care using self-completed instruments: UK validation of PHQ-9 and CORE-OM. Br J Gen Pract 57(541):650–652, 2007a 17688760

Gilbody S, Richards D, Brealey S, et al: Screening for depression in medical settings with the Patient Health Questionnaire (PHQ): a diagnostic meta-analysis. J Gen Intern Med 22(11):1596–1602, 2007b 17874169

Gilbody S, Sheldon T, House A: Screening and case-finding instruments for depression: a meta-analysis. CMAJ 178(8):997–1003, 2008 18390942

Gitlin DF, Levenson JL, Lyketsos CG: Psychosomatic medicine: a new psychiatric subspecialty. Acad Psychiatry 28(1):4–11, 2004 15140802

Goldberg DP, Blackwell B: Psychiatric illness in general practice. A detailed study using a new method of case identification. BMJ 1(5707):439–443, 1970 5420206

Hackett TP, Cassem NH, Stern TA, et al: Beginnings: psychosomatic medicine and consultation psychiatry in the general hospital, in Massachusetts General Hospital Handbook of General Hospital Psychiatry, 6th Edition. Edited by Stern TA, Fricchione GL, Cassem NH, et al. Philadelphia, PA, Saunders/Elsevier, 2010, pp 1–6

Hodges B, Inch C, Silver I: Improving the psychiatric knowledge, skills, and attitudes of primary care physicians, 1950–2000: a review. Am J Psychiatry 158(10):1579–1586, 2001 11578983

Hunkeler EM, Katon W, Tang L, et al: Long term outcomes from the IMPACT randomised trial for depressed elderly patients in primary care. BMJ 332(7536):259–263, 2006 16428253

Hyman SE, Tesar GE: The emergency psychiatric evaluation, including the mental status examination, in Manual of Psychiatric Emergencies, 3rd Edition. Edited by Hyman SE, Tesar GE. Boston, MA, Little, Brown, 1994, pp 3–11

Katon W, Gonzales J: A review of randomized trials of psychiatric consultation-liaison studies in primary care. Psychosomatics 35(3):268–278, 1994 8036256

Katon WJ, Schoenbaum M, Fan MY, et al: Cost-effectiveness of improving primary care treatment of late-life depression. Arch Gen Psychiatry 62(12):1313–1320, 2005 16330719

Katon WJ, Russo JE, Von Korff M, et al: Long-term effects on medical costs of improving depression outcomes in patients with depression and diabetes. Diabetes Care 31(6):1155–1159, 2008 18332158

Klinkman MS, Okkes I: Mental health problems in primary care. A research agenda. J Fam Pract 47(5):379–384, 1998 9834775

Koenig HG, Kuchibhatla M: Use of health services by hospitalized medically ill depressed elderly patients. Am J Psychiatry 155(7):871–877, 1998 9659849

Kontos N, Freudenreich O, Querques J, Norris E: The consultation psychiatrist as effective physician. Gen Hosp Psychiatry 25(1):20–23, 2003 12583923

Kroenke K, Spitzer RL, Williams JB: The PHQ-9: validity of a brief depression severity measure. J Gen Intern Med 16(9):606–613, 2001 11556941

Kroenke K, Spitzer RL, Williams JB: The PHQ-15: validity of a new measure for evaluating the severity of somatic symptoms. Psychosom Med 64(2):258–266, 2002 11914441

Leentjens AF, Diefenbacher A: A survey of delirium guidelines in Europe. J Psychosom Res 61(1):123–128, 2006 16813854

Leentjens AFG, Boenink AD, Sno HN, et al; Netherlands Psychiatric Association: The guideline "consultation psychiatry" of the Netherlands Psychiatric Association. J Psychosom Res 66(6):531–535, 2009 19446712

Levenson JL, Hamer RM, Rossiter LF: Relation of psychopathology in general medical inpatients to use and cost of services. Am J Psychiatry 147(11):1498–1503, 1990 2121054

Lipowski ZJ: Review of consultation psychiatry and psychosomatic medicine, II: clinical aspects. Psychosom Med 29(3):201–224, 1967 5340349

Löwe B, Kroenke K, Gräfe K: Detecting and monitoring depression with a two-item questionnaire (PHQ-2). J Psychosom Res 58(2):163–171, 2005 15820844

Mayfield D, McLeod G, Hall P: The CAGE questionnaire: validation of a new alcoholism screening instrument. Am J Psychiatry 131(10):1121–1123, 1974 4416585

Murray GB, Kontos N: Limbic music, in Massachusetts General Hospital Handbook of General Hospital Psychiatry, 6th Edition. Edited by Stern TA, Fricchione GF, Cassem NH, et al. Philadelphia, PA, Saunders/Elsevier, 2010, pp 45–51

Nasreddine ZS, Phillips NA, Bédirian V, et al: The Montreal Cognitive Assessment, MoCA: a brief screening tool for mild cognitive impairment. J Am Geriatr Soc 53(4):695–699, 2005 15817019

Perry S, Viederman M: Adaptation of residents to consultation-liaison psychiatry, I: working with the physically ill. Gen Hosp Psychiatry 3(2):141–147, 1981 7250694

Querques J, Stern TA, Cassem NH: Psychiatric consultation to medical and surgical patients, in Massachusetts General Hospital Psychiatry Update and Board Preparation, 3rd Edition. Edited by Stern TA, Herman JB, Gorrindo T. Boston, MA, Massachusetts General Hospital Psychiatry Academy, 2012, pp 525–527

Richards DA, Lovell K, Gilbody S, et al: Collaborative care for depression in UK primary care: a randomized controlled trial. Psychol Med 38(2):279–287, 2008 17803837

Rossom RC, Solberg LI, Magnan S, et al: Impact of a national collaborative care initiative for patients with depression and diabetes or cardiovascular disease. Gen Hosp Psychiatry 44:77–85, 2017 27558106

Royal Colleges of Physicians and Psychiatrists: The psychological care of medical patients: recognition of need and service provision. A joint working party report. London, Royal College of General Practitioners, 1995

Simon GE: Evidence review: efficacy and effectiveness of antidepressant treatment in primary care. Gen Hosp Psychiatry 24(4):213–224, 2002 12100832

Spitzer RL, Kroenke K, Williams JB: Validation and utility of a self-report version of PRIME-MD: the PHQ primary care study. Primary Care Evaluation of Mental Disorders. Patient Health Questionnaire. JAMA 282(18):1737–1744, 1999 10568646

Spitzer RL, Kroenke K, Williams JB, et al: A brief measure for assessing generalized anxiety disorder: the GAD-7. Arch Intern Med 166(10):1092–1097, 2006 16717171

Stern TA, Herman JB, Slavin PL (eds): Massachusetts General Hospital Guide to Primary Care Psychiatry, 2nd Edition. New York, McGraw-Hill, 2004

Tait RJ, French DJ, Hulse GK: Validity and psychometric properties of the General Health Questionnaire-12 in young Australian adolescents. Aust N Z J Psychiatry 37(3):374–381, 2003 12780478

Thombs BD, Coyne JC, Cuijpers P, et al: Rethinking recommendations for screening for depression in primary care. CMAJ 184(4):413–418, 2012 21930744

Unützer J, Katon W, Callahan CM, et al; IMPACT Investigators. Improving Mood-Promoting Access to Collaborative Treatment: Collaborative care management of late-life depression in the primary care setting: a randomized controlled trial. JAMA 288(22):2836–2845, 2002 12472325

Unützer J, Schoenbaum M, Druss BG, et al: Transforming mental health care at the interface with general medicine: report for the presidents commission. Psychiatr Serv 57(1):37–47, 2006 16399961

Worth JL, Stern TA: Benefits of an outpatient Psychiatric TeleConsultation Unit (PTCU): results of a one-year pilot. Prim Care Companion J Clin Psychiatry 5(2):80–84, 2003 15156235

CHAPTER 2

Legal and Ethical Issues

Rebecca W. Brendel, M.D., J.D.
Ronald Schouten, M.D., J.D.
Ariana Nesbit, M.D., M.B.E.
James L. Levenson, M.D.

The practice of psychosomatic medicine is grounded in science, knowledge, and the standards of ethics of the profession, and occurs in the context of applicable laws and regulations. Colleagues often ask psychiatrists for consultation when issues of law, ethics, and mental health are involved generally, and more particularly when legal, ethical, and clinical values and practices come into tension with one another. These topics may be particularly anxiety-provoking because physicians want to do the right thing, ethically and clinically, while also following the law. The different foundations of law, ethics, medicine, and psychiatry, however, mean that conflicts often do emerge. The purpose of this chapter is to explore the ethical and legal underpinnings of psychosomatic medicine practice and to provide practical guidance for psychiatrists to identify, address, and (where possible) resolve legal and ethical challenges that arise.

When psychiatrists receive a consultation request, it often involves challenges in managing a patient's affect, behavior, or cognition. These presenting symptoms themselves often raise legal and ethical concerns, especially in acute care settings, where decisions frequently need to be made under time pressure. Consulting psychiatrists often struggle to untangle the complex relationship between symptoms of psychiatric illness and the provision of medical care. Central issues at this interface include privacy and confidentiality, capacity and competency, informed consent for treatment and treatment refusal, substitute decision making and guardianship, and malpractice. Familiarity with such issues is important both to avoid unnecessary entanglements in protocol and regulation and to identify when those with expertise in ethics and law might be called on to provide guidance, counsel, and intervention. By identifying legal and ethical tensions in practice and utilizing available resources when needed, the psychosomatic psychiatrist may focus on engaging sound clinical judgment rather than misplaced overreliance on legal considerations in particular.

In this chapter, we first address general ethical considerations that may be helpful in guiding consulting psychiatrists in making recommendations about how to figure out the way forward with treatment. We then turn to the general legal framework for medical practice. Finally, we address specific topics in which law and ethics may be particularly relevant in psychiatric consultation. Other issues, including physician-assisted suicide (see Chapter 8, "Suicidality") and deceptive patients (see Chapter 12, "Deception Syndromes: Factitious Disorders and Malingering"), are addressed elsewhere in this volume.

Ethics in Psychosomatic Medicine

Psychosomatic medicine, like all medical practice, occurs in the context of the ethical standards of the profession. At the core is the ethical imperative that psychosomatic medicine psychiatrists interact respectfully with patients and colleagues in accordance with established principles of medical ethics (American Psychiatric Association 2001, 2015). In addition, consulting psychiatrists are often consulted about complicated questions with important ethical components (Roberts 2016). For example, many consultations include questions about patients' abilities for self-determination and decision making that have profound ethical implications for their autonomy and personhood. In these situations, the line between psychiatry and ethics may quickly become blurred. Sometimes a psychiatric consultation may involve an ethical or legal question or vice versa (Rosenstein and Miller 2011). In addition, when these consults arise, they may be incompletely formulated and emotionally charged (Rosenstein and Miller 2011). For this reason, consulting psychiatrists should be familiar with ethical concepts relevant to their practice and the application of those concepts to specific cases.

Different philosophers and bioethicists have proposed various moral and ethical theories and approaches to guiding ethical inquiry and methods to resolve ethical dilemmas. For example, three main traditional schools of moral theory have influenced the evolution of bioethics. *Deontological theory,* following in the tradition of Immanuel Kant, derives from the notion of duty to all human beings, by which we are required never to treat a person as merely a means to an end but rather to respect humanity as an end in itself (Beauchamp and Childress 2013; Timmons 2013). Kant's reason-based philosophy requires that we work to promote the interests of others and not employ others merely as a means to achieving our own aims. In current-day medical terms, for example, the fiduciary nature of the doctor–patient relationship reflects concepts of duty to others in medicine (Beauchamp and Childress 2013).

Another theory of ethics follows in the *utilitarian tradition* of Jeremy Bentham and John Stuart Mill, who assessed the moral value of actions by the outcome of the action. In utilitarian analysis, the ethical action is that which promotes the most good ("happiness") for the greatest number (Beauchamp and Childress 2013; Timmons 2013). A third traditional theory of ethics is *virtue ethics.* Virtue ethics, in the tradition of Aristotle, considers not just the action of the individual or the consequences of the action, but also the individual's character, disposition, and motives. Virtue ethics is more about "how to be" than what to do. Because virtues such as compassion, discernment, trustworthiness, integrity, and conscientiousness are essential aspects of the professionalism of medicine, a form of virtue ethics called "the ethics of care" has been developed. The ethics of care approach originated from feminist writers and emphasizes not only what health care providers do (e.g., withhold health information from their patients) but also "how they perform those actions, which motives and feelings underlie them, and whether their actions promote or thwart positive relationships" (Beauchamp and Childress 2013, p. 35). Finally, considerations of justice, in the tradition of John Rawls (1971), also come into play to the extent that fairness and equitably addressing disparities are central to our ever more complex care delivery systems (Beauchamp and Childress 2013).

Over time, one widespread approach to medical ethics, the *principlism* of Beauchamp and Childress, has emerged. It takes contributions from traditional theory and calls for a balancing approach between principles of biomedical ethics. Beauchamp and Childress have identified four principles based on our shared, or common, morality that they posit are sufficient to do work in bioethics: respect for autonomy, beneficence, nonmaleficence, and justice (Beauchamp and Childress 2013). The principle of respect for autonomy directs health care providers to respect their patients' autonomous choices. *Autonomous choices* are those that are intentional and made with understanding and freedom from controlling influences. The principle of *beneficence* directs providers to contribute to the welfare of others, whereas the principle of *nonmaleficence* instructs them to avoid actions that harm their patients. Together, the principles of beneficence and nonmaleficence "underlie the obligation of clinicians to assess the risk–benefit ratios of patient care" (Rosenstein and Miller 2011, p. 35). Finally, the principle of *justice* enjoins providers to provide fair and equitable health care. The consulting psychiatrist can employ these principles to lend guidance as well as to identify cases that may benefit from formal input and consideration by an ethics committee.

These principles are not absolute, but rather are in tension with one another in constituting ethical dilemmas. In addition, whereas Beauchamp and Childress identified four principles, others have added to the list, although the additional principles can be seen as logically related to one of Beauchamp and Childress's four. *Veracity* refers to truth-telling and avoiding deception (including through omission). *Fidelity* refers to serving another faithfully, as patients put their trust in providers (Roberts 2016). *Confidentiality* protects patients' privacy and dignity.

Finally, although principlism is a common and useful approach to medical ethics, it is by no means the only approach. In the narrative approach, for example, the use of stories may contextualize patients' situations and challenges in the context of their life, experiences, and meaning (Montello 2014). Consideration of culture, ethnicity, race, gender, and other factors unique to individuals is also important in addressing ethical challenges, as is learning from casuistic approaches that highlight the importance of cases (Sugarman and Sulmasy 2010; Tomlinson 2012). These approaches need not be mutually exclusive (McCarthy 2003).

No code of ethics is specific to the practice of psychosomatic medicine. The most relevant professional documents are the American Medical Association's Code of Medical Ethics (American Medical Association Council on Ethical and Judicial Affairs 2001) and the American Psychiatric Association's (APA's) annotation of this code (American Psychiatric Association 2001). The more recent "APA Commentary on Ethics in Practice" provides an approach to specific ethical challenges (e.g., sexual boundary violations, breaches of confidentiality, abandonment of patients) and is directly relevant to all areas of psychiatric practice, including subspecialties (American Psychiatric Association 2015).

Legal Issues in Psychosomatic Medicine

Medical practice occurs in a legal and regulatory context. Like ethical aspects of practice, legal concerns often emerge at the intersection of law and medicine in psychosomatic medicine. For a number of reasons, legal questions arise frequently for consultation-liaison psychiatrists, more often than in most other areas of medicine. One reason is the sensitive nature of communications made by patients to psychiatrists and the historical protections afforded to psychiatry and psychotherapy records that may raise concerns about laws related to confidentiality. A second reason is that medical and surgical practitioners may rely on psychiatric colleagues' training and expertise in understanding disorders of behavior and cognition for assistance in determining patients' ability to make medical decisions, give informed consent, or refuse recommended treatment. A third reason is that the complex balancing of individual interests against public policy considerations may lead to questions in the treatment of a particular patient in a number of contexts, including duties to third parties, mandated reporting, and malpractice liability.

For most practitioners, legal concerns are background considerations that remain largely unfocused and absent from conscious awareness in daily practice. However, as with ethical issues, when legal issues arise, they often do so in the context of particularly challenging clinical issues that may be confusing and emotionally charged. If not properly understood and considered, legal considerations may lead to obfuscation, departure from sound clinical judgment, and even bad outcomes (Schouten and Brendel 2009). It is therefore critical for clinicians to be aware of relevant legal principles and regulations pertaining to the provision of medical care in jurisdictions relevant to their practice. However, it is also critical for clinicians to appreciate that the best way of minimizing legal complications in providing care to patients is through attention to thorough and sound clinical judgment and care (Brendel and Schouten 2007; Schouten and Brendel 2004, 2009). It is important to note that this chapter refers predominantly to legal paradigms and practice in the United States.

Confidentiality

The principle of doctor–patient confidentiality was codified in the Hippocratic oath as early as 430 B.C.: "Whatever I see or hear, professionally or privately, which ought not to be divulged, I will keep secret and tell no one" (Lloyd 1983). Since that time, confidentiality has remained a central facet of the doctor–patient relationship on the rationale that it promotes the open and honest exchange of information in the interest of treatment and patient welfare (American Psychiatric Association 1978, 2001; Appelbaum 2002; Brendel and Brendel 2005). Doctor–patient confidentiality is a professional, legal, and ethical requirement. Signs in hospital hallways and elevators reminding staff to respect patient confidentiality serve as just one emblem of this responsibility of health care providers to their patients.

From an ethical perspective, confidentiality derives from the concepts of respect for persons and nonmaleficence. There are also beneficence considerations. For example, one justification for confidentiality is that it promotes trust in physicians such that patients will be truthful and thus receive better care (Beauchamp and Childress 2013).

However, the notion of total confidentiality in medicine is, in practice, arcane. Even before the recent expansion of health information systems and electronic medical records over the last decade in particular, medical information was not strictly confidential between doctor and patient in the setting of hospital treatment. For example, even more than 35 years ago, one observer detailed the large number of individuals with access to a patient's medical chart (Siegler 1982). Now, as medical charts have become increasingly electronic, questions about ownership, access, and commoditization are emerging at a rapid pace and will likely further challenge notions of confidentiality as time goes on (Hall and Schulman 2009). In addition, increasing attention has started to focus on the scope of confidentiality after a patient's death (Robinson and O'Neill 2007).

Over time, the principle of strict or absolute confidentiality between one physician and one patient has eroded beyond the sharing of medical information with hospital personnel, as described by Siegler (1982). The considerations of a complex society have increasingly led to an erosion of confidentiality as it was understood in the era of Hippocrates and subsequent centuries. Ethical considerations of justice and obligations to others have driven some of these trends. Like other ethical principles, confidentiality is not an absolute mandate, and it must give way when another ethical principle takes precedence. For example, courts and legislatures have created limitations to doctor–patient confidentiality in circumstances in which confidentiality is determined to be at odds with public safety or to be more harmful than beneficial for the patient. More recently, increased administrative and practical concerns, rather than ethical analysis, led to federal law recognizing the efficiency and effectiveness of the health care system as a consideration to be balanced against traditional management and safeguarding of protected health information under the Health Insurance Portability and Accountability Act of 1996 (HIPAA; P.L. 104-191) (Brendel and Bryan 2004).

Public Safety and Welfare Exceptions to Confidentiality

Physicians often express concern that reporting information to government authorities, social service agencies, or other third parties may violate their ethical responsibility to patients or expose them to potential liability. While protecting patient information and confidentiality is the default rule, there are several situations in which physicians have an affirmative legal duty to disclose information to authorities. These departures are generally grounded in principles of beneficence to vulnerable individuals, justice considerations and respect for the greater public health, or prevention of harm. One such example is child or elder abuse and neglect reporting. Every jurisdiction in the United States mandates that physicians report suspected child or elder abuse and neglect (Brendel 2005; Milosavljevic et al. 2012, 2016).

Four decades ago, federal law set a minimum standard for what actions and inactions constitute child abuse and neglect, respectively (Child Abuse Prevention and Treatment Act 2003). However, individual states have interpreted the federal definition in different ways, leading to variations in the definition of child abuse among

U.S. jurisdictions. As a general rule of thumb, state definitions generally incorporate the concept of "harm or substantial risk of harm" or "serious threat or serious harm" to a person younger than 18 years who is not emancipated (Milosavljevic et al. 2016). Approximately half of states have some form of emancipation law that may exempt an emancipated or mature minor younger than 18 years from being subject to a child abuse or neglect report. Physicians should be aware of the specific prevailing standards in the jurisdictions in which they practice regarding the applicable definitions and requirements for reporting. In general, liability attaches to a physician for failing to comply with a mandatory child abuse reporting statute rather than for breaching confidentiality by making a report to child protection authorities (this applies even when a report is ultimately unsubstantiated, provided that the report was made in good faith) (Milosavljevic et al. 2016).

Beginning in the 1960s, legislation emerged out of the child protection model to protect vulnerable adults, and by the mid-1970s, a federal law was passed to establish adult protective services (Milosavljevic et al. 2016). Today, every U.S. jurisdiction identifies physicians as mandated reporters of suspected elder abuse and neglect (Milosavljevic et al. 2016). Akin to the jurisdictional variations in definitions of child abuse and neglect, the definition of elder abuse and neglect varies from state to state. That being said, most states use a standard incorporating five common elements: infliction of pain or injury, infliction of emotional or psychological harm, sexual assault, material or financial exploitation, and neglect (Milosavljevic et al. 2016). Elder abuse standards may also include self-neglect, in recognition of the frequency of waning self-care abilities that accompany age-related physical and cognitive decline (Abrams et al. 2002). Unlike laws pertaining to the reporting of suspected child abuse, elder protection laws may recognize the ability of a competent elder to refuse investigation or intervention by protective services agencies.

Consultation-liaison psychiatrists should be aware of the risk factors for and manifestations of elder abuse and neglect, especially given that they may be more likely to encounter elders at risk due to their presentation with dementia and other mental status changes, as well as when hospitalized for medical consequences of neglect or abuse. Mistreatment of elderly individuals has been linked to poor emotional and physical health years later (Acierno et al. 2017), so psychiatrists' assistance in earlier identification can lead to important preventive interventions. As a whole, physicians may be inadequately trained to recognize elder mistreatment, at least in part because the manifestations of abuse and neglect may be subtle and may be masked by illness or debility (Alpert et al. 1998; Melton 2002). Simply put, elderly victims of abuse and/or neglect may appear nothing more than frail or sick to the untrained clinician (Kahan and Paris 2003), and recognition rates in emergency departments appear to be far lower than the estimated prevalence in the community (Evans et al. 2017). The psychiatric consultant is in a critically important position to detect elder mistreatment and to intervene to protect vulnerable geriatric patients, because hospitals and other health care organizations may be the only source of help for them. Therefore, practitioners should familiarize themselves with the reporting standards in the jurisdictions in which they practice. As is the case for child abuse reporting, physicians are more likely to face legal liability for *failure* to report elder abuse and neglect than for good-faith reporting of suspected abuse and/or neglect, even when reports are "screened out" or found to be unsubstantiated following investigation by elder protective services.

Duties to Third Parties and the Duty to Protect

Since the landmark California Supreme Court Decision in *Tarasoff v. Board of Regents of the University of California* in 1976, the concept of a duty to warn third parties or protect them from physical harm from patients has emerged as a well-known exception to doctor–patient confidentiality (Schouten and Brendel 2004). In this court decision, California's highest court engaged in an analysis of the complex balance between individual patient privacy and the public interest in preventing harm to hold that psychotherapists have a duty to act to protect third parties when the therapist knows or should know that a patient poses a risk of harm to a third party or parties (*Tarasoff v. Board of Regents of the University of California* 1976). In the more than four decades that have passed since this landmark decision, clinicians and lawmakers alike have debated the relative priority of patient confidentiality and public safety in defining the parameters of the duty, for which situations clinicians will face professional and/or legal responsibility, and even whether the duty to warn or protect would apply in different jurisdictions.

Unlike mandated reporting of abuse and neglect, the duty to protect is not recognized in all jurisdictions (Almason 1997; Ginsberg 2004). It is therefore critical for practitioners to familiarize themselves with the law regarding the duty to protect in the jurisdiction(s) in which they practice. In general, many states have enacted statutory laws characterizing the scope of the duty to protect, and others have narrowed the scope of or eliminated the duty (Appelbaum et al. 1989; Kachigian and Felthous 2004). State laws regarding the duty to protect generally limit the situations in which the physician's duty to protect is triggered.

Statutory methods by which the psychiatrist's duty to protect and potential liability may be circumscribed include requiring that there be a specific threat to an identified or identifiable victim, that the clinician have knowledge of the patient's past history of violence, and/or that there be a reasonable basis for anticipating violence prior to invocation of the duty to protect. In addition to defining and/or limiting the circumstances in which the duty to protect arises, state laws may also specify what measures mental health clinicians may or must take to satisfactorily comply with their duty to protect. These measures often include notifying the police or another law enforcement agency, hospitalizing the patient, or warning the potential victim. The Massachusetts statute is one that both limits the scope of the duty and defines measures by which the duty to protect can be discharged ("Duty to Warn Patient's Potential Victims; Cause of Action" 2005).

One critical aspect of the duty to protect is that this duty often applies to psychiatrists and other mental health clinicians, but not to nonpsychiatric physicians and clinicians (Brendel and Cohen 2008; Brendel and Schouten 2007). In the setting of providing consultation to medical and surgical services, psychiatrists may be subject to duties to warn and/or protect that do not apply to a physician of record or the primary treatment team and that may create competing and conflicting obligations for the consultant and the consultee.

The complex tension between doctor–patient confidentiality and protecting patient privacy on the one side and public protection and welfare on the other is not a new issue and is reflective of the tension between important ethical considerations of responsibilities to the patient and to others. In fact, the *Tarasoff* court relied on the precedent of mandated reporting of communicable diseases to public health authorities in its reasoning supporting the duty to protect third parties (*Tarasoff v. Board of Regents of the University of California* 1976). Infectious disease reporting remains a well-established exception to doctor–patient confidentiality, and individual states, as well as the federal government, have enacted laws about which contagious diseases must be reported—to state public health officials, the Centers for Disease Control and Prevention, or both. Examples of reportable communicable diseases are HIV, varicella, viral hepatitis, severe acute respiratory syndrome, influenza, and syphilis (see, e.g., Averhoff et al. 2006). Reporting requirements vary from jurisdiction to jurisdiction, both in terms of what conditions are reportable and with regard to the type and amount of information that must be reported. For example, in the case of HIV, states vary in what information must accompany a report of a positive test result, including whether the report is anonymized or de-identified and whether partner/spousal notification is to occur (Brendel and Cohen 2008; New York State Department of Health 2000, 2003). Physicians should also be aware that both before and following *Tarasoff*, doctors have faced civil liability for failure to disclose a patient's infection status that led to the infection of other individuals, highlighting how critically important it is for physicians to be aware of reporting requirements in the jurisdictions in which they practice (*Bradshaw v. Daniel* 1993; Gostin and Webber 1998; Liang 2002).

But while clinicians should be aware of the legal and regulatory requirements and constraints applicable to their practice, it is also critical that they remember to think and act like clinicians, in accordance with ethical standards of the profession. Simply put, clinicians should resist the tendency to think legally when difficult issues arise and instead should act clinically and professionally responsibly in the setting of an understanding of the law or consultation with appropriate risk management or legal resources (Schouten and Brendel 2009). From the clinical perspective, the starting point for considering the responsibilities to breach confidentiality is the paradigm of doctor–patient confidentiality. The default rule is to protect patient confidentiality and privacy, and breaches for any reason must be carefully weighed and understood. Alternatives to releasing private information (e.g., hospitalization of a patient who has made threats) should be considered before a clinician breaches confidentiality (Beck 1998). Psychiatrists should never forget their default ethical responsibility to the patient. In addition, even when a clinician is required to share patient information, only the minimum amount of information necessary to achieve the legal, regulatory, or clinical purpose should be disclosed.

Finally, circumstances may arise in which the consultation psychiatrist is asked to evaluate a patient whose legal status may draw into question the confidentiality of the interview. Examples of patients in these circumstances include individuals who are in immigration, police, or correctional custody. In these situations, it is important for the psychiatrist to take steps to maximize the privacy of the interview and also to make the patient aware of the potential limitations on confidentiality inherent in the evaluation, given the patient's custodial status. Furthermore, the psychiatrist should follow standard clinical practice regarding communication with law enforcement officials. Specifically, the clinician should consider all information gathered in the course of the interview as being covered by doctor–patient confidentiality and should limit contact with law enforcement to providing the minimum necessary to meet any mandated reporting obligations and to ensure the patient's safety. When patients are transferred from medical settings to jail or prison, psychiatrists should work to identify appropriate clinical personnel within the legal system to provide this hand-off and should avoid communicating clinical information through nonclinical personnel (Schouten and Brendel 2009). Finally, when law enforcement officials seek to interview patients, clinicians should continue to maintain their therapeutic fiduciary stance relative to the patient and should consider principles of patient autonomy, noninterference with medical care, protection of privacy, and maintenance of professional boundaries in making decisions about the appropriateness of these interviews (Jones et al. 2006).

Health Insurance Portability and Accountability Act

The paradigm of doctor–patient confidentiality often conjures up images of records in locked file cabinets and strict confidentiality for all patient information, especially in the field of psychiatry. As discussed above, however, over time, exceptions to the strict rule of doctor–patient confidentiality have emerged, because from ethical and legal perspectives, public safety and welfare considerations at times prevail over the safeguarding of private patient information by physicians. With Congress's passage of HIPAA in 1996 and subsequent adoption of the regulations promulgated to implement HIPAA, the circumstances under which medical information could be released without the patient's explicit written informed consent were substantially broadened—not just for reasons of public safety but also for the purposes of payment and health care operations. Perhaps the most common misconception about HIPAA is that it makes it harder, rather than easier, to release a patient's medical information. As will be further elucidated, rather than promoting privacy, HIPAA has had the opposite effect of expanding the situations in which patient consent is *not* required for release of patient health information. If there is a take-home message about HIPAA, it is simple: the "P" in HIPAA is for portability, not privacy (Brendel and Bryan 2004). The effect of HIPAA has been to increase the circumstances under which patient information can be released without the specific informed consent of the patient (Brendel 2005; Brendel and Bryan 2004; Feld 2005).

With the passage of HIPAA, psychiatrists in particular were concerned about the effect the act would have on the protections accorded to often-sensitive psychiatric records, protections that until the passage of HIPAA were regulated by state law. HIPAA, a federal law, applies to health care providers who perform "certain electronic transactions," and because these functions (e.g., electronic billing, eligibility determinations, claims processing) are performed by hospitals, most if not all consultation-liaison psychiatrists are covered by the provisions of HIPAA. HIPAA does not cover all information, but instead governs the management of "protected health information," a category that includes not only specific medical information about mental or physical conditions but also patient identifiers such as name, social security number, payment information, and records of treatment or services rendered (HIPAA Privacy Rule 2001).

The provisions of HIPAA with greatest relevance to psychiatric consultants relate to disclosure of medical information, patient access to information, and a category of records established and defined by HIPAA that is known as "psychotherapy notes." When lawmakers passed HIPAA, they specifically aimed to improve the "efficiency and effectiveness" of the health care system. In defining the parameters of what information should be considered protected health information under HIPAA, lawmakers attempted to strike a balance between the important principles of confidentiality and privacy and the efficient functioning of an increasingly complex health care system that requires regular sharing of information between multiple entities in order to function. HIPAA's implementation promoted efficiency by allowing the release of protected health information for treatment, payment, and health care operational purposes without specific informed consent from the patient. This move drew criticism from patient and privacy advocates who believed that abolition of the consent requirement for release of records would become just the first step in a slippery slope of furthering administrative and operational needs at the expense of doctor–patient confidentiality, a centuries-old ethical and legal cornerstone of medical treatment (Feld 2005; Friedrich 2001; Gordon 2002).

HIPAA is not a carte blanche for release of medical information. Federal regulations do limit disclosure of protected health information under HIPAA in several ways. First, under HIPAA, covered entities (such as hospitals) are required to inform patients of their practices under HIPAA in the form of privacy notices. In addition, patients may request a record of some disclosures of their protected health information. Finally, HIPAA is preempted by federal and state laws that provide greater protection than that afforded by HIPAA for protected health information, including records that are considered especially sensitive. For example, under federal law, records from alcohol and substance abuse treatment programs are considered especially sensitive, and written informed consent is specifically required for their release. Additionally, state laws vary from jurisdiction to jurisdiction but may require specific written informed consent for release of HIV testing and treatment records as well as records related to domestic violence and sexual assault (Brendel 2005; Brendel and Bryan 2004).

Prior to the passage of HIPAA, distinctions between the handling of medical and psychiatric records often caused confusion for psychiatrists. Specifically, psychiatric records were often maintained separately from the general medical record, and even when contained within the medical record, they were subject to limitations on release. For example, at our institution prior to HIPAA, psychiatric consultation notes contained within the hospital record were redacted before records were released to patients. Since the passage of HIPAA, all psychiatry entries into the medical chart are considered part of the general medical record. The implications of HIPAA's inclusion of psychiatric records in the general medical chart are several. First, under HIPAA, the records may be released for treatment, payment, and health care operations purposes without specific consent. Second, HIPAA grants patients broad rights of access to their medical records. The practical effect of this broad right of access means that a patient's access to psychiatric records and psychiatric entries in the medical record may be denied only if a licensed professional makes a determination that release of the records to the patient would harm, endanger the life, or compromise the physical safety of the patient or another person (Brendel and Bryan 2004). It is especially important for all clinicians to be aware that patients have the right to access their records and will be allowed to do so—highlighting the need for careful documentation around sensitive issues, use of nonjudgmental terms and avoidance of jargon, and thoughtful formulation, as if the patient were looking over the clinician's shoulder.

Post-HIPAA, confusion frequently arises among psychiatrists regarding psychotherapy notes. It is critical for practitioners to be aware that although HIPAA affords extra protection for psychotherapy notes in recognition of the sensitive nature of psychiatric treatment, HIPAA's definition of psychotherapy notes is extremely narrow and does not preclude the patient, or others, from accessing the notes (Maio 2003). Very few notes of psychotherapy sessions, inpatient or outpatient, would qualify as psychotherapy notes under HIPAA, which specifically defines psychotherapy notes as a clinician's notes that document or analyze the contents of conversations in private counseling sessions and are kept separate from the rest of the patient's record (what psychotherapists refer to as "process notes"). In addition, certain information that is more appropriately kept in a medical chart—such as medication information, results of tests, diagnosis, prognosis, progress, and treatment plans and goals—is not subject to the psychotherapy note protection of HIPAA (Appelbaum 2002; Brendel and Bryan 2004). Notes that qualify under the psychotherapy notes provision of HIPAA may not be released without specific authorization from the patient. In addition, although patients do not have the right to access their psychotherapy notes, there is no prohibition on allowing patients to access their psychotherapy notes. Notwithstanding HIPAA, psychotherapy notes are treated as part of the medical record for legal purposes in the event that the record is subpoenaed for litigation (Schouten and Brendel 2004).

Overall, as discussed above, HIPAA has had the effect of facilitating the release of medical information, in large part by departing from the consent requirement each time a patient's protected health information is released for treatment, payment, or health care operations purposes. In addition, HIPAA recognizes that consent is not required to release information in emergency, mandated reporting, and public safety and monitoring situations (Appelbaum 2002; Schouten and Brendel 2004).

Clinicians should also be familiar with two additional points about HIPAA. First, HIPAA sets a floor regarding the minimum requirements for the protection of health information, and states may enact laws that are more protective of patient privacy and more permissive of patient access. Second, even though HIPAA permits disclosure of protected health information without specific informed consent in many circumstances, clinicians should still use clinical judgment every time they make a disclosure and should limit the information released to the minimum amount needed to achieve the purpose of the disclosure.

Treatment Consent and Refusal

Psychiatrists are often consulted to assess a patient's ability to understand proposed medical and surgical interventions, especially in settings in which the patient is refusing treatment that the treating clinician has determined to be medically indicated. The psychiatrist's threshold clinical determination of a patient's ability to make a decision is a *capacity assessment. Capacity* refers to an individual's ability to perform a task, such as making a medical decision. *Competency* is the legal analogue of capacity and is presumed for all adults. Hence, clinicians make judgments of capacity and incapacity, and judges make determinations of competency and incompetency (Appelbaum and Roth 1981; Brendel and Schouten 2007; Schouten and Brendel 2004; Schouten and

Edersheim 2008). Consulting psychiatrists must always remain aware that determinations of capacity are likely to have ethical implications relative to patients' abilities for self-determination.

Ethically, the principle of respect for autonomy directs the heath care provider to respect patients' autonomous choices—that is, those that are intentional and made with understanding and freedom from controlling influences. The default position, legally and ethically, is to honor the decision or course of action that the patient chooses. However, there are scenarios in which the most ethical course of action is to *not* honor the patient's decision based on considerations of beneficence, nonmaleficence, justice, and obligations to others. When patients lack the ability to make capacitated or competent decisions, autonomy and beneficence direct providers to respect and even protect the patient by either acting as the patient would have acted if he or she had been able to make the decision (respect for autonomy) or, alternatively, acting in the patient's best interest (beneficence).

Capacity and incapacity may be global or specific. An example of a globally incapacitated person is an individual in a coma. More commonly, psychiatrists are asked to evaluate task-specific capacity, such as the capacity to leave the hospital against medical advice, a frequently encountered capacity determination in the general hospital. Different tasks and decisions require different abilities and levels of understanding, and therefore the first step in any evaluation of capacity is to ask the question "Capacity for what?" To assess the degree to which the patient understands the information relevant to a decision, the psychiatrist must first have an understanding of the type of decision and circumstances the patient is facing.

Capacity Assessment

A patient's decisional capacity depends on his or her understanding of the underlying illness, its prognosis, the proposed interventions, and the consequences of treatment and nontreatment. The best-established method of capacity determination for medical decision making is a practical four-pronged analysis developed by Appelbaum and Grisso (Appelbaum 2007; Appelbaum and Grisso 1988). Under this model, the four factors for consideration in determining decisional capacity are preference, factual understanding, appreciation of the facts presented (i.e., an understanding of how information relates to oneself and one's specific situation), and rational manipulation of information. All four elements must be met for the individual to demonstrate decisional capacity. In practice, a patient's decisional capacity is rarely questioned when the patient is in agreement with the proposed medical interventions.

In assessing the *preference* element of capacity, the central facet is the patient's ability to communicate a consistent preference over time. A patient who is unable to demonstrate a stable preference regarding a decision—whether because of inability or unwillingness—is said to lack decisional capacity (although this determination is not meant to preclude the patient's changing his or her mind).

The second element of the four-part capacity evaluation is an assessment of the individual's *factual understanding* of his or her condition and its proposed treatment. Factual understanding may be assessed through inquiry about the nature of the patient's illness or condition, the treatment options, the recommended treatment, the prognosis with and without treatment, and the risks and benefits of treatment. If the patient does not demonstrate a factual understanding, it is critical for the evaluator to assess why and also to determine whether the patient is capable of acquiring a factual understanding. For example, a patient may not have a factual understanding of the relevant information because the primary treaters did not provide this information to the patient, or provided it in a form the patient did not understand. Even in the United States and other developed countries, rates of functional illiteracy are high (Marcus 2006). Patients who have not been sufficiently educated about their condition and its recommended treatment cannot be expected to factually understand the relevant information. On the other hand, if efforts have been made to inform the patient of the relevant information and the patient is unable to retain it, the patient may not be capable of acquiring the requisite information in order to meet the second prong of the capacity evaluation.

The third element in capacity assessment is a determination of whether the patient *appreciates the significance of the information presented* to him or her. Appreciation goes beyond a recitation of the facts and requires a broad perspective of the implications of the medical decision. Factors that may be explored in assessing appreciation include asking the patient about the consequences both of accepting and of refusing the proposed intervention as well as the consequences of one decision or another for the individual's future. Some treatment decisions require comparisons of statistics, such as the odds of remission and response with different treatment options. Yet, it is estimated that 22% of adults in the United States lack basic "quantitative literacy," or the ability to perform fundamental quantitative tasks (Marcus 2006).

The fourth, and final, element of the standard capacity assessment for medical decision making, *rational manipulation of information,* requires the patient to demonstrate that his or her decision-making process is a rational one. The focus of inquiry and assessment is not on the final decision the patient makes, but rather on the process that the individual uses to arrive at that decision, taking into account the individual's past preferences, values, and decisions. An often-used example illustrating the importance of viewing the individual medical decision in the context of the patient's life, beliefs, and previous choices is that of a Jehovah's Witness who is faced with making a decision about whether to accept or refuse a life-saving blood transfusion. In this case, the adult individual's decision to refuse the transfusion and face certain death might seem irrational on the surface, but in the context of this individual's faith-based life decisions and belief that accepting the transfusion would be contrary to religious doctrine, the decision could meet the rationality requirement. Ethical psychiatrists may struggle when a patient's choices are inconsistent with their own values. Awareness of this discomfort is critical to ensure that psychiatrists are respecting their patients by giving full credence to patients' capacitated wishes.

Assessing the rationality of a patient's decision-making process is the key element in determining whether seriously mentally ill patients have sufficient capacity to make specific medical decisions. For example, a patient with chronic schizophrenia who refuses cancer chemotherapy because he does not think the side effects are worth the limited benefits may well have sufficient capacity to make this choice even if he is delusional about other areas of his life. However, if the reason he is refusing is that he thinks the doctors are trying to control his mind through the infusion, he would most likely be deemed to lack capacity. The question of whether mental illness has distorted a patient's thinking sufficiently to preclude capacity can also arise in nonpsychotic disorders such as major depression and can be particularly difficult when a patient has refused life-saving treatment (Sullivan and Youngner 1994).

Informed Consent

Decisional capacity is a threshold requirement for the ability to give informed consent for or refusal of treatment. In other words, a patient who is unable to make consistent and/or meaningful decisions cannot authorize, or for that matter refuse, proposed medical interventions. In ethical terms, patients' autonomy is diminished when they lack capacity. The process by which a patient agrees to permit a physician or other treater to do something to or for him or her is *informed consent.* Informed consent is required before any medical intervention because, in civil law, any unauthorized touching, including medical intervention, is considered a battery. In the treatment context, a patient must therefore give informed consent before any intervention can begin, and informed refusal if a treatment intervention is not authorized. Informed consent is an extension of broad principles of individual autonomy and has been a solid cornerstone of medical treatment since the late 1960s (Dalla-Vorgia et al. 2001; Mohr 2000).

In hospital settings, informed consent may be equated with having a signed consent form on file. Clinicians should be aware that informed consent involves not just signing a form but also engaging in a process characterized by exchange of information, communication, and an active decision by the patient to accept or refuse the treatment. Through this active process, the ethical requirement is substantiated and the legal standard of informed consent can be met. Specifically, in addition to requiring decisional capacity, the ethical and legal standard for informed consent requires that consent must be knowing (or intelligent) and voluntary (Appelbaum et al. 1987; *Salgo v. Leland Stanford Jr. University Board of Trustees* 1957; *Schloendorff v. Society of New York Hospital* 1914). The knowing/intelligent standard varies from jurisdiction to jurisdiction, with two general approaches (Schouten and Edersheim 2008). The first approach to the knowing standard is the "reasonable professional" standard, wherein the amount of information about a proposed medical intervention that must be shared with the patient beforehand is defined as what a reasonable practitioner would tell a patient in similar circumstances. A small majority of states use this clinician-centered standard. The second approach to the knowing standard defines the scope of the required disclosure as the information that an average or reasonable patient would use in coming to a decision. A substantial minority of states employ this patient-centered approach, and some states go even further and require an inquiry into what information a particular patient would find pertinent (material) or relevant in making a particular decision. This individual patient inquiry is often referred to as the *materiality standard* (Iheukwumere 2002). Two states use a hybrid approach incorporating both physician- and patient-focused inquiries in determining the amount and type of information that must be presented to the patient in order for informed consent to occur (King and Moulton 2006). From an ethical perspective, a patient-centered standard for information gives autonomy precedence, whereas a clinician-centered standard emphasizes beneficence. Pragmatically, to demonstrate true informed consent, patients should be able to repeat the information in their own words.

As stated above, the first core element of informed consent is that it must be *knowing*—in other words, the patient must possess the requisite information about the proposed intervention. As a practical guide to sound clinical practice and risk management, the more information presented to the patient and the more extensive the communication about that information between the doctor and the patient, the better. That being said, there are six broad categories of information that, if presented to the patient, are generally accepted as meeting the standard of how much information needs to be presented, regardless of the particular jurisdictional standard (King and Moulton 2006):

1. The diagnosis and the nature of the condition being treated
2. The reasonably expected benefits from the proposed treatment
3. The nature and likelihood of the risks involved
4. The inability to precisely predict results of the treatment
5. The potential irreversibility of the treatment
6. The expected risks, benefits, and results of alternative, or no, treatment

   There are limits to how much information physicians are required to share in the course of the informed consent process. Overall, the ideal of informed consent is a process incorporating a clear and frank discussion and exchange of information between doctor and patient (King and Moulton 2006). The necessity of striking a balance among patients' right to know, fairness to physicians, and public policy considerations of avoiding unreasonable burdens on clinicians has been recognized (*Precourt v. Frederick* 1985).

   The second core element of informed consent is that it must be *voluntary*. The patient must give consent freely and unencumbered by external coercive forces. A decision made under circumstances that limit the patient's ability to exercise a choice is not voluntary and does not meet the standard for informed consent (Faden and Beauchamp 1986; Keeton et al. 1984). Nonetheless, distinguishing between voluntary and coerced choices requires a complex and nuanced inquiry (Roberts 2002). For example, patients may be under pressure from family members to make certain treatment decisions, and in these situations, patients are generally determined to have acted voluntarily from both ethical and legal perspectives (although exceptions do exist) (Grisso and Appelbaum 1998; Mallary et al. 1986). However, individuals who are totally dependent on others for their care are generally (notwithstanding some debate on the issue) deemed unable to give voluntary consent to treatment or research because of the inherent inequality between the patient and the institution. Examples of individuals in this category include nursing home residents and prisoners (Gold 1974; Moser et al. 2004; National Commission for the Protection of Human Subjects of Biomedical and Behavioral Research 1976, 1978).

Exceptions to Informed Consent

There are certain narrow and circumscribed situations in which informed consent is not required for the initiation of treatment, but these situations are the exception and not the rule (Meisel 1979; Schouten and Brendel 2004; Sprung and Winick 1989). The most common and well-known exception to the informed consent requirement is the *emergency* exception. For the purposes of exemption from the informed consent requirement, an emergency is a situation in which failure to treat would result in serious and potentially irreversible deterioration of the patient's condition. Invocation of the emergency exception is ethically permissible in recognition of beneficence, but only until the patient is stabilized, at which time informed consent must be obtained. In addition, the presence of an emergency is not enough to authorize treatment if the physician has knowledge that the patient would have refused the emergency treatment if he or she were able to express his or her wishes. The patient's prior expressed wishes cannot be overridden by an emergency (Annas 1999; *Shine v. Vega* 1999).

Two additional narrow exceptions to informed consent are *waiver* and *therapeutic privilege* (Meisel 1979; Schouten and Brendel 2004; Sprung and Winick 1989). A competent patient may defer to the clinician or another party, thereby waiving his or her informed consent. In these situations, clinicians should carefully assess and thoroughly document the patient's capacity to designate a surrogate (Appelbaum et al. 1987). Therapeutic privilege applies when the consent process itself would worsen or contribute to a deterioration in the patient's condition (*Canterbury v. Spence* 1972; Dickerson 1995). In these circumstances, the physician may obtain consent for an intervention from an alternate decision maker. Therapeutic privilege does not apply, however, simply because there is a situation in which providing information to the patient could make the patient less likely to accept the proposed treatment. Over time, the justification for withholding information from a competent patient has narrowed so much that therapeutic privilege is rarely invoked (Bostick et al. 2006). In practice, however, striving to "tell the whole truth" in a single encounter simply to comply with the law deviates from the spirit of the law and does not optimize patient autonomy. Instead, for some patients, an iterative process—involving a series of discussions in which the necessary information is limited to what the patient is able to understand, remember, and handle—is more effective in achieving full informed consent (Richard et al. 2010). In sum, the default rule is to obtain informed consent for all interventions and to view therapeutic privilege and waiver as two extremely narrow exceptions that should be used in only well-defined and cautiously characterized situations.

Advance Directives and Substitute Decision Making

Decisional incapacity is highly prevalent in medical inpatient settings, with estimates as high as 40% in some studies, and is nearly ubiquitous in intensive care units (Raymont et al. 2004). When a patient lacks capacity to make medical decisions, an alternate decision maker must be identified to authorize medical intervention or to refuse treatment on behalf of the patient. This other person is referred to as a *substitute* or *surrogate decision maker.* The surrogate decision maker is charged with making decisions for the patient, and most often for making decisions according to what the patient would have wanted were he or she competent. This standard is known as the *substituted judgment standard* and reflects respect for autonomy. In the case of minors and in some limited circumstances in which substituted judgment cannot be applied, the substitute decision maker may be charged with making decisions in the patient's best interest, taking beneficence more prominently into consideration (Schouten and Edersheim 2008).

Substitute decision makers may be either informally or formally appointed. Informal appointment occurs without judicial intervention. An advance directive is one common way of appointing a substitute decision maker. An *advance directive* is a document prepared and executed by an individual at a time when he or she is competent that either gives instructions to guide decisions or appoints a substitute decision maker should the individual become incapacitated at some time in the future. Two types of advance directives are the *health care proxy* and the *durable power of attorney for health care.* Both types are characterized by a "springing clause"—that is, once crafted, they remain inactive until such time as the patient, or principal, is incapacitated. At the time of incapacity and for the duration of the incapacity, the advance directive "springs" into effect. Should the patient regain capacity at a future time, the advance directive would again become inactive.

Since the passage of the federal Patient Self-Determination Act of 1990 (1995), hospitals have been legally required to ask whether patients have an advance directive at the time patients are admitted to the hospital and additionally required to provide information about advance directives to patients. This law also required provision of education about advance directives to health care personnel and community members (Patient Self-Determination Act of 1990 [1995]). Notwithstanding passage of this law, only 26% of Americans have advance directives (Rao et al. 2014). In the absence of an advance directive, one of several pathways is generally followed. A legally recognized pathway available in some states is provided by surrogate decision-making statutes that prioritize potential surrogate decision makers according to their relationship to the patient. For example, the Illinois law prioritizes the patient's guardian (if any) and then moves on to the patient's spouse, adult child, and then parent as the order in which a surrogate decision maker should be appointed. At the bottom of the list are more distant blood relatives, followed by close friends and the guardian of the estate (Health Care Surrogate Act 2005). Most states have a provision for appointment of a default surrogate in the absence of a designated surrogate (DeMartino et al. 2017).

In the absence of an advance directive and of a state surrogate decision-making law, clinicians often defer decisions to family members at the bedside, especially in situations in which there is little or no disagreement about the course of care, about the patient's wishes, and between family members and when the proposed treatment is well established and low risk (Brendel and Cohen 2008; Schouten and Edersheim 2008). In situations in which there is less clarity about interventions, in which proposed interventions are more intrusive, and/or in which there is disagreement between potential surrogate decision makers, the second type of substitute decision maker—a formal substitute decision maker—is more likely to be appointed. Formal surrogate decision makers are court appointed and are most commonly guardians.

Appointment of guardians is governed by state law. Increasingly, states have adopted guardianship laws and standards that derive from model legislation known as the *Uniform Probate Code* (UPC). Unlike a clinical finding of incapacity triggering the use of an informal advance directive, guardianship is a legal process that may include appointment of an attorney to represent the patient's values and interests, obtaining of independent medical opinions, and a formal court hearing. In addition, the standard for guardianship requires more than a finding of decisional incapacity. For example, UPC-derived state laws generally require three elements for imposition of a guardian: a clinically diagnosed condition, decision-making inability, and functional impairment. To obtain a treatment guardian for a patient, courts may look to neurocognitive assessment and functional testing to determine the need for and scope of the guardianship (Massachusetts Probate and Family Court 2017; Massachusetts Uniform Probate Code 2009). Finally, a guardian may be required even when the treating clinicians do not believe that an intervention is intrusive. For example, under Massachusetts law, a guardian is required in order for antipsychotic medication to be given to an incapacitated person (*Rogers v. Commissioner of Department of Mental Health* 1983).

Treatment Refusal and Involuntary Treatment

Consultation-liaison psychiatrists frequently become involved when medical inpatients refuse or are uncooperative with particular interventions or decline treatment altogether. The legal criteria for involuntary medical treatment are based on capacity criteria and, where applicable, surrogate decision making, as discussed above. In other words, authorization for involuntary medical treatment is based on capacity criteria, and authorization for involuntary medical treatment depends on demonstrating that the patient does not have sufficient capacity to refuse treatment; it does not require that the patient's medical condition be life- or limb-threatening.

In contrast, the legal processes and criteria for temporary psychiatric detention and civil commitment do not as closely follow a decisional capacity–based approach (Byatt et al. 2006). Rather, although laws vary by state, the criteria for involuntary psychiatric detention in general require that the patient have a mental illness and pose a danger to self or to others because of mental illness, or that the patient be unable to perform self-care activities or maintain personal safety because of mental illness. In addition, many jurisdictions follow a bifurcated approach to detention and treatment, meaning that if a patient refuses psychiatric treatment following a psychiatric admission, treatment may proceed only after specific judicial authorization, emergently to prevent imminent harm, and/or with a second psychiatric opinion, depending on the jurisdiction. Some medically ill patients with psychiatric illness may require separate and parallel processes for authorization of medical treatment and for psychiatric admission and/or treatment.

Restraints

In psychiatry, the legal and ethical issues surrounding the use of physical restraints are complex (Annas 1999; Tardiff 1984). Restraints are a serious intrusion on the freedom of patients and come into conflict with respect for autonomy. On the other hand, their use may be justified by beneficence considerations when they allow provision of care that would be wanted by a patient if he or she were competent; by justice considerations when others are at risk; and by nonmaleficence and beneficence considerations when a patient is at risk of harming himself or herself. As for involuntary medical and psychiatric treatment, the paradigms for use of restraints for medical purposes and for psychiatric purposes are different. In the United States, the Joint Commission and the Centers for Medicare & Medicaid Services have issued some restrictive guidance regarding the use of physical restraints in medical settings. In general, the use of restraints is broadly allowable to prevent interference with medical care. It is therefore commonplace to encounter physical restraint in inpatient medical settings, especially intensive care units (Glezer and Brendel 2010).

Consultation-liaison psychiatrists can assist nonpsychiatric colleagues and nurses in determining the risks and benefits of using restraints in general hospital settings.

For example, physical restraints may be required in confused, medically unstable patients if chemical restraint is ineffective, contraindicated, or more restrictive. If restraints are not used in some patients with delirium or dementia, they may pull out intravenous or arterial lines, endotracheal tubes, or other vital interventions, and this risk often cannot be safely eliminated with sedation alone. Psychiatrists in medical settings can help explore the various options for managing the patient and address the discomfort staff may have in using restraints. It is important to bear in mind that there are clinical and legal risks inherent in using restraints as well as in failing to employ restraints for patient treatment and safety. As a general guideline, the decision about whether to use physical restraints in medical settings should ultimately be determined by what is required to safely provide necessary medical treatment while being least restrictive, and the physician and other clinical staff should document their reasoning for the decision to use physical restraints in the medical record.

In contrast to the use of physical restraints in medical settings, the use of physical restraints in psychiatric units is more limited, and many psychiatric units and facilities have adopted no-restraint policies. Generally, the use of physical restraints in psychiatric settings is legally appropriate only when a patient presents an imminent risk of harm to self or others and a less restrictive alternative is not available.

Discharges Against Medical Advice

Discharges against medical advice (AMA) account for approximately 1% of discharges for general medical patients. In a recent study at one county hospital, the rate was 2.7% (Stearns et al. 2017). AMA discharges commonly occur when patients are experiencing conflict in the doctor–patient relationship, are too anxious about their medical condition or treatment to engage in care, have personal or work pressures to leave the hospital, or have an addictive disorder that has not been adequately diagnosed or treated in the hospital (e.g., nicotine withdrawal or cocaine craving) (Alfandre 2009). In one study, patients with AMA discharges were more likely than those traditionally discharged to be young, male, and homeless (Stearns et al. 2017).

Decisions about AMA discharges generally follow the decisional capacity–based model of medical treatment refusal. Specifically, since medical patients are admitted voluntarily to a general hospital, an AMA discharge is akin to a withdrawal of the original consent to hospitalization and follows the ethical principle of autonomy. Therefore, one role of the consulting psychiatrist is to perform a capacity assessment to determine whether the patient has the requisite capacity to decide to leave the hospital AMA. In addition, the psychiatrist can explore why the patient wants to leave the hospital and, when possible and appropriate, help effect a solution leading to willingness of the patient to remain in the hospital. In other words, the psychiatrist can play a key role in depolarizing a standoff between the patient and the care team. From an ethical perspective, this role is critically important in that individuals who are discharged AMA may be particularly vulnerable.

Care providers often believe that an AMA discharge is an automatic protection from liability (Devitt et al. 2000). Too often, hospital personnel are intent on getting a patient to sign an AMA discharge form, but the form is neither necessary nor sufficient to avoid legal liability. Regardless of whether the patient signs an AMA discharge form, a clear assessment of decisional capacity should be performed, and clear and complete documentation should be made in the medical record of the capacity assessment, the recommendations given to the patient regarding the need for and nature of follow-up care, and the possible risks of premature discharge (Gerbasi and Simon 2003). Medical patients who lack decisional capacity may be kept in the hospital against their will in cases of emergency, until either judicial approval or other authorized surrogate consent can be obtained. Unlike holding a patient involuntarily for psychiatric reasons, involuntary medical hospitalization in these limited circumstances generally does not require a finding of dangerousness to self or to others.

When efforts to convince a competent patient to remain in the hospital fail, a power struggle may ensue and members of the health care team often become angry at the patient. Such anger is not clinically constructive and may contribute to legal liability. For example, some physicians believe that they should refuse to give the departing AMA patient any outpatient prescriptions, thinking that would potentially make them liable for the patient's subsequent clinical course. However, if stopping the medication would endanger the patient (e.g., a beta-blocker after an acute myocardial infarction), it may be both ethical and prudent to give the patient a time-limited prescription, even if the patient wishes to leave the hospital. The patient should be told that he is welcome to return to the hospital if he changes his mind or his symptoms get worse, and robust efforts should be made to secure and convince the patient to accept follow-up care.

Emergency Treatment Requirements and EMTALA

The Emergency Medical Treatment and Labor Act (EMTALA), a U.S. federal law enacted in 1986, obligates emergency departments of all hospitals that participate in Medicare to examine patients who seek emergency care and to either stabilize them before discharge or admit or transfer them to another willing facility if medically indicated (Quinn et al. 2002). EMTALA has the effect of preventing health care providers from discriminating against patients who need medical care but are unable to pay. From an ethical perspective, EMTALA serves justice and fidelity by protecting vulnerable, disadvantaged individuals who are acutely ill. Issues with EMTALA, however, may arise when patients who present to emergency rooms with unstable medical and psychiatric illness are uncooperative with treatment. For example, if a dialysis patient who has been banned from a hospital's outpatient dialysis program because of aggressive behavior toward staff and other patients comes to that hospital's emergency room with severe uremia or hyperkalemia, he or she must be provided with emergent dialysis nonetheless.

Conflicts may also occur between hospitals and between physicians when a patient appears too psychiatrically unstable to be treated in a medical facility and too medically unstable to be transferred to a psychiatric facility. The potential penalties for violations of the law are severe, and therefore, in these situations, emergency physicians may admit patients to either a medical or a psychiatric facility against the advice of psychiatric and medical colleagues out of fear of EMTALA liability. EMTALA applies only to emergency settings and does not apply to discharges from medical or psychiatric inpatient units, as clarified in the 2003 EMTALA rules. However, issues regarding the transfer of psychiatric patients were not addressed in the new rules (Saks 2004).

Maternal Competency

Psychiatric consultations are sometimes requested to evaluate maternal (or more rarely paternal) competency (i.e., capacity to care for a child) when it is thought that a vulnerable infant or child will be at risk if the parent is allowed to take the child home from the hospital (Nair and Morrison 2000). This occurs most commonly in situations of maternal substance abuse, severe mental disorder, child abuse or neglect, or factitious disorder imposed on another. Child protective services typically becomes involved. The courts can be asked to sever parental rights temporarily or permanently. This proceeding is not a competency evaluation in the legal senses described earlier in this chapter (see section "Capacity Assessment"); rather, it is an assessment of the parent's ability to safely care for the child. The consulting psychiatrist usually collaborates with pediatrics, obstetrics, nursing, and social work staff and may require collateral information from others, including family members. Awareness of state law and relevant local social agencies is important.

A particularly challenging area of maternal competency, from ethical, legal, and policy perspectives, is how maternal substance misuse during pregnancy should be addressed. With the nationwide opioid crisis in the United States, there has been renewed debate about how to manage opioid and other substance use during pregnancy. At a minimum, federal law requires reporting of positive drug screens in newborns to child protective services (Ho and Rovzar 2017). Beyond mandated reporting and protective services involvement, states have varied in their approaches to pregnant women with substance use disorders along a continuum from treatment-focused policies promoting the well-being of both mother and child to criminal prosecution of women on the birth of a substance-positive child (Ho and Rovzar 2017; Lollar 2017). Some convictions under these laws have been overturned in recent years, and critics have challenged the laws both on their efficacy in addressing substance use and on their disproportionate effect on women of color and low socioeconomic status (Lollar 2017). At present, there is disagreement within the medical, legal, and policy realms on how to most effectively address maternal and child well-being in the setting of substance use during pregnancy, and the debate over intervention strategies continues (Lollar 2017).

Malpractice

Fidelity and trustworthiness are important virtues for psychiatrists. From an ethical perspective, patients trust physicians to advance their treatment and health. Like all physicians, the consultation-liaison psychiatrist must meet the standard of care in treating patients from both ethical and legal perspectives. This standard is a specification of the principle of nonmaleficence—the physician should not harm the patient (Beauchamp and Childress 2013). However, the responsibility of the consultant is different from that of the treating physician. Specifically, the consultation-liaison psychiatrist's primary duty is to the consultee, or the physician who requests the consult. The consultant must provide competent consultation to the requesting physician (Brendel and Schouten 2007; Schouten and Brendel 2004). Conversely, the responsibility of the treating clinician is directly to the patient. Consultants should be careful to maintain boundaries between the role of consultant and the role of treating clinician. For example, when a psychiatrist (consultant) is requested by a treating physician (consultee) to recommend an appropriate medication to prescribe a patient, the consultant's duty is to provide appropriate recommendations and information to the consultee. But if the consultant directly enters an order for the medication to be given to the patient, the consultant will generally be held to have assumed a direct treatment role and assumed a direct responsibility to the patient. If the consultant does assume a primary treatment role (and there may be good reasons for the consultant to do so), it is important that the consultant be cognizant that he or she thereby assumes all responsibilities of a treating psychiatrist, including the responsibility to either monitor and follow up on the patient's progress or arrange for another clinician to do so.

Physicians—and the consultation-liaison psychiatrist is no exception—often fear legal liability and malpractice lawsuits. There is good reason to be concerned, given that defending a malpractice lawsuit, regardless of the outcome, is a personally and professionally burdensome endeavor (Schouten et al. 2008). That being said, the best way to avoid malpractice litigation is to exercise sound clinical judgment, engage in judicious clinical practice, document appropriately, and communicate well with consultees and patients (Schouten et al. 2008). At the same time, familiarity with the legal concept of malpractice and a basic understanding of physicians' responsibilities may help the practitioner contextualize malpractice within the provision of health care.

Malpractice is an area of tort law that covers personal injuries resulting from medical interventions (Brendel and Schouten 2007; Schouten and Brendel 2004; Schouten et al. 2008). For a claim of malpractice to be established, four elements must be met. First, a *duty* must be established, by the existence of either a direct doctor–patient relationship or a consultant–consultee relationship. In some cases, even limited or cursory interactions may be considered by the court to have constituted a doctor–patient relationship. Second, a *breach* of that duty must have occurred (i.e., a violation of the standard of care). Third, this breach must have *directly* caused harm to a patient that resulted in the fourth element, *damage* to the patient. The legal requirement for malpractice is often summarized as "the four D's": duty, dereliction of duty, direct causation, and damage. Malpractice does not require that the physician acted intentionally in causing harm to the patient. Rather, malpractice is an unintentional tort, a tort of negligence, which means that deviation from the accepted standard of care caused damage to the patient.

As a final note, studies of malpractice lawsuits have shown that only a small number of cases involving injury to patients due to medical errors actually lead to malpractice claims or litigation and that defendants prevail in the majority of cases that lead to litigation (Localio et al. 1991; Schouten et al. 2008). Notwithstanding, in a study of paid claims, no medical error was found in up to one-third of claims, highlighting the fact that even error-free practice does not insulate against malpractice liability (Schouten et al. 2008; see also Brennan et al. 1996). As a practical matter, physicians can reduce their risk of malpractice liability by recognizing individual and systemic factors contributing to errors, communicating effectively with colleagues and patients, acknowledging error and preserving relationships, maintaining good records, avoiding overlegalization and focusing on good clinical care, and consulting with colleagues (Schouten et al. 2008).

Conclusion

Issues at the interface of clinical practice, ethics, and law may often arise in the practice of psychosomatic medicine. Areas in which ethical and legal considerations frequently emerge include confidentiality and exceptions thereto, HIPAA, capacity determinations, informed consent and refusal, and concerns about malpractice liability. The best rule of thumb is for clinicians to be aware of ethical considerations, relevant legal and regulatory provisions in the jurisdictions in which they practice, and ethics and legal resources to advise on complex issues so that they may focus on providing sound, clinically informed care to patients. Finally, it is important for consulting psychiatrists to be cognizant of their specific role in patients' treatment by maintaining clarity between consultative and direct treatment roles.

References

Abrams RC, Lachs M, McAvay G, et al: Predictors of self-neglect in community-dwelling elders. Am J Psychiatry 159(10):1724–1730, 2002 12359679

Acierno R, Hernandez-Tejada MA, Anetzberger GJ, et al: The National Elder Mistreatment Study: an 8-year longitudinal study of outcomes. J Elder Abuse Negl 29(4):254–269, 2017 28837418

Alfandre DJ: "I'm going home": discharges against medical advice. Mayo Clin Proc 84(3):255–260, 2009 19252113

Almason AL: Personal liability implications of the duty to warn are hard pills to swallow: from Tarasoff to Hutchinson v Patel and beyond. J Contemp Health Law Policy 13(2):471–496, 1997 9212527

Alpert EJ, Tonkin AE, Seeherman AM, et al: Family violence curricula in U.S. medical schools. Am J Prev Med 14(4):273–282, 1998 9635071

American Medical Association Council on Ethical and Judicial Affairs: AMA Code of Medical Ethics: AMA Principles of Medical Ethics. Revised June 2001. Available at: https://www.ama-assn.org/sites/default/files/media-browser/principles-of-medical-ethics.pdf. Accessed April 5, 2018.

American Psychiatric Association: Position Statement on Confidentiality. Washington, DC, American Psychiatric Association, 1978

American Psychiatric Association: The Principles of Medical Ethics With Annotations Especially Applicable to Psychiatry. Washington, DC, American Psychiatric Association, 2001

American Psychiatric Association: Commentary on Ethics in Practice. Washington, DC, American Psychiatric Association, 2015. Available at: https://www.psychiatry.org/File%20Library/Psychiatrists/Practice/Ethics/APA-Commentary-on-Ethics-in-Practice.pdf. Accessed September 21, 2017.

Annas GJ: The last resort—the use of physical restraints in medical emergencies. N Engl J Med 341(18):1408–1412, 1999 10536135

Appelbaum PS: Privacy in psychiatric treatment: threats and responses. Am J Psychiatry 159(11):1809–1818, 2002 12411211

Appelbaum PS: Clinical practice. Assessment of patients' competence to consent to treatment. N Engl J Med 357(18):1834–1840, 2007 17978292

Appelbaum PS, Grisso T: Assessing patients' capacities to consent to treatment. N Engl J Med 319(25):1635–1638, 1988 3200278

Appelbaum PS, Roth LH: Clinical issues in the assessment of competency. Am J Psychiatry 138(11):1462–1467, 1981 7294214

Appelbaum PS, Lidz CW, Meisel A: Informed Consent: Legal Theory and Clinical Practice. New York, Oxford University Press, 1987

Appelbaum PS, Zonana H, Bonnie R, et al: Statutory approaches to limiting psychiatrists' liability for their patients' violent acts. Am J Psychiatry 146(7):821–828, 1989 2742008

Averhoff F, Zimmerman L, Harpaz R, et al; Centers for Disease Control and Prevention (CDC): Varicella surveillance practices—United States, 2004. MMWR Morb Mortal Wkly Rep 55(41):1126–1129, 2006 17060900

Beauchamp TC, Childress JF: Principles of Biomedical Ethics, 7th Edition. New York, Oxford University Press, 2013

Beck JC: Legal and ethical duties of the clinician treating a patient who is liable to be impulsively violent. Behav Sci Law 16(3):375–389, 1998 9768467

Bostick NA, Sade R, McMahon JW, et al; American Medical Association Council on Ethical and Judicial Affairs: Report of the American Medical Association Council on Ethical and Judicial Affairs: withholding information from patients: rethinking the propriety of "therapeutic privilege." J Clin Ethics 17(4):302–306, 2006 17330719

Bradshaw v Daniel, 854 SW2d 865 (Tenn 1993)

Brendel RW: An approach to forensic issues, in The Ten-Minute Guide to Psychiatric Diagnosis and Treatment. Edited by Stern TA. New York, Professional Publishing Group, 2005, pp 399–412

Brendel RW, Brendel DH: Professionalism and the doctor—patient relationship in psychiatry, in The Ten-Minute Guide to Psychiatric Diagnosis and Treatment. Edited by Stern TA. New York, Professional Publishing Group, 2005, pp 1–7

Brendel RW, Bryan E: HIPAA for psychiatrists. Harv Rev Psychiatry 12(3):177–183, 2004 15371073

Brendel RW, Cohen MA: Ethical issues, advance directives, and surrogate decision-making, in Comprehensive Textbook of AIDS Psychiatry. Edited by Cohen MA, Gorman J. New York, Oxford University Press, 2008, pp 577–584

Brendel RW, Schouten R: Legal concerns in psychosomatic medicine. Psychiatr Clin North Am 30(4):663–676, 2007 17938039

Brennan TA, Sox CM, Burstin HR: Relation between negligent adverse events and the outcomes of medical-malpractice litigation. N Engl J Med 335(26):1963–1967, 1996 8960477

Byatt N, Pinals D, Arikan R: Involuntary hospitalization of medical patients who lack decisional capacity: an unresolved issue. Psychosomatics 47(5):443–448, 2006 16959935

Canterbury v Spence, 464 F2d 772 (DC 1972)

Child Abuse Prevention and Treatment Act, P.L. 92-273; 42 USC § 5101 (2003)

Dalla-Vorgia P, Lascaratos J, Skiadas P, et al: Is consent in medicine a concept only of modern times? J Med Ethics 27(1):59–61, 2001 11233382

DeMartino ES, Dudzinski DM, Doyle CK, et al: Who decides when a patient can't? Statutes on alternate decision makers. N Engl J Med 376(15):1478–1482, 2017 28402767

Devitt PJ, Devitt AC, Dewan M: Does identifying a discharge as "against medical advice" confer legal protection? J Fam Pract 49(3):224–227, 2000 10735481

Dickerson DA: A doctor's duty to disclose life expectancy information to terminally ill patients. Clevel State Law Rev 43(2):319–350, 1995 11660488

Duty to warn patient's potential victims; cause of action. Mass Gen Laws Ch 123, § 36B (2005)

Emergency Medical Treatment and Labor Act (EMTALA), 42 USC § 1395dd (1986)

Evans CS, Hunold KM, Rosen T, et al: Diagnosis of elder abuse in US emergency departments. J Am Geriatr Soc 65(1):91–97, 2017 27753066

Faden RR, Beauchamp TL: A History and Theory of Informed Consent. New York, Oxford University Press, 1986

Feld AD: The Health Insurance Portability and Accountability Act (HIPAA): its broad effect on practice. Am J Gastroenterol 100(7):1440–1443, 2005 15984962

Friedrich MJ: Health care practitioners and organizations prepare for approaching HIPAA deadlines (medical news and perspectives). JAMA 286(13):1563–1565, 2001 11585459

Gerbasi JB, Simon RI: Patients' rights and psychiatrists' duties: discharging patients against medical advice. Harv Rev Psychiatry 11(6):333–343, 2003 14713569

Ginsberg B: Tarasoff at thirty: victim's knowledge shrinks the psychotherapist's duty to warn and protect. J Contemp Health Law Policy 21(1):1–35, 2004 15799533

Glezer A, Brendel RW: Beyond emergencies: the use of physical restraints in medical and psychiatric settings. Harv Rev Psychiatry 18(6):353–358, 2010 21080773

Gold JA: Kaimowitz v Department of Mental Health: involuntary mental patient cannot give informed consent to experimental psychosurgery. Rev Law Soc Change 4(2):207–227, 1974 11664643

Gordon S: Privacy standards for health information: the misnomer of administrative simplification. Delaware Law Review 5:23–56, 2002

Gostin LO, Webber DW: HIV infection and AIDS in the public health and health care systems: the role of law and litigation. JAMA 279(14):1108–1113, 1998 9546571

Grisso T, Appelbaum PS: Assessing Competence to Consent to Treatment: A Guide for Physicians and Other Health Professionals. New York, Oxford University Press, 1998

Hall MA, Schulman KA: Ownership of medical information. JAMA 301(12):1282–1284, 2009 19318657

Health Care Surrogate Act, 755 Ill Comp Stat 40 (2005)

HIPAA Privacy Rule, 45 CFR 164.512 (2001)

Ho JA, Rovzar AO: Preventing neonatal abstinence syndrome within the opioid epidemic: a uniform facilitative policy. Harvard J Legis 54:423–455, 2017

Iheukwumere EO: Doctor, are you experienced? The relevance of disclosure of physician experience to a valid informed consent. J Contemp Health Law Policy 18(2):373–419, 2002 12173441

Jones PM, Appelbaum PS, Siegel DM; Massachusetts Work Group on Law Enforcement Access to Hospital Patients: Law enforcement interviews of hospital patients: a conundrum for clinicians. JAMA 295(7):822–825, 2006 16478905

Kachigian C, Felthous AR: Court responses to Tarasoff statutes. J Am Acad Psychiatry Law 32(3):263–273, 2004 15515914

Kahan FS, Paris BE: Why elder abuse continues to elude the health care system. Mt Sinai J Med 70(1):62–68, 2003 12516011

Keeton WP, Dobbs DB, Keeton RE, et al: Prosser and Keeton on the Law of Torts, 5th Edition. St Paul, MN, West Publishing, 1984

King JS, Moulton BW: Rethinking informed consent: the case for shared medical decision-making. Am J Law Med 32(4):429–501, 2006 17240730

Liang BA: Medical information, confidentiality, and privacy. Hematol Oncol Clin North Am 16(6):1433–1447, 2002 12512176

Lloyd GER (ed): Hippocrates: the oath, in Hippocratic Writings. Translated by Chadwick J, Mann WN. London, Penguin, 1983, p 67

Localio AR, Lawthers AG, Brennan TA, et al: Relation between malpractice claims and adverse events due to negligence. Results of the Harvard Medical Practice Study III. N Engl J Med 325(4):245–251, 1991 2057025

Lollar CE: Criminalizing pregnancy. Indiana Law J 92:947–1005, 2017

Maio JE: HIPAA and the special status of psychotherapy notes. Lippincotts Case Manag 8(1):24–29, 2003 12555040

Mallary SD, Gert B, Culver CM: Family coercion and valid consent. Theor Med 7(2):123–126, 1986 3738841

Marcus EN: The silent epidemic—the health effects of illiteracy. N Engl J Med 355(4):339–341, 2006 16870912

Massachusetts Probate and Family Court: MPC 902 (Instructions to Clinicians for Completing the Medical Certificate for Guardianship or Conservatorship), 2017. Available at: http://www.mass.gov/courts/docs/forms/probate-and-family/mpc902-instructions-to-clinicians.pdf. Accessed September 21, 2017.

Massachusetts Uniform Probate Code, Article V (Protection of Persons Under Disability and Their Property), 2009

McCarthy J: Principlism or narrative ethics: must we choose between them? Med Humanit 29(2):65–71, 2003 15884187

Meisel A: The "exceptions" to the informed consent doctrine: striking a balance between competing values in medical decisionmaking. Wis L Rev 1979(2):413–488, 1979 11665172

Melton GB: Chronic neglect of family violence: more than a decade of reports to guide US policy. Child Abuse Negl 26(6–7):569–586, 2002 12201156

Milosavljevic N, Green A, Brendel RW: Abuse and neglect, in Massachusetts General Hospital Psychiatry Update and Board Preparation, 3rd Edition. Edited by Stern TA, Herman JB, Gorrindo T. Boston, MA, MGH Psychiatry Academy Publishing, 2012, pp 543–545

Milosavljevic N, Taylor JB, Brendel RW: Psychiatric correlates and consequences of abuse and neglect, in Comprehensive Clinical Psychiatry, 2nd Edition. Edited by Stern TA, Rosenbaum JF, Fava M, et al. New York, Elsevier, 2016, pp 904–911

Mohr JC: American medical malpractice litigation in historical perspective. JAMA 283(13):1731–1737, 2000 10755500

Montello M: Narrative ethics. Hastings Cent Rep 44 (1 suppl):S2–S6, 2014 24408701

Moser DJ, Arndt S, Kanz JE, et al: Coercion and informed consent in research involving prisoners. Compr Psychiatry 45(1):1–9, 2004 14671730

Nair S, Morrison MF: The evaluation of maternal competency. Psychosomatics 41(6):523–530, 2000 11110117

National Commission for the Protection of Human Subjects of Biomedical and Behavioral Research: Report and Recommendations: Research Involving Prisoners. Washington, DC, U.S. Government Printing Office, 1976

National Commission for the Protection of Human Subjects of Biomedical and Behavioral Research: Research Involving Those Institutionalized as Mentally Infirm: Report and Recommendations. Washington, DC, U.S. Government Printing Office, 1978

New York State Department of Health: HIV reporting and partner notification questions and answers. May 2000. Available at: https://www.health.ny.gov/diseases/aids/providers/regulations/reporting_and_notification/question_answer.htm. Accessed September 21, 2017.

New York State Department of Health AIDS Institute: Identification and ambulatory care of HIV-exposed and infected adolescents, Appendix B: summary, HIV reporting and partner notification. 2003. Available at: http://www.hivguidelines.org. Accessed September 21, 2017.

Patient Self-Determination Act of 1990, 42 USC 1395 cc(a); final rule: 60 CFR 123 at 33294 (1995)

Precourt v Frederick, 481 NE2d 1144 (Mass 1985)

Quinn DK, Geppert CM, Maggiore WA: The Emergency Medical Treatment and Active Labor Act of 1985 and the practice of psychiatry. Psychiatr Serv 53(10):1301–1307, 2002 12364679

Rao JK, Anderson LA, Lin FC, et al: Completion of advance directives among U.S. consumers. Am J Prev Med 46(1):65–70, 2014 24355673

Raymont V, Bingley W, Buchanan A, et al: Prevalence of mental incapacity in medical inpatients and associated risk factors: cross-sectional study. Lancet 364(9443):1421–1427, 2004 15488217

Rawls J: A Theory of Justice. Cambridge, MA, Harvard University Press, 1971

Richard C, Lajeunesse Y, Lussier MT: Therapeutic privilege: between the ethics of lying and the practice of truth. J Med Ethics 36(6):353–357, 2010 20530090

Roberts LW: Informed consent and the capacity for voluntarism. Am J Psychiatry 159(5):705–712, 2002 11986120

Roberts LW: A Clinical Guide to Psychiatric Ethics. Washington, DC, American Psychiatric Association Publishing, 2016

Robinson DJ, O'Neill D: Access to health care records after death: balancing confidentiality with appropriate disclosure. JAMA 297(6):634–636, 2007 17299198

Rogers v Commissioner of Department of Mental Health, 458 NE2d 308 (Mass 1983)

Rosenstein DL, Miller FG: Ethical issues, in The American Psychiatric Publishing Textbook of Psychosomatic Medicine, 2nd Edition. Washington, DC, American Psychiatric Publishing, 2011, pp 33–44

Saks SJ: Call 911: psychiatry and the new Emergency Medical Treatment and Active Labor Act (EMTALA) regulations. J Psychiatry Law 32(4):483–512, 2004 16018118

Salgo v Leland Stanford Jr. University Board of Trustees, 154 Cal App 2d 560, 317 P2d 170 (1957)

Schloendorff v Society of New York Hospital, 105 NE 92 (NY 1914)

Schouten R, Brendel RW: Legal aspects of consultation, in The Massachusetts General Hospital Handbook of General Hospital Psychiatry, 5th Edition. Edited by Stern TA, Fricchione GL, Cassem EH, et al. Philadelphia, PA, CV Mosby, 2004, pp 349–364

Schouten R, Brendel RW: Common pitfalls in giving medical-legal advice to trainees and supervisees. Harv Rev Psychiatry 17(4):291–294, 2009 19637076

Schouten R, Edersheim JG: Informed consent, competency, treatment refusal, and civil commitment, in Massachusetts General Hospital Comprehensive Clinical Psychiatry. Edited by Stern TA, Rosenbaum JF, Fava M, et al. Philadelphia, PA, Mosby/Elsevier, 2008, pp 1143–1154

Schouten R, Brendel RW, Edersheim JG: Malpractice and boundary violations, in Massachusetts General Hospital Comprehensive Clinical Psychiatry. Edited by Stern TA, Rosenbaum JF, Fava M, et al. Philadelphia, PA, Mosby/Elsevier, 2008, pp 1165–1175

Shine v Vega, 429 Mass 456, 709 NE2d 58 (Mass 1999)

Siegler M: Sounding Boards. Confidentiality in medicine—a decrepit concept. N Engl J Med 307(24):1518–1521, 1982 7144818

Sprung CL, Winick BJ: Informed consent in theory and practice: legal and medical perspectives on the informed consent doctrine and a proposed reconceptualization. Crit Care Med 17(12):1346–1354, 1989 2686937

Stearns CR, Bakamjian A, Sattar S, et al: Discharges against medical advice at a county hospital: provider perceptions and practice. J Hosp Med 12(1):11–17, 2017 28125826

Sugarman J, Sulmasy DP: Methods in Medical Ethics, 2nd Edition. Washington, DC, Georgetown University Press, 2010

Sullivan MD, Youngner SJ: Depression, competence, and the right to refuse lifesaving medical treatment. Am J Psychiatry 151(7):971–978, 1994 8010382

Tarasoff v Board of Regents of the University of California, 17 Cal3d 425 (1976)

Tardiff K (ed): The Psychiatric Uses of Seclusion and Restraint. Washington, DC, American Psychiatric Press, 1984

Timmons M: Moral Theory: An Introduction, 2nd Edition. Lanham, MD, Rowman & Littlefield Publishers, 2013

Tomlinson T: Methods in Medical Ethics: Critical Perspectives. New York, Oxford University Press, 2012

CHAPTER 3

Psychological Responses to Illness

Mark S. Groves, M.D.
Philip R. Muskin, M.D., M.A.

A central task of psychiatrists working with the medically ill is to understand patients' subjective experiences of illness to design therapeutic interventions that modulate the patients' behavioral or emotional responses, decrease their distress, and improve their medical outcomes. Physicians witness a tremendous diversity of emotional and behavioral responses to illness. Some individuals face devastating illnesses for which no cure is currently available with courage and a sense of humor (Druss and Douglas 1988). Others, facing easily treatable illnesses, have difficulty overcoming intense emotions such as anger, fear, or hopelessness. Clinical experience and research indicate that illness variables such as severity, chronicity, or organ system involvement cannot predict an individual's response to any given medical illness (Lloyd 1977; Sensky 1997). It is in the realm of the individual's subjective experience of an illness that one can begin to understand his or her emotional and behavioral responses (Lipowski 1970).

There has been considerable research investigating interindividual differences in responses to the stresses of illness (see, e.g., Ciechanowski et al. 2003; Druss 1995; Geringer and Stern 1986; Lazarus 1999; Strain and Grossman 1975). We provide a general overview of the stresses that accompany medical illness and hospitalization and review psychological, emotional, and behavioral responses that these stresses frequently elicit.

The concepts of stress, personality types, coping strategies, and defense mechanisms can be integrated into a framework that illustrates the complexity of an individual's behavioral or emotional responses to illness (Figure 3–1). This framework, adapted from the work of Lazarus and Folkman (Lazarus 1999; Lazarus and Folkman 1984), attempts to integrate the psychodynamic concepts of character style and intra-

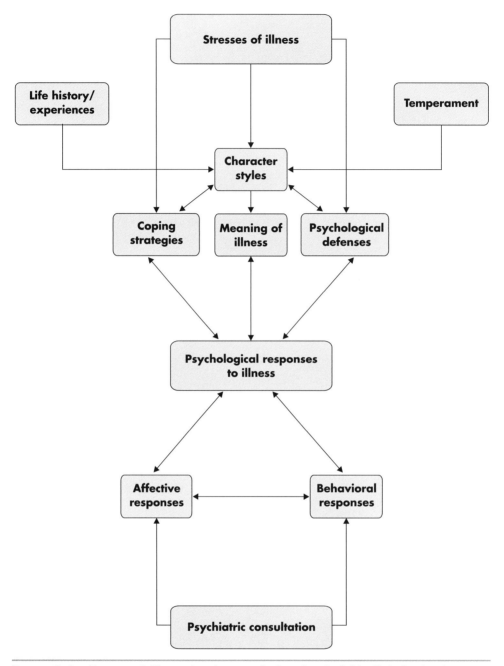

FIGURE 3–1. Framework illustrating the complexity of an individual's behavioral or emotional responses to illness.

Source.   Adapted from Lazarus 1999; Lazarus and Folkman 1984.

psychic defenses with other psychological concepts such as stress and coping. The importance of individual subjectivity is emphasized through the placement of coping styles, defense mechanisms, personality types, and the appraised meaning of illness as central mediators of the behavioral and emotional responses to the stresses of medical illness.

It is important not to limit the discussion to maladaptive responses to illness or to psychopathology. A coping strategy or defense mechanism may be relatively maladaptive or ineffective in one context but adaptive and effective in another (Penley et al. 2002). The maladaptive use of denial by a patient diagnosed with early breast cancer might lead to a long delay in seeking treatment (Fang et al. 2016; Zervas et al. 1993), while the adaptive use of denial by a man diagnosed with untreatable metastatic pancreatic cancer might enable him to maximize his quality of life in the final months of his life (Druss 1995).

Psychiatrists do not see most people who become ill, nor will most patients' responses to their illnesses concern their physicians (Patterson et al. 1993; Perry and Viederman 1981). That does not mean that there is no psychological response to the illness. An overt display of emotion may or may not be appropriate for a patient's racial and cultural background. Patients may feel or be discouraged from expressing their thoughts and feelings about their illness to family members or physicians. The determination that a psychological response to illness is problematic must be based on the effect the response has on the patient, the patient's adherence to treatment, and social functioning.

There is no one correct way to characterize psychological responses to illness. Psychodynamic formulations, coping styles, and personality types offer different perspectives that may or may not be useful in understanding the response of a particular patient. Therefore we provide an overview of the following topics without subscribing exclusively to any single theoretical framework: 1) the stresses of medical illness and hospitalization; 2) the influences of personality types, attachment styles, coping styles, and defense mechanisms on patients' subjective experiences of illness; 3) optimism and pessimism; 4) denial; 5) emotional responses to illness; and 6) behavioral responses to illness.

Stresses of Medical Illness and Hospitalization

The stresses of medical illness and hospitalization are significant and numerous (Strain and Grossman 1975). Some of the stresses accompanying illness are nearly universal, whereas others vary by illness and are more specific (Druss 1995). In this section, we discuss the most common stresses experienced by patients in medical settings.

Separate from medical illness, the hospital environment can be stressful (Gazzola and Muskin 2003; Kornfeld 1972). Many people find the hospital a frightening place associated with painful memories. Hospitalization separates patients from their usual environments and social supports. Patients are asked to wear a hospital gown, which results in deindividualization and loss of privacy (Gazzola and Muskin 2003). The machines, intravenous lines, blood withdrawals, interactions with strangers, and neighboring ill patients all contribute to the stress of hospitalization regardless of the patient's specific illness. The hospital demands that the patient be largely dependent on others for the most basic tasks—a requirement that can be very stressful (Kornfeld 1972; Muskin 1995; Perry and Viederman 1981). There are three successive (although at times overlapping) tasks that patients facing medical illness must go through: 1) acknowledgment to themselves and others that they are ill; 2) regressive dependency on others for care; and 3) resumption of normal functioning after recovery (Perry and Viederman 1981). All three tasks bring their own stresses and must be confronted for the patient to cope successfully with illness and hospitalization.

On a nearly universal level, medical illness results in narcissistic injury, i.e., it requires patients to confront their views of themselves (Strain and Grossman 1975). Although few would overtly claim that they are invulnerable to serious illness, many may hold such a belief subconsciously. Unconscious fantasies of invulnerability may be unknown until the person is injured or becomes ill. The development of a medical illness shatters any such conscious or unconscious beliefs. The sick patient may feel "defective," "weak," or less desirable to others.

One determinant of the effect of an illness is whether it is acute or chronic. Although an acute, non-life-threatening illness gives the individual little time to adapt, its effects are short term. Chronic illnesses require patients to change their self-concept more permanently. The challenges of chronic illness are ongoing and become a part of daily life. A change in identity or body image is disorienting and often anxiety producing; the patient's previously held self-concept is disturbed, shaken up, or shattered.

Separation from family or friends in the hospital or at home when one is ill produces isolation, disconnection, and stress (Heiskell and Pasnau 1991; Strain and Grossman 1975). This can precipitate conscious or unconscious fears of abandonment. The stress of separation and fear of abandonment are not only experienced by children.

The lack of privacy in the hospital environment or clinic creates additional stresses (Kornfeld 1972). Bodily exposure evokes discomfort. Given only a thin gown to wear, patients may be subjected to repeated examinations by doctors, nurses, and trainees. Exposure of the most private aspects of life can occur (Perry and Viederman 1981). A woman presenting with symptoms of a sexually transmitted disease must give a detailed account of her sexual history, and a young patient brought in with acute chest pain and hypertension is asked about use of cocaine, an illegal drug. For the vulnerable individual, such exposure experiences can evoke feelings of shame, requiring clinicians to be tactful and empathic to put the patient at ease and maintain a therapeutic alliance.

Beyond simple exposure, the medical environment often involves stressful experiences of bodily invasion (Gazzola and Muskin 2003). From the more invasive experiences of a colonoscopy, nasogastric tube insertion, or tracheal intubation to ostensibly more benign procedures such as a fine-needle biopsy of a breast lump or a rectal examination, patients' fear and discomfort are often not fully recognized by physicians, for whom such procedures have become routine. Individuals vary in their fears; e.g., victims of sexual abuse might be especially fearful of such experiences, requiring doctors to use greater care and psychological preparation than usual.

Pain should not be overlooked as a profound stressor that should be dealt with rationally (Chou et al. 2009). Even the most highly adapted patient with effective coping skills and strong social support can be taxed to the limit by extreme pain. Psychiatrists are frequently asked to evaluate patients for depression and hopelessness. If the pain is inadequately treated, the consultant can facilitate increased pain control, sometimes leading to full remission of hopelessness and depression without any additional intervention. Sleep disturbances are also extremely common in the medically ill, with significant psychological effects. A patient's outlook, emotional expression, and ability to cope may shift dramatically when insomnia is remedied.

When illness leads to disability, that becomes an additional stressor that can have a profound effect on the patient's activities of daily life (Westbrook and Viney 1982). What was previously routine and required no conscious planning can become tremendously challenging, both psychologically and practically. For example, on the acute rehabilitation unit, patients are assisted in their efforts to learn to walk again. What was previously automatic has become incredibly difficult and requires new techniques, assistive devices, and the help of others. Disabilities frequently preclude the possibility of an immediate return to work. Feelings of accomplishment, productivity, and usefulness are important to an individual's self-image; damage to one's self-esteem can result when this important source of gratification is lost.

Although only a small proportion of medical illnesses signify the imminent approach of death, forcing affected individuals to confront their mortality directly, even minor illnesses can evoke a sense of the fragility and impermanence of life (Perry and Viederman 1981). Psychiatric consultants are often called to assist patients who are experiencing difficulty facing death (or patients whose illnesses evoke these difficulties in caregivers). Patients may refuse to consent to do-not-resuscitate orders despite clear evidence that resuscitation would be futile because they equate do-not-resuscitate orders with suicide, which is morally unacceptable to them (Sullivan and Youngner 1994). Facing mortality—whether in the near future or later—can force a person to reflect deeply on life and can shatter previously held dreams of the future. This can stir up regrets and evoke numerous emotions, as described in the work of Elisabeth Kubler-Ross (1969).

Attachment Styles, Personality Types, Coping Styles, and Defense Mechanisms

There is great individual variation in responses to an environmental stressor such as receiving a diagnosis of cancer (Heim et al. 1993). Models of human behavior that involve only environmental stress and reflexive behavioral responses cannot account for such variation and are therefore considered to have limited utility and explanatory power. Richard Lazarus (1999) has reviewed the historical transition in health psychology and other disciplines from the traditional stimulus → response model to the more contemporary stimulus → organism → response model, which emphasizes the importance of understanding individuals' *subjective* experiences. Only through understanding individuals' subjective experiences can the inter-individual differences in reactions to a stressor be accounted for.

Although the medical team may readily identify the situational stressors and patients' behavioral responses, patients' subjective experiences are more elusive and require inquiry. Psychiatrists are often asked to evaluate patients with problematic behavioral or emotional reactions to the hospital setting or to their illnesses. The stated reason for consultation may identify the behavioral or emotional responses judged to be problematic, such as displaying anger or threatening to sign out against medical advice. Consulting psychiatrists seek to understand patients' subjective experiences of illness to explain their emotional and behavioral responses and to design interventions to help patients (and their caregivers).

Research investigating subjective variables that influence an individual's response to a given stressor generally has focused on several areas: attachment styles, personality types, coping styles, optimism/pessimism, and defense mechanisms. These areas are addressed separately below.

Attachment Styles

Attachment theory is a productive way of examining patients' interactions with the health care setting and their physicians. John Bowlby (1969) developed a theory that emphasized the effect of early interactions with primary caregivers on an individual's internal relationship schemas. Attachment theory has recently been applied to psychosomatic medicine.

Four predominant attachment styles have been described in the literature (secure, preoccupied, dismissing, and fearful; Bartholomew and Horowitz 1991). Each attachment style implies a view of self and other formed from early life experiences with caregivers; these internal relationship models are stable and enduring over time; thus, they would inevitably affect the patient–physician relationship (Klest and Philippon 2016). Patients with insecure attachment styles report lower degrees of trust in and satisfaction with their doctors (Holwerda et al. 2013). The individual with a secure attachment style is hypothesized to have experienced consistently responsive caregiving in early life and therefore has positive expectations and comfort in depending on others for care. Inconsistently responsive caregiving is proposed as the environmental antecedent to a preoccupied attachment style, characterized by increased effort on the part of the individual to elicit caregiving and a positive expectation of others, with a negative view of self. These individuals may be particularly vulnerable to consciously or unconsciously exaggerated illness behavior and high medical services use (Ciechanowski et al. 2002b).

The dismissing attachment style is thought to derive from early experiences with consistently unresponsive caregivers. As an adaptation to such an environment, these individuals come to dismiss their need for others, value extreme self-reliance, and have difficulty trusting others. They develop a positive view of themselves as independent and self-reliant and have negative expectations of others. Individuals with dismissing attachment styles are therefore averse to reaching out to others or disclosing their emotional experiences. They avoid engaging in psychotherapy but once engaged benefit from the experience (Fonagy et al. 1996).

Hostile, rejecting, or abusive caregiving early in life is thought to result in a fearful attachment style, characterized by negative views of self and others and a desire for support with simultaneous fears of rejection and difficulty trusting others. These individuals often alternate between help-seeking and help-rejecting behaviors and frequently demand care but are often nonadherent and miss appointments. Individuals may show characteristics of more than one attachment style, but identification of the predominant style can be useful.

Ciechanowski and colleagues' studies of diabetic individuals with various attachment styles exemplify the application of this theory to health care. These researchers found that dismissive and fearful attachment styles are associated with worse diabetes self-care, lower adherence to hypoglycemic agents, and higher blood glucose levels. They describe the difficulty such patients have in trusting and depending on others, which affects their interactions with physicians in our fragmented health care system (Ciechanowski and Katon 2006; Ciechanowski et al. 2001). Ciechanowski et al. proposed that awareness of a patient's predominant attachment style enhances understanding of patient–physician dynamics. Skilled clinicians can use this understanding to alter their approach to patients to facilitate patient engagement and treatment adherence.

Other studies have found that attachment style is an important factor associated with 1) frequency of follow-up in a pain management specialty clinic; 2) symptom reporting in primary care, health care costs, and utilization; 3) symptom perception or somatization; and 4) medically unexplained symptoms among hepatitis C patients (Ciechanowski et al. 2002a, 2002b, 2003). Reviews, such as Hunter and Maunder (2001) and Thompson and Ciechanowski (2003), provide a more detailed introduction to this research, relevant to psychosomatic medicine research and practice.

Personality Types

It is important to distinguish between the concepts of personality type or character style and personality disorder. Personality types may be understood as existing on a continuum with respective personality disorders (Oldham and Skodol 2000). In addition, most patients do not fit exclusively into one type but may show characteristics of several personality types. The characterization of discrete personality types is useful in highlighting differences and providing vivid prototypical examples. Following Kahana and Bibring's (1964) classic and still relevant paper, "Personality Types in Medical Management," we have organized our discussion around the seven personality types they described (altering their terms to fit with more commonly used modern descriptions): 1) dependent, 2) obsessional, 3) histrionic, 4) masochistic, 5) paranoid, 6) narcissistic, and 7) schizoid.

Under conditions of stress, an individual's characteristic means of adaptation are heightened (Heiskell and Pasnau 1991). Thus, when confronted with the stress of a medical illness requiring hospitalization, the mildly obsessional patient might appear overly rigid or controlling. Similarly, a moderately dependent individual may appear "clingy" or excessively needy. Patients with extreme forms of these personality types can frustrate caregivers, often evoking intense negative emotions. These countertransference responses can be useful diagnostically. The negative emotions that patients with these extreme personality types evoke in physicians and nurses may result in caregiver responses that aggravate the situation (Muskin and Epstein 2009).

Groves (1978) characterized four types of patients who most challenge physicians: dependent clingers, entitled demanders, manipulative help-rejecters, and self-destructive deniers. He described the typical countertransference responses to each type and provided helpful tips on their management. In this subsection, we integrate Groves' descriptions of these four types of challenging patients with the seven personality types described by Kahana and Bibring.

Table 3–1 summarizes each of the seven personality types including their characteristics, the meaning of illness to each type, frequent caregiver countertransference responses, and tips on management, drawing on the contributions of Geringer and Stern (1986), Groves (1978), Kahana and Bibring (1964), Muskin and Haase (2001), Leigh (2015), and others.

TABLE 3–1.   Personality types

Type	Characteristics	Meaning of illness	Countertransference responses	Tips on management
Dependent	Needy, demanding, clingy Unable to reassure self Seeks reassurance from others	Threat of abandonment	Positive: doctor feels powerful and needed Negative: doctor feels overwhelmed and annoyed; may try to avoid patient	Reassure within limits Schedule visits Mobilize other supports Reward efforts toward independence Avoid tendency to withdraw from patient
Obsessional	Meticulous, orderly Likes to feel in control Very concerned with right/wrong	Loss of control over body/emotions/impulses	May admire When extreme: anger—a "battle of wills"	Try to set routine Give patient choices to increase sense of control Provide detailed information and "homework" Foster collaborative approach/avoid "battle of wills"
Histrionic	Entertaining Melodramatic Seductive, flirtatious	Loss of love or loss of attractiveness	Anxiety, impatience, off-putting Erotic; finds patient attractive	Strike a balance between warmth and formality Maintain clear boundaries Encourage patient to discuss fears Do not confront head-on
Masochistic	"Perpetual victim" Self-sacrificing martyr	Ego-syntonic Conscious or unconscious punishment	Anger, hate, frustration Helplessness, self-doubt	Avoid excessive encouragement Share patient's pessimism Deemphasize connection between symptoms and frequent visits Suggest that patient consider treatment as another burden to endure, or emphasize treatment's positive effect on loved ones

TABLE 3–1. Personality types (continued)

Type	Characteristics	Meaning of illness	Countertransference responses	Tips on management
Paranoid	Guarded, distrustful Quick to blame or counterattack Sensitive to slights	Proof that world is against patient Medical care is invasive and exploitative	Anger, feeling attacked or accused May become defensive	Avoid defensive stance Acknowledge patient's feelings without disputing them Maintain interpersonal distance; avoid excessive warmth Do not confront irrational fears
Narcissistic	Arrogant, devaluing Vain, demanding	Threat to self-concept of perfection and invulnerability Shame evoking	Anger, desire to counterattack Activation of feelings of inferiority, or enjoyment of feeling of status of working with an important patient	Resist the desire to challenge patient's entitlement Reframe entitlement to foster treatment adherence Take a humble stance, provide opportunities for patient to show off, offer consultations if appropriate
Schizoid	Aloof, remote Socially awkward Inhibited	Fear of intrusion	Little connection to patient Difficult to engage	Respect patient's privacy Prevent patient from completely withdrawing Maintain gentle, quiet interest in patient Encourage routine and regularity

Source. Derived in large part from Geringer and Stern 1986; Kahana and Bibring 1964; Perry and Viederman 1981.

Coping Styles

How individuals cope with the stressors of illness is another rich area of investigation (Jensen et al. 1991; Lazarus 1999; Penley et al. 2002), and having problems in coping with illness is a frequent reason for psychiatric consultation (Strain et al. 1993). Health psychologists have developed the concepts of appraisal (the assignment of meaning or value to a particular thing or event) and coping (Lazarus and Folkman 1984). An extensive body of literature developed over the past few decades has examined these processes in health care settings. This psychological literature is often underrecognized by the psychiatric and medical communities but is extremely useful and can complement psychodynamic perspectives.

Coping can be defined as "thoughts and behaviors that the person uses to manage or alter the problem that is causing distress (problem-focused coping) and regulate the emotional response to the problem (emotion-focused coping)" (Folkman et al. 1993, pp. 409–410). A comprehensive review of the literature on the many defined coping strategies in medical illness is beyond the scope of this chapter. The reader is referred to the excellent reviews by Lazarus (1999) and Penley et al. (2002). Some important empirical generalizations that have emerged from research on coping are discussed in this section (Lazarus 1999).

Use of Multiple Coping Styles in Stressful Situations

Folkman et al. (1986) identified eight categories of coping styles: 1) confrontative coping (hostile or aggressive efforts to alter a situation), 2) distancing (attempts to detach oneself mentally from a situation), 3) self-controlling (attempts to regulate one's feelings or actions), 4) seeking social support (efforts to seek emotional support or information from others), 5) accepting responsibility (acknowledgment of a personal role in the problem), 6) using escape–avoidance (cognitive or behavioral efforts to escape or avoid the problem or situation), 7) planful problem solving (deliberate and carefully thought-out efforts to alter the situation), and 8) conducting positive reappraisal (efforts to reframe the situation in a positive light) (Penley et al. 2002). Research has shown that patients use multiple coping strategies in any given situation (Lazarus 1999). Individuals often prefer or habitually use certain strategies over others, but generally multiple strategies are used for a complex stressful situation such as a medical illness or hospitalization. People use some trial and error in the selection of coping styles (Lazarus 1999).

Coping as a Trait and a Process

Preferred coping styles are commonly tied to personality variables; sometimes they can be viewed as traits as well as processes (Heim et al. 1997; Lazarus 1999). Therefore, it is useful to ask patients how they previously dealt with very stressful situations. This can provide useful information because patients are likely to use strategies in the present that are similar to those they used in the past, whether they were effective or not.

Research on women with breast cancer at various stages of illness has found that coping strategies may change as the nature of the stressor changes (Heim et al. 1993, 1997). For example, on initial detection of breast cancer, a woman may seek social support from her friends and spouse to cope with the uncertainties of her situation. Later, after lumpectomy and staging, she might shift her primary coping strategy to planful problem solving—a plan to follow up regularly for chemotherapy and to adhere fully to her oncologist's prescription of tamoxifen.

Problem-Focused Coping vs. Emotion-Focused Coping

One way to organize coping styles is whether they are problem focused or emotion focused. Research has shown that patients will tend to choose problem-focused coping strategies when they appraise the situation as being changeable or within their control (Folkman et al. 1993; Richardson et al. 2017). In conditions considered out of their control, patients may choose emotion-focused coping styles (Folkman et al. 1993; Richardson et al. 2017). In the medical setting, consulting psychiatrists can help change the patient's appraisal of the situation and encourage the patient to choose more adaptive coping styles. For example, if a patient newly diagnosed with diabetes mellitus misperceives high blood glucose as out of his control, he might choose an emotion-focused coping strategy such as avoidance or denial. In educating this patient about how treatable hyperglycemia can be, the physician could encourage the patient to change his coping to a problem-focused strategy such as making dietary changes or increasing exercise.

Variations in Usefulness of Coping Strategies Over Time

Coping is a powerful mediator of how a patient responds emotionally to a given stressor (Folkman and Lazarus 1988; Lipowski 1970). Coping strategies also have been reported to have different effects on health outcomes—some positive, others negative (see Penley et al. 2002 for a meta-analysis of this research). Although some coping strategies may be considered more effective than others, they vary in usefulness depending on the situation. A strategy that is initially effective in dealing with a stressor may no longer be effective when the nature of the stressor changes (Penley et al. 2002). The discussion of maladaptive versus adaptive denial under "Denial" later in this chapter illustrates this point.

Relation Between Coping Styles and the Meaning of Illness

Lipowski (1970) described eight "illness concepts": 1) illness as challenge, 2) illness as enemy, 3) illness as punishment, 4) illness as weakness, 5) illness as relief, 6) illness as strategy, 7) illness as irreparable loss or damage, and 8) illness as value. Lipowski proposed that a patient's choice of coping strategy is partially dependent on the underlying illness concept. In a study of 205 patients with chronic physical illness, the descriptors "illness as challenge" and "illness as value" were found to be related to "adaptive coping and mental well-being." Similar concepts, "illness perception" and "illness representation," have been shown to be related to coping styles, functional status, disability, and quality of life in patients with COPD (Kaptein et al. 2008) and patients with cancer (Richardson et al. 2017).

Defense Mechanisms

Defense mechanisms are automatic psychological processes by which the mind confronts a psychological threat (e.g., the fear of death or deformity) or conflict between a wish and the demands of reality or the dictates of conscience. This psychoanalytic concept has a rich history that is beyond the scope of this chapter. Although there is some overlap of the concept of coping with that of defenses, the psychological concept of coping is more behavioral; it involves action (e.g., seeking social support or productive problem solving) and is generally a conscious experience. Defenses are usually conceptualized as intrapsychic processes that are largely out of the individual's awareness. A basic understanding of the concept of defense and various defense mechanisms can provide the psychiatrist in the medical setting with another lens through which to examine a patient and to predict or explain the patient's emotional or behavioral responses to medical illness.

Vaillant (1993) proposed a hierarchy of defense mechanisms ranked in four levels of adaptivity: psychotic, immature (or borderline), neurotic, and mature. This hierarchy is based on the degree to which each defense distorts reality and how effectively it enables the expression of wishes or needs without untoward external consequences. Patients often use many different defense mechanisms in different situations or under varying levels of stress. When a patient inflexibly and consistently uses lower-level defenses, this is often consistent with a personality disorder. Table 3–2 lists major defense mechanisms grouped into four levels.

The *psychotic defenses* are characterized by the extreme degree to which they distort external reality. Patients in psychotic states usually employ these defenses; psychotherapy is generally ineffective in altering them, and antipsychotic medication may be indicated.

The *immature defenses* are characteristic of patients with personality disorders, especially antisocial, borderline, histrionic, and narcissistic personality disorders. Vaillant (1993) emphasized how many of these defenses are irritating to others and get under other people's skin. "Those afflicted with immature defenses often transmit their shame, impulses and anxiety to those around them" (p. 58).

In contrast to the immature defenses, the *neurotic defenses* do not typically irritate others and are more privately experienced—they are less interpersonal and often involve mental inhibitions. They distort reality less than do immature or psychotic defenses and may go unnoticed by the observer. With appropriate tact and timing, neurotic defenses can be effectively interpreted in exploratory psychotherapy when it is considered appropriate by the treating psychiatrist. "Over the short haul, neurotic defenses make the user suffer; immature defenses make the observer suffer" (Vaillant 1993, p. 66).

The *mature defenses* "integrate sources of conflict…and thus require no interpretation" (Vaillant 1993, p. 67). The use of mature defenses such as humor or altruism in the confrontation of a stressor such as medical illness often earns admiration from others and can be inspirational. Such mature defenses are not interpreted by the psychiatrist but rather are praised. These defenses maximize expression of drives or wishes without negative consequences or distortion of reality.

Optimism and Pessimism

At first glance it might seem that optimism and pessimism exist on a single dimension in relation to the experience of illness and in predicting patient outcomes. People who are generally happy (i.e., have positive affect) can also have negative affect (Diener and Emmons 1984). Research generally supports the dimensional view that greater optimism relates to better health; however, individuals who are optimistic are not de-

TABLE 3–2. **Defense mechanisms**

Mature defenses

Suppression	Consciously putting a disturbing experience out of mind
Altruism	Vicarious but instinctively gratifying service to others
Humor	Overt expression of normally unacceptable feelings without unpleasant effect
Sublimation	Attenuated expression of drives in alternative fields without adverse consequences
Anticipation	Realistic planning for inevitable discomfort

Neurotic defenses

Repression	Involuntary forgetting of a painful feeling or experience
Control	Manipulation of external events to avoid unconscious anxiety
Displacement	Transfer of an experienced feeling from one person to another or to something else
Reaction formation	Expression of unacceptable impulses as directly opposite attitudes and behaviors
Intellectualization	Replacing of feelings with facts/details
Rationalization	Inventing a convincing, but usually false, reason why one is not bothered
Isolation of affect	Separating a painful idea or event from feelings associated with it
Undoing	Ritualistic "removal" of an offensive act, sometimes by atoning for it

Immature defenses

Splitting	Experiencing oneself and others as all good or all bad
Idealization	Seeing oneself or others as all-powerful, ideal, or godlike
Devaluation	Depreciating others
Projection	Attributing unacceptable impulses or ideas to others
Projective identification	Causing others to experience one's unacceptable feelings; one then fears or tries to control the unacceptable behavior in the other person
Acting out	Direct expression of an unconscious wish or impulse to avoid being conscious of the affect, and thoughts that accompany it
Passive aggression	Expressing anger indirectly and passively
Intermediate: denial	Refusal to acknowledge painful realities

Psychotic defenses

Psychotic denial	Obliteration of external reality
Delusional projection	Externalization of inner conflicts and giving them tangible reality—minimal reality testing
Schizoid fantasy	Withdrawal from conflict into social isolation and fantasizing

Source. Carlat 1999; Muskin and Haase 2001; Vaillant 1993.

void of pessimism—people can have both traits at the same time. A meta-analysis of 83 studies showed a positive relationship between optimism and physical outcomes in a variety of conditions (Rasmussen et al. 2009). People with higher levels of optimism tend to attribute successful outcomes to their own efforts and unsuccessful outcomes to external events. The reverse is true for those with lower levels of optimism. Using a scale to measure both optimism and pessimism in patients who underwent coronary artery bypass grafting, Tindle et al. (2012) found that optimism scores, but not pessimism scores, predicted treatment response for patients who were depressed. (Optimists were less likely to be rehospitalized than were pessimists). Patients who had high levels of optimism 2 weeks after admission for acute coronary syndrome were more physically active and had fewer readmissions over the next 6 months (Huffman et al. 2016). A recent review of studies of psychological functioning in patients with breast cancer found that women who were highly optimistic were more likely to use active coping styles, had higher well-being and life satisfaction, and derived more benefit/meaning from their experiences of illness (Casellas-Grau et al. 2016). Gilboa et al. (1999) found that male burn patients who displayed optimism had better psychological outcomes. Although optimism and pessimism are personality traits, confronting a patient's pessimistic beliefs and using cognitive-behavioral approaches to challenge a patient's negative views of the self and the world may lead to better outcomes.

Denial

Denial is a complex concept and a common reason for psychiatric consultation. Weisman and Hackett (1961) defined *denial* as "the conscious or unconscious repudiation of part or all of the total available meanings of an event to allay fear, anxiety, or other unpleasant affects" (p. 232). It is to be distinguished from a lack of awareness due to a cognitive deficit such as anosognosia and from the limited insight of a patient with chronic schizophrenia. Psychiatrists are often called to see a patient "in denial" about a newly diagnosed illness and may be asked to assess the patient's capacity to consent to or refuse certain treatments. Denial can be *adaptive,* protecting the patient from being emotionally overwhelmed by an illness, or *maladaptive,* preventing or delaying diagnosis, treatment, and lifestyle changes. Deniers may experience fewer symptoms and less distress following a myocardial infarction, but they are more likely to delay coming to the hospital (Fang et al. 2016).

Psychiatrists are most likely to be called on when the patient's denial makes the physician uncomfortable, but providers sometimes use the term *denial* loosely and inaccurately (Goldbeck 1997; Havik and Maeland 1988; Jacobsen and Lowery 1992). A physician's statement that a patient is "in denial" may refer to various situations: 1) the patient rejects the diagnosis, 2) the patient minimizes symptoms of the illness or does not seem to appreciate its implications, 3) the patient avoids or delays medical treatment, or 4) the patient appears to have no emotional reaction to the diagnosis or illness (Goldbeck 1997). The first task of the psychiatric consultant is to determine specifically what the referring physician means by "denial."

The severity of denial varies by the nature of what is denied, by the predominant defense mechanisms at work (e.g., suppression, repression, psychotic denial), and by the degree of accessibility to consciousness (Goldbeck 1997). Patients who use the mature defense of *suppression* in confronting an illness are not truly in denial. Rather, they have chosen to put aside their fears about illness and treatment until a later time. Their fears are not deeply unconscious but are easily accessible if patients so choose.

These patients typically accept treatment, face their illnesses with courage, and do not let their emotions overtake them. Such "denial" is considered adaptive (Druss and Douglas 1988). Many authors have proposed that some denial is perhaps necessary for very effective coping with an overwhelming illness (see discussions in Druss 1995; Ness and Ende 1994).

In contrast, the patient using *repression* as a defense is generally unaware of the internal experience (e.g., fear, thought, wish) being warded off. Repressed thoughts or feelings are not easily accessible to consciousness. Such a patient may feel very anxious without understanding why. For example, a 39-year-old man whose father died of a myocardial infarction at the age of 41 may become increasingly anxious as his 40th birthday approaches without being aware of the connection.

When it is more severe and pervasive, denial can result in patients flatly denying they are ill and not seeking medical care. If they are already in care, they decline treatment or are nonadherent. Repeated attempts by the medical team to educate them about their illness have no effect. Extreme denial may be severe enough to distort the perception of reality, sometimes described as *psychotic denial.* Most patients with pervasive denial of illness are not psychotic. Psychotic denial occurs in chronic mental illness like schizophrenia. Such patients may pay no attention to signs or symptoms of illness or may incorporate them into somatic delusions. Psychotic patients who deny illness usually do not conceal its signs; others often readily recognize they are ill. In contrast, nonpsychotic patients with pervasive denial often conceal signs of their illness from themselves and others. For example, a nonpsychotic woman with pervasive denial of a growing breast mass avoided medical care and undressing in front of others and kept a bandage over what she regarded as a bruise. Although pregnancy is not an illness, a dramatic example of pervasive (sometimes psychotic) denial is the denial of pregnancy (see Chapter 31, "Obstetrics and Gynecology").

How does one determine whether denial is adaptive or maladaptive? For the woman with a growing breast tumor, denial is clearly maladaptive because it has prevented her from receiving potentially lifesaving treatment. In other situations, denial may be quite adaptive. In determining the adaptivity of a patient's denial, it is important to answer the following questions (Goldbeck 1997):

- Does the patient's denial prevent the patient from receiving necessary treatment or lead to actions that endanger the patient's health? If so, then the denial is deemed maladaptive. In cases in which no effective treatment is available, the denial might be judged as adaptive to the extent that it decreases distress and improves quality of life, or it may be maladaptive if it prevents critical life planning (e.g., a single parent with little support and a terminal illness who has made no plans for his or her young children).
- Which component of denial—denial of the facts of illness, denial of the implications of the illness, or denial of the emotional reaction to illness—does the patient show? The latter two components of denial are not as maladaptive as the first component and may be adaptive in some situations. Denying the full implications of a disease, such as inevitable death, might be adaptive because it facilitates hope and improved quality of life. Likewise, denial of certain emotional reactions to the illness such as fear or hopelessness might enable a patient to stay motivated through a completed course of treatment.

- Is the denial a temporary means of "buying time," to accept a diagnosis gradually so that the immediate effect is not so overwhelming, or has the denial been so protracted that it has prevented adaptive action? Many patients are unable to accept a diagnosis immediately, and denial may be a way for them to adjust at their own pace.

Even when denial is adaptive for the patient, it may bother physicians or other caregivers. The following case vignette illustrates this point.

Case Vignette

A psychiatric consultation was requested for a 24-year-old man, quadriplegic after a gunshot wound to the spine. The physician was insistent that the patient's denial be "broken through" because the patient was convinced that he would walk again. The patient had a thorough understanding of his condition and maintained that hard work and faith would restore his physical abilities. The physician worried that the patient might commit suicide when he realized that there was no chance of recovery of function. Instead of forcing the patient to face the prognosis, the consultant recommended that the physician offer the patient training in the skills necessary to maintain himself in his current state because recovery, in whatever form it took, would take a considerable amount of time. The patient continued to cooperate with physical therapy, learned how to use a motorized wheelchair, and discussed plans for his living arrangements. The physician felt comfortable with this approach because it was "realistic."

All too often, physicians misjudge patients as being in denial. This tends to occur with three types of patients: 1) patients without an overt emotional reaction to an illness or a diagnosis, 2) patients whose reactions differ from those expected by their caregivers, and 3) patients who have been inadequately informed about their illness. The absence of an overt reaction to medical illness is a style of psychological response. Although it is not evident to an observer, individuals may actually be aware of their emotions and thoughts about their illness. Some physicians have a tendency to misjudge patients as being in denial who do not express an expected emotional response or who seek alternative treatments instead of those recommended by the physician (Cousins 1982). An obsessional middle-aged accountant in the coronary care unit, for example, may be acutely aware of his condition and quite concerned about it, yet he may not express the fears or anxiety that his caregivers would expect, appearing calm and hopeful. This patient is not denying his illness but may be considered to be doing so by caregivers because he "looks too relaxed and in too good a mood." Gattellari et al. (1999) found that some patients judged by their caregivers to be using denial were in reality relatively uninformed about the details of their illness or prognosis. On the other hand, some patients who say that they have not been informed have in fact been repeatedly educated by their health care professionals and really are in denial.

Some studies have reported positive effects of denial on medical outcome. Hackett and Cassem (1974) found that among patients in coronary care units after myocardial infarction, "major deniers" had better outcomes than did "minor deniers." Levenson et al. (1989) found that among patients with unstable angina, "high deniers" had fewer episodes of angina and more favorable outcomes than did "low deniers." Other studies suggest that denial is useful for specific clinical situations such as elective surgery (Cohen and Lazarus 1973) and wound healing (Marucha et al. 1998). Denial was associated with better survival rates in a small study of patients awaiting heart transplantation (Young et al. 1991).

Other studies have found a mixed or negative effect of denial on medical outcome. "Major deniers" have shorter stays in the intensive care unit but are more likely to be noncompliant after discharge (Levine et al. 1987). Greater denial was associated with worse medical outcome but decreased mood symptoms and sleep problems in patients with end-stage renal disease (Fricchione et al. 1992). Denial may be counterproductive in asthma patients (Staudenmayer et al. 1979). Croog et al. (1971) noted lower treatment adherence among deniers in their large sample of myocardial infarct patients. In a study of women scheduled for breast biopsy, those with a history of habitual use of denial were observed to have been more likely to delay medical evaluation (Greer 1974).

When denial is present and is assessed as maladaptive, interventions usually should be directed toward the underlying emotions provoking the denial (e.g., fear). Direct confrontation of denial generally should be avoided because it is counterproductive (Ness and Ende 1994; Perry and Viederman 1981). For example, a 17-year-old adolescent who is newly diagnosed with diabetes mellitus may not want to accept this diagnosis and the need for changes in his lifestyle because of his painful memories of seeing other family members suffer through complications of diabetes. The physician may be tempted to frighten the patient into compliance with a statement such as, "If you don't change your diet, measure your blood sugar, and take insulin regularly, you will wind up with complications just like your mother's." Such statements increase anxiety, which is driving the patient's use of denial in the first place. Instead, a gentle, empathic, and nonjudgmental stance is more effective (Ness and Ende 1994). Diminishing the intensity of negative affects such as anxiety through psychopharmacological or psychotherapeutic interventions also can be helpful because these affects may be driving the patient's need for denial.

In addition, the consulting psychiatrist should consider whether a patient's maladaptive denial is fostered by particular interpersonal relationships, such as those with family members, friends, a religious community, physicians, or other caregivers (Goldbeck 1997). In such cases, interventions aimed solely at the individual patient's denial without addressing the reinforcing interpersonal relationships are likely to be unsuccessful.

Emotional Responses to Medical Illness

Psychiatrists in the medical setting are frequently called on to help a patient manage emotional responses to illness and hospitalization (e.g., anger, fear, grief, shame). Often the patient's emotional response is identified in the consultation request. For example, "Please come see this 25-year-old man just diagnosed with testicular cancer who is angry and refusing treatment." The young man's internist cannot understand why this patient would refuse therapy needed to treat (and probably cure) his testicular cancer. With an understanding of the patient's subjective experience of his illness and his predominant coping styles and defense mechanisms, the consulting psychiatrist can help the patient and the internist to understand the patient's anger, facilitating an alliance within which treatment is more likely to be accepted.

Because every patient is unique, empathic listening to a patient's story of his or her illness will identify the predominant emotional response, which is a potential clue to the subjective meaning of illness for that patient (Lazarus 1999). An illness can evoke multiple emotional responses simultaneously or sequentially. The illness may have multiple meanings, and the meanings may change over the course of the illness. The predominant emotional response should not be the sole focus of the psychiatrist's attention (although it may demand the most attention). The 25-year-old man just diagnosed with testicular cancer is markedly angry and refuses treatment. One can hypothesize that it might be because he feels frightened or weakened, or that he fears he will literally be emasculated via castration. This patient is not only angry about his cancer diagnosis but is also angry with his physician as the bearer of bad news. Accepting and attempting to understand the patient's anger aids the psychiatrist in giving this man permission to express his feelings while tactfully helping him to see that he can do so without forgoing his own treatment. The patient's refusal of treatment also may be determined by fear of what the treatment will involve. The psychiatrist might also work with the oncologist and his response to the patient's anger. Education by the physicians about the treatment options and the high likelihood of cure could dramatically shift the patient's emotional and behavioral responses and evoke relief and hope. Assisting the patient in naming his emotional responses and understanding *why* they are present can help the patient feel understood. This can facilitate the acceptance of an individualized treatment plan that appropriately involves medication, psychotherapy, psychoeducation, or other interventions.

Anger

Anger is a common emotional response to medical illness and may be the most difficult emotional response for physicians to confront. This is particularly true when the anger is directed toward them or is expressed as treatment refusal. Patients with paranoid, narcissistic, borderline, or antisocial personality styles or disorders are particularly likely to express anger in the face of medical illness (Muskin and Haase 2001). Common reflexive reactions include counterattacking or distancing oneself from the patient. The skilled psychiatrist will convey appropriate empathy along with necessary limit setting for the angry patient. Many maneuvers are possible, such as a tactful redirection of the patient's anger toward more productive targets (e.g., away from refusal of treatment and toward planning with the oncologist to combat the illness through potentially curative chemotherapy). Helping the team to respond appropriately to the patient is just as important. Viewing expressed anger as natural and diffusing the intensity of affect can help to reestablish collaborative relationships with the patient.

Anxiety and Fear

Some degree of anxiety is likely to be experienced universally by patients in the medical setting (Lloyd 1977). The degree of anxiety varies by individual and by situation. Patients with premorbid anxiety disorders are more likely to experience severe anxiety when confronted with medical illness. The patient with a dependent personality style may experience acute anxiety on hospitalization when faced with separation from his or her support system. The obsessional patient is likely to become anxious if

the treatment plan or diagnosis remains unclear. The intrusiveness of the medical setting may evoke anxiety in the schizoid patient.

Psychotherapies, education about the illness and treatments, teaching breathing techniques (Brown and Gerbarg 2012), and judicious use of medication can greatly diminish the patient's anxiety (Perry and Viederman 1981). Although fear (usually involving a specific threat or danger) and anxiety (the feeling of nervousness or apprehension experienced on facing uncertain threats) are distinct emotions, their management is similar. It is important to elicit what the patient fears specifically—pain, death, abandonment, disfigurement, dependence, disability, and so forth. Blanket reassurance is usually ineffective and may actually be detrimental because the patient may perceive it as not empathic, superficial, false, or patronizing. Empathy and reassurance tailored to the patient's specific fears can offer significant relief (Perry and Viederman 1981).

Sadness

Situations in which people experience a loss evoke sadness (Lloyd 1977). Medical illness can lead to multiple types of loss: loss of physical function or social role, loss of ability to work, loss of the pursuit of a goal or dream, or loss of a part of one's body. Internal losses of organs or organ functions can be as significant as external losses such as amputation of a limb. Patients with untreated mood disorders may be more likely to develop clinically significant depression in the face of medical illness. Sadness may be the primary manifestation of an adjustment disorder, which is common in medically ill patients (Strain et al. 1998). Drawing an analogy to the process of mourning is often appropriate and helps to normalize the patient's sadness (Fitzpatrick 1999). A fact not well appreciated in medical settings is that mourning a loss takes time. It is important for the physician to convey a sense of appropriate hope. Describing true examples of other patients' positive outcomes in similar situations can often be helpful. Even when the patient's sadness represents a normal grief-like reaction, physicians are often tempted to prescribe antidepressant medication, desiring to make the patient feel better. In such cases, the psychosomatic medicine specialist can redirect the treatment plan to interventions that are more likely to be helpful, such as psychotherapy, pastoral care, and—often most important—more time speaking with the primary treating physician.

Guilt

Some patients experience illness as a punishment for real or imagined sins. Clarifying that illness is not the patient's fault—and thereby confronting the guilt—is a helpful technique. Patients also may experience guilt related to their earlier or current illness-promoting behaviors, such as smoking cigarettes, nonadherence to medication regimens, or risky sexual practices. Education of family members can be critical if they blame the patient inappropriately for the illness. If the patient is religious, counseling from a hospital chaplain or the appropriate clergy member should be considered.

Shame

Illness is universally experienced as narcissistic injury to some degree. Narcissistic patients are more susceptible to experiencing shame in the face of medical illness. Patients who view their illness as a result of earlier behaviors—such as contracting HIV through impulsive sexual liaisons or developing lung cancer after a long history of smoking—may experience shame in the medical setting. It is important for physicians to take a nonjudgmental stance and avoid blaming patients. Critical, disapproving responses are counterproductive, heighten patients' shame, and frequently lead to treatment avoidance. For example, the noncompliant diabetic patient who is repeatedly admitted to the hospital for diabetic ketoacidosis frustrates her doctors and nurses. They are often tempted to scold the patient, thinking that this is necessary to avoid colluding with her failure to take her disease seriously. Such responses are typically humiliating for the patient, are ineffective in motivating behavior change, and often worsen the vicious cycle of noncompliance.

Behavioral Responses to Illness

Patients' behavioral responses to illness vary tremendously within a spectrum ranging from maladaptive to adaptive. Adaptive responses may simply warrant encouragement or praise. Psychiatrists in the medical setting are often asked to see patients whose behavioral responses to illness or hospitalization are maladaptive and are interfering with their treatment. In understanding the patient's subjective experience, personality style, defense mechanisms, and coping strategies, one can design therapeutic interventions to help change the patient's responses to more adaptive behaviors. This section highlights a few of the common behavioral responses to illness.

Adaptive Responses

Support Seeking

Facing a new medical illness or hospitalization can be highly taxing for even the most well-adapted individual. Patients who are fortunate enough to have well-developed social support networks can benefit greatly from the support of friends and family. Social support improves quality of life, well-being, sense of purpose, and positive adjustment in women with breast cancer (Casellas-Grau et al. 2016). Patients with conflicts about dependency might have more difficulty with this task, and psychotherapy can normalize this need and assist patients in reaching out to others. Referral to patient support groups also can be helpful for many patients; they can learn from the experiences of others facing the same illness and can feel less alone or alienated from other people. Information about self-help organizations can be obtained from major national organizations such as the Alzheimer's Association and the American Cancer Society, among others.

Altruism

Altruistic behavior such as volunteering to raise money for breast cancer, becoming a transplant advocate who meets with preoperative patients and shares experiences with them, or participating in an AIDS walkathon can represent a highly adaptive response to illness. One of the common stresses of illness is the effect on an individual's self-esteem and sense of productivity. Through helping others, patients feel a sense of purpose and gratification that can help improve their mood. Generally, the consulting psychiatrist needs only to support and encourage such behaviors. For many patients with severe illnesses, voluntary participation in research can have the same effect. Particularly for those with terminal illness, participation in research can provide a sense of purpose and hope by contributing to the potential for new treatment options in the future.

Epiphany Regarding Life Priorities

Going through a serious illness can yield unexpected benefits—a "silver lining"—if the experience helps patients regain perspective on what is most important to them in life. Normal daily hassles may no longer seem as stressful, and some patients facing a serious illness experience an epiphany and dramatically change their lives for the better. Patient narratives of the life-affirming effects of illness and stories of personal growth abound in the literature (Druss 1995). At times, the consultation psychiatrist can witness and support a patient through a personal transformation.

A 47-year-old male executive recently diagnosed with a myocardial infarction may dramatically change his diet, embark on a new exercise regimen, and reconfigure his role at work to reduce emotional stress. Similarly, a woman newly diagnosed with HIV who commits herself to taking her medications regularly, seeks treatment for substance use, and rejoins her church also exemplifies this phenomenon.

"Posttraumatic growth" (Tedeschi and Calhoun 2004) after breast cancer has been shown to be related to social support seeking, cognitive reframing, positive reappraisal, engagement, gratitude, and other factors (see Casellas-Grau et al. 2016 for an excellent review). There are wonderful opportunities for effective psychotherapy in the medically ill. Patients are under tremendous stress when faced with serious medical illness, and the usual distractions of their daily lives no longer dominate their thoughts. Sometimes a therapeutic alliance can form and work can progress more rapidly than is typical in other settings (Muskin 1990).

Becoming an Expert on One's Illness

For the obsessional patient in particular, learning as much as possible about the illness can create a greater sense of control. Although the information itself may not be positive, patients often find that reality can seem more manageable than their imagined fears. However, this response to illness is not appealing to all patients. Some will prefer to put their trust in their physicians and prefer not to know everything. The psychiatrist, armed with an understanding of the patient's personality style, characteristic coping styles, and defense mechanisms, will be able to know whether increased information might reduce the patient's distress and augment a sense of control.

Maladaptive Responses: Nonadherence to Treatment Regimens

Treatment nonadherence is more common than most physicians recognize (Abegaz et al. 2017). Estimates suggest that up to 50% of patients fail to adhere to their prescribed medication regimens. Patients typically overestimate their own adherence to treatment, and physicians are often unaware of their patients' lack of adherence (Levenson 1998). Physicians working in all medical settings witness the negative effects of nonadherence, and psychiatrists are called frequently to see problem patients who are repetitively nonadherent. The psychiatric consultant is often brought in to be a disciplinarian, detective, or magician; medical colleagues may expect the psychiatrist's interventions to result in rapid change to the patient's adherence patterns. Although it is possible in some cases, this scenario is typically unrealistic. It is possible to undertake interventions that improve patient adherence when the underlying factors accounting for nonadherence are correctly identified and addressed.

Patients do not fully adhere to treatment regimens for numerous reasons. Psychiatric disorders and psychological motivations are not the only factors that may be involved. Other factors, such as cost, side effects, and treatment complexity, may play a role. It is important to determine the degree of a patient's nonadherence and its context. Is the patient occasionally or consistently nonadherent? Is the nonadherence specific to a certain medication or type of recommendation (e.g., dieting), or is it more generalized across different treatments and different physicians? Identifying the context of nonadherence can provide clues to the underlying factors involved when the patient cannot directly give the reasons for nonadherence. In this section, we identify some of the most common reasons for treatment nonadherence and offer 11 general principles for management of this common clinical problem.

Psychologically Motivated Factors in Nonadherence

Perry and Viederman (1981) outlined several distinct psychological reasons that patients do not adhere to treatment recommendations. One reason is nonadherence to defend against humiliation (Perry and Viederman 1981). Rather than accept the stigma of his illness, a patient with HIV might stop his medications, which remind him daily of his illness (Blashill et al. 2011). Active empathic work to counteract the illness concepts that cause shame can diminish this motivation for treatment nonadherence.

Another psychological motivation for nonadherence is to counteract a feeling of helplessness (Perry and Viederman 1981). An adolescent with newly diagnosed diabetes mellitus who is struggling with a developmentally appropriate desire to gain autonomy may believe that the only way to feel autonomous and in control is to rebel against her parents and caregivers by not taking insulin. Such nonadherence also may be motivated by the wish to be healthy like her peers.

Anger toward the treating physician or toward the illness or diagnosis itself may be another psychological motivator for treatment nonadherence, whether the anger is appropriate to the situation or is a product of character pathology. Various degrees of denial also may be involved. Specific interventions for clinical situations in which anger and denial are primary motivators for nonadherence were discussed earlier in this chapter.

Patients' trust in the physicians recommending their treatment is an important determinant of their likelihood of complying with the treatment regimen. Physicians must earn their patients' trust through building rapport and direct, honest communication. Patients with psychotic disorders or significant character pathology might have particular difficulty placing trust in their caregivers. Mistrust and paranoia may play a role in these patients' noncompliance with treatment regimens.

Comorbid Psychiatric Disorders and Nonadherence

Comorbid psychiatric disorders also may lead to treatment nonadherence, particularly mood disorders. Depressed patients may not have the motivation, concentration, or energy required to comply fully with treatment recommendations—for example, studies have consistently found an association between depression and worse HIV medication adherence (Blashill et al. 2011). Depressed patients might even stop treatment as an indirect means of attempting suicide. Manic patients may believe that they no longer need treatment, may abuse substances, or may become disorganized or psychotic. Psychotic disorders, anxiety disorders, substance use disorders, and cognitive disorders are other psychiatric conditions that often play a role in treatment nonadherence. Therefore, a thorough psychiatric history and comprehensive review of symptoms are essential parts of the evaluation of the noncompliant patient.

Other Factors in Nonadherence

Nonadherence may be due to reality factors rather than psychological motivations. Cost of treatment, side effects (whether feared or experienced), and complicated or inconvenient medication dosing schedules are treatment-specific factors that should be considered. Other practical barriers, such as difficulties with transportation, inflexible and lengthy work schedules, or childcare responsibilities, may preclude consistent keeping of appointments.

A lack of information about the illness or its treatment should always be ruled out as a potential contributing factor in nonadherence. Patients should understand their illness, the treatment options, and the reasons for treatment. Patient education should always be provided in the patient's primary language to ensure full understanding. To assess patient understanding, physicians should ask patients to repeat in their own words what they have been told about their illness. If possible, family members should be involved in the education. Written or visual materials may be helpful tools in patient education.

Incongruities between the health beliefs of patients and physicians can also account for nonadherence and should be identified (Gaw 2001). All physicians must make an effort to understand the cultural and religious backgrounds of their patients, paying particular attention to patients' beliefs and values about health and illness. Physicians should attempt to elicit patients' explanatory models about diseases and the effects of treatments. When possible, attempts can be made to explain treatment within patients' belief systems. At the least, mutual acknowledgment and acceptance of the differences between the explanatory models of the physician and the patient may facilitate treatment adherence and build doctor–patient rapport. When patients feel that their caregivers accept and understand their cultural, health, or religious beliefs, they will be more likely to volunteer information about their use of alternative or herbal treatments.

Interventions to Increase Treatment Adherence

The literature suggests that interventions involving dosage reduction, monitoring/feedback, and education have a positive impact on adherence, but no one approach works for all patients (Kripalani et al. 2007; Marcum et al. 2017). The following general principles may assist physicians in facilitating greater patient adherence to treatment (Becker and Maiman 1980; Chen 1991; Gaw 2001):

- Ask patients directly about their adherence, maintaining a nonjudgmental stance. Design a collaborative plan to increase adherence. Normalizing statements and questions such as *"Many patients find it difficult to take their medications on a regular basis. Have you had this experience?"* will be more effective in eliciting information about adherence than questions such as *"You've been taking your medication regularly, right?"*

- Ensure that patients are fully informed about their illness and treatments.
- Rule out cognitive deficits (e.g., intellectual disability or dementia), because they may play a role in nonadherence.
- Uncover any underlying psychological motivating factors for nonadherence, and address them specifically.
- Diagnose and treat any comorbid psychiatric disorders.
- Minimize treatment-related factors for nonadherence, such as side effects, cost, and complexity of regimens, when possible.
- Identify, acknowledge, and contend with any cultural reasons for nonadherence.
- Avoid shaming, scolding, or frightening the patient. Scolding patients or scaring them with statements such as "If you don't take your medications, you could have a heart attack and die!" is almost always counterproductive (Heiskell and Pasnau 1991). Such statements may shame patients or inflate their fears and can increase the likelihood that they will not return for treatment.
- Use positive reinforcement as a motivator when possible because it is generally more effective than negative reinforcement at facilitating behavior change.
- Involve family members in facilitating patient adherence when they are "on board" with the treatment plan.

Maladaptive Responses: Signing Out Against Medical Advice

A common reason for urgent inpatient psychiatric consultation is a patient threatening to sign out against medical advice (AMA). A recent review indicated that 2.7% of admissions to a county hospital ended with patients signing out AMA (Stearns et al. 2017). The 30-day readmission rate and overall mortality of patients who sign out AMA is higher compared with conventionally discharged patients (Alfandre 2013). Often the psychiatrist is asked to assess the decisional capacity of a patient who wants to sign out against medical advice (Kornfeld et al. 2009). Legal and ethical aspects of this assessment are discussed in Chapter 2, "Legal and Ethical Issues." The patient's threat to sign out is usually not truly motivated by a primary desire to leave, but more often reflects another agenda, intense emotion, or interpersonal friction with physicians or nursing staff. In some cases, it is a means of expressing anger or frustration toward caregivers (Albert and Kornfeld 1973).

The motivations for signing out against medical advice vary significantly and are similar to the issues motivating treatment nonadherence. Among the more common motivations are 1) anger with caregivers or dissatisfaction with the treatment received (legitimate and/or due to character pathology); 2) overwhelming fear or anxiety; 3) substance craving or withdrawal (sometimes due to the medical team's inadequate use of prophylactic medications such as benzodiazepines or nicotine patches); 4) delirium or dementia; 5) psychosis or paranoia; 6) desire to leave the hospital to attend to outside responsibilities (e.g., child care, work, court dates, or a pet at home alone); and 7) impatience with discharge planning or feeling well enough to leave. In a classic study of patients threatening to sign out against medical advice, the most common underlying motivations were overwhelming fear, anger, and psychosis or confusion (Albert and Kornfeld 1973). In most cases, there had been a progressive increase in the patient's distress that had not been recognized or addressed adequately for days before the threat to sign out (Albert and Kornfeld 1973).

Among interventions, *empathic listening* to the patient's frustrations is critical, in that it provides an opportunity for the patient to ventilate frustrations and to feel understood. Empathic listening will often have a dramatic de-escalating effect, enabling the team to re-engage the patient in treatment. The psychiatrist can also intervene in helping the team to achieve a better understanding of the patient's behavior and to diminish the patient's feelings of anger and frustration. Other guidelines for intervention are the following:

- Understand the threat as a communication—Does the patient really want to leave, or is he or she expressing frustration, anger, anxiety, or another affect?
- If the patient is justifiably angry, apologize on behalf of the system or hospital.
- Avoid scare tactics or direct confrontation of denial, because these techniques are generally counterproductive.
- Design interventions with an understanding of the patient's personality type.
- Diagnose and treat any comorbid psychiatric disorders.
- Involve social supports (if they are allied with the treatment plan).
- Ensure that the patient is adequately informed about the illness and its need for treatment.
- Assess the patient's capacity to sign out, if indicated (discussed further in Chapter 2, "Legal and Ethical Issues").
- When patients still sign out against medical advice, encourage them to return for treatment if they change their mind.

Conclusion

How does one integrate these various theoretical concepts into the consultation process? How do the psychological responses to illness guide the consultant to use his or her time efficiently, understand the situation, and make useful suggestions? We are aware of no magic formula, but we believe that experienced consultants use their knowledge of human behavior and concepts such as attachment styles, personality types, coping styles, and defense mechanisms to understand their patients and to intervene. Opportunities abound in the medical setting for psychiatric interventions, which can dramatically modify patients' psychological responses to illness. The key to these interventions lies in the development of an understanding of the patient's subjective experience of illness. A curious inquiry into the internal experience of a patient facing medical illness and the appropriate conveyance of empathy is a rewarding experience. We hope the framework, concepts, and guidelines presented in this chapter will prove useful in assisting psychiatrists who have chosen to work with patients in medical settings.

References

Abegaz TM, Shehab A, Gebreyohannes EA, et al: Nonadherence to antihypertensive drugs: a systematic review and meta-analysis. Medicine (Baltimore) 96(4):e5641, 2017 28121920

Albert HD, Kornfeld DS: The threat to sign out against medical advice. Ann Intern Med 79(6):888–891, 1973 4761912

Alfandre D: Reconsidering against medical advice discharges: embracing patient-centeredness to promote high quality care and a renewed research agenda. J Gen Intern Med 28(12):1657–1662, 2013 23818160

Bartholomew K, Horowitz LM: Attachment styles among young adults: a test of a four-category model. J Pers Soc Psychol 61(2):226–244, 1991 1920064

Becker MH, Maiman LA: Strategies for enhancing patient compliance. J Community Health 6(2):113–135, 1980 7204635

Blashill AJ, Perry N, Safren SA: Mental health: a focus on stress, coping, and mental illness as it relates to treatment retention, adherence, and other health outcomes. Curr HIV/AIDS Rep 8(4):215–222, 2011 21822626

Bowlby J: Attachment and Loss, Vol 1: Attachment. New York, Basic Books, 1969

Brown RP, Gerbarg PL: The Healing Power of the Breath. London, Shambhala, 2012

Carlat DJ: The Psychiatric Interview: A Practical Guide. Philadelphia, PA, Lippincott Williams & Wilkins, 1999

Casellas-Grau A, Vives J, Font A, Ochoa C: Positive psychological functioning in breast cancer: an integrative review. Breast 27:136–168, 2016 27113230

Chen A: Noncompliance in community psychiatry: a review of clinical interventions. Hosp Community Psychiatry 42(3):282–287, 1991 1851496

Chou R, Fanciullo GJ, Fine PG, et al; American Pain Society–American Academy of Pain Medicine Opioids Guidelines Panel: Clinical guidelines for the use of chronic opioid therapy in chronic noncancer pain. J Pain 10(2):113–130, 2009 19187889

Ciechanowski P, Katon WJ: The interpersonal experience of health care through the eyes of patients with diabetes. Soc Sci Med 63(12):3067–3079, 2006 16997440

Ciechanowski PS, Katon WJ, Russo JE, Walker EA: The patient-provider relationship: attachment theory and adherence to treatment in diabetes. Am J Psychiatry 158(1):29–35, 2001 11136630

Ciechanowski PS, Katon WJ, Russo JE, Dwight-Johnson MM: Association of attachment style to lifetime medically unexplained symptoms in patients with hepatitis C. Psychosomatics 43(3):206–212, 2002a 12075035

Ciechanowski PS, Walker EA, Katon WJ, Russo JE: Attachment theory: a model for health care utilization and somatization. Psychosom Med 64(4):660–667, 2002b 12140356

Ciechanowski P, Sullivan M, Jensen M, et al: The relationship of attachment style to depression, catastrophizing and health care utilization in patients with chronic pain. Pain 104(3):627–637, 2003 12927635

Cohen F, Lazarus RS: Active coping processes, coping dispositions, and recovery from surgery. Psychosom Med 35(5):375–389, 1973 4803347

Cousins N: Denial. Are sharper definitions needed? JAMA 248(2):210–212, 1982 7087112

Croog SH, Shapiro DS, Levine S: Denial among male heart patients. An empirical study. Psychosom Med 33(5):385–397, 1971 5125906

Diener E, Emmons RA: The independence of positive and negative affect. J Pers Soc Psychol 47(5):1105–1117, 1984 6520704

Druss RG: The Psychology of Illness: In Sickness and in Health. Washington, DC, American Psychiatric Press, 1995

Druss RG, Douglas CJ: Adaptive responses to illness and disability. Healthy denial. Gen Hosp Psychiatry 10(3):163–168, 1988 2967786

Fang XY, Albarqouni L, von Eisenhart Rothe AF, et al: Is denial a maladaptive coping mechanism which prolongs pre-hospital delay in patients with ST-segment elevation myocardial infarction? J Psychosom Res 91:68–74, 2016 27894465

Fitzpatrick MC: The psychologic assessment and psychosocial recovery of the patient with an amputation. Clin Orthop Relat Res (361):98–107, 1999 10212602

Folkman S, Lazarus RS: The relationship between coping and emotion: implications for theory and research. Soc Sci Med 26(3):309–317, 1988 3279520

Folkman S, Lazarus RS, Dunkel-Schetter C, et al: Dynamics of a stressful encounter: cognitive appraisal, coping, and encounter outcomes. J Pers Soc Psychol 50(5):992–1003, 1986 3712234

Folkman S, Chesney M, Pollack L, Coates T: Stress, control, coping, and depressive mood in human immunodeficiency virus–positive and –negative gay men in San Francisco. J Nerv Ment Dis 181(7):409–416, 1993 8320542

Fonagy P, Leigh T, Steele M, et al: The relation of attachment status, psychiatric classification, and response to psychotherapy. J Consult Clin Psychol 64(1):22–31, 1996 8907081

Fricchione GL, Howanitz E, Jandorf L, et al: Psychological adjustment to end-stage renal disease and the implications of denial. Psychosomatics 33(1):85–91, 1992 1539108

Gattellari M, Butow PN, Tattersall MH, et al: Misunderstanding in cancer patients: why shoot the messenger? Ann Oncol 10(1):39–46, 1999 10076720

Gaw AC: Concise Guide to Cross-Cultural Psychiatry. Washington, DC, American Psychiatric Publishing, 2001

Gazzola L, Muskin PR: The impact of stress and the objectives of psychosocial interventions, in Psychosocial Treatment for Medical Conditions: Principles and Techniques. Edited by Schein LA, Bernard HS, Spitz HI, et al. New York, Brunner-Routledge, 2003, pp 373–406

Geringer ES, Stern TA: Coping with medical illness: the impact of personality types. Psychosomatics 27(4):251–261, 1986 3704101

Gilboa D, Bisk L, Montag I, Tsur H: Personality traits and psychosocial adjustment of patients with burns. J Burn Care Rehabil 20(4):340–346, discussion 338–339, 1999 10425599

Goldbeck R: Denial in physical illness. J Psychosom Res 43(6):575–593, 1997 9430071

Greer S: Psychological aspects: delay in the treatment of breast cancer. Proc R Soc Med 67(6 Pt 1):470–473, 1974 4853948

Groves JE: Taking care of the hateful patient. N Engl J Med 298(16):883–887, 1978 634331

Hackett TP, Cassem NH: Development of a quantitative rating scale to assess denial. J Psychosom Res 18(2):93–100, 1974 4436841

Havik OE, Maeland JG: Verbal denial and outcome in myocardial infarction patients. J Psychosom Res 32(2):145–157, 1988 3404496

Heim E, Augustiny KF, Schaffner L, Valach L: Coping with breast cancer over time and situation. J Psychosom Res 37(5):523–542, 1993 8350294

Heim E, Valach L, Schaffner L: Coping and psychosocial adaptation: longitudinal effects over time and stages in breast cancer. Psychosom Med 59(4):408–418, 1997 9251161

Heiskell LE, Pasnau RO: Psychological reaction to hospitalization and illness in the emergency department. Emerg Med Clin North Am 9(1):207–218, 1991 2001666

Holwerda N, Sanderman R, Pool G, et al: Do patients trust their physician? The role of attachment style in the patient-physician relationship within one year after a cancer diagnosis. Acta Oncol 52(1):110–117, 2013 23113593

Huffman JC, Beale EE, Celano CM, et al: Effects of optimism and gratitude on physical activity, biomarkers, and readmissions after an acute coronary syndrome: the Gratitude Research in Acute Coronary Events Study. Circ Cardiovasc Qual Outcomes 9(1):55–63, 2016 26646818

Hunter JJ, Maunder RG: Using attachment theory to understand illness behavior. Gen Hosp Psychiatry 23(4):177–182, 2001 11543843

Jacobsen BS, Lowery BJ: Further analysis of the psychometric properties of the Levine Denial of Illness Scale. Psychosom Med 54(3):372–381, 1992 1620811

Jensen MP, Turner JA, Romano JM, Karoly P: Coping with chronic pain: a critical review of the literature. Pain 47(3):249–283, 1991 1784498

Kahana RJ, Bibring G: Personality types in medical management, in Psychiatry and Medical Practice in a General Hospital. Edited by Zinberg NE. New York, International Universities Press, 1964, pp 108–123

Kaptein AA, Scharloo M, Fischer MJ, et al: Illness perceptions and COPD: an emerging field for COPD patient management. J Asthma 45(8):625–629, 2008 18951252

Klest B, Philippon O: Trust in the medical profession and patient attachment style. Psychol Health Med 21(7):863–870, 2016 26652310

Kornfeld DS: The hospital environment: its impact on the patient. Adv Psychosom Med 8:252–270, 1972 4576878

Kornfeld DS, Muskin PR, Tahil FA: Psychiatric evaluation of mental capacity in the general hospital: a significant teaching opportunity. Psychosomatics 50(5):468–473, 2009 19855032

Kripalani S, Yao X, Haynes RB: Interventions to enhance medication adherence in chronic medical conditions: a systematic review. Arch Intern Med 167(6):540–550, 2007 17389285

Kubler-Ross E: On Death and Dying. New York, Macmillan, 1969

Lazarus RS: Stress and Emotion: A New Synthesis. New York, Springer, 1999

Lazarus RS, Folkman S: Stress, Appraisal and Coping. New York, Springer, 1984

Leigh H: The patient's personality, personality types, traits and disorders in the CL setting, in Handbook of Consultation-Liaison Psychiatry. New York, Springer, 2015, pp 345–366

Levenson JL: Psychiatric aspects of medical practice, in Clinical Psychiatry for Medical Students, 3rd Edition. Edited by Stoudemire A. Philadelphia, PA, Lippincott-Raven, 1998, pp 727–763

Levenson JL, Mishra A, Hamer RM, Hastillo A: Denial and medical outcome in unstable angina. Psychosom Med 51(1):27–35, 1989 2784580

Levine J, Warrenburg S, Kerns R, et al: The role of denial in recovery from coronary heart disease. Psychosom Med 49(2):109–117, 1987 3575599

Lipowski ZJ: Physical illness, the individual and the coping processes. Psychiatry Med 1(2):91–102, 1970 4257952

Lloyd GG: Psychological reactions to physical illness. Br J Hosp Med 18(4):352–358, 355–358, 1977 912159

Marcum ZA, Hanlon JT, Murray MD: Improving medication adherence and health outcomes in older adults: an evidence-based review of randomized controlled trials. Drugs Aging 34(3):191–201, 2017 28074410

Marucha PT, Kiecolt-Glaser JK, Favagehi M: Mucosal wound healing is impaired by examination stress. Psychosom Med 60(3):362–365, 1998 9625226

Muskin PR: The combined use of psychotherapy and pharmacotherapy in the medical setting. Psychiatr Clin North Am 13(2):341–353, 1990 2352895

Muskin PR: The medical hospital, in Psychodynamic Concepts in General Psychiatry. Edited by Schwartz HJ, Bleiberg E, Weissman SH. Washington, DC, American Psychiatric Press, 1995, pp 69–88

Muskin PR, Epstein LA: Clinical guide to countertransference. Curr Psychiatr 8(4):25–32, 2009

Muskin PR, Haase EK: Difficult patients and patients with personality disorders, in Textbook of Primary Care Medicine, 3rd Edition (Noble J, Editor in Chief). St Louis, MO, CV Mosby, 2001, pp 458–464

Ness DE, Ende J: Denial in the medical interview. Recognition and management. JAMA 272(22):1777–1781, 1994 7966927

Oldham JM, Skodol AE: Charting the future of axis II. J Pers Disord 14(1):17–29, 2000 10746202

Patterson DR, Everett JJ, Bombardier CH, et al: Psychological effects of severe burn injuries. Psychol Bull 113(2):362–378, 1993 8451340

Penley JA, Tomaka J, Wiebe JS: The association of coping to physical and psychological health outcomes: a meta-analytic review. J Behav Med 25(6):551–603, 2002 12462958

Perry S, Viederman M: Management of emotional reactions to acute medical illness. Med Clin North Am 65(1):3–14, 1981 7206897

Rasmussen HN, Scheier MF, Greenhouse JB: Optimism and physical health: a meta-analytic review. Ann Behav Med 37(3):239–256, 2009 19711142

Richardson EM, Schüz N, Sanderson K, et al: Illness representations, coping, and illness outcomes in people with cancer: a systematic review and meta-analysis. Psychooncology 26(6):724–737, 2017 27412423

Sensky T: Causal attributions in physical illness. J Psychosom Res 43(6):565–573, 1997 9430070

Staudenmayer H, Kinsman RA, Dirks JF, et al: Medical outcome in asthmatic patients: effects of airways hyperreactivity and symptom-focused anxiety. Psychosom Med 41(2):109–118, 1979 441228

Stearns CR, Bakamjian A, Sattar S, Weintraub MR: Discharges against medical advice at a county hospital: provider perceptions and practice. J Hosp Med 12(1):11–17, 2017 28125826

Strain JJ, Grossman S: Psychological reactions to medical illness and hospitalization, in Psychological Care of the Medically Ill: A Primer in Liaison Psychiatry. New York, Appleton-Century-Crofts, 1975, pp 23–36

Strain J, Hammer JS, Huertas D, et al: The problem of coping as a reason for psychiatric consultation. Gen Hosp Psychiatry 15(1):1–8, 1993 8382180

Strain JJ, Smith GC, Hammer JS, et al: Adjustment disorder: a multisite study of its utilization and interventions in the consultation-liaison psychiatry setting. Gen Hosp Psychiatry 20(3):139–149, 1998 9650031

Sullivan MD, Youngner SJ: Depression, competence, and the right to refuse lifesaving medical treatment. Am J Psychiatry 151(7):971–978, 1994 8010382

Tedeschi RG, Calhoun LG: Posttraumatic growth: conceptual foundations and empirical evidence. Psychol Inq 15(1):1–18, 2004

Thompson D, Ciechanowski PS: Attaching a new understanding to the patient-physician relationship in family practice. J Am Board Fam Pract 16(3):219–226, 2003 12755249

Tindle H, Belnap BH, Houck PR, et al: Optimism, response to treatment of depression, and rehospitalization after coronary artery bypass graft surgery. Psychosom Med 74(2):200–207, 2012 22286847

Vaillant GE: The Wisdom of the Ego. Cambridge, MA, Harvard University Press, 1993

Weisman AD, Hackett TP: Predilection to death. Death and dying as a psychiatric problem. Psychosom Med 23:232–256, 1961 13784028

Westbrook MT, Viney LL: Psychological reactions to the onset of chronic illness. Soc Sci Med 16(8):899–905, 1982 7101005

Young LD, Schweiger J, Beitzinger J, et al: Denial in heart transplant candidates. Psychother Psychosom 55(2–4):141–144, 1991 1891560

Zervas IM, Augustine A, Fricchione GL: Patient delay in cancer. A view from the crisis model. Gen Hosp Psychiatry 15(1):9–13, 1993 8436288

PART II

Symptoms and Disorders

CHAPTER 4

Delirium

Albert F.G. Leentjens, M.D., Ph.D.
David J. Meagher, M.D., MRCPsych, Ph.D.

*Some lose their senses and take no notice when spoken to;
some have a wild look; in some the eyes move from side to
side as if they were out of control; generally on the third
or fifth day delirium supervenes; many have also spasm of
sinews. Again, before death many tear off the bandages
with which their head has been bound up, and expose the
bared wound to cold.*

Aulus Cornelius Celsus (circa 25 B.C.–circa 50 A.D.),
De Medicina, Book V, Chapter 26

The word *delirium* originates from the Latin *de* (meaning "out of") and *lira* (meaning "furrow"). It was probably introduced by Aulus Cornelius Celsus, a Roman best known for his medical encyclopedia *De Medicina* (Adamis et al. 2007). In this work, the term *delirium* was used to describe the acute confusional states that could occur after wound infections or head injuries. In the modern era, the term is still used in the same sense—namely, to describe confusional states that may occur in physically ill patients.

Delirium is a neuropsychiatric disorder that occurs commonly among patients in all health care settings. It is the most prevalent psychiatric disorder in general hospital settings, with an average prevalence of greater than 20%, and it is especially common among patients who are elderly, who have preexisting brain lesions or cognitive impairment, and who are admitted to the intensive care unit (ICU) (National Institute for Health and Care Excellence 2010). In the past decade, the negative prognostic implications of delirium have become widely known. Patients with delirium have longer hospital stays, more complications, higher in-hospital mortality rates, worse functional recovery, and increased chances of developing dementia and of requiring institutionalization in a nursing home. This negative prognosis has led to renewed and increased interest in delirium, both in clinical practice and in research. Clinical research focuses mainly on early detection, effectiveness of treatment, and possible proactive interventions to prevent delirium. Basic research generated new hypotheses about the pathophysiology of delirium and potential future treatment targets.

In spite of this renewed interest, delirium is frequently not recognized and is inadequately managed in clinical practice. This, as well as the negative prognostic implications, makes delirium a major health problem for the individual patient as well as a general health care problem for society. Delirium is responsible for increased health care costs. Milbrandt et al. (2004) compared ICU costs incurred by 183 mechanically ventilated medical ICU patients with at least one delirium episode against costs incurred by nondelirious control patients. The median ICU costs for delirious patients were significantly higher than those for nondelirious patients: $22,346 versus $13,332, respectively. Total hospital costs were also higher for delirious patients than for nondelirious patients: $41,836 versus $27,106, respectively. Inouye et al. (1999) calculated the total direct 1-year health care costs in the United States attributable to delirium as somewhere between $143 billion and $152 billion. Implementing a multicomponent delirium prevention program can substantially reduce health care costs. The Hospital Elder Life Program saved an average of $831 per patient in annual acute hospital costs and $9,446 per patient in long-term nursing home costs (Leslie et al. 2005; Rizzo et al. 2001). In a study of children admitted to a pediatric ICU (PICU), delirium was associated with an 85% increase in PICU costs after controlling for patient age, gender, severity of illness, and PICU length of stay (Traube et al. 2016). (Delirium in children is discussed in detail in Chapter 32, "Pediatrics.") Implementation of adequate care for hospitalized patients with delirium may lead to better outcomes for these patients as well as large cost savings. For these reasons, it has been advocated that delirium care be considered an indicator of hospital care quality (Schofield 2008; Young et al. 2008).

Clinical Features and Classification

Symptoms

Delirium is a complex neuropsychiatric syndrome that can include a wide range of cognitive and psychiatric features. These include disturbances in consciousness, awareness of the immediate environment, thinking, language, perception, affective regulation, sleep–wake cycle, and motor behavior. These disturbances can be grouped into three core domains: cognitive, circadian (e.g., altered sleep–wake cycle and motor activity levels), and higher-order thinking (e.g., disorganization of thought processes, language abnormalities, and impaired comprehension) (Franco et al. 2013).

In terms of cognitive features, delirium involves generalized impairment of cognitive abilities, but with particular disturbance to consciousness and attention. Consciousness can be affected qualitatively ("clouding") as well as quantitatively in terms of arousal, with both reduced arousal and hyperarousal states possible. A level of arousal that renders formal testing of cognition impossible is considered to be evidence of severe inattention and thus is consistent with a diagnosis of delirium (American Psychiatric Association 2013; European Delirium Association and American Delirium Society 2014). It should be noted that this rule does not apply in patients who are untestable by virtue of being comatose, as this state is considered a phenomenon separate from delirium. The primary cognitive disturbance in delirium is in the ability to focus, sustain, and shift attention, as evidenced by difficulty in orienting to salient stimuli, poor concentration, reduced vigilance, distractibility, and impaired awareness of the immediate environment. Attentional abilities are disproportionately affected, but typically there are disturbances in other cognitive abilities, including orientation, visuospatial processing, executive function, and short-term memory, which can usually be demonstrated with simple bedside tests.

A variety of neuropsychiatric symptoms can also occur, including disrupted circadian integrity (sleep and motor function) and disturbances in thinking, perception, affect, and behavior. More than 40% of patients with delirium have psychotic features (Webster and Holroyd 2000). Delusions are typically simple and persecutory in character and relate to the immediate surroundings (e.g., the delusion that the hospital is a prison). Perceptual disturbances include illusions and hallucinations, which are most commonly visual or tactile. Affective lability, with unpredictable shifts in mood, anger, and/or irritability, is common, but some patients present with a more sustained lowering of mood that is easily mistaken for depressive illness.

Motor Subtypes

Although delirium is considered to be a unitary syndrome of acute generalized cognitive impairment, the presentation in terms of patterns of motor activity can vary considerably. Two principal patterns have been recognized since the time of Hippocrates: *phrenitus*, now termed *hyperactive* or agitated delirium, and *lethargus*, now termed *hypoactive* or somnolent delirium. In addition, a third, mixed subtype accounts for patients who experience elements of both increased and decreased motor activity within short time frames. Studies comparing the clinical profiles of these presentations indicate similar levels of disturbance across neuropsychological domains, but with differing patterns in terms of underlying etiology. Hyperactive presentations are more common in delirium occurring in younger patients and delirium related to substance use, whereas hypoactive delirium is more common in patients with organ failure and patients with preexisting dementia. Moreover, detection rates differ: compared with hyperactive delirium, the diagnosis of hypoactive delirium is more frequently missed or delayed. Finally, outcomes are different: patients with hypoactive presentations have a poorer prognosis (Meagher 2009). Inconsistent approaches to defining these motor subtypes limit the comparability of studies, but the Delirium Motor Subtype Scale (DMSS) provides a reliable and validated method for rapid identification of subtypes, both for clinical practice and for research (Meagher et al. 2014a). Future work can clarify the extent to which patients with different motor presentations differ in terms of underlying pathophysiology and therapeutic response.

Course

Delirium typically develops over a short period of time, usually hours to a few days, and tends to fluctuate over the day, with symptoms worsening in the evening and at night, when external anchoring stimuli decrease (DSM-5; American Psychiatric Association 2013). DSM-5 notes that in hospital settings, delirium usually lasts about 1 week, but it may sometimes persist for longer periods of time and may even still be evident at the time the patient is discharged from the hospital to home or to long-term care. A subtype of chronic delirium is now recognized in DSM-5. However, persistent delirium is not rare. Especially in elderly individuals and those with dementia, delirium may develop gradually and follow a chronic course. In a systematic review by Cole et al. (2009), delirious symptoms persisted in 45% of elderly hospitalized patients at discharge, and symptoms were still present in 33% of elderly patients after 1 month, in 26% after 3 months, and in 21% after 6 months. In a study by Miu et al. (2016), 78% of elderly patients were still delirious at discharge, and 55% were still delirious at 3-month follow-up. In another study, delirium persisted in 56% of patients 1 month after admission to postacute care; this rate declined to 32% at 6 months (Anderson et al. 2012; Kiely et al. 2009).

Risk factors for persistence of delirium, as identified by the meta-analysis conducted for the National Institute for Health and Care Excellence (NICE) clinical guideline (National Institute for Health and Care Excellence 2010), are cognitive impairment (odds ratio [OR]=2.3; 95% confidence interval [CI]=1.41–3.74), vision impairment (OR=2.10; 95% CI=1.34–3.29), a Charlson Comorbidity Index score >3 (OR=1.7; 95% CI=1.11–2.61), and the use of physical restraints (OR=3.20; 95% CI= 1.93–5.29). Another systematic review identified a greater number of medical conditions, increased severity of delirium, hypoactive symptoms, and hypoxic illnesses as additional risk factors for delirium persistence (Dasgupta and Hillier 2010). Increased duration of delirium, or persistent delirium, has consistently been associated with a number of negative outcomes, including increased mortality, more complications, worse cognitive and functional recovery, and higher risk of unplanned hospital readmission or nursing home placement (Anderson et al. 2012; Cole et al. 2009; Kiely et al. 2009; Miu et al. 2016; National Institute for Health and Care Excellence 2010).

DSM-5 and ICD-10 Diagnostic Criteria

Delirium involves a generalized disturbance of brain function that occurs in the context of physical illness. It thus provides an excellent example of the interface between brain and bodily well-being. Hippocrates used about 16 different words to refer to and name the clinical syndrome that we now call delirium, and a plethora of labels appear in the modern literature, including terms such as acute confusional state, acute brain failure, toxic or metabolic encephalopathy, and ICU psychosis (Adamis et al. 2007). Delirium was introduced in DSM-III (American Psychiatric Association 1980) as an umbrella diagnostic term to account for all acute/subacute generalized brain syndromes. This clarity of definition has promoted more coherent management in clinical practice and more focused research efforts. Subsequent DSM definitions of delirium, including the current DSM-5 criteria (American Psychiatric Association 2013; Table 4–1), have further refined the definition of delirium as an acute neurocognitive disorder characterized by prominent disturbance of attention, awareness, and other cognitive and perceptual functions. Although these features are not specific to delirium, the time course and context are distinctive: developing over a short time (hours or days), tending to fluctuate, and having temporal links to medical illness or other physical insults such as drug effects. The diagnostic criteria further specify that

TABLE 4-1.	DSM-5 diagnostic criteria for delirium

A. A disturbance in attention (i.e., reduced ability to direct, focus, sustain, and shift attention) and awareness (reduced orientation to the environment).

B. The disturbance develops over a short period of time (usually hours to a few days), represents a change from baseline attention and awareness, and tends to fluctuate in severity during the course of a day.

C. An additional disturbance in cognition (e.g., memory deficit, disorientation, language, visuospatial ability, or perception).

D. The disturbances in Criteria A and C are not better explained by another preexisting, established, or evolving neurocognitive disorder and do not occur in the context of a severely reduced level of arousal, such as coma.

E. There is evidence from the history, physical examination, or laboratory findings that the disturbance is a direct physiological consequence of another medical condition, substance intoxication or withdrawal (i.e., due to a drug of abuse or to a medication), or exposure to a toxin, or is due to multiple etiologies.

Specify whether:

Substance intoxication delirium: This diagnosis should be made instead of substance intoxication when the symptoms in Criteria A and C predominate in the clinical picture and when they are sufficiently severe to warrant clinical attention.

Substance withdrawal delirium: This diagnosis should be made instead of substance withdrawal when the symptoms in Criteria A and C predominate in the clinical picture and when they are sufficiently severe to warrant clinical attention.

Medication-induced delirium: This diagnosis applies when the symptoms in Criteria A and C arise as a side effect of a medication taken as prescribed.

Delirium due to another medical condition: There is evidence from the history, physical examination, or laboratory findings that the disturbance is attributable to the physiological consequences of another medical condition.

Delirium due to multiple etiologies: There is evidence from the history, physical examination, or laboratory findings that the delirium has more than one etiology (e.g., more than one etiological medical condition; another medical condition plus substance intoxication or medication side effect).

Specify if:

Acute: Lasting a few hours or days.

Persistent: Lasting weeks or months.

Specify if:

Hyperactive: The individual has a hyperactive level of psychomotor activity that may be accompanied by mood lability, agitation, and/or refusal to cooperate with medical care.

Hypoactive: The individual has a hypoactive level of psychomotor activity that may be accompanied by sluggishness and lethargy that approaches stupor.

Mixed level of activity: The individual has a normal level of psychomotor activity even though attention and awareness are disturbed. Also includes individuals whose activity level rapidly fluctuates.

the disturbances must not be attributable to other neurocognitive disorders, such as dementia, although the high comorbidity between delirium and dementia means that distinguishing between the two is often challenging (as discussed in the next subsection, "Differential Diagnosis"). The clinical rule of thumb is that such disturbances should be attributed to delirium in the first instance because it is typically a more urgent diagnosis.

The ICD-10 criteria are largely comparable to those of DSM-5, with clouding of consciousness and disturbance of cognition being the principal features (World Health Organization 1992). In contrast to DSM, in which psychomotor disturbances became part of the delirium criteria only with the publication of DSM-5 in 2013 and sleep–wake cycle abnormalities in delirium are not explicitly mentioned, both psychomotor disturbances and sleep–wake cycle abnormalities were already included in the ICD delirium criteria in 1992. In ICD-10, psychomotor disturbances refer not only to hypoarousal and hyperarousal states but also to increased reaction time, increased or decreased flow of speech, and an enhanced startle reaction. Moreover, sleep–wake cycle abnormalities refer not only to nighttime insomnia with daytime drowsiness but also to nocturnal worsening of symptoms and disturbing dreams or nightmares, which may continue as hallucinations or illusions after awakening. Compared with a DSM diagnosis, an ICD diagnosis of delirium requires the presence of a greater number of features, thereby excluding many patients whose presentations would typically be considered as delirium. For this reason, the ICD criteria are less commonly used among clinicians and researchers (Morandi et al. 2013).

Differential Diagnosis

Because delirium encompasses so many potential symptoms and can easily be mistaken for other neurocognitive and neuropsychiatric disorders, such as dementia, depression, or psychotic disorders, its differential diagnosis is broad. Accurate diagnosis requires careful history taking, augmented by a collateral source where possible, aligned with thorough examination, cognitive assessment, and investigation for acute medical conditions. Importantly, delirium can be the first presentation of serious medical illness, such as stroke or septicemia, and, as such, should take diagnostic precedence. In practical terms, the clinical rule of thumb is that *acute changes in mental status should be considered as possible delirium until proven otherwise.*

The most difficult differential diagnosis for delirium is dementia, the other cause of generalized cognitive impairment. Although these conditions are classically distinguished by their acuity of onset and temporal course, many dementias, such as vascular dementia, may also have a relatively acute presentation; Lewy body dementia can present with a very similar clinical picture to delirium, with fluctuation of symptom severity, visual hallucinations, attentional impairment, alteration of consciousness, and delusions (Gore et al. 2015). Moreover, more than 50% of cases of delirium occur in the setting of comorbid dementia (Bellelli et al. 2016), a circumstance that further complicates accurate diagnosis and highlights the considerable overlap between these major neurocognitive disorders. Similarly, there is considerable overlap in presentation between hypoactive delirium and depression with psychomotor retardation, because both states include reduced amounts and speed of activity and speech. Not surprisingly, delirium and depression are commonly misdiagnosed in clinical practice (O'Sullivan et al. 2014). Distinction from psychotic states can also sometimes be problematic, as both delirium and psychotic disorders such as schizophrenia and psychotic depression can include disturbed thinking and perception. In rare cases, severe mania may also closely resemble delirium, a condition referred to as "delirious mania." This condition is usually characterized by the absence of physical disease (Jacobowski et al. 2013).

However, careful consideration of the symptom profile can usually distinguish delirium from these other states. Abrupt onset and fluctuating course are highly indicative of delirium. In addition, consciousness and attention are invariably disturbed in delirium but remain relatively intact in mood disorders, psychotic disorders, and dementia. More recent studies have highlighted tests of attention, vigilance, and visuospatial function that can distinguish delirious patients, including those with comorbid dementia, from nondelirious patients (Leonard et al. 2016). Disorganized or illogical thinking with diminished awareness and grasp of the immediate environment are very suggestive of delirium. In addition, the pattern of disruption in the sleep–wake cycle, often including severe fragmentation or reversal of the cycle, can help to distinguish delirium from other states. The pattern of affective change typically involves affective lability rather than sustained lowering of mood (as occurs in depression). Careful assessment of the context of symptoms can facilitate more accurate attribution, because delirium is typically more acute in onset and more likely to be linked to acute physical illness, whereas depressive symptoms typically develop more gradually (over weeks) and are linked to psychological stressors. The character of psychotic symptoms also differs—psychotic features in delirium are often simple and persecutory and relate to the immediate environment, whereas psychotic features in mood disorders classically include complex mood-congruent psychotic symptoms involving themes of guilt and nihilism or grandiosity. In contrast to hallucinations in psychotic disorders, hallucinations in delirium tend to be visual or tactile rather than auditory, and so-called Schneiderian features are rare.

When presentations are more challenging, or when greater diagnostic precision is needed (e.g., in research studies), tools such as the Delirium Rating Scale—Revised–98 (DRS-R-98) (Trzepacz et al. 2001) and the Cognitive Test for Delirium (CTD) (Hart et al. 1996) can help distinguish delirium from other neuropsychiatric presentations. Moreover, the short version of the Informant Questionnaire on Cognitive Decline in the Elderly (Short IQCODE) (Jorm 2004) can reliably identify long-standing disturbances of dementia as long as a reliable informant is available. The Cornell Scale for Depression in Dementia (CSDD) (Alexopoulos et al. 1988) can also assist in reliably identifying depressive illness in patients with significant cognitive difficulties, including those with dementia. On occasion, electroencephalography (EEG) can further assist, because the presence of diffuse slowing is more indicative of delirium.

Assessment Tools

Delirium is underdetected in clinical practice, with around 50% of cases missed or diagnosed late (O'Hanlon et al. 2014). For this reason, the use of standardized approaches to assessment can assist in delirium detection in both research settings and everyday clinical practice. Although both DSM and ICD provide formal diagnostic criteria, DSM-IV (American Psychiatric Association 1994)—and, increasingly, DSM-5—criteria are most commonly applied because of their relative simplicity. Typically, diagnosis is achieved by a two-step process, with initial screening followed by a more detailed application of diagnostic criteria for patients who screen positive. In research settings, a delirium diagnosis is made according to formal DSM or ICD criteria, supported by general clinical judgment or sometimes by more formal operationalized algorithms (Meagher et al. 2014b).

Screening and Diagnostic Instruments

A variety of tools are available for delirium screening. These differ principally in terms of their emphasis on observed behaviors versus elicited cognitive impairments (De and Wand 2015). The Confusion Assessment Method (CAM) (Inouye et al. 1990) has been the preferred screening tool over much of the past two decades. It is based on DSM-III-R (American Psychiatric Association 1987) criteria and consists of a diagnostic algorithm in which the rater administers a cognitive test and obtains an informant history. A delirium diagnosis requires the presence of 1) acute change or fluctuating course *and* 2) inattention with *either* 3) disorganized thinking *or* 4) altered level of consciousness. The CAM requires specific training and takes approximately 10 minutes to complete. The CAM-ICU version is anchored by formal tests taken from the CTD to enhance its standardization (Ely et al. 2001). In a meta-analysis of 22 studies, the pooled sensitivities and specificity for the CAM were 82% and 99%, respectively, and those for the CAM-ICU were 81% and 98%, respectively (Shi et al. 2013). However, the accuracy of the CAM is lower when used by nonexpert assessors, and it has not been rigorously validated in distinguishing delirium from dementia or other psychiatric disorders. The 3D-CAM is a new adaptation of the CAM that is more structured and requires 3 minutes to administer (Marcantonio et al. 2014), with initial work indicating improved sensitivity compared with the CAM-ICU (Kuczmarska et al. 2016).

The 4AT, a rapid assessment test for delirium (www.the4AT.com), is designed for routine use by nonspecialists and does not require specific training. It takes 1–2 minutes to complete and includes items for level of arousal, orientation, attention (listing months of the year backward), and acute onset or fluctuating course. The test's sensitivity and specificity are 89.7% and 84.1%, respectively, for DSM-IV–defined delirium in acute geriatric and rehabilitation service inpatients, and it maintains good accuracy in comorbid delirium–dementia cases as well (Bellelli et al. 2014). Similarly, its sensitivity and specificity are 87% and 80%, respectively, for DSM-5–defined delirium in geriatric inpatients with mixed neuropsychiatric and cultural backgrounds (De et al. 2017). A Thai version of the 4AT has demonstrated sensitivity and specificity of 83% and 86%, respectively, for delirium in hospitalized elderly patients with acute medical illnesses (Kuladee and Prachason 2016).

The Richmond Agitation and Sedation Scale (RASS) was not designed as a delirium severity scale; rather, it focuses on level of consciousness as evidenced by alertness and arousal (Sessler et al. 2002). It is a one-item observational scale consisting of 10 points ranging from –5 (unrousable) to +4 (combative), with a score of 0 equated with being alert and calm. Patients with a RASS score of –3 or less should have their sedation decreased or modified to achieve a RASS score of –2 to 0. Patients with a

RASS score of 2–4 are insufficiently sedated and should be assessed for pain, anxiety, and delirium. The RASS is often used to quantify the level of agitation in delirious patients. It has demonstrated usefulness as an ultrabrief measure for detecting delirium, including delirium superimposed on dementia, with a sensitivity of 70.4% and a specificity of 84.8% for comorbid delirium and dementia in elderly patients in ICU, emergency department, and rehabilitation settings (Morandi et al. 2016).

The Nursing Delirium Screening Scale (Nu-DESC) is an observational instrument designed especially for nurses, which has been validated in four different languages (Gaudreau et al. 2005). The scale assesses five items—orientation, behavior, communication, illusions/hallucinations, and psychomotor retardation—each rated on a two-point scale. The total score ranges between zero and 10, where zero indicates no symptoms, and a score greater than 2 indicates probable delirium. The Nu-DESC items are ideally assessed three times per day during each shift (morning, day, and evening), and screening can be completed in less than 2 minutes. Four studies (Leung et al. 2008; Lingehall et al. 2013; Luetz et al. 2010; Neufeld et al. 2013) have indicated a sensitivity of 32%–96% and a specificity of 69%–92% for DSM-IV–defined delirium. However, there is uncertainty as to the optimal cutoff score, with higher sensitivity evident when a cutoff score of >0 was applied (Leung et al. 2008).

The Delirium Observation Screening (DOS) scale is a 13-item observational scale developed for use by nurses. It requires approximately 5 minutes to administer (Schuurmans et al. 2003), ideally during morning, day, and evening shifts. Studies to date indicate high sensitivity (89%–100%) and specificity (87%–97%) for DSM-IV–defined delirium (Koster et al. 2009; Van Gemert and Schuurmans 2007).

The "recognizing acute delirium as part of your routine" (RADAR) scale is an ultrabrief (typically requiring <10 seconds) screening scale designed for use by nurses during drug administration rounds. It assesses three components—drowsiness, inability to follow instructions, and slowed actions—each of which is rated as present or absent, with any positive rating considered indicative of possible delirium. To date, a single study has demonstrated a sensitivity of 73% and a specificity of 67% for DSM-IV–defined delirium, with good inter-rater reliability between research assistants and nurses, ranging from 82% to 98% (Voyer et al. 2015).

Severity Rating Scales

More-detailed instruments used for assessing severity of delirium include the Memorial Delirium Assessment Scale (MDAS) and the DRS-R-98.

The DRS-R-98 is an adaptation of the original Delirium Rating Scale (DRS) (Trzepacz et al. 1989). It is designed to assist physicians and trained researchers in detecting and assessing individual symptoms of delirium. It typically takes 15–20 minutes to conduct and has been validated for use in multiple languages. The scale consists of 16 items, of which three items are primarily intended for diagnosis, with the others covering the range of cognitive and neuropsychiatric symptoms that occur in delirium. Scores range from 0 to 46 points. Different cutoff scores can be applied for delirium detection, depending on the population studied, but in general, a score of 18 or higher indicates delirium. Studies indicate a sensitivity of 56%–93% and a specificity of 82%–98%, with high inter-rater reliability (0.92–1.00). The DRS-R-98 has demonstrated discriminatory ability for delirium and dementia and has been used extensively in the phenomenological assessment of delirium and for monitoring changing delirium severity in treatment studies (Trzepacz et al. 2009).

The MDAS is a 10-item severity rating scale (Breitbart et al. 1997) designed for obtaining repeated ratings within a 24-hour period, as occurs in treatment studies. Available in multiple languages, it includes a wide range of delirium symptoms and has been used extensively in studies of delirium in palliative care. However, the MDAS is less useful for diagnosis, because there is a lack of clarity as to optimal diagnostic cutoff scores, and it has not been studied in terms of its ability to discriminate delirium from other neuropsychiatric conditions, such as dementia or depression.

Epidemiology

Prevalence and Incidence

The prevalence and incidence of delirium depend on the setting and the age of the study sample, as well as on the diagnostic criteria used. It is known that DSM-IV criteria are less restrictive than ICD-10 criteria, the latter requiring the presence of a greater number of mandatory features for a delirium diagnosis. Because of this difference, studies using ICD-10 criteria will generally report lower prevalences of delirium than those using DSM-IV criteria. This is illustrated in a cohort study of elderly medical hospital patients and nursing home residents with a mean age of 88.4 years, in which 24.9% met DSM-IV diagnostic criteria for delirium, whereas only 10.1% met ICD-10 criteria (Laurila et al. 2004). Most studies have been conducted in the setting of general or academic hospitals. Fewer studies have been performed in the general population or in long-term care facilities such as nursing homes.

A systematic review of delirium in older people identified eight studies conducted in the general population (representing a total of 90,258 patients ages 65 years and older, with sample sizes in individual studies varying from 199 to 76,688), which reported delirium prevalences ranging from 0.5% to 34.5% (de Lange et al. 2013). Low prevalences were found in studies that excluded persons suffering from dementia. Higher prevalences were found in studies that had older study samples (e.g., studies enrolling only participants ages 75 or 85 years and older). A longer observation period produced higher period prevalences. Age-specific prevalences in the community were reported in the Eastern Baltimore Mental Health Survey: 0.4% for people older than 18 years of age, 1.1% for those older than 55 years, and 13.6% for those older than 85 years (Folstein et al. 1991).

The NICE clinical guideline on delirium contained an extensive systematic review and meta-analysis of studies examining prevalence and incidence of delirium in the hospital setting (National Institute for Health and Care Excellence 2010). This meta-analysis was based on 75 studies, including 2 randomized controlled trials, 68 prospective cohort studies, and 5 cross-sectional studies. Most studies ($n=32$) were conducted in the United States, 13 in Canada, and 18 in Northern European countries, with the remaining studies conducted in other countries. On the basis of quality criteria, 4 studies were excluded from the analysis. The meta-analysis was performed separately for different settings within the hospital: general medicine, surgery, orthopedics, ICU, and so forth. Both incidence and prevalence data were reported, as well as "occurrence" of delirium when data permitted. The term *occurrence* was used when both incident and prevalent cases were included. The results are summarized in Table 4–2.

As shown in Table 4–2, delirium is especially common in ICUs. The highest reported occurrence was in medical ICUs, at 80%. The trauma ICU, surgical ICU, and general ICU had lower occurrence rates (59%, 44%, 32%, respectively), followed by orthopedic wards (28%), wards for cardiac and vascular surgery (21% and 31%, respectively), and wards for neurosurgery (15%). A low occurrence rate (2.8%, from a single study) was reported for delirium in a general hospital psychiatric ward.

Only a few studies have reported data on the prevalence of delirium in nursing homes and long-term care facilities. A systematic review of delirium in older people identified 15 studies conducted in nursing home or long-term care populations (representing a total of 55,598 patients, with sample sizes in individual studies varying from 74 to 35,721), which reported widely varying prevalences, ranging from 1.4% to 70.3% (de Lange et al. 2013). The prevalence depended on the type of facility, the age of the included patient group, and the diagnostic criteria used. Delirium prevalence was higher in patients who were institutionalized than in those who attended day care facilities. The highest prevalences were seen in populations in which dementia was common.

Etiology and Risk Factors

Delirium has a wide variety of etiologies, which may occur alone or in combination. DSM-5 includes specifiers for coding etiological subtype: delirium due to substance intoxication or withdrawal, medication-induced delirium, delirium due to another medical condition, and delirium due to multiple etiologies (American Psychiatric Association 2013). Single-etiology delirium, however, is the exception; most cases involve contributions from multiple factors, often sequentially, thus making regular rigorous reassessment of causation essential in management (Meagher and Leonard 2008). This multifactorial nature has been underemphasized in research settings, where etiological attributions typically are based on clinical impressions that are not standardized (e.g., the most likely cause identified by the referring physician) or that are oversimplified (e.g., by the practice of assigning only one etiology for each case).

The clinical model developed by Inouye (1999) distinguishes predisposing factors, or a priori risk factors, and precipitating or etiological factors. Predisposing factors constitute a baseline risk for delirium. The relationship between predisposing and precipitating factors is shown in Figure 4–1 (Inouye et al. 2014b). Patients with high vulnerability, for example, with some level of cognitive decline, severe underlying illness, or visual or hearing impairment, may develop delirium with a relatively minor insult, such as a subclinical urinary tract infection. Conversely, patients with low vulnerability would require serious and/or multiple noxious insults to develop delirium. This model is attractive not only because it explains the relation between predisposing and precipitating factors but also because it allows identification of targets for preventive measures for elective hospital admissions or surgical procedures, because predisposing factors can be identified upon admission.

The NICE clinical guideline (National Institute for Health and Care Excellence 2010) made no distinction between predisposing and precipitating factors; rather, it distinguished modifiable and nonmodifiable risk factors. According to the meta-

TABLE 4–2.   Prevalence, incidence, and occurrence of delirium across hospital settings

Hospital ward	Number of studies	Prevalence (%)	Incidence (%)	Occurrence[a] (%)
General medicine	16	21.4	15.2	22.0
Stroke unit	2	12.0		24.3
General surgery	5			11.4
Orthopedic surgery (acute)	10	22.0	30.3	28.3
Orthopedic surgery (elective)	3			13.6
Cardiac surgery	5			21.0
Vascular surgery	2			31.1
Neurosurgery	1			14.9
Gynecology	1			17.5
Psychiatry	1			2.8
Emergency department	4			59.0
General ICU	3			31.8
Medical ICU	7	36.6	24.4	80.0
Surgical ICU	4			43.5
Trauma ICU	1			59.0

Note.   ICU=intensive care unit.
[a]The term *occurrence* was used when both incident and prevalent cases (delirium present at admission) were included.

Source.   Adapted from National Institute for Health and Care Excellence 2010.

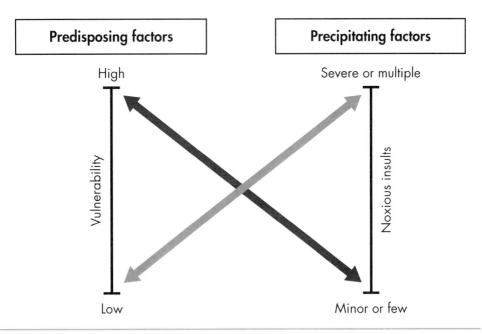

FIGURE 4–1. The multifactorial model for delirium.

The development of delirium involves a complex interrelationship between baseline patient vulnerability (*left axis*) and precipitating factors or noxious insults (*right axis*). A patient with high vulnerability may develop delirium with a relatively benign insult (*dark arrow*). Conversely, a patient with low vulnerability would be relatively resistant and require multiple noxious insults to develop delirium (*light arrow*).

Source. Adapted from Inouye SK, Westendorp RG, Saczynski JS: "Delirium in Elderly People." *The Lancet* 383(9920):911–922, 2014b. Copyright 2014, Elsevier. Used with permission.

analysis in the NICE guideline, established risk factors include higher age, cognitive decline, visual impairment, higher disease severity, and a fracture at admission to the hospital. In this review, there was inconsistent evidence for hearing impairment, polypharmacy, and dehydration as risk factors for delirium. Additional risk factors for developing delirium were a history of delirium, depression, history of transient ischemic attacks or stroke, and alcohol abuse (Inouye et al. 2014b). An overview of risk factors and their relative risk for developing delirium is given in Table 4–3.

There are many factors that can cause delirium. To be considered causal, an etiology should be a recognized possible cause of delirium and be temporally related in onset and course to delirium presentation; also, the delirium should not be better accounted for by other factors. A single etiology is identified in fewer than 50% of cases (Camus et al. 2000; O'Keeffe and Lavan 1999). In frail elderly patients, Laurila et al. (2008) identified a mean of three etiologies per delirious patient, in addition to a mean of 5.2 predisposing factors. Etiological factors include primary cerebral disorders, systemic disturbances that affect cerebral function, drug and toxin exposure (including substance intoxication and withdrawal), and a range of factors that can contribute to delirium but have an uncertain etiological role by themselves (including psychological and environmental factors). An overview of etiological factors in delirium is shown in Table 4–4.

Some causes of delirium are more frequently encountered in particular populations. Delirium in children and adolescents involves the same categories of etiology

TABLE 4–3.   **Risk factors for incident delirium and odds ratios for the development of delirium**

Risk factor	Odds ratio (95% confidence interval)
High confidence	
Age over 65 years	3.03 (1.19–7.71)
Age over 80 years	5.22 (2.61–8.23)
Cognitive impairment	6.30 (2.89–13.74)
Vision impairment	1.70 (1.01–2.85)
Illness severity (APACHE II score)	3.49 (1.48–8.23)
Infection	2.96 (1.42–6.15)
Fracture on admission	6.57 (2.23–19.33)
Less confidence	
Vascular surgery	2.70 (1.72–4.24)
Comorbidity (>3 diseases)	15.94 (4.60–55.27)
Uncertain	
Polypharmacy (>3 medications)	33.60 (1.90–591.6)
Polypharmacy (>7 medications)	1.90 (1.11–3.24)
Dehydration	2.02 (0.72–5.64)
Electrolyte disturbance	2.40 (1.09–5.27)
Depression	2.43 (0.93–6.35)
Bladder catheter	2.70 (1.44–5.05)

Note.   APACHE II = Acute Physiology and Chronic Health Evaluation, version II (Knaus et al. 1985).

Source.   Adapted from National Institute for Health and Care Excellence 2010.

as in adults, although frequencies of specific causes differ. Delirium related to the use of illicit drugs is more common in younger populations, whereas delirium due to prescribed drugs and polypharmacy is more common in older populations. Cerebral hypoxia is common at age extremes: chronic obstructive airway disease, myocardial infarction, and stroke are more frequent in older patients, whereas instances of hypoxia due to foreign-body inhalation, drowning, and asthma are more frequent in younger patients. Poisonings are more common in children than in adults, and young adults have the highest rates of head trauma.

Prognostic Implications

The occurrence of delirium in hospital settings is associated with a number of negative outcomes, both during the hospital stay and after discharge. However, not all patients who experience delirium have poor outcomes. A systematic review identified 18 predictors of poor outcomes among patients with delirium (Jackson et al. 2016). Delirium-related predictors of poorer prognosis were hypoactive motor subtype and increased duration and severity of delirium and (in an emergency department population) a missed diagnosis of delirium. Among patient factors, psychiatric comorbidity, most importantly dementia and depression, was a predictor of worse outcomes.

TABLE 4–4.   Selected etiologies of delirium

Central nervous system (CNS) disease

Stroke

Seizures

CNS tumor

Subarachnoid hemorrhage

Cerebral edema

Meningitis, encephalitis

Hypertensive encephalopathy

Eclampsia

CNS vasculitis

CNS paraneoplastic syndrome

CNS HIV infection

Drug intoxication

Alcohol and other drugs of abuse

Sedative-hypnotics

Opioids, especially meperidine

Anticholinergics

Antihistamines

Corticosteroids

Drug withdrawal

Alcohol

Sedative-hypnotics

Hyperthermia

Heatstroke

Neuroleptic malignant syndrome

Malignant hyperthermia

Serotonin syndrome

Metabolic and endocrine disturbance

Hypoglycemia or hyperglycemia

Severe electrolyte disturbance

Acidosis or alkalosis

Hypoxia

Hypercapnia

Uremia

Severe endocrinopathy

Hepatic failure

Refeeding syndrome

Other metabolic disorders (e.g., porphyria, carcinoid syndrome)

Systemic conditions

Sepsis, bacteremia

Minor infection in dementia (e.g., urinary tract infection)

Acute graft rejection

Acute graft-versus-host disease

Shock

Postoperative state

Disseminated intravascular coagulation and other hypercoagulable states

Trauma

Traumatic brain injury

Subdural hematoma

Fat emboli

Infection

Pneumonia

Urinary tract infection

Wound infection

Other patient-related predictors were frailty, organ failure, hypoxia, acute kidney injury, and worse baseline functioning (Jackson et al. 2016).

These negative prognostic implications have been known for a long time, and several reviews have been published. The NICE clinical guideline reported findings from a meta-analysis examining outcomes in delirium, as well as prognostic factors related to delirium severity and duration (Table 4–5).

Hospitalized patients who experience delirium have longer hospital stays, higher numbers of hospital-acquired complications, and higher mortality rates. Cognitive impairment from delirium may persist beyond hospital discharge, increasing the risks for a subsequent diagnosis of dementia, functional deterioration with loss of independence, and nursing home admission. The relation between delirium and cognitive decline has been a topic of much discussion. Delirium could be a marker of vulnerability for dementia, or it may unmask unrecognized dementia. It may be that the effects of delirium on cognitive symptoms are solely due to effects of its underlying etiology, or delirium may itself cause neuronal damage (Fong et al. 2015). It is well established that cognitive decline and dementia are important and independent risk factors for delirium (Fong et al. 2015; National Institute for Health and Care Excellence 2010). Alternatively, delirium appears to be a risk factor for dementia (Fong et al. 2015). Clinically, the occurrence of delirium is often a first indicator of cognitive decline. It is often advised that cognitive screening should take place in patients not previously known to have cognitive deterioration after remission of delirium. In patients with Alzheimer's disease, delirium can result in a marked increase in cognitive dysfunction that seems to be irreversible (Fong et al. 2012, 2015).

Pathophysiology

Pathophysiological Hypotheses

Delirium is considered a unitary syndrome in which a variety of different etiological insults produce a relatively consistent syndrome of generalized disturbance in brain function that is thought to reflect widespread disturbance of neural networks. This heterogeneity in terms of causation suggests that delirium involves pathophysiological underpinnings that reflect complex interactions among direct brain insults, aberrant stress responses, and neuroinflammatory mechanisms (Maclullich et al. 2008; Maldonado 2013). Direct brain insults such as those caused by hypoxia, hypoglycemia, hypercapnia, hyponatremia, drug effects, stroke, and trauma directly disrupt brain functioning. However, delirium also results from peripheral disturbances (e.g., urinary tract infection) in which there is no obvious direct insult to the brain. In such cases, delirium is thought to represent an abnormal and exaggerated stress response that is possibly mediated through cytokines, dysregulation of the hypothalamic-pituitary-adrenal (HPA) axis and glucocorticoid levels, vagal transmission, and communication routes between the brain and the periphery. Such aberrant responses are more common in the aging or diseased brain; the two most potent constitutional risk factors for delirium are older age and preexisting dementia.

The delirious state is characterized by elevated cortisol levels; exogenous glucocorticoids are also known to precipitate delirium. Higher and more sustained elevations

TABLE 4–5. **Prognostic consequences of delirium**

Consequence	Odds ratio (95% confidence interval)	Follow-up
Presence or incidence of delirium		
Length of hospital stay	1.4 (1.1–1.9)	In hospital
Mortality	2.6 (0.7–6.2)	In hospital
Hospital-acquired complications	2.3 (1.7–5.0)	In hospital
Institutional placement	2.6 (0.8–8.5)	At discharge
Diagnosis of dementia	6.0 (1.8–19.5)	Assessed 3 years after discharge
Increased duration of delirium		
Length of hospital stay[a]	1.2 (1.1–1.3)	In hospital
Mortality[a]	1.1 (1.0–1.2)	6 months after discharge
Functional decline[a]	1.2 (1.0–1.4)	Assessed 6 months after discharge
Increased severity of delirium		
Mortality[a]	1.9 (1.1–3.1)	1 year after discharge

[a] Based on a single study.

Source.   Adapted from National Institute for Health and Care Excellence 2010.

of cortisol occur in older patients when they are confronted with acute stressors such as infection. Elevated glucocorticoids are thought to be linked to delirium through their interactions with monoaminergic neurotransmission, whereas the longer-term disturbances that are noted in many patients experiencing delirium may reflect the neurotoxic effects of sustained activation of the stress axis, which can cause or accelerate neurodegeneration (Maclullich et al. 2008).

Altered central nervous system immunoreactivity is also thought to be linked to delirium pathogenesis, whereby the combination of high levels or persistence of proinflammatory cytokines and reduced cerebral reserve is associated with delirium proneness (Androsova et al. 2015). Corroboration of this hypothesis is provided by the finding that delirium in children and older adults commonly occurs in response to relatively minor precipitating illnesses. Delirium often occurs in infectious states in which elevated cytokines are present, and therapeutic use of cytokines can also cause delirium. A further hypothesis is that cytokines exert their effects indirectly through activation of the HPA axis, resulting in the release of glucocorticoids, occupation of the low-affinity glucocorticoid receptor, and downregulation of inflammatory responses (Maclullich et al. 2008).

From a neurochemical perspective, the principal disturbances that are linked to delirium involve reduced cholinergic function and an absolute or relative excess of dopaminergic activity. Intoxication with dopaminergic drugs can cause delirium; elevated levels of plasma homovanillic acid (a dopaminergic metabolite) have been found during the delirious state (Ramirez-Bermudez et al. 2008). Dopamine-blocking antipsychotics are the most commonly used pharmacological intervention for delirium (Meagher et al. 2013). Similarly, in terms of cholinergic function, medications with anticholinergic effects are among the most common drug-related causes of delirium (Clegg and Young 2011), whereas delirium can sometimes be reversed by treatment with physostigmine (Dawson and Buckley 2016). Cholinergic function is reduced in states of hypoxia and hypoglycemia, which are recognized causes of delirium. Age-associated reductions in cholinergic function may underpin the increased delirium incidence with advanced age; dementia is characterized by reduced brain cholinergic activity. Dopaminergic and cholinergic mechanisms also interact, whereby D_2 receptor activation can inhibit cholinergic activity. There is also evidence for involvement of a variety of other neurochemical systems (e.g., γ-aminobutyric acid [GABA]ergic, glutamatergic, adrenergic) in delirium (Egberts et al. 2015; Fitzgerald et al. 2013), such that simple explanations are unlikely to provide a comprehensive account of the neurochemical mechanisms that underpin delirium.

Other studies have considered the potential influence of apolipoprotein E (ApoE) genotype as a risk factor for the development of delirium in elderly medical inpatients in ICU, surgery, and other medical settings, with conflicting results. A recent meta-analysis of eight studies (Adamis et al. 2016) found no relationship between ApoE and delirium.

Neuroimaging

A number of studies indicate that localized brain insults are associated with delirium. Early studies of electroconvulsive therapy–induced delirium in depressed elderly patients identified structural changes in the basal ganglia and white matter using magnetic resonance imaging (Figiel et al. 1990). More recent neuroimaging studies demonstrate the involvement of subcortical areas and indicate that white matter hyperintensities may be associated with delirium (Hatano et al. 2013; Morandi et al. 2012; Naidech et al. 2016; Omiya et al. 2015; Root et al. 2013). By contrast, other work points to the involvement of the brain cortex in delirium (Caeiro et al. 2004; Fong et al. 2006; Koponen et al. 1989). Given that cortical and subcortical areas of the brain are interconnected with long pathways, precise anatomical localization of delirium is difficult. Similarly, given that the clinical symptoms of delirium include disturbances of attention, arousal, and thought; cognitive problems; and disruption of the sleep–wake cycle, widespread involvement of both cortical and subcortical structures can be expected. A study by Choi et al. (2012) showed that reductions in functional connectivity of subcortical regions with frontal and prefrontal cortex may underlie the pathophysiology of delirium. An increased duration of delirium has also been associated with smaller frontal lobe and hippocampal volumes and worsening cognitive performance at 3- and 12-month follow-up (Gunther et al. 2012).

Electroencephalography and Evoked Potentials

For decades it has been known that the electroencephalogram shows generalized slowing of background activity during delirium (Jacobson et al. 1993). However, this pattern is also evident during sleep and in patients with dementia. Findings from studies that apply quantitative measures indicate that EEG profiling can differentiate dementia plus delirium from dementia alone with almost 90% accuracy (Thomas et al. 2008) and that EEG profiling can differentiate delirious from nondelirious subjects with up to 100% sensitivity and 96% specificity (van der Kooi et al. 2012, 2015). In a study using evoked potentials, Trzepacz et al. (1989) found evidence suggesting that the underlying pathophysiology of delirium may reside at the subcortical level. More recently, methods have been developed for monitoring the level of consciousness during anesthesia to ensure optimal dosing of anesthetic agents in order to reduce the risk of postoperative delirium. These methods include intraoperative measurement of EEG burst suppression (Fritz et al. 2016; Radtke et al. 2013) and brain monitoring with the Bispectral Index (Chan et al. 2013; Whitlock et al. 2014). The usefulness of EEG monitoring in everyday practical management of patients experiencing or at risk of developing delirium remains to be clarified.

Prevention of Delirium

Delirium is a highly predictable occurrence such that a variety of patient-, illness-, and treatment-related factors can allow for the identification of those who are most at risk. Table 4–6 provides a list of risk factors, many of which are highly modifiable (e.g., polypharmacy, active infection), whereas the presence of others (e.g., age, dementia) can inform the assessment of the risk–benefit balance of surgical and other interventions in deciding on optimal care. Awareness of these factors can also help to identify patients who require particularly close monitoring for emergent delirium and thus allows for early intervention in order to limit the secondary consequences of active delirium.

TABLE 4–6.   **Key considerations in the investigation of suspected delirium**

1. **Careful history and physical examination**

2. **Collateral history**
   Baseline cognition
   Presence of sensory impairments
   Exposure to risk factors
   Review of medications, procedures, tests, intraoperative data

3. **First-line investigations**
   Complete blood count
   Electrolytes, Mg, Ca, and PO_4 tests
   Liver function tests
   Urinalysis
   Electrocardiogram
   Erythrocyte sedimentation rate
   Blood glucose measurement
   Chest radiograph
   Urinalysis

4. **Second-line investigations (as indicated)**
   Drug screen
   Blood cultures
   Cardiac enzyme measurement
   Blood gas measurement
   Serum folate/B_{12} measurement
   Electroencephalography
   Cerebrospinal fluid examination
   Computed tomography of the brain
   Magnetic resonance imaging of the brain
   Prolactin level
   HIV antibodies test
   Syphilis serology
   Urinary porphyrins test

A variety of studies have demonstrated that improving staff awareness of the importance of delirium through proactive education—combined with formalized approaches to amelioration of identified risk factors, systematic screening for delirium, and patient-tailored treatment of emergent delirium—can reduce delirium incidence and, when delirium does occur, can lower its severity and duration, thereby reducing overall delirium-related mortality (Akunne et al. 2012). Of note, both pharmacological and nonpharmacological measures appear to be more effective in patients without dementia than in patients with dementia; however, the evidence to support a positive impact on longer-term outcomes, such as independence and mortality at 1-year follow-up, is relatively lacking.

Nonpharmacological Interventions

Primary prevention of delirium using nonpharmacological risk-reduction strategies has been demonstrated in elderly medical and surgical populations (Siddiqi et al. 2016). Moreover, when delirium occurs despite these efforts, it tends to be less severe and of shorter duration. Because a complex range of factors are involved in delirium causation, simple interventions (e.g., consensus guidelines, educational approaches) have limited impact compared with multifaceted interventions. A recent meta-analysis of 14 studies of multicomponent nonpharmacological interventions found that these strategies reduced delirium incidence by 44%, with significant reductions in falls and with a trend toward decreased lengths of hospital stay and reduced need for institutionalization (Hshieh et al. 2015). These interventions typically include efforts to assist in orientation, enhance sensory efficacy (e.g., encouraging patient to use their glasses or hearing aids), promote sleep, minimize pain, optimize physiological parameters (e.g., electrolytes, hydration), and foster physical therapy/mobilization. Many of these components are elements that should ideally be addressed as part of standard medical and nursing care; however, given the many competing pressures in modern health care, protocolization of these elements can enhance the quality of routine care provided in real-world settings.

Proactive reviews by specialist nurses, geriatricians, or geriatric or psychosomatic psychiatrists can further assist in ensuring that efforts are made to achieve optimal delirium-friendly care. The success of complex delirium prevention programs is linked to the degree of actual implementation of the various elements along with a variety of systems factors that include involvement of clinical leaders and support from senior management, integration of activities into everyday routines, and monitoring to promote continued adherence. These interventions are most successful when supported by activities that promote enthusiasm, support implementation, remove barriers, and allow for monitoring of progress (Yanamadala et al. 2013).

Pharmacological Prophylaxis

A series of studies have explored the impact of antipsychotic/antidopaminergic and procholinergic agents in prevention of delirium in high-risk populations. Some prospective work indicates that prophylactic use of low-dose typical or atypical antipsychotics may reduce delirium incidence, may reduce transition from subsyndromal delirium to full delirium, and/or may result in significantly shorter and less severe episodes when delirium does occur (Fok et al. 2015). However, the NICE clinical guideline concluded that evidence for pharmacological prevention was lacking (National Institute for Health and Care Excellence 2010). A recent review (Inouye et al. 2014a) likewise concluded that evidence for a positive impact of antipsychotic treatment on longer-term outcomes, such as duration of hospital stay and mortality rate, was lacking. Moreover, recent studies of prophylactic use of antipsychotics in ICU patients have not demonstrated a preventive effect on delirium (Al-Qadheeb et al. 2016; Page et al. 2013). Studies of cholinesterase inhibitors in delirium prevention trials also have not demonstrated benefit. Preliminary evidence supports the use of the α_2-adrenergic agonist dexmedetomidine as a less deliriogenic means of sedation, as well as the use of melatonin in elderly inpatients with medical illness, both of which strategies have been linked with reduced delirium incidence (Djaiani et al. 2016). Careful management of analgesia and/or sedation using protocolized care can also reduce delirium incidence (Dale et al. 2014; Skrobik et al. 2010).

Overall, the potential of pharmacological prophylaxis is appealing, but evidence to date does not yet support routine use, because of uncertainties in usefulness across patient populations, including high-risk elderly medical inpatients and patients with comorbid dementia.

Management of Delirium

General Principles

Delirium is a complex and multifaceted condition that requires collaboration between primary physicians, nursing staff, family/caregivers, and delirium specialists to achieve optimal outcomes. A fundamental challenge is to identify and treat the underlying causes of the episode while also addressing any problematic delirium symptoms, because both the severity of underlying physical morbidity and the severity of delirium symptoms are key predictors of outcome.

Identifying Underlying Causes

Identifying and treating the underlying causes of delirium are at the core of delirium care. Delirium is usually multifactorial, with typically three to four significant causative factors being relevant during any single episode that interact and overlap sequentially to produce or sustain delirium symptoms. Evaluation of a delirious patient thus requires a comprehensive assessment for multiple causes, beginning with a thorough history and examination, a collateral history to clarify baseline status and course of symptoms, and a review of recent medication exposure. The most common causes are infection, polypharmacy, and metabolic abnormalities (Laurila et al. 2008). No identifiable cause is detected in 10% of cases. Table 4–6 lists investigations that should be considered in all delirious patients, as well as other second-line investigations that are appropriate where clinical assessment and findings from preliminary tests suggest.

Nonpharmacological Management Strategies

The key principles of ward management of delirious patients include the following: 1) ensuring the safety of the patient and of those in his or her immediate environment; 2) minimizing the potential for complications such as falls, self-injury, and hypostasis; 3) simplifying the care environment to avoid excessive sensory stimulation; 4) minimizing the impact of any sensory impediments while promoting patient self-efficacy in terms of orientation and functional abilities; 5) promoting healthy sleep–wake patterns; and 6) minimizing pain. Communication with delirious patients should include simple language spoken in a clearly audible, slow-paced voice. The use of orienting techniques (e.g., calendars, night-lights, reorientation by staff) and familiar objects (e.g., family photographs) can make the environment easier to comprehend. Recovered delirium patients report that simple but firm communications, reality orientation, a visible clock, and the presence of a relative contributed to a heightened sense of control (Schofield 1997). Engaging family members in care can also help in clarifying changes from baseline status and understanding the meaning of symptoms, but it is important that relatives be educated about delirium and its management, given that ill-informed, critical, or anxious caregivers can add to patient burden. The challenges of providing an optimal care environment require a careful balance between the need to minimize risk and the provision of individualized, patient-focused care that promotes autonomy and dignity. For example, efforts to ensure the safety of delirious patients at risk of falls and wandering can result in restrictive care practices that inhibit reorientation, mobility, and self-efficacy. Less restrictive care can be facilitated by electronic alarms and pressure mats to monitor patient behavior and alert staff when vulnerable patients are at risk of wandering or falls.

Whereas many of the key elements of nonpharmacological interventions reflect careful attention to nursing care along with focused interdisciplinary collaboration, the highly pressurized environments of modern health care require specific formalized efforts to ensure that these practices are implemented. The application of both pharmacological and nonpharmacological interventions is more common in hyperactive than in hypoactive patients who present with problematic and challenging behaviors, which are more disruptive to patient care than the core cognitive disturbances of delirium. Hypoactive patients warrant particular concern given the evidence that these patients experience poorer outcomes (Meagher 2009).

Ensuring an optimal care environment for the delirious patient has obvious benefits in terms of maximizing the likelihood of achieving a full recovery and minimizing the deleterious impact of delirium on patients, their loved ones, and care providers. However, evidence that nonpharmacological interventions have an impact on established delirium is much less convincing than evidence for primary prevention. Existing research indicates that nonpharmacological treatments modestly influence the duration of delirium and possibly the length of inpatient stay, but longer-term outcomes such as discharge to independent living and mortality rates appear unaltered (Abraha et al. 2015). Much of this work has focused on delirium in frail elderly medical populations, in which the course of delirium may be less modifiable because of high rates of comorbid dementia. The degree of implementation of strategies is important, considering a recent meta-analysis finding that interventions for delirium that involve six or more strategies are most likely to reduce length of hospital stay and mortality (Trogrlić et al. 2017). Other studies have focused on the use of specialist delirium care units to manage more difficult or prolonged delirium. Preliminary findings suggest a positive impact on patient and caregiver experience, but without necessarily affecting outcomes such as length of hospital stay (Goldberg et al. 2013).

Pharmacological Interventions

Data on the pharmacological management of delirium in everyday practice are both controversial and highly inconsistent. Most suggested treatments derive from clinical experience with psychotropic agents used in the management of other neuropsychiatric conditions, especially psychotic disorders and dementia. The principal agents that have been studied are antipsychotics (both typical and atypical), benzodiazepines, procholinergics, and dexmedetomidine. The best evidence is for the use of antipsychotic agents, which remain the clinical standard and are mostly supported in treatment guidelines.

Antipsychotics

The use of antipsychotics is supported by a sizable number of prospective studies, which suggest that around 75% of delirious patients who receive short-term low-dose antipsychotic treatment experience clinical response (Meagher et al. 2013). Because delirium is a highly fluctuating, typically multifactorial condition that frequently re-mits with resolution of the primary insult, placebo-controlled studies are especially important in determining the value of interventions. However, such evidence is lack-ing in the variable findings of the four existing placebo-controlled studies; findings range from more rapid resolution of delirium in two small studies of quetiapine use in the ICU (Devlin et al. 2010) and in elderly medicine populations (Tahir et al. 2010) to no benefit from haloperidol and ziprasidone in an ICU setting (Girard et al. 2010) to poorer survival without any positive impact from either haloperidol or risperidone in a palliative care–based study (Agar et al. 2017).

There is a lack of high-quality evidence demonstrating benefits of antipsychotic use in terms of medium- and longer-term outcomes. In addition, antipsychotics are asso-ciated with a variety of risks, including sedation, hypotension, extrapyramidal side effects (EPS), and cardiotoxicity (e.g., QTc prolongation), as well as an increased risk of stroke in patients with dementia. As a consequence, decisions about medication use must be made on a case-by-case basis according to the needs of the individual patient.

Therefore, the use of antipsychotics in highly morbid patients with delirium re-quires careful consideration of the balance between likely benefits and risks of ad-verse effects. The actual documented rate of significant adverse effects in controlled studies is relatively low. A review of prospective studies of delirium treatment with antipsychotics concluded that the frequency of EPS was low, rising to 8% in studies that included a validated instrument (Meagher et al. 2013). In a retrospective analysis of 10 years of experience using haloperidol and quetiapine for delirium treatment in a cardiac care unit, Naksuk et al. (2017) found elevated mortality in patients with de-lirium, but this was not related to antipsychotic use, and they did not find any evi-dence of changes to mean QTc interval duration. In general, cardiac effects are rare when cumulative daily dosages of intravenous haloperidol remain lower than 2 mg, unless patients have additional risk factors for QTc prolongation (Meyer-Massetti et al. 2011). Other work has highlighted improvements in outcome when the care of de-lirious patients is protocolized to include dosage titration with regular monitoring of arousal, cardiac status, and EPS (Dale et al. 2014; Skrobik et al. 2010; Sullinger et al. 2017). Other effects are poorly studied; there are no systematic reports on the fre-quency of cerebrovascular incidents or metabolic effects.

Of note, there are uncertainties about the mechanism of action of antipsychotics in delirium. Antipsychotic treatment is more frequently used in patients with behav-ioral difficulties or hyperactivity, because many clinicians perceive the primary ther-apeutic effect of these agents as being sedative or antipsychotic, even though patient response is not closely linked to these actions (Meagher et al. 2010). The NICE clinical guideline recommended cautious use of olanzapine or haloperidol (Young et al. 2010), and such interventions are justified when a patient is experiencing severe agi-tation or psychosis or when a patient's delirium symptoms are impeding provision of optimal care in terms of essential treatments, as well as in situations involving signif-icant risk of physical harm to the patient or others.

Although studies do not suggest significant differences in efficacy between haloperidol and atypical antipsychotics, haloperidol is associated with a higher rate of EPS. Commonly used agents include risperidone (starting dosage 0.25 mg/day), olanzapine (starting dosage 2.5 mg/day), quetiapine (starting dosage 12.5 mg/day), and haloperidol (starting dosage 0.5 mg/day). Of these agents, quetiapine is relatively more sedating, whereas haloperidol offers more flexibility of administration, with both oral and parenteral formulations available. The option to administer haloperidol intravenously represents an important advantage over the atypical antipsychotics. Best-practice recommendations are to "start low and go slow," with dosage titration according to response and adverse effects. Only rarely do patients require extremely high doses of haloperidol. Treatment is short-term and is typically discontinued after 3–5 days.

Other Agents

Benzodiazepines are the first-line treatment for delirium caused by alcohol or sedative withdrawal states or seizures, but they are otherwise best avoided, as they can perpetuate delirium, cloud ongoing cognitive assessment, and lead to falls, oversedation, and respiratory depression (Clegg and Young 2011; Lonergan et al. 2009). Procholinergic treatments have theoretical appeal, given the link between delirium and hypocholinergic states, but cholinesterase inhibitors do not appear to be effective in the management of acute delirium episodes (van Eijk et al. 2010). A recent review of seven trials of cholinesterase inhibitors found that in five of the studies, there was no benefit from the medications for either prevention or management of delirium (Tampi et al. 2016). Preliminary evidence suggests that dexmedetomidine, an α_2-adrenergic agonist, may be useful as a rescue drug for treating delirium-related agitation in nonintubated patients in whom haloperidol has failed (Carrasco et al. 2016).

Patient Perspectives

Recently, there has been more interest in the patients' subjective experience of delirium and the challenges that patients face coping with delirium once it has resolved. There also has been more interest in the experience of family members. Better understanding of these experiences may lead to more empathic, and possibly more effective, care of patients.

The Delirium Experience

One-third to one-half of patients who experience delirium can recall the delirious episode afterward (Breitbart et al. 2002; Grover et al. 2015; Morandi et al. 2015). Recall of delirium is associated with increased severity of delirious symptoms, notably visual hallucinations and language disturbances (Grover et al. 2015). Patients who do recall the episode describe a highly distressing and fearful experience. Symptoms that are reported as most distressing are anxiety and fear, disorientation, (paranoid) delusions, and hypokinesia (Morandi et al. 2015). Some patients will develop acute or posttraumatic stress disorder after remission of the delirium. The reported incidence of posttraumatic stress disorder after a delirium episode varies widely among studies, from no increased incidence to up to 14% of patients (O'Malley et al. 2008; Svenningsen et al. 2015).

In qualitative research, several themes consistently emerge that characterize patients' feelings, thoughts, and experiences during the delirious state (Lingehall et al. 2015; Pollard et al. 2015; Whitehorne et al. 2015). The first of these themes involves *concerns about fear and safety.* Delirious patients often cannot understand what is going on around them and may refuse interventions. They may become paranoid and distrustful, both toward hospital staff and toward family members. Interventions are sometimes perceived by patients as part of a plot to harm them. Such perceptions can lead patients to actively oppose necessary treatment by refusing medication or removing catheters, lines, or tubes, or even by trying to escape from the hospital. Second, because of problems with concentrating and thinking clearly, as well as hallucinations and delusions, patients may have *problems differentiating between what is real and what is not.* They can become preoccupied with trying to "get things straight," and their ability to communicate can be reduced, which increases feelings of distrust and forms a barrier to seeking explanations from staff or family members. Often patients search for cues in the environment to help them understand where they are and what is happening. Finally, many patients describe delirium as a very *solitary experience.* Patients feel disconnected or separated from others who are around them. Not only are they physically separated from loved ones because of the hospital admission, but they also feel that they are not understood, especially when staff and family members do not go along with their delusional thoughts or hallucinations. Sometimes feelings of disconnection are increased by intubation, tracheotomy, or restraints. Patients can feel powerless and overwhelmed.

Coping With the Aftermath of Delirium

After remission of the delirium, many patients feel embarrassment or shame about their behavior and try to make sense of it. They frequently stress that they would normally not behave like they did and try to distance themselves from their behavior (Pollard et al. 2015). They often have the urge to apologize to staff and family members for their behavior and have feelings of guilt, even though they know that their behavior was not intentional but was due to the delirium. Sometimes patients cannot remember which staff members they offended and do not know to whom they might apologize, a dilemma that is experienced as especially embarrassing.

Memories of the delirium experience may come back in "flashes." Such recollections can lead patients to worry about being perceived as weird or abnormal or to fear that the experience is indicative of a "mental condition." Patients also dread a recurrence of delirium and may avoid, or plan to avoid, situations that might trigger a further episode. Because of such reactions, patients may fear future surgery or may avoid or refuse certain medications, such as sleeping pills (Whitehorne et al. 2015). Discussions with medical and/or nursing staff can help patients to accurately understand what has happened and its significance for ongoing care.

The Caregiver Experience

Partners, caregivers, and family members of patients find the experience of delirium in their loved one to be very stressful. They do not recognize their loved one's demeanor and behavior, which may be bizarre and out of character. They may fear that the patient has "gone mad" or will develop a permanent psychiatric disorder or dementia. Family members may feel confused or challenged about how to respond to the sudden changes in the patient's behavior. They may want to help the patient by being close and supportive, but despite this need for human contact, the meaning of interactions is often distorted or impaired, which can make the family feel frustrated or powerless (Whitehorne et al. 2015). Also, after remission of the delirium, there may be extended worries of recurrence.

Helping Patients and Families Cope

Given the distressing nature of delirium for all concerned, information and support from clinicians may help patients and family members to cope with the experience of delirium. Patients at risk of delirium may benefit from receiving both oral and written information about delirium before elective admissions or prior to surgery. Early recognition and treatment of delirium may reduce the severity of delirious symptoms and thus reduce levels of distress. When patients become delirious, they may benefit from (repeated) explanations about delirium. Family members may also benefit from information as well as guidance on how to deal with the most distressing symptoms. After recovering from delirium, patients should be given the opportunity to discuss their experience with their doctor or the nursing staff. Such conversations should be supportive, and discussions about feelings of shame and guilt should not be avoided. Worries of recurrence should also be addressed. Follow-up appointments should be offered for patients with continuing emotional distress or persistent cognitive symptoms (Pollard et al. 2015).

Organizing Care for Delirium

Given the high prevalence and the negative prognostic and financial consequences of delirium, identification and treatment of delirium warrants a systematic and hospital-wide approach. Such an approach requires active collaboration and communication between nurses and physicians, and it is essential that clear agreement exists about each discipline's responsibilities. Nurses will usually play the most important role in screening and initial identification of delirium, as well as administering nonpharmacological treatment, providing information, and supporting patients and their relatives. Physicians will usually confirm the diagnosis, investigate and treat underlying conditions, and take responsibility for pharmacological treatment. Both nurses and physicians will be responsible for following up with delirious patients. Where available, nurse practitioners or physician assistants may assume some of the physicians' responsibilities. The organization of delirium care may be different across institutions and settings.

Whereas clinical guidelines provide recommendations on screening and identification, as well as on nonpharmacological and pharmacological treatment of delirium, they provide little guidance on how best to implement these recommendations in daily clinical routines. A recent systematic appraisal of clinical practice guidelines identified "applicability" as the weakest component of guidelines. *Applicability* in this context refers to identification of facilitators of and barriers to implementation, provision of implementation tools, dissemination of advice on how to put the recommendations into practice, consideration of resource implications, and implementation of monitoring and/or audit recommendations (Bush et al. 2017).

Barriers to Guideline Implementation

Factors recognized as barriers to implementation of guideline recommendations include knowledge deficits and lack of skills; lack of motivation; workload concerns and documentation burden; professional role opinions; lack of communication and collaboration, especially between doctors and nurses; and insufficient resources (Balas et al. 2013; Collinsworth et al. 2016; Trogrlić et al. 2017; van de Steeg et al. 2014). Knowledge about delirium and the use of delirium rating scales differs across different professions and settings. Especially in nurses, Trogrlić et al. (2017) reported low familiarity with delirium guidelines and disbelief that patients would receive optimal care when adhering to guidelines, lack of trust in delirium screening tools, and the belief that delirium is not preventable. Some nurses felt inadequately confident administering delirium screening instruments. Studies also show that nurses may lack the motivation to systematically use these screening instruments because of a lack of clarity about the goals and benefits of screening (Trogrlić et al. 2017; van de Steeg et al. 2014). In such circumstances, nursing staff may view screening as yet another imposed administrative registration or checklist. They also expect that screening will increase their workload (Balas et al. 2013; van de Steeg et al. 2014). Thus, screening procedures are the first activities that are omitted when time is short (van de Steeg et al. 2014). With respect to the professional role of nurses, it is reported that they may not consider screening as part of essential care for (older) patients (van de Steeg et al. 2014) and may feel that using screening instruments limits their autonomy. However, other nurses reported that the use of a delirium screening instrument, such as the DOS scale, strengthened their position when communicating with doctors. This increased credibility could be a facilitator of implementation (van de Steeg et al. 2014). Doctor–patient communication was also mentioned as a potential barrier, as well as nurse dissatisfaction with physician-prescribed delirium management (Balas et al. 2013; Trogrlić et al. 2017).

Facilitating Implementation

Studies that have examined factors that can facilitate implementation of guideline recommendations report remarkably similar findings. Guidelines can be more successfully implemented when all relevant stakeholders are involved in the development of both the guideline and its implementation plan. Agreement about assignment of tasks and responsibilities to certain disciplines should be obtained and spelled out in a local protocol. Multidisciplinary collaboration is essential to better appreciate the contribution and diverse expertise between disciplines and to increase respect among disciplines. Such collaboration can be achieved through engagement of staff from different backgrounds as project leaders (e.g., nurses, physicians, pharmacy staff, rehabilitation staff), formation of a multidisciplinary treatment team, and use of interdisciplinary rounds in which delirium screening results are discussed and a joint care plan is made for delirious patients.

Moreover, studies stress the importance of sustained and diverse educational efforts (Balas et al. 2013; Davies et al. 2008; Trogrlić et al. 2017; van de Steeg et al. 2014). Education can address faulty beliefs about the prognosis of delirium, the efficacy of prevention strategies, the evidence base of guidelines, and the validity of delirium screening tools. The organization should support staff attendance at educational sessions by providing staff replacement time. Education may take different forms, including classical teaching sessions, e-learning modules, and bedside teaching (Davies et al. 2008). Ongoing audits with feedback to staff may increase awareness of the benefits of using screening tools and of following guidelines and may help sustain motivation for long-term adherence. Finally, concerns about increased workload and registration burden should be addressed, and when possible, changes should be facilitated. Software adjustments can reduce workloads, and in particular can remove the need for duplicate data entry of the same information (e.g., first screening with paper and pencil before entering data in the electronic medical record).

Conclusion

Delirium is the most prevalent psychiatric syndrome in general hospitals. Historically understudied, in recent times, delirium has received increasing attention, both in clinical practice and in research. Progress has been made in understanding the epidemiology, etiology, course and prognosis, prevention, and treatment of delirium. Evidence-based guidelines are available that summarize current knowledge and facilitate a rational approach to recognition and treatment. In spite of this increased attention, many basic and clinical aspects of delirium remain poorly understood. Although a number of biomarkers have been associated with delirium, delirium's fundamental pathophysiological basis remains obscure. The biggest challenge clinically is how to incorporate preventive measures, screening procedures, and early treatment into routine clinical practice in an efficacious and cost-effective way. In particular, regular formal screening for delirium can allow for more timely recognition in everyday practice. Further research is needed to compare the efficacy of different approaches in order to improve clinical practice and to study whether long-term complications, such as cognitive decline, can be prevented.

References

Abraha I, Trotta F, Rimland JM, et al: Efficacy of non-pharmacological interventions to prevent and treat delirium in older patients: a systematic overview. The SENATOR project ONTOP Series. PLoS One 10(6):e0123090, 2015 26062023

Adamis D, Treloar A, Martin FC, et al: A brief review of the history of delirium as a mental disorder. Hist Psychiatry 18(72 Pt 4):459–469, 2007 18590023

Adamis D, Meagher D, Williams J, et al: A systematic review and meta-analysis of the association between the apolipoprotein E genotype and delirium. Psychiatr Genet 26(2):53–59, 2016 26901792

Agar MR, Lawlor PG, Quinn S, et al: Efficacy of oral risperidone, haloperidol, or placebo for symptoms of delirium among patients in palliative care: a randomized clinical trial. JAMA Intern Med 177(1):34–42, 2017 27918778

Akunne A, Murthy L, Young J: Cost-effectiveness of multi-component interventions to prevent delirium in older people admitted to medical wards. Age Ageing 41(3):285–291, 2012 22282171

Alexopoulos GS, Abrams RC, Young RC, et al: Cornell Scale for Depression in Dementia. Biol Psychiatry 23(3):271–284, 1988 3337862

Al-Qadheeb NS, Skrobik Y, Schumaker G, et al: Preventing ICU subsyndromal delirium conversion to delirium with low-dose IV haloperidol: a double-blind, placebo-controlled pilot study. Crit Care Med 44(3):583–591, 2016 26540397

American Psychiatric Association: Diagnostic and Statistical Manual of Mental Disorders, 3rd Edition. Washington, DC, American Psychiatric Association, 1980

American Psychiatric Association: Diagnostic and Statistical Manual of Mental Disorders, 3rd Edition, Revised. Washington, DC, American Psychiatric Association, 1987

American Psychiatric Association: Diagnostic and Statistical Manual of Mental Disorders, 4th Edition, Revised. Washington, DC, American Psychiatric Association, 1994

American Psychiatric Association: Diagnostic and Statistical Manual of Mental Disorders, 5th Edition. Arlington, VA, American Psychiatric Association, 2013

Anderson CP, Ngo LH, Marcantonio ER: Complications in postacute care are associated with persistent delirium. J Am Geriatr Soc 60(6):1122–1127, 2012 22646692

Androsova G, Krause R, Winterer G, et al: Biomarkers of postoperative delirium and cognitive dysfunction. Front Aging Neurosci 7:112, 2015 26106326

Balas MC, Burke WJ, Gannon D, et al: Implementing the awakening and breathing coordination, delirium monitoring/management, and early exercise/mobility bundle into everyday care: opportunities, challenges, and lessons learned for implementing the ICU Pain, Agitation, and Delirium Guidelines. Crit Care Med 41 (9 suppl 1):S116–S127, 2013 23989089

Bellelli G, Morandi A, Davis DH, et al: Validation of the 4AT, a new instrument for rapid delirium screening: a study in 234 hospitalised older people. Age Ageing 43(4):496–502, 2014 24590568

Bellelli G, Morandi A, Di Santo SG, et al; Italian Study Group on Delirium (ISGoD): "Delirium Day": a nationwide point prevalence study of delirium in older hospitalized patients using an easy standardized diagnostic tool. BMC Med 14:106, 2016 27430902

Breitbart W, Rosenfeld B, Roth A, et al: The Memorial Delirium Assessment Scale. J Pain Symptom Manage 13(3):128–137, 1997 9114631

Breitbart W, Gibson C, Tremblay A: The delirium experience: delirium recall and delirium-related distress in hospitalized patients with cancer, their spouses/caregivers, and their nurses. Psychosomatics 43(3):183–194, 2002 12075033

Bush SH, Marchington KL, Agar M, et al: Quality of clinical practice guidelines in delirium: a systematic appraisal. BMJ Open 7(3):e013809, 2017 28283488

Caeiro L, Ferro JM, Albuquerque R, et al: Delirium in the first days of acute stroke. J Neurol 251(2):171–178, 2004 14991351

Camus V, Gonthier R, Dubos G, et al: Etiologic and outcome profiles in hypoactive and hyperactive subtypes of delirium. J Geriatr Psychiatry Neurol 13(1):38–42, 2000 10753006

Carrasco G, Baeza N, Cabré L, et al: Dexmedetomidine for the treatment of hyperactive delirium refractory to haloperidol in nonintubated ICU patients: a nonrandomized controlled trial. Crit Care Med 44(7):1295–1306, 2016 26925523

Chan MT, Cheng BC, Lee TM, Gin T; CODA Trial Group: BIS-guided anesthesia decreases postoperative delirium and cognitive decline. J Neurosurg Anesthesiol 25(1):33–42, 2013 23027226

Choi SH, Lee H, Chung TS, et al: Neural network functional connectivity during and after an episode of delirium. Am J Psychiatry 169(5):498–507, 2012 22549209

Clegg A, Young JB: Which medications to avoid in people at risk of delirium: a systematic review. Age Ageing 40(1):23–29, 2011 21068014

Cole MG, Ciampi A, Belzile E, et al: Persistent delirium in older hospital patients: a systematic review of frequency and prognosis. Age Ageing 38(1):19–26, 2009 19017678

Collinsworth AW, Priest EL, Campbell CR, et al: A review of multifaceted care approaches for the prevention and mitigation of delirium in intensive care units. J Intensive Care Med 31(2):127–141, 2016 25348864

Dale CR, Kannas DA, Fan VS, et al: Improved analgesia, sedation, and delirium protocol associated with decreased duration of delirium and mechanical ventilation. Ann Am Thorac Soc 11(3):367–374, 2014 24597599

Dasgupta M, Hillier LM: Factors associated with prolonged delirium: a systematic review. Int Psychogeriatr 22(3):373–394, 2010 20092663

Davies B, Edwards N, Ploeg J, et al: Insights about the process and impact of implementing nursing guidelines on delivery of care in hospitals and community settings. BMC Health Serv Res 8:29, 2008 18241349

Dawson AH, Buckley NA: Pharmacological management of anticholinergic delirium—theory, evidence and practice. Br J Clin Pharmacol 81(3):516–524, 2016 26589572

De J, Wand AP: Delirium screening: a systematic review of delirium screening tools in hospitalized patients. Gerontologist 55(6):1079–1099, 2015 26543179

De J, Wand AP, Smerdely PI, Hunt GE: Validating the 4A's test in screening for delirium in a culturally diverse geriatric inpatient population. Int J Geriatr Psychiatry 32(12):1322–1329, 2017 27766672

de Lange E, Verhaak PF, van der Meer K: Prevalence, presentation and prognosis of delirium in older people in the population, at home and in long term care: a review. Int J Geriatr Psychiatry 28(2):127–134, 2013 22513757

Devlin JW, Roberts RJ, Fong JJ, et al: Efficacy and safety of quetiapine in critically ill patients with delirium: a prospective, multicenter, randomized, double-blind, placebo-controlled pilot study. Crit Care Med 38(2):419–427, 2010 19915454

Djaiani G, Silverton N, Fedorko L, et al: Dexmedetomidine versus propofol sedation reduces delirium after cardiac surgery: a randomized controlled trial. J Am Soc Anesthesiol 124(2):362–368, 2016 26575144

Egberts A, Fekkes D, Wijnbeld EH, et al: Disturbed serotonergic neurotransmission and oxidative stress in elderly patients with delirium. Dement Geriatr Cogn Dis Extra 5(3):450–458, 2015 26955379

Ely EW, Margolin R, Francis J, et al: Evaluation of delirium in critically ill patients: validation of the Confusion Assessment Method for the Intensive Care Unit (CAM-ICU). Crit Care Med 29(7):1370–1379, 2001 11445689

European Delirium Association, American Delirium Society: The DSM-5 criteria, level of arousal and delirium diagnosis: inclusiveness is safer. BMC Med 12:141, 2014 25300023

Figiel GS, Coffey CE, Djang WT, et al: Brain magnetic resonance imaging findings in ECT-induced delirium. J Neuropsychiatry Clin Neurosci 2(1):53–58, 1990 2136061

Fitzgerald JM, Adamis D, Trzepacz PT, et al: Delirium: a disturbance of circadian integrity? Med Hypotheses 81(4):568–576, 2013 23916192

Fok MC, Sepehry AA, Frisch L, et al: Do antipsychotics prevent postoperative delirium? A systematic review and meta-analysis. Int J Geriatr Psychiatry 30(4):333–344, 2015 25639958

Folstein MF, Bassett SS, Romanoski AJ, et al: The epidemiology of delirium in the community: the Eastern Baltimore Mental Health Survey. Int Psychogeriatr 3(2):169–176, 1991 1811771

Fong TG, Bogardus ST Jr, Daftary A, et al: Cerebral perfusion changes in older delirious patients using 99mTc HMPAO SPECT. J Gerontol A Biol Sci Med Sci 61(12):1294–1299, 2006 17234823

Fong TG, Jones RN, Marcantonio ER, et al: Adverse outcomes after hospitalization and delirium in persons with Alzheimer disease. Ann Intern Med 156(12):848–856, W296, 2012 22711077

Fong TG, Davis D, Growdon ME, et al: The interface between delirium and dementia in elderly adults. Lancet Neurol 14(8):823–832, 2015 26139023

Franco JG, Trzepacz PT, Meagher DJ, et al: Three core domains of delirium validated using exploratory and confirmatory factor analyses. Psychosomatics 54(3):227–238, 2013 23218057

Fritz BA, Kalarickal PL, Maybrier HR, et al: Intraoperative electroencephalogram suppression predicts postoperative delirium. Anesth Analg 122(1):234–242, 2016 26418126

Gaudreau JD, Gagnon P, Harel F, et al: Fast, systematic, and continuous delirium assessment in hospitalized patients: the Nursing Delirium Screening Scale. J Pain Symptom Manage 29(4):368–375, 2005 15857740

Girard TD, Pandharipande PP, Carson SS, et al; MIND Trial Investigators: Feasibility, efficacy, and safety of antipsychotics for intensive care unit delirium: the MIND randomized, placebo-controlled trial. Crit Care Med 38(2):428–437, 2010 20095068

Goldberg SE, Bradshaw LE, Kearney FC, et al; Medical Crises in Older People Study Group: Care in specialist medical and mental health unit compared with standard care for older people with cognitive impairment admitted to general hospital: randomised controlled trial (NIHR TEAM trial). BMJ 347:f4132, 2013 23819964

Gore RL, Vardy ER, O'Brien JT: Delirium and dementia with Lewy bodies: distinct diagnoses or part of the same spectrum? J Neurol Neurosurg Psychiatry 86(1):50–59, 2015 24860139

Grover S, Ghosh A, Ghormode D: Experience in delirium: is it distressing? J Neuropsychiatry Clin Neurosci 27(2):139–146, 2015 25162511

Gunther ML, Morandi A, Krauskopf E, et al: The association between brain volumes, delirium duration and cognitive outcomes in intensive care unit survivors: a prospective exploratory cohort magnetic resonance imaging study. Crit Care Med 40:2022–2032, 2012 22710202

Hart RP, Levenson JL, Sessler CN, et al: Validation of a cognitive test for delirium in medical ICU patients. Psychosomatics 37(6):533–546, 1996 8942204

Hatano Y, Narumoto J, Shibata K, et al: White-matter hyperintensities predict delirium after cardiac surgery. Am J Geriatr Psychiatry 21(10):938–945, 2013 24029014

Hshieh TT, Yue J, Oh E, et al: Effectiveness of multicomponent nonpharmacological delirium interventions: a meta-analysis. JAMA Intern Med 175(4):512–520, 2015 25643002

Inouye SK: Predisposing and precipitating factors for delirium in hospitalized older patients. Dement Geriatr Cogn Disord 10(5):393–400, 1999 10473946

Inouye SK, van Dyck CH, Alessi CA, et al: Clarifying confusion: the confusion assessment method. A new method for detection of delirium. Ann Intern Med 113(12):941–948, 1990 2240918

Inouye SK, Schlesinger MJ, Lydon TJ: Delirium: a symptom of how hospital care is failing older persons and a window to improve quality of hospital care. Am J Med 106(5):565–573, 1999 10335730

Inouye SK, Marcantonio ER, Metzger ED: Doing damage in delirium: the hazards of antipsychotic treatment in elderly persons. Lancet Psychiatry 1(4):312–315, 2014a 25285270

Inouye SK, Westendorp RG, Saczynski JS: Delirium in elderly people. Lancet 383(9920):911–922, 2014b 23992774

Jackson TA, Wilson D, Richardson S, et al: Predicting outcome in older hospital patients with delirium: a systematic literature review. Int J Geriatr Psychiatry 31(4):392–399, 2016 26302258

Jacobowski NL, Heckers S, Bobo WV: Delirious mania: detection, diagnosis, and clinical management in the acute setting. J Psychiatr Pract 19(1):15–28, 2013 23334676

Jacobson SA, Leuchter AF, Walter DO: Conventional and quantitative EEG in the diagnosis of delirium among the elderly. J Neurol Neurosurg Psychiatry 56(2):153–158, 1993 8437004

Jorm AF: The Informant Questionnaire on cognitive decline in the elderly (IQCODE): a review. Int Psychogeriatr 16(3):275–293, 2004 15559753

Kiely DK, Marcantonio ER, Inouye SK, et al: Persistent delirium predicts greater mortality. J Am Geriatr Soc 57(1):55–61, 2009 19170790

Knaus WA, Draper EA, Wagner DP, Zimmerman JE: APACHE II: a severity of disease classification system. Crit Care Med 13(10):818–829, 1985 3928249

Koponen H, Hurri L, Stenbäck U, et al: Computed tomography findings in delirium. J Nerv Ment Dis 177(4):226–231, 1989 2703827

Koster S, Hensens AG, Oosterveld FG, et al: The delirium observation screening scale recognizes delirium early after cardiac surgery. Eur J Cardiovasc Nurs 8(4):309–314, 2009 19285452

Kuczmarska A, Ngo LH, Guess J, et al: Detection of delirium in hospitalized older general medicine patients: a comparison of the 3D-CAM and CAM-ICU. J Gen Intern Med 31(3):297–303, 2016 26443577

Kuladee S, Prachason T: Development and validation of the Thai version of the 4 'A's Test for delirium screening in hospitalized elderly patients with acute medical illnesses. Neuropsychiatr Dis Treat 24:437–443, 2016 26966365

Laurila JV, Pitkala KH, Strandberg TE, et al: Impact of different diagnostic criteria on prognosis of delirium: a prospective study. Dement Geriatr Cogn Disord 18(3–4):240–244, 2004 15286453

Laurila JV, Laakkonen M-L, Tilvis RS, et al: Predisposing and precipitating factors for delirium in a frail geriatric population. J Psychosom Res 65(3):249–254, 2008 18707947

Leonard M, McInerney S, McFarland J, et al: Comparison of cognitive and neuropsychiatric profiles in hospitalised elderly medical patients with delirium, dementia and comorbid delirium-dementia. BMJ Open 6(3):e009212, 2016 26956160

Leslie DL, Zhang Y, Bogardus ST, et al: Consequences of preventing delirium in hospitalized older adults on nursing home costs. J Am Geriatr Soc 53(3):405–409, 2005 15743281

Leung Jl, Leung Vc, Leung CM, et al: Clinical utility and validation of two instruments (the Confusion Assessment Method Algorithm and the Chinese version of Nursing Delirium Screening Scale) to detect delirium in geriatric inpatients. Gen Hosp Psychiatry 30(2):171–176, 2008 18291299

Lingehall HC, Smulter N, Engström KG, et al: Validation of the Swedish version of the Nursing Delirium Screening Scale used in patients 70 years and older undergoing cardiac surgery. J Clin Nurs 22(19–20):2858–2866, 2013 24033713

Lingehall HC, Smulter N, Olofsson B, et al: Experiences of undergoing cardiac surgery among older people diagnosed with postoperative delirium: one year follow-up. BMC Nurs 14:17, 2015 25866476

Lonergan E, Luxenberg J, Areosa Sastre A: Benzodiazepines for delirium. Cochrane Database Syst Rev (4):CD006379, 2009 19821364

Luetz A, Heymann A, Radtke FM, et al: Different assessment tools for intensive care unit delirium: which score to use? Crit Care Med 38(2):409–418, 2010 20029345

Maclullich AM, Ferguson KJ, Miller T, et al: Unravelling the pathophysiology of delirium: a focus on the role of aberrant stress responses. J Psychosom Res 65(3):229–238, 2008 18707945

Maldonado JR: Neuropathogenesis of delirium: review of current etiologic theories and common pathways. Am J Geriatr Psychiatry 21(12):1190–1222, 2013 24206937

Marcantonio ER, Ngo LH, O'Connor M, et al: 3D-CAM: derivation and validation of a 3-minute diagnostic interview for CAM-defined delirium: a cross-sectional diagnostic test study. Ann Intern Med 161(8):554–561, 2014 25329203

Meagher D: Motor subtypes of delirium: past, present and future. Int Rev Psychiatry 21(1):59–73, 2009 19219713

Meagher DJ, Leonard M: The active management of delirium: improving detection and treatment. Advances in Psychiatric Treatment 14(4):292–301, 2008

Meagher DJ, Leonard M, Donnelly S, et al: A comparison of neuropsychiatric and cognitive profiles in delirium, dementia, comorbid delirium-dementia and cognitively intact controls. J Neurol Neurosurg Psychiatry 81(8):876–881, 2010 20587481

Meagher DJ, McLoughlin L, Leonard M, et al: What do we really know about the treatment of delirium with antipsychotics? Ten key issues for delirium pharmacotherapy. Am J Geriatr Psychiatry 21(12):1223–1238, 2013 23567421

Meagher D, Adamis D, Leonard M, et al: Development of an abbreviated version of the delirium motor subtyping scale (DMSS-4). Int Psychogeriatr 26(4):693–702, 2014a 24429062

Meagher DJ, Morandi A, Inouye SK, et al: Concordance between DSM-IV and DSM-5 criteria for delirium diagnosis in a pooled database of 768 prospectively evaluated patients using the delirium rating scale-revised-98. BMC Med 12:164, 2014b 25266390

Meyer-Massetti C, Vaerini S, Rätz Bravo AE, et al: Comparative safety of antipsychotics in the WHO pharmacovigilance database: the haloperidol case. Int J Clin Pharm 33(5):806–814, 2011 21809143

Milbrandt EB, Deppen S, Harrison PL, et al: Costs associated with delirium in mechanically ventilated patients. Crit Care Med 32(4):955–962, 2004 15071384

Miu DK, Chan CW, Kok C: Delirium among elderly patients admitted to a post-acute care facility and 3-months outcome. Geriatr Gerontol Int 16(5):586–592, 2016 26044170

Morandi A, Rogers BP, Gunther ML, et al; VISIONS Investigation, VISualizing Icu SurvivOrs Neuroradiological Sequelae: The relationship between delirium duration, white matter integrity, and cognitive impairment in intensive care unit survivors as determined by diffusion tensor imaging: the VISIONS prospective cohort magnetic resonance imaging study. Crit Care Med 40(7):2182–2189, 2012 22584766

Morandi A, Davis D, Taylor JK, et al: Consensus and variations in opinions on delirium care: a survey of European delirium specialists. Int Psychogeriatr 25(12):2067–2075, 2013 23962713

Morandi A, Lucchi E, Turco R, et al: Delirium superimposed on dementia: a quantitative and qualitative evaluation of informal caregivers and health care staff experience. J Psychosom Res 79(4):272–280, 2015 26286892

Morandi A, Han JH, Meagher D, et al: Detecting delirium superimposed on dementia: evaluation of the diagnostic performance of the Richmond Agitation and Sedation Scale. J Am Med Dir Assoc 17(9):828–833, 2016 27346621

Naidech AM, Polnaszek KL, Berman MD, et al: Hematoma locations predicting delirium symptoms after intracerebral hemorrhage. Neurocrit Care 24(3):397–403, 2016 26503511

Naksuk N, Thongprayoon C, Park JY, et al: Editor's Choice—Clinical impact of delirium and antipsychotic therapy: 10-year experience from a referral coronary care unit. Eur Heart J Acute Cardiovasc Care 6(6):560–668, 2017 26124454

National Institute for Health and Care Excellence: Delirium: Prevention, Diagnosis and Management. NICE Clinical Guideline 103. London, National Institute for Health and Care Excellence, 2010. Available at: https://www.nice.org.uk/guidance/cg103/evidence/full-guideline-pdf-134653069. Accessed November 10, 2017.

Neufeld KJ, Leoutsakos JS, Sieber FE, et al: Evaluation of two delirium screening tools for detecting post-operative delirium in the elderly. Br J Anaesth 111(4):612–618, 2013 23657522

O'Hanlon S, O'Regan N, Maclullich AM, et al: Improving delirium care through early intervention: from bench to bedside to boardroom. J Neurol Neurosurg Psychiatry 85(2):207–213, 2014 23355807

O'Keeffe ST, Lavan JN: Clinical significance of delirium subtypes in older people. Age Ageing 28(2):115–119, 1999 10350406

O'Malley G, Leonard M, Meagher D, et al: The delirium experience: a review. J Psychosom Res 65(3):223–228, 2008 18707944

Omiya H, Yoshitani K, Yamada N, et al: Preoperative brain magnetic resonance imaging and postoperative delirium after off-pump coronary artery bypass grafting: a prospective cohort study. Can J Anaesth 62(6):595–602, 2015 25652160

O'Sullivan R, Inouye SK, Meagher D: Delirium and depression: inter-relationship and clinical overlap in elderly people. Lancet Psychiatry 1(4):303–311, 2014 26360863

Page VJ, Ely EW, Gates S, et al: Effect of intravenous haloperidol on the duration of delirium and coma in critically ill patients (Hope-ICU): a randomised, double-blind, placebo-controlled trial. Lancet Respir Med 1(7):515–523, 2013 24461612

Pollard C, Fitzgerald M, Ford K: Delirium: the lived experience of older people who are delirious post-orthopaedic surgery. Int J Ment Health Nurs 24(3):213–221, 2015 25976839

Radtke FM, Franck M, Lendner J, et al: Monitoring depth of anaesthesia in a randomized trial decreases the rate of postoperative delirium but not postoperative cognitive dysfunction. Br J Anaesth 110 (suppl 1):i98–i105, 2013 23539235

Ramirez-Bermudez J, Ruiz-Chow A, Perez-Neri I, et al: Cerebrospinal fluid homovanillic acid is correlated to psychotic features in neurological patients with delirium. Gen Hosp Psychiatry 30(4):337–343, 2008 18585537

Rizzo JA, Bogardus ST Jr, Leo-Summers L, et al: Multicomponent targeted intervention to prevent delirium in hospitalized older patients: what is the economic value? Med Care 39(7):740–752, 2001 11458138

Root JC, Pryor KO, Downey R, et al: Association of pre-operative brain pathology with post-operative delirium in a cohort of non-small cell lung cancer patients undergoing surgical resection. Psychooncology 22(9):2087–2094, 2013 23457028

Schofield I: A small exploratory study of the reaction of older people to an episode of delirium. J Adv Nurs 25(5):942–952, 1997 9147199

Schofield I: Delirium: challenges for clinical governance. J Nurs Manag 16(2):127–133, 2008 18269542

Schuurmans MJ, Shortridge-Baggett LM, Duursma SA: The Delirium Observation Screening Scale: a screening instrument for delirium. Res Theory Nurs Pract 17(1):31–50, 2003 12751884

Sessler CN, Gosnell MS, Grap MJ, et al: The Richmond Agitation-Sedation Scale: validity and reliability in adult intensive care unit patients. Am J Respir Crit Care Med 166(10):1338–1344, 2002 12421743

Shi Q, Warren L, Saposnik G, Macdermid JC: Confusion assessment method: a systematic review and meta-analysis of diagnostic accuracy. Neuropsychiatr Dis Treat 9:1359–1370, 2013 24092976

Siddiqi N, Harrison JK, Clegg A, et al: Interventions for preventing delirium in hospitalised non-ICU patients. Cochrane Database Syst Rev (3):CD005563, 2016 26967259

Skrobik Y, Ahern S, Leblanc M, et al: Protocolized intensive care unit management of analgesia, sedation, and delirium improves analgesia and subsyndromal delirium rates. Anesth Analg 111(2):451–463, 2010 20375300

Sullinger D, Gilmer A, Jurado L, et al: Development, implementation, and outcomes of a delirium protocol in the surgical trauma intensive care unit. Ann Pharmacother 51(1):5–12, 2017 27630190

Svenningsen H, Egerod I, Christensen D, et al: Symptoms of posttraumatic stress after intensive care delirium. Biomed Res Int 2015:876947, 2015 26557708

Tahir TA, Eeles E, Karapareddy V, et al: A randomized controlled trial of quetiapine versus placebo in the treatment of delirium. J Psychosom Res 69(5):485–490, 2010 20955868

Tampi RR, Tampi DJ, Ghori AK: Acetylcholinesterase inhibitors for delirium in older adults. Am J Alzheimers Dis Other Demen 31(4):305–310, 2016 26646113

Thomas C, Hestermann U, Walther S, et al: Prolonged activation EEG differentiates dementia with and without delirium in frail elderly patients. J Neurol Neurosurg Psychiatry 79(2):119–125, 2008 17519320

Traube C, Mauer EA, Gerber LM, et al: Cost associated with pediatric delirium in the ICU. Crit Care Med 44(12):e1175–e1179, 2016 27518377

Trogrlić Z, Ista E, Ponssen HH, et al: Attitudes, knowledge and practices concerning delirium: a survey among intensive care unit professionals. Nurs Crit Care 22(3):133–140, 2017 26996876

Trzepacz PT, Sclabassi RJ, van Thiel DH: Delirium: a subcortical phenomenon? J Neuropsychiat Clin Neurosci 1:283–290, 1989 2521072

Trzepacz PT, Mittal D, Torres R, et al: Validation of the Delirium Rating Scale–revised–98: comparison with the delirium rating scale and the cognitive test for delirium. J Neuropsychiatry Clin Neurosci 13(2):229–242, 2001 11449030

Trzepacz PT, Maldonado JR, Kean J, et al: The Delirium Rating Scale–Revised–98 (DRS-R-98) Administration Manual: A Guide to Increase Understanding of How to Solicit Delirium Symptoms to Administer the DRS-R-98. Indianapolis, IN, Paula Trzepacz, 2009

van der Kooi AW, Leijten FS, van der Wekken RJ, et al: What are the opportunities for EEG-based monitoring of delirium in the ICU? J Neuropsychiatry Clin Neurosci 24(4):472–477, 2012 23224454

van der Kooi AW, Zaal IJ, Klijn FA, et al: Delirium detection using EEG: what and how to measure. Chest 147(1):94–101, 2015 25166725

van de Steeg L, Langelaan M, Ijkema R, et al: Improving delirium care for hospitalized older patients. A qualitative study identifying barriers to guideline adherence. J Eval Clin Pract 20(6):813–819, 2014 25081423 van Eijk MM, Roes KC, Honing ML, et al: Effect of rivastigmine as an adjunct to usual care with haloperidol on duration of delirium and mortality in critically ill patients: a multicentre, double-blind, placebo-controlled randomised trial. Lancet 376(9755):1829–1837, 2010 21056464

Van Gemert LA, Schuurmans MJ: The Neecham Confusion Scale and the Delirium Observation Screening Scale: capacity to discriminate and ease of use in clinical practice. BMC Nurs 6:3, 2007 17394635

Voyer P, Champoux N, Desrosiers J, et al: Recognizing acute delirium as part of your routine [RADAR]: a validation study. BMC Nurs 14:19, 2015 25844067

Webster R, Holroyd S: Prevalence of psychotic symptoms in delirium. Psychosomatics 41(6):519–522, 2000 11110116

Whitehorne K, Gaudine A, Meadus R, et al: Lived experience of the intensive care unit for patients who experienced delirium. Am J Crit Care 24(6):474–479, 2015 26523004

Whitlock EL, Torres BA, Lin N, et al: Postoperative delirium in a substudy of cardiothoracic surgical patients in the BAG-RECALL clinical trial. Anesth Analg 118(4):809–817, 2014 24413548

World Health Organization: The ICD-10 Classification of Mental and Behavioural Disorders: Diagnostic Criteria for Research. Geneva, World Health Organization, 1992. Available at: www.who.int/classifications/icd/en/GRNBOOK.pdf. Accessed February 1, 2018.

Yanamadala M, Wieland D, Heflin MT: Educational interventions to improve recognition of delirium: a systematic review. J Am Geriatr Soc 61(11):1983–1993, 2013 24219200

Young J, Leentjens AFG, George J, et al: Systematic approaches to the prevention and management of patients with delirium. J Psychosom Res 65(3):267–272, 2008 18707950

Young J, Murthy L, Westby M, et al; Guideline Development Group: Diagnosis, prevention, and management of delirium: summary of NICE guidance. BMJ 341:c3704, 2010 20667955

CHAPTER 5

Dementia

Antonio Lobo, M.D., Ph.D.

Pedro Saz, M.D., Ph.D.

Miguel Ángel Quintanilla, M.D., Ph.D.

Patricia Gracia-Garcia, M.D., Ph.D.

Concern is increasing about the worldwide epidemic and consequences of dementia. The high prevalence of dementing conditions in medical settings, often undiagnosed, and the association of dementia with longer hospital stays and greater use of health resources have direct implications for psychosomatic medicine and consultation-liaison psychiatry. The psychiatric consultant is an invaluable collaborator with other health care professionals in the identification, evaluation, treatment, management, discharge planning, placement, and rehabilitation of the patient with dementia. In this chapter, we focus on the general clinical approach to dementia and its common causes. Some of these and other causes of dementia are also discussed elsewhere in this book: those disorders that are particularly likely to present with other neurological symptoms in Chapter 30, "Neurology and Neurosurgery"; HIV and other infections in Chapter 26, "Infectious Diseases"; alcohol and other substance use in Chapter 16, "Substance-Related Disorders"; toxic/metabolic conditions in Chapter 21, "Endocrine and Metabolic Disorders," and Chapter 35, "Medical Toxicology"; rheumatological/inflammatory conditions in Chapter 24, "Rheumatology"; traumatic brain injury in Chapter 33, "Physical Medicine and Rehabilitation"; and paraneoplastic syndromes in Chapter 22, "Oncology."

We gratefully acknowledge research grants from the Gobierno de Aragón, European Union; Centro de Investigación Biomédica en Red de Salud Mental (CIBERSAM), Ministry of Science and Innovation, Spain. We also wish to thank Isabel Rabanaque for her help in the development of this chapter.

Concept of Dementia and Clinical Approach

Dementia is traditionally defined as a syndrome of global deterioration of intellectual function occurring in clear consciousness and caused by brain disease. It is a paradigm of the disease model in psychiatry (McHugh and Slavney 1998). The notion of deterioration emphasizes the acquired nature of the impairment in dementia, to distinguish it from intellectual disability, and the requirement of clear consciousness underlines the differentiation from delirium, if dementia is the only diagnosis. Dementia is now subsumed under the new category *major neurocognitive disorder* in DSM-5 (American Psychiatric Association 2013), but the traditional name persists in clinical practice (Table 5–1). To qualify for the diagnosis, the deterioration must be severe enough to adversely affect performance of activities of daily living (ADLs). Social or occupational activities may also be impaired.

Deterioration in personality and noncognitive psychopathological symptoms are almost universal in dementia (Lyketsos et al. 2002; Steinberg et al. 2008) and are most important for psychiatrists. Although the diagnostic criteria are based on cognitive psychopathology, inclusion of noncognitive psychopathological symptoms has been advocated, particularly the negative symptoms in view of their frequency and relative specificity (Saz et al. 2009). Persistence of the syndrome is important for the diagnosis, and some international committees require that symptoms be present for at least 6 months (World Health Organization 1992). However, exceptions occur and are important in the general hospital setting. Whereas progression of the syndrome is the norm in most cases of dementia, this aspect is not included in the concept because some cases of dementia are stable and potentially reversible.

Mild cognitive impairment is conceptualized as a possible transitional state between the cognitive changes of normal aging and dementia (Petersen 2004). According to DSM-5 criteria, *mild neurocognitive disorder* may be a similar construct. Several studies have shown that persons without dementia who have modest cognitive impairment are at greater risk of developing dementia. However, mild cognitive impairment is a heterogeneous category (Wahlund et al. 2003), and most cases, including mild neurocognitive disorder cases, do not progress to dementia, even after a follow-up period of 5 years (Marcos et al. 2016).

Epidemiology, Etiology, and Risk Factors

Dementia has been etiologically associated with numerous heterogeneous conditions, as listed in Table 5–2. The adjusted prevalence has been estimated at 8.2% for all dementias in the U.S. population older than 65 years (Koller and Bynum 2015), with dementia of the Alzheimer's type (DAT)—the most common neurodegenerative disorder—accounting for 43.5% of dementia cases (Goodman et al. 2017). Similar rates have been reported in Europe and other countries (Wu et al. 2017).

Estimates of dementia incidence show that DAT rates rise with age, from 2.8 per 1,000 person-years in individuals ages 65–69 years to 56.1 per 1,000 person-years in those older than 90 years (Kukull et al. 2002). These data are consistent with data in comparable studies in countries outside the United States (Fratiglioni et al. 2000). In

TABLE 5–1.   **The dementia syndrome**

A.   Global deterioration of intellectual function (learning and memory, complex attention, language, executive function, perceptual–motor abilities, social cognition)

B.   Clear consciousness (rule out delirium)

C.   Impairment in performance of personal activities of daily living and social or occupational activities due to the decline in intellectual function

D.   Noncognitive psychopathological symptoms and/or deterioration in emotional control, motivation, or personality frequently present but not necessary for diagnosis

E.   Duration of at least 6 months (with important exceptions, such as in the general hospital)

Source.   Lobo A: *Manual de Psiquiatría General.* Madrid, Editorial Panamericana S.A., 2013.

all of these population studies, both the prevalence and the incidence rates of dementia, and of DAT in particular, increased dramatically with age, doubling approximately every 5 years.

The huge global impact of dementia has been documented (Prince et al. 2015). Total U.S. health care payments in 2014 for elderly people with dementia were estimated at more than $200 billion (Langa 2015). Predictions for the future should be based on the expected increase of the aged populations, particularly in developing countries. However, the Zaragoza study (Lobo et al. 2007) and more recent studies have shown that the prevalence and/or the incidence of dementia, and of DAT, have stabilized or declined in recent years (Wu et al. 2016).

DAT and vascular dementia are reported to be the most prevalent types of dementia in population studies (Fratiglioni et al. 2000; van der Flier and Scheltens 2005). However, mixtures of dementia-related lesions in the same patient are common, including co-occurrence of DAT and vascular-type lesions (Neuropathology Group of the Medical Research Council Cognitive Function and Ageing Study 2001; White et al. 2005), as well as co-occurrence of dementia with Lewy bodies (DLB) with frontotemporal dementia (FTD) in cases with earlier onset (Campbell et al. 2001).

Dementia is also commonly found in general hospitals. One study found that the prevalence of dementia among patients discharged from medical wards was 3.9%, but prevalence was dependent on age, ranging from 2.6% in individuals ages 60–64 years to 8.9% in those 85 years and older (Lyketsos et al. 2000). Prevalence estimates of mild cognitive impairment have ranged from 3% to 19% in population studies in individuals 65 years and older (Gauthier et al. 2006), and the prevalence of DSM-5 mild neurocognitive disorder was found to be almost 4% in subjects ages 55 years and older (Lopez-Anton et al. 2015).

Epidemiological studies also have suggested that noncognitive psychopathological symptoms—sometimes called behavioral and psychological symptoms of dementia (BPSDs)—are common in dementia (Saz et al. 2009). Lyketsos et al. (2002), in their population-based study, found that the most common disturbances among individuals with dementia were apathy (36%), depression (32%), and agitation or aggression (30%). The prevalence of depression among persons with dementia varies according to the diagnostic criteria used. A study using National Institute of Mental Health criteria reported a depression prevalence of 44% (Teng et al. 2008). Symptoms of depression in elderly patients with dementia may differ from symptoms in elderly patients

TABLE 5–2.   Disorders and conditions that may produce dementia syndromes

Degenerative disorders

Cortical

   Alzheimer's disease

   Frontotemporal lobar degeneration

   Dementia with Lewy bodies

Subcortical

   Parkinson's disease

   Huntington's disease

Vascular dementias

Vascular disease

Hydrocephalic dementias

CNS infection–associated dementias

HIV-associated dementia

Neurosyphilis

Prion disease

Dementias due to another medical condition

Metabolic dementias

Neoplastic dementias

Substance/medication-induced dementias

Dementias due to trauma

Traumatic brain injury

Dementias due to multiple etiologies

Note.   CNS=central nervous system.

without dementia. Depression frequently has negative consequences for both patients and caregivers (Lyketsos and Lee 2004). Psychotic symptoms are also frequent in DAT and are associated with rapid cognitive deterioration (Ropacki and Jeste 2005).

Table 5–3 summarizes the results of recent sophisticated analytic epidemiological research (Gottesman et al. 2017; Medina et al. 2017; Reitz and Mayeux 2014), including case–control studies in incident cases. Confirmed risk factors for DAT are scarce and are limited to age, unalterable genetic factors (the apolipoprotein E epsilon4 [*APOE* ε4] allele), and mild cognitive impairment. Mild cognitive impairment may have important clinical and also preventive implications (Marcos et al. 2016; Modrego et al. 2005). Clinically significant depression was recently confirmed as a risk factor for DAT (Gracia-García et al. 2015), and recent epidemiological research has emphasized that among the identified risk factors for dementia/DAT, the following are potentially preventable: low education, hypertension, obesity, diabetes, tobacco use, physical inactivity, and depression. The relevant implication is that appropriate primary-prevention measures might decrease by one-third the prevalence of dementia (Norton et al. 2014). Proposed explanations for findings of stabilized/decreased prevalence and incidence of dementia/DAT in five recent community studies have cited improvements in general health, cardiovascular risk factors, and/or educational levels in the past decades (Wu et al. 2016).

Although the preventive potential of moderate alcohol consumption has stirred considerable interest (Peters et al. 2008), it remains controversial (E. Lobo et al. 2010).

Risk factors for vascular dementia are also listed in Table 5–3 and include hyperhomocysteinemia and low serum folate levels, which are potentially reversible and can be identified early.

Genetics

Genetic knowledge about dementia pathophysiology may be summarized as follows. Huntington's disease is inherited as an autosomal dominant trait with complete penetrance, the mutation responsible being in an elongated and unstable trinucleotide (CAG) repeat on the short arm of chromosome 4 (Haskins and Harrison 2000). In DAT, particularly with early onset, several well-documented reports (Medina et al. 2017) suggested that the disorder is transmitted in families through an autosomal dominant gene, although such transmission is rare. Genetic loci for familial DAT were documented in chromosomes 21 (the amyloid precursor protein [APP] gene), 14 (the presenilin-1 gene), and 1 (the presenilin-2 gene) (Medina et al. 2017).

A significant proportion of the liability for DAT with onset after age 65 years may be explained by genetic factors, and more than 20 loci have been considered to be robustly associated with DAT (Deming et al. 2017)

Advances in the genetics of other dementias include identification of *tau* gene mutations on chromosome 17 in some familial cases of FTD and identification of genetic loci in other neurodegenerative disorders, such as Pick's disease and certain forms of Parkinson's disease. Classification of the dementias is evolving with advances in the genetics of dementia. Observations of tau aggregates and alpha-synucleinopathy aggregates in neurodegenerative disorders have generated the concepts of tauopathies and alpha-synucleinopathies, respectively, to differentiate them from amyloidopathies such as DAT. Most cases of FTD now tend to be classified as tauopathies related to mutations in the tau gene, with a large clinical spectrum that includes Pick's disease, progressive supranuclear palsy, and corticobasal degeneration (Lebert et al. 2002). Alpha-synucleinopathies include DLB and Parkinson's disease (Rcom-H'cheo-Gauthier et al. 2016), but identification of both types of pathological aggregates in several other diseases has led to disagreement on classifications (Iseki et al. 2003).

General Clinical Features

The Dementia Syndrome

The clinical picture may differ widely according to the type and severity of dementia, and the characteristics are important in the differential diagnosis. In most cases of degenerative processes—in particular, DAT, some types of vascular dementia, and dementias due to endocrinopathies, brain tumors, metabolic disorders, and abuse of medications—the onset of symptoms is gradual, and the signs of the dementia syn-

TABLE 5–3.   **Risk factors in dementias**

	Strength of association[a]
Risk factors for dementia of the Alzheimer's type	
Older age	++
Female sex	+
Low education	+
First-degree relative with Alzheimer's	+
Down syndrome	+
Head trauma	+
Apolipoprotein ε4 allele	++
High aluminum levels	+/−
Cigarette smoking	+
Hypertension	+
Hyperhomocysteinemia	+/−
Depression	+
Mild cognitive impairment	++
Social isolation	+
Risk factors for vascular dementia	
Age >60 years	+
Male sex	+
Previous stroke	++
Stroke risk factors	
Hypertension	++
Heart disease/atrial fibrillation	+
Cigarette smoking	++
Diabetes mellitus	++
Excessive alcohol consumption (>3 drinks/day)	+
Hyperlipidemia	+
Hyperhomocysteinemia, low serum folate levels	+
Previous mental decline	+/−

[a]Strength of association: ++=confirmed; +=probable; +/−=controversial.

Source.   Gottesman et al. 2017; Medina et al. 2017; Reitz and Mayeux 2014.

drome are subtle and may at first be ignored by both the patient and his or her relatives. In contrast, the onset may be abrupt after severe cerebral infarcts, head trauma,
cardiac arrest with cerebral hypoxia, or encephalitis.

The full dementia syndrome progresses through severity levels in degenerative
processes and is very characteristic in DAT (Table 5–4). The earliest manifestations,
such as impairment of memory, may be very subtle. Individuals with dementia also
show impairment in thinking and in capacity for reasoning, but the earliest difficulties
can be mistakenly disregarded or explained away as the expression of fatigue, distraction, or discouragement. The deficits may become apparent in the face of more complex problems or when specifically tested, but patients often attempt to compensate
for defects by using strategies to avoid showing failures in intellectual performance.

TABLE 5–4. **Clinical findings in patients with dementia of the Alzheimer's type, by severity level**

Mild (MMSE score=18–23; duration of disease=1–3 years)

Impaired registration and recent memory (early sign); remote recall mildly impaired

Defective temporal orientation

Mild impairment in thinking; bewilderment in the face of complexity

Impoverishment of language; naming problems

Mild apraxia for complex tasks

Agnosia not evident unless tested

Difficulties in planning, sequencing, and executing instrumental activities of daily living

Frequent personality changes: irritability, less apparent concern about issues of daily life and effects of their behavior on others

Depression in approximately 20% of patients; mild apathy; loss of initiative; lack of energy

Frequent misinterpretations; psychotic phenomena rare

Urinary incontinence in fewer than 10%

Other neurological signs and primitive reflexes rare

Moderate (MMSE score=12–17; duration of disease=2–8 years)

Recent memory and remote recall more severely impaired

Severe temporal disorientation, moderate spatial disorientation

Obvious impairment of thinking; catastrophic reactions if pressured

Fluent aphasia, anomia, paraphasic errors, empty quality of language, perseveration

Praxis difficulties (in managing dressing, feeding, manipulations)

Agnosia evident: failure to identify objects, including familiar faces

Difficulties in planning, sequencing, and executing extend to basic activities of daily living

Evident personality changes: marked irritability; marked lack of concern about issues of daily life and effects of their behavior on others

Dysphoric mood, depression less frequent; apathy; loss of initiative

Frequent psychotic phenomena (delusions, illusions, hallucinations)

Restlessness, pacing, wandering occasionally, agitation, sporadic aggressiveness

Urinary incontinence frequent; fecal incontinence rare

Gait disorder and frequent primitive reflexes

Severe (MMSE score <12; duration of disease=7–12 years)

Memory: only earliest learned information retained

Total disorientation

Severe impairment of thinking; indifference in the face of failures

Extreme impoverishment of language; communication impossible

Complete incapacity to manage dressing, feeding, simple manipulations

Severe agnosia: cannot identify close relatives

Total dependence for even basic activities of daily living

Total disconnection from environment

Affective indifference; severe apathy; loss of initiative

Double incontinence (urinary and fecal)

Motor system rigidity and flexion contractures of all limbs; final stage of decortication

Note. MMSE=Mini-Mental State Examination.

Although cognitive symptoms are the hallmark of dementia, BPSDs often dominate both the presentation and the course of the disease. These symptoms occur in clusters or syndromes identified as psychosis (delusions and hallucinations), agitation (e.g., arguing, pacing, crying out), aggression (physical or verbal); depression (or dysphoria); anxiety, apathy, disinhibition (socially and sexually inappropriate behaviors), motor disturbance (wandering, rummaging), nighttime behaviors (getting up at night), and appetite and eating disturbances. One-third of dementia care costs have been attributed to the management of these symptoms, and BPSDs are also associated with faster disease progression and adverse effects on caregivers, including reduced quality of life and worse health (Kales et al. 2015). The course of BPSDs does not always parallel cognitive and functional deterioration in DAT patients. For instance, depression and anxiety are common phenomena among patients with mild disease, whereas aggression, agitation, and apathy are more frequent among patients with more advanced dementia. BPSDs have been observed in the prodromal stage of dementia, before any cognitive or functional decline is apparent (Stella 2014). These prodromal signs have been termed *mild behavioral impairment* (Ismail et al. 2016).

The course of the syndrome varies according to the type of dementia and has implications for the differential diagnosis. An incrementally worsening or stepwise course is common in vascular dementia, whereas the deficits may be stable in other types of dementia, such as that related to head trauma. Furthermore, regression of symptoms following treatment initiation is a possibility in dementias caused by potentially reversible disorders.

Reversible dementias are considered by some authors to be rare. Michel and Sellal (2011) estimated that only 1.5% of all dementias are reversible, although other studies have reported a reversibility prevalence of 7.3% (Muangpaisan et al. 2012). The most common potentially reversible etiologies are those that can be neurosurgically addressed, such as benign tumors, normal-pressure hydrocephalus, or subdural hematoma. Other potentially reversible dementias are due to infectious diseases (syphilis, HIV), an endocrine disorder, or a vitamin deficiency. Whereas treatment of a reversible cause of dementia does not always allow full recovery, it is important to systematically look for reversible conditions even in patients with a degenerative dementia, because such conditions can contribute to the worsening of the irreversible disease in nearly 25% of dementia cases (Michel and Sellal 2011).

Clinicopathological Correlations

Certain clinical characteristics suggest the involvement of specific brain areas, with implications for diagnosis and course as well as for understanding the underlying pathology of cognitive and noncognitive phenomena (McHugh and Folstein 1979). The term *cortical dementia* refers to dementia in which the preponderance of dysfunction is in the cortex. The most characteristic signs of cortical dementia are amnesia (which is not helped by cues to remember), aphasia, apraxia, and agnosia, which are often designated "the four *A*s" (Table 5–5).

Subcortical dementia describes dementia with the predominant involvement of the white and deep gray matter, such as basal ganglia, thalamus, and their frontal lobe projections. McHugh and Folstein (1975) were among the first to emphasize that parts of the brain other than the cortex have a role in cognition. They described the distinc-

TABLE 5–5. **Clinical characteristics of cortical and subcortical dementia syndromes**

	Cortical	Subcortical
Aphasia	Early	No
Agnosia	Late	No
Apraxia	Rather early	Rare
Alexia	Rather late	No
Apathy, inertia	Rare or late	Very marked, early
Loss of initiative	Frequent, late	Marked
Psychomotor retardation	Rare or late	Very marked, early
Amnesia	Recall and recognition not aided by cues to remember	Recognition better preserved, may be aided by cues to remember
Gait	Normal until late	Abnormal, early
Extrapyramidal signs	Rare or late	Very marked, early
Primitive reflexes (e.g., grasp, snout, suck)	Late	Rare
Affective syndromes	Less frequent	Frequent, severe

tive combination of three features in "subcortical dementia syndrome": 1) a slowly progressive dilapidation of all cognitive powers; 2) prominent psychic apathy and inertia that may worsen to akinetic mutism; and 3) absence of aphasia, alexia, and agnosia (see Table 5–5). The same authors also emphasized the early appearance in subcortical dementias of prominent BPSDs, particularly depression and other affective disturbances, considered to be a direct consequence of the cerebral pathology. Rabins et al. (1999) designated four specific features of subcortical dementia as "the four Ds": dysmnesia (memory impairment; patients may benefit from cues to remember), dysexecutive (related to troubles with decision making), delay (related to slowed thinking and moving), and depletion (related to reduced complexity of thought).

In dementia in which both cortical and subcortical regions are involved, the clinical characteristics include signs of cortical dementia, such as aphasia and apraxia, together with the apathetic state characteristic of subcortical lesions.

Clinical Types and Pathophysiology of Dementia

Cortical Dementias

Alzheimer's Disease

Most cases of Alzheimer's disease start after age 65 years, but an earlier onset is not uncommon. The characteristic general dementia syndrome has been described and includes cortical signs (see Table 5–5). Typically, patients present with prominent impairment in memory and learning. The insidious onset and the slowly worsening, relentless course are very characteristic and are crucial in making the diagnosis.

Other characteristic clinical signs and symptoms include 1) a "hippocampal type" of memory difficulty, which is not reliably aided by cues on memory testing and involves a high number of intrusions and false recognitions; 2) language difficulties, including a fluent aphasia with anomia, paraphasic errors, and a tendency toward perseveration; 3) in many cases, a continued capability to recognize objects and to use them appropriately, even when the patient can no longer name them accurately; and 4) agnosia for faces, including family faces in late stages of the disease. Gait disorder in the middle stage is also common, as are frontal signs such as grasping and sucking reflexes, along with changes in muscular tone.

The neuropathology of Alzheimer's disease is its defining characteristic (Schneider et al. 2012), and the extent and severity of neuropathological changes correlate with the type and severity of the cognitive signs and symptoms. Cortical atrophy occurs, leading to widened sulci and ventricular enlargement. The most severe changes occur in the medial temporal lobe, including the hippocampus. Areas of the association cortex in the parietal and temporal lobes, and to a lesser degree in the frontal lobes, are also involved. Characteristic microscopic findings are neuronal loss; synaptic loss, particularly in the cortex; senile plaques with a core of amyloid peptide; neurofibrillary tangles containing abnormally phosphorylated tau proteins; granulovacuolar degeneration of the neurons; and amyloid angiopathy. The locations and abundance of microscopic findings determine the postmortem histological diagnosis of Alzheimer's disease (Cummings et al. 1998). The cause of DAT is not well understood. According to the amyloid hypothesis, amyloid beta ($A\beta$) deposition is an "upstream" event in the cascade that is associated with "downstream" pathological changes in synaptic function, including degeneration and eventual neuronal loss in cholinergic, serotonergic, and dopaminergic neurons. A temporal lag of approximately a decade between deposition of $A\beta$ and appearance of the clinical syndrome of dementia has been postulated (Sperling et al. 2011).

Several studies have supported the cholinergic deficit hypothesis in DAT, including specific degeneration of cholinergic neurons in the nucleus basalis of Meynert; decreases in acetylcholine and choline acetyltransferase concentrations in the brain; and observations about the role of cholinergic agonists and antagonists. Evidence also indicates that the excitatory activity of L-glutamate plays a role in the pathogenesis of DAT. However, some research suggests that vascular factors may have an important influence on the rate of progression of DAT (Mielke et al. 2007). In fact, the neurobiology of this complex brain disorder has been conceptualized in terms of progressive failures in an array of interconnected complex systems or neural networks, rather than the result of a unitary etiological factor (Khachaturian 2012).

Dementia With Lewy Bodies

DLB is a condition of uncertain nosological status, with cortical signs suggesting DAT alongside the classic extrapyramidal features of Parkinson's disease (Gomperts 2016). However, the typical neuropathological findings of DAT are much less common in this condition. Both DLB and Parkinson's disease dementia (PD) are now called Lewy body dementia (LBD) because they share the same pathophysiology, with hallmark alpha-synuclein neuronal inclusions (Lewy bodies). Cholinergic dysfunction has been found in both conditions. DLB differs from PD in the sequence of onset of dementia and parkinsonism (Walker et al. 2015). Patients with DLB have similar free recall but better delayed-recognition memory compared with patients with DAT. The core features of DLB are fluctuating cognition, recurrent well-formed visual hallucinations, and parkinsonism. Other suggestive features are rapid eye movement (REM) sleep behavior disorder, severe sensitivity to antipsychotic-induced extrapyramidal side effects, and low dopamine transporter uptake in the basal ganglia. In general, DLB has a more variable course and worse prognosis than DAT.

Frontotemporal Dementia

FTD is an umbrella term encompassing a group of neurodegenerative diseases characterized by progressive changes in behavior, executive function, and language. The features that are most important in distinguishing FTD from DAT are personality changes and neuropsychiatric symptoms, which may be quite marked and may precede cognitive decline by several years. Psychiatric symptoms in FTD include behavioral disinhibition; apathy or inertia; loss of sympathy or empathy toward family members and friends; stereotyped, compulsive behaviors; and hyperorality or changes in eating (e.g., binge eating, increased consumption of sweets or alcohol). Executive dysfunction is a frequent early sign of the disease. Neuron motor disease may develop in about 15% of patients with FTD, and early parkinsonism is present in up to 20% of patients. Disease onset occurs earlier in FTD than in DAT, usually between the ages of 45 and 64 years. Survival after symptom onset is 6–11 years.

Neuronal loss, gliosis, and microvacuolar changes in the frontotemporal areas define this type of neurodegenerative dementia. Several types of FTD have been described, each of which is associated with a characteristic pattern of abnormal protein deposition. The most common subtypes of FTD are Pick's disease, corticobasal degeneration, and progressive supranuclear palsy. Pick's disease, characterized by the presence of distinctive intraneuronal Pick bodies and ballooned Pick cells on microscopic examination, may be diagnosed in up to 30% of cases (Bang et al. 2015). Primary progressive aphasia is a clinical variant of FTD that involves progressive language impairment. Aphasia is the most prominent deficit and the main cause of functional impairment during the first 2 years of the disease.

Subcortical Dementias

Huntington's Disease

Huntington's disease (HD) has the three main characteristics of the subcortical dementia syndrome (Folstein and McHugh 1983), together with the classic choreoathetoid movement disorder and a positive family history. Huntington's disease usually has its onset between 30 and 50 years. The mean duration of the disease is 17–20 years, and the most common cause of death is pneumonia, followed by suicide. Both cognitive and noncognitive psychopathology may appear before the movement abnormalities. The cognitive changes are particularly notable in executive function. All psychomotor processes become severely retarded. Psychiatric symptoms are commonly present in the early stage of the disease, with depression the most frequent symptom. Low self-esteem, feelings of guilt, and anxiety are common. Suicide occurs more frequently in early symptomatic individuals and also in asymptomatic gene carriers (Roos 2010). Obsessions and compulsions are distressing and can lead to irritability and aggression. Psychosis is common in the later stages of the disease, in most cases parallel to cognitive decline. HD can resemble schizophrenia, with paranoid and auditory hallucinations (Roos 2010).

Neuropathological features in Huntington's disease include atrophy of the caudate nucleus and corticostriatal pathway and loss of γ-aminobutyric acid (GABA) interneurons (Bunner and Rebec 2016).

Parkinson's Disease

A typical subcortical, progressive dementia syndrome may occur in patients with Parkinson's disease. The risk of dementia increases with duration of disease and reaches 50% 10 years after diagnosis. The typical cognitive profile is similar to that of DLB. The presence of behavioral features such as apathy, depressed or anxious mood, hallucinations, delusions, and/or excessive daytime sleepiness increases the likelihood that dementia is developing.

Braak et al. (2003) proposed a pathological staging of PD, with Lewy bodies spreading rostrally in the brain stem (substantia nigra, basal ganglia), then to the limbic system, and finally to the neocortex (Walker et al. 2015).

Wilson's Disease

Wilson's disease is caused by an inherited defect in the copper-carrying serum protein ceruloplasmin that leads to excessive copper deposition in the liver, corneas, and basal ganglia. Onset is usually during adolescence or early adulthood and is heralded by dystonia, parkinsonism, or cerebellar ataxia. Cognitive impairment is relatively mild in the early stages; however, depression, irritability, disinhibition, personality changes, and poor impulse control are common, with severity paralleling the severity of the neurological signs (Shanmugiah et al. 2008).

Normal-Pressure Hydrocephalus

Normal-pressure hydrocephalus (NPH) is a very characteristic neuropsychiatric syndrome, presenting as a triad of clinical symptoms combining motoric and psychopathological features (Folstein and McHugh 1983; McHugh 1966): 1) an early gait disturbance resembling the stiff steps of spastic paraparesis, 2) subcortical dementia with particularly severe apathetic features, and 3) urinary incontinence that may not appear until late in the disease course. In the early stages of NPH, the cognitive profile is characterized mainly by impairment of attention, psychomotor speed, and memory, suggesting frontal involvement. NPH is considered to be a potentially reversible dementia, and the treatment of choice is shunt surgery, which can help to reduce cognitive impairment, especially if performed during the early stage of deterioration (Picascia et al. 2015). In chronic hydrocephalus, the mechanical pressure on the subcortical tissue surrounding the lateral and third ventricles may lead to exhaustion of the normal elasticity of brain tissue and eventually to tissue destruction. "Probable" or "possible" NPH has been associated with increased risk of dementia and excess mortality (Jaraj et al. 2017).

Mixed Dementia and Dementia in Disseminated Brain Diseases

Vascular Dementia

Vascular dementia (VaD) is defined as dementia resulting from ischemic, ischemic–hypoxic, or hemorrhagic brain lesions arising from cerebrovascular or cardiovascular pathology. The term *vascular dementia* is controversial, and some authors prefer the term *vascular cognitive impairment* in a more dimensional approach. The course of multi-infarct dementia has classically been described as stepwise and patchy; however, VaD may also have a clinical course as gradual and smooth as that in patients with DAT, and pathological and neuroimaging studies show that subcortical small-vessel disease (previously known as Binswanger's disease), rather than large cortical infarcts, accounts for most cases of VaD. Mortality is higher in VaD than in DAT, with a mean survival of 3–5 years.

Cognitive changes in vascular dementia are more variable than those in DAT and are dependent on the particular neural substrates affected by the vascular pathology. Because subcortical pathology is common, interrupting frontostriatal circuits, deficits in attention, information processing, and executive function are predominantly seen. Noncognitive symptoms are also common, with depression and apathy particularly prominent. Accurate diagnosis of VaD requires the presence of sufficient cerebrovascular disease on brain imaging to plausibly account for the degree of cognitive impairment (O'Brien and Thomas 2015).

Prion Dementias

Prion dementias are uncommon diseases that are now considered to be caused by an abnormal form of prion, a cerebral protein. This protein is encoded by a gene on chromosome 20, the prion-related protein gene (PRNP). Because prion diseases are transmissible by transferring the altered prion proteins, they act like infectious agents. Sporadic Creutzfeldt-Jakob disease (sCJD) is the most common form of human prion disease. It has a mean survival of about 6 months, with 90% of patients dying within 1 year (Geschwind 2015). The peak age at onset is 55–75 years, with a mean age at onset of about 64 years. The classical clinical phenotype of sCJD is an insidious-onset, rapidly progressive dementia accompanied by behavioral abnormalities, ataxia, extrapyramidal signs, and eventually myoclonus. Because sCJD affects many regions of the brain, its presentation can mimic many other neurological or psychiatric conditions, making diagnosis difficult. Pathological findings are widespread in both the cortex and subcortical structures. Spongiform changes in neurons are characteristic, and neuronal loss and astrocytic proliferation occur.

A new variant of Creutzfeldt-Jakob disease (vCJD) was first detected in Europe. Compared with sCJD, vCJD may have an earlier onset, typically before age 40 years Both forms of Creutzfeldt-Jakob disease (CJD) are discussed in greater detail in Chapter 26, "Infectious Diseases." Despite a successful reduction in incidence of vCJD, in part related to decreases in bovine spongiform encephalopathy, risk remains of acquiring vCJD through transmission in blood products or tissues derived from vCJD-infected donors. An autosomal-dominant familial type of prion disease known as Gerstmann-Straussler-Scheinker syndrome typically presents as a slowly progressive ataxic or motoric (parkinsonian) disorder with late-onset dementia, although rapidly progressive and amyotrophic cases occur as well (Geschwind 2015).

Infection-Associated Dementias

Dementias caused by infectious agents are described in detail in Chapter 26, "Infectious Diseases."

HIV-associated dementia. HIV-associated dementia, formerly called AIDS dementia complex, is now the most common dementia caused by an infectious disease.

Cognitive dysfunction may be the earliest or the only clinical manifestation of AIDS. However, with use of antiretroviral therapy in developed countries, it is estimated that fewer than 5% of infected individuals will develop full criteria for dementia during their life-course. HIV-associated dementia is a subcortical dementia, with prominent executive dysfunction, psychomotor slowing, and difficulty with tasks that require high levels of attention and learning. This type of dementia is considered to be caused directly by HIV, through activation of neurotoxic elements in the immune system.

Noncognitive psychopathology (apathy, emotional blunting, and inappropriate or aggressive affect) is also common in patients infected with HIV.

In HIV-infected patients who present with an abrupt change in mental status or exhibit heterogeneous cognitive impairment, with occurrence of both cortical and subcortical features, an opportunistic infection (common in advanced stages of illness) or other AIDS-related central nervous system (CNS) condition (primary CNS lymphoma, progressive multifocal leukoencephalopathy) should be suspected.

Neurosyphilis.   Neurosyphilis is a serious complication of syphilis that can develop at any time during the course of the disease. Whereas the early forms occur within a few months to a few years after infection and affect the meninges and blood vessels, the late forms occur years to decades after infection and affect the brain if left untreated. Early in the course of syphilitic dementia, patients are forgetful and manifest personality changes (disinhibition, indifference, or poor judgment). With time, they may develop psychiatric symptoms, such as mania, depression, or psychosis. Syphilitic dementia, also called *general paresis,* is accompanied by characteristic neurological signs, such as pupillary abnormalities; intention tremor of the face, tongue, and hands; and facial and limb hypotonia (Marra 2015).

Herpes simplex encephalitis.   Herpes simplex encephalitis may cause major neurological and cognitive sequelae. Because herpes encephalitis has a predilection for the temporal lobes, amnestic and aphasic syndromes are common, but dementia also can be seen.

Metabolic and Toxic Dementias

Metabolic and toxic dementias (see also Chapter 21, "Endocrine and Metabolic Disorders," and Chapter 35, "Medical Toxicology") form a heterogeneous group of diseases (see Table 5–2) that are of special interest to the consultant psychiatrist because they are relatively common in medical settings and are potentially reversible. Dementia in these conditions has predominantly subcortical features but may have mixed characteristics. Whether the metabolic and toxic encephalopathies are best conceptualized as reversible dementias or as chronic deliria is unclear, and perhaps the distinction is primarily semantic, particularly in cases of hepatic, renal, and cardiopulmonary failure. The diagnosis is supported if cognitive impairment improves or stabilizes with treatment of the medical condition.

The neuropathology in these conditions is not well understood. Hippocampal neurons are probably the most vulnerable to anoxic injury but are also vulnerable to severe hypercholesterolemia and to repeated or severe episodes of hypoglycemia. Vitamin B_{12} deficiency, as seen in pernicious anemia, has been associated with disseminated degeneration in areas of cortical white matter, the optic tracts, and the cerebellar peduncles. In pellagra, deficiency in nicotinic acid and probably other B vitamins may lead to neuronal destruction.

Alcoholic dementia, one possible complication of chronic alcoholism, is more common after age 50 years and is likely multifactorial in etiology. The pathophysiology of alcoholic dementia is not fully understood, but the disorder is thought to be caused by the combination of alcohol neurotoxicity and thiamine and other vitamin B deficiencies. Multiple traumatic brain injuries contribute in some cases. Neuropathological changes include cortical atrophy and nerve-fiber disintegration with dissolution of myelin sheaths. Dementing syndromes are also seen in distinct brain diseases related to chronic alcoholism, such as Marchiafava-Bignami disease, characterized by degeneration of the corpus callosum and anterior commissure.

Dementing syndromes also may occur in chronic intoxication with medications, which can be either prescribed or abused by patients. The onset of medication-intoxication dementia is insidious, and the course is progressive; physicians should be alert to the possibility of this reversible dementia, given that deficits can improve or stabilize after an abstinence period. Benzodiazepines, including those with high potency and a short half-life, are known to cause anterograde amnesia and impairment of memory consolidation and subsequent memory retrieval. Elderly patients are more vulnerable than younger patients to developing benzodiazepine-related dementia. Finally, syndromes of cognitive deterioration have been reported in abusers of cocaine, methamphetamine, or inhalants (see also Chapter 16, "Substance-Related Disorders").

Neoplastic-Associated Dementias

Neoplastic disease can affect any part of the brain and can produce essentially any kind of neuropsychiatric symptoms, depending on tumor location and extent, as well as on the tumor's rapidity of growth and propensity to cause increased intracranial pressure (see Chapter 22, "Oncology," and Chapter 30, "Neurology and Neurosurgery"). Dementia in cancer patients may be due to primary or metastatic tumors in the CNS, or occur as a paraneoplastic syndrome.

Dementia Following Traumatic Brain Injury

A variety of cognitive difficulties are very common after traumatic brain injury (TBI) (see Chapter 33, "Physical Medicine and Rehabilitation"). Symptoms vary depending on the site of the lesions. Focal injuries usually occur in the orbitofrontal, temporal polar, and occipital regions. By contrast, diffuse TBI is widespread throughout the brain and involves widely dispersed axonal injury, brain swelling, and hypoxia. Moreover, TBI initiates a process that induces changes contributing to ongoing neuronal damage and death over time, so that patients have an increased risk of developing neurodegenerative disorders such as DAT in later stages of life (Gupta and Sen 2016). Common cognitive difficulties include dysmnesia, persistent personality changes, dysphasia, attentional disturbances, and impairments suggestive of frontal lobe damage, particularly executive dysfunction. Dementia also occurs in a minority of TBI cases and may be accompanied by seizures and neurological deficits, as well as secondary psychiatric syndromes, including depression, mania, and psychosis. Chronic traumatic encephalopathy, or *dementia pugilística*, affects individuals with a history of repeated closed-head injuries, most often occurring in career boxers. The onset is typically insidious, with symptoms progressing slowly over decades to dementia (Gupta and Sen 2016). Extradural and subdural hematomas, potentially reversible causes of dementia, are commonly seen after TBI.

Depression

The relation between dementia and depression is complex. Cognitive dysfunction, particularly executive dysfunction, is common in late life depression (LLD). Some older adults with LLD may develop a dementia syndrome (delirium superimposed on dementia [DSD]; previously called pseudodementia). These patients usually manifest severe symptoms of depression (psychomotor retardation and other melancholic symptoms, and sometimes psychotic features) and a mild dementia syndrome (Morimoto et al. 2015). Cortical signs such as language disturbances are uncommon, and in DSD, in contrast to DAT, prompting and organization of material tend to improve memory performance (O'Brien et al. 2001). DSD may be reversible and tends to disappear with successful treatment of the depression. However, cognitive monitoring and follow-up are recommended because a persistent dementia syndrome may develop in a significant proportion of cases (Chen et al. 2008). Moreover, a longitudinal increased risk of dementia has been found in subjects with severe forms of clinical depression (Gracia-García et al. 2015). In addition, the "vascular depression" hypothesis posits that cerebrovascular disease may predispose a person to symptoms of both depression and cognitive impairment, and studies have proposed inflammatory and hypoperfusion hypotheses for the development of cognitive impairment and depression (Taylor et al. 2013).

Diagnosis and Differential Diagnosis

Early detection of dementia can play an important role in managing both the social and the health care aspects of the disease (Wimo et al. 2013). A number of brief interviews can detect the dementia syndrome with reasonable accuracy (Lin et al. 2013) and can be taught to nonpsychiatrists. Dementia should be suspected in patients at risk who are referred to psychiatrists, particularly elderly medical patients with delirium or unexpected behavioral disturbances; it should also be suspected in patients who are referred by primary care physicians because of subjective complaints or observations by relatives of memory problems or loss of intellectual efficiency. In both cases, the clinical approach to diagnosis follows a classic sequence: first, identify characteristic signs and symptoms of cognitive impairment; second, document whether the signs and symptoms cluster in a defined syndrome (Table 5–6); third, eliminate false-positive cases; and finally, determine the etiological type of dementia. A search for associated medical conditions, neuropsychiatric symptoms, and special social needs completes the evaluation process. The DSM-5 criteria for major neurocognitive disorder (equivalent to dementia) are similarly defined: evidence of significant cognitive decline (in one or more cognitive domains) that interferes with independence in everyday activities, does not occur exclusively in the context of delirium, and is not better explained by another mental disorder (American Psychiatric Association 2013, p. 602).

TABLE 5–6.   **Neurocognitive domains potentially affected in dementia**

Domain	Subdomains
Complex attention	Sustained attention; divided attention; selective attention; processing speed
Executive function	Planning; decision making; working memory; responding to feedback; inhibition; flexibility
Perceptual–motor function	Visual perception; visuoconstructional reasoning; perceptual–motor coordination; praxis or motor planning; gnosia or perceptual recognition
Language	Object naming; word finding; verbal fluency; grammar and syntax; receptive language
Learning and memory	Free recall; cued recall; recognition memory; semantic and autobiographical long-term memory; implicit learning
Social cognition	Recognition of emotions; theory of mind; insight

Source.   American Psychiatric Association 2013; Sachdev et al. 2014.

Clinical History

A clinical history corroborated by reliable caregivers and a systematic mental status examination are the foundations of the diagnostic process (Rabins et al. 2007). In taking the history, it is important to search for specific evidence of deterioration in memory and other cognitive functions (summarized in Table 5–6). Specific, convincing examples should be required as support for the diagnosis of dementia. Furthermore, the consultant must assess the presence, extent, and consequences of the cognitive problems in occupational activities and ADLs. An outside informant is crucial for obtaining data about decline in cognitive function measured against premorbid abilities. The Informant Questionnaire on Cognitive Decline in the Elderly (IQCODE; Jorm and Jacomb 1989)—and in particular the short form (Jorm 1994)—is suggested as a useful, simple questionnaire that has good reliability and validity. The onset and pattern of progression of the cognitive difficulties also should be carefully documented. Insidious diseases such as DAT can easily go undetected for years before becoming apparent. Finally, it is important to determine whether changes in personality and behavior have accompanied the cognitive difficulties and whether psychopathological signs and symptoms, including negative-type symptoms such as apathy, are present.

Mental Status Examination

A systematic basic bedside or office mental status examination is a minimum requirement in each case of suspected dementia. Cognitive assessment is relatively easy to complete and should include all relevant domains. Table 1–4 ("Detailed assessment of cognitive domains") in Chapter 1, "Psychiatric Assessment and Consultation," summarizes the cognitive areas to cover in the assessment. Figure 5–1 shows performance by patients with dementia on specific construction tasks. Even two simple questions about patients' age and year of birth can be useful in ruling out cases of dementia (negative predictive value=98.2%) (Ventura et al. 2013). In-depth examination requires assessment of the neurocognitive domains potentially affected in dementia (see Table 5–6).

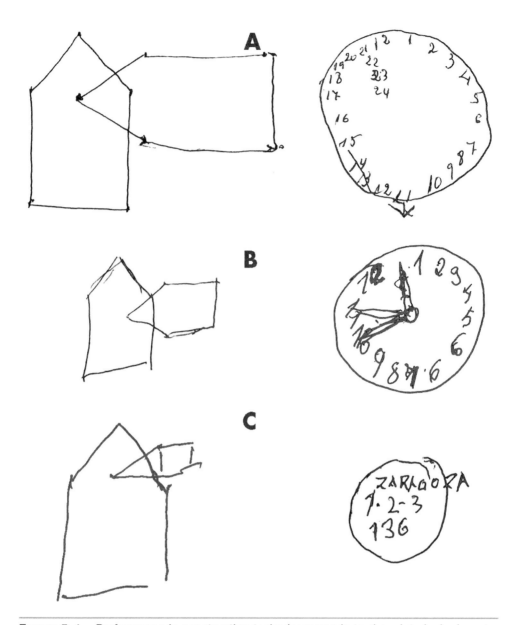

FIGURE 5–1.   Performance in construction tasks (commands to draw interlocked pentagons and a clock) by patients with increasing levels of dementia severity.

Impairment in performance appears earlier in clock drawing than in pentagon construction and increases with severity level of dementia. **(A) Clock A** (Mini-Mental State Examination [MMSE] score=18) shows executive deficits in planning and organization; construction deficits to place the numbers; probable perseveration (24 hours); and deficits in judgment to correct errors and to place the hands indicating the time (11:10). **Pentagon A** shows nominal construction deficit. **(B) Clock B** (MMSE score=15) shows subtle construction deficits (mild deviation of numbers, but spacing is correct); executive deficits in planning and judgment to indicate the time; and unsuccessful executive attempts to correct errors (in placing number 6; in placing the hands). **Pentagon B** shows mild construction deficit. **(C) Clock C** (MMSE score=14) shows deficits both in remembering and in understanding the command and probable "stimulus dependence syndrome" (the pen in the patient's hand acts as a stimulus and writes inappropriately inside the circle). **Pentagon C** shows construction and visuomotor coordination deficits.

It is strongly recommended that the clinician be familiar with a standard validated assessment method. Although no standardized instrument is a substitute for sound clinical assessment, some assessment instruments can be quite helpful, provided that their limitations are kept in mind.

The Mini-Mental State Examination (MMSE) (Folstein et al. 1975) is a useful instrument for screening purposes (National Institute for Health and Care Excellence 2016a). Considerable evidence supports the accuracy of this brief scale in detection of dementia (Lin et al. 2013), and it is considered to be the standard screening measure in most clinical and research studies (Gray and Cummings 2002). The MMSE fares very well in different cultures, if the standardization has been adequate (Lobo et al. 1999). Available data on the efficiency of individual items in the MMSE, remarkable in items such as temporal orientation, may help the consultant in interpreting the results of the test (Lobo et al. 1999).

The Modified Mini-Mental State (Teng and Chui 1987) and the Montreal Cognitive Assessment (MoCA) (Nasreddine et al. 2005) are more sensitive to mild cognitive impairment and subcortical dementia. Executive functions, which are not well covered in the MMSE, may be easily assessed at bedside with the Frontal Assessment Battery (Dubois et al. 2000) or the clock drawing test (van der Burg et al. 2004).

Neuropsychological testing is valuable as an adjunct to the clinical examination, particularly in differentiating early dementia from milder cognitive syndromes or normal aging or in differentiating subtypes of dementia. However, neuropsychological testing, which can take a full day, is not necessary in most cases. Standardized assessment scales also may be recommended for cases of severe dementia (Rabins and Steele 1996), for noncognitive symptoms (Neuropsychiatric Inventory [NPI]; Cummings et al. 1994), and specifically for depression (Cornell Scale for Depression in dementia; Alexopoulos et al. 1988).

Dementia Rating Scales

Instruments for specific purposes have been designed, such as the Alzheimer's Disease Assessment Scale (ADAS; Rosen et al. 1984). Global staging instruments, such as the Clinical Dementia Rating (CDR; Hughes et al. 1982), have come into wide use. A variety of assessments are also available for documenting functional deficits, such as the classic instruments of Lawton and Brody (1969), the Katz Index (Katz et al. 1970), and the Functional Assessment Staging (FAST) procedure, which can be used in conjunction with the Global Deterioration Scale (GDS) staging system (Reisberg et al. 1993). The degree of functional impairment documented with these scales may help in the classification of DSM-5 dementia severity as mild (impairment on instrumental ADLs), moderate (impairment on basic ADLs), or severe (complete impairment on ADLs). The International Dementia Alliance (IDEAL) scale for the staging of "care needs" in dementia (Semrau et al. 2015) is a more recent development.

Neurological Examination

The neurological examination is an integral part of, and informs, the diagnosis and differential diagnosis of dementia. The examination should be standard but may focus on the assessment of neurological signs described in the clinical section, including specific gait difficulties, apraxia, and primitive reflexes. Other testing should be included if warranted by clinical information.

Differential Diagnosis

Differential diagnosis starts by ruling out false-positive cases of dementia—namely, previous intellectual disability; amnestic syndromes (such as Korsakoff's psychosis) lacking the global deficits required for the diagnosis of dementia; cognitive difficulties due to general physical frailty, particularly in elderly patients; and age-related memory impairment (or benign senescent forgetfulness), characterized by a minor degree of memory problems observed as a normal part of aging and not significantly interfering with a person's social or occupational functioning. Pseudodementia syndromes may be the result of motivational or emotional factors that interfere with performance. Such factors include acute psychotic episodes, conversion or dissociative disorders, factitious disorder (e.g., Ganser's syndrome), and malingering (suggested by reports of relatives, examination, or evidence of primary and/or secondary gains). Chronic schizophrenia may present special diagnostic difficulties, both because of emotional and psychotic features and because of cognitive deficits (Zakzanis et al. 2003).

Depressive disorders in elderly patients should be considered, because these patients may have memory difficulties, slowed thinking, and lack of spontaneity, which suggest dementia (see discussion of DSD earlier in this chapter in the "Depression" subsection).

If present, delirium makes it very difficult to determine whether concurrent dementia is present, and delirium without fluctuating levels of consciousness may be very difficult to distinguish from dementia. The diagnosis of delirium is suggested when global cognitive disturbance (including immediate and recent memory) is accompanied by rapid onset, fluctuating level of consciousness, impairment of attention, incoherence of thought, visual illusions or hallucinations or other perceptual disturbances, and disturbances of the sleep–wake cycle, all in the presence of a severe medical condition. Definitive diagnosis often must be postponed until evaluation after recovery from the acute medical illness.

Mild cognitive impairment (MCI), as described in the "Concept of Dementia and Clinical Approach" section earlier in this chapter, merits special consideration because of its high prevalence and the considerable rate of progression to dementia. The DSM-5 category *mild neurocognitive disorder* is equivalent to MCI. This diagnosis requires cognitive decline in one or more domains, but to a milder degree than does the diagnosis of dementia (i.e., decline on test performance in the range of one to two standard deviations below appropriate norms). In contrast to the cognitive deficits in dementia, the cognitive deficits in MCI are insufficient to interfere with the capacity for independence in everyday activities.

Once false-positive cases are ruled out and the presence of a dementia syndrome is confirmed, the clinical characteristics of cortical, subcortical, or mixed type (see Table 5–5), as described in the previous sections, are defined. The onset and progression of the cognitive difficulties, the presence of other psychopathological features, and the presence of another medical condition will give further clues as to the type of dementia. (For diagnostic purposes, clinical differences between types of dementia are detailed in the "Clinical Types and Pathophysiology of Dementia" section earlier in this chapter.) The search for potentially reversible types of dementia due to medical conditions or toxic effects remains an important step in the diagnostic process. Such conditions are more common in general hospital patients, although identification of truly reversible causes is less common today than in the past, and true reversibility often depends on early treatment of causes. Workup recommendations for the diagnosis of dementia are available (Knopman et al. 2001; Small et al. 1997). Table 5–7 lists a screening battery of tests that are commonly used to identify conditions associated with dementia, such as infectious, metabolic, and neoplastic diseases and substance-induced dementia. The specific tests used should be determined by various factors, including the patient's age, medical comorbidities, history, and physical examination.

TABLE 5–7. **Laboratory tests and other diagnostic procedures used in the assessment of dementia**

Screening battery[a]
Complete blood cell count with differential cell type count
Erythrocyte sedimentation rate
Blood glucose
Blood urea nitrogen
Electrolytes, calcium, magnesium
Thyrotropin
Vitamin B_{12} and folate levels
Urinalysis
Fluorescent treponemal antibody absorption[b]
Liver and renal function tests

Neuroimaging
Computed tomography (CT) head scan
Magnetic resonance imaging (MRI) head scan[c]
Single photon emission computed tomography[b,c]

Other tests and procedures[a]
Blood tests
   Arterial blood gases
   Blood and urine screens for alcohol, drugs, and heavy metals
   Serum HIV test[b,c]
   Homocysteine level
   Antinuclear antibody, C3, C4, anti-double-stranded DNA, anticardiolipin antibody
Other
   Chest X ray
   Electrocardiogram
   Disease-specific tests (e.g., serum copper and ceruloplasmin for Wilson's disease)
   Lumbar puncture[c] (usually after CT or MRI)

[a]Tests may be selected on the basis of patient age.
[b]May require special consent and counseling.
[c]Tests selected on the basis of specific symptoms (history and physical examination) or patient populations.

Neuroimaging and Electroencephalography

Neuroimaging has revolutionized the ability of clinicians to diagnose dementia. It is a useful adjunct to clinical diagnosis and is considered to be mandatory in some stringent diagnostic systems (McKhann et al. 2011). However, neuroimaging may be unnecessary in cases involving advanced symptoms and a long history of the disease. Computed tomography (CT) and magnetic resonance imaging (MRI) are very useful in ruling out reversible conditions such as NPH, subdural hematoma, and brain tumors. Therefore, these imaging modalities should be routinely considered in patients with a history or findings suggesting those conditions.

In DAT, both CT and MRI are helpful diagnostic tools (Table 5–8). However, the findings are not specific (particularly for general atrophy, which may be found in elderly patients without dementia). Imaging views of enlarged ventricles are considered to be better discriminators. Early findings in the disease may be CT—and particularly MRI—views of disproportionate atrophy in the medial, basal, and lateral temporal lobes and in the medial parietal cortex (McKhann et al. 2011). Single photon emission computed tomography (SPECT) may be particularly useful in early cases of FTD or DLB to detect changes in blood flow. Positron emission tomography (PET) is also a promising technique (see Table 5–8), although not all hospitals have adequate facilities. Decreased fluorodeoxyglucose uptake on PET in the temporoparietal cortex and positive PET amyloid imaging have been accepted as major biomarkers of DAT. At present, the cerebral amyloid burden, as imaged with PET, may help to exclude the presence of DAT as well as forecast its possible onset (Del Sole et al. 2016). However, the costs of tests, and whether the results will make a difference in management of the patient, should be considered before routine recommendation in clinical practice.

In vascular dementia, neuroimaging can provide strong support for the diagnosis, especially the MRI finding of large-artery strokes, strategic infarcts (e.g., angular gyrus, thalamus, anterobasal regions of brain), many lacunar infarcts, substantial burden (>25%) of confluent white matter lesions (leukoaraiosis), or combinations thereof. The overlap between vascular and degenerative Alzheimer's pathology has prompted a search for common pathophysiological pathways (O'Brien and Thomas 2015). In CJD, brain MRI has high diagnostic utility, particularly diffusion-weighted imaging, with the apparent diffusion coefficient mapping sequences showing restricted diffusion in the cortical or deep gray matter nuclei (Geschwind 2015).

The electroencephalogram (EEG) has limited utility in the differential diagnosis of dementia because abnormalities are frequent but nonspecific. Slow-wave activity characteristic of delirium does not appear until late in the course of DAT, but it is a supportive feature of DLB (McKeith et al. 2005). EEG was the earliest diagnostic test for CJD, showing 1 Hz to 2 Hz periodic sharp-wave (often biphasic and triphasic) complexes. These abnormalities, however, do not appear until CJD is quite advanced (Geschwind 2015). EEG might also be useful in patients with some metabolic dementias, such as hepatic encephalopathy (triphasic waves), although such findings are not pathognomonic.

Cerebrospinal Fluid Analysis

Lumbar puncture is not routinely part of a dementia workup but should be considered for patients with early-onset, rapidly progressive dementia or atypical clinical

TABLE 5–8. **Neuroimaging findings in dementia syndromes**

Syndrome and findings	Neuroimaging modalities
Dementias treatable by surgical procedures	
Normal-pressure hydrocephalus, brain tumors, subdural hematoma	CT, MRI
Dementia of the Alzheimer's type	
Enlarged ventricles	CT, MRI
General atrophy	CT, MRI
Medial temporal lobe or hippocampus atrophy (early markers)	CT, MRI (combined with SPECT)
Temporoparietal (and sometimes frontal) hypoperfusion	SPECT
Temporoparietal (and sometimes frontal) hypometabolism; relative sparing of visual and sensorimotor cortex	PET
Absence of signs of vascular dementia	CT, MRI
Vascular dementia	
Leukoaraiosis in white matter (very frequent)	CT
Areas of infarct (very characteristic, only half the cases)	CT
Hyperintensities in white matter (more sensitive)	MRI
Frontotemporal dementia	
Frontal (and temporal) atrophy	CT, MRI
Frontal (and temporal) hypoperfusion	SPECT
Normal-pressure hydrocephalus	
Very enlarged ventricles	CT, MRI
Huntington's disease	
Atrophy of caudate nucleus	CT, MRI
Alcoholic dementia	
Enlarged ventricles and atrophy	CT, MRI
HIV dementia	
Atrophy	CT, MRI
Demyelination of subcortical white matter	MRI
Hypermetabolism of thalamus and basal ganglia	PET
Depression	
Frontal hypometabolism, asymmetric (reversible)	PET
Mild cognitive impairment	
Hippocampal and entorhinal volume reduction	MRI, CT
Hypoperfusion or hypometabolism	SPECT, PET

Note.   Structural imaging: CT=computed tomography; MRI=magnetic resonance imaging. Functional imaging: PET=positron emission tomography; SPECT=single photon emission computed tomography.

features, as well as for patients with positive syphilis serology or suspected hydro-cephalus, CNS infection, vasculitis, immunosuppression, or metastatic cancer.

The core cerebrospinal fluid biomarkers of neurodegeneration (decreased $A\beta_{1-42}$ together with increased total tau [T-tau] or phosphorylated tau [P-tau]) have shown a strong association with Alzheimer's disease (Dubois et al. 2014; Olsson et al. 2016). These biomarkers have recently been incorporated in new diagnostic guidelines for DAT, such as those published by the National Institute on Aging and the Alzheimer's Association (NIA/AA; McKhann et al. 2011), and are also recommended for use in diagnosing high-risk presymptomatic Alzheimer's disease (Dubois et al. 2014).

Clinical Course, Prognosis, and Outcome

The course and prognosis of dementia are generally disease specific but may be influenced by a variety of factors. Timely surgical treatment, before irreversible brain damage occurs, may have spectacular results in subdural hematoma or brain tumors, depending on type and location. Classic studies suggest the improvement of patients with NPH after shunt surgery, although the beneficial effects are typically in gait and continence rather than in cognition (Klassen and Ahlskog 2011).

Medical comorbidity may be present in two-thirds of DAT patients and is strongly associated with greater impairment in cognition and in self-care (Doraiswamy et al. 2002). Optimal management of medical illnesses may improve cognition in Alzheimer's disease. Dementias associated with infections have disease-specific prognoses. Untreated HIV dementia generally progresses quickly (over months) to severe global dementia, mutism, and death. However, with careful antiretroviral treatment, patients may survive for years. Adequate treatment with dopamine agonists and other standard treatments significantly improves the prognosis of dementia in Parkinson's disease. Early treatment with thiamine is vital in alcoholic patients with cognitive dysfunction (Rees and Gowing 2013).

Important events or changes in a patient's routine may precipitate episodes of behavioral disturbance. Medical illness (most often urinary tract infection or pneumonia) or the use of benzodiazepines or anticholinergics also may precipitate episodes of delirium. Patients with good premorbid adjustment and greater intelligence and education are in general more able to compensate for intellectual deficit. Support from family and caregivers may determine to an important extent the presence or absence of affective and other psychological symptoms, as well as the course of dementia.

Studies suggest that median survival after the onset of DAT is much shorter than had previously been estimated, with a median time from diagnosis to death of 3.8 years reported in a U.S. study (James et al. 2014). No important differences in mean survival have been found between DAT and vascular dementia (Wolfson et al. 2001).

The relative risk of death is three to four times higher among persons with DAT compared with those without DAT (James et al. 2014). Women and persons with early or very late dementia onset experience a faster deterioration, even though there is significant variability in individual decline (Rabins et al. 2013; Tschanz et al. 2011). The presence of the *APOEε4* allele may increase the speed of progression, although findings are variable (Rabins et al. 2013). Some studies found that early appearance of disruptive symptoms or the presence of apathy, depression, or psychotic symptoms can predict faster cognitive deterioration (Jones 2013; Rabins et al. 2013; Scarmeas et al. 2007).

Functional impairment in DAT is highly correlated with severity of cognitive impairment (Mohs et al. 2000). Instrumental ADLs demand a higher level of cognitive functioning than do basic ADLs, and, as expected, the former are impaired earlier. Nursing home placement has consistently been related not only to severity of dementia but also to severity of functional impairment and neuropsychiatric symptoms (Luppa et al. 2008). Strong evidence suggests that caring for patients with dementia has negative effects on caregivers, and that these effects are often more severe than the effects of caring for a person with physical disabilities (Morris et al. 1988). The ability of caregivers to tolerate neuropsychiatric symptoms reduces the probability of nursing home placement (Luppa et al. 2008).

Considerably less evidence is available regarding the course of degenerative diseases other than Alzheimer's, but clinical experience and some reports suggest that disease progression is similar to that in DAT. Survival after onset of DLB ranges from 1.8 to 9.5 years (Walker et al. 2000). Patients with early-onset DLB may show more rapid deterioration, and some DLB patients may have a rapidly fatal course (McKeith et al. 2004).

A faster rate of deterioration in executive functions, but not of other cognitive functions, has been reported in patients with FTD compared with those with DAT (Galasko et al. 2000). Over time, patients with FTD develop global cognitive impairment and motor deficits (Bang et al. 2015), and they usually die about 3–5 years after the diagnosis (Chow et al. 2006).

In the late stages of subcortical dementias such as Huntington's disease, apathy may be quite severe and may cause profound self-neglect; the patient's condition may resemble akinetic mutism. Survival after disease onset varies from 5–10 years in progressive supranuclear palsy to 10–15 years in Huntington's disease. Survival in Parkinson's disease may be 12–14 years, provided that the treatment is adequate. Patients with Wilson's disease may have a normal survival time if their symptoms are adequately treated with chelation before irreversible liver and brain damage occurs.

There is considerable individual variation in the course of vascular dementia; whereas some patients have a nonprogressive course (as long as they do not have a new stroke), other patients decline rapidly (Kimchi and Lyketsos 2016). Although average rates of cognitive decline in vascular dementia might be similar to those in DAT, mortality is higher in vascular dementia, with a mean survival of 3–5 years (Kua et al. 2014).

Treatment

General Principles

Principles of dementia treatment are summarized in Table 5–9. Extensive clinical guidelines for care of patients with dementia are available (Rabins et al. 2007). In addition to neuropsychiatric symptoms and the social needs that accompany cognitive deterioration, patients with dementia very often have a broad range of medical prob-

---

TABLE 5–9.   **General principles for treatment of dementia and bases for consultation-liaison programs**

Use a multimodal treatment plan and individualize it for each patient.

Adjust treatment to stage of disease.

Provide adequate care for emergencies.

Evaluate for suicidal potential, self-harm (e.g., falling or wandering), or accidents (e.g., fires).

Treat agitation and potential for violence.

Initiate early treatment of potentially reversible medical or surgical conditions etiologically related to dementia (e.g., hypothyroidism, subdural hematoma).

See patient on a regular basis.

Schedule frequent visits when starting therapy; see for routine follow-up every 4–6 months thereafter (more frequent visits may be required in special circumstances).

Ensure adequate medical care.

Maintain the patient's physical health: nutritious diet, proper exercise.

Identify and treat comorbid medical conditions: cardiopulmonary dysfunction, pain, urinary tract infections, decubitus ulcers, visual and auditory problems, etc.

Provide care for iatrogenic events (e.g., pressure sores, aspiration pneumonia, fecal impaction).

Exert stringent control of unnecessary drugs taken for other medical disorders.

Try to control underlying disease and slow progression in nonreversible dementias.

Prevent and treat vascular risk factors (in both vascular dementia and dementia of the Alzheimer's type): hypertension, hyperlipidemia, obesity, cardiac disease, diabetes, alcohol dependence, smoking, etc.

Treat cognitive loss: pharmacological, other measures.

Use other general measures.

Use general health measures: recreational and activity therapies, etc.

Restrict driving and use of other dangerous equipment.

Identify neuropsychiatric symptoms and treat as needed.

Provide psychological support and treatment for patient.

Provide orientation aids (calendars, clocks, television).

Assess activities of daily living and provide assistance as needed.

Use special techniques: stimulation-oriented, reminiscence therapy, cognitive or reality therapy.

Provide social treatment.

Educate family caregivers.

Give advice regarding arrangements for wills, power of attorney, and general estate matters.

Suggest support groups, community organizations.

Provide support for caregivers and treatment if needed (e.g., for depression).

Arrange long-term treatment and coordinate with care organizations.

Arrange sessions at a memory clinic.

Research community resources, geriatric day hospitals.

Consider multidisciplinary rehabilitation in an outpatient setting.

TABLE 5–9. **General principles for treatment of dementia and bases for consultation-liaison programs** *(continued)*

Arrange long-term treatment and coordinate with care organizations *(continued).*

Encourage participation in support groups (e.g., Alzheimer's Association).

Provide regular respite care for family caregivers.

Arrange care in a long-term facility (including nursing homes, hospice) if home caregivers are not available.

Maintain vigilance regarding neglect or abuse.

Incorporate health care strategies.

Support public awareness campaigns (e.g., campaigns for early detection and treatment of dementia).

---

lems (Lyketsos et al. 2006). For this reason, dementia care requires a multimodal plan adapted to the individual and to the specific stage of the disease (Samus et al. 2014). Specific treatment recommendations are discussed in the following sections.

Pharmacological Treatment

General guidelines for psychotropic medication use in frail elderly patients are applicable (Spar and La Rue 2002). Specific suggestions for dementia patients are summarized in Table 5–10. Because of the increased risks associated with use of medications to treat neuropsychiatric symptoms, clinicians should consider using nonpharmacological interventions as first-line therapy (Kimchi and Lyketsos 2016; National Institute for Health and Care Excellence 2016a). Systematic evidence to support the effectiveness of particular psychotropic drugs in dementia patients is limited. Therefore, choice of drug class may be based on clinical evidence, and choice of agent is often based on the side-effect profiles of medications and on the characteristics of the given patient. Noncognitive, psychopathological, and behavioral manifestations in patients with dementia may be early targets for psychiatric intervention.

Treatment of Psychosis and Agitation

Antipsychotics have traditionally been used for treating psychotic symptoms and agitation in patients with dementia, but now, because of evidence of their association with increased mortality and limited randomized controlled trial evidence of their efficacy, antipsychotics are no longer recommended for routine use (Corbett et al. 2014). The U.S. Food and Drug Administration (FDA) has issued a black box warning (U.S. Food and Drug Administration 2005, 2008). Antipsychotics may be used in cases of intense agitation or severe psychotic symptoms in which the patient's or caregiver's safety is at risk, or in which the patient does not respond to other interventions (Press and Alexander 2017). Treatment should be initiated at a low dosage, with gradual titration up to the minimum effective dosage. Treatment should be maintained only in the case of a beneficial response. There should be periodic discontinuation trials, considering the risk of relapse and the possible side effects (Declercq et al. 2013; Reus et al. 2016; Seitz et al. 2013). Risperidone and olanzapine have been shown to modestly improve some psychiatric symptoms (Sultzer et al. 2008). In patients with Parkinson's disease or DLB, conventional antipsychotics should be avoided because

TABLE 5–10.   **Suggested guidelines for psychotropic medication use**

Consider whether agitation and/or behavioral disturbances might be caused by:

A medical condition, pain, other psychiatric condition, or sleep loss, which could resolve with treatment of the primary condition.

Hunger, constipation, stressful atmosphere, change in living conditions, or interpersonal difficulties.

Use strategies to minimize the total amount of medication required.

Instruct caregivers to appropriately administer sedatives when warranted.

Mild symptoms or limited risk often may resolve with support, reassurance, and distraction.

Remember that dementia patients are often physically frail and have decreased renal clearance and slowed hepatic metabolism.

Be specific in selecting target symptoms.

Use low initial dosages (one-quarter to one-third of usual initial dosage); dosage increments should be smaller and between-dose intervals longer. Seek the lowest effective dosage.

Avoid polypharmacy.

Keep especially alert to:

Medical conditions and drug interactions.

Frequent and worrying side effects (orthostatic hypotension and central nervous system sedation, which may worsen cognition and cause falls; susceptibility to extrapyramidal side effects).

Idiosyncratic drug effects (mental confusion; restlessness; increased sedation; vulnerability to anticholinergic effects of psychotropic medication).

If extrapyramidal effects occur, reduce the dosage or switch to another drug rather than adding anticholinergic drugs.

Reassess risks and benefits of psychotropic treatment on an ongoing basis.

---

of these patients' extreme sensitivity to extrapyramidal effects, but pimavanserin, clozapine, or quetiapine are possible options (Hunter et al. 2015; Kimchi and Lyketsos 2016; Walker et al. 2015).

The use of cholinesterase inhibitors—namely, donepezil, rivastigmine, and galantamine—is considered to be an appropriate pharmacological strategy for management of psychotic symptoms and agitation in patients with dementia. Substantial clinical experience with these agents is available (Wang et al. 2015), although evidence of their efficacy is still limited (Ballard et al. 2009). Use of memantine to treat dementia-related psychosis or agitation is controversial (Ballard et al. 2009; Wang et al. 2015).

Among the antidepressants, only citalopram has been found to have significant benefit for agitation (Seitz et al. 2011). There is limited evidence for use of anticonvulsants (Gallagher and Herrmann 2014). Although there is considerable clinical experience with other medications, such as trazodone or buspirone, in cases of agitated behavior, there is little empirical support for use of these agents (Brown et al. 2015). When using benzodiazepines, low dosages of relatively short-acting drugs, such as lorazepam, for brief periods of time, are preferred.

Treatment of Depression

Psychological interventions may be an option in treating depression in mild cognitive impairment (Orgeta et al. 2014). Despite limited evidence for the efficacy of antidepressants in treatment of depressive syndromes in patients with dementia, some authors and clinical organizations recommend their use (Kimchi and Lyketsos 2016). The selective serotonin reuptake inhibitors (SSRIs) are widely considered to be the first-line choice, and they should be preferentially used because of their favorable side-effect profile (Sepehry et al. 2012). Other antidepressants, such as venlafaxine or mirtazapine, may also be used (Press and Alexander 2017). Because of their adverse-event profile (e.g., orthostatic hypotension, cardiac conduction delays, anticholinergic effects), tricyclic antidepressants are difficult to use in dementia, although nortriptyline and desipramine may be the best-tolerated agents in this class (Press and Alexander 2017).

Apathy in patients with dementia is common, underrecognized, and undertreated. Cholinesterase inhibitors are considered an appropriate option. There is some evidence of efficacy for memantine and psychostimulants, but less evidence for calcium antagonists, antipsychotics, antidepressants, and anticonvulsants (Berman et al. 2012; Rosenberg et al. 2013).

Treatment of Insomnia

Sleep disturbances, which are common in patients with dementia, should primarily be managed with nonpharmacological strategies (Gitlin et al. 2012). When sleep disturbances occur in patients with other neuropsychiatric symptoms requiring psychotropic treatment, a drug with sedating properties, given at bedtime, probably should be selected. Otherwise, trazodone (50–100 mg, once at bedtime) is often prescribed, with good results (Camargos et al. 2014).

Short-term use of low-dose zolpidem or zopiclone can be helpful. Clonazepam is recommended by some clinicians for patients with frequent awakening or nocturnal wandering. However, all hypnotics have the potential to cause nocturnal confusion, daytime sedation, tolerance, rebound insomnia, worsening of cognition, disinhibition, and delirium (Press and Alexander 2017). Diphenhydramine should not be used in patients with dementia because of its anticholinergic properties, which may exacerbate confusion and also counteract the effects of cholinesterase inhibitors (Press and Alexander 2017). There is no evidence that melatonin is beneficial for patients with sleep problems and moderate to severe dementia (McCleery et al. 2004).

Treatment of Cognitive Deficits

Pharmacological treatment of DAT also should aim at improving cognitive function and mitigating associated functional losses (Farlow and Boustani 2009). Currently, the main drugs approved for this purpose—donepezil, rivastigmine, and galantamine—act by inhibiting acetylcholinesterase, thus providing cholinergic augmentation. These agents may improve cognitive and behavioral symptoms, as well as functional ADLs, although the degree of benefit achieved is limited (see Cochrane reviews listed in Table 5–11; Birks and Harvey 2006), with little proven effect on ultimate outcomes. Unfortunately, these agents neither reverse nor halt the degenerative process (Kimchi and Lyketsos 2016).

TABLE 5–11.   Drug treatments for cognitive and functional losses in dementia of the Alzheimer's type (DAT): Cochrane reviews

| Drug | Evidence[a] | | | | Indications in DAT | Dosage | Mechanism of action | Side effects |
	Effectiveness	Cognitive	Behavioral	ADLs				
Donepezil[b]	++	++	++	++	All stages	5–10 mg once daily	AChE inhibitor	Nausea, vomiting, diarrhea
Rivastigmine[c]	++	++	++	++	Mild or moderate	3–6 mg twice daily	AChE, BChE inhibitor	Nausea, vomiting, diarrhea
					All stages	4.6–13.3 mg/day skin patch		
Galantamine[d]	++	++	++	++	Mild or moderate	8–24 mg once daily	AChE inhibitor	Nausea, vomiting, diarrhea
Memantine[e]	+	++	+	+	Moderate or severe	10–20 mg twice daily	NMDA antagonist	Agitation, urinary incontinence

Note.   AChE=acetylcholinesterase; ADLs=activities of daily living; BChE=butyrylcholinesterase; NMDA=*N*-methyl-D-aspartate.
[a]Evidence: ++=evidence considerable; +=some evidence/limited number of controlled trials.
[b]Birks 2006; Birks and Harvey 2006.
[c]Birks et al. 2015.
[d]Birks and Harvey 2006; Loy and Schneider 2006.
[e]Areosa Sastre et al. 2004; McShane et al. 2006.

Donepezil, rivastigmine, and galantamine, the agents approved for the treatment of mild to moderate DAT, appear to have comparable efficacy (Kimchi and Lyketsos 2016). A range of formulations (including a transdermal patch for rivastigmine and an extended-release capsule for galantamine) make these three drugs equally easy to use. In the event of intolerance or unsatisfactory response, switching to another agent is a valid option (Burns et al. 2006; Massoud et al. 2011). Because of some evidence that these drugs improve cognition and functionality in patients with DAT, even at late stages (Herrmann et al. 2013), donepezil and rivastigmine (in patches) have also been approved for use in severe cognitive impairment (Kimchi and Lyketsos 2016). There is debate about how much time patients should continue to receive cholinesterase inhibitors (Kimchi and Lyketsos 2016), given that discontinuation of these agents can be followed by rapid symptomatic deterioration (Scarpini et al. 2011; Schwarz et al. 2012).

Memantine (see Table 5–11), a drug that blocks the excitotoxic effects of glutamate in stimulating the *N*-methyl-D-aspartate receptor, has been shown to modestly delay deterioration in cognition and ADLs (Mulsant and Pollock 2015), and has received FDA approval for the treatment of moderate to severe DAT. It should be considered as an alternative to cholinesterase inhibitors in moderate cases of DAT in which the first-line agents are contraindicated or ineffective (National Institute for Health and Care Excellence 2016b; Schwarz et al. 2012).

Combining cholinesterase inhibitors with memantine to theoretically potentiate their benefits is a common clinical strategy, but evidence to support this practice is mixed (Jones 2013; National Institute for Health and Care Excellence 2016b; Schwarz et al. 2012).

Positive results in DAT treatment have been reported for a wide variety of agents, with systematic reviews supporting the benefits of nimodipine (90 mg/day), a calcium channel blocker (Birks and López-Arrieta 2002); naftidrofuryl, a vasodilator (Lu et al. 2011); nicergoline, an ergot derivative (Fioravanti and Flicker 2001); and selegiline, a monoamine oxidase–B inhibitor (Birks and Flicker 2003).

Development of vaccines directed against the formation and accumulation of amyloid plaques via active or passive immunotherapeutic approaches has been attempted (Folch et al. 2016). Unfortunately, many promising compounds have undergone numerous unsuccessful trials (Wisniewski and Goñi 2015). For this reason, there is increasing interest in the possibility that a tau aggregation inhibitor could have therapeutic utility in DAT (Wischik et al. 2015), and other strategies are also being studied (Godyń et al. 2016).

Drug treatment of MCI is controversial, because supporting evidence remains limited (Cooper et al. 2013). We recommend follow-up and monitoring of individuals with MCI, especially when neuroimaging or biomarkers suggest a high probability of conversion to DAT (see subsection "Neuroimaging and Electroencephalography" earlier in this chapter).

Vascular dementia has no standard treatment. A meta-analysis of studies using cholinesterase inhibitors and memantine suggested certain benefits for cognition, but these agents lacked a clear clinical benefit (Birks et al. 2013). However, these agents may be useful in cases of mixed dementia (vascular and DAT) (O'Brien and Thomas 2015). Similarly, limited evidence supports the use of nicergoline (Fioravanti and Flicker 2001), nimodipine (Birks and López-Arrieta 2002), cerebrolysin (Chen et al.

2013), and huperzine A (Hao et al. 2009) in vascular dementia. No single pharmacological strategy (antiplatelet agents, antihypertensives, antidiabetics, or statins) has sufficient evidence on its own for primary or secondary prevention of vascular dementia, but these pharmacological strategies are effective in treatment of vascular dementia risk factors (O'Brien and Thomas 2015).

Cholinesterase inhibitors have shown some promise in the treatment of other dementias. A Cochrane review found statistically significant improvements in dementia in Parkinson's disease, but not in DLB (Rolinski et al. 2012). The FDA has approved rivastigmine for use in Parkinson's disease (Rabins et al. 2007). Memantine can be useful in DLB and in Parkinson's dementia, although the evidence is conflicting (Kimchi and Lyketsos 2016; Matsunaga et al. 2015). Neither the cholinesterase inhibitors nor memantine has been found to be useful in FTD (Bang et al. 2015). There is limited evidence supporting the efficacy of cholinesterase inhibitors and memantine in other types of dementia, such as dementia associated with corticobasal degeneration, Huntington's disease, prion disease (Li et al. 2015), and Down syndrome (Hanney et al. 2012; Mohan et al. 2009).

Psychological Treatment

Two main goals may be identified in the psychological treatment of dementia: providing support and modifying behavior. Although few psychological treatments have been subjected to systematic evaluation, some research, including single case studies, along with clinical experience, supports their effectiveness. Supportive techniques are based on the recognition that deterioration in cognitive function and sense of identity has significant psychological meaning for patients with dementia and may cause high levels of distress. There is some overlap with cognitive-behavioral techniques, because support is often accompanied by educational measures in which the nature and course of the illness are clearly explained. Psychiatrists also can help patients and teach other staff to find ways to maximize functioning in preserved areas and to compensate for the impaired functions. Strategies include simple maneuvers, such as taking notes for memory problems or making schedules to help structure activities into a daily routine. In this way, patients with dementia may have a predictable schedule and avoid undue distress, including catastrophic reactions when confronted with unfamiliar activities or environments.

Behavioral treatments are often focused on specific cognitive deficits, and different strategies have been devised. Reality orientation involves presentation of information about the patient's environment (e.g., time-, place-, and person-related), which is thought to provide the person with a greater understanding of his or her surroundings. A systematic review found evidence that reality orientation provided benefit for both cognition and behavior in dementia (Spector et al. 2000a). Cognitive stimulation therapy has been reported to be beneficial for cognition and to potentially be more cost-effective than treatment as usual (Woods et al. 2012). Observational studies provide some support for other strategies, such as recreational activity, art therapy, dance therapy, and pet therapy. Reminiscence therapy tries to stimulate the patient to talk about the past. Beneficial effects on the patient's mood and/or behavior have been reported with this technique, but evidence in systematic reviews is limited (Chung et al. 2002; Spector et al. 2000b).

Family Support and Social Care

The care received by dementia patients is determined to a large extent by their social framework (Organization for Economic Cooperation and Development 2015). Patients should ideally receive optimal nutrition and hydration, some variety of activities and socializing, and support in their everyday routine (Kimchi and Lyketsos 2016). The majority (60%–70%) of elderly patients with dementia live within the community and are cared for by family members or close others (Theis et al. 2013). Psychiatrists and other providers should pay attention to family and social structures as well as community supports and should monitor the potential need for residential treatment. Strong evidence suggests that informal (i.e., family) caregivers very frequently have psychiatric morbidity and possibly also medical morbidity related to the burden of caring for patients with dementia (Schneider et al. 1999). Caregivers have unmet needs for support (Black et al. 2013). The effectiveness of techniques aimed at improving caregivers' coping strategies and effectiveness in managing their loved one with dementia has been reported (Brodaty and Donkin 2009). Referral to support groups is often indicated, and associations of families of patients with dementia exist in many countries and can provide critical support. Education, counseling, and support for family caregivers of DAT patients have been shown to improve the lives of both caregivers and patients (Olin and Schneider 2002) and to decrease the likelihood that the loved one will need to be placed in a nursing home (Brodaty and Donkin 2009). One book that has been very helpful for family members and other caregivers is *The 36-Hour Day* (Mace and Rabins 2006).

Care Provision

Mental health care facilities that specialize in treating dementia are varied. Psychiatrists should participate in supporting access to quality care, but no consensus currently exists about what constitutes quality care and how to assess care provision (Innes 2002). Social service referrals are indicated to inform the family about available resources. Special care units for patients with dementia may offer models of optimal care, but no empirical evidence indicates that this type of unit achieves better outcomes than do traditional facilities.

Among the various types of ambulatory facilities providing care for dementia patients, the memory clinic is the most commonly used (Colvez et al. 2002). Such clinics gain value when attached to a psychosomatic medicine/consultation-liaison service, particularly when liaison is developed with primary care (Lobo and Saz 2004). Community resources include home health services, day care, and nursing homes. Shortages of nursing home beds are reported in most countries, so residential care remains important and in demand (Organization for Economic Cooperation and Development 2015). Geriatric day hospitals provide multidisciplinary rehabilitation in an outpatient setting. A review of studies documented a significant difference in favor of day hospital attendance when compared with no comprehensive elderly care (Forster et al. 2000). However, the general move toward an increased emphasis on community care is also dependent on the availability of informal caregivers. Respite services are considered very important for informal caregivers, although data on their effectiveness remain inconclusive.

Long-term care of patients with dementia presents special problems. Delirium, a frequent complication in institutionalized elderly patients with dementia, is discussed in Chapter 4, "Delirium." DAT patients may place themselves at risk by wandering, creating difficult challenges for caregivers and institutional staff. Traditional interventions to prevent wandering include restraints, drugs, and locked doors. New techniques that incorporate knowledge about how cognitively impaired patients respond to environmental stimuli include the design of visual and other selective barriers, such as mirrors and grids or stripes of tape. However, a systematic review found no evidence that these techniques are effective (Price et al. 2000).

Overuse of medication in long-term institutionalized patients can lead to worsening of dementia and to harmful side effects. Available alternatives, such as the search for medical, psychiatric, or environmental factors that may be causing agitation or behavior problems, as discussed earlier in this chapter (see the section "Epidemiology, Etiology, and Risk Factors"), should be pursued. However, if a patient's behavior is dangerous, psychotropic medications should be used, and additional measures may be needed if the dangerous behavior cannot be managed with medication. Use of physical restraints should be limited to situations in which patients are at imminent risk of physically harming themselves or others; such measures should be used only after other measures have been exhausted (or pose greater risk to the patient) and only until more definitive treatment can be provided. Good clinical practice and legal regulations in some countries require careful consideration and documentation of the indications for and available alternatives to use of restraints; monitoring of the response; and reassessment of the need for treatment. Structured educational programs for staff may help reduce the misuse of tranquilizers and physical restraints in the institutionalized elderly.

Conclusion

In a context of increasing concern about the frequency and negative consequences of dementia, the psychiatric consultant working with other health care professionals may have a crucial role in the early identification of cases, as well as in the treatment, discharge planning, referral, and placement of patients.

References

Alexopoulos GS, Abrams RC, Young RC, et al: Cornell scale for depression in dementia. Biol Psychiatry 23(3):271–284, 1988 3337862

American Psychiatric Association: Diagnostic and Statistical Manual of Mental Disorders, 5th Edition. Arlington, VA, American Psychiatric Association, 2013

Areosa Sastre A, McShane R, Sherriff F: Memantine for dementia. Cochrane Database Syst Rev (4):CD003154, 2004 15495043

Ballard CG, Gauthier S, Cummings JL, et al: Management of agitation and aggression associated with Alzheimer disease. Nat Rev Neurol 5(5):245–255, 2009 19488082

Bang J, Spina S, Miller BL: Frontotemporal dementia. Lancet 386(10004):1672–1682, 2015 26595641

Berman K, Brodaty H, Withall A, Seeher K: Pharmacologic treatment of apathy in dementia. Am J Geriatr Psychiatry 20(2):104–122, 2012 21841459

Birks J: Cholinesterase inhibitors for Alzheimer's disease. Cochrane Database Syst Rev (1):CD005593, 2006 16437532

Birks J, Flicker L: Selegiline for Alzheimer's disease. Cochrane Database Syst Rev (1):CD000442, 2003 12535396

Birks J, Harvey RJ: Donepezil for dementia due to Alzheimer's disease. Cochrane Database Syst Rev (1):CD001190, 2006 16437430

Birks J, López-Arrieta J: Nimodipine for primary degenerative, mixed and vascular dementia. Cochrane Database Syst Rev (3):CD000147, 2002 12137606

Birks J, McGuinness B, Craig D: Rivastigmine for vascular cognitive impairment. Cochrane Database Syst Rev (5):CD004744, 2013 23728651

Birks JS, Chong LY, Grimley Evans J: Rivastigmine for Alzheimer's disease. Cochrane Database Syst Rev (9):CD001191, 2015 26393402

Black BS, Johnston D, Rabins PV, et al: Unmet needs of community-residing persons with dementia and their informal caregivers: findings from the maximizing independence at home study. J Am Geriatr Soc 61(12):2087–2095, 2013 24479141

Braak H, Del Tredici K, Rüb U, et al: Staging of brain pathology related to sporadic Parkinson's disease. Neurobiol Aging 24(2):197–211, 2003 12498954

Brodaty H, Donkin M: Family caregivers of people with dementia. Dialogues Clin Neurosci 11(2):217–228, 2009 19585957

Brown R, Howard R, Candy B, et al: Opioids for agitation in dementia. Cochrane Database Syst Rev (5):CD009705, 2015 25972091

Bunner KD, Rebec GV: Corticostriatal dysfunction in Huntington's disease: the basics. Front Hum Neurosci 10:317, 2016 27445757

Burns A, O'Brien J, BAP Dementia Consensus group, et al: Clinical practice with anti-dementia drugs: a consensus statement from British Association for Psychopharmacology. J Psychopharmacol 20(6):732–755, 2006 17060346

Camargos EF, Louzada LL, Quintas JL, et al: Trazodone improves sleep parameters in Alzheimer disease patients: a randomized, double-blind, and placebo-controlled study. Am J Geriatr Psychiatry 22(12):1565–1574, 2014 24495406

Campbell S, Stephens S, Ballard C: Dementia with Lewy bodies: clinical features and treatment. Drugs Aging 18(6):397–407, 2001 11419914

Chen R, Hu Z, Wei L, et al: Severity of depression and risk for subsequent dementia: cohort studies in China and the UK. Br J Psychiatry 193(5):373–377, 2008 18978315

Chen N, Yang M, Guo J, et al: Cerebrolysin for vascular dementia. Cochrane Database Syst Rev (1):CD008900, 2013 23440834

Chow TW, Hynan LS, Lipton AM: MMSE scores decline at a greater rate in frontotemporal degeneration than in AD. Dement Geriatr Cogn Disord 22(3):194–199, 2006 16899996

Chung JCC, Lai CKY, Chung PMB, et al: Snoezelen for dementia. Cochrane Database Syst Rev (4):CD003152, 2002 12519587

Colvez A, Joël ME, Ponton-Sanchez A, et al: Health status and work burden of Alzheimer patients' informal caregivers: comparisons of five different care programs in the European Union. Health Policy 60(3):219–233, 2002 11965332

Cooper C, Li R, Lyketsos C, Livingston G: Treatment for mild cognitive impairment: systematic review. Br J Psychiatry 203(3):255–264, 2013 [Erratum in: Br J Psychiatry 204(1):81, 2014] 24085737

Corbett A, Burns A, Ballard C: Don't use antipsychotics routinely to treat agitation and aggression in people with dementia. BMJ 349:g6420, 2014 25368388

Cummings JL, Mega M, Gray K, et al: The Neuropsychiatric Inventory: comprehensive assessment of psychopathology in dementia. Neurology 44(12):2308–2314, 1994 7991117

Cummings JL, Vinters HV, Cole GM, et al: Alzheimer's disease: etiologies, pathophysiology, cognitive reserve, and treatment opportunities. Neurology 51 (1 suppl 1):S2–S17, discussion S65–S67, 1998 9674758

Declercq T, Petrovic M, Azermai M, et al: Withdrawal versus continuation of chronic antipsychotic drugs for behavioural and psychological symptoms in older people with dementia. Cochrane Database Syst Rev (3):CD007726, 2013 23543555

Del Sole A, Malaspina S, Magenta Biasina A: Magnetic resonance imaging and positron emission tomography in the diagnosis of neurodegenerative dementias. Funct Neurol 31(4):205–215, 2016 28072381

Deming Y, Li Z, Kapoor M, et al: Genome-wide association study identifies four novel loci associated with Alzheimer's endophenotypes and disease modifiers. Acta Neuropathol 133(5):839–856, 2017 28247026

Doraiswamy PM, Leon J, Cummings JL, et al: Prevalence and impact of medical comorbidity in Alzheimer's disease. J Gerontol A Biol Sci Med Sci 57(3):M173–M177, 2002 11867654

Dubois B, Slachevsky A, Litvan I, Pillon B: The FAB: a Frontal Assessment Battery at bedside. Neurology 55(11):1621–1626, 2000 11113214

Dubois B, Feldman HH, Jacova C, et al: Advancing research diagnostic criteria for Alzheimer's disease: the IWG-2 criteria. Lancet Neurol 13(6):614–629, 2014 24849862

Farlow MR, Boustani M: Pharmacological treatment of Alzheimer disease and mild cognitive impairment, in The American Psychiatric Publishing Textbook of Alzheimer Disease and Other Dementias. Edited by Weiner MF, Lipton AM. Washington, DC, American Psychiatric Publishing, 2009, pp 317–331

Fioravanti M, Flicker L: Efficacy of nicergoline in dementia and other age associated forms of cognitive impairment. Cochrane Database Syst Rev (4):CD003159, 2001 11687175

Folch J, Petrov D, Ettcheto M, et al: Current research therapeutic strategies for Alzheimer's disease treatment. Neural Plast 2016:8501693, 2016 26881137

Folstein MF, McHugh PR: The neuropsychiatry of some specific brain disorders, in Handbook of Psychiatry 2, Mental Disorders and Somatic Illness. Edited by Lader MH. London, Cambridge University Press, 1983, pp 107–118

Folstein MF, Folstein SE, McHugh PR: "Mini-mental state": a practical method for grading the cognitive state of patients for the clinician. J Psychiatr Res 12(3):189–198, 1975 1202204

Forster A, Young J, Langhorne P: Medical day hospital care for the elderly versus alternative forms of care. Cochrane Database Syst Rev (2):CD001730, 2000 10796660

Fratiglioni L, Launer LJ, Andersen K, et al; Neurologic Diseases in the Elderly Research Group: Incidence of dementia and major subtypes in Europe: a collaborative study of population-based cohorts. Neurology 54 (11 suppl 5):S10–S15, 2000 10854355

Galasko DR, Gould RL, Abramson IS, et al: Measuring cognitive change in a cohort of patients with Alzheimer's disease. Stat Med 19(11–12):1421–1432, 2000 10844707

Gallagher D, Herrmann N: Antiepileptic drugs for the treatment of agitation and aggression in dementia: do they have a place in therapy? Drugs 74(15):1747–1755, 2014 25239267

Gauthier S, Reisberg B, Zaudig M, et al; International Psychogeriatric Association Expert Conference on Mild Cognitive Impairment: Mild cognitive impairment. Lancet 367(9518):1262–1270, 2006 16631882

Geschwind MD: Prion diseases. Continuum (Minneap Minn) 21(6 Neuroinfectious Disease):1612–1638, 2015 26633779

Gitlin LN, Kales HC, Lyketsos CG: Nonpharmacologic management of behavioral symptoms in dementia. JAMA 308(19):2020–2029, 2012 23168825

Godyń J, Jończyk J, Panek D, et al: Therapeutic strategies for Alzheimer's disease in clinical trials. Pharmacol Rep 68(1):127–138, 2016 26721364

Gomperts SN: Lewy body dementias: dementia with Lewy bodies and Parkinson disease dementia. Continuum (Minneap Minn) 22(2 Dementia):435–463, 2016 27042903

Goodman RA, Lochner KA, Thambisetty M, et al: Prevalence of dementia subtypes in United States Medicare fee-for-service beneficiaries, 2011–2013. Alzheimers Dement 13(1):28–37, 2017 27172148

Gottesman RF, Albert MS, Alonso A, et al: Associations between midlife vascular risk factors and 25-year incident dementia in the Atherosclerosis Risk in Communities (ARIC) cohort. JAMA Neurol 74(10):1246–1254, 2017 28783817

Gracia-García P, de-la-Cámara C, Santabárbara J, et al: Depression and incident Alzheimer disease: the impact of disease severity. Am J Geriatr Psychiatry 23(2):119–129, 2015 23791538

Gray KF, Cummings JL: Dementia, in The American Psychiatric Publishing Textbook of Consultation-Liaison Psychiatry: Psychiatry in the Medically Ill, 2nd Edition. Edited by Wise MG, Rundell JR. Washington, DC, American Psychiatric Publishing, 2002, pp 273–306

Gupta R, Sen N: Traumatic brain injury: a risk factor for neurodegenerative diseases. Rev Neurosci 27(1):93–100, 2016 26352199

Hanney M, Prasher V, Williams N, et al; MEADOWS trial researchers: Memantine for dementia in adults older than 40 years with Down's syndrome (MEADOWS): a randomised, double-blind, placebo-controlled trial. Lancet 379(9815):528–536, 2012 22236802

Hao Z, Liu M, Liu Z, et al: Huperzine A for vascular dementia. Cochrane Database Syst Rev (2):CD007365, 2009 19370686

Haskins BA, Harrison MB: Huntington's Disease. Curr Treat Options Neurol 2(3):243–262, 2000 11096752

Herrmann N, Lanctôt KL, Hogan DB: Pharmacological recommendations for the symptomatic treatment of dementia: the Canadian Consensus Conference on the Diagnosis and Treatment of Dementia 2012. Alzheimers Res Ther 5 (suppl 1):S5, 2013 24565367

Hughes CP, Berg L, Danziger WL, et al: A new clinical scale for the staging of dementia. Br J Psychiatry 140:566–572, 1982 7104545

Hunter NS, Anderson KC, Cox A: Pimavanserin. Drugs Today (Barc) 51(11):645–652, 2015 26744739

Innes A: The social and political context of formal dementia care provision. Ageing Soc 22(4):483–499, 2002

Iseki E, Togo T, Suzuki K, et al: Dementia with Lewy bodies from the perspective of tauopathy. Acta Neuropathol 105(3):265–270, 2003 12557014

Ismail Z, Smith EE, Geda Y, et al; ISTAART Neuropsychiatric Symptoms Professional Interest Area: Neuropsychiatric symptoms as early manifestations of emergent dementia: provisional diagnostic criteria for mild behavioral impairment. Alzheimers Dement 12(2):195–202, 2016 26096665

James BD, Leurgans SE, Hebert LE, et al: Contribution of Alzheimer disease to mortality in the United States. Neurology 82(12):1045–1050, 2014 24598707

Jaraj D, Wikkelsø C, Rabiei K, et al: Mortality and risk of dementia in normal-pressure hydrocephalus: a population study. Alzheimers Dement 13(8):850–857, 2017 28238737

Jones RW: Pharmacological treatment of dementia, in Oxford Textbook of Old Age Psychiatry, 2nd Edition. Edited by Dening T, Alan T. New York, Oxford University Press, 2013, pp 439–442

Jorm AF: A short form of the Informant Questionnaire on Cognitive Decline in the Elderly (IQCODE): development and cross-validation. Psychol Med 24(1):145–153, 1994 8208879

Jorm AF, Jacomb PA: The Informant Questionnaire on Cognitive Decline in the Elderly (IQCODE): socio-demographic correlates, reliability, validity and some norms. Psychol Med 19(4):1015–1022, 1989 2594878

Kales HC, Gitlin LN, Lyketsos CG: Assessment and management of behavioral and psychological symptoms of dementia. BMJ 350:h369, 2015 25731881

Katz S, Downs TD, Cash HR, Grotz RC: Progress in development of the index of ADL. Gerontologist 10(1):20–30, 1970 5420677

Khachaturian ZS: Perspectives on Alzheimer's disease: past, present, and future, in Alzheimer's Disease: Modernizing Concept, Biological Diagnosis, and Therapy. Edited by Hampel H, Carrillo MC. New York, Karger, 2012, pp 179–188

Kimchi EZ, Lyketsos CG: Dementia and mild neurocognitive disorders, in The American Psychiatric Publishing Textbook of Geriatric Psychiatry, 5th Edition. Edited by Steffens DC, Blazer DG, Thakur ME. Washington, DC, American Psychiatric Publishing, 2016, pp 177–242

Klassen BT, Ahlskog JE: Normal pressure hydrocephalus: how often does the diagnosis hold water? Neurology 77(12):1119–1125, 2011 21849644

Knopman DS, DeKosky ST, Cummings JL, et al: Practice parameter: diagnosis of dementia (an evidence-based review). Report of the Quality Standards Subcommittee of the American Academy of Neurology. Neurology 56(9):1143–1153, 2001 11342678

Koller D, Bynum JP: Dementia in the USA: state variation in prevalence. J Public Health (Oxf) 37(4):597–604, 2015 25330771

Kua EH, Ho E, Tan HH, et al: The natural history of dementia. Psychogeriatrics 14(3):196–201, 2014 25323961

Kukull WA, Higdon R, Bowen JD, et al: Dementia and Alzheimer disease incidence: a prospective cohort study. Arch Neurol 59(11):1737–1746, 2002 12433261

Langa KM: Is the risk of Alzheimer's disease and dementia declining? Alzheimers Res Ther 7(1):34, 2015 25815064

Lawton MP, Brody EM: Assessment of older people: self-maintaining and instrumental activities of daily living. Gerontologist 9(3):179–186, 1969 5349366

Lebert F, Delacourte A, Pasquier F: Treatment of frontotemporal dementia, in Alzheimer's Disease and Related Disorders Annual 2002. Edited by Gauthier S, Cummings JL. London, Taylor & Francis, 2002, pp 171–182

Li Y, Hai S, Zhou Y, et al: Cholinesterase inhibitors for rarer dementias associated with neurological conditions. Cochrane Database Syst Rev (3):CD009444, 2015 25734590

Lin JS, O'Connor E, Rossom RC, et al: Screening for cognitive impairment in older adults: an evidence update for the U.S. Preventive Services Task Force. Evidence Syntheses, No 107. Agency for Healthcare Research and Quality, Nov 2013. Available at: https://www.ncbi.nlm.nih.gov/books/NBK174643/. Accessed April 17, 2017.

Lobo A: Manual de Psiquiatría General. Madrid, Editorial Panamericana S.A., 2013

Lobo A, Saz P: Clínica de la memoria y unidad de demencias: un programa de enlace con atención primaria (A memory clinic and dementia unit: a liaison program with primary care). Cuadernos de Medicina Psicosomática 69/70:115–123, 2004

Lobo A, Saz P, Marcos G, et al: [Revalidation and standardization of the cognition mini-exam (first Spanish version of the Mini-Mental Status Examination) in the general geriatric population] [in Spanish]. Med Clin (Barc) 112(20):767–774, 1999 10422057

Lobo A, Saz P, Marcos G, et al; ZARADEMP Workgroup: Prevalence of dementia in a southern European population in two different time periods: the ZARADEMP Project. Acta Psychiatr Scand 116(4):299–307, 2007 17803760

Lobo E, Dufouil C, Marcos G, et al: Is there an association between low-to-moderate alcohol consumption and risk of cognitive decline? Am J Epidemiol 172(6):708–716, 2010 20699263

Lopez-Anton R, Santabárbara J, De-la-Cámara C, et al: Mild cognitive impairment diagnosed with the new DSM-5 criteria: prevalence and associations with non-cognitive psychopathology. Acta Psychiatr Scand 131(1):29–39, 2015 24893954

Loy C, Schneider L: Galantamine for Alzheimer's disease and mild cognitive impairment. Cochrane Database Syst Rev (1):CD001747, 2006 16437436

Lu D, Song H, Hao Z, et al: Naftidrofuryl for dementia. Cochrane Database Syst Rev (12):CD002955, 2011 22161372

Luppa M, Luck T, Brähler E, et al: Prediction of institutionalisation in dementia. A systematic review. Dement Geriatr Cogn Disord 26(1):65–78, 2008 18617737

Lyketsos CG, Lee HB: Diagnosis and treatment of depression in Alzheimer's disease. A practical update for the clinician. Dement Geriatr Cogn Disord 17(1–2):55–64, 2004 14564126

Lyketsos CG, Sheppard JM, Rabins PV: Dementia in elderly persons in a general hospital. Am J Psychiatry 157(5):704–707, 2000 10784461

Lyketsos CG, Lopez O, Jones B, et al: Prevalence of neuropsychiatric symptoms in dementia and mild cognitive impairment: results from the cardiovascular health study. JAMA 288(12):1475–1483, 2002 12243634

Lyketsos CG, Colenda CC, Beck C, et al; Task Force of American Association for Geriatric Psychiatry: Position statement of the American Association for Geriatric Psychiatry regarding principles of care for patients with dementia resulting from Alzheimer disease. Am J Geriatr Psychiatry 14(7):561–572, 2006 16816009

Mace NL, Rabins PV: The 36-Hour Day, 4th Edition: A Family Guide to Caring for People With Alzheimer Disease, Other Dementias, and Memory Loss in Later Life. Baltimore, MD, Johns Hopkins University Press, 2006

Marcos G, Santabárbara J, Lopez-Anton R, et al; ZARADEMP Workgroup: Conversion to dementia in mild cognitive impairment diagnosed with DSM-5 criteria and with Petersen's criteria. Acta Psychiatr Scand 133(5):378–385, 2016 26685927

Marra CM: Neurosyphilis. Continuum (Minneap Minn) 21(6 Neuroinfectious Disease):1714–1728, 2015 26633785

Massoud F, Desmarais JE, Gauthier S: Switching cholinesterase inhibitors in older adults with dementia. Int Psychogeriatr 23(3):372–378, 2011 21044399

Matsunaga S, Kishi T, Iwata N: Memantine for Lewy body disorders: systematic review and meta-analysis. Am J Geriatr Psychiatry 23(4):373–383, 2015 24406251

McCleery J, Cohen DA, Sharpley AL: Pharmacotherapies for sleep disturbances in Alzheimer's disease. Cochrane Database Syst Rev (3):CD009178, 2004 24659320

McHugh PR: Hydrocephalic dementia. Bull N Y Acad Med 42(10):907–917, 1966 5231976

McHugh PR, Folstein MF: Psychiatric syndromes of Huntington's chorea: a clinical and phenomenologic study, in Psychiatric Aspects of Neurologic Disease. Edited by Benson DF, Blumer D. New York, Grune & Stratton, 1975, pp 267–285

McHugh PR, Folstein MF: Psychopathology of dementia: implications for neuropathology, in Congenital and Acquired Cognitive Disorders. Edited by Katzman R. New York, Raven, 1979, pp 17–30

McHugh PR, Slavney PR: The Perspectives of Psychiatry. Baltimore, MD, Johns Hopkins University Press, 1998

McKeith I, Mintzer J, Aarsland D, et al; International Psychogeriatric Association Expert Meeting on DLB: Dementia with Lewy bodies. Lancet Neurol 3(1):19–28, 2004 14693108

McKeith IG, Dickson DW, Lowe J, et al; Consortium on DLB: Diagnosis and management of dementia with Lewy bodies: third report of the DLB Consortium. Neurology 65(12):1863–1872, 2005 16237129

McKhann GM, Knopman DS, Chertkow H, et al: The diagnosis of dementia due to Alzheimer's disease: recommendations from the National Institute on Aging–Alzheimer's Association workgroups on diagnostic guidelines for Alzheimer's disease. Alzheimers Dement 7(3):263–269, 2011 21514250

McShane R, Areosa Sastre A, Minakaran N: Memantine for dementia. Cochrane Database Syst Rev (2):CD003154, 2006 16625572

Medina M, Khachaturian ZS, Rossor M, et al: Toward common mechanisms for risk factors in Alzheimer's syndrome. Alzheimers Dement (N Y) 3(4):571–578, 2017 29124116

Michel JM, Sellal F: ["Reversible" dementia in 2011] [in French]. Geriatr Psychol Neuropsychiatr Vieil 9(2):211–225, 2011 21690030

Mielke MM, Rosenberg PB, Tschanz J, et al: Vascular factors predict rate of progression in Alzheimer disease. Neurology 69(19):1850–1858, 2007 17984453

Modrego PJ, Fayed N, Pina MA: Conversion from mild cognitive impairment to probable Alzheimer's disease predicted by brain magnetic resonance spectroscopy. Am J Psychiatry 162(4):667–675, 2005 15800137

Mohan M, Carpenter PK, Bennett C: Donepezil for dementia in people with Down syndrome. Cochrane Database Syst Rev (1):CD007178, 2009 19160328

Mohs RC, Schmeidler J, Aryan M: Longitudinal studies of cognitive, functional and behavioural change in patients with Alzheimer's disease. Stat Med 19(11–12):1401–1409, 2000 10844705

Morimoto SS, Kanellopoulos D, Manning KJ, et al: Diagnosis and treatment of depression and cognitive impairment in late life. Ann N Y Acad Sci 1345:36–46, 2015 25655026

Morris RG, Morris LW, Britton PG: Factors affecting the emotional wellbeing of the caregivers of dementia sufferers. Br J Psychiatry 153:147–156, 1988 3076489

Muangpaisan W, Petcharat C, Srinonprasert V: Prevalence of potentially reversible conditions in dementia and mild cognitive impairment in a geriatric clinic. Geriatr Gerontol Int 12(1):59–64, 2012 21794050

Mulsant BH, Pollock BG: Psychopharmacology, in The American Psychiatric Publishing Textbook of Geriatric Psychiatry, 5th Edition. Edited by Steffens DC, Blazer DG, Thakur ME. Washington, DC, American Psychiatric Publishing, 2015, pp 527–587

Nasreddine ZS, Phillips NA, Bédirian V, et al: The Montreal Cognitive Assessment, MoCA: a brief screening tool for mild cognitive impairment. J Am Geriatr Soc 53(4):695–699, 2005 15817019

National Institute for Health and Care Excellence: Dementia: supporting people with dementia and their carers in health and social care. Clinical Guideline 42. Published date: November 2006; last updated: September 2016a. Available at: https://www.nice.org.uk/guidance/CG42/chapter/1-Guidance#diagnosis-and-assessment-of-dementia. Accessed August 17, 2017.

National Institute for Health and Care Excellence: Donepezil, galantamine, rivastigmine and memantine for the treatment of Alzheimer's disease. Technology Appraisal Guidance TA217. Published date: 23 March 2011; last updated: 11 May 2016b. Available at: https://www.nice.org.uk/guidance/Ta217. Accessed April 17, 2017.

Neuropathology Group of the Medical Research Council Cognitive Function and Aging Study: Pathological correlates of late-onset dementia in a multicentre, community-based population in England and Wales. Lancet 357(9251):169–175, 2001 11213093

Norton S, Matthews FE, Barnes DE, et al: Potential for primary prevention of Alzheimer's disease: an analysis of population-based data. Lancet Neurol 13(8):788–794, 2014 25030513

O'Brien JT, Thomas A: Vascular dementia. Lancet 386(10004):1698–1706, 2015 26595643

O'Brien J, Thomas A, Ballard C, et al: Cognitive impairment in depression is not associated with neuropathologic evidence of increased vascular or Alzheimer-type pathology. Biol Psychiatry 49(2):130–136, 2001 11164759

Olin J, Schneider L: Galantamine for Alzheimer's disease. Cochrane Database Syst Rev (3):CD001747, 2002 12137632

Olsson B, Lautner R, Andreasson U, et al: CSF and blood biomarkers for the diagnosis of Alzheimer's disease: a systematic review and meta-analysis. Lancet Neurol 15(7):673–684, 2016 27068280

Organization for Economic Cooperation and Development: Addressing Dementia: The OECD Response. Paris, OECD Health Policy Studies, 2015. Available at: http://www.oecd.org/health/addressing-dementia-9789264231726-en.htm. Accessed October 25, 2017.

Orgeta V, Qazi A, Spector AE, et al: Psychological treatments for depression and anxiety in dementia and mild cognitive impairment. Cochrane Database Syst Rev (1):CD009125, 2014 24449085

Peters R, Peters J, Warner J, et al: Alcohol, dementia and cognitive decline in the elderly: a systematic review. Age Ageing 37(5):505–512, 2008 18487267

Petersen RC: Mild cognitive impairment as a diagnostic entity. J Intern Med 256(3):183–194, 2004 15324362

Picascia M, Zangaglia R, Bernini S, et al: A review of cognitive impairment and differential diagnosis in idiopathic normal pressure hydrocephalus. Funct Neurol 30(4):217–228, 2015 26727700

Press D, Alexander M: Management of neuropsychiatric symptoms of dementia. UpToDate, January 18, 2017. Available at: http://www.uptodate.com/contents/management-of-neuropsychiatric-symptoms-of-dementia. Accessed April 17, 2017.

Price JD, Hermans DG, Grimley Evans J: Subjective barriers to prevent wandering of cognitively impaired people. Cochrane Database Syst Rev (4):CD001932, 2000 11034735

Prince M, Wimo A, Guerchet M, et al: World Alzheimer Report 2015: The global impact of dementia: an analysis of prevalence, incidence, cost and trends. Alzheimer's Disease International, 2015. Available at: https://www.alz.co.uk/research/world-report-2015. Accessed April 17, 2017.

Rabins PV, Steele CD: A scale to measure impairment in severe dementia and similar conditions. Am J Geriatr Psychiatry 4(3):247–251, 1996 28531083

Rabins PV, Lyketsos CG, Steele C: Practical Dementia Care. New York, Oxford University Press, 1999

Rabins PV, Blacker D, Rovner BW, et al: American Psychiatric Association practice guideline for the treatment of patients with Alzheimer's disease and other dementias, second edition. Am J Psychiatry 164 (12 suppl):5–56, 2007 18340692

Rabins PV, Schwartz S, Black BS, et al: Predictors of progression to severe Alzheimer's disease in an incidence sample. Alzheimers Dement 9(2):204–207, 2013 23123228

Rcom-H'cheo-Gauthier AN, Osborne SL, Meedeniya AC, Pountney DL: Calcium: alpha-synuclein interactions in alpha-synucleinopathies. Front Neurosci 10:570, 2016 28066161

Rees E, Gowing LR: Supplementary thiamine is still important in alcohol dependence. Alcohol Alcohol 48(1):88–92, 2013 23161892

Reisberg B, Sclan SG, Franssen E, et al: Clinical stages of normal aging and Alzheimer's disease: the GDS staging system. Neurosci Res Commun 13 (suppl 1):S551–S554, 1993

Reitz C, Mayeux R: Alzheimer disease: epidemiology, diagnostic criteria, risk factors and biomarkers. Biochem Pharmacol 88(4):640–651, 2014 24398425

Reus VI, Fochtmann LJ, Eyler AE, et al: The American Psychiatric Association practice guideline on the use of antipsychotics to treat agitation or psychosis in patients with dementia. Am J Psychiatry 173(5):543–546, 2016 27133416

Rolinski M, Fox C, Maidment I, et al: Cholinesterase inhibitors for dementia with Lewy bodies, Parkinson's disease dementia and cognitive impairment in Parkinson's disease. Cochrane Database Syst Rev (3):CD006504, 2012 22419314

Roos RA: Huntington's disease: a clinical review. Orphanet J Rare Dis 5:40, 2010 21171977

Ropacki SA, Jeste DV: Epidemiology of and risk factors for psychosis of Alzheimer's disease: a review of 55 studies published from 1990 to 2003. Am J Psychiatry 162(11):2022–2030, 2005 16263838

Rosen WG, Mohs RC, Davis KL: A new rating scale for Alzheimer's disease. Am J Psychiatry 141(11):1356–1364, 1984 6496779

Rosenberg PB, Lanctôt KL, Drye LT, et al; ADMET Investigators: Safety and efficacy of methylphenidate for apathy in Alzheimer's disease: a randomized, placebo-controlled trial. J Clin Psychiatry 74(8):810–816, 2013 24021498

Sachdev PS, Blacker D, Blazer DG, et al: Classifying neurocognitive disorders: the DSM-5 approach. Nat Rev Neurol 10(11):634–642, 2014 25266297

Samus QM, Johnston D, Black BS, et al: A multidimensional home-based care coordination intervention for elders with memory disorders: the maximizing independence at home (MIND) pilot randomized trial. Am J Geriatr Psychiatry 22(4):398–414, 2014 24502822

Saz P, López-Antón R, Dewey ME, et al: Prevalence and implications of psychopathological non-cognitive symptoms in dementia. Acta Psychiatr Scand 119(2):107–116, 2009 19053966

Scarmeas N, Brandt J, Blacker D, et al: Disruptive behavior as a predictor in Alzheimer disease. Arch Neurol 64(12):1755–1761, 2007 18071039

Scarpini E, Bruno G, Zappalà G, et al: Cessation versus continuation of galantamine treatment after 12 months of therapy in patients with Alzheimer's disease: a randomized, double blind, placebo controlled withdrawal trial. J Alzheimers Dis 26(2):211–220, 2011 21606568

Schneider J, Murray J, Banerjee S, et al: EUROCARE: a cross-national study of co-resident spouse carers for people with Alzheimer's disease, I: factors associated with carer burden. Int J Geriatr Psychiatry 14(8):651–661, 1999 10489656

Schneider JA, Montine TJ, Sperling RA, et al: Neuropathological basis of Alzheimer's disease and Alzheimer's disease diagnosis, in Alzheimer's Disease: Modernizing Concept, Biological Diagnosis, and Therapy. Edited by Hampel H, Carrillo MC. New York, Karger, 2012, pp 49–70

Schwarz S, Froelich L, Burns A: Pharmacological treatment of dementia. Curr Opin Psychiatry 25(6):542–550, 2012 22992546

Seitz DP, Adunuri N, Gill SS, et al: Antidepressants for agitation and psychosis in dementia. Cochrane Database Syst Rev (2):CD008191, 2011 21328305

Seitz DP, Gill SS, Herrmann N, et al: Pharmacological treatments for neuropsychiatric symptoms of dementia in long-term care: a systematic review. Int Psychogeriatr 25(2):185–203, 2013 23083438

Semrau M, Burns A, Djukic-Dejanovic S, et al; International Dementia Alliance (IDEAL) study group: Development of an international schedule for the assessment and staging of care for dementia. J Alzheimers Dis 44(1):139–151, 2015 25182744

Sepehry AA, Lee PE, Hsiung GY, et al: Effect of selective serotonin reuptake inhibitors in Alzheimer's disease with comorbid depression: a meta-analysis of depression and cognitive outcomes. Drugs Aging 29(10):793–806, 2012 23079957

Shanmugiah A, Sinha S, Taly AB, et al: Psychiatric manifestations in Wilson's disease: a cross-sectional analysis. J Neuropsychiatry Clin Neurosci 20(1):81–85, 2008 18305288

Small GW, Rabins PV, Barry PP, et al: Diagnosis and treatment of Alzheimer disease and related disorders: consensus statement of the American Association for Geriatric Psychiatry, the Alzheimer Association, and the American Geriatrics Society. JAMA 278(16):1363–1371, 1997 9343469

Spar JE, La Rue A: Concise Guide to Geriatric Psychiatry, 3rd Edition. Washington, DC, American Psychiatric Publishing, 2002

Spector A, Orrell M, Davies S, et al: Reality orientation for dementia. Cochrane Database Syst Rev (2):CD001119, 2000a 10796602

Spector A, Orrell M, Davies S, et al: Reminiscence therapy for dementia. Cochrane Database Syst Rev (2):CD001120, 2000b 11034700

Sperling RA, Aisen PS, Beckett LA, et al: Toward defining the preclinical stages of Alzheimer's disease: recommendations from the National Institute on Aging–Alzheimer's Association workgroups on diagnostic guidelines for Alzheimer's disease. Alzheimers Dement 7(3):280–292, 2011 21514248

Steinberg M, Shao H, Zandi P, et al; Cache County Investigators: Point and 5-year period prevalence of neuropsychiatric symptoms in dementia: the Cache County Study. Int J Geriatr Psychiatry 23(2):170–177, 2008 17607801

Stella F: Neuropsychiatric symptoms in Alzheimer's disease patients: improving the diagnosis. Journal of Alzheimers Disease & Parkinsonism 4(3):146, 2014

Sultzer DL, Davis SM, Tariot PN, et al; CATIE-AD Study Group: Clinical symptom responses to atypical antipsychotic medications in Alzheimer's disease: phase 1 outcomes from the CATIE-AD effectiveness trial. Am J Psychiatry 165(7):844–854, 2008 18519523

Taylor WD, Aizenstein HJ, Alexopoulos GS: The vascular depression hypothesis: mechanisms linking vascular disease with depression. Mol Psychiatry 18(9):963–974, 2013 23439482

Teng EL, Chui HC: The Modified Mini-Mental State (3MS) examination. J Clin Psychiatry 48(8):314–318, 1987 3611032

Teng E, Ringman JM, Ross LK, et al; Alzheimer's Disease Research Centers of California–Depression in Alzheimer's Disease Investigators: Diagnosing depression in Alzheimer disease with the National Institute of Mental Health provisional criteria. Am J Geriatr Psychiatry 16(6):469–477, 2008 18515691

Theis W, Bleiler L; Alzheimer's Association: 2013 Alzheimer's disease facts and figures. Alzheimers Dement 9(2):208–245, 2013 23507120

Tschanz JT, Corcoran CD, Schwartz S, et al: Progression of cognitive, functional, and neuropsychiatric symptom domains in a population cohort with Alzheimer dementia: the Cache County Dementia Progression study. Am J Geriatr Psychiatry 19(6):532–542, 2011 21606896

U.S. Food and Drug Administration: FDA Public Health Advisory: Death With Antipsychotics in Elderly Patients With Behavioral Disturbances, April 11, 2005. Available at: https://www.fda.gov/Drugs/DrugSafety/PostmarketDrugSafetyInformationforPatientsandProviders/ucm053171.htm. Accessed April 17, 2017.

U.S. Food and Drug Administration: FDA Alert: Information for Healthcare Professionals: Conventional Antipsychotics, June 2008. Available at: http://www.fda.gov/Drugs/DrugSafety/ucm124830.htm. Accessed April 17, 2017.

van der Burg M, Bouwen A, Stessens J, et al: Scoring clock tests for dementia screening: a comparison of two scoring methods. Int J Geriatr Psychiatry 19(7):685–689, 2004 15254925

van der Flier WM, Scheltens P: Epidemiology and risk factors of dementia. J Neurol Neurosurg Psychiatry 76 (suppl 5):v2–v7, 2005 16291918

Ventura T, De-la-Cámara C, Lopez-Anton R, et al: Usefulness of 2 questions about age and year of birth in the case-finding of dementia. J Am Med Dir Assoc 14(8):627.e7–627.e12, 2013 23773305

Wahlund LO, Pihlstrand E, Jönhagen ME: Mild cognitive impairment: experience from a memory clinic. Acta Neurol Scand Suppl 179:21–24, 2003 12603246

Walker Z, Allen RL, Shergill S, et al: Three years survival in patients with a clinical diagnosis of dementia with Lewy bodies. Int J Geriatr Psychiatry 15(3):267–273, 2000 10713586

Walker Z, Possin KL, Boeve BF, et al: Lewy body dementias. Lancet 386(10004):1683–1697, 2015 26595642

Wang J, Yu JT, Wang HF, et al: Pharmacological treatment of neuropsychiatric symptoms in Alzheimer's disease: a systematic review and meta-analysis. J Neurol Neurosurg Psychiatry 86(1):101–109, 2015 24876182

White L, Small BJ, Petrovitch H, et al: Recent clinical-pathologic research on the causes of dementia in late life: update from the Honolulu-Asia Aging Study. J Geriatr Psychiatry Neurol 18(4):224–227, 2005 16306244

Wimo A, Jönsson L, Bond J, et al; Alzheimer Disease International: The worldwide economic impact of dementia 2010. Alzheimers Dement 9(1):1.e3–11.e3, 2013 23305821

Wischik CM, Staff RT, Wischik DJ, et al: Tau aggregation inhibitor therapy: an exploratory phase 2 study in mild or moderate Alzheimer's disease. J Alzheimers Dis 44(2):705–720, 2015 25550228

Wisniewski T, Goñi F: Immunotherapeutic approaches for Alzheimer's disease. Neuron 85(6):1162–1176, 2015 25789753

Wolfson C, Wolfson DB, Asgharian M, et al; Clinical Progression of Dementia Study Group: A reevaluation of the duration of survival after the onset of dementia. N Engl J Med 344(15):1111–1116, 2001 11297701

Woods B, Aguirre E, Spector AE, et al: Cognitive stimulation to improve cognitive functioning in people with dementia. Cochrane Database Syst Rev (2):CD005562, 2012 22336813

World Health Organization: The ICD-10 Classification of Mental and Behavioural Disorders: Clinical Descriptions and Diagnostic Guidelines. Geneva, World Health Organization, 1992

Wu YT, Fratiglioni L, Matthews FE, et al: Dementia in western Europe: epidemiological evidence and implications for policy making. Lancet Neurol 15(1):116–124, 2016 26300044

Wu YT, Beiser AS, Breteler MMB, et al: The changing prevalence and incidence of dementia over time—current evidence. Nat Rev Neurol 13(6):327–339, 2017 28497805

Zakzanis KK, Andrikopoulos J, Young DA, et al: Neuropsychological differentiation of late-onset schizophrenia and dementia of the Alzheimer's type. Appl Neuropsychol 10(2):105–114, 2003 12788685

CHAPTER 6

Aggression and Violence

Elizabeth A. Wise, M.D.

Constantine G. Lyketsos, M.D., M.H.S.

Chiadi U. Onyike, M.D., M.H.S.

In this chapter, we cover aggression associated with psychiatric, neurological, and general medical conditions. The focus is on hostile behaviors that threaten or inflict harm. Definitions of aggression, violence, and related terms used in this chapter are in Table 6–1. Although most aggression involves intent to harm, the definition we use does not require it because clinically important aggressive behavior can occur in the absence of demonstrable intent—such as in patients with cognitive disorders. We set aside behaviors that may be characterized as agitation, such as yelling, screaming, and other nonthreatening outbursts; oppositional and resisting behaviors; intrusiveness; and fidgeting, pacing, and other hyperkinetic actions. We also do not address community violence or criminality.

Psychiatrists mainly encounter aggression and violence when patients present for treatment in acutely ill states. Aggression may present as a complication of delusional psychoses, dementia, delirium, intoxication, personality disorders, and even adjustment disorder. It may complicate nonpsychiatric illnesses because it can develop when patients feel disregarded, dissatisfied, frustrated, confused, frightened, disenfranchised, thwarted, or angered by perceived mistreatment. Aggression can be perpetrated by men or women and by individuals of any age (except early infancy). It is seen in all patient care settings—outpatient clinics, inpatient units, rehabilitation programs, residential and custodial care facilities, nursing homes, and emergency departments (EDs). Aggressive behavior can result in involuntary confinement (in hospitals and jails), disruption of clinical and custodial care environments, longer hospital stays, and physical injury to patients, their caregivers, and their health care providers. Family members, home health aides, and health professionals who are repeatedly exposed to aggression generally experience demoralization, which adversely affects the quality of care the patient receives.

TABLE 6–1. **Terms used in this chapter**

Aggression	Hostile, threatening, and violent actions directed at person(s) or object(s), sometimes with no (or trivial) provocation
Violence	Overtly aggressive actions directed at person(s) or object(s)
Domestic violence	Behaviors directed against an intimate partner, ranging from verbal abuse to threats and intimidation to sexual assault and violence
Agitation	A state of pathologically intense emotional arousal and motor restlessness
Disinhibition	A state in which the individual's capacity for preemptive evaluation and restraint of behavioral responses is decreased or lost
Impulsivity	A state characterized by a proneness to act without thought or self-restraint; a habitual tendency toward "hair-trigger" actions
Irritability	A state of abnormally low tolerance in which the individual is easily provoked to anger and hostility

In this chapter, we focus on aggression and violence in the medically ill, beginning with the frequency, correlates, risk factors, and causes of aggressive and violent behaviors in diverse clinical settings, with reference to the *host, agent,* and *environment* causal model. We also discuss elder abuse and intimate partner violence, which are not necessarily manifestations of illness but are important causes and correlates of psychiatric and medical morbidity (we do not address child abuse). We review the evaluation, case formulation, and differential diagnosis of aggression and the management of aggressive behavior in the general hospital, including the ED.

Epidemiology

Epidemiological data demonstrate a relationship between violence and psychiatric illness. A 1990 community study (Swanson et al. 1990) found that 8.9%–21.1% of the men and 3.3%–21.7% of the women who had a psychiatric diagnosis self-reported violent behavior, in contrast to 2.7% of the men and 1.1% of the women who did not have a psychiatric diagnosis. The association was strongest for substance use disorders, DSM-III (American Psychiatric Association 1980) major affective disorders (i.e., major depressive disorder and bipolar disorder), and schizophrenia. Data from the National Comorbidity Survey show that rates of violence in adults with psychiatric illness are two to eight times higher than rates in the general population (Corrigan and Watson 2005). These observations should not be taken to mean that violence is the inevitable outcome of mental illness. Longitudinal data from the National Epidemiologic Survey on Alcohol and Related Conditions showed that mental illness alone did not predict violent behavior (Elbogen and Johnson 2009). Violence (measured by self-report) was instead associated with various clinical factors (e.g., substance use, perceived threats), demographic factors (e.g., age, sex, income), historical factors (e.g., past violence, juvenile detention, physical abuse, parental arrests), and social factors (e.g., recent divorce, unemployment, history of victimization). It appears that violence among individuals with mental illness is not merely a product of the illness, and that causal relationships are "complex, indirect, and embedded in a web" of pertinent personal and contextual factors (Elbogen and Johnson 2009). It has also been shown that individuals with severe mental illness are more frequently the *victims* of violence rather than the perpetrators (Desmarais et al. 2014). A meta-analytic review of violence and victimization in people with serious mental illness showed that victimization was strongly associated with homelessness, substance misuse, and violence perpetration (Khalifeh et al. 2016). Lack of social integration for individuals with serious mental illness may leave them vulnerable to victimization. In addition, individuals who abuse recreational substances and those with personality disorders may be both victims and perpetrators of violence through processes of "provocation, retaliation, or chronic relationship conflict" (Roaldset and Bjørkly 2015).

Whereas most mental illness does not result in violent behavior, violence has been described in individuals with schizophrenia (and other primary psychoses), substance use disorders, and personality disorders (specifically, the antisocial, borderline, paranoid, and narcissistic types) (Elbogen and Johnson 2009; Pulay et al. 2008). Violent behavior has been observed in primary dementia (Kalunian et al. 1990) and in cognitive disorder resulting from head trauma (Rao et al. 2009). Violence is also associated with confusion, substance intoxication, akathisia, fearfulness, agitation, paranoid delusions, and command hallucinations (McNiel et al. 2000; Swanson et al. 2006). Psychotic illness concurrent with substance use can amplify the risk of violent behavior (Elbogen and Johnson 2009; Witt et al. 2013).

Men generally are more likely than women to engage in aggressive behavior. However, the gender gap in aggression frequency and severity narrows among individuals with major mental illness and may disappear among psychiatric inpatients and individuals recently evaluated in the ED (Lam et al. 2000; Newhill et al. 1995). There is evidence that a gender gap may exist for serious violence, such as assault, but not for lesser forms of aggression, such as threats (Hiday et al. 1998). In a study of involuntarily admitted patients with schizophrenia, women exhibited aggressive behavior more frequently, whereas men committed the most severe aggressive acts (Nawka et al. 2013).

Other correlates of aggression include childhood conduct disorders (Hodgins et al. 2008; Swanson et al. 2008), onset of psychiatric illness at a younger age, previous violence, longer duration of hospitalization (Amore et al. 2008; Bobes et al. 2009; Pinna et al. 2016), and treatment nonadherence, particularly among patients with psychotic illness (Ehmann et al. 2001; Swartz et al. 1998). Overcrowding, sensory overload, provocation by other patients, high staff anxiety, poor staff training, and insensitive staff attitudes and communication styles can predispose psychiatric inpatients to anger and violence (Flannery 2005; Hamrin et al. 2009).

Aggression has been observed in ambulatory, hospital, and custodial (or residential) settings, with the frequency generally varying according to the specific population (e.g., diagnostic mix) and the characteristics of the setting (e.g., crowding, low staffing levels). Aggression is especially common in emergency care settings, where a confluence of risk factors promote its development. Emergency medical services (EMS) personnel must stabilize and transport patients to the ED and are therefore at high risk of exposure to violence. It has been estimated that 8.5% of EMS encounters involve aggression (Grange and Corbett 2002); about 50% of incidents of aggression involve violence, with patients responsible for 90% of these incidents and relatives and other bystanders responsible for the remainder. In a survey of EMS providers, up to 95% reported having had to restrain a patient, and more than 60% reported having been assaulted by a patient (with 25% suffering injury) (Furin et al. 2015).

Aggression in the ED may manifest as threats, belligerent confrontations, and/or assaults, and it is especially common in large EDs (i.e., those with volumes of 60,000 or more cases annually) (Behnam et al. 2011). Surveys of such large EDs have shown that staff are threatened by patients every day, that use of restraints is frequently necessary, and that nearly 50% of these facilities have one or more staff members assaulted each month (resulting in injury in 25% of cases) (Blanchard and Curtis 1999). For many patients, the aggressive or violent behavior may be the reason they are in the ED; others develop such behaviors in the ED setting as a result of their condition worsening or other factors. Some patients are carrying guns, knives, or other weapons (Kansagra et al. 2008), which signals a general predisposition to violence. Although health professionals (especially nurses) are the typical victims of patient aggression, sometimes a visitor or another patient is assaulted. At times, a family member or other visitor is the perpetrator of aggression. Assailants are more likely to be males, repeat offenders, residents of deprived communities, and intoxicated (James et al. 2006). Other contributing factors include involuntary transport to the ED; negative perceptions of the staff; inadequately trained and/or overextended staff; adverse ED conditions such as crowding, noise, discomfort, and long waits; and inadequate ED security.

Aggression is common beyond the ED. An estimated 20% of general hospital staff are assaulted by patients annually, with up to 90% of incidents occurring in inpatient units (Whittington et al. 1996). In hospitalized patients, aggressive acts may arise from confusion associated with serious illness (e.g., thyroid storm, head injuries, hypoxia, encephalitis), treatments (e.g., benzodiazepines, corticosteroids), or co-occurring mental illness. On surgical units, aggression may result from confusion during the immediate postoperative period, undiagnosed alcohol withdrawal, or inadequately controlled postoperative pain. Aggression in the general hospital may also evolve from dissatisfaction with care, from frustration about unfulfilled expectations, or during conflicts between patient and staff.

In a survey of intensive care units (ICUs) in England and Wales, nurses were subjected to verbal hostility from patients in 87% of the ICUs and from patients' relatives in 74% (Lynch et al. 2003). Nurses were assaulted by patients in 77% of the ICUs, and by patients' relatives in 17%; rates of hostility and assault directed at physicians were lower. Illness severity was associated with aggressive acts committed by patients, whereas emotional distress, alcohol abuse, and sociopathic traits were associated with aggressive acts committed by relatives.

Individuals are more likely to show negative affect and personality traits during times of high stress, including serious medical illness; thus, patients with personality styles characterized by impulsivity, distrust, and aggressiveness may be more likely to commit violent acts during hospitalization. Substance users experiencing withdrawal symptoms or intense cravings are frequent perpetrators of in-hospital aggression. Although unlikely to directly cause violence, nicotine withdrawal and craving can provoke or inflame conflict between patients and staff.

Aggression has serious consequences for patients and for those who care for them. Such consequences include disruption of the care environment, longer duration of hospitalization, higher treatment costs, and stigmatization of the mentally ill and their caregivers (Cheng et al. 2016; Greenfield et al. 1989). Patients may sustain injuries from punching walls or glass, handling dangerous objects, falling, fighting with other patients, or resisting restraint. In addition, inpatients who are prone to impulsive aggressive acts tend to be at higher risk of flight (Bowers et al. 2000) and impulsive suicidal acts (Giegling et al. 2009).

Although all health care personnel are at risk of injury, nurses and clinical assistants are the most likely to be injured by violent patients (Gillespie et al. 2017). Patient aggression results in demoralization, physical and psychological disability, absenteeism (as a result of sick days and disability), and job departures among nurses (Ferri et al. 2016; Gerberich et al. 2004; Nachreiner et al. 2007), as well as higher administrative costs and litigation exposure for the facility. Violence can cause staff members to adopt negative attitudes toward their work and their patients, resulting in impaired job performance, poor patient–staff relationships, and patient dissatisfaction with care (Arnetz and Arnetz 2001).

Mechanisms of Aggression

Aggression and violence can be categorized as impulsive or instrumental. *Impulsive* aggression is spontaneous behavior that is typically reactive, emotion laden, and sometimes explosive, whereas *instrumental* (or *premeditated*) aggression is purposeful, controlled behavior that may be predatory (i.e., committed for material or strategic advantage) or pathological (i.e, a deliberated response to misperceptions or delusions). In general, clinical aggression is either predominantly impulsive or predominantly instrumental. Impulsive aggression may be associated with cognitive deficits, psychotic states, and high emotional sensitivity and is usually accompanied by autonomic arousal (Nelson and Trainor 2007; Siever 2008). Instrumental aggression, on the other hand, may be associated with low sensitivity and low autonomic arousal, as in antisocial personality disorder (Nelson and Trainor 2007). Impulsive aggression is not necessarily unintentional; rather, it occurs on a *continuum of intention,* depending on the coalescence of individual susceptibility and context, ranging from entirely unintentional reflexive behaviors (e.g., ill-directed shoving and swinging in a patient with postictal confusion) to vigorous resistance (e.g., thrashing and biting during placement of lines or tubes by an agitated patient with delirium) and spur-of-the-moment intentional behaviors (e.g., throwing of a telephone at a scolding nurse by a patient with borderline personality disorder).

From a pathogenetic perspective, aggression is a heterogeneous behavior associated with background genetic, familial, and social determinants. These include unfavorable prenatal, perinatal, and/or rearing experiences (e.g., childhood neglect or abuse); genetic susceptibilities; low education; and negative cultural and peer influences (Volavka 1999). These factors and others acquired, such as DSM-IV (American Psychiatric Association 1994) Axis I conditions, brain injury syndromes, and personality disorders, can be viewed as coalescing in the individual to yield a *host* with a baseline propensity for aggression who reacts to specific provocations (*agents*) that occur in the environment (*circumstances*) to produce aggression. Examples of *agents* include threats by others, misperceptions, conflicts, or physical discomfort. *Circumstances* are contexts, such as intense (or distant) interpersonal relationships, personal

losses, or hospitalization for a serious illness, that are captured in a narrative that reveals a vulnerable patient's maladaptive interactions with his or her environment.
Consider the following illustrations:

- Episodes of aggression and violence are relatively frequent during the first 2 days after admission among inpatients with acute psychosis and/or a history of substance misuse (Barlow et al. 2000; Sheridan et al. 1990). A rapid decline in the risk of aggression was reported to occur a few days after admission among patients with schizophrenia (Binder and McNiel 1990). The fact that aggression and acute psychosis demand more intensive treatment efforts may help explain these observations.
- Substance users may become aggressive soon after admission as a result of withdrawal-related irritability. This risk is minimized by anticipating and preemptively treating withdrawal.
- Patient and staff conflicts—especially those that involve enforcement of rules, denial of requests (e.g., discharge, change in medications), or involuntary admission—can precipitate aggressive acts and violence (Iozzino et al. 2015; Papadopoulos et al. 2012).

The role of the prefrontal cortex in maintaining self-control and prosocial behavior has been recognized since John Martyn Harlow's description of Phineas Gage's personality change (i.e., coarse manner, jocularity, impulsivity, and aggressive outbursts) after sustaining an orbitofrontal cortical injury from a projectile (Harlow 1848, 1868). With frontotemporal dementia, patients frequently manifest a similar phenotype. Acquired antisocial behavior and aggressive behavior have also been observed in adults who sustained injuries of the prefrontal cortex in childhood (Siever 2008). Abnormalities in working memory, abstract thinking, moral reasoning, affective regulation, and behavioral inhibition have been noted in impulsively aggressive patients with antisocial personality disorder or frontal lobe injuries (Brower and Price 2001; Coccaro and Siever 2002; Davidson et al. 2000).

Evaluation of Aggression

Violence of psychiatric interest typically arises from a specific clinical circumstance—the *setting*—which leads to a *sequence* of events and an *outcome:* aggressive behavior. Several factors influence the expression of aggression in the clinic or hospital: aggression may follow specific symptoms, adverse effects of medicines, dissatisfaction with care, or conflicts with staff. However, aggression can be prevented, its intensity reduced, or its consequences avoided or minimized by prompt intervention. The clinical progression of aggressive behavior in the general hospital is depicted in Figure 6–1. The choice of intervention depends on the specific situation as well as the case formulation.

Clarification of *setting–sequence–outcome* involves describing the specific behavior, the sequence of events preceding it, and the symptoms and factors that may be influencing its expression. This approach has been referred to as a "define and decode" strategy (Lyketsos 2000). The effects of the patient's behavior should be noted by inquiring about injury to the patient or others, disruption of the milieu, and so on. Pre-

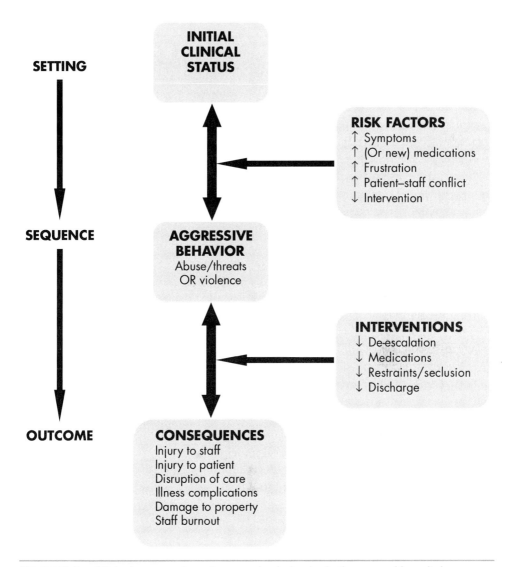

SETTING

INITIAL CLINICAL STATUS

RISK FACTORS
↑ Symptoms
↑ (Or new) medications
↑ Frustration
↑ Patient–staff conflict
↓ Intervention

SEQUENCE

AGGRESSIVE BEHAVIOR
Abuse/threats
OR violence

INTERVENTIONS
↓ De-escalation
↓ Medications
↓ Restraints/seclusion
↓ Discharge

OUTCOME

CONSEQUENCES
Injury to staff
Injury to patient
Disruption of care
Illness complications
Damage to property
Staff burnout

FIGURE 6–1. Clinical progression of aggressive behavior in the general hospital.

cipitants such as unsatisfied demands or staff–patient conflicts should be carefully sought, and the history also should describe the setting in which the behavior has occurred and the temporal relation of the aggressive behavior to any co-occurring symptoms. It is important to note whether the patient is febrile, confused, in pain, craving an addicting substance, cognitively impaired, anxious or fearful, hallucinating, delusional or paranoid, or postictal. The psychiatrist should systematically search for symptoms that require urgent intervention, such as acute confusion, akathisia, or agitation.

Also important is an inventory of the patient's concurrent illnesses; medications (both prescribed and over-the-counter); personal and family history; substance use; and personality disorder and psychiatric status. General physical, neurological, cognitive, and mental status examinations are focused on the systems implicated in the patient's history, but they should also include important "inspections," such as checking of vital signs, airway, and cardiovascular status; exclusion of injuries; and assessment and monitoring of alertness, reality testing, and dangerousness.

In the general hospital, blood tests facilitate detection of infections, anemia, electrolyte disturbances, and other abnormalities that may explain delirium. Toxicology screens and serum drug concentrations facilitate detection of acute intoxication and chronic substance use. Urinalysis, blood and urine cultures, and chest X ray may be helpful in certain circumstances (e.g., in immunosuppressed patients or patients with dementia). If seizures are a possibility, an electroencephalogram (EEG) should be performed. When obtundation, head wounds, or other reasons to suspect acute intracranial injury are present, brain imaging should be obtained. In most circumstances, obtaining computed tomography (CT) of the head is adequate. A high index of suspicion for intracranial hemorrhage (especially subdural hematoma) is appropriate, because perpetrators are themselves at heightened risk of being victims of violence.

Integration of the clinical data leads to a case formulation and differential diagnosis, as well as a summary narrative that lays out the *setting–sequence–outcome* chain. The formulation addresses the following questions:

- Does the patient have a mental illness, a vulnerability of temperament or disposition, a cognitive impairment, or another condition that predisposes him or her to aggressive behavior?
- Is the aggression linked to specific aspects of illness, such as psychomotor agitation, disinhibition, command hallucinations, aphasia, or acute pain?
- Can the aggression be explained by medications that bring about confusion, akathisia, or intoxication?
- Is the aggression associated with a specific activity or with interpersonal conflicts?
- How is the environment contributing to the behavior?

It is also important for psychiatrists to remember that many impulsively aggressive patients have a relatively high risk of suicidal behavior. Thus, the evaluation also must include an assessment of the risk of self-injury and suicide.

Disorders Associated With Aggressive Behavior

Many disorders can manifest with aggression and violence in the general hospital (Table 6–2). The psychiatrist's task will include consideration of these disorders in the differential diagnosis of violent behaviors.

Psychoses and Chronic Serious Mental Illness

Irritable patients with mania, depression, schizophrenia, or other psychoses may commit impulsive violence. This risk is greatest during acute presentations and is particularly high when patients have been brought to treatment against their will. Clinicians should maintain high levels of vigilance when evaluating irritable psychotic patients, especially in the ED or soon after involuntary hospitalization.

Premeditated violence can arise from psychotic disorders—usually as a response to delusional beliefs—but generally, the content of psychotic patients' delusions is focused on people in the patients' daily life or imaginary persecutors rather than on the

---

TABLE 6–2. **Differential diagnosis of aggressive and violent behavior**

Psychoses (mania, depression, schizophrenia, delusional disorder)

Personality disorders (antisocial, borderline, paranoid, narcissistic)

Other behavioral disorders or syndromes (intermittent explosive disorder, hypothalamic–limbic rage syndrome)

Substance use disorders (alcohol, phencyclidine, stimulants, cocaine)

Epilepsy

Delirium

Executive dysfunction syndromes

Dementia

Neurodevelopmental disorders (intellectual disability, XYY genotype)

---

providers caring for them. Up to 20% of the assaults observed in the psychiatric ward may be motivated by delusions and hallucinations (Nolan et al. 2003). It is also to be noted that many patients with chronic mental illness have maladaptive coping, resulting in a predisposition to violent reactions to conflicts and other stressors. Therefore, a crucial aspect of the psychiatrist's role is educating the physicians, nurses, and others caring for these patients. When patients with major mental illness are admitted to nonpsychiatric settings, the psychiatrist's role as consultant should include educating the medical team about the illness (its current status and treatment) and the fact that most such patients can communicate their concerns and symptoms, will cooperate with care, and are nonviolent (even when psychotic). Treatment recommendations should include ways of approaching the patient (e.g., from within his or her line of sight so as not to startle, calling out a greeting to signal good faith, and so forth), ensuring that the current psychotropic regimen is prescribed, and pointing out known habits or preferences so that they can be accommodated (e.g., preferred meals, favorite music or television shows). The patient's physicians and nurses should be educated about early signs of agitation, such as pacing, restlessness, staring, and refusal of medications. Contingency plans for managing these symptoms or states should be specified—what behavioral approaches (usually involving positive reinforcement and pacification) and tranquilization strategies should be used and how the psychiatrist can be contacted when urgently needed.

Personality Disorders

Antisocial personality disorder is the personality disorder most likely to be associated with habitual aggression. Patients with antisocial personality disorder often present to the ED with injuries resulting from violence (e.g., stab and gunshot wounds) and with medical complications of substance use (e.g., intoxication, wound infection, head injury, hepatitis). Antisocial patients who are intoxicated can become dangerous because of their mood instability, lowered frustration tolerance, and behavioral disinhibition. While in the hospital, they may become aggressive when their demands are not met.

Many antisocial patients are repeatedly hospitalized for treatment of problems arising from their lifestyle (e.g., medical complications of addictions and risk-taking behaviors). These repeated admissions often arouse resentment in staff, who see their efforts to care for the patient as unappreciated and futile. Such patients will have earned notoriety during earlier hospitalizations, which places them at risk for angry exchanges with and retaliatory responses from health care professionals, such as provision of suboptimal care, inadequate pain treatment, and premature discharge. Because these circumstances can increase the risk of missed diagnoses and medical errors, psychiatrists involved in the care of such patients need to know their reputation on the unit and the feelings of the staff caring for them. One of the psychiatrist's responsibilities with such patients is to help physicians, nurses, and other staff manage their resentments and frustrations properly, avoiding overreaction (e.g., berating patients, precipitous discharge) as well as underreaction (e.g., failing to set limits, failing to discharge when indicated). Antisocial patients are not immune to other conditions that may explain aggression, such as delirium, substance withdrawal, and psychosis. Therefore, psychiatrists should pursue a systematic psychiatric and general medical assessment whenever antisocial patients are encountered in nonpsychiatric settings.

Borderline personality disorder is characterized by intense emotionality, intense relationships, rejection sensitivity, manipulative behaviors, impulsiveness, low self-regard, irritability, and a tendency toward extreme reactions. The violent acts of borderline patients usually are impulsive and typically occur during interpersonal conflict. These individuals also have a high potential for self-injury and suicidal acts, for which they are often seen in the ED. They may obstruct their own care by demanding specific conditions or providers before submitting to interview or examination. They are capable of angrily refusing care and of violent tantrums. Thus, for clinicians, the highest priorities in caring for these patients are creating an effective relationship, maintaining behavior limits, and managing the intense countertransference that these individuals can trigger.

Individuals with borderline personality disorder seen in the ED should be screened for depression, substance use, and domestic violence, because these conditions are highly comorbid. On medical units, patients with borderline personality disorder can become disruptive when their expectations are not met. Psychiatrists should educate physician and nurse colleagues about the need to define behavior limits, meet expectations agreed on with the patient, and maintain a consistent approach to the patient's care. Such education is best provided in the context of an interdisciplinary care conference, with the psychiatrist assisting the staff in constructing a treatment contract to be negotiated with and signed by the patient.

Other personality disorders are less frequently associated with violent behavior, although narcissistic individuals may lash out in retaliation for perceived slights or to satiate their sense of entitlement, and individuals with paranoid personality disorder may become aggressive in response to perceived mistreatment.

Intermittent Explosive Disorder and Hypothalamic–Limbic Rage Syndrome

The terms *intermittent explosive disorder, episodic dyscontrol syndrome,* and *hypothalamic–limbic rage syndrome* describe disturbances characterized by explosive episodes of aggression and violence. *Intermittent explosive disorder,* as defined by DSM-5 (American Psychiatric Association 2013), is a disturbance characterized by recurrent episodes of explosive anger that cannot be explained by psychosis or another mental disorder.

Although rare, rage attacks in association with neoplastic and surgical lesions of the hypothalamus and amygdala have been described (Demaree and Harrison 1996; Tonkonogy and Geller 1992). These attacks, which have been reproduced in experimental animals, have been termed *hypothalamic rage attacks* or *hypothalamic–limbic rage syndrome.* These syndromes involve provoked and unprovoked episodes of uncontrollable rage and may represent an acquired form of intermittent explosive disorder. In addition to rage attacks, patients may have symptoms such as hyperphagia, polydipsia, excessive weight gain, or obesity; clinical findings suggesting thyroid, adrenal, or pituitary disease; a history of recently diagnosed pituitary, midbrain, or temporal lobe tumor; or recent brain surgery. Treatment involves correction of the underlying condition (including surgical resection of tumors) and use of behavioral and pharmacological interventions targeted at aggression.

Substance Use Disorders

Alcohol is the psychoactive substance most often associated with violence. Alcohol-related violence may result from a severely intoxicated state that produces gross impairment of judgment. Pathological intoxication, seen in vulnerable individuals who have had modest amounts of alcohol, may be associated with disorganized behavior, emotional lability, and violent outbursts. In severe cases, it may be accompanied by delirium with hyperarousal, hallucinations, and delusions, followed by amnesia after recovery. Alcohol withdrawal can be accompanied by irritability and low frustration tolerance, which predispose individuals to directed aggression. Alcohol withdrawal can also result in seizures that are followed by aggression during the postictal state. Patients who develop delirium tremens may show poorly coordinated resistive or preemptive violence.

Cocaine and amphetamine use can produce impulsive, disinhibited intoxicated states during which violence may occur. Patients undergoing opioid, sedative, or cocaine withdrawal experience anxious tension and irritability that can result in violent behavior. Phencyclidine intoxication can manifest as severe, impulsively directed violence. By contrast, violence is far less common in intoxication from hallucinogens; in these cases, the aggressive behavior appears to relate to the severe perceptual disturbances. Violence as a consequence of anticholinergic intoxication is rare, and is most often associated with acute delirium. In recent years, violent behavior has been observed during intoxication with novel psychoactive substances, particularly synthetic cannabis and stimulants. High doses of stimulant bath salts can induce combative behavior (Vazirian et al. 2015). In a recent study, more than one-third of patients presenting to the ED following intoxication with synthetic cannabinoids displayed severe agitation (Rowley et al. 2017); of these patients, 25% required tranquilizers and 5% required physical restraints (see also Chapter 16, "Substance-Related Disorders").

Epilepsy

In evaluating episodes of aggression in patients with epilepsy (see also Chapter 30, "Neurology and Neurosurgery"), consultation-liaison psychiatrists must carefully consider whether the episode is directly related to a seizure, to mental state changes associated with seizures, or to a complication of other conditions that increase the risk of aggressive behavior. In addition, psychiatrists must be aware that certain types of seizures can be misinterpreted as intentional violent behavior. Violent behavior may be observed during complex partial seizures, but never during generalized tonic-clonic seizures.

Ictal violence is rare, and most cases are characterized by spontaneous, undirected, stereotyped aggressive behaviors. Typically, the patient's consciousness is impaired, and the aggressive behavior is poorly directed and not purposeful (Marsh and Krauss 2000). In practice, it can be difficult to determine whether a violent act can be attributed to a seizure event. This determination requires integration of findings from the interview, clinical history, and in some cases video EEG monitoring. Abnormal nonseizure EEG phenomena (such as sharp waves) are nonspecific findings and should not be used as evidence that violence is ictal. Criteria for attributing a specific violent act to an epileptic seizure have been developed (Treiman 1986) and are presented in Table 6–3.

Although uncommon, a prodromal state of affective instability preceding a seizure episode by several hours or days may be associated with directed aggression (Marsh and Krauss 2000). The affective symptoms may be specific to the preictal state or an exacerbation of interictal phenomena; these states and their aggressive features usually resolve after the seizure.

Violent behavior in epilepsy usually occurs in postictal confusional states, which are typically brief but vary in duration, shaped by the type and severity of the preceding seizures. Abnormal mood, paranoia, hallucinations, and delirium may occur and result in violence by heightening aggressive propensities or distorting perceptions of environmental stimuli. In general, episodes of postictal violence are longer in duration than episodes of ictal violence, are associated with amnesia for the event, and are out of character for the individual. In some males, stereotypic episodes of severe postictal aggression can occur after clusters of seizures (Gerard et al. 1998). Postictal delirium can be detected clinically by assessing the patient's level of consciousness and awareness and evaluating EEG patterns for evidence of diffuse slowing in the absence of ictal activity. Typically, the delirium is brief, and a gradual return to normal consciousness follows, but prolonged or repetitive seizures can extend the duration of delirium. Violence during postictal delirium is usually undirected; resistive violence is fairly common, occurring when attempts are made to help or restrain the patient.

Sometimes postictal violence is motivated by a postictal psychosis. The psychosis may emerge from postictal confusion or a lucid state and tends to follow a psychosis-free interval of several hours to a few days after a seizure (or cluster of complex partial seizures) (Marsh and Krauss 2000). Postictal psychosis usually manifests as an affective state (featuring mood-congruent delusions), but some patients with psychosis present with thought disorder, hallucinations, and paranoid ideational psychoses reminiscent of schizophrenia. Although usually no longer than several hours in duration, these states may extend over several weeks. Postictal psychosis has a tendency to recur and may become chronic. Violence is more likely to occur in individuals with postictal psychosis compared with those with interictal psychosis or postictal confusion (Kanemoto et al. 2010). Most episodes of postictal psychosis resolve spontaneously or following treatment with low doses of an antipsychotic, and improved control of the epilepsy then becomes the treatment focus (see also Chapter 9, "Psychosis, Mania, and Catatonia," and Chapter 30).

TABLE 6–3. **Criteria for determining whether a violent act resulted from an epileptic seizure**

1. Diagnosis of epilepsy established by an expert neurologist[a]

2. Epileptic automatisms documented by clinical history and closed-circuit-television electroencephalogram

3. Aggression during epileptic automatisms documented on closed-circuit-television electroencephalogram

4. Determination that the violent behavior is characteristic of the patient's habitual seizures

5. Clinical judgment by the neurologist that the behavior was part of a seizure

[a]A neurologist with special competence in epilepsy.

Source. Adapted from Treiman 1986.

Most violent behaviors in patients with epilepsy have no particular association with ictal or postictal states. They typically occur around other people and are purposeful, nonstereotyped, and highly coordinated. The aggression usually can be "explained" by the situation at hand, is associated with the buildup of negative emotions concerning some circumstance, and may be of relatively prolonged duration. Brain injury and cognitive impairment are important risk factors for interictal aggressive behavior. Interictal psychiatric phenomena, such as depression, hallucinations and delusions, and sociopathic personality traits, also predispose patients with epilepsy to aggressive behavior.

Delirium

States of heightened arousal often accompany the confusion and fluctuating alertness of delirium and may predispose patients to violent behavior. Hallucinations and delusions increase the potential for violence. The presence of delirium in an aggressive patient should prompt a thorough search for an underlying cause. When ambiguity exists about the presence of delirium, the diagnosis can be established by noting high variability in scores on the Montreal Cognitive Assessment or Mini-Mental State Examination (or other short cognitive battery) within a relatively short period (several hours) or by observing slowed cerebral activity on the EEG. A more detailed discussion of delirium is presented in Chapter 4, "Delirium."

Executive Dysfunction Syndromes

Executive dysfunction syndromes (Lyketsos et al. 2004), more commonly called *frontal lobe syndromes,* are manifestations of brain injury characterized by varying combinations of inattention, impulsivity, disinhibition, absence of insight, impairments of judgment and temperament, and diminished initiative and vitality. These syndromes, which reflect injury principally affecting the frontal and temporal lobes and subcortical nuclei, result from a range of etiologies, including trauma, infection, neoplasm, stroke, and neurodegenerative disease. Explosive violence may be manifested by patients in whom disinhibition or affective dysregulation predominates, although violent behavior in these patients is usually reactive. In many individuals with habitual impulsive violence, formal neuropsychological testing indicates deficits in executive cognition (see section "Mechanisms of Aggression" earlier in this chapter); these individuals may be viewed as having occult executive dysfunction syndromes (see also Chapter 30).

Dementia

Aggression is a common complication of dementia, with the frequency rising with dementia severity, concurrent medical illness or pain, provocative environmental stimuli, stressed patient–caregiver relationships, and disordered sleep (Kales et al. 2015). Aggression in patients with dementia is most commonly encountered during routine care, where it complicates activities such as bathing, grooming, and toileting. In these situations, the aggressive behavior may result from adversarial interactions with caregivers.

The presence of motor restlessness, depression, hallucinations, or delusions in patients with dementia should alert the clinician to the risk of aggressive behavior. Dementia type appears to have limited influence on the likelihood of aggression, although patients with vascular dementia or Huntington's disease who exhibit aggressive behavior may be less cognitively impaired than their counterparts with other forms of dementia.

In dementia, aggression generally manifests as relatively simple behaviors such as throwing objects, pushing, kicking, pinching, biting, and scratching (Cohen-Mansfield and Billig 1986). Destruction of property is uncommon. Intrusive, aggressive sexual behaviors have been reported, particularly in residential care settings, and intimacy-seeking behaviors can also be complicated by reactive aggression when the patient is thwarted (de Medeiros et al. 2008). It is unusual for elderly persons with dementia to have well-coordinated and goal-directed physical aggression. When such violence does occur, it is often associated with distorted perceptions, illusions, or hallucinations that give rise to persecutory delusions. This violence can be serious, especially when enacted by individuals with combat training or with early-onset dementia. Careful identification of environmental or caregiver factors that may be triggering the aggressive behavior can facilitate removal or modification of these factors (see also Chapter 5, "Dementia").

Neurodevelopmental Disorders

Violent behavior has been observed in neurodevelopmental disorders and syndromes. On the whole, few patients with intellectual disability are habitually or impulsively aggressive. However, many individuals with severe communication or language deficiencies are prone to outbursts, tantrums, and violence when frustrated or experiencing physical discomfort. These persons are also at increased risk of psychiatric symptoms, such as irritability, impulsivity, disinhibition, and low frustration tolerance, and of affective and psychotic conditions, which sometimes contribute to aggressive behavior.

Domestic Aggression Presenting in Medical Settings

Elder Abuse

In elderly individuals, mistreatment, in the form of abuse or neglect, may provoke aggression from the victim. Mistreatment begets aggression, but aggressive elders also are more likely to be mistreated by caregivers, whether at home or in an institutional setting. Screening for mistreatment is indicated if an elderly person presents with an unusual pattern of agitated behavior—for example, aggression directed at a particular caregiver or restricted to a particular context (e.g., while being bathed or dressed)—or if there are physical signs of mistreatment, such as unexplained or recurring bruising or skin tears. For a comprehensive discussion of elder mistreatment, including screening and management, the reader is referred to the recent review of Pillemer et al. (2016).

Intimate Partner Violence

Intimate partner abuse refers to emotional, psychological, physical, and/or sexual coercion within an intimate relationship, and *intimate partner violence* (IPV) denotes battery of an intimate partner (McHugh and Frieze 2006).

The U.S. National Intimate Partner and Sexual Violence Survey estimated that 36% of women and 29% of men have experienced an episode of IPV in their lifetime (Black et al. 2011). It is estimated that 10%–20% of women have experienced IPV from more than one partner (Thompson et al. 2006), and the frequency of IPV is especially high for younger women, single mothers, those who are poorly educated, and those with a history of childhood abuse. IPV is a pervasive, cross-cultural, worldwide problem (Stewart et al. 2016). Alcohol abuse is common among both perpetrators and victims of severe IPV (McKinney et al. 2010). Perpetrators also tend to have high rates of exposure to IPV during childhood (Ernst et al. 2009) and high rates of psychopathology (Stanford et al. 2008).

IPV results in high utilization of health care services (Bonomi et al. 2009b), particularly for mental health. These patients are seen in a variety of ambulatory care settings, in the general hospital, and in psychiatry wards. Victims of IPV experience adverse health outcomes besides injury (and death), such as cigarette smoking, asthma, musculoskeletal disease, complications of pregnancy and childbirth, sexually transmitted diseases, substance use, somatoform disorders, anxiety, and depression (Bonomi et al. 2009a). Exposed children sustain emotional injury living in an environment of domestic aggression and may themselves be victims of accidental or intentional violence. Many of these children show a wide range of psychopathology later in life and are prone to becoming victims or perpetrators themselves.

Many IPV cases go undetected. Factors contributing to lack of detection include inadequate physician training in recognition and management of IPV, physicians' feelings of discomfort and powerlessness, and pressures on physicians to spend less time with patients. Patients' reluctance to discuss IPV may derive from negative past experiences, pessimism, low self-confidence, fear of retaliation, or financial dependence.

Behavioral patterns that facilitate detection include repeat visits for vague or minor complaints or chronic pain (especially pelvic), evasive and anxious behavior, inability to recall events leading to the presenting problem, inadequate or baffling explanations for injuries, domineering and obstructive behavior in the partner, and unexplained nonadherence to treatment plans (Eisenstat and Bancroft 1999). In addition, certain physical findings suggest the possibility of battery: injuries to the head, neck, or mouth; bruises in various stages of healing; defensive injuries of the forearms; dental trauma; and genital injuries. It is prudent to screen for IPV in patients with depression, anxiety, substance use, or somatic symptom disorders, as well as in those with suicidal ideation or a suicide attempt.

Routine screening of all women, recommended by many advocacy organizations and professional associations, is controversial. Although the U.S. Preventive Services Task Force recommends that all women of childbearing age be screened for IPV, evidence is lacking that such screening leads to increased referrals to and women's engagement with support services, reduced violence, or improvements in women's health (O'Doherty et al. 2015; Rabin et al. 2009). Victims may prefer self-completed questionnaires to face-to-face questioning (MacMillan et al. 2006). Computer-based screening approaches can improve rates of detection in the ED (Trautman et al. 2007), but they are not likely to be widely implemented. A simpler strategy is to incorporate probe questions into the clinical interview. Ultimately, screening must be coupled with individualized psychosocial and mental health interventions to be effective.

Table 6–4 lists sample questions that may be used to initiate the screening process. Incorporating screening questions into the routine interview process can minimize physician and patient discomfort. When abuse or IPV is identified, descriptions of current, recent, and past battery, including dates and circumstances, should be elicited and carefully documented. Legal intervention may rely on this documentation, so the findings should be described in precise language, using quotations from the patient when possible. A complete history and thorough examination should be performed, all injuries should be carefully described, and photographs should be taken if the patient consents. Strict confidentiality of the disclosure is needed to protect the patient from retaliation; this may require restricted access or sequestration of the disclosure records. On completion of the medical evaluation, a social work evaluation, a safety plan, and referrals to shelters and services such as the National Domestic Violence Hotline (1-800-799-SAFE) and local advocacy organizations should follow. It is usually best for the physician to respect the patient's wishes regarding when to report the violence to legal authorities and when to flee the situation. However, in some states, the physician is required by law to make a report (see also Chapter 2, "Legal and Ethical Issues").

Management of Aggressive Behavior

Education and Relationship Building

Education of health care providers and staff in management of aggression in the general hospital is a major component of the psychiatrist's liaison role. It can be provided through seminars, bedside teaching, care conferences, and continuing education. Important content includes training in recognition of warning signs (e.g., restlessness,

TABLE 6–4.	Helpful screening questions for intimate partner abuse

1. Do you and your partner argue a lot? Does it ever get physical? Has either one of you ever hit the other? Has either one of you ever injured the other?

2. Do you ever feel unsafe at home?

3. Has anyone ever hit you or tried to injure you in any way?

4. Has anyone ever threatened you or tried to control you?

5. Have you ever felt afraid of your partner or ex-partner?

6. Is there anything particularly stressful going on now? How are things at home?

7. I see patients in my practice who are being hurt or threatened by their partner. Is this happening to you? Has this ever happened to you?

Source. Questions are adapted: question 1 from J.L. Levenson (personal communication, October 2003); questions 2–5 from Eisenstat and Bancroft 1999; and questions 6 and 7 from Gerbert et al. 2000.

staring, pacing) and in behavioral interventions, including verbal de-escalation techniques (i.e., speaking calmly, using gentle eye contact, adopting a problem-solving stance, knowing when to disengage), and guidance on when and how to use a "show of force," pharmacological tranquilization, and physical restraint. This teaching serves to broaden the skill set of the medical team and to increase their confidence in their ability to manage these patients.

Safety of the Environment

The safety of the environment should be ensured before any aggressive patient is evaluated. The psychiatrist should check that weapons, such as guns and knives, and potential weapons, such as scissors and belts, have been removed. In the ED, this is often accomplished by routinely using hand searches and metal detectors and by keeping discovered items safely locked away. On inpatient units, monitoring and controlling what the patient can keep, conducting periodic room searches, and providing plastic utensils for meals are common interventions. A safe environment also should allow for the examiner's easy escape, as well as observation and easy entry by other health care personnel. The psychiatrist should use what information is available to anticipate what precautions and emergency interventions may be needed before starting the evaluation, and should make sure that the medical team is ready to intervene if the patient becomes severely agitated or violent. It is also prudent to separate potentially violent patients from other patients to reduce stimulation and avoid escalation (Tishler et al. 2013).

Psychiatric Evaluation

Effective management requires a comprehensive psychiatric evaluation, ultimately leading to identification of potentially modifiable factors and a specific psychiatric diagnosis for targeted intervention. However, in many aggressive patients, the psychiatric diagnosis only partially explains the behavior and does not fully indicate what the appropriate treatment strategy should be. This situation is typical in patients with personality disorders, brain injury, or dementia, and is frequently true for patients with major mental disorders.

Positive Therapeutic Alliance

The first step in the management of the aggressive patient is to forge a positive therapeutic alliance (Beauford et al. 1997). It is crucial to actively seek the patient's collaboration in the treatment process. A positive therapeutic alliance facilitates the patient's compliance with behavioral expectations and with prescribed treatments and makes it easier to mediate patient–staff conflicts and de-escalate aggressive episodes. A positive alliance also enables a psychotherapeutic relationship that may allow the psychiatrist to work toward a lasting reduction in the patient's propensity to violent responses (O'Connor 2003).

Behavioral Approaches

Communication-based de-escalation techniques (shown in Table 6–5) are often effective for controlling and terminating mild to moderate aggression (threats and belligerence). Although verbal de-escalation should be conceptualized as a semistructured intervention, in practice it is often deployed as an instinctive, commonsense reaction to the patient's behavior rather than as a systematic intervention. The basic goal of de-escalation is to bring a supportive and problem-solving stance and to balance acknowledgment of the patient's autonomy with boundary and limit setting (Price and Baker 2012). Verbal de-escalation techniques are most useful in situations that involve patient–staff conflict, but they also can be used to manage pathological aggression and to set the stage for pharmacological interventions.

Other behavioral approaches typically used in the management of chronic aggression incorporate (to varying degrees) the following: validation therapy, activity programs, manipulation of ambient light and/or sound and other environment modifications, behavioral analysis, operant conditioning, and differential reinforcement strategies (Lyketsos 2000).

Seclusion and Restraint

It is not unusual for de-escalation and other behavioral techniques to fail, particularly in acute care settings. In some settings, de-escalation techniques may be impractical because the patient is unable to communicate meaningfully (e.g., because of confusion, cognitive impairment, or communication disorders), is known to be explosive, or is already engaging in violent behavior. In such cases, the use of physical restraint—which may involve *manual restraint* (wherein the patient is restrained by several health care workers) and/or *mechanical restraint* (wherein an appliance is used to restrain the patient)—may be needed to terminate the dangerous behavior. Sometimes physical restraint is required to allow administration of tranquilizers or to protect other medical interventions (e.g., to keep the patient from pulling out intravenous or other vital lines or tubes). For a brief period immediately after the application of physical restraints (or the administration of tranquilizers), it is prudent to observe patients in isolation (in their own room or a designated safe room) to ensure that the violent episode and its consequences and triggers have been successfully managed. Because improper use of restraints can result in injury to the patient or to staff, use of restraints should be directed and implemented only by experienced personnel. Train-

---

TABLE 6–5.   Communication-based de-escalation techniques

Communication

Nonverbal

    Maintain a safe distance.

    Maintain a neutral posture.

    Do not stare; eye contact should convey sincerity.

    Do not touch the patient.

    Stay at the same height as the patient.

    Avoid sudden movements.

Verbal

    Speak in a calm, clear tone.

    Personalize yourself.

    Avoid confrontation; offer to solve the problem.

Tactics

Debunking

    Acknowledge the patient's grievance.

    Acknowledge the patient's frustration.

    Shift focus to discussion of how to solve the problem.

Aligning goals

    Emphasize common ground.

    Focus on the big picture.

    Find ways to make small concessions.

Monitoring

    Be acutely aware of progress.

    Know when to disengage.

    Do not insist on having the last word.

---

ing courses in the use of manual and physical restraints are widely supported, and many jurisdictions have developed certification programs.

During the past two decades, the use of seclusion and physical restraints has come under intense criticism. As a result, governmental and judicial regulation of restraint use has steadily increased (see also Chapter 2). The Academy of Psychosomatic Medicine guidelines state the following:

> Constant observation and restraints should be implemented for the shortest possible time with the least restrictive, though effective, means available; these interventions must not be made solely for the convenience of medical staff. Assessment and treatment of underlying psychiatric conditions that contribute to the patient's need for these measures should be expeditiously undertaken. (Bronheim et al. 1998, p. S20)

These guidelines are consistent with guidelines developed by other medical associations, with regulatory standards, and with the general opinion of the courts. The standards for the clinical use of restraints are as follows: 1) restraints should be used only when necessary to protect the patient or others from harm; 2) restraints should not be used solely to coerce the patient to accept treatments or remain in the treatment setting; and 3) restraint use should be accompanied by close monitoring and frequent reassessment of the patient's condition. The clinical and regulatory issues involved in the use of restraints are complex; thus, it is often necessary for psychiatrists to help other medical colleagues explore the various options for managing an aggressive patient and to address any staff discomfort with the use of restraints, keeping in view the clinical and legal risks involved.

Pharmacological Approaches

Pharmacotherapy of aggression is based more on contemporary intuitions about the neurotransmitters thought to modulate the expression of aggressive behavior and less on evidence from controlled trials. Medications are prescribed for impulsive and pathological forms of aggression. In general, treatment of clinically relevant aggression follows two approaches: 1) treatment of aggression as a *syndrome*, separate from the larger diagnostic context, and 2) treatment of conditions that manifest aggression as a *symptom*, such as schizophrenia, delusional disorders, and delirium. The discussion that follows focuses on the treatment of aggression as a syndrome; treatments for specific conditions are covered in other chapters of this volume.

Pharmacological agents are prescribed for both acute and chronic aggression. For acute aggression, the treatment goal is typically rapid tranquilization. A survey of U.S. psychiatrists who specialize in emergency psychiatry found that benzodiazepines (particularly lorazepam) were the preferred agents for treating acute aggression (Allen et al. 2005) because they are relatively free of the adverse effects typically associated with antipsychotics, such as acute dystonia, akathisia, and parkinsonism. Antipsychotics, especially haloperidol, were considered first-line agents as well, particularly for acute aggression associated with psychosis. Risperidone has effects similar to those of haloperidol and can be safely used—alone or in combination with a benzodiazepine—in many situations. Intramuscular olanzapine is another option when parenteral administration is necessary. Data on newer agents are more limited compared with data on haloperidol.

A broad range of medicines are used for the treatment of chronic aggression. Antipsychotics are the most widely used medication class. The relative dearth of evidence from placebo-controlled trials and the heterogeneity of aggression may explain the diversity of agents used. It is noteworthy that some controlled trials of treatments for agitation and aggression in elderly patients have reported placebo response rates as high as 60%, a finding that underscores the importance of rigorous methodology in the evaluation of treatments (Lyketsos 2000). However, considerable empirical support exists for the use of specific psychotropic classes in treating aggression.

Antipsychotics are the preferred agents for treating agitation and aggression in the general medical setting, especially in patients with delirium or a psychotic disorder (Ostinelli et al. 2017). Tranquilization may terminate an episode of aggression but has no effect on the frequency or severity of future episodes of impulsive aggression.

Clinical trials of typical antipsychotics for the treatment of impulsive aggression in patients with personality disorders have yielded mixed results. Antipsychotics are also used to treat aggression in patients with brain diseases. In multicenter trials in patients with dementia, risperidone and olanzapine were found useful in reducing aggression (Ballard and Waite 2006; Lyketsos 2000), but results from the Clinical Antipsychotic Trials of Intervention Effectiveness Alzheimer's disease study (CATIE-AD) indicated that their beneficial effects were modest and were offset by adverse effects (Schneider et al. 2006), including cerebrovascular events, extrapyramidal symptoms, and increased mortality in dementia. Clinicians must balance these agents' modest efficacy and associated risks against the risks of untreated aggression (Salzman et al. 2008). It is prudent to reserve antipsychotics for cases of severe aggression that pose significant risk or cause marked distress. In cases of dementia-related aggression that are successfully treated with an antipsychotic, planned withdrawal of the drug after 3 months is recommended (Ballard et al. 2008; Onyike 2008). There is a growing consensus among specialists that behavioral interventions should be the first-line treatments for aggression in dementia, with pharmacological interventions reserved for behavioral emergencies and refractory cases (Tampi et al. 2016).

Animal studies showing that serotonin neurotransmission can reduce aggression provided support for treating impulsive human aggression with selective serotonin reuptake inhibitors (SSRIs), lithium, buspirone, or other drugs that may enhance central serotonin levels. In addition, SSRIs, lithium, and buspirone have been effective in small placebo-controlled trials in reducing impulsive nonviolent aggression in patients with personality disorders, autism spectrum disorder, or depressive disorders (Coccaro and Siever 2002), although this effect is not consistently observed (Lee et al. 2008). Lithium was shown in a recent study to reduce the risk of self-harm and unintentional injury (Hayes et al. 2016).

Anticonvulsants may be effective in reducing impulsive aggression. A Cochrane review (Huband et al. 2010) concluded that valproate/divalproex, carbamazepine, oxcarbazepine, and phenytoin can reduce recurrent impulsive aggression in a broad spectrum of patients, including male psychiatric outpatients, prison inmates, and adults with personality disorders. Another review concluded that topiramate and lamotrigine may reduce impulsive aggression in adults with personality disorders (Stanford et al. 2009). A third review found evidence of significant reductions in aggression with phenytoin, lithium, carbamazepine, or oxcarbazepine, but not with valproic acid or levetiracetam (Jones et al. 2011). In regard to treatment of agitation and aggression in patients with dementia, a controlled trial found that valproate was ineffective and poorly tolerated (Herrmann et al. 2007). In a few small placebo-controlled trials, carbamazepine was shown to reduce aggression in patients with dementia (Olin et al. 2001; Tariot et al. 1998), but oxcarbazepine did not reduce aggression in dementia in another trial (Sommer et al. 2009). Small trials suggest that topiramate might reduce aggression in individuals with borderline personality disorder (e.g., Nickel and Loew 2008).

Because noradrenergic overactivity has been implicated in the expression of aggression, β-adrenergic blockade has emerged as another therapeutic strategy. The agents most commonly used are propranolol, pindolol, and nadolol. Clinical trials have found beta-blockers to be effective in patients with traumatic brain injury, dementia, or psychosis (Caspi et al. 2001; Ratey et al. 1992). Beta-blockers may cause hypotension and bradycardia and therefore should be used with caution.

Progesterone and leuprolide have been used in some patients with aggressive sexual behavior. In routine practice, psychiatrists often use combinations of medications from different classes because the response to single-agent therapy is usually modest.

Conclusion

Aggression is a major clinical and public health problem. It is a difficult, disruptive, and dangerous problem for psychiatrists, other physicians, nurses, and other health care workers. A careful description of the aggressive episode, in the context of a comprehensive psychiatric examination, informs clinical management. Out of the clinical examination comes an appreciation of the fundamental nature of the problem, including whether the aggression is impulsive or premeditated, the factors that have produced and/or sustained it, and individualized treatment strategies.

Psychiatric diagnosis alone is often not enough to inform the treatment; an individualized approach is required. For most patients, aggression is managed with a combination of approaches. In the general hospital, the management of aggressive patients involves active collaboration among psychiatrists, other physicians, nurses, and other health care workers. Collaboration works best when the ground has been prepared beforehand through the liaison efforts of the psychiatrist; these efforts will maximize the effectiveness of interventions while minimizing the risk of injury to patients and staff.

Finally, it is important to keep in mind that many aggressive patients, particularly those with impulsive aggression, are at risk of suicidal behavior and require suicide risk assessment and appropriate interventions. Research has yielded much insight into the neurobiology of aggression and violence, but more work is needed to develop predictive methods and more effective preventive and treatment modalities.

References

Allen MH, Currier GW, Carpenter D, et al; Expert Consensus Panel for Behavioral Emergencies 2005: The expert consensus guideline series. Treatment of behavioral emergencies 2005. J Psychiatr Pract 11 (suppl 1):5–108; quiz 110–112, 2005 16319571

American Psychiatric Association: Diagnostic and Statistical Manual of Mental Disorders, 3rd Edition. Washington, DC, American Psychiatric Association, 1980

American Psychiatric Association: Diagnostic and Statistical Manual of Mental Disorders, 4th Edition, Revised. Washington, DC, American Psychiatric Association, 1994

American Psychiatric Association: Diagnostic and Statistical Manual of Mental Disorders, 5th Edition. Arlington, VA, American Psychiatric Association, 2013

Amore M, Menchetti M, Tonti C, et al: Predictors of violent behavior among acute psychiatric patients: clinical study. Psychiatry Clin Neurosci 62(3):247–255, 2008 18588583

Arnetz JE, Arnetz BB: Violence towards health care staff and possible effects on the quality of patient care. Soc Sci Med 52(3):417–427, 2001 11330776

Ballard C, Waite J: The effectiveness of atypical antipsychotics for the treatment of aggression and psychosis in Alzheimer's disease. Cochrane Database Syst Rev (1):CD003476, 2006 16437455

Ballard C, Lana MM, Theodoulou M, et al; Investigators DART AD: A randomised, blinded, placebo-controlled trial in dementia patients continuing or stopping neuroleptics (the DART-AD trial). PLoS Med 5(4):e76, 2008 18384230

Barlow K, Grenyer B, Ilkiw-Lavalle O: Prevalence and precipitants of aggression in psychiatric inpatient units. Aust N Z J Psychiatry 34(6):967–974, 2000 11127627

Beauford JE, McNiel DE, Binder RL: Utility of the initial therapeutic alliance in evaluating psychiatric patients' risk of violence. Am J Psychiatry 154(9):1272–1276, 1997 9286188

Behnam M, Tillotson RD, Davis SM, et al: Violence in the emergency department: a national survey of emergency medicine residents and attending physicians. J Emerg Med 40(5):565–579, 2011 20133103

Binder RL, McNiel DE: The relationship of gender to violent behavior in acutely disturbed psychiatric patients. J Clin Psychiatry 51(3):110–114, 1990 2307664

Black MC, Basile KC, Breiding MJ, et al: The National Intimate Partner and Sexual Violence Survey: 2010 summary report. National Center for Injury Prevention and Control, Centers for Disease Control and Protection, 2011

Blanchard JC, Curtis KM: Violence in the emergency department. Emerg Med Clin North Am 17(3):717–731, viii, 1999 10516849

Bobes J, Fillat O, Arango C: Violence among schizophrenia out-patients compliant with medication: prevalence and associated factors. Acta Psychiatr Scand 119(3):218–225, 2009 19178395

Bonomi AE, Anderson ML, Reid RJ, et al: Medical and psychosocial diagnoses in women with a history of intimate partner violence. Arch Intern Med 169(18):1692–1697, 2009a 19822826

Bonomi AE, Anderson ML, Rivara FP, et al: Health care utilization and costs associated with physical and nonphysical-only intimate partner violence. Health Serv Res 44(3):1052–1067, 2009b 19674432

Bowers L, Jarrett M, Clark N, et al: Determinants of absconding by patients on acute psychiatric wards. J Adv Nurs 32(3):644–649, 2000 11012807

Bronheim HE, Fulop G, Kunkel EJ, et al; The Academy of Psychosomatic Medicine: The Academy of Psychosomatic Medicine practice guidelines for psychiatric consultation in the general medical setting. Psychosomatics 39(4):S8–S30, 1998 9691717

Brower MC, Price BH: Neuropsychiatry of frontal lobe dysfunction in violent and criminal behaviour: a critical review. J Neurol Neurosurg Psychiatry 71(6):720–726, 2001 11723190

Caspi N, Modai I, Barak P, et al: Pindolol augmentation in aggressive schizophrenic patients: a double-blind crossover randomized study. Int Clin Psychopharmacol 16(2):111–115, 2001 11236069

Cheng JE, Shumway M, Leary M, et al: Patient factors associated with extended length of stay in the psychiatric inpatients of a large urban county hospital. Community Ment Health J 52(6):658–661, 2016 26883829

Coccaro EF, Siever LJ: Pathophysiology and treatment of aggression, in Neuropsychopharmacology: The Fifth Generation of Progress. Edited by Davis KL, Charney D, Coyle JT, et al. Philadelphia, PA, Lippincott, Williams & Wilkins, 2002, pp 1709–1723

Cohen-Mansfield J, Billig N: Agitated behaviors in the elderly, I: a conceptual review. J Am Geriatr Soc 34(10):711–721, 1986 3531296

Corrigan PW, Watson AC: Findings from the National Comorbidity Survey on the frequency of violent behavior in individuals with psychiatric disorders. Psychiatry Res 136(2–3):153–162, 2005 16125786

Davidson RJ, Putnam KM, Larson CL: Dysfunction in the neural circuitry of emotion regulation—a possible prelude to violence. Science 289(5479):591–594, 2000 10915615

Demaree HA, Harrison DW: Case study: topographical brain mapping in hostility following mild closed head injury. Int J Neurosci 87(1–2):97–101, 1996 8913823

de Medeiros K, Rosenberg PB, Baker AS, et al: Improper sexual behaviors in elders with dementia living in residential care. Dement Geriatr Cogn Disord 26(4):370–377, 2008 18931496

Desmarais SL, Van Dorn RA, Johnson KL, et al: Community violence perpetration and victimization among adults with mental illnesses. Am J Public Health 104(12):2342–2349, 2014 24524530

Ehmann TS, Smith GN, Yamamoto A, et al: Violence in treatment resistant psychotic inpatients. J Nerv Ment Dis 189(10):716–721, 2001 11708673

Eisenstat SA, Bancroft L: Domestic violence. N Engl J Med 341(12):886–892, 1999 10486421

Elbogen EB, Johnson SC: The intricate link between violence and mental disorder: results from the National Epidemiologic Survey on Alcohol and Related Conditions. Arch Gen Psychiatry 66(2):152–161, 2009 19188537

Ernst AA, Weiss SJ, Hall J, et al: Adult intimate partner violence perpetrators are significantly more likely to have witnessed intimate partner violence as a child than nonperpetrators. Am J Emerg Med 27(6):641–650, 2009 19751620

Ferri P, Silvestri M, Artoni C, et al: Workplace violence in different settings and among various health professionals in an Italian general hospital: a cross-sectional study. Psychol Res Behav Manag 9:263–275, 2016 27729818

Flannery RB Jr: Precipitants to psychiatric patient assaults on staff: review of empirical findings, 1990–2003, and risk management implications. Psychiatr Q 76(4):317–326, 2005 16217626

Furin M, Eliseo LJ, Langlois B, et al: Self-reported provider safety in an urban emergency medical system. West J Emerg Med 16(3):459–464, 2015 25987930

Gerard ME, Spitz MC, Towbin JA, et al: Subacute postictal aggression. Neurology 50(2):384–388, 1998 9484358

Gerberich SG, Church TR, McGovern PM, et al: An epidemiological study of the magnitude and consequences of work related violence: the Minnesota Nurses' Study. Occup Environ Med 61(6):495–503, 2004 15150388

Gerbert B, Moe J, Caspers N, et al: Simplifying physicians' response to domestic violence. West J Med 172(5):329–331, 2000 10832426

Giegling I, Olgiati P, Hartmann AM, et al: Personality and attempted suicide. Analysis of anger, aggression and impulsivity. J Psychiatr Res 43(16):1262–1271, 2009 19481222

Gillespie GL, Pekar B, Byczkowski TL, et al: Worker, workplace, and community/environmental risk factors for workplace violence in emergency departments. Arch Environ Occup Health 72(2):79–86, 2017 26980080

Grange JT, Corbett SW: Violence against emergency medical services personnel. Prehosp Emerg Care 6(2):186–190, 2002 11962565

Greenfield TK, McNiel DE, Binder RL: Violent behavior and length of psychiatric hospitalization. Hosp Community Psychiatry 40(8):809–814, 1989 2759570

Hamrin V, Iennaco J, Olsen D: A review of ecological factors affecting inpatient psychiatric unit violence: implications for relational and unit cultural improvements. Issues Ment Health Nurs 30(4):214–226, 2009 19363726

Harlow JM: Passage of an iron rod through the head. Boston Med Surg J 39:389–393, 1848. Available at: https://neuro.psychiatryonline.org/doi/full/10.1176/jnp.11.2.281. Accessed April 12, 2018.

Harlow JM: Recovery from the passage of an iron rod through the head. Publications of the Massachusetts Medical Society 2:327–347, 1868

Hayes JF, Pitman A, Marston L, et al: Self-harm, unintentional injury, and suicide in bipolar disorder during maintenance mood stabilizer treatment: a UK population-based electronic health records study. JAMA Psychiatry 73(6):630–637, 2016 27167638

Herrmann N, Lanctôt KL, Rothenburg LS, et al: A placebo-controlled trial of valproate for agitation and aggression in Alzheimer's disease. Dement Geriatr Cogn Disord 23(2):116–119, 2007 17148938

Hiday VA, Swartz MS, Swanson JW, et al: Male-female differences in the setting and construction of violence among people with severe mental illness. Soc Psychiatry Psychiatr Epidemiol 33 (suppl 1):S68–S74, 1998 9857782

Hodgins S, Cree A, Alderton J, et al: From conduct disorder to severe mental illness: associations with aggressive behaviour, crime and victimization. Psychol Med 38(7):975–987, 2008 17988416

Huband N, Ferriter M, Nathan R, et al: Antiepileptics for aggression and associated impulsivity. Cochrane Database Syst Rev (2):CD003499, 2010 20166067

Iozzino L, Ferrari C, Large M, et al: Prevalence and risk factors of violence by psychiatric acute inpatients: a systematic review and meta-analysis. PLoS One 10(6):e0128536, 2015 26061796

James A, Madeley R, Dove A: Violence and aggression in the emergency department. Emerg Med J 23(6):431–434, 2006 16714500

Jones RM, Arlidge J, Gillham R, et al: Efficacy of mood stabilisers in the treatment of impulsive or repetitive aggression: systematic review and meta-analysis. Br J Psychiatry 198(2):93–98, 2011 21282779

Kales HC, Gitlin LN, Lyketsos CG: Assessment and management of behavioral and psychological symptoms of dementia. BMJ 350:h369, 2015 25731881

Kalunian DA, Binder RL, McNiel DE: Violence by geriatric patients who need psychiatric hospitalization. J Clin Psychiatry 51(8):340–343, 1990 2380159

Kanemoto K, Tadokoro Y, Oshima T: Violence and postictal psychosis: a comparison of postictal psychosis, interictal psychosis, and postictal confusion. Epilepsy Behav 19(2):162–166, 2010 20727827

Kansagra SM, Rao SR, Sullivan AF, et al: A survey of workplace violence across 65 U.S. emergency departments. Acad Emerg Med 15(12):1268–1274, 2008 18976337

Khalifeh H, Oram S, Osborn D, et al: Recent physical and sexual violence against adults with severe mental illness: a systematic review and meta-analysis. Int Rev Psychiatry 28(5):433–451, 2016 27645197

Lam JN, McNiel DE, Binder RL: The relationship between patients' gender and violence leading to staff injuries. Psychiatr Serv 51(9):1167–1170, 2000 10970922

Lee R, Kavoussi RJ, Coccaro EF: Placebo-controlled, randomized trial of fluoxetine in the treatment of aggression in male intimate partner abusers. Int Clin Psychopharmacol 23(6):337–341, 2008 18854722

Lyketsos CG: Aggression, in The American Psychiatric Press Textbook of Geriatric Neuropsychiatry. Edited by Coffey E, Cummings JL. Washington, DC, American Psychiatric Press, 2000, pp 477–488

Lyketsos CG, Rosenblatt A, Rabins P: Forgotten frontal lobe syndrome or "Executive Dysfunction Syndrome." Psychosomatics 45(3):247–255, 2004 15123852

Lynch J, Appelboam R, McQuillan PJ: Survey of abuse and violence by patients and relatives towards intensive care staff. Anaesthesia 58(9):893–899, 2003 12911365

MacMillan HL, Wathen CN, Jamieson E, et al; McMaster Violence Against Women Research Group: Approaches to screening for intimate partner violence in health care settings: a randomized trial. JAMA 296(5):530–536, 2006 16882959

Marsh L, Krauss GL: Aggression and violence in patients with epilepsy. Epilepsy Behav 1(3):160–168, 2000 12609149

McHugh MC, Frieze IH: Intimate partner violence: new directions. Ann N Y Acad Sci 1087:121–141, 2006 17189502

McKinney CM, Caetano R, Rodriguez LA, et al: Does alcohol involvement increase the severity of intimate partner violence? Alcohol Clin Exp Res 34(4):655–658, 2010 20102574

McNiel DE, Eisner JP, Binder RL: The relationship between command hallucinations and violence. Psychiatr Serv 51(10):1288–1292, 2000 11013329

Nachreiner NM, Gerberich SG, Ryan AD, et al: Minnesota nurses' study: perceptions of violence and the work environment. Ind Health 45(5):672–678, 2007 18057810

Nawka A, Kalisova L, Raboch J, et al: Gender differences in coerced patients with schizophrenia. BMC Psychiatry 13:257, 2013 24118928

Nelson RJ, Trainor BC: Neural mechanisms of aggression. Nat Rev Neurosci 8(7):536–546, 2007 17585306

Newhill CE, Mulvey EP, Lidz CW: Characteristics of violence in the community by female patients seen in a psychiatric emergency service. Psychiatr Serv 46(8):785–789, 1995 7583478

Nickel MK, Loew TH: Treatment of aggression with topiramate in male borderline patients, part II: 18-month follow-up. Eur Psychiatry 23(2):115–117, 2008 18024088

Nolan KA, Czobor P, Roy BB, et al: Characteristics of assaultive behavior among psychiatric inpatients. Psychiatr Serv 54(7):1012–1016, 2003 12851439

O'Connor S: Violent behavior in chronic schizophrenia and inpatient psychiatry. J Am Acad Psychoanal Dyn Psychiatry 31(1):31–44, 2003 12722886

O'Doherty L, Hegarty K, Ramsay J, et al: Screening women for intimate partner violence in healthcare settings. Cochrane Database Syst Rev (7):CD007007, 2015 26200817

Olin JT, Fox LS, Pawluczyk S, et al: A pilot randomized trial of carbamazepine for behavioral symptoms in treatment-resistant outpatients with Alzheimer disease. Am J Geriatr Psychiatry 9(4):400–405, 2001 11739066

Onyike CU: Neuroleptic discontinuation during dementia care: a recent trial and its implications for practice. Nat Clin Pract Neurol 4(10):528–529, 2008 18725920

Ostinelli EG, Brooke-Powney MJ, Li X, et al: Haloperidol for psychosis-induced aggression or agitation (rapid tranquillisation). Cochrane Database Syst Rev (7):CD009377, 2017 28758203

Papadopoulos C, Ross J, Stewart D, et al: The antecedents of violence and aggression within psychiatric in-patient settings. Acta Psychiatr Scand 125(6):425–439, 2012 22268678

Pillemer K, Burnes D, Riffin C, et al: Elder abuse: global situation, risk factors, and prevention strategies. Gerontologist 56 (suppl 2):S194–S205, 2016 26994260

Pinna F, Tusconi M, Dessì C, et al: Violence and mental disorders. A retrospective study of people in charge of a community mental health center. Int J Law Psychiatry 47:122–128, 2016 27180213

Price O, Baker J: Key components of de-escalation techniques: a thematic synthesis. Int J Ment Health Nurs 21(4):310–319, 2012 22340073

Pulay AJ, Dawson DA, Hasin DS, et al: Violent behavior and DSM-IV psychiatric disorders: results from the national epidemiologic survey on alcohol and related conditions. J Clin Psychiatry 69(1):12–22, 2008 18312033

Rabin RF, Jennings JM, Campbell JC, et al: Intimate partner violence screening tools: a systematic review. Am J Prev Med 36(5):439–445.e4, 2009 19362697

Rao V, Rosenberg P, Bertrand M, et al: Aggression after traumatic brain injury: prevalence and correlates. J Neuropsychiatry Clin Neurosci 21(4):420–429, 2009 19996251

Ratey JJ, Sorgi P, O'Driscoll GA, et al: Nadolol to treat aggression and psychiatric symptomatology in chronic psychiatric inpatients: a double-blind, placebo-controlled study. J Clin Psychiatry 53(2):41–46, 1992 1347291

Roaldset JO, Bjørkly S: Comparison of patients who were violent, victimized and violent-victimized during the first year after discharge from emergency psychiatry. Psychiatry Res 230(3):978–981, 2015 26616305

Rowley E, Benson D, Tiffee A, et al: Clinical and financial implications of emergency department visits for synthetic marijuana. Am J Emerg Med 35(10):1506–1509, 2017 28457767

Salzman C, Jeste DV, Meyer RE, et al: Elderly patients with dementia-related symptoms of severe agitation and aggression: consensus statement on treatment options, clinical trials methodology, and policy. J Clin Psychiatry 69(6):889–898, 2008 18494535

Schneider LS, Tariot PN, Dagerman KS, et al; CATIE-AD Study Group: Effectiveness of atypical antipsychotic drugs in patients with Alzheimer's disease. N Engl J Med 355(15):1525–1538, 2006 17035647

Sheridan M, Henrion R, Robinson L, et al: Precipitants of violence in a psychiatric inpatient setting. Hosp Community Psychiatry 41(7):776–780, 1990 2365311

Siever LJ: Neurobiology of aggression and violence. Am J Psychiatry 165(4):429–442, 2008 18346997

Sommer OH, Aga O, Cvancarova M, et al: Effect of oxcarbazepine in the treatment of agitation and aggression in severe dementia. Dement Geriatr Cogn Disord 27(2):155–163, 2009 19182483

Stanford MS, Houston RJ, Baldridge RM: Comparison of impulsive and premeditated perpetrators of intimate partner violence. Behav Sci Law 26(6):709–722, 2008 19039796

Stanford MS, Anderson NE, Lake SL, et al: Pharmacologic treatment of impulsive aggression with antiepileptic drugs. Curr Treat Options Neurol 11(5):383–390, 2009 19744405

Stewart DE, Vigod S, Riazantseva E: New developments in intimate partner violence and management of its mental health sequelae. Curr Psychiatry Rep 18(1):4, 2016 26711508

Swanson JW, Holzer CE 3rd, Ganju VK, et al: Violence and psychiatric disorder in the community: evidence from the Epidemiologic Catchment Area surveys. Hosp Community Psychiatry 41(7):761–770, 1990 [Erratum in: Hosp Community Psychiatry 42(9):954–955, 1991] 2142118

Swanson JW, Swartz MS, Van Dorn RA, et al: A national study of violent behavior in persons with schizophrenia. Arch Gen Psychiatry 63(5):490–499, 2006 16651506

Swanson JW, Van Dorn RA, Swartz MS, et al: Alternative pathways to violence in persons with schizophrenia: the role of childhood antisocial behavior problems. Law Hum Behav 32(3):228–240, 2008 17602288

Swartz MS, Swanson JW, Hiday VA, et al: Taking the wrong drugs: the role of substance abuse and medication noncompliance in violence among severely mentally ill individuals. Soc Psychiatry Psychiatr Epidemiol 33 (suppl 1):S75–S80, 1998 9857783

Tampi RR, Tampi DJ, Balachandran S, et al: Antipsychotic use in dementia: a systematic review of benefits and risks from meta-analyses. Ther Adv Chronic Dis 7(5):229–245, 2016 27583123

Tariot PN, Erb R, Podgorski CA, et al: Efficacy and tolerability of carbamazepine for agitation and aggression in dementia. Am J Psychiatry 155(1):54–61, 1998 9433339

Thompson RS, Bonomi AE, Anderson M, et al: Intimate partner violence: prevalence, types, and chronicity in adult women. Am J Prev Med 30(6):447–457, 2006 16704937

Tishler CL, Reiss NS, Dundas J: The assessment and management of the violent patient in critical hospital settings. Gen Hosp Psychiatry 35(2):181–185, 2013 23260370

Tonkonogy JM, Geller JL: Hypothalamic lesions and intermittent explosive disorder. J Neuropsychiatry Clin Neurosci 4(1):45–50, 1992 1627961

Trautman DE, McCarthy ML, Miller N, et al: Intimate partner violence and emergency department screening: computerized screening versus usual care. Ann Emerg Med 49(4):526–534, 2007 17276547

Treiman DM: Epilepsy and violence: medical and legal issues. Epilepsia 27 (suppl 2):S77–S104, 1986 3720715

Vazirian M, Jerry JM, James J, et al: Bath salts in the emergency department: a survey of emergency clinicians' experience with bath salts-intoxicated patients. J Addict Med 9(2):94–98, 2015 25525943

Volavka J: The neurobiology of violence: an update. J Neuropsychiatry Clin Neurosci 11(3):307–314, 1999 10440006

Whittington R, Shuttleworth S, Hill L: Violence to staff in a general hospital setting. J Adv Nurs 24(2):326–333, 1996 8858437

Witt K, van Dorn R, Fazel S: Risk factors for violence in psychosis: systematic review and meta-regression analysis of 110 studies. PLoS One 8(2):e55942, 2013 23418482

CHAPTER 7

Depression

Madeline Li, M.D., Ph.D., FRCPC

Joshua Rosenblat, M.D.

Gary Rodin, M.D., FRCPC

The risk of developing depressive disorders is increased in most chronic medical conditions, and reciprocally, depression can be a risk factor for the development of medical illnesses (Ramasubbu et al. 2012). There are multiple nonspecific factors, such as disability and physical suffering, that may increase the risk of depression in serious medical illnesses. There is also speculation about whether specific biological mechanisms account for the comorbidity of depression with particular medical conditions.

Depression is frequently underdiagnosed and untreated in medical settings, despite its frequency, negative effects on health, and responsiveness to treatment. This diagnostic and therapeutic neglect may be due to underreporting of symptoms because of stigma, difficulty distinguishing normative from pathological distress, physical symptom overlap between depression and medical illness, and lack of sufficient caregiver training in or comfort with mental health inquiry. There may also be mistaken beliefs among both providers and patients about the untreatability of depression that is "understandable." Untreated depression is of concern in medical populations because it is associated with greater somatic symptom burden (Katon et al. 2007) and worse quality of life (Katon 2003) in common medical disorders. Depression is also associated with higher rates of health care utilization, such that the cost of medical care for depressed medical patients is 50% higher than that for nondepressed medical patients; depressed patients also tend to be less compliant with medical treatment and to have less functional capacity and less occupational productivity (Unützer et al. 2009). Paradoxically, depression is also overdiagnosed in medical settings, with unnecessary prescription of antidepressant medication for nonpathological sadness or grief or diagnoses based solely on scores on depression screening instruments.

In this chapter we review the prevalence and clinical features of depression in the medically ill; discuss approaches to depression screening, diagnosis, and treatment;

and explore mechanisms that may account for the etiology, course, and outcome of depression in the medical setting. We do not attempt to provide in-depth information on depression in particular diseases; for details on the effects of comorbid depression in various medical conditions, readers are referred to the chapters on specific disorders in this textbook.

The Continuum of Depression: From Experience to Disorder

Sadness is a normal, expectable response to the adverse effects of a serious medical illness, including changes in bodily appearance and functioning; pain and physical distress; limitations in the capacity to work and to engage in pleasurable activities; perceived alteration in the anticipated life trajectory; fears of disability and dependency; and alterations in intimate relationships, family life, social relationships, and other activities. Nonpathological sadness and grief lie at one end of the continuum of depression in medical populations. In the middle lie subthreshold depressions (Rodríguez et al. 2012), which are the most prevalent depressive presentations among medically ill patients (Gellis 2010). At the more severe end are depressive symptoms that clearly meet diagnostic criteria for major depressive disorder as specified in DSM-5 (American Psychiatric Association 2013). These categorical distinctions have heuristic and communicative value, although the boundaries that demarcate and distinguish them from one another are somewhat arbitrary and often difficult to determine, particularly in medically ill patients.

The eight major categories of depressive disorders specified in DSM-5 are major depressive disorder (MDD), persistent depressive disorder (PDD; formerly dysthymia), substance/medication-induced depressive disorder, depressive disorder due to another medical condition, disruptive mood dysregulation disorder (applicable only in children), premenstrual dysphoric disorder, other specified depressive disorder (formerly minor or subsyndromal depression), and unspecified depressive disorder (when insufficient information is available to make a specific diagnosis). Subthreshold disorders, including PDD and the other specified and unspecified depressive disorder categories, may substantially reduce quality of life and result in moderate functional impairment (Rowe and Rapaport 2006). At least 10%–20% of subthreshold depressions progress to MDD (Lyness et al. 2006).

DSM-5 no longer excludes recent bereavement from a diagnosis of MDD, although it should be noted that normative and nonpathological grief following a loss may meet all diagnostic criteria for a depressive episode (Horwitz and Wakefield 2007). Indeed, it may be argued that the onset, exacerbation, or progression of a serious medical illness may be experienced as a loss that can be at least as distressing as the loss of a loved one.

Notably, a diagnosis of adjustment disorder, which in DSM-5 is reconceptualized as one of the trauma- and stressor-related disorders, can be applied when a patient has symptoms of depression in reaction to a stressor, such as medical illness, that do not meet criteria for MDD or PDD. The operational criteria for this diagnosis, including what constitutes an "excessive" response to the multiple and chronic stressors of medical illness, are not clear. However, despite this ambiguity, the heuristic and non-stigmatizing appeal of the category of adjustment disorder contribute to its being one of the most common psychiatric diagnoses made in medical patients (Li et al. 2010).

Epidemiology

Depressive disorders are extremely common in the general population, with up to 17% of adults in the United States having had at least one episode of MDD during their lifetime (Kessler et al. 2003) and 2%–4% suffering from a current MDD (Ferrari et al. 2013). Medical illness has consistently been shown to be a risk factor for depression (Patten et al. 2018). PDD and subthreshold depression are the most common depressive syndromes in medical populations, reported in up to 26% of medical outpatients, a rate several times higher than that in the general population (Rowe and Rapaport 2006). The prevalence of MDD varies by population, with rates of 2%–4% in community samples, 5%–10% in primary care settings, and 6%–14% in medical inpatient settings; these progressive increases presumably are based on differences in medical disease severity (Burvill 1995). Similarly, the risk of a depressive episode in patients in primary care (Barkow et al. 2002) and in the community (Wilhelm et al. 1999) rises with the number of comorbid medical diseases. The reported prevalence rates of depressive disorders in specific medical conditions, including cancer, diabetes, cardiovascular disease, chronic obstructive pulmonary disease (COPD)/asthma, HIV/AIDS, stroke, epilepsy, multiple sclerosis, Alzheimer's disease, and Parkinson's disease, are listed in Table 7–1.

Etiology

Increased rates of depressive symptoms and depressive disorders have been found in virtually all chronic medical conditions in which depression has been studied (Patten et al. 2018). It has been hypothesized that illness-specific biological mechanisms lay the foundations for depression in certain medical conditions, including hypothyroidism, stroke, Parkinson's disease, diabetes, and some types of cancer. Although specificity for depression has not been substantiated in any of these conditions, each is associated with multiple nonspecific risk factors that may increase the prevalence of depression. In fact, depression in the context of medical illness is a prime example of the biopsychosocial model of disease, with interacting pathophysiological and psychosocial factors contributing to comorbidity. The final common pathway to depression—resulting from the interaction of disease-related, psychological, and social risk and protective factors—is shown in Figure 7–1.

Potential biological contributors to depression in medical illness include the physical effects of illness and treatment, medications, neurological involvement, genetic vulnerability, and systemic inflammation. In this regard, greater pain and treatment intensity (Patten et al. 2018), more advanced disease (Manne et al. 2001), and proximity to death (Lo et al. 2011) have all been shown to increase the risk of depression. Individuals with a genetic vulnerability to depression are also more likely to develop it in the context of medical illness (Levinson 2006), and common genetic vulnerabilities

TABLE 7–1. Prevalence of depression in selected medical illnesses

Medical illness	Prevalence of MDD (%)	MDD vs. subthreshold depression (%)	References
Cancer	8–24	15 vs. 22	Mitchell et al. 2011
Diabetes	9–26	14 vs. 32	Musselman et al. 2003; Roy and Lloyd 2012
	Type 2: 6–33		
	Type 1: 6–44		
Heart disease	17–27	18 vs. 27	Rudisch and Nemeroff 2003; Schleifer et al. 1989
COPD/asthma	20–50	28 vs. 40	Van Lieshout et al. 2009
HIV/AIDS	18–50	22 vs. 45	Arseniou et al. 2014
Stroke	15–31	14 vs. 18	Morris et al. 1990; Robinson and Jorge 2016
Epilepsy	20–29	23 vs. 29	Fiest et al. 2013
Multiple sclerosis	26–35	30 vs. 33	Boeschoten et al. 2017
Alzheimer's disease	13–22	22 vs. 27	Chi et al. 2015; Lyketsos et al. 1997
Parkinson's disease	18–27	23 vs. 30	Goodarzi et al. 2016b

Note. COPD=chronic obstructive pulmonary disease; MDD=major depressive disorder.

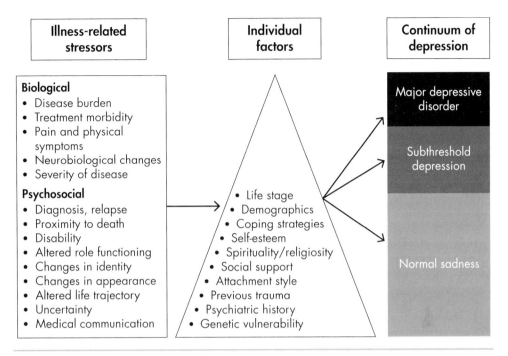

FIGURE 7–1. Pathways to depression.

Although depression is often regarded as a discrete disorder, it can also be considered as a final common pathway of distress that arises from the interaction of biological, psychological and social factors. Biological factors interact with the psychological impact of the disease which is filtered through the prism of individual and interpersonal strengths to result in a range of depressive responses from normal sadness to major depressive disorder.

may account for the frequent comorbidity of depression and Alzheimer's disease (Kim et al. 2002), Parkinson's disease (Mössner et al. 2001), and coronary artery disease (Su et al. 2009). Immune-activated systemic inflammation (Miller et al. 2009), manifesting as cytokine-induced "sickness behavior," is another proposed common pathophysiological mechanism that may underlie depression in a wide range of medical disorders, including cancer (Raison and Miller 2003), cardiovascular disease (Parissis et al. 2007), diabetes (Musselman et al. 2003), Alzheimer's disease (Leonard 2007), stroke (Arbelaez et al. 2007), multiple sclerosis (Wallin et al. 2006), asthma (Van Lieshout et al. 2009), and infectious diseases such as HIV/AIDS (Leserman 2003). This association has led some to posit the existence of a specific subtype of depression—inflammatory cytokine-associated depression (ICAD) (Lotrich 2015), characterized by more neurovegetative and fewer core psychological symptoms (Capuron et al. 2009; Pasquini et al. 2008)—that is more common in individuals with medical conditions associated with inflammation (Dantzer et al. 2008).

It has been suggested that medication-induced depression is symptomatically different from MDD, with less prominent and milder depression and atypical features more characteristic of ICAD (Patten and Barbui 2004). The association of depression with medications such as L-dopa, calcium channel blockers, analgesics, nonsteroidal anti-inflammatory drugs, isotretinoin, and phenobarbital has largely been based on case reports, with few high-quality studies. Valid evidence linking medications to atypical depressive syndromes has been found only for corticosteroids, interferon-α, interleukin-2, gonadotropin-releasing hormone agonists, mefloquine, and progestin-releasing implanted contraceptives (Patten and Barbui 2004). Most of these drugs and their psychiatric side effects are discussed in other chapters of this textbook.

Psychosocial factors that may contribute to the development of a comorbid depressive disorder in medical illness include the stigma and personal meaning of the medical condition, illness-related disability (Talbot et al. 1999), maladaptive coping styles (Wallin et al. 2006), low self-esteem, impaired spiritual well-being (Rodin et al. 2007), and reduced capacity to express affect (Classen et al. 2008). Low social support (Lewis 2001) and poor communication with medical caregivers (Gurevich et al. 2004) also increase the likelihood of a comorbid depressive disorder. Additionally, expectations of support and the capacity for flexible use of social support, captured in the construct of *attachment security,* may provide protection against the emergence of depressive symptoms in medically ill patients (Rodin et al. 2007).

Age is inversely related to the severity of depressive symptoms (Gottlieb et al. 2004). Although depression in the general population has been strongly associated with female gender (Lucht et al. 2003), this gender difference has not been found consistently in depression in medical populations (Miller et al. 2011; Rodin et al. 2007). It may be that the overriding common stressors related to the medical illness obliterate gender-related differences that would otherwise emerge.

Clinical Features and Diagnosis

The diagnosis of depressive disorders in medical populations is fraught with difficulties that include the following:

1. Many physical symptoms of medical illness (e.g., fatigue, anorexia, weight loss, insomnia, psychomotor retardation, diminished concentration) resemble those of depression. In addition, a variety of emotional disturbances, such as "emotionalism," pathological crying, apathy, and fatigue in poststroke patients (Bogousslavsky 2003) or in patients with multiple sclerosis (Chwastiak and Ehde 2007), can be mistaken for depression. It may also be difficult to distinguish depression from the apathy associated with hypoactive delirium or dementia, or from akinesia and masked facies in Parkinson's disease.
2. Thoughts of death and the desire for death in patients with advanced medical disease have been associated with depression and demoralization in the terminally ill (Breitbart et al. 2000). However, such thoughts must be distinguished from adaptive death acceptance or an attempt at cognitive mastery that does not reflect depression (Nissim et al. 2009).
3. Physical suffering and disability, in the absence of comorbid depression, may diminish the capacity to experience pleasure in many formerly enjoyable activities. Depressed mood or withdrawal from social or physical activities that is disproportionate to physical disability increases the likelihood that the loss of pleasure is secondary to depression.
4. In medical populations, depressive symptoms may manifest in atypical or masked forms, including amplification of somatic symptoms (Katon et al. 2007) and non-

compliance with or refusal of medical treatment (DiMatteo et al. 2000). These symptoms or behaviors may not be recognized as manifestations of depression, leading to underdiagnosis of depression.

5. The categories of MDD, substance/medication-induced depressive disorder, and depressive disorder due to another medical condition may overlap in the context of medical illness. The latter two diagnoses imply that the etiology of the depression is a direct physiological consequence of the specified general medical condition or substance, whereas the causation of depression is most often multifactorial.

Various approaches have been proposed to diminish the confounding effect of medical symptoms in the diagnosis of MDD. In DSM-5, it is acknowledged that there are no "infallible guidelines" to follow in determining when depression is secondary to another medical condition but that the index of suspicion should be raised by 1) a temporal association between symptoms and the onset, exacerbation, or remission of a medical condition, and 2) an age at onset, course, or absence of family history that is atypical for a primary mood disorder. The criteria for determining which symptoms are due to a medical illness and which are due to other factors unrelated to the medical illness are unclear and are left to "the clinician's best judgment" (American Psychiatric Association 2013).

A combined "exclusive" and "etiological" approach to the diagnosis of depression in patients with medical illness was previously advocated, with exclusion of symptoms judged by the clinician to be etiologically related to a general medical condition or not more frequent in depressed than nondepressed patients with such conditions (Bukberg et al. 1984). This approach was intended to avoid attributing symptoms of physical illness to a depressive syndrome. The exclusive approach is usually applied only to the somatic symptoms of depression, although this does not take into account that depressed medical patients report significantly more physical symptoms than matched nondepressed medical patients (Fitzgerald et al. 2015).

Evaluating the rates of depression in hospitalized elderly medical patients according to six different diagnostic schemes, Koenig et al. (1997) found no overall advantage of one diagnostic scheme over others. In cases in which the diagnosis remains unclear, a focus on the qualitative differences of psychological features on the continuum of depression (Table 7–2), along with a trial of treatment as appropriate, may be the most practical means of resolving the question.

Health Outcomes

The bidirectional comorbidity between depression and medical illness is evidenced by the increased risk of acquiring certain medical conditions in patients with a prior history of depression. MDD has been shown to increase the risk of coronary artery disease 1.5- to 2-fold (Van der Kooy et al. 2007), stroke 1.8-fold (Ramasubbu and Patten 2003), cancer 1.9-fold (Gross et al. 2010), diabetes 1.4-fold (Yu et al. 2015), epilepsy 4- to 6-fold (Hesdorffer et al. 2000), and Alzheimer's disease 2.1-fold (Green et al. 2003). These risk increases may be mediated by biological mechanisms as well as by unhealthy behaviors related to medical compliance, self-care, diet, or exercise (Katon 2003).

TABLE 7–2.   Psychological features on the continuum of depression

Normal sadness	Subthreshold depression	DSM-5 major depressive disorder
• Maintenance of intimacy and connection • Belief that things will get better • Capacity to enjoy happy memories • Sense of self-worth fluctuating with thoughts of cancer • Capacity to look forward to the future • Retention of capacity for pleasure • Maintenance of will to live	• Low mood presentation similar to major depressive disorder but not meeting full criteria for symptom number or duration • Potentially transient and self-limited, including mood episodes lasting <2 weeks • Includes persistent depressive disorder if >2 years' duration	• Feeling of isolation • Feeling of permanence • Excessive guilt and regret • Self-critical ruminations/loathing • Constant, pervasive, and nonreactive sadness • Sense of hopelessness • Loss of interest in activities • Suicidal thoughts/behavior

Source.   Adapted with permission from Li M., Kennedy E.B., Byrne N., et al.: *The Management of Depression in Patients With Cancer: A Quality Initiative of the Program in Evidence-Based Care (PEBC), Cancer Care Ontario (CCO).* Guideline #19–4. Toronto, ON, Canada, Cancer Care Ontario, 2016.

The World Health Organization (WHO) recently reported that depression is the leading cause of disability worldwide, with more than 320 million people affected globally (World Health Organization 2017). Remarkably, the WHO World Health Survey (Moussavi et al. 2007) found that depression reduces overall health significantly more than do chronic diseases such as coronary artery disease, arthritis, asthma, and diabetes and that the comorbid state of depression plus medical illness worsens health more than any combination of chronic diseases without depression. Comorbid depression is associated with a significant economic burden, including almost twofold higher rates of health care utilization and workplace disability (Stein et al. 2006), longer inpatient lengths of stay (Saravay et al. 1996), and at least a twofold increase in emergency room visits (Himelhoch et al. 2004). Comorbid depression is also associated with a threefold greater risk of nonadherence to medical treatment, thereby contributing to increased morbidity and mortality (DiMatteo et al. 2000). Such noncompliance may include not taking treatments that are prescribed, not following diet or lifestyle recommendations, and not appearing for medical appointments.

Comorbid depression and medical illness have been shown to be associated with worse medical outcomes and higher mortality rates in a number of medical conditions, but specific causal relationships between depression and such outcomes have not been confirmed (Cuijpers et al. 2014). Depression has been associated with more rapid progression of HIV disease (Leserman 2003) and with increased all-cause mortality in cardiovascular disease (Carney and Freedland 2017), cancer (Batty et al. 2017; Pinquart and Duberstein 2010), organ transplant (Dew et al. 2015), and diabetes (Park et al. 2013). This increased mortality rate, which persists even after factors such as smoking, disease severity, and alcohol consumption (Schulz et al. 2000) are controlled for, may be attributable to several different factors. Biological mechanisms in depression may increase mortality rates in the medically ill via effects on the autonomic nervous system and on related cardiac outcomes. The association of suicide with depression may also increase mortality rates in medical populations, a finding that has been demonstrated in medical conditions such as cancer (Steel et al. 2007), multiple sclerosis (Stenager et al. 1996), and Huntington's disease (Almqvist et al. 1999). Depression may be associated with other health risk behaviors—such as cigarette smoking, overeating, physical inactivity, obesity, and excess alcohol consumption—that increase the prevalence of associated medical illness and affect its course adversely.

Screening for Depression

Obstacles to Diagnosis in Medical Settings

Depression and other forms of distress are commonly underdiagnosed and undertreated in medical settings (Fallowfield et al. 2001). A U.K. study suggested that fewer than one-half of cases of depression are correctly diagnosed by general practitioners (Mitchell et al. 2009). This finding warrants concern, because a missed diagnosis of MDD may represent a lost opportunity to improve quality of life, decrease the risk of suicide, shorten hospital stay, and improve treatment compliance in the medically ill. There are many explanations for the low rate of detection of clinical depression in medical settings. The structure of medical care—with medical visits often lasting less than 15 minutes, with multiple clinical concerns that may need to be addressed during each visit, and the frequent lack of privacy in clinic and hospital settings—may inhibit disclosure or elaboration of symptoms. Furthermore, some clinicians avoid emotional inquiry because they fear that they lack sufficient time or skill to manage emotional reactions. Some patients are reluctant to disclose depressive symptoms because of perceived stigma or anticipated lack of interest of their medical caregivers. However, most patients welcome the opportunity to discuss psychosocial issues that are raised by their health care providers (Rodin et al. 2009). In some cases, both patients and clinicians have difficulty differentiating the somatic symptoms of depression from those of medical disease. Even when clinically significant depression is recognized as being present, it may be perceived as an "understandable" reaction to medical illness and therefore not worth treating.

Paradoxically, time-pressured medical clinic visits that preclude adequate assessment of mood can lead to the overdiagnosis of depression and unnecessary pharmacotherapy. This may be a result of misattribution of the symptoms of physical illness to depression and use of low diagnostic thresholds for depression, with an overreadiness to prescribe antidepressant medications and/or to refer for specialized psychiatric assessment (Boland et al. 1996) because of inadequate resources or training to explore or manage psychological distress (Aragonès et al. 2006). More appropriate utilization of limited specialized psychiatric resources may be facilitated by routine use of validated depression screening tools in medical settings (Cahill et al. 2015; Caruso et al. 2017; Gill et al. 2017; Hermanns et al. 2013; McCollister 2011; Moraes et al. 2017; Quittner et al. 2016; Swartz et al. 2016), as has been recommended for primary care by the U.S. Preventive Services Task Force, "with adequate systems in place to ensure accurate diagnosis, effective treatment, and appropriate follow-up" (O'Connor et al. 2016).

Screening Process

General Considerations

Screening for depression may be particularly helpful in medical settings, where routine assessment of mood might otherwise not occur. The ideal screening instrument would be easy to administer and score, acceptable to patients, and, most importantly, accurate. However, the utility of screening for depression depends not only on the measure used but also on whether screening results are routinely assessed by medical caregivers and followed up with appropriate and effective intervention. Failure to ensure that such a response loop is implemented partially contributes to the paucity of evidence that depression screening results in improved depression outcomes (Canadian Task Force on Preventive Health Care et al. 2013; Thombs et al. 2014). The WHO's principles of screening for disease (Andermann et al. 2008) require that medical screening tests demonstrate evidence of effectiveness, with benefits outweighing harms. Screening for depression differs from screening for conditions such as cancer because of the recurrent nature of depression, where early identification may not necessarily reduce incidence in the context of chronic medical illness. Furthermore, positive primary screening tests only identify individuals with a high risk for a medical condition and must be followed by appropriate secondary assessment to make a diagnosis. When positive depression screens automatically trigger intervention, inappropriate use of mental health resources or overprescription of antidepressants may occur. The goal of depression screening should be to initiate a clinical assessment by the health care provider (Li et al. 2016b).

Screening Instruments Commonly Used in Medical Populations

There is no true gold standard for the diagnosis of depression, particularly in the context of medical illness, but clinical interviews have traditionally been used to confirm diagnoses and to establish prevalence rates. Such interviews may be unstructured, utilizing an inclusive or substitutive approach to counting symptoms, or more structured, utilizing diagnostic instruments such as the Structured Clinical Interview for DSM-5 Disorders—Clinician Version (SCID-5-CV; First et al. 2016), the Composite International Diagnostic Interview (CIDI; World Health Organization 1997), the Mini-International Neuropsychiatric Interview (MINI; Sheehan et al. 1998), the Present State Examination (PSE; Hall et al. 1999), or the Primary Care Evaluation of Mental Disorders (PRIME-MD; Spitzer et al. 1999).

Depression rating scales can be used to screen patients to identify those who require clinical diagnostic assessment or to measure depression severity and symptom change over time. Numerous psychometric measures have been developed to measure depressive symptoms, with criterion validity and optimal cutoff scores usually established with some form of clinical interview (Wakefield et al. 2015). The cutoff scores selected determine the sensitivity and specificity of the measure and, therefore, the proportion of false-negative and false-positive cases. Use of higher cutoffs that avoid false positives may be preferable for research purposes and for determining resource allocation in more severe cases. Lower thresholds may be preferable in well-resourced treatment settings in which a premium is placed on avoiding false negatives and on detecting subthreshold disorders. In the following paragraphs we briefly discuss four commonly used self-report instruments that have been validated in medical populations: Center for Epidemiologic Studies—Depression Scale (CES-D; Radloff 1977), Hospital Anxiety and Depression Scale (HADS; Zigmond and Snaith 1983), Beck Depression Inventory–II (BDI-II; Beck et al. 1996), and Patient Health Questionnaire–9 (PHQ-9; Kroenke et al. 2001). The HADS and the BDI-II are copyrighted instruments, while the CES-D and the PHQ-9 are available in the public domain.

The CES-D is a 20-item self-report measure of depressive symptoms, in which only 4 of the 20 items are somatic. Originally designed as a measure of depressive distress in community samples, the CES-D has also been extensively used in medically ill samples, with evidence of good psychometric properties. A cutoff score of 17 was originally recommended to identify clinically significant depression (Radloff 1977), but the low positive predictive value of the CES-D suggests that it might be a better measure of general distress than of depression. Reported cutoff scores in a variety of medical populations have varied between 14 and 23. Depending on cutoffs and medical illness, sensitivity ranges from 73% to 100% and specificity from 61% to 89%.

The HADS is a 14-item self-report scale specifically designed for use in the medically ill, with separate 7-item subscales for anxiety and depression. The depression subscale emphasizes anhedonia and does not include somatic items. The HADS is highly acceptable to patients and has been extensively used in the medically ill, with reported cutoff scores ranging from 8 to 16. Depending on cutoffs and medical illness, sensitivity ranges from 39% to 87% and specificity from 64% to 95%. The HADS does not discriminate well between depression and anxiety, and like the CES-D, it may be better used as a measure of emotional distress (Cosco et al. 2012; Norton et al. 2013).

The BDI-II was originally developed as a 21-item self-report measure of symptom severity in psychiatric patients, but this instrument has been used in numerous studies in the medically ill. Concerns have been raised about its validity in patients with medical illness because of its preponderance of somatic items and about the acceptability to patients of its forced-choice format and complex response alternatives (Koenig et al. 1992). However, there are many studies of the BDI-II as a screening instrument in medically ill samples that have found it to be an accurate self-report measure (Wang and Gorenstein 2013). The cutoff scores recommended in the medically ill have ranged widely, from 7 to 22, providing sensitivity ranging from 45% to 100% and specificity ranging from 64% to 100%, depending on the medical condition (Wang and Gorenstein 2013).

The PHQ-9, the 9-item depression module of the self-administered Patient Health Questionnaire, has been studied in thousands of primary care and medical specialty outpatients in the United States, Europe, and China. The PHQ-9 measures each of the nine DSM-5 criteria for a major depressive episode, with scores ranging from 0 (not at all) to 3 (nearly every day). Reported cutoff scores used in medical populations have ranged from 5 to 10. Depending on cutoffs and medical illness, sensitivity ranges from 52% to 97% and specificity from 73% to 97% (Levis et al. 2017). Of note, Levis et al. (2017) identified significant reporting bias in studies using the PHQ-9, as primary study authors often only selectively report results from cutoffs that perform well in their study.

Single-Item and Very Brief Screening Scales

Single-item screening tests for depression have wide appeal to health care providers and patients, but not surprisingly, they have poor positive predictive value in medical settings (Mitchell 2007; Mitchell and Coyne 2007).

Kroenke et al. (2001) evaluated the two-item PHQ-2, which was derived from the PHQ-9. Meta-analytic studies using the PHQ-2 have reported sensitivity and specificity estimates of 89.3% and 75.9%, respectively, in a primary care population (Mitchell et al. 2016), and 91.8% and 67.7%, respectively, in a geriatric population (Tsoi et al. 2017).

The lower specificity of single-item or ultra-brief self-report measures of depression limits their utility, although measures such as the PHQ-2, which focuses on the core features of depressed mood and/or anhedonia, may be useful, particularly in a step-wise fashion. However, the most common shortcoming in the detection of depression is not in the nature of the instrument used or in the questions posed, but rather in the failure to screen for depression using *any* method.

Treatment Outcomes

Although the negative impact of depression on illness is unequivocal and the bidirectional relationship between depression and medical illness is strong, evidence that treatment of depression improves disease-specific medical outcomes is less clear. In an analysis of studies evaluating the benefits of a screen-and-treat strategy for depression in diabetes, heart failure, and coronary artery disease, Sharkey et al. (2013) found no evidence of improved chronic disease outcomes. However, Katon et al. (2010) demonstrated in a randomized controlled trial (RCT) that patients with depression and chronic illness (poorly controlled diabetes, coronary artery disease, or both) receiving collaborative care had greater overall 12-month improvements in hemoglobin A1c, low-density lipoprotein cholesterol, systolic blood pressure, and depression scores compared with those receiving usual care. The question of whether treatment of depression improves medical outcomes has been most extensively investigated in cardiovascular disease and cancer, in which several studies have explored the relationship between treatment of depression and survival.

In cardiovascular disease, no beneficial effects on cardiac outcomes were found in studies of psychotherapeutic interventions such as the Montreal Heart Attack Readjustment Trial (M-HART; Frasure-Smith 1995) and the Enhancing Recovery in Coronary Heart Disease Patients (ENRICHD; Berkman et al. 2003) trial, although these studies may have been underpowered to detected significant differences, given the modest effectiveness of treatment. Randomized trials of pharmacological treatment for depression in cardiovascular disease, such as the Sertraline Antidepressant Heart Attack Randomized Trial (SADHART; Glassman et al. 2002) and a related trial regarding congestive heart failure, SADHART-CHF (O'Connor et al. 2010), and the Myocardial INfarction and Depression—Intervention Trial (MIND-IT; van den Brink et al. 2002) of mirtazapine, also failed to demonstrate a statistically significant reduction in risk for cardiac events, although these studies similarly demonstrated little reduction in depression. However, in a subanalysis of subjects in the ENRICHD trial, there was reduced risk of death or nonfatal myocardial infarction in subjects who received antidepressants, particularly selective serotonin reuptake inhibitors (SSRIs) (adjusted hazard ratio=0.57). Similarly, secondary analysis of the subgroup of patients in the SADHART-CHF trial who achieved clinical remission of depression demonstrated a statistically significant reduction in cardiovascular events compared with the nonremission group (1.34±1.86 vs. 1.93±2.71; adjusted $P=0.01$) (Jiang et al. 2011). Beneficial pleiotropic effects of SSRIs, such as reduction in platelet activity (Serebruany et al. 2003) and improvement in heart rate variability (Yeragani et al. 2002), may account for these findings. Notably, one large study of enhanced depression treatment in patients with acute coronary syndrome demonstrated a reduction in major adverse cardiac events in intervention patients compared with usual-care patients (Davidson et al. 2010). Unique aspects of this study were a flexible treatment model in which patients could choose problem-solving therapy and/or antidepressants and selection for persistent (>3 months) depression. A better understanding of the temporal and mechanistic relationships between depression and coronary artery disease is needed to clarify potential medical effects of antidepressant treatment (Dickens et al. 2007; see also Chapter 17, "Heart Disease").

Studies have yet to be published on medical outcomes associated with treatment of MDD in cancer patients, although such outcomes have been assessed in studies in which threshold depression was not an inclusion criterion. In an RCT of a 6-month course of fluoxetine versus placebo in early-stage breast cancer patients undergoing adjuvant therapy, Navari et al. (2008) reported that fluoxetine reduced depressive symptoms, improved quality of life, and increased the likelihood of completion of adjuvant treatment. The question of whether psychotherapy can improve survival in cancer has been a hotly debated one (Coyne et al. 2009; Kraemer et al. 2009), with better-designed trials demonstrating that psychosocial interventions that are effective in reducing depressive symptoms do not confer a survival benefit in metastatic cancer patients (Jassim et al. 2015; Kissane et al. 2007; see also Chapter 22, "Oncology").

It may be that the effectiveness of currently available treatments for depression in medical illness is too limited to shift the physiological disease burden of advanced illness enough to alter survival outcomes. More effective treatments may be needed to determine whether alleviation of depression in medical illness has a significant impact on survival and to identify biologically plausible mechanisms that could account for such an effect. Emphasis instead should be on improving quality of life.

Treatment

Several studies have reported that both pharmacological and psychotherapeutic interventions are effective in treating depression in patients with medical disorders, although these effects may be less robust than those in individuals with MDD without medical comorbidity (Iosifescu 2007). The latter finding may be due not only to a difference in the response of MDD to treatment but also to the more prevalent subthreshold presentations in medical populations, which tend not to respond to antidepressant medications (Baumeister 2012) and for which optimal treatment approaches are less clear (Rowe and Rapaport 2006).

The primary evidence base for the effectiveness of treatment of depression in specific medical conditions is limited. Most systematic reviews and meta-analyses have demonstrated modest benefit in illnesses including diabetes (Baumeister et al. 2014), coronary artery disease (Baumeister et al. 2011), COPD (Panagioti et al. 2016), cancer (Li et al. 2017), HIV infection and AIDS (Sherr et al. 2011), chronic kidney disease (Grigoriou et al. 2015), stroke (Nabavi et al. 2014), multiple sclerosis (Fiest et al. 2016), dementia (Ford and Almeida 2017), and Parkinson's disease (Troeung et al. 2013). All such reviews comment on the limited evidence base and the need for more RCTs of depression treatments. Most current disease-specific depression treatment guidelines recommend the use of both pharmacological and psychotherapeutic interventions, based on pooled evidence of benefit in medical populations and extrapolation from effectiveness in primary psychiatric populations (Goodarzi et al. 2016a; Li et al. 2016a; Lichtman et al. 2008; Relf et al. 2013; Towfighi et al. 2017). The National Institute for Health and Care Excellence (NICE) has synthesized the available evidence on the treatment of depression in adults with a chronic physical health problem (National Collaborating Centre for Mental Health [UK] 2010). Updated guidelines published in November 2015 identified a few new treatment trials, but none that altered NICE's recommendations for a stepped-care approach to depression management (National Institute for Health and Care Excellence 2015). Stepped care is a framework for care delivery in which treatment is graded to the severity of depression (Figure 7–2). All patients with depression are provided with basic assessment, support, psychoeducation, monitoring, and referral (Step 1). Based on evidence that the risk–benefit ratio does not support the use of antidepressant medications in subthreshold depression,

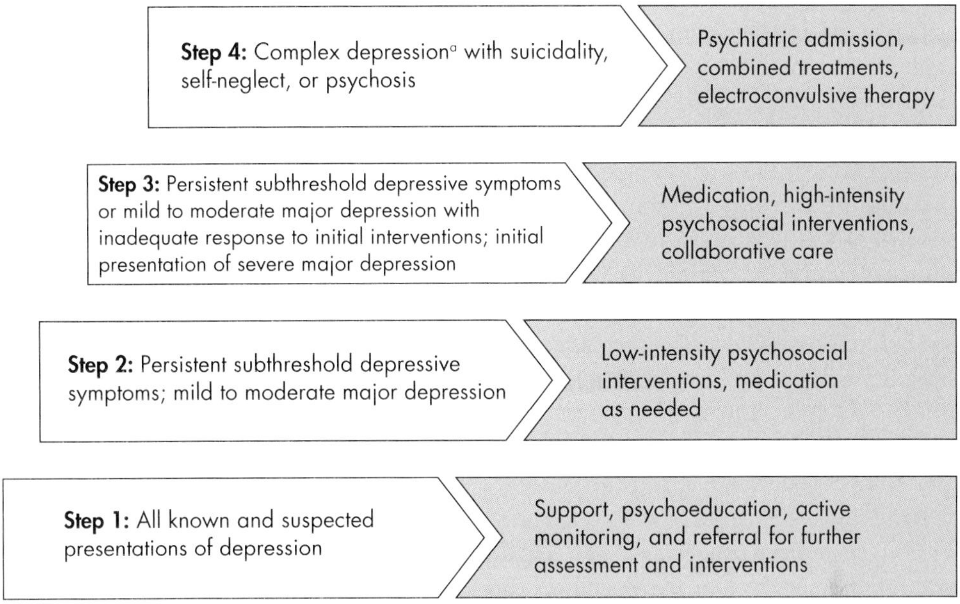

Step 4: Complex depression[a] with suicidality, self-neglect, or psychosis → Psychiatric admission, combined treatments, electroconvulsive therapy

Step 3: Persistent subthreshold depressive symptoms or mild to moderate major depression with inadequate response to initial interventions; initial presentation of severe major depression → Medication, high-intensity psychosocial interventions, collaborative care

Step 2: Persistent subthreshold depressive symptoms; mild to moderate major depression → Low-intensity psychosocial interventions, medication as needed

Step 1: All known and suspected presentations of depression → Support, psychoeducation, active monitoring, and referral for further assessment and interventions

FIGURE 7–2. Stepped-care model of depression care, with treatment intensity corresponding to depression severity.

[a]*Complex depression* includes depression that shows an inadequate response to multiple treatments, is complicated by psychotic symptoms, and/or is associated with significant psychiatric comorbidity or psychosocial factors.

Source. Reprinted from Li M, Kennedy EB, Byrne N, et al.: "Management of Depression in Patients With Cancer: A Clinical Practice Guideline." *Journal of Oncology Practice* 12(8):747–756, 2016; content from National Institute for Health and Care Excellence 2015.

less intrusive and low-intensity psychological or psychosocial interventions are provided first (Step 2), with progression to the next step of medications and/or high-intensity psychological interventions (Step 3), which may be delivered within a collaborative care model (Archer et al. 2012) if there is inadequate response to initial treatment. Complex depression involving suicide risk, psychosis, or severe psychosocial risk may require inpatient admission and/or brain stimulation therapies. The components of these interventions are described more fully below.

Psychotherapeutic Treatment

The full range of psychosocial interventions designed to treat depression in medical populations is discussed in more detail in Chapter 37 ("Psychotherapy") and in the chapters on specific disorders in this textbook. The stepped-care model suggests use of low-intensity psychosocial interventions for persistent subthreshold depressive symptoms or mild to moderate depression. Low-intensity interventions include structured group physical activity programs, group-based peer support or self-help programs, individual guided self-help programs based on cognitive-behavioral therapy (CBT), and computerized CBT. Such group-based therapies may protect patients from depression by diminishing stigma and feelings of isolation and by promoting self-efficacy and a sense of mastery. Patients with inadequate response to treatment or with initial presentations of moderate to severe depression should be offered high-intensity psychosocial interventions that are professionally facilitated. Such interventions include individual or group CBT or behavioral couples' therapy. A Cochrane review of psychotherapy for depression in patients with incurable cancer concluded that psychotherapy was effective in decreasing depressive symptoms, although no studies were identified that focused specifically on patients with MDD (Akechi et al. 2008).

Although the preponderance of research evidence supports cognitive-behavioral approaches to treatment of depression in medical illness (Baumeister et al. 2014; Hummel et al. 2017; Jassim et al. 2015; Orgeta et al. 2015; Ski et al. 2016), such approaches are rarely adopted in routine clinical practice. More commonly, an individualized eclectic approach is used, combining elements of psychoeducation, behavioral activation, problem solving, interpersonal therapy, mindfulness-based therapy, and supportive–expressive psychotherapy delivered on an individual or a group basis. The relationship with the primary medical caregiver may be the most important psychotherapeutic tool to prevent or treat depression for many patients with a serious medical illness. Specific psychological therapies may alleviate or prevent depression, without the risk of physical side effects or drug interactions, and may help to modify health behaviors that adversely affect disease outcomes. The indication to refer to a mental health professional for psychotherapy will depend on the severity of the depression and on the skill and availability of practitioners. The specific psychotherapeutic intervention selected should also take into account the available support network and the patient's capacity to learn new coping strategies and/or to engage in a process that may involve introspection and the expression of feelings. Unique features of psychotherapy in the medically ill are the importance of collaborative relationships between the therapist and the medical caregivers, the likelihood of frequent disruptions in treatment due to complications of the disease, and the need for flexible treatment goals that accommodate shifts in the patient's physical well-being and capacity to participate. In more advanced disease, issues related to hope, existential well-being, and advance care planning may be prominent (Rodin et al. 2009).

Replicated evidence has demonstrated moderate antidepressant effects of psychotherapeutic interventions for patients with cardiovascular disease (Ski et al. 2016; Whalley et al. 2011), diabetes (Baumeister et al. 2012; Musselman et al. 2003), cognitive impairment (Orgeta et al. 2015), HIV/AIDS (van Luenen et al. 2018), multiple sclerosis (Fiest et al. 2016; Wallin et al. 2006), heart failure (Freedland et al. 2015), hemodialysis (Xing et al. 2016), and stroke (Stalder-Lüthy et al. 2013). Numerous systematic reviews and meta-analyses of psychosocial interventions in cancer have found treatment effects for depressive symptoms (Williams and Dale 2006), and systematic reviews of psychosocial interventions for categorical diagnoses of MDD (Li et al. 2016a; Williams and Dale 2006) also demonstrate a treatment effect in RCTs, although the number of studies in these reviews is small. Newly emerging therapies, including Meaning-Centered Psychotherapy (Breitbart et al. 2012), Dignity Therapy (Chochinov et al. 2011), and CALM Therapy (Lo et al. 2014, 2016), have shown benefit in reducing depressive symptoms in patients with advanced cancer, although the effectiveness of these therapies in treating MDD has yet to be demonstrated.

In summary, studies of psychotherapeutic interventions to treat depression in a variety of medical populations indicate some degree of effectiveness, which is often improved in more severe depression when psychotherapy is combined with antidepressant medication. Numerous other nonspecific psychotherapeutic and educational interventions also may be effective in reducing and preventing depressive symptoms.

Psychopharmacological Treatment

SSRIs, heterocyclic antidepressants and tricyclic antidepressants (TCAs), novel antidepressants, and psychostimulants have been evaluated in the treatment of depression comorbid with medical illness. All antidepressants are discussed fully in Chapter 36 ("Psychopharmacology"); here we summarize key points.

SSRIs are generally regarded as the first-line pharmacological treatment for depression in medically ill patients because of their tolerability and relative safety, although mixed-action antidepressants have become increasingly popular in this population because of the potential for dual benefits arising from their receptor-targeting profiles. Venlafaxine is effective for hot flashes in breast cancer (Loprinzi et al. 2000); venlafaxine, duloxetine, and milnacipran are effective for the treatment of pain syndromes (Jann and Slade 2007); mirtazapine may be useful in treating nausea, insomnia, and anorexia (de Boer 1996); and bupropion may be particularly useful in treating patients with prominent neurovegetative symptoms, such as fatigue (Raison et al. 2005). Vortioxetine and vilazodone are multimodal serotonin modulator and stimulator antidepressants recently approved for use in the treatment of MDD. Vortioxetine may have procognitive effects (Rosenblat et al. 2015), but they have yet to be evaluated in medical populations. TCAs such as amitriptyline and nortriptyline have been shown to be effective as analgesics in the treatment of chronic pain syndromes and insomnia (see Chapter 34, "Pain"). Psychostimulants such as methylphenidate and modafinil (Ballon and Feifel 2006) have been reported to rapidly alleviate depressive symptoms in a range of medical conditions, including stroke (Grade et al. 1998), HIV disease (Fernandez et al. 1995), and cancer (Andrew et al. 2017; Conley et al. 2016). Many consider psychostimulants to be the antidepressants of choice in the palliative care setting because of their rapid onset of action (Wilson et al. 2000); however, the evidence remains mixed, with both positive (Ng et al. 2014) and negative (Centeno et al. 2012; Sullivan et al. 2017) trials in palliative care. A Cochrane review (Candy et al. 2008) suggested that the improvement in depression that occurs with psychostimulants may not be clinically significant. Atypical antipsychotics such as olanzapine and quetiapine are effective as augmenting agents in the treatment of MDD in the general population, although this effect has not been studied in medical populations. However, antipsychotics used for this purpose may have additional benefits by stimulating appetite, relieving chemotherapy-induced nausea, improving sleep, and alleviating perceptual disturbances associated with delirium.

Brain Stimulation Therapies

Electroconvulsive therapy (ECT) is sometimes used in the medically ill to treat severe or refractory depression (Beale et al. 1997). It has been shown to be effective in improving depression in Parkinson's disease and also may improve the symptoms of the Parkinson's disease itself (Borisovskaya et al. 2016); it has also been shown to improve poststroke depression and depression associated with multiple sclerosis, endocrine disorders, and renal failure (Krystal and Coffey 1997). ECT has been associated with improvements in cognition and mood in patients with dementia (Rao and

Lyketsos 2000) and is considered safe for epilepsy patients with severe or refractory depression (Lambert and Robertson 1999). ECT should be considered early in the course of depression with psychosis or catatonia, and for depression associated with severe suicidal ideation or failure to maintain adequate nutritional status. ECT and its risks are reviewed in detail in Chapter 38 ("Electroconvulsive Therapy and Other Brain Stimulation Therapies").

Similarly, repetitive transcranial magnetic stimulation (rTMS), which does not produce the short-term memory impairment associated with ECT, is sometimes used as an alternative to pharmacotherapy, with growing evidence supporting its use in the medically ill. Replicated evidence (i.e., more than 80 RCTs) supports a robust antidepressant effect of rTMS for depression alone and in specific medical populations (Brunoni et al. 2017). In a recent meta-analysis, Shen et al. (2017) identified 22 RCTs, all in China (N=1,764 patients), of rTMS for poststroke depression. The results demonstrated that rTMS had a positive effect, with high antidepressant response and remission rates and improvement in activities of daily living. Likewise, in a meta-analysis of eight RCTs (N=312) evaluating the effects of rTMS for depression in Parkinson's disease, Xie et al. (2015) found a positive pooled antidepressant effect for rTMS versus sham rTMS and an equivocal antidepressant effect for rTMS versus SSRIs. Furthermore, patients who received rTMS showed improvement in symptoms of Parkinson's disease and in performance of activities of daily living compared with patients who received sham rTMS or SSRIs. Taken together, there is growing evidence to support the use of rTMS for depression in medically ill patients, particularly those with neurological disorders (McIntyre et al. 2016).

Collaborative Care

At a systems level of care, there is now strong evidence to support the effectiveness of collaborative care models for the treatment of depression in cancer (Sharpe et al. 2014; Walker et al. 2014), coronary artery disease (Atlantis et al. 2014), diabetes (Tully and Baumeister 2015), multiple sclerosis (Ehde et al. 2016), and hepatitis C (Kanwal et al. 2016). Whereas the stepped-care model suggests use of collaborative care for either refractory or moderate to severe depression, recent studies have supported the clinical and cost effectiveness of collaborative care for subthreshold depression as well (Gilbody et al. 2017; Lewis et al. 2017). (For further information on collaborative care, see Chapter 37, "Psychotherapy.")

Conclusion

Clinical depression is common in the medically ill and is associated with impaired quality of life, decreased compliance with medical treatment, and increased medical morbidity and mortality. The elevated prevalence of depression in the medically ill is most often the result of multiple risk factors, although there is continued speculation that specific biological mechanisms operate in certain medical conditions. The diagnosis of depressive disorders in medical patients is complicated by the frequent overlap between symptoms of depression and those of medical illness. This overlap may contribute to underdiagnosis when symptoms of depression are assumed to be features of the medical condition, or to overdiagnosis when symptoms of a medical illness are attributed to depressed mood. However, the neglect of simple inquiry about the symptoms of depression may be the most common reason that the diagnosis of depression is overlooked in medical patients. Screening tests may be useful for drawing the attention of clinicians to these symptoms and identifying patients in medical settings who are most likely to have depressive disorders. Psychopharmacological and psychotherapeutic approaches are both effective in the treatment of depressive disorders in the medically ill and are often even more effective when used together in collaborative care models.

References

Akechi T, Okuyama T, Onishi J, et al: Psychotherapy for depression among incurable cancer patients. Cochrane Database Syst Rev (2):CD005537, 2008 18425922

Almqvist EW, Bloch M, Brinkman R, et al: A worldwide assessment of the frequency of suicide, suicide attempts, or psychiatric hospitalization after predictive testing for Huntington disease. Am J Hum Genet 64(5):1293–1304, 1999 10205260

American Psychiatric Association: Diagnostic and Statistical Manual of Mental Disorders, 5th Edition. Arlington, VA, American Psychiatric Publishing, 2013

Andermann A, Blancquaert I, Beauchamp S, Déry V: Revisiting Wilson and Jungner in the genomic age: a review of screening criteria over the past 40 years. Bull World Health Organ 86(4):317–319, 2008 18438522

Andrew B, Ng CG, Jaafar NR: The use of methylphenidate in cancer patients: a review. Curr Drug Targets March 17, 2017 [Epub ahead of print] 28322161

Aragonès E, Piñol JL, Labad A: The overdiagnosis of depression in non-depressed patients in primary care. Fam Pract 23(3):363–368, 2006 16461446

Arbelaez JJ, Ariyo AA, Crum RM, et al: Depressive symptoms, inflammation, and ischemic stroke in older adults: a prospective analysis in the cardiovascular health study. J Am Geriatr Soc 55(11):1825–1830, 2007 17916124

Archer J, Bower P, Gilbody S, et al: Collaborative care for depression and anxiety problems. Cochrane Database Syst Rev (10):CD006525, 2012 23076925

Arseniou S, Arvaniti A, Samakouri M: HIV infection and depression. Psychiatry Clin Neurosci 68(2):96–109, 2014 24552630

Atlantis E, Fahey P, Foster J: Collaborative care for comorbid depression and diabetes: a systematic review and meta-analysis. BMJ Open 4(4):e004706, 2014 24727428

Ballon JS, Feifel D: A systematic review of modafinil: potential clinical uses and mechanisms of action. J Clin Psychiatry 67(4):554–566, 2006 16669720

Barkow K, Maier W, Ustün TB, et al: Risk factors for new depressive episodes in primary health care: an international prospective 12-month follow-up study. Psychol Med 32(4):595–607, 2002 12102374

Batty GD, Russ TC, Stamatakis E, et al: Psychological distress in relation to site specific cancer mortality: pooling of unpublished data from 16 prospective cohort studies. BMJ 356:j108, 2017 28122812

Baumeister H: Inappropriate prescriptions of antidepressant drugs in patients with subthreshold to mild depression: time for the evidence to become practice. J Affect Disord 139(3):240–243, 2012 21652081

Baumeister H, Hutter N, Bengel J: Psychological and pharmacological interventions for depression in patients with coronary artery disease. Cochrane Database Syst Rev (9):CD008012, 2011 21901717

Baumeister H, Hutter N, Bengel J: Psychological and pharmacological interventions for depression in patients with diabetes mellitus and depression. Cochrane Database Syst Rev (12):CD008381, 2012 23235661

Baumeister H, Hutter N, Bengel J: Psychological and pharmacological interventions for depression in patients with diabetes mellitus: an abridged Cochrane review. Diabet Med 31(7):773–786, 2014 24673571

Beale MD, Kellner CH, Parsons PJ: ECT for the treatment of mood disorders in cancer patients. Convuls Ther 13(4):222–226, 1997 9437566

Beck AT, Steer RA, Brown GK: Manual for Beck Depression Inventory–II. San Antonio, TX, Psychological Corporation, 1996

Berkman LF, Blumenthal J, Burg M, et al; Enhancing Recovery in Coronary Heart Disease Patients Investigators (ENRICHD): Effects of treating depression and low perceived social support on clinical events after myocardial infarction: the Enhancing Recovery in Coronary Heart Disease Patients (ENRICHD) randomized trial. JAMA 289(23):3106–3116, 2003 12813116

Boeschoten RE, Braamse AMJ, Beekman ATF, et al: Prevalence of depression and anxiety in multiple sclerosis: a systematic review and meta-analysis. J Neurol Sci 372:331–341, 2017 28017241

Bogousslavsky J: William Feinberg lecture 2002: emotions, mood, and behavior after stroke. Stroke 34(4):1046–1050, 2003 12649523

Boland RJ, Diaz S, Lamdan RM, et al: Overdiagnosis of depression in the general hospital. Gen Hosp Psychiatry 18(1):28–35, 1996 8666210

Borisovskaya A, Bryson WC, Buchholz J, et al: Electroconvulsive therapy for depression in Parkinson's disease: systematic review of evidence and recommendations. Neurodegener Dis Manag 6(2):161–176, 2016 27033556

Breitbart W, Rosenfeld B, Pessin H, et al: Depression, hopelessness, and desire for hastened death in terminally ill patients with cancer. JAMA 284(22):2907–2911, 2000 11147988

Breitbart W, Poppito S, Rosenfeld B, et al: Pilot randomized controlled trial of individual meaning-centered psychotherapy for patients with advanced cancer. J Clin Oncol 30(12):1304–1309, 2012 22370330

Brunoni AR, Chaimani A, Moffa AH, et al: Repetitive transcranial magnetic stimulation for the acute treatment of major depressive episodes: a systematic review with network meta-analysis. JAMA Psychiatry 74(2):143–152, 2017 28030740

Bukberg J, Penman D, Holland JC: Depression in hospitalized cancer patients. Psychosom Med 46(3):199–212, 1984 6739680

Burvill PW: Recent progress in the epidemiology of major depression. Epidemiol Rev 17(1):21–31, 1995 8521939

Cahill MC, Bilanovic A, Kelly S, et al: Screening for depression in cardiac rehabilitation: a review. J Cardiopulm Rehabil Prev 35(4):225–230, 2015 25622216

Canadian Task Force on Preventive Health Care, Joffres M, Jaramillo A, et al: Recommendations on screening for depression in adults. Can Med Assoc J 185(9):775–782, 2013 23670157

Candy M, Jones L, Williams R, et al: Psychostimulants for depression. Cochrane Database Syst Rev (2):CD006722, 2008 18425966

Capuron L, Fornwalt FB, Knight BT, et al: Does cytokine-induced depression differ from idiopathic major depression in medically healthy individuals? J Affect Disord 119(1–3):181–185, 2009 19269036

Carney RM, Freedland KE: Depression and coronary heart disease. Nat Rev Cardiol 14(3):145–155, 2017 27853162

Caruso R, Nanni MG, Riba M, et al: Depressive spectrum disorders in cancer: prevalence, risk factors and screening for depression: a critical review. Acta Oncol 56(2):146–155, 2017 28140731

Centeno C, Sanz A, Cuervo MA, et al: Multicentre, double-blind, randomised placebo-controlled clinical trial on the efficacy of methylphenidate on depressive symptoms in advanced cancer patients. BMJ Support Palliat Care 2(4):328–333, 2012 24654216

Chi S, Wang C, Jiang T, et al: The prevalence of depression in Alzheimer's disease: a systematic review and meta-analysis. Curr Alzheimer Res 12(2):189–198, 2015 25654505

Chochinov HM, Kristjanson LJ, Breitbart W, et al: Effect of dignity therapy on distress and end-of-life experience in terminally ill patients: a randomised controlled trial. Lancet Oncol 12(8):753–762, 2011 21741309

Chwastiak LA, Ehde DM: Psychiatric issues in multiple sclerosis. Psychiatr Clin North Am 30(4):803–817, 2007 17938046

Classen CC, Kraemer HC, Blasey C, et al: Supportive-expressive group therapy for primary breast cancer patients: a randomized prospective multicenter trial. Psychooncology 17(5):438–447, 2008 17935144

Conley CC, Kamen CS, Heckler CE, et al: Modafinil moderates the relationship between cancer-related fatigue and depression in 541 patients receiving chemotherapy. J Clin Psychopharmacol 36(1):82–85, 2016 26658264

Cosco TD, Doyle F, Ward M, et al: Latent structure of the Hospital Anxiety And Depression Scale: a 10-year systematic review. J Psychosom Res 72(3):180–184, 2012 22325696

Coyne JC, Stefanek M, Thombs BD, et al: Time to let go of the illusion that psychotherapy extends the survival of cancer patients: reply to Kraemer, Kuchler, and Spiegel (2009). Psychological Bulletin 135(2):179–182, 2009

Cuijpers P, Vogelzangs N, Twisk J, et al: Comprehensive meta-analysis of excess mortality in depression in the general community versus patients with specific illnesses. Am J Psychiatry 171(4):453–462, 2014 24434956

Dantzer R, Capuron L, Irwin MR, et al: Identification and treatment of symptoms associated with inflammation in medically ill patients. Psychoneuroendocrinology 33(1):18–29, 2008 18061362

Davidson KW, Rieckmann N, Clemow L, et al: Enhanced depression care for patients with acute coronary syndrome and persistent depressive symptoms: coronary psychosocial evaluation studies randomized controlled trial. Arch Intern Med 170(7):600–608, 2010 20386003

de Boer T: The pharmacologic profile of mirtazapine. J Clin Psychiatry 57 (suppl 4):19–25, 1996 8636062

Dew MA, Rosenberger EM, Myaskovsky L, et al: Depression and mortality as risk factors for morbidity and mortality after organ transplantation: a systematic review and meta-analysis. Transplantation 100(5):988–1003, 2015 26492128

Dickens C, McGowan L, Percival C, et al: Depression is a risk factor for mortality after myocardial infarction: fact or artifact? J Am Coll Cardiol 49(18):1834–1840, 2007 17481442

DiMatteo MR, Lepper HS, Croghan TW: Depression is a risk factor for noncompliance with medical treatment: meta-analysis of the effects of anxiety and depression on patient adherence. Arch Intern Med 160(14):2101–2107, 2000 10904452

Ehde D, Alschuler K, Fann J, et al: Collaborative care for improving pain and depression care in a multiple sclerosis specialty clinic: implementation and preliminary findings from a randomized controlled trial (abstract 538). J Pain 17 (4 suppl):S109, 2016

Fallowfield L, Ratcliffe D, Jenkins V, et al: Psychiatric morbidity and its recognition by doctors in patients with cancer. Br J Cancer 84(8):1011–1015, 2001 11308246

Fernandez F, Levy JK, Samley HR, et al: Effects of methylphenidate in HIV-related depression: a comparative trial with desipramine. Int J Psychiatry Med 25(1):53–67, 1995 7649718

Ferrari AJ, Somerville AJ, Baxter AJ, et al: Global variation in the prevalence and incidence of major depressive disorder: a systematic review of the epidemiological literature. Psychol Med 43(3):471–481, 2013 22831756

Fiest KM, Dykeman J, Patten SB, et al: Depression in epilepsy: a systematic review and meta-analysis. Neurology 80(6):590–599, 2013 23175727

Fiest KM, Walker JR, Bernstein CN, et al; CIHR Team Defining the Burden and Managing the Effects of Psychiatric Comorbidity in Chronic Immunoinflammatory Disease: Systematic review and meta-analysis of interventions for depression and anxiety in persons with multiple sclerosis. Mult Scler Relat Disord 5:12–26, 2016 26856938

First M, Williams JBW, Karg RS, Spitzer RL: Structured Clinical Interview for DSM-5 Disorders—Clinician Version (SCID-5-CV). Arlington, VA, American Psychiatric Association Publishing, 2016

Fitzgerald P, Lo C, Li M, et al: The relationship between depression and physical symptom burden in advanced cancer. BMJ Support Palliat Care 5(4):381–388, 2015 24644172

Ford AH, Almeida OP: Management of depression in patients with dementia: is pharmacological treatment justified? Drugs Aging 34(2):89–95, 2017 28074409

Frasure-Smith N: The Montreal Heart Attack Readjustment Trial. J Cardiopulm Rehabil 15(2):103–106, 1995 8542512

Freedland KE, Carney RM, Rich MW, et al: Cognitive behavior therapy for depression and self-care in heart failure patients: a randomized clinical trial. JAMA Intern Med 175(11):1773–1782, 2015 26414759

Gellis ZD: Depression screening in medically ill homecare elderly. Best Practices Ment Health 6(1):1–16, 2010 21743801

Gilbody S, Lewis H, Adamson J, et al: Effect of collaborative care vs usual care on depressive symptoms in older adults with subthreshold depression: the CASPER randomized clinical trial. JAMA 317(7):728–737, 2017 28241357

Gill SJ, Lukmanji S, Fiest KM, et al: Depression screening tools in persons with epilepsy: a systematic review of validated tools. Epilepsia 58(5):695–705, 2017 28064446

Glassman AH, O'Connor CM, Califf RM, et al; Sertraline Antidepressant Heart Attack Randomized Trial (SADHEART) Group: Sertraline treatment of major depression in patients with acute MI or unstable angina. JAMA 288(6):701–709, 2002 12169073

Goodarzi Z, Mele B, Guo S, et al: Guidelines for dementia or Parkinson's disease with depression or anxiety: a systematic review. BMC Neurol 16(1):244, 2016a 27887589

Goodarzi Z, Mrklas KJ, Roberts DJ, et al: Detecting depression in Parkinson disease: a systematic review and meta-analysis. Neurology 87(4):426–437, 2016b 27358339

Gottlieb SS, Khatta M, Friedmann E, et al: The influence of age, gender, and race on the prevalence of depression in heart failure patients. J Am Coll Cardiol 43(9):1542–1549, 2004 15120809

Grade C, Redford B, Chrostowski J, et al: Methylphenidate in early poststroke recovery: a double-blind, placebo-controlled study. Arch Phys Med Rehabil 79(9):1047–1050, 1998 9749682

Green RC, Cupples LA, Kurz A, et al: Depression as a risk factor for Alzheimer disease: the MIRAGE Study. Arch Neurol 60(5):753–759, 2003 12756140

Grigoriou SS, Karatzaferi C, Sakkas GK: Pharmacological and non-pharmacological treatment options for depression and depressive symptoms in hemodialysis patients. Health Psychol Rev 3(1):1811, 2015 26973957

Gross AL, Gallo JJ, Eaton WW: Depression and cancer risk: 24 years of follow-up of the Baltimore Epidemiologic Catchment Area sample. Cancer Causes Control 21(2):191–199, 2010 19885645

Gurevich M, Devins GM, Wilson C, et al: Stress response syndromes in women undergoing mammography: a comparison of women with and without a history of breast cancer. Psychosom Med 66(1):104–112, 2004 14747644

Hall A, A'Hern R, Fallowfield L: Are we using appropriate self-report questionnaires for detecting anxiety and depression in women with early breast cancer? Eur J Cancer 35(1):79–85, 1999 10211092

Hermanns N, Caputo S, Dzida G, et al: Screening, evaluation and management of depression in people with diabetes in primary care. Prim Care Diabetes 7(1):1–10, 2013 23280258

Hesdorffer DC, Hauser WA, Annegers JF, et al: Major depression is a risk factor for seizures in older adults. Ann Neurol 47(2):246–249, 2000 10665498

Himelhoch S, Weller WE, Wu AW, et al: Chronic medical illness, depression, and use of acute medical services among Medicare beneficiaries. Med Care 42(6):512–521, 2004 15167319

Horwitz AV, Wakefield JC: The Loss of Sadness: How Psychiatry Transformed Normal Sorrow Into Depressive Disorder. New York, Oxford University Press, 2007

Hummel J, Weisbrod C, Boesch L, et al: AIDE–Acute Illness and Depression in Elderly patients. Cognitive behavioral group psychotherapy in geriatric patients with comorbid depression: a randomized controlled trial. J Am Med Dir Assoc 18(4):341–349, 2017 27956074

Iosifescu DV: Treating depression in the medically ill. Psychiatr Clin North Am 30(1):77–90, 2007 17362805

Jann MW, Slade JH: Antidepressant agents for the treatment of chronic pain and depression. Pharmacotherapy 27(11):1571–1587, 2007 17963465

Jassim GA, Whitford DL, Hickey A, et al: Psychological interventions for women with non-metastatic breast cancer. Cochrane Database Syst Rev (5):CD008729, 2015 26017383

Jiang W, Krishnan R, Kuchibhatla M, et al; SADHART-CHF Investigators: Characteristics of depression remission and its relation with cardiovascular outcome among patients with chronic heart failure (from the SADHART-CHF Study). Am J Cardiol 107(4):545–551, 2011 21295172

Kanwal F, Pyne JM, Tavakoli-Tabasi S, et al: Collaborative care for depression in chronic hepatitis C clinics. Psychiatr Serv 67(10):1076–1082, 2016 27364808

Katon WJ: Clinical and health services relationships between major depression, depressive symptoms, and general medical illness. Biol Psychiatry 54(3):216–226, 2003 12893098

Katon W, Lin EH, Kroenke K: The association of depression and anxiety with medical symptom burden in patients with chronic medical illness. Gen Hosp Psychiatry 29(2):147–155, 2007 17336664

Katon WJ, Lin EHB, Von Korff M, et al: Collaborative care for patients with depression and chronic illnesses. N Engl J Med 363(27):2611–2620, 2010 21190455

Kessler RC, Berglund P, Demler O, et al; National Comorbidity Survey Replication: The epidemiology of major depressive disorder: results from the National Comorbidity Survey Replication (NCS-R). JAMA 289(23):3095–3105, 2003 12813115

Kim JM, Shin IS, Yoon JS: Apolipoprotein E among Korean Alzheimer's disease patients in community-dwelling and hospitalized elderly samples. Dement Geriatr Cogn Disord 13(3):119–124, 2002 11893833

Kissane DW, Grabsch B, Clarke DM, et al: Supportive-expressive group therapy for women with metastatic breast cancer: survival and psychosocial outcome from a randomized controlled trial. Psychooncology 16(4):277–286, 2007 17385190

Koenig HG, Cohen HJ, Blazer DG, et al: A brief depression scale for use in the medically ill. Int J Psychiatry Med 22(2):183–195, 1992 1517023

Koenig HG, George LK, Peterson BL, Pieper CF: Depression in medically ill hospitalized older adults: prevalence, characteristics, and course of symptoms according to six diagnostic schemes. Am J Psychiatry 154(10):1376–1383, 1997 9326819

Kraemer HC, Kuchler T, Spiegel D: Use and misuse of the consolidated standards of reporting trials (CONSORT) guidelines to assess research findings: comment on Coyne, Stefanek, and Palmer (2007). Psychol Bull 135(2):173–178, discussion 179–182, 2009 19254073

Kroenke K, Spitzer RL, Williams JB: The PHQ-9: validity of a brief depression severity measure. J Gen Intern Med 16(9):606–613, 2001 11556941

Krystal AD, Coffey CE: Neuropsychiatric considerations in the use of electroconvulsive therapy. J Neuropsychiatry Clin Neurosci 9(2):283–292, 1997 9144111

Lambert MV, Robertson MM: Depression in epilepsy: etiology, phenomenology, and treatment. Epilepsia 40 (suppl 10):S21–S47, 1999 10609603

Leonard BE: Inflammation, depression and dementia: are they connected? Neurochem Res 32(10):1749–1756, 2007 17705097

Leserman J: HIV disease progression: depression, stress, and possible mechanisms. Biol Psychiatry 54(3):295–306, 2003 12893105

Levinson DF: The genetics of depression: a review. Biol Psychiatry 60(2):84–92, 2006 16300747

Levis B, Benedetti A, Levis AW, et al: Selective cutoff reporting in studies of diagnostic test accuracy: a comparison of conventional and individual-patient-data meta-analyses of the Patient Health Questionnaire-9 depression screening tool. Am J Epidemiol 185(10):954–964, 2017 28419203

Lewis L: Mood disorders: diagnosis, treatment, and support from a patient perspective. Psychopharmacol Bull 35(4):186–196, 2001 12397865

Lewis H, Adamson J, Atherton K, et al: CollAborative care and active surveillance for Screen-Positive EldeRs with subthreshold depression (CASPER): a multicentred randomised controlled trial of clinical effectiveness and cost-effectiveness. Health Technol Assess 21(8):1–196, 2017 28248154

Li M, Hales S, Rodin G: Adjustment disorders, in Psycho-Oncology, 2nd Edition. Edited by Holland JC. New York, Oxford University Press, 2010, pp 303–310

Li M, Kennedy EB, Byrne N, et al: Management of depression in patients with cancer: a clinical practice guideline. J Oncol Pract 12(8):747–756, 2016a 27382000

Li M, Macedo A, Crawford S, et al: Easier said than done: keys to successful implementation of the Distress Assessment and Response Tool (DART) program. J Oncol Pract 12(5):e513–e526, 2016b 27048610

Li M, Kennedy EB, Byrne N, et al: Systematic review and meta-analysis of collaborative care interventions for depression in patients with cancer. Psychooncology 26(5):573–587, 2017 27643388

Lichtman JH, Bigger JT Jr, Blumenthal JA, et al; American Heart Association Prevention Committee of the Council on Cardiovascular Nursing; American Heart Association Council on Clinical Cardiology; American Heart Association Council on Epidemiology and Prevention; American Heart Association Interdisciplinary Council on Quality of Care and Outcomes Research; American Psychiatric Association: Depression and coronary heart disease: recommendations for screening, referral, and treatment: a science advisory from the American Heart Association Prevention Committee of the Council on Cardiovascular Nursing, Council on Clinical Cardiology, Council on Epidemiology and Prevention, and Interdisciplinary Council on Quality of Care and Outcomes Research: endorsed by the American Psychiatric Association. Circulation 118(17):1768–1775, 2008 18824640

Lo C, Hales S, Zimmermann C, et al: Measuring death-related anxiety in advanced cancer: preliminary psychometrics of the Death and Dying Distress Scale. J Pediatr Hematol Oncol 33 (suppl 2):S140–S145, 2011 21952572

Lo C, Hales S, Jung J, et al: Managing Cancer And Living Meaningfully (CALM): phase 2 trial of a brief individual psychotherapy for patients with advanced cancer. Palliat Med 28(3):234–242, 2014 24170718

Lo C, Hales S, Chiu A, et al: Managing Cancer And Living Meaningfully (CALM): randomised feasibility trial in patients with advanced cancer. BMJ Support Palliat Care January 19, 2016 [Epub ahead of print] 26787360

Loprinzi CL, Kugler JW, Sloan JA, et al: Venlafaxine in management of hot flashes in survivors of breast cancer: a randomised controlled trial. Lancet 356(9247):2059–2063, 2000 11145492

Lotrich FE: Inflammatory cytokine-associated depression. Brain Res 1617:113–125, 2015 25003554

Lucht M, Schaub RT, Meyer C, et al: Gender differences in unipolar depression: a general population survey of adults between age 18 to 64 of German nationality. J Affect Disord 77(3):203–211, 2003 14612220

Lyketsos CG, Steele C, Baker L, et al: Major and minor depression in Alzheimer's disease: prevalence and impact. J Neuropsychiatry Clin Neurosci 9(4):556–561, 1997 9447496

Lyness JM, Heo M, Datto CJ, et al: Outcomes of minor and subsyndromal depression among elderly patients in primary care settings. Ann Intern Med 144(7):496–504, 2006 16585663

Manne S, Glassman M, Du Hamel K: Intrusion, avoidance, and psychological distress among individuals with cancer. Psychosom Med 63(4):658–667, 2001 11485120

McCollister DH: Screening pulmonary hypertension patients for depression. Int J Clin Pract Suppl 174(174):4–5, 2011 22171816

McIntyre A, Thompson S, Burhan A, et al: Repetitive Transcranial Magnetic Stimulation for depression due to cerebrovascular disease: a systematic review. J Stroke Cerebrovasc Dis 25(12):2792–2800, 2016 27743927

Miller AH, Maletic V, Raison CL: Inflammation and its discontents: the role of cytokines in the pathophysiology of major depression. Biol Psychiatry 65(9):732–741, 2009 19150053

Miller S, Lo C, Gagliese L, et al: Patterns of depression in cancer patients: an indirect test of gender-specific vulnerabilities to depression. Soc Psychiatry Psychiatr Epidemiol 46(8):767–774, 2011 20574846

Mitchell AJ: Pooled results from 38 analyses of the accuracy of distress thermometer and other ultra-short methods of detecting cancer-related mood disorders. J Clin Oncol 25(29):4670–4681, 2007 17846453

Mitchell AJ, Coyne JC: Do ultra-short screening instruments accurately detect depression in primary care? A pooled analysis and meta-analysis of 22 studies. Br J Gen Pract 57(535):144–151, 2007 17263931

Mitchell AJ, Vaze A, Rao S: Clinical diagnosis of depression in primary care: a meta-analysis. Lancet 374(9690):609–619, 2009 19640579

Mitchell AJ, Chan M, Bhatti H, et al: Prevalence of depression, anxiety, and adjustment disorder in oncological, haematological, and palliative-care settings: a meta-analysis of 94 interview-based studies. Lancet Oncol 12(2):160–174, 2011 21251875

Mitchell AJ, Yadegarfar M, Gill J, et al: Case finding and screening clinical utility of the Patient Health Questionnaire (PHQ-9 and PHQ-2) for depression in primary care: a diagnostic meta-analysis of 40 studies. BJPsych Open 2(2):127–138, 2016 27703765

Moraes GP, Lorenzo L, Pontes GA, et al: Screening and diagnosing postpartum depression: when and how? Trends Psychiatry Psychother 39(1):54–61, 2017 28403324

Morris PLP, Robinson RG, Raphael B: Prevalence and course of depressive disorders in hospitalized stroke patients. Int J Psychiatry Med 20(4):349–364, 1990 2086522

Mössner R, Henneberg A, Schmitt A, et al: Allelic variation of serotonin transporter expression is associated with depression in Parkinson's disease. Mol Psychiatry 6(3):350–352, 2001 11326308

Moussavi S, Chatterji S, Verdes E, et al: Depression, chronic diseases, and decrements in health: results from the World Health Surveys. Lancet 370(9590):851–858, 2007 17826170

Musselman DL, Betan E, Larsen H, et al: Relationship of depression to diabetes types 1 and 2: epidemiology, biology, and treatment. Biol Psychiatry 54(3):317–329, 2003 12893107

Nabavi SF, Turner A, Dean O, et al: Post-stroke depression therapy: where are we now? Curr Neurovasc Res 11(3):279–289, 2014 24852795

National Collaborating Centre for Mental Health (UK): Depression in adults with a chronic physical health problem: treatment and management. Leicester, UK, British Psychological Society, 2010

National Institute for Health and Care Excellence (NICE): Surveillance report—depression in adults with a chronic physical health problem (2009) NICE guideline CG91. November 2015. Available at: https://www.nice.org.uk/guidance/cg91/evidence/surveillance-review-decision-november-2015-2183644621. Accessed October 4, 2017.

Navari RM, Brenner MC, Wilson MN: Treatment of depressive symptoms in patients with early stage breast cancer undergoing adjuvant therapy. Breast Cancer Res Treat 112(1):197–201, 2008 18064563

Ng CG, Boks MP, Roes KC, et al: Rapid response to methylphenidate as an add-on therapy to mirtazapine in the treatment of major depressive disorder in terminally ill cancer patients: a four-week, randomized, double-blinded, placebo-controlled study. Eur Neuropsychopharmacol 24(4):491–498, 2014 24503279

Nissim R, Gagliese L, Rodin G: The desire for hastened death in individuals with advanced cancer: a longitudinal qualitative study. Soc Sci Med 69(2):165–171, 2009 19482401

Norton S, Cosco T, Doyle F, et al: The Hospital Anxiety and Depression Scale: a meta confirmatory factor analysis. J Psychosom Res 74(1):74–81, 2013 23272992

O'Connor CM, Jiang W, Kuchibhatla M, et al: Safety and efficacy of sertraline for depression in patients with heart failure: results of the SADHART-CHF (Sertraline Against Depression and Heart Disease in Chronic Health Failure) trial. J Am Coll Cardiol 56(9):692–699, 2010 20723799

O'Connor E, Rossom RC, Henninger M, et al: Screening for depression in adults: an updated systematic evidence review for the U.S. Preventative Services Task Force (Report No 14-05208-EF-1). Rockville, MD, Agency for Healthcare Research and Quality, 2016

Orgeta V, Qazi A, Spector A, et al: Psychological treatments for depression and anxiety in dementia and mild cognitive impairment: systematic review and meta-analysis. Br J Psychiatry 207(4):293–298, 2015 26429684

Panagioti M, Bower P, Kontopantelis E, et al: Association between chronic physical conditions and the effectiveness of collaborative care for depression: an individual participant data meta-analysis. JAMA Psychiatry 73(9):978–989, 2016 27602561

Parissis JT, Fountoulaki K, Filippatos G, et al: Depression in coronary artery disease: novel pathophysiologic mechanisms and therapeutic implications. Int J Cardiol 116(2):153–160, 2007 16822560

Park M, Katon WJ, Wolf FM: Depression and risk of mortality in individuals with diabetes: a meta-analysis and systematic review. Gen Hosp Psychiatry 35(3):217–225, 2013 23415577

Pasquini M, Speca A, Mastroeni S, et al: Differences in depressive thoughts between major depressive disorder, IFN-alpha-induced depression, and depressive disorders among cancer patients. J Psychosom Res 65(2):153–156, 2008 18655860

Patten SB, Barbui C: Drug-induced depression: a systematic review to inform clinical practice. Psychother Psychosom 73(4):207–215, 2004 15184715

Patten SB, Williams JVA, Lavorato DH, et al: Patterns of association of chronic medical conditions and major depression. Epidemiol Psychiatr Sci 27(1):42–50, 2018 27784343

Pinquart M, Duberstein PR: Depression and cancer mortality: a meta-analysis. Psychol Med 40(11):1797–1810, 2010 20085667

Quittner AL, Abbott J, Georgiopoulos AM, et al; International Committee on Mental Health; EPOS Trial Study Group: International committee on mental health in cystic fibrosis: Cystic Fibrosis Foundation and European Cystic Fibrosis Society consensus statements for screening and treating depression and anxiety. Thorax 71(1):26–34, 2016 26452630

Radloff L: The CES-D Scale: a self-report depression scale for research in the general population. Applied Psychological Measurement 1(3):385–401, 1977

Raison CL, Miller AH: Depression in cancer: new developments regarding diagnosis and treatment. Biol Psychiatry 54(3):283–294, 2003 12893104

Raison CL, Demetrashvili M, Capuron L, et al: Neuropsychiatric adverse effects of interferon-alpha: recognition and management. CNS Drugs 19(2):105–123, 2005 15697325

Ramasubbu R, Patten SB: Effect of depression on stroke morbidity and mortality. Can J Psychiatry 48(4):250–257, 2003 12776392

Ramasubbu R, Taylor VH, Samaan Z, et al; Canadian Network for Mood and Anxiety Treatments (CANMAT) Task Force: The Canadian Network for Mood and Anxiety Treatments (CANMAT) task force recommendations for the management of patients with mood disorders and select comorbid medical conditions. Ann Clin Psychiatry 24(1):91–109, 2012 22303525

Rao V, Lyketsos CG: The benefits and risks of ECT for patients with primary dementia who also suffer from depression. Int J Geriatr Psychiatry 15(8):729–735, 2000 10960885

Relf MV, Eisbach S, Okine KN, et al: Evidence-based clinical practice guidelines for managing depression in persons living with HIV. J Assoc Nurses AIDS Care 24 (1 suppl):S15–S28, 2013 23290374

Robinson RG, Jorge RE: Post-stroke depression: a review. Am J Psychiatry 173(3):221–231, 2016 26684921

Rodin G, Walsh A, Zimmermann C, et al: The contribution of attachment security and social support to depressive symptoms in patients with metastatic cancer. Psychooncology 16(12):1080–1091, 2007 17464942

Rodin G, Mackay JA, Zimmermann C, et al: Clinician-patient communication: a systematic review. Support Care Cancer 17(6):627–644, 2009 19259706

Rodríguez MR, Nuevo R, Chatterji S, et al: Definitions and factors associated with subthreshold depressive conditions: a systematic review. BMC Psychiatry 12:181, 2012 23110575

Rosenblat JD, Kakar R, McIntyre RS: The cognitive effects of antidepressants in major depressive disorder: a systematic review and meta-analysis of randomized clinical trials. Int J Neuropsychopharmacol 19(2):1–13, 2015 26209859

Rowe SK, Rapaport MH: Classification and treatment of sub-threshold depression. Curr Opin Psychiatry 19(1):9–13, 2006 16612172

Roy T, Lloyd CE: Epidemiology of depression and diabetes: a systematic review. J Affect Disord 142 (suppl):S8–S21, 2012 23062861

Rudisch B, Nemeroff CB: Epidemiology of comorbid coronary artery disease and depression. Biol Psychiatry 54(3):227–240, 2003 12893099

Saravay SM, Pollack S, Steinberg MD, et al: Four-year follow-up of the influence of psychological comorbidity on medical rehospitalization. Am J Psychiatry 153(3):397–403, 1996 8610829

Schleifer SJ, Macari-Hinson MM, Coyle DA, et al: The nature and course of depression following myocardial infarction. Arch Intern Med 149(8):1785–1789, 1989 2788396

Schulz R, Beach SR, Ives DG, et al: Association between depression and mortality in older adults: the Cardiovascular Health Study. Arch Intern Med 160(12):1761–1768, 2000 10871968

Serebruany VL, Glassman AH, Malinin AI, et al; Sertraline AntiDepressant Heart Attack Randomized Trial Study Group: Platelet/endothelial biomarkers in depressed patients treated with the selective serotonin reuptake inhibitor sertraline after acute coronary events: the Sertraline AntiDepressant Heart Attack Randomized Trial (SADHART) Platelet Substudy. Circulation 108(8):939–944, 2003 12912814

Sharkey S, Agnew T, Bhattacharrya O, et al; Health Quality Ontario: Screening and management of depression for adults with chronic diseases: an evidence-based analysis. Ont Health Technol Assess Ser 13(8):1–45, 2013 24133570

Sharpe M, Walker J, Holm Hansen C, et al; SMaRT (Symptom Management Research Trials) Oncology-2 Team: Integrated collaborative care for comorbid major depression in patients with cancer (SMaRT Oncology-2): a multicentre randomised controlled effectiveness trial. Lancet 384(9948):1099–1108, 2014 25175478

Sheehan DV, Lecrubier Y, Sheehan KH, et al: The Mini-International Neuropsychiatric Interview (M.I.N.I.): the development and validation of a structured diagnostic psychiatric interview for DSM-IV and ICD-10. J Clin Psychiatry 59 (suppl 20):22–33; quiz 34–57, 1998 9881538

Shen X, Liu M, Cheng Y, et al: Repetitive transcranial magnetic stimulation for the treatment of post-stroke depression: a systematic review and meta-analysis of randomized controlled clinical trials. J Affect Disord 211:65–74, 2017 28092847

Sherr L, Clucas C, Harding R, et al: HIV and depression—a systematic review of interventions. Psychol Health Med 16(5):493–527, 2011 21809936

Ski CF, Jelinek M, Jackson AC, et al: Psychosocial interventions for patients with coronary heart disease and depression: a systematic review and meta-analysis. Eur J Cardiovasc Nurs 15(5):305–316, 2016 26475227

Spitzer RL, Kroenke K, Williams JB: Validation and utility of a self-report version of PRIME-MD: the PHQ primary care study. Primary Care Evaluation of Mental Disorders. Patient Health Questionnaire. JAMA 282(18):1737–1744, 1999 10568646

Stalder-Lüthy F, Messerli-Bürgy N, Hofer H, et al: Effect of psychological interventions on depressive symptoms in long-term rehabilitation after an acquired brain injury: a systematic review and meta-analysis. Arch Phys Med Rehabil 94(7):1386–1397, 2013 23439410

Steel JL, Geller DA, Gamblin TC, et al: Depression, immunity, and survival in patients with hepatobiliary carcinoma. J Clin Oncol 25(17):2397–2405, 2007 17557953

Stein MB, Cox BJ, Afifi TO, et al: Does co-morbid depressive illness magnify the impact of chronic physical illness? A population-based perspective. Psychol Med 36(5):587–596, 2006 16608557

Stenager EN, Koch-Henriksen N, Stenager E: Risk factors for suicide in multiple sclerosis. Psychother Psychosom 65(2):86–90, 1996 8711087

Su S, Miller AH, Snieder H, et al: Common genetic contributions to depressive symptoms and inflammatory markers in middle-aged men: the Twins Heart Study. Psychosom Med 71(2):152–158, 2009 19073752

Sullivan DR, Mongoue-Tchokote S, Mori M, et al: Randomized, double-blind, placebo-controlled study of methylphenidate for the treatment of depression in SSRI-treated cancer patients receiving palliative care. Psychooncology 26(11):1763–1769, 2017 27429350

Swartz RH, Bayley M, Lanctôt KL, et al: Post-stroke depression, obstructive sleep apnea, and cognitive impairment: rationale for, and barriers to, routine screening. Int J Stroke 11(5):509–518, 2016 27073189

Talbot F, Nouwen A, Gingras J, et al: Relations of diabetes intrusiveness and personal control to symptoms of depression among adults with diabetes. Health Psychol 18(5):537–542, 1999 10519470

Thombs BD, Ziegelstein RC, Roseman M, et al: There are no randomized controlled trials that support the United States Preventive Services Task Force Guideline on screening for depression in primary care: a systematic review. BMC Med 12:13, 2014 24472580

Towfighi A, Ovbiagele B, El Husseini N, et al; American Heart Association Stroke Council; Council on Cardiovascular and Stroke Nursing; and Council on Quality of Care and Outcomes Research: Poststroke depression: a scientific statement for healthcare professionals from the American Heart Association/American Stroke Association. Stroke 48(2):e30–e43, 2017 27932603

Troeung L, Egan SJ, Gasson N: A meta-analysis of randomised placebo-controlled treatment trials for depression and anxiety in Parkinson's disease. PLoS One 8(11):e79510, 2013 24236141

Tsoi KK, Chan JY, Hirai HW, et al: Comparison of diagnostic performance of Two-Question Screen and 15 depression screening instruments for older adults: systematic review and meta-analysis. Br J Psychiatry 210(4):255–260, 2017 28209592

Tully PJ, Baumeister H: Collaborative care for comorbid depression and coronary heart disease: a systematic review and meta-analysis of randomised controlled trials. BMJ Open 5(12):e009128, 2015 26692557

Unützer J, Schoenbaum M, Katon WJ, et al: Healthcare costs associated with depression in medically ill fee-for-service Medicare participants. J Am Geriatr Soc 57(3):506–510, 2009 19175438

van den Brink RH, van Melle JP, Honig A, et al: Treatment of depression after myocardial infarction and the effects on cardiac prognosis and quality of life: rationale and outline of the Myocardial INfarction and Depression-Intervention Trial (MIND-IT). Am Heart J 144(2):219–225, 2002 12177637

Van der Kooy K, van Hout H, Marwijk H, et al: Depression and the risk for cardiovascular diseases: systematic review and meta analysis. Int J Geriatr Psychiatry 22(7):613–626, 2007 17236251

Van Lieshout RJ, Bienenstock J, MacQueen GM: A review of candidate pathways underlying the association between asthma and major depressive disorder. Psychosom Med 71(2):187–195, 2009 19073754

van Luenen S, Garnefski N, Spinhoven P, et al: The benefits of psychosocial interventions for mental health in people living with HIV: a systematic review and meta-analysis. AIDS Behav 22(1):9–42, 2018 28361453

Wakefield CE, Butow PN, Aaronson NA, et al; International Psycho-Oncology Society Research Committee: Patient-reported depression measures in cancer: a meta-review. Lancet Psychiatry 2(7):635–647, 2015 26303561

Walker J, Hansen CH, Martin P, et al; SMaRT (Symptom Management Research Trials) Oncology-3 Team: Integrated collaborative care for major depression comorbid with a poor prognosis cancer (SMaRT Oncology-3): a multicentre randomised controlled trial in patients with lung cancer. Lancet Oncol 15(10):1168–1176, 2014 25175097

Wallin MT, Wilken JA, Turner AP, et al: Depression and multiple sclerosis: review of a lethal combination. J Rehabil Res Dev 43(1):45–62, 2006 16847771

Wang YP, Gorenstein C: Assessment of depression in medical patients: a systematic review of the utility of the Beck Depression Inventory-II. Clinics (Sao Paulo) 68(9):1274–1287, 2013 24141845

Whalley B, Rees K, Davies P, et al: Psychological interventions for coronary heart disease. Cochrane Database Syst Rev (8):CD002902, 2011 21833943

Wilhelm K, Parker G, Dewhurst-Savellis J, Asghari A: Psychological predictors of single and recurrent major depressive episodes. J Affect Disord 54(1–2):139–147, 1999 10403157

Williams S, Dale J: The effectiveness of treatment for depression/depressive symptoms in adults with cancer: a systematic review. Br J Cancer 94(3):372–390, 2006 16465173

Wilson K, Chochinov HM, de Fay B, et al: Diagnosis and management of depression in palliative care, in Handbook of Psychiatry in Palliative Medicine. Edited by Chochinov HM, Breitbart W. New York, Oxford University Press, 2000, pp 25–40

World Health Organization: Composite International Diagnostic Interview, Version 2.1. Geneva, Switzerland, World Health Organization, 1997

World Health Organization (WHO): Depression fact sheet. http://www.who.int/mediacentre/factsheets/fs369/en/. February 2017. Accessed October 4, 2017.

Xie CL, Chen J, Wang XD, et al: Repetitive transcranial magnetic stimulation (rTMS) for the treatment of depression in Parkinson disease: a meta-analysis of randomized controlled clinical trials. Neurol Sci 36(10):1751–1761, 2015 26209930

Xing L, Chen R, Diao Y, et al: Do psychological interventions reduce depression in hemodialysis patients? A meta-analysis of randomized controlled trials following PRISMA. Medicine (Baltimore) 95(34):e4675, 2016 27559971

Yeragani VK, Pesce V, Jayaraman A, et al: Major depression with ischemic heart disease: effects of paroxetine and nortriptyline on long-term heart rate variability measures. Biol Psychiatry 52(5):418–429, 2002 12242058

Yu M, Zhang X, Lu F, et al: Depression and risk for diabetes: a meta-analysis. Can J Diabetes 39(4):266–272, 2015 25773933

Zigmond AS, Snaith RP: The hospital anxiety and depression scale. Acta Psychiatr Scand 67(6):361–370, 1983 6880820

CHAPTER 8

Suicidality

John Michael Bostwick, M.D.

James L. Levenson, M.D.

Common requests received by all psychiatrists, including psychosomatic medicine specialists, are suicidality evaluations. Suicidal ideation, ubiquitous in medical settings, challenges psychiatrists to discern what drives patients' suicidal statements. Compared with suicidal ideation, completed suicide is rare in psychiatric patients and rarer still in the medically ill. Many risk factors are recognized, but none has shown high positive predictive value (Mann 1987). Given suicide's low base rate, suicide risk screening yields a high rate of false-positive results. Demographic risk factors alone will identify many more subjects who are potentially at risk than who are imminently in danger of dying (Goldberg 1987).

Despite hundreds of studies over decades, drawing dozens of epidemiological correlations between suicide and particular descriptors, no effective screening paradigm has emerged. This situation is no different with suicidality in medical illness. Qin et al. (2013) compared 27,262 Danish subjects who died by suicide with 468,007 living control subjects and found that 63.5% of suicide cases versus 44.5% of control cases involved a history of hospitalization for physical illness, and that physical illness more than doubled the suicide risk. Risk increased not only with frequency and recency of hospitalization but also with involvement of more than one organ or organ system. Nevertheless, given the rarity of completed suicide, these increased rates are usually too low to make medical illness a useful predictor, generally or specifically, of suicide potential. Moreover, medical comorbidity does not take into account an individual's suicide intent—the essential, highly personal variable in suicide prediction (Davidson 1993). Fortunately, the field of suicidology has shifted from trying to predict individual suicides to a more realistic goal of estimating probabilities of risk for particular subpopulations (Hughes and Kleespies 2001). Such data can then be used to generally inform a psychiatric assessment while also considering the personal meaning of the patient's communication and warning signs of impending suicidal actions.

A focus on risk probabilities and general psychiatric symptoms rather than individual diagnoses lends itself well to understanding suicidality in the medically ill. Medical illness alone rarely determines suicide potential. Comorbid factors drive what are best understood as multidetermined acts (Hughes and Kleespies 2001). Shneidman (1989) conceptualized a cubic model of suicidal states, incorporating *perturbation* (the state of being stirred up or upset), *pain* (psychological pain resulting from frustrated psychological needs), and *press* (genetic and developmental susceptibility to particular events). Mościcki (1995) envisioned two distinct but interactive groups of risk factors, with recent events—"proximal factors"—unfolding on a substrate of underlying "distal factors," as did Mann (1998), whose "stress" resembles Mościcki's proximal factors and whose "diathesis" correlates with Mościcki's distal factors. According to all of these models, a suicide assessment for a medically ill person—as is the case for any suicidal person—demands attention not only to current events but also to characterological, temperamental, and experiential features that propel the person toward suicide. Acute psychosocial or medical events may be superimposed on a tendency toward impulsive or suicidal behavior stemming from genetic predisposition, early life experience, or long-term effects of chronic physical illness or substance misuse (Mann 1998). Extreme stress alone, which Mann defined as acute psychiatric or medical illness, intoxication, or family and social stresses, is not typically enough to impel suicidal behavior without a predisposition, or diathesis, on which the stress is superimposed (Mann 1998).

In medical settings, psychiatrists encounter acute intrinsic psychiatric illness in the form of dementia, depression, delirium, and anxiety. Acute substance use disorder may present as an intoxication or withdrawal syndrome. Acute medical illness includes not only the disease itself but also its treatment effects. Acute family and social stresses can include fears of becoming a burden, financial consequences such as treatment expenses and lost income, and disruption in family members' lives.

In this chapter we first review the general epidemiology of suicide and suicide attempts, including the roles of psychodynamic and social factors. We then discuss management of the medical and surgical consequences of a suicide attempt and the care of high-risk patients on medical inpatient units. Specific aspects of suicide in the medically ill are considered next, as exemplified by a focus on cancer and AIDS, with a final section addressing physician-assisted suicide.

Epidemiology

Suicide assessment begins with demographic clues to the patient's relative risk of suicide. Both descriptive and dynamic risk factors are important. In this section, we review descriptive risk factors—comparatively static characteristics of the individual. As the subsequent sections make clear, however, changes in psychiatric status coupled with recent life events are crucial in understanding suicidality in the medically ill.

Completed Suicide

In 2015, suicide was the tenth leading cause of death in the United States (44,193 suicides, accounting for 1.6% of all deaths) (Drapeau and McIntosh 2016). At 13.8 cases per 100,000 population, the U.S. annual suicide rate in 2015 (Drapeau and McIntosh

2016) was only slightly higher than it was in 1900 (Monk 1987). The suicide rate in 2015 was 3.4 times higher for men than for women, and the rate for nonwhite Americans was less than half the rate for white Americans (Drapeau and McIntosh 2016).

Over the course of the life cycle, men and women show different suicide patterns. For men, suicide rates rise gradually from adolescence onward. In 2014, the rate was 18.2 suicides per 100,000 population for men ages 15–24 years, jumping to 24.3 per 100,000 for men ages 25–44 years and 29.7 per 100,000 for men ages 45–64 years, dipping slightly to 26.6 per 100,000 for men ages 65–74 years, and culminating in a dramatic leap to 38.8 per 100,000 in men ages 75 years and older. For women, suicide rates start low, peak in midlife, and then decline. In 2014, the rate was 4.6 suicides per 100,000 population for women ages 15–24 years, jumping to 9.8 per 100,000 for women in midlife (ages 45–64 years), and then gradually declining to 4.0 per 100,000 for women 75 years and older (Curtin et al. 2016). Compared with methods used by females, the suicide methods used by males tend to be more violent and lethal: hanging, drowning, and shooting. Women attempters more often survive because of their preference for less lethal methods such as wrist-cutting and overdose (Kaplan and Klein 1989; Morgan 1989). Attempters are more likely to be younger, female, and married and to use pills, whereas completers are more likely to be older, male, and single and to use violent means (Fawcett and Shaughnessy 1988). However, anyone at any age may contemplate or execute suicide.

A history of suicide attempts is an important predictor of future suicide risk (Pokorny 1983). One in 100 survivors of a suicide attempt will die by suicide within a year of the index attempt, a mortality risk approximately 100 times that in the general population (Hawton 1992). Twenty-five percent of chronically self-destructive or suicidal individuals will eventually kill themselves (Litman 1989). One study found that among suicide completers, 25%–50% had made previous attempts (Patterson et al. 1983). A Danish study of 207 patients admitted to a psychiatric unit after a suicide attempt reported that 12% died by suicide over the next 5 years, with 75% of suicides occurring less than 6 months after discharge from the unit (Nielsen et al. 1990). Bostwick and Pankratz (2000) reported a lifetime suicide prevalence of 8.6% among patients with depression who had ever been hospitalized for suicidal ideation or a suicide attempt. Palmer et al. (2005) found that three-fourths of suicides in patients with schizophrenia occurred within 10 years of the initial diagnosis or first admission. In an observational cohort study of Minnesota residents who had attempted suicide, Bostwick et al. (2016) reported that 60% died in the index attempt (i.e., first lifetime attempt reaching medical attention), and that a high proportion of these suicides were coroner cases, which usually are not included in studies of completed suicide after a suicide attempt. Among survivors of the initial attempt, 80% subsequently killed themselves within a year. Therefore, on either the initial or a subsequent attempt, a total of 81 (5.4%) of the 1,490 cohort members—1 in 9 males and 1 in 50 females—died by suicide within the study period. Gunshot death had an odds ratio (OR) of 140 compared with all other methods.

Active alcohol and other substance use disorders figure prominently in many suicides. An Australian study of completed suicides by methods other than overdose found evidence of alcohol use in 41% and illicit drug use in 20% (Darke et al. 2009). Although individuals who abuse alcohol may kill themselves at any age, particularly when acute intoxication clouds their judgment and disinhibits them, those with chronic alcoholism tend to commit suicide in response to an acute personal crisis, after relationships, work performance, and health have already deteriorated. A study of persons with chronic alcoholism who had committed suicide found that alcoholic individuals often had numerous suicide risk factors, many resulting from their substance abuse, including comorbid major depressive disorder, estrangement from family, lack of social supports, unemployment, homelessness, and serious medical illness (Murphy et al. 1992). People who abuse other psychoactive substances also have high suicide rates. For example, over the past 18 years (a period coinciding with the emergence of the American opioid epidemic), the annual death rate from suicide by opiate poisoning has doubled, from 0.3 per 100,000 population in 1999 to 0.6 per 100,000 in 2014 (Braden et al. 2017), with opioids a contributing cause in 4.4% of all U.S. suicides.

Attempted Suicide

Based on a 25:1 ratio of attempted to completed suicides, an estimated 1,100,000 suicide attempts occurred in the United States in 2015 (Drapeau and McIntosh 2016). Attempted suicides overlap with completed ones, particularly in the medically ill. Attempts occur across spectra of lethality of intent and effect, which may or may not coincide. Some patients deliberately plan death but naively choose nonlethal methods (e.g., benzodiazepine overdose), whereas others intend only gestures but unwittingly select fatal methods (e.g., acetaminophen overdose). At the more severe end of the spectrum, suicide attempters resemble completers. In a New Zealand study comparing completers with survivors of serious attempts, Beautrais (2001) found that the two groups shared the same predictors, including current psychiatric disorder, previous suicide attempts, previous psychiatric contact, social disadvantage, and exposure to recent stressful life events.

A prominent characteristic distinguishing suicide completers from surviving attempters is method. Patients who have overdosed are more likely to survive because they often have time to reconsider their action (or be found) and to undergo medical treatment, options less likely after a jump or a gunshot wound. As with completed suicides, demographics for suicide attempts change over the life cycle. The ratio of attempts to deaths in the young is 25:1; by old age, the ratio has narrowed precipitously, to 4:1 (American Foundation for Suicide Prevention 2015). Medical illness is common among suicide attempters admitted to general psychiatry units. In a year-long study of patients sequentially admitted to a Danish psychiatry unit after a suicide attempt, 52% carried a somatic diagnosis and 21% took daily analgesic medications for pain. Patients in the somatic group were older, with most having neurological or musculoskeletal conditions in conjunction with depression more severe than in the nonsomatic group (Stenager et al. 1994). Hall et al. (1999) found that among 100 serious suicide attempters, 41% had a chronic, deteriorating medical illness and 9% had recently been diagnosed with a life-threatening illness.

Psychodynamic and Social Factors

Litman (1989) described a *presuicidal syndrome*—a change in cognitive set that confers heightened risk for lethal attempts and completed suicides. Presuicidal patients in crisis are emotionally agitated and physically tense. They perceive themselves as having constricted choices and fantasize that death will relieve their distress. Hopelessness may be combined with help rejection and distrust. These patients may have a long-term disposition toward impulsive action, an all-or-nothing approach to problems, and a characterological attitude of "my way or no way."

Klerman (1987) opined that presuicidal patients have lost the capacity for rational thought. The hopelessness and helplessness of severe depression may have reached irrational proportions. Auditory hallucinations may command self-harm. Clouded sensorium, impaired judgment, and the disinhibition and misperceptions that accompany delirium, intoxication, or substance withdrawal may drive self-destructive acts.

Berger (1995) observed that rational-seeming suicides were unusual in the medically ill and that suicides in this population were correlated with maladaptive emotional reactions. Describing the role of hopelessness in the thinking of terminally ill cancer patients desiring hastened death, Breitbart et al. (2000) noted that hopelessness accompanied pessimistic cognitive styles rather than accurate assessments of prognosis. That is, patients wished to speed death not because of mortal illness but because of chronic pessimism. A similar conclusion came from Goodwin and Olfson's (2002) study of suicidal ideation in nearly 2,600 patients with physical illness diagnoses. Perceived poor health and diminished hope of recovery significantly predicted suicidal ideation, even after the study authors controlled for the effects of psychiatric disorders, physical conditions, and other factors.

One conclusion of these studies is that attribution of hopelessness to a disease on the part of patients and medical providers—the proximal factor—may preemptively curtail further investigation, resulting in failure to recognize the mental disorder or personality type—the distal condition—that is actually speaking. "There has been a tendency to regard the suicide of a victim of severe medical illness, such as cancer, as a rational alternative to the distress caused by the disease," noted Suominen et al. (2002, p. 412) after analyzing a year's worth of Finnish suicides. "On the other hand, most suicide victims with physical illness have suffered from concurrent mental disorder.... Mental disorders may thus have a mediating role between medical disorder and suicide."

Suicide can be a response to a loss, real or imagined. To help assess the meaning of suicidal ideation or behavior, psychiatrists must inquire about recent or anticipated losses and coping strategies the patient has used with past losses (Davidson 1993). A patient's degree of autonomy and extent of dependence on external sources of emotional support can shed light on the level of psychic resilience (Buie and Maltsberger 1989). In medical settings, a part of oneself may be lost. It may be tangible—an organ, a limb, sexual potency—or intangible—a sense of youthfulness, health, or invincibility. Glickman (1980) believed that a suicidal patient cannot be judged safe until he or she has regained the lost object, accepted its loss, or replaced it with a new object.

A social history that explores the patient's social and interpersonal context will likely identify remediable contributors to suicidal states. Not unexpectedly, physical illness—particularly pain and increased physical dependence—contributes to suicidal behaviors, as do interpersonal issues, including conflict with or health worries about a loved one, and bereavement—both the recent death of a loved one and long-term social problems resulting from that death. Lesser contributors include impending nursing home relocation, financial distress, and occupational or retirement concerns (Harwood et al. 2006). Once again, separate from whether these stressors independently predict suicide, they help create the setting for a suicidal crisis.

Psychiatrists must examine countertransference responses both in themselves and in their fellow medical providers. These include classic "countertransference hate" reactions (Maltsberger and Buie 1974), in which (conscious or unconscious) aversion to suicidal patients fuels acting out by physicians, either with anger or with aloof withdrawal, both of which can increase suicide risk for their patients. Countertransference-driven responses to seriously ill patients may lead psychiatrists and other providers to express excessive pessimism or to offer false reassurances when reality lies somewhere in between.

Suicide in the Medically III

White et al. (1995) subdivided suicidal medically ill patients into three general categories: 1) patients admitted to medical–surgical beds after suicide attempts, 2) patients with delirium-associated agitation and impulsivity, and 3) patients with chronic medical illness causing frustration or hopelessness. Inpatient suicides are rare. One Finnish study found that about 2% of suicides in that country occurred in medical or surgical inpatient settings (Suominen et al. 2002). In a study of suicides occurring in Montreal, Quebec, over a 5-year period, about 3% took place in general hospitals, with one-third of these occurring on medical–surgical units (Proulx et al. 1997). During a 10-year period in a 3,000-bed Chinese medical hospital, 75 self-destructive acts occurred, only 15 of which proved fatal (Hung et al. 2000).

Hundreds of studies have linked a seemingly arbitrary list of medical conditions with increased suicide risk. In a review of this literature, Harris and Barraclough (1994) identified 63 conditions associated with potentially elevated risk but concluded that the only disorders with actual increased risk were HIV/AIDS, Huntington's disease, cancer (particularly head and neck), multiple sclerosis, peptic ulcer disease, end-stage renal disease, spinal cord injuries, and systemic lupus erythematosus. A Canadian study showed elevated ORs for completed suicide in cancer (1.73), prostate disease (1.70), and chronic pulmonary disease (1.86) (Quan et al. 2002). A 2003 study drawing on data from the U.S. National Comorbidity Survey identified 12 general medical diagnostic categories with statistically significantly elevated adjusted ORs for suicide attempts, most ranging from 1.1 to 3.2, except for AIDS, which had an adjusted OR of 44.1 (a rate that is lower now) (Goodwin et al. 2003). A Danish study examining the association between 39 physical diseases and death by suicide in adults ages 65 years and older found up to four times the risk of suicide within 3 years of diagnosis for more than 20 medical conditions (Erlangsen et al. 2015). Elevated ORs notwithstanding, diagnosis alone is rarely helpful in estimating suicide risk. Even though the ORs in each of the 12 categories in the Goodwin et al. (2003) study achieved statistical significance, the suicide rates—except in AIDS—were only slightly higher than suicide's very low base rate, thereby offering minimal help in clinical decision making.

What *is* useful is evidence that suicides in the medically ill—as in the general population—appear to be related to frequently unrecognized comorbid psychiatric illnesses (Davidson 1993; Kellner et al. 1985; Nock et al. 2010). In their study of the role of physical disease in 416 Swedish suicides, Stensman and Sundqvist-Stensman (1988) concluded that although somatic disease factored into suicidal acts, psychiatric conditions such as depression and alcohol abuse played even more significant roles.

Suicidality may vary across an illness course. For example, suicidal ideation is particularly prominent at two points in Huntington's disease: 1) when the patient first becomes aware of neurological changes without yet having a confirmed diagnosis, and 2) when cognitive and physical symptoms have advanced enough to curtail independent living (Paulsen et al. 2005). A Danish study of suicide risk in epilepsy revealed an overall relative risk of 3.17 compared with risk in the general population, with risk particularly high, at 5.35, in the 6-month period after diagnosis. The presence of standard risk factors may predict suicidality more reliably than particular disease characteristics. In U.S. dialysis patients, advanced age, male sex, white or Asian race, substance dependence, geographic region of the country, and recent psychiatric hospitalization all reached significance as independent predictors of completed suicide (Kurella et al. 2005). In patients with chronic pain, family history of suicide and access to potentially lethal medications, in addition to abdominal pain, were significantly associated with both passive and active suicidal ideation, whereas pain severity and depression severity were not (Smith et al. 2004). In the Danish epilepsy study, comorbid psychiatric illness raised the relative risk of suicide to 13.7, with particularly high risk (more than doubled, at 29.2) during the first 6 months after diagnosis (Christensen et al. 2007).

Therefore, rather than focusing on particular medical diagnoses, medical psychiatrists will find it more fruitful to determine whether suicide-prone psychiatric conditions are present, whether patients are at emotionally difficult times in their illness courses, and whether secondary effects of medical illnesses—pain, physical disfigurement, cognitive dysfunction, and disinhibition—are augmenting risk. Much can be done to help. In a review of the literature on suicide in chronic pain patients, Tang and Crane (2006) identified specific pain-induced risk factors, including sleep-onset insomnia, hopelessness, catastrophizing, desire for escape, and problem-solving deficits, all of which respond to psychological interventions.

Patients labeled as "suicidal" may actually be struggling with other phenomena that afflict the medically or terminally ill. A model developed by Bostwick and Cohen (2009)—which focuses on presence or absence of intent to die and presence or absence of collaboration with physicians and significant others in deciding whether to die—can be useful in distinguishing frank suicide from life-ending acts such as noncompliance and treatment withdrawal; physician-assisted suicide; and end-of-life decision making in palliative care situations. The model proceeds from the premise that lumping diverse entities under the rubric of suicide obscures the complexities of end-of-life decision making and inflames critical conversations best undertaken with rational appreciation for distinctions between specifically suicidal exit strategies from life and look-alike entities (Bostwick 2015).

According to Brown et al. (1986), most terminally ill patients do not develop severe depression and associated suicidality. In a study in 97 terminally ill cancer patients, Breitbart et al. (2000) found that only 17% expressed a desire for hastened death, with depression and hopelessness being the strongest predictors of this desire. Feeling oneself to be a burden on others is an underestimated contributor to suicidality in the terminally ill (Wilson et al. 2005). A Canadian study in terminally ill patients found that the will to live fluctuated as depression, anxiety, hypoxia, and sense of well-being waxed and waned (Chochinov et al. 1999). It must be emphasized that no matter how horrific the medical condition, significant suicide risk is not the rule. When suicidality does emerge, it is frequently linked to specific illness stages or mental states.

We next discuss the diagnosis of cancer to illustrate these points further, with the understanding that principles common to cancer are applicable to the breadth of diagnoses encountered in medical settings. The history of the HIV/AIDS epidemic is also explored in some detail to illustrate that although suicide risk dropped as the illness became treatable, risk remained in relation to the social and behavioral factors that contributed to acquiring HIV infection in the first place.

Cancer

Population studies confirm what has been known for decades: cancer patients have an elevated suicide risk compared with the general population. Among medical illnesses, cancer may even have a singular relationship to suicide. In a study using conditional logistic regression to analyze data from a U.S. sample of 1,408 individuals ages 65 years and older, cancer (with an OR of 2.3) was the only medical diagnosis that retained an association with suicide in adjusted analyses (Miller et al. 2008). However, all cancers do not manifest suicide risk similarly. Risk level varies based on cancer type, time since diagnosis, cancer prognosis, co-occurring psychiatric disease, and diagnosis-specific morbidity. In a U.S. cohort of nearly 3.6 million individuals diagnosed with cancer between 1973 and 2002, the standardized mortality ratio (SMR) for suicide in cancer patients relative to the general population was 1.9 (Misono et al. 2008). The highest risks were associated with lung and bronchial (SMR= 5.74), stomach (SMR=4.68), oral–pharyngeal (SMR=3.66), and laryngeal cancer (SMR=2.83). As is the case for suicide risk in the general population, older white men were at particularly high risk. In a U.S. sample of 1.3 million cancer patients, Kendal (2007) found that males had 6.2 times the suicide risk of females, a difference again mirroring that seen in the general population.

In an Australian study examining incidence and risk of suicide among cancer patients (Dormer et al. 2008), suicide risk in the poor-prognosis group (SMR=3.39) was nearly four times the risk in the good-prognosis group (SMR=0.86). Risk was highest during the first 3 months after diagnosis, with particularly marked lethality as the poor-prognosis group confronted the lack of treatment for their conditions. A second period of increased suicide risk occurred at 12–14 months, the likeliest time of recurrence or acknowledgment of treatment failure. Consistent with the Australian study, Björkenstam et al. (2005) in Sweden demonstrated a reciprocal relationship between cancer prognosis and suicide risk. The lower the survival rate of the cancer, the higher the suicide rate, with the highest rates found in pancreatic, esophageal, hepatocellular, and pulmonary cancers, conditions known for being particularly painful and destructive of quality of life. A recent Austrian study of more than 900,000 individuals diagnosed with cancer over an 18-year period reported an SMR of 1.23, although suicide risk in the cancer cohort, compared with risk in the general population, was more than doubled in the year after diagnosis (SMR=3.17) and was more than tripled when metastatic disease was present (SMR=4.07). Lung cancer (SMR=3.86) and central nervous system cancer (SMR=2.86) had the highest suicide risks (Vyssoki et al. 2015). A

Korean study found an elevated suicide risk in the first year after diagnosis when the cancer was diagnosed at an advanced stage (Ahn et al. 2015).

In a U.S. study of 871,320 cases of lung cancer diagnosed between 1973 and 2008, Urban et al. (2013) found an overall SMR of 4.95, with suicide risk dramatically heightened, at 13.4, within the first 3 months after diagnosis but dropping to 3.8 thereafter. Although the highest SMRs were associated with metastatic disease, higher-grade tumors, advanced age, male sex, and treatment refusal, more than half of the suicides occurred in patients with localized, potentially curable disease. The authors attributed the suicides of these patients to acute overwhelming fear and cognitive overload despite their hopeful prognosis. Fears about pain, disfigurement, and loss of function and autonomy that cancer evokes in patients' imaginations can precipitate suicide, especially early in the disease course, even with a good prognosis. In a large Italian cohort of cancer patients, suicide accounted for only 0.2% of the deaths, but the relative risk during the first 6 months after diagnosis was 27.7 (Crocetti et al. 1998). Additional important contributors may include excessive pessimism and nihilism about treatment and prognosis, exaggerated impressions of anticipated suffering, and fear of loss of control. Patients may dread loss of dignity or compromised privacy, or may feel guilt about unhealthy habits that caused their disease. Surgical treatments may be disfiguring, chemotherapy debilitating, and side effects defeminizing or emasculating (Filiberti et al. 2001). It is notable that the majority of patients who have opted for physician-assisted suicide to date have been cancer patients (Emanuel et al. 2016).

Nonetheless, as cancer patients live longer with their disease, most adjust, becoming less frightened and less susceptible to suicide, with those in remission having suicide risk factors similar to those in the general population. Allebeck et al. (1989) observed in a Swedish cohort that the longer the time since diagnosis of cancer, the lower the relative risk for suicide. In the first year after cancer diagnosis, relative risk was 16.0 for men and 15.4 for women. From 1 to 2 years, the SMR decreased to 6.5 for men and 7.0 for women. By 3–6 years, the SMR was 2.1 for men and 3.2 for women. Ten years after diagnosis, the rate was 0.4, less than one-half the general population rate. A study in Japanese cancer patients found that suicide risk was highest soon after hospital discharge, with elevated relative risk persisting for 5 years before disappearing (Tanaka et al. 1999).

Ultimately, cancer patients who die by suicide are psychiatrically similar to non-cancer patients. In a case–control study of 60 suicides in individuals with cancer and 60 suicides in age- and sex-matched comparison subjects without a cancer history, Henriksson et al. (1995) found a diagnosable psychiatric disorder in most of the patients—and most of the control subjects—who committed suicide. Investigators have speculated that lung cancer's particularly high suicide rate is related more to the high prevalence of preexisting psychiatric disorders known to increase risk than to the cancer itself (Kessler et al. 1999). Moreover, major mental illnesses such as schizophrenia and mood disorders are associated with high rates of smoking, which adds its own independent contribution to suicide risk (Bronisch et al. 2008).

HIV/AIDS

Although suicide risk has plummeted over the past 30 years as HIV/AIDS has evolved from an almost inevitably terminal illness to a chronic one, HIV/AIDS patients continue to have increased suicide risk. In New York City during the first, terror-ridden years of the AIDS epidemic, Marzuk et al. (1988) found that the suicide rate in men with AIDS was 36 times the rate in an age-matched sample of men without AIDS. In California in 1986, the suicide rate among men with AIDS was 21 times higher than the rate in the general population (Kizer et al. 1988).

Early data were primarily based on men engaging in sex with men (MSM) prior to the introduction of antiretroviral agents, a time when an AIDS diagnosis was a virtual death sentence. In the years since that period of profound fear and hopelessness, much has changed, including advances in medical care, improved access to psychiatric care, and diminished social stigma. The contributions of comorbid risk factors for suicide in populations at highest risk for HIV/AIDS—MSM, injection drug users, and poor minority heterosexual women—have become evident. Each of these risk factors—substance abuse, psychiatric illness, and intimate partner violence—contributes independently to elevated suicide risk.

Tracking the association between the debut of highly active antiretroviral therapy (HAART) in 1996 and suicide rates in patients with HIV/AIDS, Gurm et al. (2015) found that suicides in British Columbia declined more than 300-fold after the introduction of effective treatment, from a peak of 961 per 100,000 person-years in 1998 to 2.81 per 100,000 person-years in 2010. They noticed, however, that the suicide rate among persons with HIV/AIDS remained three times that in the general population, an elevation they attributed to untreated mental illness, injection drug use, and inadequately integrated care (Gurm et al. 2015). Schwarcz et al. (2014) found that deaths from drug overdose and suicide contributed disproportionately to mortality in a San Francisco cohort of persons with HIV/AIDS.

Longitudinal studies reflect both the changing demographics of HIV/AIDS and the interplay between HIV-positive status and stable classic risk factors for suicidality. Although the vast majority of HIV-related suicides in the United States in the late 1980s were in men (Coté et al. 1992), nearly one-third of patients attempting suicide a decade later were young women. Both male and female attempters were more likely to report a family history of suicidal behavior, childhood trauma, and/or comorbid depression (Roy 2003).

In a sample of 611 women, Gielen et al. (2005) compared the rates of suicidal thoughts and attempts, anxiety, and depression among four subgroups based on HIV status and experience of intimate partner violence (IPV). HIV-negative women who had not experienced IPV were least likely to report ever having had suicidal ideation, suicide attempts, or either anxiety or depression. Relative to HIV-positive women, women who had experienced IPV were more likely to report a history of suicide attempts, depression, and anxiety and were equally likely to report suicidal ideation. Women who were HIV-positive and had experienced IPV outstripped the other three subgroups on all four mental health indicators, with three times the rate of suicidal ideation, eight times the rate of suicide attempts, four times the rate of anxiety, and three times the rate of depression compared with HIV-negative women who had not experienced IPV. In a study of 2,909 HIV-positive individuals (75% male), 19% reported having had suicidal ideation within the previous week (Carrico et al. 2007). Suicidal ideation was unevenly distributed, however, with its likelihood increased in persons self-identifying as nonheterosexual, those experiencing more severe HIV-related symptoms and medication side effects, those who used marijuana regularly, and those who were depressed. Individuals who reported being in stable romantic relationships and those describing themselves as having good coping skills expressed less suicidal ideation.

Cooperman and Simoni (2005) identified specific periods of risk in the course of the illness. Since being diagnosed, 26% of the sample had made a suicide attempt, 42% of these within a month of diagnosis and 27% within a week. As with cancer, earlier studies showed increases in suicide attempts around the time that physical symptoms first appeared and around the time that full-blown AIDS emerged, with the rate dropping for those living long-term with AIDS (McKegney and O'Dowd 1992; O'Dowd et al. 1993).

Finally, several studies have underscored the possibility that the contribution of HIV/AIDS status to suicidality is incidental or minimal in comparison with the contribution of more robust population-specific factors. Studies in Italy (Grassi et al. 2001) and Brazil (Malbergier and de Andrade 2001) found that psychiatric morbidity and suicidal ideation or suicide attempts were equally common in HIV-positive and HIV-negative intravenous drug users. A Swiss study in MSM found high rates of suicide attempts in both HIV-negative and HIV-positive individuals, with moderately more suicidal ideation in the HIV-positive subjects (Cochand and Bovet 1998). In a comparison of 4,147 HIV-positive and 12,437 HIV-negative U.S. military service applicants who were disqualified from service because of other medical conditions, Dannenberg et al. (1996) found that relative risks for suicide in the two groups were similar: 2.08 in HIV-positive and 1.67 in HIV-negative applicants. All of these studies reinforce the point that psychopathology is implicated more potently in suicidality than is HIV status.

Prevention and Treatment

The first priority in preventing suicide in the medically ill is early detection and treatment of comorbid psychiatric disorders, which are covered throughout this volume. Patient and family education about a disease and its treatment can help prevent excessive fear and pessimism. Direct questions and frank discussion about suicidal thoughts can reduce suicidal pressures. Nonpsychiatric physicians often fail to recognize medically ill patients who are at high risk of suicide—for example, by misattributing severe vegetative symptoms to medical illness and missing suicidal depression (Copsey Spring et al. 2007). One important role for psychiatrists is to discourage other physicians from automatically prescribing antidepressants for every medically ill patient who expresses a wish to die, particularly without also recommending psychotherapy to address cognitive misconceptions that may be encouraging hopelessness or impulsivity (Mann et al. 2005). Overdiagnosis of depression can lead to inappropriate pharmacotherapy, pathologizing of normal feelings, or neglect of relevant personality traits potentially amenable to psychotherapeutic intervention. Soliciting patients' wishes and preferences regarding pain management and end-of-life care may reduce the fear of loss of control of their dying that lures some patients toward suicide.

Psychiatrists can help elicit fears, guilt, impulses, and history that patients may be reluctant to share with their primary physicians. In addition to treating psychiatric symptoms, psychiatrists can monitor for illicit drug use, medication side effects, and emergent neuropsychiatric complications of the underlying medical illness. Psychotherapy can facilitate the exploration and expression of grief and help restore a sense of meaning in life (Chochinov 2002; Frierson and Lippmann 1988; see also Chapter 37, "Psychotherapy," and Chapter 39, "Palliative Care"). Palliative care for the terminally ill is essential in offering relief to those for whom life has become (or is expected to become) unbearable. Psychotherapy also may be psychoeducational, reinforcing patients' and family members' accurate knowledge about the disease. Attention to patients' spiritual needs is very important as well; spiritual well-being offers some protection against end-of-life despair (McClain et al. 2003). Finally, for both patients and family, support groups and other community resources may make the difference between feeling that life is worth living and giving up.

Management of Suicidality in Medical Inpatient Settings

For a survivor of a recent suicide attempt, the emergency department is usually the first stop for assessment and triage. After medical clearance, a mental health professional—ideally a psychiatrist—evaluates the patient and decides whether inpatient or outpatient management is most appropriate. When self-induced injuries are severe enough to require admission for additional medical care, psychiatrists may become involved early on or later when the medical team considers the patient to be stable enough for psychiatric transfer. Whatever the setting, psychiatrists should form their own judgments about whether patients are truly medically stable for discharge or transfer. Countertransference reactions to suicidal patients may cause physicians to minimize medical instability and prematurely "clear" patients. Once a patient is labeled "psychiatric," an appropriate medical workup may be precluded, with unresolved medical issues potentially missed.

A case–control study of eight patients making suicide attempts while medically hospitalized found that attempters were significantly more likely than control patients to have made previous attempts ($P=0.049$) and to have had psychiatric consultations during the current hospitalization ($P=0.02$). A stressor—poorly controlled pain, insomnia, agitation, delirium, or psychosocial issues—was identified for each attempt, only one of which proved fatal (Shekunov et al. 2013). Patients who are admitted to medical–surgical beds after a suicide attempt represent a particularly dangerous subset of suicidal patients. Considering data from all of New Zealand's public hospitals, Conner et al. (2003) showed that individuals hospitalized with self-induced injuries had a relative risk of 105.4 for suicide within the next year and a relative risk of 175.7 for subsequent self-injury hospitalizations.

During a medical–surgical stay, staff must create and maintain a safe space until the patient is stable enough for psychiatric transfer (Bostwick and Rackley 2007). The impulsivity common to diagnoses as divergent as delirium, psychosis, personality disorder, and intoxication and withdrawal syndromes must be anticipated and managed. Warning signs of imminent risk—agitation, extreme hopelessness, and stated intent to die—should receive immediate psychiatric attention. Rudd's concept of warning signs, observable behaviors manifesting in current functioning, assumes clinical relevance in the acute setting that risk factors do not have (Rudd 2008). What subjective evidence is visible to staff that would suggest that a patient may be prone to sudden self-endangering action or is actually contemplating suicide?

Cultures of medical and psychiatric inpatient units differ. On medical units, staff assume that patients are fundamentally compliant (Kelly et al. 1999). Early reports of suicide in hospitals focused on jumping, a then readily available and frequently lethal means of suicide in medically hospitalized patients (Tishler and Reiss 2009). Staff should therefore prevent access to open stairwells, roofs, and balconies and should secure all windows (Bostwick and Rackley 2007). With suicide prevention in mind, modern hospitals are deliberately constructed without open stairwells and windows that open or break easily; however, many older buildings remain in service, warranting vigilance.

Staff must also secure patients' immediate surroundings. In doing so, they must "think like a suicide" (Bostwick and Lineberry 2009)—that is, anything potentially usable for self-injury must be removed. Luggage and possessions should be searched with a suspicious eye and a morbid imagination. Staff must ferret out sharp objects, lighters, belts, caches of pills—anything that could be used to inflict damage in either an impulsive or a deliberate way. Special attention should be paid to items that could be used for self-strangulation, such as drapery cords, belts, shoelaces, ties, and other clothing items (Tishler and Reiss 2009). Imported objects (e.g., phlebotomists' needles, pop-tops from soft drink cans, custodians' disinfectants, meal utensils) should be regarded as potential hazards. Rooms in general medical hospitals often lack safeguards that are now routine on inpatient psychiatric units, such as locked unit entrances, secured windows, and collapsible shower heads, curtain rods, and light fixtures. Scissors and a variety of paraphernalia that can be "creatively" used for self-harm are easily accessible.

Constant observation by one-to-one sitters is indicated for patients at high risk of impulsive self-harm. Use of such monitoring may require compromising patients' privacy. Patients permitted to use the bathroom unobserved have been known to hang or cut themselves behind closed doors. A moment of privacy granted out of misplaced civility, or a few minutes of sitter inattention or absence, may be enough time to execute a suicide plan. All staff guarding suicidal patients should know how to summon security personnel as reinforcements when they perceive that they have lost control of a situation. Despite the absence of published data examining whether constant observation reduces risk (Jaworowski et al. 2008), prudent risk management supports its deployment while avoiding its overuse or underuse (Cardell and Pitula 1999). In a cost-cutting era, consultants may feel pressure to limit the use of one-on-one observation. Economizing on sitters could mean losing a suicidal patient's life, however. On the other hand, staff anxiety can lead to overuse of this measure, with sitters ordered for every patient who expresses suicidal thoughts. In addition to wasting resources, overuse of sitters may desensitize them to the constant awareness needed in their role. When suicidal or impulsive patients are deemed too medically ill for a general psychiatry unit, a medical–psychiatry unit may be the ideal disposition. In the absence of such a specialty unit, intensive care units are better equipped than general medical/surgical units to provide one-to-one nursing care and constant observation.

Once the environment is secured, medical psychiatrists should search for reversible contributors to impulsive states, including delirium (see Chapter 4, "Delirium"), acute medical illness, or medications that may affect mood (see Chapter 7, "Depression"), anxiety (see Chapter 10, "Anxiety Disorders"), or psychotic disorders (see Chapter 9, "Psychosis, Mania, and Catatonia").

Agitation and active suicide attempts in the hospital may require use of restraints. Antipsychotics should be used in patients with hyperactive delirium or psychosis, and antipsychotics and/or benzodiazepines in nonpsychotic but agitated anxious patients. In rare cases, physical restraints may be required if other measures prove inadequate. In some cases, emergency electroconvulsive therapy may be necessary (see Chapter 38, "Electroconvulsive Therapy and Other Brain Stimulation Therapies").

Physician-Assisted Suicide

End-of-life care encompasses a spectrum of options (described in items 1–6 below) ranging from making the dying process as comfortable as possible without deliberately speeding it up (option 1) to actively participating in hastening death (option 6) (Quill et al. 2016):

1. Provision of symptom-directed care to help patients and their loved ones face death as comfortably as possible without hastening its arrival (i.e., the basis of palliative care).
2. Withholding or withdrawing of life-extending technologies, epitomized in discontinuation of dialysis treatment, a practice now so common that at least a quarter of American dialysis patients die this way (Gessert et al. 2013).
3. Prescribing of potentially deadly sedatives and analgesics to combat intractable pain or distress, a practice defensible under St. Thomas Aquinas's 850-year-old doctrine of double effect, in which an action causing a harmful side effect is justified if the actor's intent was to do good (McIntyre 2004).
4. Recommending that the patient voluntarily stop eating and drinking, a practice leading to death in 1–3 weeks that is increasingly being recognized as medically and ethically appropriate (Pope and West 2014).
5. Physician-assisted suicide (PAS), or passive euthanasia, in which a physician prescribes a lethal dose of medication for the patient to self-administer in order to hasten death—a practice legal in five states and the District Columbia in the United States and in five other countries (Emanuel et al. 2016).
6. Active euthanasia, in which the physician him- or herself administers medication with the intent to kill—a practice illegal in all U.S. jurisdictions but legal in the Netherlands, Belgium, Luxembourg, Canada, and Colombia (Emanuel et al. 2016; Ganzini and Back 2016; Kennedy Institute of Ethics 2017).

Options 1–4 in the list above have become normative end-of-life management. PAS (option 5) has remained at the forefront of ethics discussions about end-of-life decision making for more than two decades.

Even before PAS was legal in any jurisdiction in the United States, McHugh (1994) argued that assisted suicides and "naturalistic" ones occur in different groups of people. Moreover, Quill et al. (2016) recently argued that use of the term "suicide" in conjunction with physician-assisted death is pejorative, connoting mental illness–driven wanton self-destruction. They prefer the term "hastening death" for what they describe as a patient-driven issue that "reflects fundamental concern of patients living with serious illnesses who feel they are being destroyed by their illness; they are seeking what they regard as a small measure of self-preservation" (p. 246). For purposes of this discussion, we will refer to these death-hastening measures as PAS, given the term's current widespread use in law and medicine.

Conceptually, PAS depends on a rational request from a competent, hopelessly ill patient whose decision-making ability is not compromised by psychiatric illness. In a pair of unanimous 1997 decisions, the U.S. Supreme Court ruled that no constitutional right to PAS exists and that states can prohibit physician conduct in which the primary purpose is to hasten death (Burt 1997). At the same time, however, it endorsed making palliative care more available and acknowledged the legal acceptability of providing pain relief, even if it hastened death (Burt 1997; Quill et al. 1997). The Court also permitted the states wide latitude in legislating their own statutes regarding PAS (Gostin and Roberts 2016). While voters or legislatures in many states have rejected PAS ballot measures, five states and the District of Columbia have legalized PAS. Oregon was the first, with its Death with Dignity Act enacted in 1994 and implemented in 1997, and with its first PAS occurring that same year, followed by Washington (2008), Vermont (2013), California (2016), Colorado (2016), and the District of Columbia (2017). With its first PAS death in April 2017, Colorado joined Oregon, Washington, and Vermont as U.S. jurisdictions in which PAS has actually occurred (Powell 2017). Montana's Supreme Court ruled in 2009 that state law did not forbid physicians from prescribing lethal medication to a terminally ill patient, but the state has failed to enact an actual statute (Death with Dignity 2017).

Four European countries (the Netherlands, Belgium, Luxembourg, and Switzerland), one South American nation (Colombia), and one North American nation (Canada) permit variations of PAS (Dyer et al. 2015). In contrast to the U.S. Supreme Court's ruling that because no constitutional right for PAS exists, states can decide for themselves whether they want to permit it within their borders, Canada's Supreme Court legalized PAS for the entire nation in 2015, providing a year-long grace period for the 10 provincial governments to work with the medical profession so that all Canadians who wish it can "choose to die with a doctor's help" (Attaran 2015). In the buildup to the Canadian supreme court decision, Schafer (2013) had opined that the high degree of public support for PAS emanated from a predominant Canadian national belief that "important life decisions, including decisions about how and when to end one's life (with assistance if necessary), should be left to the autonomous decision of competent adults." In mid-2016, the grace period expired, and the Canadian parliament legalized both passive and active euthanasia across the entire nation (Emanuel et al. 2016). In a recent article describing the early experience at University Health Network (UHN) in Toronto, Li et al. (2017) noted that the Department of Supportive Care, the entity overseeing MAiD (Medical Assistance in Dying), made a deliberate decision to offer only active euthanasia. "This decision was based on the predictability of the outcome with this method, the lower complication rate than with oral administration of drugs, and the structure of medical care at UHN, which is largely hospital-based" (p. 2083).

In the United States, the Oregon law contains specific mandates meant to standardize the PAS process and provide safeguards against abuses. It requires supplicants to have the capacity to make their own health care decisions. They must have an illness expected to kill them within 6 months and must petition their physicians via one written and two oral statements separated by 15 days from each other. A second physician must agree with the first that the patient has capacity and a terminal prognosis. Either can refer the patient for an optional mental health evaluation if psychopathology appears to be compromising the patient's judgment. In practice, such referrals are rare. In 2016 in Oregon, for example, physicians wrote 204 prescriptions but made only five mental health referrals (Oregon Health Authority Public Health Division 2017). In what Ganzini considered "the most important component of the competency evaluation," the primary physician is required to inform the patient of all feasible options, such as comfort care, hospice care, and pain management (Ganzini 2014, p. 10). Only then can the patient be given a lethal prescription (Chin et al. 1999). The law specifically forbids active euthanasia. PAS is thereby denied to patients who lack the motor capacity to self-administer a lethal medication dose (e.g., those with advanced amyotrophic lateral sclerosis [ALS]; Rowland 1998), although they may still desire PAS. Ganzini et al. (2002) reported that one-third of ALS patients discussed wanting assisted suicide in the last month of life, particularly those with greater distress at being a burden and those with more insomnia, pain, and other discomfort.

Although the annual rate of PAS has continued its gradual rise since the inception of the Death with Dignity Act, PAS accounted for less than 1 in 260 Oregon deaths in 2015 (Oregon Public Empowerment News 2016). Likewise, despite increases in the number of prescriptions written annually (from 24 in 1998 to 218 in 2015), Oregon physicians have written a total of only 1,545 prescriptions, with 991 individuals using legally prescribed medication to hasten death (Blanke et al. 2017). Blanke et al. (2017) found that nearly equal percentages of men and women in Oregon had died after ingesting legally prescribed medication, with about two-thirds of those obtaining prescriptions declining to use them. The average age was 71 years, and 94% died at home. More than three-quarters suffered from cancer, followed by ALS (8%), lung disease (4.5%), heart disease (5.3%), and HIV/AIDS (0.9%). Concerns that patients would not avail themselves of hospice care have not been borne out, with 92.2% in care at the time of their deaths (Blanke et al. 2017). Likewise, concerns of ethicists and disability rights activists that the law would target the elderly, the physically disabled, the chronically physically or mentally ill, the uninsured, people of color, and other marginalized people have not been supported (Coombs Lee 2014). The vast majority of PAS recipients were white and had insurance (Blanke et al. 2017). The fact that statutes require extensive physician documentation is postulated to prevent threats to vulnerable populations (Cain 2016). With 213 requests for lethal medication and 166 deaths by the end of 2015, Washington State data mirror the Oregon statistics (Washington State Department of Health 2016).

Survey research by Ganzini et al. (2009) refutes the notion that current physical discomfort or interpersonal issues drive patients' interest in PAS. For 56 Oregonians who had expressed interest in PAS at end of life, the most important motivations were desire to control the timing and location of death and desire to avoid loss of independence. Worries about future pain, compromised quality of life, and dependence on others for care came next. Least important were limited supports or current physical or mental symptoms. The overall portrait of a typical PAS requester was of a rugged individualist determined to be in charge of his or her destiny, even unto the moment of death. More recent data similarly show that the most common reasons—actual or feared—for desiring PAS are loss of enjoyment of life (89.7%), loss of autonomy (91.6%), and loss of dignity (78.7%), trailed distantly by inadequate pain control (25.2%) (Blanke et al. 2017). The Canadian data from UHN mirror those from Oregon, both in demographics of requesters and in reasons given and not given for seeking MAiD (Li et al. 2017).

The psychiatrist's role in PAS is to be available for consultation, specifically if depression, cognitive impairment, or other psychiatric factors may be interfering with patient capacity. In that psychiatrists are almost never primary care providers for terminally ill patients other than dementia patients, who, by definition, lack capacity and are thus not eligible for PAS, Oregon psychiatrists have not been writing lethal prescriptions (L. Ganzini, personal communication, 2017). Despite expressed concerns by forensic psychiatrists that primary care physicians—let alone general psychiatrists—are not adequately trained to tease out factors confounding a truly informed decision to take an active role in the timing of one's own death (Ganzini et al. 2000), only 5.3% of the 991 patients who died by PAS between 1998 and 2006 were referred for psychiatric capacity evaluations. Hicks (2006) expressed concern that requests for PAS could potentially be influenced by coercion, particularly in geriatric patients, or could be affected by unconscious and unexamined motives in physicians, caregivers, and patients themselves. An additional concern was the possibility that PAS requests could be honored inappropriately, given the high rate of depression—often underrecognized by physicians—in terminally ill patients that can influence their decision making.

Before PAS was legal anywhere in the United States, Block and Billings (1995) outlined five key clinical questions for psychiatrists to explore in the process of clarifying decision-making capacity in terminally ill patients who request euthanasia or assisted suicide:

1. Does the patient have physical pain that is undertreated or uncontrolled?
2. Does the patient have psychological distress driven by inadequately managed psychiatric symptoms?
3. Does the patient have social disruption resulting from interpersonal relationships strained by fears of burdening others, losing independence, or exacting revenge?
4. Does the patient have spiritual despair in the face of taking the measure of a life nearing its end while coming to terms with personal beliefs about the presence or absence of God?
5. Does the patient have iatrogenic anxiety about the dying process itself and the physician's availability as death encroaches?

The questions Block and Billings raised have been subsumed within the ethos and practice of palliative care. It is universally agreed that if the patient is seeking PAS to avoid physical pain, mental anguish, strained interpersonal relationships, spiritual uncertainty, or the dying process itself, these should be addressed prior to considering PAS. Thought leaders opining on the appropriate deployment of PAS since its inception now concur that "patients with serious illness wish to have control over their own bodies, their own lives, and concern about future physical and psychosocial distress" (Quill et al. 2016, p. 246). In other words, existential concerns rather than physical distress usually motivate requests for hastened death (Herx 2015). Much of what drives contemporary PAS requests may not be ameliorated with palliative interventions. A study comparing PAS requesters and nonrequesters—both groups with advanced illness—identified greater depression and hopelessness in the requesters but also more tenuous attachment to others and less belief in a higher meaning for their lives (spirituality). Their independence and self-reliance characterized a lifelong style that never brooked others—including God—deciding the hour of their death (Smith et al. 2015). A related study described how "requests for physician-assisted death may often be the culmination of a person's lifelong pattern of concern with issues such as control, autonomy, self-sufficiency, distrust of others, and avoidance of intimacy" (Oldham et al. 2011, p. 123).

Despite the fact that PAS remains illegal in 45 states, Block and Billings (1995) argued that physicians nonetheless will receive requests for PAS, and they explicitly acknowledged in a case example—as others have done in notorious publications ("A Piece of My Mind: It's Over, Debbie" 1988; Quill 1991)—that some physicians participate in extralegal PAS. They enjoined psychiatrists to perform several functions for nonpsychiatric colleagues wrestling with such requests, including "offering a second opinion on the patient's psychological status, providing a sophisticated evaluation of the patient's decision-making capacity, validating that nothing treatable is being missed, and helping create a setting in which the primary physician and team can formulate a thoughtful decision about how to respond" (Block and Billings 1995, pp. 454–455).

Making time and space for a comprehensive mental health assessment for the presence of a treatable psychiatric disorder can result in a patient deciding to live longer and withdraw the PAS request (Hendin and Klerman 1993), particularly if "the demoralizing triad" of depression, anxiety, and preoccupation with death is confronted and addressed. The Oregon experience has shown that offering palliative interventions can result in patients deciding not to pursue PAS. Only 1 in 6 requests resulted in the physician issuing a prescription, and only 1 in 10 individuals initially requesting PAS ultimately used the medication to hasten death (Ganzini et al. 2001).

The distinctions among—and propriety of—PAS, active euthanasia, and passive euthanasia remain controversial and are beyond the scope of this chapter, but some clarifications should be noted. At present, all 50 states in the United States continue to outlaw active euthanasia. Some have worried that making PAS legal would undermine the availability of appropriate care, partly driven by financial exigencies such as strained health care resources. In the Netherlands, the availability of euthanasia appears to have stunted the evolution of palliative care (Cohen-Almagor 2002), but in Oregon, the reverse appears to have occurred. The availability of PAS coincided there with a dramatic increase in the use of hospice. In 1994, when voters approved PAS, 22% of Oregonians died in hospice care. By 1999, that figure had risen to 35% without any appreciable increase in the geographic distribution or number of hospice beds (Ganzini et al. 2001). The fear that PAS would become a ubiquitous way of prematurely disposing of Oregon's dying patients also appears not to have been borne out: In the first 19 years of legal PAS (1998–2016), 1,127 PAS deaths occurred, and even though the annual number has continued to slowly rise, the 133 PAS deaths in 2016 represented only 0.37% of the total Oregon deaths that year (Oregon Health Authority Public Health Division 2017). Another concern among the public is whether allowing patients to decide to die through refusal of fluids and nutrition will cause undue suffering. The evidence clearly shows that this is not the case (Ganzini et al. 2003).

Psychiatrists will continue to be consulted when patients request withdrawal of treatment or assisted suicide. Evaluation of the patient's capacity for decision making follows the same principles as for other medical decisions (see Chapter 2, "Legal and Ethical Issues"), but psychiatrists should strive to distinguish individuals who wish to die despite having remediable contributing factors in their despair from those who primarily find the burdens of treatment outweighing the offered benefits. As with any "competency consultation," the psychiatrist should always broaden the scope of examination to a full understanding of the patient and his or her predicament.

Conclusion

Compared with suicidal ideation, completed suicide is rare in psychiatric patients and rarer still in the medically ill. Although identifiable demographic factors are associated with increased suicide risk, these factors by themselves will identify many more persons potentially at risk than imminently in danger of dying. Many medical illnesses have been associated with increased suicide attempts, but medical illness by itself is rarely the sole determinant of suicide potential. The assessment of a suicidal medically ill person—as with any suicidal person—demands attention to the role played by characterological, temperamental, or experiential features in the individual's immediate push toward suicide. Management begins with a search for reversible contributors to impulsivity, such as delirium, psychosis, and intoxication. A priority in preventing suicide in the medically ill is the early detection and treatment of comorbid psychiatric disorders.

One of the most frequent reasons for psychiatric consultation in medical hospitals is for evaluation for transfer of care of patients who have made suicide attempts. Because countertransference issues not infrequently lead nonpsychiatric physicians to prematurely "clear" patients, it is critical for psychiatrists to form their own judgments about whether patients are truly medically stable enough for transfer out of the medical setting. If a suicidal patient must remain on a medical floor, the psychiatric consultant should keep in mind that general medical units may lack safeguards routinely found on inpatient psychiatric units. Constant observation by a one-to-one sitter is indicated for patients judged to be at high risk.

Suicide is not synonymous with refusal of lifesaving treatment or with requests to hasten death in terminal illness. Psychiatrists are frequently consulted when patients request withdrawal of treatment or assisted suicide; in these situations, the clinician should evaluate the patient's capacity for decision making, the adequacy of pain management, and the role that treatable psychiatric illness may be playing in the request. Psychological distress, social disruption of interpersonal relationships, and spiritual despair must also be explored and addressed. Responding to these issues with concern and comfort may transform a desire for hastened death into a wish for a graceful and timely exit from life.

References

Ahn MH, Park S, Lee HB, et al: Suicide in cancer patients within the first year of diagnosis. Psychooncology 24(5):601–607, 2015 25336020

Allebeck P, Bolund C, Ringbäck G: Increased suicide rate in cancer patients. A cohort study based on the Swedish Cancer-Environment Register. J Clin Epidemiol 42(7):611–616, 1989 2760653

American Foundation for Suicide Prevention: Suicide statistics. 2015. Available at: https://afsp.org/about-suicide/suicide-statistics. Accessed June 4, 2017.

A piece of my mind: it's over, Debbie (case report). JAMA 259:272, 1988 3339794

Attaran A: Unanimity on death with dignity—legalizing physician-assisted dying in Canada. N Engl J Med 372(22):2080–2082, 2015 26017821

Beautrais AL: Suicides and serious suicide attempts: two populations or one? Psychol Med 31(5):837–845, 2001 11459381

Berger D: Suicide risk in the general hospital. Psychiatry Clin Neurosci 49 (suppl 1):S85–S89, 1995 9179950

Björkenstam C, Edberg A, Ayoubi S, Rosén M: Are cancer patients at higher suicide risk than the general population? Scand J Public Health 33(3):208–214, 2005 16040462

Blanke C, LeBlanc M, Hershman D, et al: Characterizing 18 years of the Death With Dignity Act in Oregon. JAMA Oncol 3(10):1403–1406, 2017 28384683

Block SD, Billings JA: Patient requests for euthanasia and assisted suicide in terminal illness. The role of the psychiatrist. Psychosomatics 36(5):445–457, 1995 7568652

Bostwick J: When suicide is not suicide: self-inducing morbidity and mortality in the general hospital. Rambam Maimonides Med J 6(2):e0013, 2015 25973265

Bostwick JM, Cohen LM: Differentiating suicide from life-ending acts and end-of-life decisions: a model based on chronic kidney disease and dialysis. Psychosomatics 50(1):1–7, 2009 19213966

Bostwick JM, Lineberry TW: Editorial on "Inpatient suicide: preventing a common sentinel event." Gen Hosp Psychiatry 31(2):101–102, 2009 19269528

Bostwick JM, Pankratz VS: Affective disorders and suicide risk: a reexamination. Am J Psychiatry 157(12):1925–1932, 2000 11097952

Bostwick JM, Rackley SJ: Completed suicide in medical/surgical patients: who is at risk? Curr Psychiatry Rep 9(3):242–246, 2007 17521522

Bostwick JM, Pabbati C, Geske JR, McKean AJ: Suicide attempt as a risk factor for completed suicide: even more lethal than we knew. Am J Psychiatry 173(11):1094–1100, 2016 27523496

Braden JB, Edlund MJ, Sullivan MD: Suicide deaths with opioid poisoning in the United States: 1999–2014. Am J Public Health 107(3):421–426, 2017 28103068

Breitbart W, Rosenfeld B, Pessin H, et al: Depression, hopelessness, and desire for hastened death in terminally ill patients with cancer. JAMA 284(22):2907–2911, 2000 11147988

Bronisch T, Höfler M, Lieb R: Smoking predicts suicidality: findings from a prospective community study. J Affect Disord 108(1–2):135–145, 2008 18023879

Brown JH, Henteleff P, Barakat S, Rowe CJ: Is it normal for terminally ill patients to desire death? Am J Psychiatry 143(2):208–211, 1986 3946656

Buie D, Maltsberger J: The psychological vulnerability to suicide, in Suicide: Understanding and Responding. Edited by Jacobs D, Brown H. Madison, CT, International Universities Press, 1989, pp 59–71

Burt RA: The Supreme Court speaks—not assisted suicide but a constitutional right to palliative care. N Engl J Med 337(17):1234–1236, 1997 9337388

Cain C: Implementing Aid in Dying in California: experiences from other states indicates the need for strong implementation guidance. Health Policy Brief, UCLA Center for Health Policy Research, 2016

Cardell R, Pitula CR: Suicidal inpatients' perceptions of therapeutic and nontherapeutic aspects of constant observation. Psychiatr Serv 50(8):1066–1070, 1999 10445656

Carrico AW, Johnson MO, Morin SF, et al; NIMH Healthy Living Project Team: Correlates of suicidal ideation among HIV-positive persons. AIDS 21(9):1199–1203, 2007 17502730

Chin AE, Hedberg K, Higginson GK, Fleming DW: Legalized physician-assisted suicide in Oregon—the first year's experience. N Engl J Med 340(7):577–583, 1999 10021482

Chochinov HM: Dignity-conserving care—a new model for palliative care: helping the patient feel valued. JAMA 287(17):2253–2260, 2002 11980525

Chochinov HM, Tataryn D, Clinch JJ, Dudgeon D: Will to live in the terminally ill. Lancet 354(9181):816–819, 1999 10485723

Christensen J, Vestergaard M, Mortensen PB, et al: Epilepsy and risk of suicide: a population-based case-control study. Lancet Neurol 6(8):693–698, 2007 17611160

Cochand P, Bovet P: HIV infection and suicide risk: an epidemiological inquiry among male homosexuals in Switzerland. Soc Psychiatry Psychiatr Epidemiol 33(5):230–234, 1998 9604673

Cohen-Almagor R: Dutch perspectives on palliative care in the Netherlands. Issues Law Med 18(2):111–126, 2002 12479156

Conner KR, Langley J, Tomaszewski KJ, Conwell Y: Injury hospitalization and risks for subsequent self-injury and suicide: a national study from New Zealand. Am J Public Health 93(7):1128–1131, 2003 12835197

Coombs Lee B: Oregon's experience with aid in dying: findings from the death with dignity laboratory. Ann N Y Acad Sci 1330:94–100, 2014 25082569

Cooperman NA, Simoni JM: Suicidal ideation and attempted suicide among women living with HIV/AIDS. J Behav Med 28(2):149–156, 2005 15957570

Copsey Spring TR, Yanni LM, Levenson JL: A shot in the dark: failing to recognize the link between physical and mental illness. J Gen Intern Med 22(5):677–680, 2007 17443378

Coté TR, Biggar RJ, Dannenberg AL: Risk of suicide among persons with AIDS. A national assessment. JAMA 268(15):2066–2068, 1992 1404744

Crocetti E, Arniani S, Acciai S, et al: High suicide mortality soon after diagnosis among cancer patients in central Italy. Br J Cancer 77(7):1194–1196, 1998 9569062

Curtin S, Warner M, Hedegaard H: Increase in suicide in the United States, 1999–2014. NCHS Data Brief No 241. DHHS Publ No 2016–1209. Hyattsville, MD, National Center for Health Statistics, Centers for Disease Control and Prevention, April 2016. Available at: https://www.cdc.gov/nchs/data/databriefs/db241.pdf. Accessed July 26, 2017.

Dannenberg AL, McNeil JG, Brundage JF, Brookmeyer R: Suicide and HIV infection. Mortality follow-up of 4147 HIV-seropositive military service applicants. JAMA 276(21):1743–1746, 1996 8940323

Darke S, Duflou J, Torok M: Drugs and violent death: comparative toxicology of homicide and non-substance toxicity suicide victims. Addiction 104(6):1000–1005, 2009 19466923

Davidson L: Suicide and aggression in the medical setting, in Psychiatric Care of the Medical Patient. Edited by Stoudemire A, Fogel B. New York, Oxford University Press, 1993, pp 71–86

Death with Dignity (Web site): Montana. 2017. Available at: https://www.deathwithdignity.org/states/montana. Accessed June 4, 2017.

Dormer NR, McCaul KA, Kristjanson LJ: Risk of suicide in cancer patients in Western Australia, 1981–2002. Med J Aust 188(3):140–143, 2008 18241168

Drapeau CW, McIntosh JL: U.S.A. Suicide: 2015 Official Final Data. Washington, DC, American Association of Suicidology, 2016. Available at: http://www.suicidology.org/Portals/14/docs/Resources/FactSheets/2015/2015datapgsv1.pdf?ver=2017-01-02-220151-870. Accessed July 26, 2017.

Dyer O, White C, Rada A: Assisted dying: law and practice around the world. BMJ 351:h4481, 2015 26290517

Emanuel EJ, Onwuteaka-Philipsen BD, Urwin JW, Cohen J: Attitudes and practices of euthanasia and physician-assisted suicide in the United States, Canada, and Europe. JAMA 316(1):79–90, 2016 27380345

Erlangsen A, Stenager E, Conwell Y: Physical diseases as predictors of suicide in older adults: a nationwide, register-based cohort study. Soc Psychiatry Psychiatr Epidemiol 50(9):1427–1439, 2015 25835959

Fawcett J, Shaughnessy R: The suicidal patient, in Psychiatry: Diagnosis and Therapy. Edited by Flaherty J, Channon R, Davis J. Norwalk, CT, Appleton & Lange, 1988, pp 49–56

Filiberti A, Ripamonti C, Totis A, et al: Characteristics of terminal cancer patients who committed suicide during a home palliative care program. J Pain Symptom Manage 22(1):544–553, 2001 11516596

Frierson RL, Lippmann SB: Suicide and AIDS. Psychosomatics 29(2):226–231, 1988 3368568

Ganzini L: Psychiatric evaluations for individuals requesting assisted death in Washington and Oregon should not be mandatory. Gen Hosp Psychiatry 36(1):10–12, 2014 24091255

Ganzini L, Back AL: The challenge of new legislation on physician-assisted death. JAMA Intern Med 176(4):427–428, 2016 26927872

Ganzini L, Leong GB, Fenn DS, et al: Evaluation of competence to consent to assisted suicide: views of forensic psychiatrists. Am J Psychiatry 157(4):595–600, 2000 10739419

Ganzini L, Nelson HD, Lee MA, et al: Oregon physicians' attitudes about and experiences with end-of-life care since passage of the Oregon Death with Dignity Act. JAMA 285(18):2363–2369, 2001 11343484

Ganzini L, Silveira MJ, Johnston WS: Predictors and correlates of interest in assisted suicide in the final month of life among ALS patients in Oregon and Washington. J Pain Symptom Manage 24(3):312–317, 2002 12458112

Ganzini L, Goy ER, Miller LL, et al: Nurses' experiences with hospice patients who refuse food and fluids to hasten death. N Engl J Med 349(4):359–365, 2003 12878744

Ganzini L, Goy ER, Dobscha SK: Oregonians' reasons for requesting physician aid in dying. Arch Intern Med 169(5):489–492, 2009 19273779

Gessert C, Haller I, Johnson B: Regional variation in care at the end of life: discontinuation of dialysis. BMC Geriatr 13:39, 2013 23635315

Gielen AC, McDonnell KA, O'Campo PJ, Burke JG: Suicide risk and mental health indicators: do they differ by abuse and HIV status? Womens Health Issues 15(2):89–95, 2005 15767199

Glickman L: Psychiatric Consultation in the General Hospital. New York, Marcel Dekker, 1980

Goldberg RJ: The assessment of suicide risk in the general hospital. Gen Hosp Psychiatry 9(6):446–452, 1987 3692151

Goodwin R, Olfson M: Self-perception of poor health and suicidal ideation in medical patients. Psychol Med 32(7):1293–1299, 2002 12420898

Goodwin RD, Marusic A, Hoven CW: Suicide attempts in the United States: the role of physical illness. Soc Sci Med 56(8):1783–1788, 2003 12639594

Gostin LO, Roberts AE: Physician-assisted dying: a turning point? JAMA 315(3):249–250, 2016 26784764

Grassi L, Mondardini D, Pavanati M, et al: Suicide probability and psychological morbidity secondary to HIV infection: a control study of HIV-seropositive, hepatitis C virus (HCV)–seropositive and HIV/HCV-seronegative injecting drug users. J Affect Disord 64(2–3):195–202, 2001 11313086

Gurm J, Samji H, Nophal A, et al: Suicide mortality among people accessing highly active antiretroviral therapy for HIV/AIDS in British Columbia: a retrospective analysis. CMAJ Open 3(2):E140–E148, 2015 26389091

Hall RC, Platt DE, Hall RC: Suicide risk assessment: a review of risk factors for suicide in 100 patients who made severe suicide attempts: evaluation of suicide risk in a time of managed care. Psychosomatics 40(1):18–27, 1999 9989117

Harris EC, Barraclough BM: Suicide as an outcome for medical disorders. Medicine (Baltimore) 73(6):281–296, 1994 7984079

Harwood DM, Hawton K, Hope T, et al: Life problems and physical illness as risk factors for suicide in older people: a descriptive and case-control study. Psychol Med 36(9):1265–1274, 2006 16734947

Hawton K: Suicide and attempted suicide, in Handbook of Affective Disorders. Edited by Paykel E. New York, Guilford, 1992, pp 635–650

Hendin H, Klerman G: Physician-assisted suicide: the dangers of legalization. Am J Psychiatry 150(1):143–145, 1993 8417557

Henriksson MM, Isometsä ET, Hietanen PS, et al: Mental disorders in cancer suicides. J Affect Disord 36(1–2):11–20, 1995 8988260

Herx L: Physician-assisted death is not palliative care. Curr Oncol 22(2):82–83, 2015 25908906

Hicks MH: Physician-assisted suicide: a review of the literature concerning practical and clinical implications for UK doctors. BMC Fam Pract 7:39, 2006 16792812

Hughes D, Kleespies P: Suicide in the medically ill. Suicide Life Threat Behav 31 (suppl):48–59, 2001 11326759

Hung CI, Liu CY, Liao MN, et al: Self-destructive acts occurring during medical general hospitalization. Gen Hosp Psychiatry 22(2):115–121, 2000 10822098

Jaworowski S, Raveh D, Lobel E, et al: Constant observation in the general hospital: a review. Isr J Psychiatry Relat Sci 45(4):278–284, 2008 19439833

Kaplan A, Klein R: Women and suicide, in Suicide: Understanding and Responding. Edited by Jacobs D, Brown H. Madison, CT, International Universities Press, 1989, pp 257–282

Kellner CH, Best CL, Roberts JM, Bjorksten O: Self-destructive behavior in hospitalized medical and surgical patients. Psychiatr Clin North Am 8(2):279–289, 1985 3895192

Kelly M, Mufson M, Rogers M: Medical settings and suicide, in The Harvard Medical School Guide to Suicide Assessment and Intervention. Edited by Jacobs D. San Francisco, CA, Jossey-Bass, 1999, pp 491–519

Kendal WS: Suicide and cancer: a gender-comparative study. Ann Oncol 18(2):381–387, 2007 17053045

Kennedy Institute of Ethics: Euthanasia Regulations Around the World. Kennedy Institute of Ethics, Georgetown University. 2017. Available at https://ethicslab.georgetown.edu/euthanasia-map/text.html. Accessed June 4, 2017.

Kessler RC, Borges G, Walters EE: Prevalence of and risk factors for lifetime suicide attempts in the National Comorbidity Survey. Arch Gen Psychiatry 56(7):617–626, 1999 10401507

Kizer KW, Green M, Perkins CI, et al: AIDS and suicide in California (letter). JAMA 260(13):1881, 1988 3418847

Klerman GL: Clinical epidemiology of suicide. J Clin Psychiatry 48 (suppl):33–38, 1987 3320035

Kurella M, Kimmel PL, Young BS, Chertow GM: Suicide in the United States end-stage renal disease program. J Am Soc Nephrol 16(3):774–781, 2005 15659561

Li M, Watt S, Escaf M, et al: Medical assistance in dying—implementing a hospital-based program in Canada. N Engl J Med 376(21):2082–2088, 2017 28538128

Litman R: Suicides: what do they have in mind? in Suicide: Understanding and Responding. Edited by Jacobs D, Brown H. Madison, CT, International Universities Press, 1989, pp 143–154

Malbergier A, de Andrade AG: Depressive disorders and suicide attempts in injecting drug users with and without HIV infection. AIDS Care 13(1):141–150, 2001 11177471

Maltsberger JT, Buie DH: Countertransference hate in the treatment of suicidal patients. Arch Gen Psychiatry 30(5):625–633, 1974 4824197

Mann JJ: Psychobiologic predictors of suicide. J Clin Psychiatry 48 (suppl):39–43, 1987 3320036

Mann JJ: The neurobiology of suicide. Nat Med 4(1):25–30, 1998 9427602

Mann JJ, Apter A, Bertolote J, et al: Suicide prevention strategies: a systematic review. JAMA 294(16):2064–2074, 2005 16249421

Marzuk PM, Tierney H, Tardiff K, et al: Increased risk of suicide in persons with AIDS. JAMA 259(9):1333–1337, 1988 3339837

McClain CS, Rosenfeld B, Breitbart W: Effect of spiritual well-being on end-of-life despair in terminally-ill cancer patients. Lancet 361(9369):1603–1607, 2003 12747880

McHugh PR: Suicide and medical afflictions. Medicine (Baltimore) 73(6):297–298, 1994 7984080

McIntyre A: The double life of double effect. Theor Med Bioeth 25(1):61–74, 2004 15180096

McKegney FP, O'Dowd MA: Suicidality and HIV status. Am J Psychiatry 149(3):396–398, 1992 1536281

Miller M, Mogun H, Azrael D, et al: Cancer and the risk of suicide in older Americans. J Clin Oncol 26(29):4720–4724, 2008 18695256

Misono S, Weiss NS, Fann JR, et al: Incidence of suicide in persons with cancer. J Clin Oncol 26(29):4731–4738, 2008 18695257

Monk M: Epidemiology of suicide. Epidemiol Rev 9:51–69, 1987 2445596

Morgan A: Special issues of assessment and treatment of suicide risk in the elderly, in Suicide: Understanding and Responding. Edited by Jacobs D, Brown H. Madison, CT, International Universities Press, 1989, pp 239–255

Mościcki EK: Epidemiology of suicide. Int Psychogeriatr 7(2):137–148, 1995 8829423

Murphy GE, Wetzel RD, Robins E, McEvoy L: Multiple risk factors predict suicide in alcoholism. Arch Gen Psychiatry 49(6):459–463, 1992 1599370

Nielsen B, Wang AG, Brille-Brahe U: Attempted suicide in Denmark, IV: a five-year follow-up. Acta Psychiatr Scand 81(3):250–254, 1990 2343748

Nock MK, Hwang I, Sampson NA, Kessler RC: Mental disorders, comorbidity and suicidal behavior: results from the National Comorbidity Survey Replication. Mol Psychiatry 15(8):868–876, 2010 19337207

O'Dowd MA, Biderman DJ, McKegney FP: Incidence of suicidality in AIDS and HIV-positive patients attending a psychiatry outpatient program. Psychosomatics 34(1):33–40, 1993 8426889

Oldham RL, Dobscha SK, Goy ER, Ganzini L: Attachment styles of Oregonians who request physician-assisted death. Palliat Support Care 9(2):123–128, 2011 24468479

Oregon Health Authority Public Health Division: Oregon Death with Dignity Act: data summary 2016. February 10, 2017. Available at: http://www.oregon.gov/oha/ph/ProviderPartnerResources/EvaluationResearch/DeathwithDignityAct/Documents/year19.pdf. Accessed June 4, 2017.

Oregon Public Empowerment News (OregonPEN): Death With Dignity reaches adulthood. Oregon PEN, Vol 2, No 9. April 16, 2016. Available at: https://oregonpen.org/death-with-dignity-reaches-adulthood. Accessed June 4, 2017.

Palmer BA, Pankratz VS, Bostwick JM: The lifetime risk of suicide in schizophrenia: a reexamination. Arch Gen Psychiatry 62(3):247–253, 2005 15753237

Patterson WM, Dohn HH, Bird J, Patterson GA: Evaluation of suicidal patients: the SAD PERSONS scale. Psychosomatics 24(4):343–345, 348–349, 1983 6867245

Paulsen JS, Hoth KF, Nehl C, Stierman L: Critical periods of suicide risk in Huntington's disease. Am J Psychiatry 162(4):725–731, 2005 15800145

Pokorny AD: Prediction of suicide in psychiatric patients. Report of a prospective study. Arch Gen Psychiatry 40(3):249–257, 1983 6830404

Pope TM, West A: Legal briefing: voluntarily stopping eating and drinking. J Clin Ethics 25(1):68–80, 2014 24779321

Powell E: Colorado woman ends her life under physician-assisted suicide law. April 18, 2017. 9News: Colorado's News Leader. Available at: http://www.9news.com/news/local/next/colorado-woman-ends-her-life-under-physician-assisted-suicide-law/423477964. Accessed June 4, 2017.

Proulx F, Lesage AD, Grunberg F: One hundred in-patient suicides. Br J Psychiatry 171:247–250, 1997 9337978

Qin P, Webb R, Kapur N, Sørensen HT: Hospitalization for physical illness and risk of subsequent suicide: a population study. J Intern Med 273:48–58, 2013 22775487

Quan H, Arboleda-Flórez J, Fick GH, et al: Association between physical illness and suicide among the elderly. Soc Psychiatry Psychiatr Epidemiol 37(4):190–197, 2002 12027246

Quill TE: Death and dignity. A case of individualized decision making. N Engl J Med 324(10):691–694, 1991 1994255

Quill TE, Lo B, Brock DW: Palliative options of last resort: a comparison of voluntarily stopping eating and drinking, terminal sedation, physician-assisted suicide, and voluntary active euthanasia. JAMA 278(23):2099–2104, 1997 9403426

Quill TE, Back AL, Block SD: Responding to patients requesting physician-assisted death: physician involvement at the very end of life. JAMA 315(3):245–246, 2016 26784762

Rowland LP: Assisted suicide and alternatives in amyotrophic lateral sclerosis. N Engl J Med 339(14):987–989, 1998 9753716

Roy A: Characteristics of HIV patients who attempt suicide. Acta Psychiatr Scand 107(1):41–44, 2003 12558540

Rudd MD: Suicide warning signs in clinical practice. Curr Psychiatry Rep 10(1):87–90, 2008 18269900

Schafer A: Physician assisted suicide: the great Canadian euthanasia debate. Int J Law Psychiatry 36(5–6):522–531, 2013 23856180

Schwarcz SK, Vu A, Hsu LC, Hessol NA: Changes in causes of death among persons with AIDS: San Francisco, California, 1996–2011. AIDS Patient Care STDS 28(10):517–523, 2014 25275657

Shekunov J, Geske JR, Bostwick JM: Inpatient medical-surgical suicidal behavior: a 12-year case-control study. Gen Hosp Psychiatry 35(4):423–426, 2013 23597876

Shneidman E: Overview: a multidimensional approach to suicide, in Suicide: Understanding and Responding. Edited by Jacobs D, Brown H. Madison, CT, International Universities Press, 1989, pp 1–30

Smith KA, Harvath TA, Goy ER, Ganzini L: Predictors of pursuit of physician-assisted death. J Pain Symptom Manage 49(3):555–561, 2015 25116913

Smith MT, Edwards RR, Robinson RC, Dworkin RH: Suicidal ideation, plans, and attempts in chronic pain patients: factors associated with increased risk. Pain 111(1–2):201–208, 2004 15327824

Stenager EN, Stenager E, Jensen K: Attempted suicide, depression and physical diseases: a 1-year follow-up study. Psychother Psychosom 61(1–2):65–73, 1994 8121978

Stensman R, Sundqvist-Stensman UB: Physical disease and disability among 416 suicide cases in Sweden. Scand J Soc Med 16(3):149–153, 1988 3194726

Suominen K, Isometsä E, Heilä H, et al: General hospital suicides—a psychological autopsy study in Finland. Gen Hosp Psychiatry 24(6):412–416, 2002 12490343

Tanaka H, Tsukuma H, Masaoka T, et al: Suicide risk among cancer patients: experience at one medical center in Japan, 1978–1994. Jpn J Cancer Res 90(8):812–817, 1999 10543251

Tang NK, Crane C: Suicidality in chronic pain: a review of the prevalence, risk factors and psychological links. Psychol Med 36(5):575–586, 2006 16420727

Tishler CL, Reiss NS: Inpatient suicide: preventing a common sentinel event. Gen Hosp Psychiatry 31(2):103–109, 2009 19269529

Urban D, Rao A, Bressel M, et al: Suicide in lung cancer: who is at risk? Chest 144(4):1245–1252, 2013 23681288

Vyssoki B, Gleiss A, Rockett IR, et al: Suicide among 915,303 Austrian cancer patients: who is at risk? J Affect Disord 175:287–291, 2015 25661393

Washington State Department of Health: 2015 Death With Dignity Act Report: Executive Summary (DOH 422-109 2015). March 25, 2016. Available at: http://www.doh.wa.gov/portals/1/Documents/Pubs/422-109-DeathWithDignityAct2015.pdf. Accessed June 4, 2017.

White RT, Gribble RJ, Corr MJ, Large MM: Jumping from a general hospital. Gen Hosp Psychiatry 17(3):208–215, 1995 7649465

Wilson KG, Curran D, McPherson CJ: A burden to others: a common source of distress for the terminally ill. Cogn Behav Ther 34(2):115–123, 2005 15986788

CHAPTER 9

Psychosis, Mania, and Catatonia

Oliver Freudenreich, M.D.

Andrew Francis, Ph.D., M.D.

Gregory L. Fricchione, M.D.

Psychosis, mania, and catatonia can greatly hamper the ability of patients to care for themselves and of medical staff to care for them. We discuss psychosis, mania, and catatonia in three subsections as if they were separate entities, with one of the symptoms dominating (and when the symptom is not the result of delirium or dementia; see Chapter 4 "Delirium," and Chapter 5 "Dementia"). In clinical practice, the distinction cannot always be made: patients with mania can be psychotic, or catatonia may occur in a manic or psychotic patient. In each of the subsections, we use the "primary/secondary" distinction even though it is not officially sanctioned by our current classification system (i.e., DSM-5 [American Psychiatric Association 2013]). Clinicians, however, base their diagnostic approach on this distinction: Are psychiatric symptoms attributable to a primary psychiatric syndrome, or are they secondary to medical diseases, substance use, or medication intoxication? In this chapter, we focus on management principles for medically hospitalized patients who are psychotic, manic, or catatonic, and place particular emphasis on the etiologies of secondary psychosis, mania, and catatonia. Psychotic symptoms due to toxic exposures are covered in Chapter 35, "Medical Toxicology."

Psychosis in the Medically Ill

Epidemiology and Risk Factors

The prevalence and etiology of psychosis in the general hospital setting depend on the diagnostic criteria used and on the specifics of the hospital setting and its geographic location. In surgical settings, particularly if elderly patients are treated, delirium and dementia are often accompanied by psychosis. When a young patient presents to an inner-city emergency department with psychosis, illicit drug use is a likely etiology. In an otherwise healthy, young patient who is evaluated in a first-episode psychosis outpatient program, the likelihood that a primary psychotic disorder is present is fairly high. In the seminal Northwick Park study, fewer than 6% of cases referred for a first episode of psychosis were thought to have an "organic" ailment (Johnstone et al. 1987).

Risk factors for the development of psychosis, particularly paranoid symptoms in an elderly patient, include cognitive problems and social isolation (Forsell and Henderson 1998) as well as hearing loss (Thewissen et al. 2005). The prevalence of any psychotic symptom in the general population of dementia-free individuals older than 85 years is about 10% (Ostling and Skoog 2002).

Clinical Features

The hallmarks of psychotic disorder due to another medical condition according to DSM-5 (American Psychiatric Association 2013) are prominent hallucinations and delusions. Hallucinations can occur in any sensory modality, but they lack diagnostic specificity (Carter 1992). If patients retain their insight into the abnormal nature of their hallucinations, the term *pseudohallucinations* is sometimes used (Berrios and Dening 1996). A good example of hallucinations that occur in patients who remain insightful (and as a consequence hesitant to divulge information about the experience unless specifically asked for fear of being labeled as insane) is the Charles Bonnet syndrome (Menon 2005). In this syndrome, generally pleasant, complex visual hallucinations occur in visually impaired individuals who are cognitively intact. Another example of complex visual hallucinations is peduncular hallucinosis, in which vivid, scenic images can emerge after focal damage to the thalamus or mesencephalic structures (Benke 2006; Mocellin et al. 2006). Some hallucinations occur only under very specific conditions. For example, auditory hallucinations heard only when the air conditioner is running are called functional hallucinations. Hypnagogic or hypnopompic hallucinations occur only in the transition to sleep or awakening, respectively.

The second hallmark of psychosis, delusions, can be fleeting and poorly formed or rather elaborate and entrenched. Delusions are often classified by their content (e.g., persecutory). Some delusional syndromes are best known by their eponyms, such as delusions of infidelity (Othello syndrome) or delusions of nihilism (Cotard's syndrome) (Freudenreich 2007). As with hallucinations, however, the type of delusion lacks diagnostic specificity. For example, although the morbid jealousy in the Othello syndrome is traditionally associated with male alcoholic patients, it can occur as both a primary psychiatric disorder and a manifestation of organic etiology (Yusim et al. 2008). Kurt Schneider described classic psychotic experiences in patients with schizophrenia. His so-called Schneiderian first-rank symptoms include delusional perception; passivity experiences; and thought insertion, withdrawal, or broadcasting. In patients with first-episode psychosis, first-rank symptoms are common; in one representative sample, only 16% of the patients did not experience any first-rank symptoms (Thorup et al. 2007). The presence of a belief in duplicates and replacements is typical for a group of delusions known as *delusional misidentification syndromes* (Weinstein 1994). For example, in the Capgras delusion, a patient believes that a family member or close friend has been replaced by an exact double.

The course and prognosis of secondary psychosis are determined to a large extent by the underlying illness. It can reasonably be expected that a pure drug-induced or medication-induced psychosis resolves once the inciting agent is removed. However, in some cases such as phencyclidine (PCP) psychosis, prolonged psychosis lasting several weeks can result. Some underlying diseases are treatable but require prolonged treatment with the very medication that caused the psychosis in the first place (e.g., steroids for systemic lupus erythematosus [SLE] or interferon for cancer). Unfortunately, many illnesses in which psychosis emerges are degenerative, progressive, and incurable. The emergence of psychosis in a degenerative disorder greatly complicates its management. For example, in a patient with Alzheimer's disease and psychosis, caregivers are more distressed, and patients are more likely to be transferred to a nursing home (Ballard et al. 2008). A more optimistic picture emerged in the only longitudinal follow-up study that used the DSM-IV (American Psychiatric Association 1994) diagnosis of psychosis due to a general medical condition (Feinstein and Ron 1998). In this cohort of 44 patients with various neurological conditions who were followed up for an average of 4 years, most required only brief, intermittent treatment with antipsychotics, and none required maintenance treatment with antipsychotics.

Diagnosis and Assessment

Psychotic symptoms in a medically hospitalized patient fall into one of three possibilities:

1. Primary psychiatric illness
   - New-onset or an acute exacerbation of psychiatric illness associated with psychosis
2. Secondary psychosis
   - Psychosis due to a general medical condition (systemic or brain-based)
   - Substance-induced psychosis
   - Medication-induced psychosis
3. "Secondary on primary"
   - A patient with a primary psychotic disorder has psychosis unrelated to his or her primary psychotic disorder

The first step in the evaluation of any new-onset psychosis requires an assessment of the patient's safety and then a careful analysis of the longitudinal history of symptoms and the cross-sectional symptom profile, taking into account the clinical context. A preadmission baseline should be established with the help of collateral sources. A physical examination that identifies abnormal vital signs or focal neurological findings often points toward a secondary cause of psychosis. The possibility of unacknowledged drug abuse (withdrawal or drug use while in the hospital) should always be considered. A chart review should focus on medications administered during the hospitalization.

Determining that psychosis is present if the patient is not cooperating sufficiently during the interview is not always straightforward. A patient might be too suspicious to answer questions. Unless a patient is able to cooperate, cognitive limitations might not be apparent, and a delirium may be overlooked. Patients with a preexisting psychosis pose particular difficulties because psychosis in and of itself might not indicate an "organic" etiology, and exacerbations resulting from intercurrent illnesses that lead to secondary psychosis are missed. Repeat examinations over the course of the day and a comprehensive survey of psychotic phenomena, including first-rank symptoms, hallucinations in all modalities, and misidentification syndromes, may be necessary to make the diagnosis.

Unfortunately, no pathognomonic signs or symptoms differentiate primary from secondary psychosis or allow clinicians to determine the presence of a secondary psychosis on clinical grounds alone. For example, the presence of Schneiderian first-rank symptoms has been reported in a wide variety of "organic" conditions, particularly epilepsy and endocrine disturbances (Marneros 1988). In a chart review of 1,698 patients diagnosed with "organic mental disorder," first-rank symptoms were seen in 7% of the patients (Marneros 1988). Conversely, visual hallucinations, which many clinicians regard as indicative of "organicity," are clearly also part of the symptom spectrum in schizophrenia, bipolar disorder, and psychotic depression (Baethge et al. 2005).

Considering the phenomenology of the reported experience, including the presence or absence of first-rank symptoms (Heinz et al. 2016), content of delusions, or modality of hallucinations, is nevertheless valuable. In an emergency department study that examined differences between substance-induced psychosis and primary psychosis, the presence of visual hallucinations on arrival at the emergency department was one of three key predictors of substance-induced psychosis, as opposed to a primary psychotic disorder (Caton et al. 2005). The other two predictors of substance-induced psychosis were parental substance abuse and dependence on any substance. Patients who experience gustatory or olfactory hallucinations, particularly if they have no associated delusions, might have organic problems, including paroxysmal disorders such as epilepsy or migraines. Delusional misidentification syndromes are possible in those with primary psychiatric disorders but strongly suggest a neurodegenerative process. Josephs (2007) reported that 81% of patients with Capgras syndrome had a neurodegenerative disorder, mostly Lewy body disease. Even the remaining 19% of the patients with a nondegenerative disorder experienced delusions secondary to methamphetamine abuse or had just had a stroke in addition to primary psychotic disorders.

The extent of the medical evaluation of psychosis in medically ill patients is guided by likely etiologies. It is important to eliminate causes of a delirium. Therefore, most patients who develop psychosis in the hospital will need a basic laboratory evaluation to assess gross organ dysfunction and infections. The information obtained from a lumbar puncture can be lifesaving. For example, N-methyl-D-aspartate (NMDA) receptor encephalitis is a treatable disease if recognized; however, a lumbar puncture is required for its diagnosis because serum antibodies are not as sensitive as central nervous system (CNS) antibodies (Gresa-Arribas et al. 2014). If seizures are considered high on the list of potential causes, then an electroencephalogram (EEG) is indicated. A normal EEG result is indicative of a primary psychiatric cause. Also, a computed tomography (CT) or magnetic resonance imaging (MRI) scan is indicated if brain pathology is suspected. Syphilis and human immunodeficiency virus (HIV) infection are crucial to exclude. If no culprit is found on the basis of history and the initial evaluation, less common medical causes should be considered (e.g., thyrotoxicosis) before making a diagnosis of schizophrenia, which is a diagnosis of exclusion (Table 9–1 lists components of the initial medical evaluation of secondary psychosis, mania, or catatonia).

However, even if a medical disease, substance, or medication that can be associated with psychosis is discovered, establishing causality is not straightforward. Slater and Beard (1963) discussed this problem of causation in comorbid conditions in a classic essay on the psychosis of epilepsy. They outlined three levels of association: epilepsy and psychosis occurring together by chance; epilepsy precipitating schizophrenia; or epilepsy producing schizophrenia-like symptoms.

Etiology and Differential Diagnosis

Secondary psychosis can be caused by many medical conditions, illicit drugs, toxins, and medications. The diagnostic challenge lies not only in the sheer number of possible conditions that can cause psychosis but also in the possibility that rare diseases (rare because of low absolute incidence or because of low local prevalence) that most clinicians will be unfamiliar with can present with psychosis, either typically (e.g., West African sleeping sickness) or atypically (e.g., adult-onset Niemann-Pick disease type C) (Bonnot et al. 2015; Freudenreich et al. 2009). Inborn errors of metabolism rarely present with psychosis as the sole symptom in the absence of other organic or neurological signs (Bonnot et al. 2014). Table 9–2 provides a comprehensive compilation of disorders that have been associated with psychosis.

Both systemic infections and infections of the brain (e.g., recurrent and chronic meningitides) can cause psychosis in the absence of a frank delirium. The exact pathogens will vary depending on geography, travel history, and immune status and include infective agents leading to tuberculosis, cerebral malaria, toxoplasmosis, Lyme disease, and neurocysticercosis. Herpes simplex, neurosyphilis, and HIV are important considerations for any hospitalized patients with unexplained psychosis. In one case series in the antibiotic era, neuropsychiatric symptoms alone were seen in 51% of confirmed cases of neurosyphilis (Timmermans and Carr 2004). (See also Chapter 26, "Infectious Diseases.")

Endocrine diseases can be accompanied by psychotic symptoms. Affective symptoms are most common, but psychosis can also occur. The classic example is thyrotoxicosis (Brownlie et al. 2000). As a special case, in a woman presenting with postpartum psychosis, postpartum thyroiditis must be ruled out (Bokhari et al. 1998). However, psychosis has been reported with a wide variety of endocrine diseases, including hypothyroidism ("myxedema madness"), Addison's disease, Cushing's disease, hyper- and hypoparathyroidism, and hypoglycemia. (See also Chapter 21, "Endocrine and Metabolic Disorders.")

Many neurological conditions can be accompanied by psychosis. Epilepsy and psychosis share a long history, with psychosis potentially occurring ictally, postictally, or interictally (Sachdev 1998; Toone 2000). Temporal lobe epilepsy is most likely to lead to psychosis, but psychosis also can occur with frontal lobe seizures (Lauten-

TABLE 9–1.   **Initial medical evaluation for secondary psychosis, mania, and catatonia**

Laboratory evaluation

Complete blood count

Electrolytes including calcium and phosphate

Blood urea nitrogen/creatinine

Glucose

Thyrotropin (TSH)

Liver function tests

Erythrocyte sedimentation rate

Antinuclear antibody

Human immunodeficiency virus test

Fluorescent treponemal antibody absorption (FTA-ABS) test for syphilis (rapid plasma reagin not sufficient)

Vitamin B_{12} and folate

Serum cortisol level

Ceruloplasmin

Urinalysis

Serum toxicology screen

Drug levels of prescribed medications, if indicated

Blood cultures

Urine culture

Brain imaging

Magnetic resonance imaging (generally preferred over computed tomography)

Electroencephalogram

If seizures or delirium is suspected

Note.   This list of tests is based on the medical evaluation of a first episode of psychosis and is neither mandatory nor exhaustive. Other tests should be considered if the clinical history and the clinical picture suggest that they might be useful diagnostically (e.g., arterial blood gases, chest X ray, lumbar puncture, genetic testing). Note the overlap with a delirium evaluation.

Other tests such as a serum pregnancy test and an electrocardiogram (to monitor QTc) might need to be added to safely administer treatment.

Source.   Based on Freudenreich et al. 2007.

schlager and Förstl 2001). Postictal psychosis typically occurs close in time to a seizure, with psychosis emerging a day or several days after the seizure. Interictal psychosis typically occurs in patients with poorly controlled seizures, after a decade or more of seizures. Dementing illnesses are frequently accompanied by neuropsychiatric symptoms, including psychosis. In Alzheimer's dementia, psychosis emerges in 31% and 16% of patients as delusions and hallucinations, respectively (Zhao et al. 2016). The severity of cognitive impairment is a risk factor for psychosis. Delusions are typically concrete and simple. If seen in the context of cognitive difficulties, delusions are understandable (e.g., delusions of theft in the elderly person who forgot where he put an item, misidentification delusions, or delusions of infidelity) (Klimstra and Mahgoub 2009). In Lewy body dementia, recurrent and well-formed visual hallucinations are a core feature (McKeith et al. 2005). Rarely, stroke can lead to post-

TABLE 9–2. **Selected causes of secondary psychosis**

Psychomotor seizures

Head trauma (history of)

Dementias
Alzheimer's disease
Pick's disease
Lewy body disease

Stroke, including CADASIL (cerebral autosomal dominant arteriopathy with subcortical infarcts and leukoencephalopathy)

Space-occupying lesions and structural brain abnormalities
Primary brain tumors
Secondary brain metastases
Brain abscesses and cysts
Tuberous sclerosis
Midline abnormalities (e.g., corpus callosum agenesis, cavum septi pellucidi)
Cerebrovascular malformations (e.g., involving the temporal lobe)

Hydrocephalus

Demyelinating diseases
Multiple sclerosis
Leukodystrophies (e.g., metachromatic leukodystrophy, X-linked adrenoleukodystrophy, Marchiafava-Bignami syndrome)
Schilder's disease

Neuropsychiatric disorders
Huntington's disease
Wilson's disease
Parkinson's disease
Friedreich's ataxia

Autoimmune disorders
Systemic lupus erythematosus and other forms of CNS vasculitis
NMDA receptor encephalitis
Other paraneoplastic and autoimmune encephalitis

Infections
Viral encephalitis
Neurosyphilis
HIV infection
CNS-invasive parasitic infections (e.g., cerebral malaria, toxoplasmosis, neurocysticercosis)
Lyme disease
Tuberculosis
Sarcoidosis
Cryptococcal meningoencephalitis
Prion diseases (e.g., Creutzfeldt-Jakob disease)

TABLE 9–2.   **Selected causes of secondary psychosis** *(continued)*

Endocrinopathies

Hypoglycemia

Addison's disease

Cushing's disease

Hyper- and hypothyroidism

Hyper- and hypoparathyroidism

Hypopituitarism

Narcolepsy

Nutritional deficiencies

Magnesium deficiency

Vitamin A deficiency

Niacin deficiency (pellagra)

Thiamine deficiency

Vitamin B_{12} deficiency (pernicious anemia)

Metabolic disorders

Amino acid metabolism (e.g., Hartnup disease, homocystinuria, phenylketonuria)

Porphyrias (e.g., acute intermittent porphyria, porphyria variegata, hereditary
coproporphyria)

GM_2 gangliosidosis

Fabry's disease

Niemann-Pick disease type C

Gaucher's disease, adult type

Chromosomal abnormalities

Sex chromosomes (e.g., Klinefelter's syndrome, XXX syndrome)

Fragile X syndrome

Velocardiofacial syndrome

Note.   CNS=central nervous system; HIV=human immunodeficiency virus; NMDA=N-methyl-D-aspartate.

Source.   Adapted from Freudenreich et al. 2016.

stroke psychosis, although the possibility of complicating seizures should be considered (Chemerinski and Robinson 2000). Interestingly, among the demyelinating disorders, rare leukodystrophies are more frequently associated with psychosis than is the prototypical demyelinating disease multiple sclerosis (Ghaffar and Feinstein 2007). Basal ganglia disorders are also a cause of psychosis (Rosenblatt and Leroi 2000), although in Parkinson's disease, the effects of treatment with dopamine agonists must be considered.

Numerous legal and illegal drugs including potent designer drugs can cause psychosis. Some drugs produce psychosis reliably in most people (e.g., PCP). Cannabis used to rarely lead to anything more than mild, transient paranoia. However, the tetrahydrocannabinol (THC) content in cannabis products has increased, and more severe intoxications with psychosis are now encountered in emergency rooms (Hudak et al. 2015). In susceptible individuals, cannabis is considered a component cause for the emergence of schizophrenia (Murray et al. 2016). Psychosis in alcoholic individuals has a large differential diagnosis, including alcohol withdrawal, delirium tremens, alcoholic hallucinosis, Wernicke-Korsakoff syndrome, pellagra, hepatic encephalopathy, Marchiafava-Bignami syndrome, central pontine myelinolysis, and alcohol-associated dementia (Greenberg and Lee 2001). Paranoia and morbid jealousy that can reach delusional conviction (i.e., the Othello syndrome) are well-recognized complications of severe alcoholism (Michael et al. 1995). (See also Chapter 16, "Substance-Related Disorders.")

Among prescription medications, certain drugs are clearly associated with the potential for inducing psychosis—for example, high-dose steroids, dopamine agonists, and interferons. Table 9–3 provides a list of more common offending agents.

Effects of Psychosis on Medical Disorders

The presence of psychosis can greatly jeopardize the cooperation necessary for a successful hospital stay. Psychosis can be disruptive because of ancillary symptom clusters (e.g., fear or agitation) or because of its thought content (e.g., a patient refusing cooperation with surgery because of conspiracy theories). Because patients who are overtly psychotic and agitated may pose a risk to themselves and others on the ward, staff might be rightly afraid and limit interactions. However, patients also can be quietly psychotic and appear withdrawn (i.e., secondary negative symptoms). Patients who are suspicious, mildly disorganized, or apathetic can get "blamed" for their inability to conform to ward routines or to participate in their own treatment (Freudenreich and Stern 2003). Lack of insight into the need for psychiatric treatment can require legal intervention, resulting in treatment delays. In any patient who requests discharge against medical advice (AMA), a psychotic process should be ruled out.

In the outpatient setting, poorly controlled psychosis is a major impediment to medical care and contributes to premature death in patients with schizophrenia (Colton and Manderscheid 2006). The emergence of psychosis is a major cause of nursing home admissions in patients with dementia who were being cared for at home (Ballard et al. 2008).

Treatment of Secondary Psychosis

General Principles of Management

Safety for all parties, identification of the etiology, and treatment of psychosis are the three initial goals in the care of psychotic patients in the hospital. Patients who are psychotic can be quite agitated and restless; they often require a sitter or restraints to prevent injury. Involuntary treatment can be required. Even when the etiology seems clear, additional causes should be considered and unnecessary CNS-active medications discontinued. In the early phase of treatment, frequent reassessment is required to determine the best course of action and to assess the efficacy and ongoing necessity of interventions. Although benzodiazepines are routinely used as an ancillary treatment to calm patients with primary psychotic disorders, they should be used cautiously in medically compromised patients because they might paradoxically worsen agitation.

TABLE 9–3.   **Selected medications that can cause psychosis at therapeutic doses**

Important offenders

Anticholinergics and antihistaminics

Dopaminergic drugs (e.g., L-dopa, amantadine)

Interferon

Stimulants

Corticosteroids

Others

Cardiovascular drugs: antiarrhythmics, digitalis

Anesthetics

Antimalaria drugs: mefloquine

Antituberculous drugs: D-cycloserine, ethambutol, isoniazid

Antibiotics: ciprofloxacin

Antivirals: human immunodeficiency virus medications (e.g., acyclovir; efavirenz at high plasma levels)

Anticonvulsants (high doses)

Antineoplastics (especially ifosfamide)

Sympathomimetics (including over-the-counter preparations)

Pain medications: opioids (especially meperidine, pentazocine), indomethacin

Miscellaneous: baclofen, disulfiram, cyclosporine, tacrolimus, ephedra-containing dietary supplements

Discharge planning should take into account dangerousness and iatrogenic morbidity and mortality. Dangerousness to self or others must be considered when the patient has command hallucinations, and dangerousness to other people must be considered if the patient has delusions such as the Othello syndrome or delusional misidentification syndromes (Leong et al. 1994; Silva et al. 1994). Discharge planning also should consider the long-term risks of antipsychotics, particularly the risk for tardive dyskinesia (TD) and metabolic problems. Given the age-related increase in TD risk (Jeste et al. 1995), the cumulative dosage of antipsychotics should be minimized for all patients, but particularly for elderly individuals. Patients successfully treated with an antipsychotic for delirium or secondary psychosis who do not require long-term antipsychotic maintenance treatment should have a clear plan in place for the discontinuation of the antipsychotic (if this has not been accomplished prior to transfer).

Specific Treatment Considerations for Secondary Psychosis

Often, antipsychotics are needed to treat secondary psychosis. Antipsychotics may be withheld if psychosis is mild and expected to resolve within hours (e.g., substance-induced psychosis). Instead, benzodiazepines such as diazepam (10 mg orally) can be given to alleviate distress. However, in instances when distress from psychosis is severe; when psychosis can be expected to last longer than a few hours; or when psychosis jeopardizes the medical treatment and safety of patients, staff, or visitors, antipsychotics are the treatment of choice. Depending on the underlying cause, treatment strategies other than antipsychotics are sometimes indicated. For example, in dementia of the Lewy body type, rivastigmine has been shown in a controlled trial to have beneficial behavioral effects, perhaps through reversing a proposed cholinergic deficit (McKeith et al. 2000). If psychosis is the result of alcohol or sedative withdrawal, benzodiazepines are the treatment of choice. Thiamine must be administered when Wernicke's encephalopathy arises and should always be given before glucose. Valproate was effective for alcoholic hallucinosis in one controlled treatment trial (Aliyev and Aliyev 2008). Clozapine and quetiapine have traditionally been used for psychosis in Parkinson's patients, but side effect management in the former and questionable antipsychotic efficacy in the latter have created treatment challenges. Pimavanserin is a nondopaminergic inverse agonist of the serotonin 2A receptor that has become available for the treatment of psychosis in Parkinson's disease (Cummings et al. 2014). More experience with the drug will be necessary, but if it is found to be effective in Parkinson's, it may be useful to evaluate its potential benefit in psychoses related to other neurodegenerative diseases.

In the ideal situation, the medical team will effectively treat the medical disease responsible for the psychosis, and the psychiatrist will control psychosis until the medical condition is alleviated. With time, psychosis resolves, and the antipsychotic can be reduced and discontinued. In some instances, control of the medical condition alone, without use of antipsychotics, might resolve the psychosis—as, for example, in the case of seizures (Nadkarni et al. 2007), although the best course of action for psychosis in epilepsy is not well established (Farooq and Sherin 2008). If the underlying medical disease (e.g., a degenerative condition) cannot be cured, then a decision must be made as to the duration of antipsychotic treatment. Interestingly, in the earlier-mentioned longitudinal study of patients diagnosed with psychosis due to a general medical condition, no temporal association between the neurological illness and psychosis was seen, and intermittent but not maintenance treatment was sufficient for the treatment of psychosis (Feinstein and Ron 1998).

The choice of an antipsychotic should be determined by the specifics of the situation (including urgency, access, medical comorbidities, and tolerability). Tolerability of antipsychotics is often a concern in medically complex patients with secondary psychosis, such as patients with HIV infection. Antipsychotics might not be effective and safe for all instances of psychosis, either (Ray et al. 2009). For example, they have been shown to be relatively ineffective in treating the neurobehavioral problems associated with Alzheimer's disease (Schneider et al. 2006). Some but not all studies (e.g., Rafaniello et al. 2014) show an increased risk of death in patients with dementia who are prescribed antipsychotics (Maust et al. 2015). The combination drug dextromethorphan/quinidine, although not an antipsychotic, has recently shown some promise in the management of agitation in demented patients, as has the selective serotonin reuptake inhibitor (SSRI) citalopram (Cummings and Zhong 2015). Use of these medications in agitated psychotic patients with dementia may at least reduce the antipsychotic dosage requirement.

In all patients, but particularly in the elderly, treatments that increase anticholinergic burden (e.g., low-potency first-generation antipsychotics or high-potency antipsychotics requiring ancillary anticholinergics) are to be avoided to reduce the risk of delirium or anticholinergic-associated cognitive problems.

Mania in the Medically Ill

Mania has been associated with a variety of conditions. It was not, however, until Kraut-hammer and Klerman's (1978) classic article on secondary mania that a category was created to separate this condition from "functional" primary bipolar mood disorder.

Epidemiology and Risk Factors

No studies have used formal instruments to report the incidence or prevalence of mania in the medically ill. In a retrospective chart review of 755 patients evaluated by a psychiatry consultation service in a general hospital, Rundell and Wise (1989) found that in a 1-year period, 13 of the 15 (87%) patients diagnosed with mania met criteria for secondary mania. A positive family or personal history of bipolar illness might steer clinicians toward diagnosing primary mania, but such a history could merely indicate an increased susceptibility for secondary mania. Postpartum mania might be considered a special case of secondary mania in which sudden hormonal changes induce a manic episode in a patient with increased (genetic) susceptibility to mood episodes. Vascular disease is a risk factor that seems to predispose some elderly to late-onset mania (Subramaniam et al. 2007).

Clinical Features

The clinical features of secondary mania mimic those of mania in bipolar disorder and often develop in stages, potentially extending from mild hypomania to delirious psychotic mania (Carlson and Goodwin 1973). Early symptoms in secondary mania include mood lability, feeling "high," and disrupted sleep. As in primary mania, grandiosity, racing thoughts, euphoria, irritability, and hostility may appear, and progression to flight of ideas, gross disorganization, and frank psychosis may occur.

The course and prognosis of secondary mania depend in part on the underlying illness. When secondary mania is caused by drugs such as methamphetamine, cocaine, or methylenedioxymethamphetamine, the behavior and mood changes generally resolve once the offending agent is stopped. However, when mania arises via CNS injury, infections, neoplasm, or neurodegenerative processes, symptoms may persist. In addition, medications to treat the underlying illness also may precipitate secondary mania, often presenting treatment dilemmas, because their continued use may be required for ongoing care (e.g., interferon for cancer, steroids for organ transplantation or autoimmune disorders). In these cases, the consultation psychiatrist may play a critical role in controlling the symptoms of secondary mania to ensure that optimal medical treatment can be delivered safely.

Diagnosis and Assessment

Although the symptoms of secondary mania are the same as those seen in primary mania, a DSM-5 diagnosis of secondary mania requires only a prominent and persistently elevated, expansive, or irritable mood. DSM-5 makes no mention of number or duration of symptoms. Because delirium and mania have similar clinical presentations, their differentiation can be difficult. Both syndromes are abrupt in onset and have accompanying symptoms of inattention, agitation, erratic sleep, and the presence of paranoia and psychosis. The waxing and waning course of delirium, along with decreased arousal and clouding of consciousness, should help differentiate it from secondary mania. To make matters more complicated, there is the possibility of delirious mania, which some equate with catatonic excitement. Delirious mania has a sudden onset; is marked by excessive purposeless and sometimes bizarre motor activity not caused by external stimuli; and is often associated with disorganized and pressured speech, flight of ideas, disorientation, and confabulation. This state can take on a dreamlike quality and is usually short lived in comparison with manic excitement (Jacobowski et al. 2013).

Once new-onset mania is diagnosed, the differentiation between primary and secondary mania should be attempted. Secondary mania often develops within a short period (e.g., hours or days) after the physiological insult and may occur throughout the life span. In contrast, episodes due to bipolar disorder typically occur during the first three decades of life, and new-onset primary mania tends to be rare after age 50 years (Oostervink et al. 2009). The diagnosis of secondary mania is more likely when cognitive dysfunction or focal neurological signs are present, no personal history or family history of bipolar disorder exists, or treatment of the mood disorder with standard interventions is ineffective (Arora and Daughton 2007).

As with psychosis, the clinical history, physical examination, and laboratory evaluations are important elements in distinguishing primary and secondary mania (see Table 9–1 for laboratory evaluation).

Although the evaluation of mania is based on a clinical assessment, rating scales can track the severity of symptoms. A well-accepted scale often used in clinical trials is the 11-item Young Mania Rating Scale (YMRS; Young et al. 1978).

Etiology and Differential Diagnosis

Secondary mania has been ascribed to numerous conditions (Table 9–4). Many of these conditions are reported as cases linked temporally to the development of mania, but some have proven to be more consistently associated with the development of manic syndromes and are discussed in more detail below.

Mania Secondary to Neurological Diseases

Cerebrovascular injury.   Poststroke mania occurs in about 1% of strokes (Jorge et al. 1993; Starkstein et al. 1989). Manic syndromes have been reported following cerebrovascular lesions in multiple areas of the brain, with most but not all cases attributed to right-sided infarcts (Santos et al. 2011).

Traumatic brain injury.   Up to 50% of all patients with traumatic brain injury (TBI) may develop posttraumatic depression (Mendez 2000), whereas mania tends to be relatively infrequent. In a study of 66 patients with a head injury, 41% had symptoms of depression, 9% developed mania, and one patient was diagnosed with bipolar disorder within 1 year of the injury (Jorge et al. 1993). Compared with patients whose mania was not secondary to a brain injury, patients with post-TBI mania were typically less euphoric and less likely to have depressive episodes, with 85% of patients manifesting irritability and 70% manifesting aggressiveness (Jorge et al. 1993; Shukla et al. 1987).

TABLE 9–4. Selected causes of secondary mania

Neurological conditions	Medications and substances of abuse
Tumors (gliomas, meningiomas, thalamic metastasis)	Amantadine
Cerebrovascular lesions (right hemispheric)	Amphetamines
Multiple sclerosis	Anabolic steroids
Traumatic brain injury	Antidepressants
Complex partial seizures	Baclofen (administration and withdrawal)
Viral encephalitis (acute and postinfectious)	Buspirone
Human immunodeficiency virus infection	Captopril
Cryptococcal meningoencephalitis	Cimetidine
Neurosyphilis	Clonidine withdrawal
Huntington's disease	Cocaine
Parkinson's disease (including treatment with deep brain stimulation)	Corticosteroids/corticosteroid withdrawal
Frontotemporal dementia	Didanosine
Wilson's disease	Hallucinogens
Fahr's disease	Isoniazid
Klinefelter's syndrome	L-Dopa
Kleine-Levin syndrome	Methylphenidate
Systemic conditions	Phencyclidine
Cushing's disease	Procainamide
Vitamin B_{12} deficiency	Thyroxine
Niacin deficiency	Zidovudine
Antiphospholipid antibody syndrome	
Hyponatremia	
Carcinoid syndrome	
Hyperthyroidism	

Neurodegenerative processes.   Dementing processes also have been associated with the development of mania. Although mania tends to be rare in Alzheimer's disease, it has been reported to occur in greater frequency in patients with frontotemporal dementia (FTD) (Arciniegas 2006; Gálvez-Andres et al. 2007; Woolley et al. 2007). Emotional changes (such as depression, mania, irritability, lability, and anger) are common in patients with FTD, as are obsessive symptoms. Neurodegenerative movement disorders also have been associated with mania. Manic episodes have been shown to occur in 2%–12% of patients with Huntington's disease, and often the mood change may precede the appearance of a movement disorder (Folstein 1989; Mendez 1994). Symptoms of mania also have been described in Fahr's disease (idiopathic basal ganglia calcification), Wilson's disease, and postencephalitic Parkinson's disease, along with a case report of mania following treatment of Parkinson's symptoms with subthalamic nucleus stimulation (Krauthammer and Klerman 1978; Raucher-Chéné et al. 2008; Rosenblatt and Leroi 2000).

Epilepsy.   Although depression is more common in those with epilepsy, mania also may arise. Investigators have reported a frequency of bipolar illness of 3%–22% (Robertson 1992) in depressed patients with epilepsy, and these disorders occasionally can be clinically difficult to distinguish from primary bipolar disorder (Himmelhoch 1984). Mania may follow right temporal lobe epileptiform discharges (Hurwitz et al. 1985) and tends to occur with an increase in seizures or intermittent epileptiform activity (Barczak et al. 1988; Ramchandani and Riggio 1992). Mania associated with epilepsy also may present with compulsive behavior and elements of psychosis (such as thought insertion and hallucinations) (Himmelhoch 1984). In one retrospective review of patients seen by psychiatric consultants, two of four manic epileptic patients had peri-ictal mania and poor seizure control (Lyketsos et al. 1993). In addition, patients in the immediate postictal state may show intermixed epileptiform activity without clinical signs of seizures (Mendez and Grau 1991). Patients may experience postictal psychosis with features of mania 12–48 hours after a burst of seizures, which may continue for weeks or even months, but this is rare (Chakrabarti et al. 1999; Mendez and Grau 1991). Mania is a potential adverse effect of anticonvulsants as well.

Mania Secondary to Infectious Diseases

Several infections involving the CNS may produce manic syndromes. Mania may be the first manifestation of neurosyphilis, cryptococcal meningoencephalitis, or viral encephalitides, including herpes simplex encephalitis (Mendez 2000). Mania also may occur as a postencephalitic process following recovery from the acute stage of illness. Patients with secondary mania attributed to advanced HIV disease were described as having more irritability and cognitive deficits and being less likely to have a family history of bipolar disorder compared with those with primary mania (Lyketsos et al. 1997). Mania has also been reported as a side effect of several antiretroviral drugs and antibiotics (see Chapter 26, "Infectious Diseases").

Mania Secondary to Endocrine Diseases

Several endocrine diseases have been associated with the development of manic states, including Cushing's disease and hyperthyroidism (Clower 1984; Lee and Hutto 2008; Villani and Weitzel 1979) and in rare cases hypothyroidism (Stowell and Barnhill 2005).

Treatment with corticosteroids is likely the most common cause of secondary mania (Rundell and Wise 1989). In a prospective study by Naber et al. (1996), of 50 patients with ophthalmic conditions being administered high-dose corticosteroids for 8 days, 13 patients (26%) developed symptoms of (mild) mania, and 5 patients (10%) developed depression. Most mood-related symptoms developed early in the course of treatment, typically within 3 days of starting corticosteroids.

Effects of Mania on Medical Disorders

Like patients with psychotic disorders, patients with bipolar disorder have medical comorbidity (Kilbourne et al. 2004) that can complicate treatment. Because of its unpredictable nature, bipolar illness may cause significant periods in which the patient has little or no contact with providers, especially during a manic episode. This lack of contact may lead to poor adherence, social instability, and increased medical comorbidity. Manic and hypomanic episodes can increase the risk of infectious diseases (e.g., cervical cancer, hepatitis C, HIV infection) through sexual indiscretions or drug use (el-Serag et al. 2002).

During an inpatient hospitalization, the development of mania may cause refusal of medical care. If secondary hypomania or mania is not suspected, the medical team may attribute the patient's behavior to personality or to being "difficult," often causing a schism between the patient and providers, potentially jeopardizing the necessary medical evaluation and care.

Treatment of Secondary Mania

General Principles of Management

Similar to the management of psychotic patients, ensuring the safety of the patient and staff is of paramount importance and is the initial goal of care for the acutely manic patient. Patients with mania are unpredictable, disinhibited, and easily agitated, especially in an unknown medical environment with an overabundance of stimuli (e.g., ancillary staff, frequent vital sign checks, laboratory blood draws, medical procedures). The psychiatry consultant can assess the patient's medical and neuropsychiatric condition and help to minimize any unnecessary interventions (including medications with CNS effects that may contribute to or exacerbate the patient's symptoms). Once safety has been addressed, the focus should be helping to elucidate the underlying etiology of secondary mania.

Psychopharmacology

Medications used for the treatment of secondary mania are generally the same as those used in primary bipolar illness. The choice of medication is based on the severity of mania, the patient's willingness or ability to receive oral medications, the etiology of the mania, and the patient's comorbid medical illnesses. For example, lithium may be difficult to administer safely in patients with fluid shifts, electrolyte abnormalities, acute or chronic renal dysfunction, or already established thyroid dysfunction. Valproate may be relatively contraindicated in patients with hepatic disease or a history of pancreatitis. Carbamazepine also may pose difficulties in patients with hepatic disease and is associated with potential hematological toxicity (e.g., leukopenia or aplastic anemia), antidiuretic actions, and quinidine-like effects on cardiac con-duction. In addition, carbamazepine is a potent inducer of cytochrome P450 enzymes. Although benzodiazepines may provide rapid symptom reduction, they may also po-tentiate CNS depression by decreasing respiratory drive, and their use is relatively contraindicated in patients with chronic obstructive pulmonary disease who are at risk for carbon dioxide retention. In addition, paradoxical disinhibition may occur, especially in patients with a TBI. Antipsychotics are often used for the treatment of secondary mania, particularly in agitated patients. Second-generation antipsychotics are generally preferred for short-term treatment of secondary mania because of their lower propensity to cause EPS. Nevertheless, monitoring for neuroleptic-induced catatonia is still warranted. If long-term use of antipsychotics for the management of secondary mania is contemplated, potential morbidity and mortality risks associated with antipsychotics should be considered (e.g., risk for metabolic syndrome or TD).

Electroconvulsive Therapy

Electroconvulsive therapy (ECT) has been used in the management of acute mania and may be especially helpful to treat mania and marked physical activity that is poorly responsive to pharmacological interventions. There are few reports of ECT specifically in secondary mania. ECT may present higher risk in some medically ill patients (see Chapter 38, "Electroconvulsive Therapy and Other Brain-Stimulation Therapies").

Catatonia in the Medically Ill

Initially described in Kahlbaum's 1874 monograph, catatonia has long been associ-ated with psychiatric, neurological, and medical disorders (Kahlbaum 1973). Modern theorists view catatonia as a syndrome of motor signs in association with disorders of affect, thought, and behavior. Some motor features are classic but infrequent (e.g., echopraxia and waxy flexibility), whereas others are common in psychiatric patients (e.g., agitation and withdrawal) but denoted as catatonic because of their duration and severity. The sometimes subtle presentation of catatonia may go undetected, which could account for the impression of a declining incidence. For example, in one study, clinicians diagnosed catatonia in only 2% of 139 patients, whereas a research team identified it in 18% (van der Heijden et al. 2005).

Epidemiology and Risk Factors

The rate of catatonia in the psychiatric population varies according to study design and diagnostic criteria. In a series of prospective studies of patients hospitalized with acute psychotic episodes, the incidence of catatonia was within the 7%–17% range (Caroff et al. 2004). When mood disorders were the focus, rates ranged from 13% to 31%. Catatonia secondary to medical illness with a variety of "organic" etiologies ac-counts for 4%–46% of cases in various series, underscoring the need for a thorough medical evaluation when catatonic signs are present. In pediatric settings, catatonia is sometimes reported in patients with mental retardation and autistic spectrum dis-orders (Wing and Shah 2006). The co-occurrence of delirium and catatonia is gaining recognition (Grover et al. 2014).

Certain conditions may increase the risk of developing neuroleptic malignant syndrome (NMS)—an important iatrogenic form of catatonia (Mann et al. 1994). A history of simple catatonia is a major risk factor for progression to NMS (White and Robins 1991). Other risk factors include schizophrenia, mood disorders, neurological disorders, and alcohol and substance use disorders. Agitation, dehydration, and exhaustion also may increase the risk for NMS. Up to one-third of patients who have had NMS will have a subsequent episode when rechallenged with neuroleptics.

Clinical Features

Stupor, mutism, negativism, motoric immobility, catalepsy, posturing, but also excitement are the core clinical features of catatonia. These features are the same regardless of whether the condition occurs in the context of a mood, psychotic, or medical state. Catatonia may have rapid or insidious onset and may be associated with high morbidity and mortality. Diametrically opposed subtypes of catatonia have been described. Catatonic withdrawal, with posturing, rigidity, mutism, and repetitive actions, is the most commonly recognized form, and the term *catatonia* is sometimes used as shorthand for this retarded motor state, occasionally referred to as "Kahlbaum's syndrome" (Fink and Taylor 2009). Patients with severe catatonia will be stuporous and may even present with low Glasgow Coma Scale scores. However, patients also can present with hyperactivity, pressured speech, and restless, agitated behavior accompanied by catatonic features (bizarre stereotypies, mannerisms, grimacing, echo phenomena, perseveration) and an acute confusional state. Catatonic excitement has at times been called "delirious mania" or "Bell's mania" (Bell 1849).

In 1934, Stauder (1934) described a syndrome of "lethal catatonia." It was marked by the acute onset of a manic delirium, high fever, and catatonic stupor and a mortality rate of greater than 50%. Because not all cases are lethal, Philbrick and Rummans (1994) suggested the term *malignant catatonia* to describe critically ill cases marked by autonomic instability or hyperthermia, in contrast to cases of "simple, nonmalignant catatonia."

The prognosis in catatonia reflects the nature and severity of the underlying etiology of the catatonia. Those with catatonia secondary to a mood disorder often do better than those with underlying schizophrenia; and those with catatonia secondary to toxic–metabolic disorders often have better prognoses than those with catatonia secondary to brain lesions. When the catatonia becomes chronic, as it does in certain cases of catatonic schizophrenia, the prognosis is poorer.

Diagnosis and Assessment

The signs and symptoms of the catatonic syndrome based on the Bush-Francis Catatonia Rating Scale (BFCRS) are listed in Table 9–5 (Bush et al. 1996a).

The BFCRS 23-item rating scale operationally defines each catatonic sign, rates its severity, and provides a standardized schema for clinical examination (Table 9–6), leading to reliable ratings that are sensitive to change (Bush et al. 1996b).

With the BFCRS, a case is defined by the presence of at least 2 of the first 14 items from this scale. However, the number of signs and symptoms required to make a diagnosis of catatonia is controversial, and the structure of catatonia remains to be defined (Wilson et al. 2015). DSM-5 requires the presence of three or more catatonic

TABLE 9–5. **Catatonic symptoms (based on the Modified Bush-Francis Catatonia Rating Scale)**

Catatonia can be diagnosed by the presence of 2 or more of the first 14 signs listed below.

1. **Excitement**—Severe hyperactivity and constant motor unrest, which is manifestly purposeless (not to be attributed to akathisia or goal-directed agitation)

2. **Immobility/stupor**—Severe hypoactivity, immobility, and minimal response to stimuli

3. **Mutism**—Verbal unresponsiveness or minimal responsiveness

4. **Staring**—Fixed gaze, little or no visual scanning of the environment, and decreased eye blink

5. **Posturing/catalepsy**—Spontaneous maintenance of posture(s), including everyday ones (e.g., sitting/standing for long periods without reacting)

6. **Grimacing**—Maintenance of bizarre facial expressions

7. **Echolalia/echopraxia**—Mimicking of an examiner's speech and/or movements

8. **Stereotypy**—Perseverative, non-goal-directed, not inherently abnormal motor activity (e.g., playing with fingers, or repetitively touching, patting, or rubbing oneself)

9. **Mannerisms**—Bizarre, inherently abnormal movements (e.g., hopping or walking on tiptoe, saluting those passing by, or exaggerating caricatures of mundane movements)

10. **Verbigeration**—Repetition of phrases (like a scratched record)

11. **Rigidity**—Maintenance of a rigid posture despite examiner's efforts to reposition; exclude if cogwheeling or tremor is present

12. **Negativism**—Seemingly motiveless resistance to instructions or attempts to move or examine the patient; patient does the exact opposite of the instruction

13. **Waxy flexibility**—During repositioning, patient first offers resistance before allowing repositioning (similar to that of a bending candle)

14. **Withdrawal**—Refusal to eat, drink, do activities of daily living, or make eye contact

15. **Impulsivity**—Sudden inappropriate behaviors (e.g., running down a hallway, screaming, or taking off clothes) without provocation and without appropriate explanation

16. **Automatic obedience**—Exaggerated cooperation with the examiner's request or spontaneous continuation of the movement requested

17. *Mitgehen*—Exaggerated arm raising in response to light pressure of finger, despite instructions to the contrary; like an "Anglepoise lamp"

18. *Gegenhalten*—Resistance to passive movement that is proportional to the strength of the stimulus; appears automatic rather than willful

19. **Ambitendency**—Appearance of being "stuck" in indecisive, hesitant movement

20. **Grasp reflex**—As in the neurological examination

21. **Perseveration**—Repeatedly returning to the same topic or persistence with movement

22. **Combativeness**—Aggressive in an undirected manner, with no or only inadequate or inappropriate explanation afterward

23. **Fever and autonomic abnormality**—Abnormal temperature, blood pressure, pulse, or respiratory rate, and diaphoresis

Note.   The full 23-item Bush-Francis Catatonia Rating Scale (BFCRS) measures the severity of 23 signs on a 0–3 continuum for each sign. The first 14 signs combine to form the Bush-Francis Catatonia Screening Instrument (BFCSI). The BFCSI measures only the presence or absence of the first 14 signs, and it is used for case detection. Item definitions on the two scales are the same.

Source.   Modified from the BFCRS (Bush et al. 1996a; Fricchione et al. 2004).

TABLE 9–6.   **Bedside examination for catatonia**

This standardized method is used to complete the 23-item Bush-Francis Catatonia Rating Scale (BFCRS) and the 14-item Bush-Francis Catatonia Screening Instrument (BFCSI). Item definitions on the two scales are the same. The BFCSI measures only the presence or absence of the first 14 signs.

Ratings are based on observed behaviors during the examination, with the exception of completing the items for "withdrawal" and "autonomic abnormality," which may be based on directly observed behavior or chart documentation.

Generally, only those items that are clearly present should be rated. If uncertain about the presence of an item, it should be rated as "0."

Procedure

1. Observe the patient while attempting to involve him or her in conversation.

2. Scratch your head in an exaggerated manner, and note whether patient imitates this action.

3. Examine the patient's arm for cogwheeling. Attempt to reposition, and instruct the patient to "keep your arm loose." Move the arm with alternating lighter and heavier force.

4. Ask the patient to extend his or her arm. Place one finger under patient's hand and state, "Do *not* let me raise your arm," and try to raise the arm slowly.

5. Extend your hand to the patient, stating, "Do *not* shake my hand."

6. Reach into your pocket and state, "Stick out your tongue. I want to stick a pin in it."

7. Evaluate patient for grasp reflex.

8. Review patient's chart for reports from the previous 24-hour period. Check for oral intake, vital signs, and any incidents.

9. Evaluate the patient indirectly, at least for a brief period each day, regarding the following:

   - Activity level
   - Abnormal movements
   - Abnormal speech
   - Echopraxia
   - Rigidity
   - Negativism
   - Waxy flexibility
   - *Gegenhalten*
   - *Mitgehen*
   - Ambitendency
   - Automatic obedience
   - Grasp reflex

Source.   Adapted from Bush et al. 1996a; Fricchione et al. 2004.

symptoms to make a diagnosis of catatonic disorder due to another medical condition if evidence confirms a medical etiology. A nosological difficulty with DSM-5 is that the "due to another medical condition" diagnosis cannot be used for an episode that occurs "exclusively during the course of a delirium."

A general evaluation to exclude secondary catatonia is provided in Table 9–1. Other entities to consider in the differential diagnosis that are not secondary catatonia but may be mistaken for it include stiff-person syndrome (Lockman and Burns 2007), malignant hyperthermia (Ali et al. 2003), locked-in syndrome (Smith and Delargy 2005), and other hyperkinetic and hypokinetic states (Fink and Taylor 2003). Akinetic Parkinson's disease can produce a catatonia-like state (i.e., mute, immobilized), but it occurs well after the diagnosis of Parkinson's disease. Selective mutism and conversion disorder are psychiatric conditions that can be confused with catatonia.

TABLE 9–7. **Clinical classification of catatonia**

Based on etiology

Primary catatonia

    Due to mood disorder

    Due to psychotic disorder

    Due to other psychiatric disorder

Secondary catatonias

    Due to neurological condition

    Due to medical condition

    Due to substance toxicity[a]

Based on severity

Simple (nonmalignant) catatonia[b]

Malignant ("lethal") catatonia[c]

[a]Neuroleptic malignant syndrome is an iatrogenic cause of a secondary malignant catatonia (i.e., antipsychotic-induced malignant catatonia).
[b]Kahlbaum's syndrome is a hypokinetic form of nonmalignant catatonia.
[c]Not all cases of "lethal" catatonia are deadly.

Source. Based on Philbrick and Rummans 1994; Taylor and Fink 2003.

Diffuse, nonspecific changes on the EEG will be found most often in patients with secondary catatonias. An EEG read as normal would be most consistent with primary catatonia, although psychiatric patients may have abnormal EEG findings. Generalized slowing that is consistent with encephalopathy is found in approximately half of NMS cases. Occasionally, EEG evidence of nonconvulsive status epilepticus is found in catatonic patients (Louis and Pflaster 1995). Neuroimaging, especially MRI of the brain, should be obtained, although a negative result does not rule out an "organic" etiology. Brain imaging is important because strokes, hematomas, and space-occupying lesions can all present with new-onset catatonia, and these conditions may worsen with prolonged benzodiazepine treatment (Carroll and Goforth 2004).

Etiology and Differential Diagnosis

Catatonia erroneously became exclusively associated with schizophrenia through the influence of Kraepelin and Bleuler despite long-standing linkage of catatonia to affective disorders and to organic conditions (Gelenberg 1976). Some have advocated a separate nosology for catatonia based on the syndromic nature of the diagnosis and its unique treatment with lorazepam and ECT (Taylor and Fink 2003). DSM-5 did not follow this suggestion; rather, it treats catatonia as a specifier that can be attached to psychiatric or medical conditions (American Psychiatric Association 2013). Clinically, the catatonic syndrome is perhaps best divided into primary (psychiatric) and secondary ("organic") varieties on the basis of etiology, as well as into simple and malignant types on the basis of severity (Table 9–7).

The numerous causes of catatonia are summarized in Table 9–8 (Carroll et al. 1994; Fricchione et al. 2004; Philbrick and Rummans 1994).

TABLE 9–8. **Selected causes of catatonia**

Primary

Acute psychoses

Conversion disorder

Dissociative disorders

Mood disorders

Obsessive-compulsive disorder

Personality disorders

Schizophrenia

Secondary

Cerebrovascular causes

Arterial aneurysms

Arteriovenous malformations

Arterial and venous thrombosis

Bilateral parietal infarcts

Temporal lobe infarct

Subarachnoid hemorrhage

Subdural hematoma

Third ventricle hemorrhage

Hemorrhagic infarcts

CNS vasculitis (e.g., SLE)

Other CNS disorders

Akinetic mutism

Alcoholic degeneration and WE

Cerebellar degeneration

Cerebral anoxia

Cerebromacular degeneration

Traumatic brain injury

Frontal lobe atrophy

Multiple sclerosis and ADEM

Hydrocephalus

Lesions of thalamus and globus pallidus

Narcolepsy

NMDA receptor encephalitis

Parkinsonism

Postencephalitic states

Seizure disorders*

Tuberous sclerosis

Toxins

Coal gas

Organic fluorides

Tetraethyl lead poisoning

Tumors

Angioma

Frontal lobe tumors

Gliomas

Langerhans' carcinoma

Paraneoplastic encephalopathy
(e.g., oat cell carcinoma, teratomas)

Periventricular diffuse pinealoma

*Infections**

Bacterial meningoencephalitis

Bacterial sepsis

Hepatic amoebiasis

HIV/AIDS

Cerebral malaria

Subacute sclerosing panencephalitis

Tertiary syphilis

Typhoid fever

Viral encephalitis (especially herpes)

*Metabolic causes**

Acute intermittent porphyria

Addison's disease

Cushing's disease

Diabetic ketoacidosis

Hepatic encephalopathy

Hereditary coproporphyria

Homocystinuria

Hyperparathyroidism

Pellagra

Uremia

TABLE 9–8. **Selected causes of catatonia** *(continued)*

Secondary *(continued)*

Drug-induced causes	*Drug withdrawal–related causes*
Antipsychotics* (both typical and atypical have been associated)	Dopaminergic agents: levodopa-carbidopa; bromocriptine, lisuride, etc.
Antidepressants (tricyclics, monoamine oxidase inhibitors, and others)	GABAergic agents: benzodiazepines, barbiturates, alcohol, etc.
Anticonvulsants (e.g., carbamazepine, primidone)	Sedative-hypnotics
Disulfiram*	Clozapine
Efavirenz	
Metoclopramide	
Dopamine depleters (e.g., tetrabenazine)	
Hallucinogens (e.g., mescaline, phencyclidine,* and LSD)	
Lithium carbonate	
Corticosteroids*	
Baclofen	
Stimulants (e.g., amphetamines, methylphenidate, and possibly cocaine)	

Note. ADEM=acute disseminated encephalomyelitis; CNS=central nervous system; GABA=γ-aminobutyric acid; LSD=lysergic acid diethylamide; NMDA=*N*-methyl-D-aspartate; SLE=systemic lupus erythematosus; WE=Wernicke's encephalopathy.
*Signifies most common medical conditions associated with catatonic disorder from literature review done by Carroll et al. 1994.

Source. Adapted from Fricchione et al. 2004; Philbrick and Rummans 1994.

When catatonic stupor occurs in the setting of delirium, limbic encephalitis should be considered in the differential diagnosis (Ali et al. 2008). Limbic encephalitis can present acutely or subacutely with confusion, cognitive impairment, seizures, and catatonia. Infectious, autoimmune, paraneoplastic, and idiopathic etiologies of limbic encephalitis should be ruled out (Eker et al. 2008; Foster and Caplan 2009; Tüzün and Dalmau 2007). Autoimmune encephalopathies include NMDA receptor encephalitis as well as other autoimmune diseases in which pathogenic autoantibodies against synaptic proteins are formed (Leypoldt et al. 2015).

Effects of Catatonia on Medical Disorders

Major medical complications that frequently occur in patients with persistent catatonic stupor require close monitoring and management (Clinebell et al. 2014). Some of this risk stems from the challenge of diagnosing medical conditions in patients who are mute, rigid, and unable to cooperate. But the risk is sometimes compounded by "therapeutic nihilism," when catatonic patients are viewed as hopeless or demented. In addition, those in chronic catatonic states often wind up in long-term care centers such as nursing homes or state facilities without the proper medical resources to adequately address their conditions.

Pulmonary Complications

Aspiration is the most common pulmonary complication of catatonia. It can result in pneumonitis or pneumonia. Risk factors for pneumonia include atelectasis, malnutrition, poor respiratory effort, and institutional settings, which also make nosocomial infections with antibiotic-resistant organisms more likely. Prophylactic antibiotics are not beneficial in patients who are considered at high risk for aspiration. Prophylactic administration of antacids, H_2 blockers, or proton pump inhibitors is also not recommended, since those measures may promote colonization by pathogenic organisms. Respiratory failure may result when respiratory effort is severely inadequate (Boyarsky et al. 1999). Immobile, catatonic patients are also more susceptible to pulmonary emboli (Larsen et al. 2011). Prophylactic measures such as hydration, physical therapy, support hose, and anticoagulation can be helpful.

Dehydration, Malnutrition, and Gastrointestinal Complications

Catatonia leads to dehydration and malnutrition. Infection, skin breakdown, constipation, and ileus may be sequelae (Kaufmann et al. 2006; Thomas 2001). Persistent catatonia may necessitate the use of enteral feeding, which can result in complications from the feeding tubes.

Oral and Cutaneous Complications

Dental caries, oral infections, and gum disease are common in chronic catatonia. Skin breakdown and decubitus ulcers are very common as a result of immobility and pressure (Thomas 2001).

Genitourinary Tract Complications

Urinary retention, urinary incontinence, and urinary tract and vaginal infections are frequent complications in the persistently catatonic patient.

Neuromuscular Complications

The immobility of catatonia can result in flexion contractures and nerve palsies. Mobilization through physical therapy can help prevent these complications. Muscle breakdown as a result of immobilization may lead to rhabdomyolysis, particularly in malignant catatonias.

Treatment of Catatonia

When properly treated, catatonia typically resolves completely. Benzodiazepines and ECT are the most frequently recommended treatments. Although no published randomized controlled trials for acute catatonia are available, many case series and prospective open trials over the past three decades with parenteral or oral benzodiazepines (such as lorazepam) showed a response rate of 60%–80% within hours or days (Rosebush and Mazurek 2004; Rosebush et al. 1990). Given the consistent reported benefit with low risk, a benzodiazepine given parenterally has been advocated as an appropriate initial treatment for catatonia (Bush et al. 1996b; Rosebush and Mazurek 2004). Arguments favoring benzodiazepines include familiarity in contemporary psychiatric practice, a favorable therapeutic index, and the availability of flumazenil, a specific antagonist for benzodiazepines. Initial dosages of 2–6 mg/day of lorazepam by any route of administration are recommended, but some patients may require higher doses.

Benzodiazepines are effective for both simple and malignant catatonia attributed to primary psychiatric illness, neuroleptic toxicity, and a variety of other secondary conditions. Treatment response is not predicted by age, sex, or severity of catatonia, although underlying chronic schizophrenia may predict a poorer response (Bush et al. 1996b). Because underlying psychiatric disorders are difficult to assess in mute catatonic patients, specific treatment may need to be delayed until resolution of the catatonic state.

ECT is the most effective treatment for catatonia. Clinical experience and case series have determined that ECT produces remission of catatonia even when other treatments such as lorazepam have failed (Girish and Gill 2003). An added benefit of ECT is its effectiveness for the mood or psychotic disorders frequently associated with the catatonic syndrome. A synergism between ECT and lorazepam has been reported in the treatment of catatonia; therefore, embarking on an ECT course does not preclude continued lorazepam use (Petrides et al. 1997). (See also Chapter 38, "Electroconvulsive Therapy and Other Brain Stimulation Therapies.")

One damaging consequence of the nosological error linking catatonia prominently to schizophrenia was the reflexive use of neuroleptic medication in catatonic patients. Many patients have been pushed into NMS as a result. The use of antipsychotics for catatonia requires caution because of the risk of transforming a simple catatonia into a malignant one. Several reports indicated that both the older high-potency agents, such as haloperidol, and the second-generation antipsychotics failed to improve catatonia, induced or worsened catatonia, or led to progression from catatonia to NMS (Lopez-Canino and Francis 2004; Rosebush and Mazurek 2004; White and Robins 1991). Nevertheless, second-generation antipsychotics may have a role in the treatment of catatonia (Van Den Eede et al. 2005). If antipsychotic medications are prescribed for psychotic patients with current or recent catatonia, consideration should be given to coadministration of lorazepam to prevent progression to malignant catatonia or recurrence of catatonia.

Unfortunately, ECT may not be available or permitted, and the clinician may be motivated to consider use of second-generation antipsychotics. Use of antipsychotic agents in the treatment of malignant catatonia is contraindicated because of the risk of exacerbation, and instead prompt use of ECT is advocated (Mann et al. 2004). In a review of 18 cases of malignant catatonia, 11 of 13 patients who received ECT survived, whereas only 1 of 5 who did not receive ECT lived (Mann et al. 2004). In another series, 16 of 19 patients who had received ECT within 5 days of symptom onset survived, whereas none of the 14 patients who had received ECT after 5 days did (Philbrick and Rummans 1994). Thus, when a patient presents with malignant catatonia of any type, ECT should be used expeditiously (i.e., within 5 days if possible) if a medication trial is unsuccessful.

Conclusion

Secondary psychosis, mania, and catatonia can occur in a wide range of medical diseases and toxic states. Prompt recognition of these neuropsychiatric complications allows for specific syndromal treatments that can lead to a complete resolution of the psychiatric symptoms, even if the underlying illness cannot be cured. If the neuropsychiatric symptoms are not recognized or poorly treated, substantial morbidity or even death can result.

References

Ali SZ, Taguchi A, Rosenberg H: Malignant hyperthermia. Best Pract Res Clin Anaesthesiol 17(4):519–533, 2003 14661655

Ali S, Welch CA, Park LT, et al: Encephalitis and catatonia treated with ECT. Cogn Behav Neurol 21(1):46–51, 2008 18327024

Aliyev ZN, Aliyev NA: Valproate treatment of acute alcohol hallucinosis: a double-blind, placebo-controlled study. Alcohol Alcohol 43(4):456–459, 2008 18495806

American Psychiatric Association: Diagnostic and Statistical Manual of Mental Disorders, 4th Edition, Revised. Washington, DC, American Psychiatric Association, 1994

American Psychiatric Association: Diagnostic and Statistical Manual of Mental Disorders, 5th Edition. Arlington, VA, American Psychiatric Association, 2013

Arciniegas DB: New-onset bipolar disorder in late life: a case of mistaken identity. Am J Psychiatry 163(2):198–203, 2006 16449470

Arora M, Daughton J: Mania in the medically ill. Curr Psychiatry Rep 9(3):232–235, 2007 17521520

Baethge C, Baldessarini RJ, Freudenthal K, et al: Hallucinations in bipolar disorder: characteristics and comparison to unipolar depression and schizophrenia. Bipolar Disord 7(2):136–145, 2005 15762854

Ballard C, Day S, Sharp S, et al: Neuropsychiatric symptoms in dementia: importance and treatment considerations. Int Rev Psychiatry 20(4):396–404, 2008 18925489

Barczak P, Edmunds E, Betts T: Hypomania following complex partial seizures. A report of three cases. Br J Psychiatry 152:137–139, 1988 3167324

Bell L: On a form of disease resembling some advanced stages of mania and fever. Am J Insanity 6(2):97–127, 1849

Benke T: Peduncular hallucinosis: a syndrome of impaired reality monitoring. J Neurol 253(12):1561–1571, 2006 17006630

Berrios GE, Dening TR: Pseudohallucinations: a conceptual history. Psychol Med 26(4):753–763, 1996 8817710

Bokhari R, Bhatara VS, Bandettini F, et al: Postpartum psychosis and postpartum thyroiditis. Psychoneuroendocrinology 23(6):643–650, 1998 9802134

Bonnot O, Klünemann HH, Sedel F, et al: Diagnostic and treatment implications of psychosis secondary to treatable metabolic disorders in adults: a systematic review. Orphanet J Rare Dis 9:65, 2014 24775716

Bonnot O, Herrera PM, Tordjman S, et al: Secondary psychosis induced by metabolic disorders. Front Neurosci 9:177, 2015 26074754

Boyarsky BK, Fuller M, Early T: Malignant catatonia-induced respiratory failure with response to ECT. J ECT 15(3):232–236, 1999 10492863

Brownlie BE, Rae AM, Walshe JW, et al: Psychoses associated with thyrotoxicosis—"thyrotoxic psychosis." A report of 18 cases, with statistical analysis of incidence. Eur J Endocrinol 142(5):438–444, 2000 10802519

Bush G, Fink M, Petrides G, et al: Catatonia, I: rating scale and standardized examination. Acta Psychiatr Scand 93(2):129–136, 1996a 8686483

Bush G, Fink M, Petrides G, et al: Catatonia, II: treatment with lorazepam and electroconvulsive therapy. Acta Psychiatr Scand 93(2):137–143, 1996b 8686484

Carlson GA, Goodwin FK: The stages of mania. A longitudinal analysis of the manic episode. Arch Gen Psychiatry 28(2):221–228, 1973 4684288

Caroff SN, Mann SC, Campbell EC, et al: Epidemiology in catatonia: from psychopathology to neurobiology, in Catatonia: From Psychopathology to Neurobiology. Edited by Caroff SN, Mann SC, Francis A, et al. Washington, DC, American Psychiatric Publishing, 2004, pp 15–31

Carroll BT, Goforth HW: Medical catatonia, in Catatonia: From Psychopathology to Neurobiology. Edited by Caroff SN, Mann SC, Francis A, et al. Washington, DC, American Psychiatric Publishing, 2004, pp 121–127

Carroll BT, Anfinson TJ, Kennedy JC, et al: Catatonic disorder due to general medical conditions. J Neuropsychiatry Clin Neurosci 6(2):122–133, 1994 8044033

Carter JL: Visual, somatosensory, olfactory, and gustatory hallucinations. Psychiatr Clin North Am 15(2):347–358, 1992 1603728

Caton CL, Drake RE, Hasin DS, et al: Differences between early-phase primary psychotic disorders with concurrent substance use and substance-induced psychoses. Arch Gen Psychiatry 62(2):137–145, 2005 15699290

Chakrabarti S, Aga VM, Singh R: Postictal mania following primary generalized seizures. Neurol India 47(4):332–333, 1999 10625913

Chemerinski E, Robinson RG: The neuropsychiatry of stroke. Psychosomatics 41(1):5–14, 2000 10665263

Clinebell K, Azzam PN, Gopalan P, et al: Guidelines for preventing common medical complications of catatonia: case report and literature review. J Clin Psychiatry 75(6):644–651, 2014 25004188

Clower CG: Organic affective syndromes associated with thyroid dysfunction. Psychiatr Med 2(2):177–181, 1984 6571621

Colton CW, Manderscheid RW: Congruencies in increased mortality rates, years of potential life lost, and causes of death among public mental health clients in eight states. Prev Chronic Dis 3(2):A42, 2006 16539783

Cummings J, Zhong K: Trial design innovations: clinical trials for treatment of neuropsychiatric symptoms in Alzheimer's disease. Clin Pharmacol Ther 98(5):483–485, 2015 26206713

Cummings J, Isaacson S, Mills R, et al: Pimavanserin for patients with Parkinson's disease psychosis: a randomised, placebo-controlled phase 3 trial. Lancet 383(9916):533–540, 2014 24183563

Eker A, Saka E, Dalmau J, et al: Testicular teratoma and anti-N-methyl-D-aspartate receptor-associated encephalitis. J Neurol Neurosurg Psychiatry 79(9):1082–1083, 2008 18708569

el-Serag HB, Kunik M, Richardson P, et al: Psychiatric disorders among veterans with hepatitis C infection. Gastroenterology 123(2):476–482, 2002 12145801

Farooq S, Sherin A: Interventions for psychotic symptoms concomitant with epilepsy. Cochrane Database Syst Rev (4):CD006118, 2008 18843704

Feinstein A, Ron M: A longitudinal study of psychosis due to a general medical (neurological) condition: establishing predictive and construct validity. J Neuropsychiatry Clin Neurosci 10(4):448–452, 1998 9813791

Fink M, Taylor MA: Catatonia: A Clinician's Guide to Diagnosis and Treatment. Cambridge, UK, Cambridge University Press, 2003

Fink M, Taylor MA: The catatonia syndrome: forgotten but not gone. Arch Gen Psychiatry 66(11):1173–1177, 2009 19884605

Folstein S: Huntington's Disease: A Disorder of Families. Baltimore, MD, Johns Hopkins University Press, 1989

Forsell Y, Henderson AS: Epidemiology of paranoid symptoms in an elderly population. Br J Psychiatry 172:429–432, 1998 9747406

Foster AR, Caplan JP: Paraneoplastic limbic encephalitis. Psychosomatics 50(2):108–113, 2009 19377018

Freudenreich O: Psychotic Disorders: A Practical Guide. Baltimore, MD, Lippincott Williams & Wilkins, 2007

Freudenreich O, Stern TA: Clinical experience with the management of schizophrenia in the general hospital. Psychosomatics 44(1):12–23, 2003 12515833

Freudenreich O, Holt DJ, Cather C, et al: The evaluation and management of patients with first-episode schizophrenia: a selective, clinical review of diagnosis, treatment, and prognosis. Harv Rev Psychiatry 15(5):189–211, 2007 17924256

Freudenreich O, Schulz SC, Goff DC: Initial medical work-up of first-episode psychosis: a conceptual review. Early Interv Psychiatry 3(1):10–18, 2009 21352170

Freudenreich O, Brown HE, Holt DJ: Psychosis and schizophrenia, in Massachusetts General Hospital Comprehensive Clinical Psychiatry, 2nd Edition. Edited by Stern TA, Fava M, Wilens TE, et al. Philadelphia, PA, Elsevier, 2016, pp 307–323

Fricchione GL, Huffman JC, Stern TA, et al: Catatonia, neuroleptic malignant syndrome, and serotonin syndrome, in Massachusetts General Hospital Handbook of General Hospital Psychiatry, 5th Edition. Edited by Stern TA, Fricchione GL, Cassem NH, et al. Philadelphia, PA, Mosby/Elsevier, 2004, pp 513–530

Gálvez-Andres A, Blasco-Fontecilla H, González-Parra S, et al: Secondary bipolar disorder and Diogenes syndrome in frontotemporal dementia: behavioral improvement with quetiapine and sodium valproate. J Clin Psychopharmacol 27(6):722–723, 2007 18004150

Gelenberg AJ: The catatonic syndrome. Lancet 1(7973):1339–1341, 1976 58326

Ghaffar O, Feinstein A: The neuropsychiatry of multiple sclerosis: a review of recent developments. Curr Opin Psychiatry 20(3):278–285, 2007 17415083

Girish K, Gill NS: Electroconvulsive therapy in lorazepam non-responsive catatonia. Indian J Psychiatry 45(1):21–25, 2003 21206808

Greenberg DM, Lee JW: Psychotic manifestations of alcoholism. Curr Psychiatry Rep 3(4):314–318, 2001 11470038

Gresa-Arribas N, Titulaer MJ, Torrents A, et al: Antibody titres at diagnosis and during follow-up of anti-NMDA receptor encephalitis: a retrospective study. Lancet Neurol 13(2):167–177, 2014 24360484

Grover S, Ghosh A, Ghormode D: Do patients of delirium have catatonic features? An exploratory study. Psychiatry Clin Neurosci 68(8):644–651, 2014 24521083

Heinz A, Voss M, Lawrie SM, et al: Shall we really say goodbye to first rank symptoms? Eur Psychiatry 37:8–13, 2016 27429167

Himmelhoch J: Major mood disorders related to epileptic changes, in Psychiatric Aspects of Epilepsy. Edited by Blumer D. Washington, DC, American Psychiatric Press, 1984, pp 271–294

Hudak M, Severn D, Nordstrom K: Edible cannabis-induced psychosis: intoxication and beyond. Am J Psychiatry 172(9):911–912, 2015 26324307

Hurwitz TA, Wada JA, Kosaka BD, et al: Cerebral organization of affect suggested by temporal lobe seizures. Neurology 35(9):1335–1337, 1985 4022380

Jacobowski NL, Heckers S, Bobo WV: Delirious mania: detection, diagnosis, and clinical management in the acute setting. J Psychiatr Pract 19(1):15–28, 2013 23334676

Jeste DV, Caligiuri MP, Paulsen JS, et al: Risk of tardive dyskinesia in older patients. A prospective longitudinal study of 266 outpatients. Arch Gen Psychiatry 52(9):756–765, 1995 7654127

Johnstone EC, Macmillan JF, Crow TJ: The occurrence of organic disease of possible or probable aetiological significance in a population of 268 cases of first episode schizophrenia. Psychol Med 17(2):371–379, 1987 3602229

Jorge RE, Robinson RG, Starkstein SE, et al: Secondary mania following traumatic brain injury. Am J Psychiatry 150(6):916–921, 1993 8494069

Josephs KA: Capgras syndrome and its relationship to neurodegenerative disease. Arch Neurol 64(12):1762–1766, 2007 18071040

Kahlbaum K: Catatonia. Baltimore, MD, Johns Hopkins University Press, 1973

Kaufmann RM, Schreinzer D, Strnad A, et al: Case report: intestinal atonia as an unusual symptom of malignant catatonia responsive to electroconvulsive therapy. Schizophr Res 84(1):178–179, 2006 16624527

Kilbourne AM, Cornelius JR, Han X, et al: Burden of general medical conditions among individuals with bipolar disorder. Bipolar Disord 6(5):368–373, 2004 15383128

Klimstra S, Mahgoub N: Psychosis of Alzheimer's disease. Psychiatric Annals 39(1):10–14, 2009

Krauthammer C, Klerman GL: Secondary mania: manic syndromes associated with antecedent physical illness or drugs. Arch Gen Psychiatry 35(11):1333–1339, 1978 757997

Larsen HH, Ritchie JC, McNutt MD, et al: Pulmonary embolism in a patient with catatonia: an old disease, changing times. Psychosomatics 52(4):387–391, 2011 21777724

Lautenschlager NT, Förstl H: Organic psychosis: insight into the biology of psychosis. Curr Psychiatry Rep 3(4):319–325, 2001 11470039

Lee CS, Hutto B: Recognizing thyrotoxicosis in a patient with bipolar mania: a case report. Ann Gen Psychiatry 7:3, 2008 18284661

Leong GB, Silva JA, Garza-Treviño ES, et al: The dangerousness of persons with the Othello syndrome. J Forensic Sci 39(6):1445–1454, 1994 7815024

Leypoldt F, Armangue T, Dalmau J: Autoimmune encephalopathies. Ann N Y Acad Sci 1338:94–114, 2015 25315420

Lockman J, Burns TM: Stiff-person syndrome. Curr Treat Options Neurol 9(3):234–240, 2007 17445501

Lopez-Canino A, Francis A: Drug induced catatonia, in Catatonia: From Psychopathology to Neurobiology. Edited by Caroff SN, Mann SC, Francis A, et al. Washington, DC, American Psychiatric Publishing, 2004, pp 129–140

Louis ED, Pflaster NL: Catatonia mimicking nonconvulsive status epilepticus. Epilepsia 36(9):943–945, 1995 7649135

Lyketsos CG, Stoline AM, Longstreet P, et al: Mania in temporal lobe epilepsy. Neuropsychiatry Neuropsychol Behav Neurol 6(1):19–25, 1993

Lyketsos CG, Schwartz J, Fishman M, et al: AIDS mania. J Neuropsychiatry Clin Neurosci 9(2):277–279, 1997 9144109

Mann SC, Caroff SN, Keck PE, et al: Neuroleptic Malignant Syndrome and Related Conditions, 2nd Edition. Washington, DC, American Psychiatric Press, 1994

Mann SC, Caroff SN, Fricchione GL, et al: Malignant catatonia, in Catatonia: From Psychopathology to Neurobiology. Edited by Caroff SN, Mann SC, Francis A, et al. Washington, DC, American Psychiatric Publishing, 2004, pp 105–120

Marneros A: Schizophrenic first-rank symptoms in organic mental disorders. Br J Psychiatry 152:625–628, 1988 3167434

Maust DT, Kim HM, Seyfried LS, et al: Antipsychotics, other psychotropics, and the risk of death in patients with dementia: number needed to harm. JAMA Psychiatry 72(5):438–445, 2015 25786075

McKeith I, Del Ser T, Spano P, et al: Efficacy of rivastigmine in dementia with Lewy bodies: a randomised, double-blind, placebo-controlled international study. Lancet 356(9247):2031–2036, 2000 11145488

McKeith IG, Dickson DW, Lowe J, et al; Consortium on DLB: Diagnosis and management of dementia with Lewy bodies: third report of the DLB Consortium. Neurology 65(12):1863–1872, 2005 16237129

Mendez MF: Huntington's disease: update and review of neuropsychiatric aspects. Int J Psychiatry Med 24(3):189–208, 1994 7890478

Mendez MF: Mania in neurologic disorders. Curr Psychiatry Rep 2(5):440–445, 2000 11122994

Mendez MF, Grau R: The postictal psychosis of epilepsy: investigation in two patients. Int J Psychiatry Med 21(1):85–92, 1991 1906057

Menon GJ: Complex visual hallucinations in the visually impaired: a structured history-taking approach. Arch Ophthalmol 123(3):349–355, 2005 15767477

Michael A, Mirza S, Mirza KA, et al: Morbid jealousy in alcoholism. Br J Psychiatry 167(5):668–672, 1995 8564326

Mocellin R, Walterfang M, Velakoulis D: Neuropsychiatry of complex visual hallucinations. Aust N Z J Psychiatry 40(9):742–751, 2006 16911748

Murray RM, Quigley H, Quattrone D, et al: Traditional marijuana, high-potency cannabis and synthetic cannabinoids: increasing risk for psychosis. World Psychiatry 15(3):195–204, 2016 27717258

Naber D, Sand P, Heigl B: Psychopathological and neuropsychological effects of 8 days' corticosteroid treatment. A prospective study. Psychoneuroendocrinology 21(1):25–31, 1996 8778901

Nadkarni S, Arnedo V, Devinsky O: Psychosis in epilepsy patients. Epilepsia 48 (suppl 9):17–19, 2007 18047594

Oostervink F, Boomsma MM, Nolen WA; EMBLEM Advisory Board: Bipolar disorder in the elderly: different effects of age and of age of onset. J Affect Disord 116(3):176–183, 2009 19087895

Ostling S, Skoog I: Psychotic symptoms and paranoid ideation in a nondemented population-based sample of the very old. Arch Gen Psychiatry 59(1):53–59, 2002 11779282

Petrides G, Divadeenam KM, Bush G, et al: Synergism of lorazepam and electroconvulsive therapy in the treatment of catatonia. Biol Psychiatry 42(5):375–381, 1997 9276078

Philbrick KL, Rummans TA: Malignant catatonia. J Neuropsychiatry Clin Neurosci 6(1):1–13, 1994 7908547

Rafaniello C, Lombardo F, Ferrajolo C, et al: Predictors of mortality in atypical antipsychotic-treated community-dwelling elderly patients with behavioural and psychological symptoms of dementia: a prospective population-based cohort study from Italy. Eur J Clin Pharmacol 70(2):187–195, 2014 24145814

Ramchandani D, Riggio S: Periictal mania. A case report. Psychosomatics 33(2):229–231, 1992 1557492

Raucher-Chéné D, Charrel CL, de Maindreville AD, et al: Manic episode with psychotic symptoms in a patient with Parkinson's disease treated by subthalamic nucleus stimulation: improvement on switching the target. J Neurol Sci 273(1–2):116–117, 2008 18597786

Ray WA, Chung CP, Murray KT, et al: Atypical antipsychotic drugs and the risk of sudden cardiac death. N Engl J Med 360(3):225–235, 2009 19144938

Robertson MM: Affect and mood in epilepsy: an overview with a focus on depression. Acta Neurol Scand Suppl 140:127–132, 1992 1441907

Rosebush P, Mazurek M: Pharmacotherapy, in Catatonia: From Psychopathology to Neurobiology. Edited by Caroff SN, Mann SC, Francis A, et al. Washington, DC, American Psychiatric Publishing, 2004, pp 141–150

Rosebush PI, Hildebrand AM, Furlong BG, et al: Catatonic syndrome in a general psychiatric inpatient population: frequency, clinical presentation, and response to lorazepam. J Clin Psychiatry 51(9):357–362, 1990 2211547

Rosenblatt A, Leroi I: Neuropsychiatry of Huntington's disease and other basal ganglia disorders. Psychosomatics 41(1):24–30, 2000 10665265

Rundell JR, Wise MG: Causes of organic mood disorder. J Neuropsychiatry Clin Neurosci 1(4):398–400, 1989 2521090

Sachdev P: Schizophrenia-like psychosis and epilepsy: the status of the association. Am J Psychiatry 155(3):325–336, 1998 9501741

Santos CO, Caeiro L, Ferro JM, et al: Mania and stroke: a systematic review. Cerebrovasc Dis 32(1):11–21, 2011 21576938

Schneider LS, Tariot PN, Dagerman KS, et al; CATIE-AD Study Group: Effectiveness of atypical antipsychotic drugs in patients with Alzheimer's disease. N Engl J Med 355(15):1525–1538, 2006 17035647

Shukla S, Cook BL, Mukherjee S, et al: Mania following head trauma. Am J Psychiatry 144(1):93–96, 1987 3799847

Silva JA, Leong GB, Weinstock R, et al: Delusional misidentification syndromes and dangerousness. Psychopathology 27(3–5):215–219, 1994 7846240

Slater E, Beard AW: The schizophrenia-like psychoses of epilepsy, V: discussion and conclusions. Br J Psychiatry 109:143–150, 1963

Smith E, Delargy M: Locked-in syndrome. BMJ 330(7488):406–409, 2005 15718541

Starkstein SE, Berthier ML, Lylyk PL, et al: Emotional behavior after a Wada test in a patient with secondary mania. J Neuropsychiatry Clin Neurosci 1(4):408–412, 1989 2521093

Stauder K: Die tödliche Katatonie. Arch Psychiatr Nervenkr 102:614–634, 1934

Stowell CP, Barnhill JW: Acute mania in the setting of severe hypothyroidism. Psychosomatics 46(3):259–261, 2005 15883148

Subramaniam H, Dennis MS, Byrne EJ: The role of vascular risk factors in late onset bipolar disorder. Int J Geriatr Psychiatry 22(8):733–737, 2007 17146839

Taylor MA, Fink M: Catatonia in psychiatric classification: a home of its own. Am J Psychiatry 160(7):1233–1241, 2003 12832234

Thewissen V, Myin-Germeys I, Bentall R, et al: Hearing impairment and psychosis revisited. Schizophr Res 76(1):99–103, 2005 15927803

Thomas DR: Prevention and treatment of pressure ulcers: what works? what doesn't? Cleve Clin J Med 68(8):704–707, 710–714, 717–722, 2001 11510528

Thorup A, Petersen L, Jeppesen P, et al: Frequency and predictive values of first rank symptoms at baseline among 362 young adult patients with first-episode schizophrenia: results from the Danish OPUS study. Schizophr Res 97(1–3):60–67, 2007 17698323

Timmermans M, Carr J: Neurosyphilis in the modern era. J Neurol Neurosurg Psychiatry 75(12):1727–1730, 2004 15548491

Toone BK: The psychoses of epilepsy. J Neurol Neurosurg Psychiatry 69(1):1–3, 2000 10864594

Tüzün E, Dalmau J: Limbic encephalitis and variants: classification, diagnosis and treatment. Neurologist 13(5):261–271, 2007 17848866

Van Den Eede F, Van Hecke J, Van Dalfsen A, et al: The use of atypical antipsychotics in the treatment of catatonia. Eur Psychiatry 20(5–6):422–429, 2005 15964746

van der Heijden FM, Tuinier S, Arts NJ, et al: Catatonia: disappeared or under-diagnosed? Psychopathology 38(1):3–8, 2005 15714008

Villani S, Weitzel WD: Secondary mania. Arch Gen Psychiatry 36(9):1031, 1979 582361

Weinstein EA: The classification of delusional misidentification syndromes. Psychopathology 27(3–5):130–135, 1994 7846227

White DA, Robins AH: Catatonia: harbinger of the neuroleptic malignant syndrome. Br J Psychiatry 158:419–421, 1991 1674666

Wilson JE, Niu K, Nicolson SE, et al: The diagnostic criteria and structure of catatonia. Schizophr Res 164(1–3):256–262, 2015 25595653

Wing L, Shah A: A systematic examination of catatonia-like clinical pictures in autism spectrum disorders. Int Rev Neurobiol 72:21–39, 2006 16697289

Woolley JD, Wilson MR, Hung E, et al: Frontotemporal dementia and mania. Am J Psychiatry 164(12):1811–1816, 2007 18056235

Young RC, Biggs JT, Ziegler VE, et al: A rating scale for mania: reliability, validity and sensitivity. Br J Psychiatry 133:429–435, 1978 728692

Yusim A, Anbarasan D, Bernstein C, et al: Normal pressure hydrocephalus presenting as Othello syndrome: case presentation and review of the literature. Am J Psychiatry 165(9):1119–1125, 2008 18765494

Zhao QF, Tan L, Wang HF, et al: The prevalence of neuropsychiatric symptoms in Alzheimer's disease: systematic review and meta-analysis. J Affect Disord 190:264–271, 2016 26540080

CHAPTER 10

Anxiety Disorders

Ted S. Liao, M.D.
Steven A. Epstein, M.D.

Anxiety is an extremely common problem in primary care and specialty medical settings. Because the 1-year prevalence rate of any anxiety disorder in the general population is approximately 22.2% (Kessler et al. 2012), many medically ill patients will have concurrent anxiety. The presence of anxiety disorders in such patients leads to less favorable medical outcomes and increased healthcare costs. Unfortunately, medical professionals often neglect to identify these treatable disorders. Even when they recognize distressing anxiety, some practitioners minimize its significance by considering it to be a "normal" response to the uncertainty and adversity associated with having a disease.

Understanding the interplay between anxiety and medical illness is key to effective psychiatric evaluation and treatment. Although a patient's anxiety may be due to a primary anxiety or other mental disorder, it is also important to consider whether anxiety is a symptom of a medical illness, a side effect of medication, a psychological reaction to the experience of illness, or a combination. Likewise, it is important to consider medical comorbidity when designing treatment plans.

In this chapter, we review general issues in clinical presentation, diagnosis, etiology, and treatment of anxiety in the medically ill. For detailed reviews of anxiety in specific medical disorders, the reader is referred to the corresponding chapters in this text.

General Features and Diagnostic Considerations

Individuals with chronic medical conditions are more likely to have anxiety disorders (Sareen et al. 2006), and many patients with anxiety do not present to mental health providers. Of all anxiety disorder visits in the National Ambulatory Medical Care Survey in 1998, 48% were to primary care physicians (Harman et al. 2002). Yet the majority of patients with anxiety disorders have their disorders go undiagnosed; for instance, a study of more than 20,000 primary care patients found that only 34% of patients with generalized anxiety disorder (GAD) were correctly diagnosed (Wittchen et al. 2002). An interview in which DSM-5 (American Psychiatric Association 2013) criteria are used is the gold standard for diagnosis of an anxiety disorder. In primary care settings, it is often useful to ask brief screening questions to determine whether a full diagnostic assessment is necessary. A seven-item anxiety inventory, the Generalized Anxiety Disorder–7 (GAD-7) scale, has been reported to be an effective screen for GAD, panic, posttraumatic stress disorder (PTSD), and social phobia (Herr et al. 2014; Kroenke et al. 2007). The Hospital Anxiety and Depression Scale (HADS; Bjelland et al. 2002), a 14-item scale, and the Patient Health Questionnaire–4 (PHQ-4; Kroenke et al. 2009), a 4-item scale, have also been shown to be valid screening instruments for both anxiety and depression.

Distinguishing between normal and pathological anxiety is crucial for accurate diagnosis of any anxiety disorder and requires the assessment of whether the symptoms are causing significant functional impairment. Anxiety disorders have clearly been shown to impair functioning among individuals with chronic medical conditions (Kessler et al. 2003; Sherbourne et al. 1996). Severe medical illnesses complicate the determination of functional impairment, since they (or related medical treatments) can themselves cause significant disability. In patients with disability due to medical illness, assessing the functional impact of anxiety can often be achieved by assessing its effect on treatment adherence.

Although depression is more clearly a predictor of poor adherence to medical treatment (DiMatteo et al. 2000), excessive anxiety may also reduce adherence (García-Llana et al. 2014) and may even cause patients to refuse diagnostic procedures or surgery and/or sign out of the hospital against medical advice. Such behavior suggests the presence of an anxiety disorder and can result in negative medical outcomes (Batty et al. 2017) and increased health care costs (Ketterer et al. 2010; Stundner et al. 2013).

Causes of Anxiety in the Medically Ill

When one is evaluating an anxious patient who is also medically ill, it is essential to consider the full range of potential etiologies of anxiety, which are here grouped into four categories:

1. Anxiety due to a primary anxiety or other mental disorder
2. Anxiety due to the effects of medical illness
3. Anxiety due to the effects of a substance/medication
4. Anxiety due to the patient's psychological reaction to the experience of illness

It is important to note the distinction between anxiety that is physiologically secondary to another medical condition and anxiety due to a primary anxiety disorder or an anxious reaction to the medical condition. For example, hyperthyroidism appears to biologically cause anxiety, whereas diabetes mellitus usually does not. The DSM-5 diagnosis of anxiety due to another medical condition refers to the former, not the latter. This difference can be confusing due to the assumption of causality when there is an epidemiological association between anxiety and a particular medical condition. For example, anxiety disorders are common among individuals with migraine (Torelli and D'Amico 2004), but the onset of the anxiety disorder generally precedes that of migraine (Merikangas and Stevens 1997). It is important to keep in mind that for many medically ill patients, the etiology of anxiety is multifactorial and may vary with the course of illness.

Primary Anxiety Disorders and Other Mental Disorders

In patients with medical illnesses who present with anxiety, it is fundamental to consider the possibility of a primary anxiety or other mental disorder as an etiology of their symptoms. These disorders are disproportionately prevalent among medically ill patients and, if left undiagnosed and untreated, can interfere with medical treatment, adversely impact outcomes, and increase morbidity and mortality.

Specific mental disorders in which anxiety is a prominent feature are reviewed below. (For a more comprehensive review of anxiety disorders and their relation to medical illnesses, see Roy-Byrne et al. 2008.)

Generalized Anxiety Disorder

Although the 12-month prevalence rate of GAD in community samples is approximately 2.0% (Kessler et al. 2012), an international study found the 1-month prevalence rate in primary care to be 7.9% (Maier et al. 2000). GAD may lead to excess health care use (Jones et al. 2001). GAD somatic symptoms, such as fatigue, muscle tension, and insomnia, often lead patients to present initially to a primary care physician. As with depression, it is important for physicians to consider GAD in the differential diagnosis. Recognizing and treating GAD is particularly important, as it has been shown to be independently associated with poorer medical outcomes; for example, GAD has been associated with a nearly twofold increased risk of mortality over the subsequent 10 years after myocardial infarction (Celano et al. 2016).

Panic Disorder

Primary care patients with panic attacks are high utilizers of medical care (Roy-Byrne et al. 1999). In particular, many patients who present with chest pain are found to have panic disorder. Researchers estimate that at least one-third of individuals with chest pain and normal coronary arteries have panic disorder (e.g., Bringager et al. 2008). These rates contrast with the 12-month prevalence rates of 2.4% found in the National Comorbidity Survey Replication (Kessler et al. 2012). Panic attacks may be difficult to distinguish symptomatically from paroxysmal atrial tachycardia; both occur frequently in young, otherwise healthy women and are frequently comorbid. Patients who present for evaluation of dizziness also have elevated rates of panic disorder (Wiltink et al. 2009), and panic disorder also has significant comorbidity with irritable bowel syndrome (Kumano et al. 2004; Sugaya et al. 2008). For further discussion of panic disorder in cardiac patients, see Chapter 17, "Heart Disease."

Specific Phobias

Although specific phobias are quite common, they rarely come to the attention of physicians. Exceptions include blood-injection-injury phobias and claustrophobia. Blood-injection-injury phobias, which have been reported to occur in 9% of adolescents in the United States (Burstein et al. 2012), may lead to fainting during medical procedures or to avoidance of injections and blood tests. Claustrophobia comes to medical attention most commonly when individuals need a magnetic resonance imaging (MRI) procedure. In a recent study of 6,500 patients undergoing MRI, the claustrophobic event rate was 10% (Napp et al. 2017); such events can necessitate the use of behavioral techniques such as relaxation exercises, or of sedation (e.g., with a short-acting benzodiazepine).

Other Mental Disorders

PTSD was reclassified from the anxiety disorders to the new category of "trauma- and stressor-related disorders" in DSM-5 (American Psychiatric Association 2013); still, it remains a common cause of anxiety in the medically ill. The National Comorbidity Survey Replication estimated the 12-month prevalence of PTSD in the general population to be 3.7% (Kessler et al. 2012). Prevalence in medical settings may be higher. For example, in a recent systematic review, PTSD prevalence in primary care patients ranged from 2% to 39%, and PTSD was associated with functional impairment or disability (Greene et al. 2016). Trauma victims and individuals with PTSD are frequent users of health care (Seng et al. 2006). PTSD also has been linked to adverse medical outcomes. For example, in a study of 637 veterans with known coronary artery disease, PTSD was associated with presence and severity of coronary atherosclerosis and predicted mortality independent of age, gender, and conventional risk factors (Ahmadi et al. 2011).

Like PTSD, obsessive-compulsive disorder (OCD) was reclassified in DSM-5 (American Psychiatric Association 2013) from the anxiety disorders to a new category, "obsessive-compulsive and related disorders," which also includes excoriation (skin-picking) disorder. These disorders can adversely impact treatment of dermatological and other medical illnesses. In a 2015 study of 2,145 adults, the prevalence of excoriation disorder was 5.4%, with the prevalence of OCD being markedly elevated in those with excoriation disorder versus those without (Leibovici et al. 2015).

Finally, anxiety can be an important aspect of the presentation of other mental disorders. For a discussion of the role of anxiety in these disorders, see Chapters 4 through 16.

Anxiety Due to Another Medical Condition

Many medical disorders have been reported to cause anxiety, but data are limited to case reports for many associations. Nonetheless, it is particularly important to consider medical causes of anxiety when the history is atypical for a primary anxiety disorder (e.g., lack of personal or family history, lack of psychosocial stressors) and when the onset of anxiety is at a later age. It is also important to evaluate medical causes when the anxiety is accompanied by disproportionate physical symptoms (e.g., marked dyspnea, tachycardia, tremor) or atypical ones (e.g., syncope, confusion, focal neurological symptoms).

The medical evaluation of the anxious patient should begin with a thorough history and physical examination, including neurological examination. Further components of the evaluation—including laboratory tests, imaging, and other diagnostic studies—should be determined by the patient's specific medical symptoms. For example, a patient with seizure-like episodes will likely require a neurological consultation and an electroencephalogram. In the absence of other findings suggestive of rare medical etiologies of anxiety, it is not advisable to routinely screen for them (e.g., pheochromocytoma or carcinoid tumors).

Next, we discuss common medical conditions that are associated with anxiety for which data are strongly supportive of a causal relation, organized by system: endocrine/metabolic, cardiovascular, respiratory, and neurological.

Endocrine Disease and Metabolic Disturbances

Anxiety symptoms commonly occur among individuals with hyperthyroidism, and thyroid function tests are routinely checked in psychiatric patients (Dickerman and Barnhill 2012). The adrenergic overreactivity that accompanies hyperthyroidism provides a ready explanation for its association with anxiety. Patients with subclinical and clinical hyperthyroidism have been shown to have elevated anxiety levels (Gulseren et al. 2006; Sait Gönen et al. 2004). Hyperthyroidism causing anxiety may be difficult to distinguish from a primary anxiety disorder; other signs of hyperthyroidism, such as persistent tachycardia or heat intolerance, help identify the former. However, differentiating the two can be challenging (see Iacovides et al. 2000)—for example, beta-blockers alleviate symptoms of both hyperthyroidism and anxiety. Improvement in anxiety usually parallels successful treatment of hyperthyroidism.

Other examples of endocrinopathies that cause anxiety include pheochromocytoma, hypoglycemia, and hyperadrenalism. Metabolic disturbances also should be considered as a possible etiology in medically ill patients presenting with anxiety—for example, hypercalcemia may present with anxiety and other neuropsychiatric symptoms. For a more complete discussion, see Chapter 21, "Endocrine and Metabolic Disorders."

Cardiovascular Disorders

Cardiovascular disorders are highly associated with anxiety. For example, there is a 26% lifetime prevalence of GAD in patients with coronary artery disease, far higher than the 3%–7% lifetime prevalence in the general population (Tully and Cosh 2013). Heart failure and cardiac arrhythmias have also demonstrated clear associations with anxiety. Anxiety and cardiac disease share some common pathophysiology; elevated inflammatory markers such as interleukin-6, dysfunction in the endovascular endothelium, platelet dysfunction, and disrupted autonomic stability are features of both cardiac disease and anxiety (Celano et al. 2016).

Cardiovascular disease experiences can traumatize patients and result in PTSD. Myocardial infarction is followed by PTSD with significant frequency (Gander and von Känel 2006), and the PTSD associated with implantable cardioverter defibrillators (ICDs) has been shown to increase long-term mortality risk (Ladwig et al. 2008). See below for further discussion of other medical treatments that cause PTSD. For a fuller discussion of anxiety in cardiovascular disorders, see Chapter 17, "Heart Disease."

Respiratory Illness

Patients with pulmonary disease often experience anxiety. For example, the adjusted odds of GAD in a Canadian population of more than 11,000 individuals was found to be four times higher for patients with chronic obstructive pulmonary disease (COPD) than for patients without COPD (Fuller-Thomson and Lacombe-Duncan 2016), and asthma and anxiety have been shown to be independent risk factors for each other in a nationwide population-based study in Taiwan (Lee et al. 2016). Although the psychological stress and uncertainty of living with asthma or COPD certainly contribute to this association, intrinsic physiological factors do as well. For example, both hypercapnia and hyperventilation may lead to panic attack symptoms. Anxiety is associated with more frequent COPD exacerbations, thereby contributing to a vicious circle in which pulmonary and anxiety symptoms exacerbate each other (Montserrat-Capdevila et al. 2017). Several asthma medications may cause anxiety as well (see Table 10–1 later in this chapter).

In addition to asthma and COPD, other respiratory illnesses are associated with anxiety. Pulmonary emboli may present with symptoms of anxiety (Tapson 2007), and if the emboli are small, they may be misdiagnosed as panic attacks. For a more complete discussion about anxiety and respiratory illness, see Chapter 18, "Lung Disease."

Neurological Illness

A recent systematic review and meta-analysis found the prevalence of anxiety disorders in Parkinson's disease to be 31% (Broen et al. 2016), which is higher than in the general population. Anxiety often appears after the manifestations of Parkinson's disease symptoms and may be due to the uncertainty with respect to both day-to-day functioning and long-term prognosis. The neurobiology of anxiety in Parkinson's disease has not been clearly delineated, but functional imaging studies have revealed an inverse correlation between dopaminergic density in the caudate and putamen and the severity of anxiety (Wen et al. 2016). The dopaminergic neural circuits implicated in Parkinson's disease have intimate connections with systems involved with anxiety (e.g., the serotonergic system). Anxiety also may be caused by medications used to treat Parkinson's disease, such as L-dopa (see Table 10–1 later in this chapter).

Anxiety disorders are frequent in epilepsy; a recent French study found 34% of patients with generalized seizures had symptoms that met criteria for GAD (Micoulaud-Franchi et al. 2016). Complex partial seizures may be accompanied by symptoms of panic disorder, including fear, depersonalization, derealization, dizziness, and paresthesias (Kim et al. 2007). Animal models have demonstrated that the underlying neurobiological mechanisms behind anxiety and epilepsy share similarities (Brandt and Mula 2016). The discharge of excitatory currents occurs in both anxiety symptoms and epilepsy, and the pathophysiology of both center around the amygdala and hippocampus (Kwon and Park 2014). Accordingly, several medications—benzodiazepines in particular—are utilized in the treatment of both anxiety and seizure disorders.

There are numerous other neurological causes of anxiety, including central nervous system (CNS) neoplasms, vestibular dysfunction, and encephalitis. For further discussion of anxiety in neurological disorders, see Chapter 30, "Neurology and Neurosurgery."

Other Conditions

Many other medical conditions cause anxiety symptoms beyond those covered above. Like myocardial infarction (discussed above), other life-threatening illnesses, such as cancer, can precipitate PTSD. While the DSM-5 reclassification of PTSD has highlighted the need to distinguish it from adjustment disorders in oncology patients

(Kangas 2013), a recent meta-analysis underscored that cancer survivors frequently develop PTSD based on the trauma of their experience with cancer (Abbey et al. 2015). However, this trauma is different from more usual PTSD stressors such as rape in two principal ways: the threat arises from one's own body; and once the patient has been treated, the ongoing stressor is often not the memory of past events but rather the fear of recurrence (Green et al. 1997). As is the case with other medical illnesses, severity of cancer is not a strong predictor of the development of PTSD.

As with ICDs mentioned above, other medical interventions can be experienced by patients as traumatic. For example, receiving treatment in intensive care units (ICUs) has been associated with development of PTSD (Davydow et al. 2008; Hatch et al. 2011), and there have been numerous studies of PTSD following organ transplantation. A recent systematic literature review found that the cumulative incidence of clinician-ascertained transplant-specific PTSD ranged from 10% to 17% (Davydow et al. 2015). For a more detailed discussion of organ transplantation, see Chapter 29, "Organ Transplantation."

Substance/Medication-Induced Anxiety

In evaluating the anxious medical patient, it is important to consider whether medications or their withdrawal might be contributory. Because they can be obtained without prescriptions, caffeine and over-the-counter sympathomimetics are common causes of anxiety in the general population. Caffeine may be present in significant quantities in coffee, tea, caffeinated soda, and other caffeinated beverages, as well as over-the-counter preparations for alertness (e.g., NoDoz), weight loss, and headache (e.g., Excedrin). Over-the-counter sympathomimetics used as decongestants (e.g., pseudoephedrine) frequently cause anxiety, and tachyphylaxis develops rapidly. Similarly, the widely used herbal preparation ephedra also may cause anxiety.

The most important drug classes that are associated with anxiety are summarized in Table 10–1, which includes examples of specific substances in each class. Where appropriate, notes have been added for further clarification. General references in this area are *The Medical Letter on Drugs and Therapeutics* ("Drugs That May Cause Psychiatric Symptoms" 2008) and *Goodman and Gilman's The Pharmacological Basis of Therapeutics* (Brunton et al. 2011). A significant number of substances beyond those listed in Table 10–1 may cause delirium, which can produce symptoms that overlap with those of anxiety. For further information about deliriogenic substances, see Chapter 4, "Delirium."

Anxiety as a Psychological Reaction to the Experience of Illness

The importance of one's health added to the oftentimes unavoidable uncertainty associated with medical illness leads many medically ill patients to feel anxious. Particularly for individuals with a predisposition to anxiety, the psychosocial stress of illness may be sufficient to induce an anxiety disorder. Psychiatrists should avoid making assumptions regarding the cause of anxiety in an individual patient; for example, it is easy to assume that the patient who is awaiting cardiac surgery is afraid of dying, when in fact the patient might actually be more concerned about potential disability.

TABLE 10–1.   Substances/medications that may cause anxiety

Class	Example(s)	Notes
Anticholinergics	Atropine, benztropine, dicyclomine, oxybutynin, scopolamine, diphenhydramine, ipratropium	At toxic doses
Antidepressants	Bupropion, SNRIs, SSRIs, tricyclics	Anxiety may also result from withdrawal
Antiepileptics	Zonisamide	Especially at supratherapeutic doses
Antimalarial agents	Mefloquine	
Antinarcolepsy agents	Modafinil, armodafinil	
Antineoplastic agents	Vinblastine	
Antipsychotics	Haloperidol, risperidone	Anxiety may be secondary to akathisia
Antiviral agents	Amantadine, efavirenz	
Beta-adrenergic agonists	Albuterol, terbutaline	
Cannabinoids	Cannabis, prescribed (dronabinol) and recreational ("K2," "Spice") synthetic forms	See Gunderson et al. 2012
Cathinones	Khat, synthetic forms ("bath salts")	See Gregg and Rawls 2014
Class I antiarrhythmics	Lidocaine, quinidine	
Corticosteroids	Methylprednisolone, prednisone	
Dopaminergic agents	Carbidopa-levodopa	
Estrogens	Hormone replacement therapy (oral, transdermal, topical, intravaginal) and breast cancer therapies (including antiestrogen therapy—e.g., tamoxifen)	Anxiety less common with contraceptives

TABLE 10–1. Substances/medications that may cause anxiety *(continued)*

Class	Example(s)	Notes
Interferons	Interferon-alpha, interferon-beta	
Methylxanthines	Caffeine, theophylline	
Nonsteroidal anti-inflammatory drugs	Indomethacin and COX-2 inhibitors	
Opiates	Morphine, hydromorphone, methadone, heroin, etc.	Anxiety can occur with withdrawal
Opioid antagonists	Naloxone, naltrexone	Can precipitate opiate withdrawal
Phenethylamines	Ephedrine, epinephrine, pseudoephedrine	
Phenothiazines	Prochlorperazine, promethazine	Anxiety may be secondary to akathisia
Prokinetic agents	Metoclopramide	Anxiety may be secondary to akathisia
Psychostimulants	Cocaine, MDMA, dextroamphetamine, methylphenidate, methamphetamine	
Sedative-hypnotics	Alcohol, barbiturates, benzodiazepines	Anxiety occurs with withdrawal

Note. COX-2=cyclo-oygenase–2; MDMA=3,4-methylenedioxymethamphetamine; SNRI=serotonin-norepinephrine reuptake inhibitor; SSRI=selective serotonin reuptake inhibitor.

When approaching the anxious patient, the psychiatrist should consider all potential psychological causes of anxiety. The following discussion reviews the major varieties of anxious reactions in the medically ill. For seminal discussions of this topic, the reader is referred to the work of Strain and Grossman (1975) and Kahana and Bibring (1964) (see also Chapter 3, "Psychological Responses to Illness").

Uncertainty Regarding Medical Diagnosis

Some individuals worry excessively that they might have a serious illness (see Chapter 11, "Somatic Symptom Disorder and Illness Anxiety Disorder"). Routine evaluations may cause anxiety, especially in those with a personal or family history of illness. For example, a woman with a family history of breast cancer might become quite anxious in the period preceding routine mammography. Anxiety also may occur during the period between initial evaluation and receipt of the definitive result—for example, after the physician tells the patient, "It's probably nothing, but let's perform a brain MRI just to be sure." Prolonged uncertainty regarding diagnosis is even more anxiety-provoking, such as when the patient is told, "Your PSA [prostate-specific antigen] is elevated, but at this point we should wait and reevaluate your level in a few months." Although physicians are well aware that there is significant uncertainty inherent in medical diagnoses, patients are generally not reassured by this fact.

Uncertainty Regarding Medical Prognosis

For many medical illnesses and procedures, prognosis is uncertain. Many patients will experience ongoing fears of recurrence, especially when they have illnesses that frequently do recur (e.g., arrhythmias, cancer, multiple sclerosis). Similarly, many fear that their treatments will fail, even if they are initially successful (e.g., rejection of a transplanted organ). It is important to keep in mind that even patients who have favorable prognoses often experience anxiety. For example, a 95% cure rate is reassuring to many patients, but some will have difficulty coping with the prospect of a 5% recurrence rate. Complicating the problem is the fact that patients may search online and find inaccurate information. Reassuring patients effectively requires addressing misinformation.

Anxiety About One's Body

Many individuals experience anxiety about the future effects of illness on their bodies (see Strain and Grossman 1975). Patients may fear that they will lose body parts (e.g., due to amputation). Ongoing fears of amputation are particularly problematic in some diseases (e.g., diabetes mellitus and peripheral vascular disease). Others may fear that they will lose functional capacities or that they will become overly dependent on others. For example, individuals with diabetes mellitus may fear eventual blindness, patients with COPD may fear "being hooked to a breathing machine," and men with prostate cancer may fear impotence and incontinence. Others are afraid of the experience of pain; for example, patients with metastatic cancer are often afraid that they will have unremitting, severe pain. Knowledge of these fears can help the physician to provide targeted reassurance (e.g., that pain will be aggressively treated).

Fear of Death

All individuals, regardless of their physical health, fear death at some time in their lives; the experience of physical illness often heightens that fear. Physicians must explore specific reasons for fear of death (e.g., a patient may fear death from childbirth because that occurred many years earlier to a close relative); identifying an irrationally high estimate of risk of death may lead to straightforward reassurance. Assessment of death anxiety also should include the opportunity for patients to discuss existential thoughts about dying (e.g., reflections about the meaning of one's life [Adelbratt and Strang 2000]). Physicians should assess for particular fears related to dying. For example, a patient may actually be at peace with dying but may be afraid that her family will not be able to survive without her. In that case, involvement of the patient's family may lead to reassurance and a more peaceful dying process (see also Chapter 39, "Palliative Care").

Anxiety About the Effect of Illness on Identity and Livelihood

Even if illness alone is not sufficient to cause anxiety, patients may be concerned about the potential effect of illness on their ability to work and perform household functions, and its financial impact. Uncertainties about medical reimbursement may make even insured individuals worried. Patients who are uninsured are often so anxious about how they or their families can pay for treatment that they decline treatment or avoid seeking health care. In these situations, meetings with family members, social workers, and financial counselors may help.

Anxiety About Strangers and Being Alone in the Hospital

Medically ill patients become anxious even when their own personal physician performs a medical procedure, so it is not surprising that acutely ill patients become intensely anxious when asked to trust their lives to physicians they have just met in the emergency department or ICU. Patients who are so anxious that they refuse treatment may be labeled as help-rejecting when fear is actually the underlying explanation. As noted by Muskin (1995), acceptance of the involvement of unfamiliar clinicians may be particularly difficult for individuals with preexisting problems with trust (e.g., those with paranoia or borderline personality disorder). Similarly, it is often difficult for some patients to tolerate being alone in the hospital. Because many individuals regress while hospitalized, it is not surprising that patients with dependency needs might become unduly anxious when left alone in an unfamiliar environment.

Anxiety About Negative Reactions From Physicians

Many patients worry about their physician's opinion of them. Excessive concern may lead to reluctance to seek health care. Those who feel guilty for not following their physician's recommendations might cancel appointments for fear of being scolded (e.g., for failure to lose weight, stop smoking, or check blood sugar levels more reliably). Similarly, some patients' anxiety might lead them to deny or fail to disclose important information (e.g., regarding sexual risk factors or level of alcohol intake). Anxiety may be particularly prominent among patients who have caused or aggravated their own illness. Physicians should be vigilant for clues that a patient might be experiencing excessive anxiety. Awareness of negative countertransference is essential; it is appropriate to provide consistent, firm reminders of the need for proper medical care, but excessive criticism is unwarranted and may contribute to poor adherence.

Treatment of Anxiety in the Medically Ill

Treatment of anxiety disorders has been shown to be safe and effective. Treatment of anxiety associated with medical illness can also improve physical symptoms, decrease disability, lower high rates of frequent medical use, and improve quality of life (Roy-Byrne et al. 2008). Most people with anxiety disorders seek care from their primary care physicians, complaining of the physical symptoms of anxiety such as pain, insomnia, or gastrointestinal distress, and often not recognizing the underlying emotional disorder. Collaboration between psychiatrists and primary care providers is important to ensure effective treatment. In a Cochrane review, collaborative care was found to be effective for anxiety (Archer et al. 2012). Several current models of collaborative care and stepped care interventions in primary care treatment of anxiety and depression show cost-effective outcomes and improved patient satisfaction (Katon et al. 2002; Simon et al. 2004; van't Veer-Tazelaar et al. 2009). Collaborative care for anxiety in primary care has been shown to be effective even in the presence of multiple medical comorbidities (Campbell-Sills et al. 2013).

Psychotherapy

An overemphasis on psychopharmacology in the care of medically ill patients sometimes results in overlooking the value of psychotherapy. The first step in treatment is to spend time listening to and talking with the patient. Just as in psychotherapy with any patient, empathic listening is a powerful tool to relieve distress. With medically ill patients, the goal is to help patients understand and discuss their emotional reactions to their illness so that they can then manage these feelings by using their own coping mechanisms. Psychotherapeutic approaches include supportive, cognitive-behavioral, and psychodynamic therapies.

Supportive Therapy

Supportive therapy involves listening and providing reassurance, sympathy, education about the medical process and the underlying illness, advice, and suggestions. The process includes listening for fears and misperceptions about illness or its treatment and giving patients appropriate information so that they can be as prepared as possible (House and Stark 2002). In supportive work, the psychotherapist promotes the patient's adaptive defenses and challenges only those defenses that are clearly maladaptive. It is also helpful to give patients as much choice in their treatment decisions as possible so that they feel they have some control over the course of their treatment.

Reassurance is an important skill that all physicians use in treating patients. In some highly anxious patients, however, simplistic reassurance can actually cause increased anxiety and lead to a cycle of maladaptive behavior. For example, if a patient who has been told that a procedure is "nothing to worry about" subsequently experiences pain or untoward results, the resulting anxiety can lead to more reassurance-seeking behavior, mistrust, and decreased cooperation. Many anxious patients tend to interpret bodily symptoms as evidence of serious disease, and as a result, they may seek multiple consultations for reassurance. Understanding the patient's beliefs, concerns, and perceptions can be helpful in challenging misperceptions, educating the patient about his or her illness, and devising a realistic plan to monitor symptoms. Having a realistic plan to help patients differentiate minor symptoms from those that may need medical attention will reduce anxiety and decrease the excessive need for reassurance (Stark and House 2000). It is also important that the physician not assume that a patient's anxiety is due to fear of dying. When reassurance is directed at the wrong fear, it may accentuate anxiety and lead patients to believe that their physician does not understand them.

Another important aspect of supportive therapy is the involvement of the patient's support system of family, friends, and spiritual/religious community. Some patients may need assistance in expanding their support network (e.g., to reach out to friends with whom they may have lost contact). Some family members may need supportive psychotherapy to reduce their anxieties about the patient's medical condition. Hospital staff such as nurses and chaplains can be instrumental in reducing the patient's fears.

Patients confronting life-threatening or terminal illnesses such as cancer may experience death anxiety (Yalom 1980). Open discussions with patients about death help to reduce anxiety and distress (Spiegel et al. 1981), and psychological interventions alone can help patients manage their death anxiety (Payne and Massie 2000). Maintaining hope is an important aspect of minimizing anxiety, although the primary goal can change from full recovery to having more time for specific short-term accomplishments. Helping patients find meaning and value in their lives, despite their illness and suffering, helps to relieve emotional distress (Frankl 1987). For example, anxiety can be reduced when patients see that they are still important to their families or that they still have unfinished business to address. Dignity-oriented therapy has extended this approach to the care of terminally ill patients (Thompson and Chochinov 2008). The hospice movement has been instrumental in helping provide relief for many patients (Byock 1997). (See Chapter 39, "Palliative Care," for further discussion.)

Supportive group interventions have been shown to be effective in reducing anxiety and distress in medically ill individuals. They can be quite helpful in providing emotional support, improving coping skills, and providing information about health promotion and wellness (Sherman et al. 2007). Internet support groups can also be extremely beneficial. See Chapter 37 ("Psychotherapy") for further discussion and Brenner (2012) for a general reference on supportive psychotherapy.

Cognitive-Behavioral Therapy

Cognitive-behavioral therapy (CBT) has been proven to be as effective as medication in treating many anxiety disorders, including GAD, PTSD, and panic disorder ("Generalized Anxiety Disorder: Toxic Worry" 2003; Stanley et al. 2009). It has been shown to be effective for anxiety and depression symptoms in primary care (Twomey et al. 2015). Cognitive techniques are used to uncover and correct misinterpretations and irrational thoughts that lead to increased anxiety and distress. Behavioral techniques can be used to help overcome fears that can interfere with effective treatment, such as claustrophobia during MRI (Munn and Jordan 2012). A brief course of CBT can have long-lasting effects, but occasional "booster" sessions may be needed.

A variety of therapies that involve teaching self-awareness and self-regulation of body functions have been found effective in reducing anxiety and physical symptoms in medically ill patients. These include muscle relaxation techniques (e.g., Jacobson's progressive muscle relaxation), autogenic training (e.g., biofeedback, which uses technology to control internal processes), and relaxation techniques (e.g., meditation, breathing exercises, self-hypnosis). Stress management interventions may improve quality of life (e.g., by decreasing anxiety in the course of medical treatments [Antoni et al. 2006]). Relaxation techniques may help to wean patients from the ventilator as well as to reduce dyspnea and anxiety in patients with COPD (Volpato et al. 2015). A review of studies that have examined efficacy of meditation and relaxation techniques indicates that these techniques are safe and may have some benefit in reducing anxiety in medically ill patients (Arias et al. 2006).

Mindfulness-based stress reduction is widely utilized to improve well-being among patients with many medical and psychiatric problems. Often given in a group format, it may incorporate mindfulness meditation, body scanning, and yoga. This approach has been shown to be effective for patients with medical conditions, including chronic pain and cancer (Gotink et al. 2015; Piet et al. 2012).

Psychodynamic Therapy

For patients who are not too ill and who have sufficient emotional resilience, brief dynamic psychotherapy can be useful in uncovering the conscious and unconscious meaning of the illness to the patient. Understanding patients' developmental history, interpersonal dynamics, and defense mechanisms can help the psychiatrist to assist them in finding healthier ways to cope with medical illness (Viederman 2000). What coping strategies have helped in the past? When did the individual feel most fulfilled in his or her life? How can those memories and skills be used now, even in the presence of significant medical illness? Psychotherapy can uncover areas leading to increased distress, such as real or imagined guilt, unhealthy coping strategies such as avoidance and denial, and recognition of past conflicted relationships that may be repeated in the current doctor–patient relationship. An understanding of the patient's underlying dynamics can help identify and resolve conflicts with the treatment team that may be interfering with recovery. An understanding of psychodynamic principles can also help psychiatrists in working with the primary treatment team that is caring for the anxious patient.

Countertransference reactions can cause problems for care providers of anxious patients. For example, physicians may overidentify with their patients, leading to frustration because of lack of progress or poor prognosis. As a result, they may then overcompensate by offering excessive reassurance, or they may minimize or overlook symptoms in an unconscious attempt to reduce their own anxiety. Caregivers also may become withdrawn and distant, providing care mechanically with little empathy or awareness of the emotional needs of the patient. Psychiatrists can play a role in helping the health care team to be cognizant of these defenses so that they do not interfere with the provision of optimal patient care. (See Chapter 37, "Psychotherapy," for further discussion of psychotherapy for the medically ill.)

Pharmacotherapy

Psychotherapeutic techniques are often not sufficient to manage anxiety in the medically ill. An increasingly broad range of psychopharmacological agents can be used safely with this population. (For further details, see Chapter 36, "Psychopharmacology," as well as discussions in the context of specific diseases in Chapters 17–35.) The risks in pregnancy of each of the drug classes reviewed here are discussed in Chapter 31, "Obstetrics and Gynecology."

Benzodiazepines and Hypnotics

For acute anxiety symptoms, the most immediately effective and frequently used agents are the benzodiazepines (Table 10–2). Diazepam and chlordiazepoxide were among the first of these to be used. They also have established efficacy for other conditions (e.g., diazepam as an anticonvulsant and muscle relaxant and chlordiazepoxide for alcohol detoxification). Newer benzodiazepines have better safety profiles and shorter half-lives, so they tend to be used more frequently.

Alprazolam works rapidly and is eliminated quickly, but as a result there may be rebound anxiety and withdrawal symptoms. Because lorazepam can be given orally, intravenously, or intramuscularly and does not have an active metabolite, it is often a preferred medication in hospitalized patients. Lorazepam can be given in an intravenous bolus or drip, but as doses increase to provide sedation and treat delirium tremens, respiratory status must be watched closely. Lorazepam and oxazepam are metabolized through conjugation, and temazepam is metabolized almost exclusively through conjugation (Trevor and Way 2007). As a result, those benzodiazepines may be less problematic in patients with liver disease than are other benzodiazepines, which are oxidatively metabolized (Crone et al. 2006). Midazolam, a benzodiazepine with a very short half-life that can only be given intravenously or intramuscularly, is used for short-term procedures such as bone marrow biopsies, endoscopies, and MRI scans in claustrophobic patients. For patients who need long-term benzodiazepines, it is often helpful to change to a medication with a longer half-life, such as clonazepam.

All benzodiazepines can cause excessive sedation. They may also cause motor and cognitive disturbances, especially in older persons and individuals with impaired cognition (due to, e.g., dementia, head injury, or intellectual disabilities). Therefore, they should be used with caution, if at all, in these patients. Anxiety in delirious patients may be better treated with antipsychotics than with benzodiazepines (Breitbart et al. 1996), but data are sparse (e.g., in palliative care [Candy et al. 2012]). Benzodiazepines can cause respiratory suppression, so they should be used cautiously in persons with pulmonary disease who retain carbon dioxide or in patients with severe sleep apnea. All benzodiazepines can lead to tolerance and dependence, so they should be avoided or used judiciously (e.g., for detoxification) in persons with a substance abuse history. It is important to use extreme caution in prescribing benzodiazepines to patients on long-term opiates, because the combination may lead to respiratory depression and death (U.S. Food and Drug Administration 2016). In persons who are conscientious and do not have a history of chemical dependence, benzodiazepines often can be used safely for years without causing problems or tolerance. Their risks should be reevaluated as patients age. Similarly, long-term benzodiazepine use may need to be reduced or discontinued among patients who develop specific medical conditions (e.g., advanced liver disease, dementia, COPD, cerebellar dysfunction).

Hypnotics are commonly used in medically ill patients who are kept awake by their anxiety (see Chapter 14, "Sleep Disorders").

TABLE 10–2.   Selected benzodiazepines used for anxiety in the medically ill

Medication	Route of administration	Dosage	Elimination half-life (hours)	Comments
Alprazolam	Oral	0.5–6 mg daily	12–15	Rapid onset. Interdose withdrawal a problem; lower risk with extended-release.
Chlordiazepoxide	Oral, intramuscular	5–25 mg qid	28–100 (including metabolites)	Useful for alcohol withdrawal.
Clonazepam	Oral	0.25–1 mg bid–tid	18–50	Also used for absence seizures, periodic leg movements, and neuropathic pain.
Diazepam	Oral, intravenous	2–10 mg bid–qid	30–100 (including metabolites)	Also used as anticonvulsant and muscle relaxant.
Lorazepam	Oral, intramuscular, intravenous	0.5–2.0 mg up to qid	10–20	Intravenous availability is an advantage. Metabolized by conjugation. Also approved for chemotherapy-related nausea and vomiting.
Midazolam	Intramuscular, intravenous	Intramuscular: 5 mg single dose Intravenous: 0.02–0.04 mg/kg	1–4	Used for preoperative sedation and intravenous induction.
Oxazepam	Oral	10–30 mg tid–qid	5–20	Metabolized by conjugation. May also be useful for alcohol withdrawal.

Note.   bid=twice a day; qid=four times a day; tid=three times a day.

Source.   Adapted from Procyshyn et al. 2015; Epocrates Drug Reference (https://online.epocrates.com).

Antidepressants

The pharmacological first-line treatments for GAD, panic disorder, PTSD, OCD, and social anxiety disorder are the selective serotonin reuptake inhibitors (SSRIs): fluoxetine, sertraline, paroxetine, citalopram, escitalopram. Fluvoxamine should be avoided because of its multiple drug–drug interactions. These medications have few side effects and therefore are generally quite safe for the medically ill; they do not result in cardiac conduction problems, orthostatic hypotension, or physical dependence. Because antidepressants may take 2–6 weeks to relieve anxiety, the patient may need initial treatment with benzodiazepines. Once the patient has been stabilized on the antidepressant, the benzodiazepines usually can be gradually withdrawn without recurrence of anxiety. The SSRI should be used for at least 3–6 months before it is stopped, and it should be tapered to avoid discontinuation symptoms. SSRIs can be used safely on a long-term basis if the anxiety disorder relapses.

The potential for drug interactions is important in the medically ill; fluoxetine and paroxetine are cytochrome P450 2D6 inhibitors, and fluvoxamine inhibits 1A2, 3A4, and 2D6. For medically ill patients taking multiple medications, the SSRIs with the fewest drug interactions—sertraline, citalopram, and escitalopram—are preferred.

Serotonin–norepinephrine reuptake inhibitors (SNRIs), including venlafaxine, duloxetine, and desvenlafaxine, also may be useful for anxiety (Katzman et al. 2014). Venlafaxine and duloxetine have been approved for treatment of some anxiety disorders and, based on their mechanism of action, are probably effective agents for treating all anxiety disorders.

Mirtazapine—an alpha-adrenergic receptor antagonist and an antagonist at serotonin 5-HT_{2A}, 5-HT_{2C}, and 5-HT_3 receptors—may be helpful in reducing anxiety. It may be particularly useful in selected medically ill patients for two reasons: 1) it has few drug interactions, and 2) its side effects of sedation and increased appetite may be helpful in patients who have insomnia and anorexia with weight loss (Cankurtaran et al. 2008). Tricyclic antidepressants (TCAs) and monoamine oxidase inhibitors (MAOIs) are well established as effective treatments for anxiety disorders and for depression. They carry greater risks in the medically ill but have particular useful niches (e.g., TCAs in diarrhea-predominant irritable bowel syndrome, and MAOIs in Parkinson's disease). The main reasons these medications are currently not used frequently as first-line treatment are their numerous side effects and their toxicity in overdose.

Antipsychotics

Antipsychotic medications are not approved for the treatment of anxiety, although limited data support their efficacy (Kreys and Phan 2015). Consultation-liaison psychiatrists often find them to be efficacious and safe to use in the short term for selected medical populations. Because antipsychotics do not cause confusion or respiratory compromise, they may be preferable to benzodiazepines for the more severe anxiety associated with agitation or delirium or in patients with respiratory compromise. For example, antipsychotics may be helpful in assisting the anxious patient who is being weaned from a ventilator (Rosenthal et al. 2007). The antipsychotic used most often in medically ill patients is haloperidol, which can be given orally, intramuscularly, or intravenously. If a high-potency typical antipsychotic such as haloperidol is used in treating anxiety, it is important to monitor for akathisia, because it can be mistaken for worsening anxiety.

Atypical antipsychotics such as olanzapine, risperidone, quetiapine, ziprasidone, and aripiprazole are also used selectively in the management of anxiety, especially in lower doses. Ziprasidone, olanzapine, and aripiprazole are available in intramuscular formulation. The intramuscular formulations may be helpful in those with severe anxiety or agitation, especially if they are unable to take oral medications. Olanzapine, risperidone, and aripiprazole are available as orally disintegrating tablets, which may be useful for patients who cannot swallow pills.

Buspirone

Buspirone is a partial serotonin agonist that may be effective in the treatment of anxiety (Lee et al. 2005). It may be useful in treating anxiety in medically ill patients because it has few drug interactions and does not cause respiratory depression. It can be used safely in patients with substance use disorders because it does not cause dependence, and its metabolism is not greatly affected by liver disease. The main drawbacks with buspirone are that it may take 2–4 weeks to become effective, and its benefits are modest.

Beta-Blockers

Beta-adrenergic blockers produce anxiolytic effects by blocking autonomic hyperarousal (elevated pulse, elevated blood pressure, sweating, tremors) associated with anxiety. They work best for specific anxiety-producing situations, such as performance anxiety and public speaking. All beta-blockers are contraindicated in persons with asthma or COPD (Dulohery et al. 2016). Patients with type 1 diabetes should not be prescribed nonselective beta-blockers because they block the sympathetic nervous system response to hypoglycemia, resulting in lack of awareness of symptoms (Kaplan 2007). Beta-blockers are not likely to cause depression, but there may be some risk with lipophilic ones like propranolol (Verbeek et al. 2011).

Antihistamines

Sedating histamine H_1 receptor blockers are sometimes used to treat anxiety and insomnia. Hydroxyzine may be effective for generalized anxiety (Guaiana et al. 2010) and is preferred over other antihistamines because it does not have anticholinergic effects. Diphenhydramine, which is often used to treat insomnia, is available in over-the-counter preparations. Because these medications are not addictive, many physicians consider them to be benign. However, they can cause dizziness, excessive sedation, incoordination, and confusion, especially when used with alcohol or other CNS depressants. Elderly patients and those with brain disease or injury are more sensitive to these medications and may become delirious even with low doses. Despite these risks, these medications are still an option when benzodiazepines must be avoided because of concerns about dependence or respiratory depression.

Anticonvulsants

Anticonvulsants may be beneficial for some individuals with anxiety. Divalproex sodium may be helpful in calming agitated, anxious patients, especially those with brain injury, intellectual disability, or dementia. Gabapentin and pregabalin have shown some promise in treating anxiety symptoms and may prove to have some role in treating anxiety in medically ill patients (Generoso et al. 2017; Lavigne et al. 2012) They may be particularly helpful in individuals with coexisting neuropathic pain.

Conclusion

The experience of medical illness often leads to clinically significant anxiety symptoms. Although many individuals with medical illnesses have anxiety disorders, these disorders are often underrecognized and undertreated. Both psychotherapy and pharmacotherapy can significantly ameliorate anxiety symptoms, even among patients with severe medical problems. Thus, careful assessment and treatment of anxiety disorders are important components of the psychiatric care of the medically ill.

References

Abbey G, Thompson SB, Hickish T, et al: A meta-analysis of prevalence rates and moderating factors for cancer-related post-traumatic stress disorder. Psychooncology 24(4):371–381, 2015 25146298

Adelbratt S, Strang P: Death anxiety in brain tumour patients and their spouses. Palliat Med 14(6):499–507, 2000 11219880

Ahmadi N, Hajsadeghi F, Mirshkarlo HB, et al: Post-traumatic stress disorder, coronary atherosclerosis, and mortality. Am J Cardiol 108(1):29–33, 2011 21530936

American Psychiatric Association: Diagnostic and Statistical Manual of Mental Disorders, 5th Edition. Arlington, VA, American Psychiatric Association, 2013

Antoni MH, Wimberly SR, Lechner SC, et al: Reduction of cancer-specific thought intrusions and anxiety symptoms with a stress management intervention among women undergoing treatment for breast cancer. Am J Psychiatry 163(10):1791–1797, 2006 17012691

Archer J, Bower P, Gilbody S, et al: Collaborative care for depression and anxiety problems. Cochrane Database Syst Rev (10):CD006525, 2012 23076925

Arias AJ, Steinberg K, Banga A, et al: Systematic review of the efficacy of meditation techniques as treatments for medical illness. J Altern Complement Med 12(8):817–832, 2006 17034289

Batty GD, Russ TC, Stamatakis E, Kivimäki M: Psychological distress in relation to site specific cancer mortality: pooling of unpublished data from 16 prospective cohort studies. BMJ 356:j108, 2017 28122812

Bjelland I, Dahl AA, Haug TT, et al: The validity of the Hospital Anxiety and Depression Scale. An updated literature review. J Psychosom Res 52(2):69–77, 2002 11832252

Brandt C, Mula M: Anxiety disorders in people with epilepsy. Epilepsy Behav 59:87–91, 2016 27116536

Breitbart W, Marotta R, Platt MM, et al: A double-blind trial of haloperidol, chlorpromazine, and lorazepam in the treatment of delirium in hospitalized AIDS patients. Am J Psychiatry 153(2):231–237, 1996 8561204

Brenner AM: Teaching supportive psychotherapy in the twenty-first century. Harv Rev Psychiatry 20(5):259–267, 2012 23030214

Bringager CB, Friis S, Arnesen H, et al: Nine-year follow-up of panic disorder in chest pain patients: clinical course and predictors of outcome. Gen Hosp Psychiatry 30(2):138–146, 2008 18291295

Broen MP, Narayen NE, Kuijf ML, et al: Prevalence of anxiety in Parkinson's disease: a systematic review and meta-analysis. Mov Disord 31(8):1125–1133, 2016 27125963

Brunton L, Chabner B, Knollman B (eds): Goodman and Gilman's The Pharmacological Basis of Therapeutics, 12th Edition. New York, McGraw-Hill Medical, 2011

Burstein M, Georgiades K, He JP, et al: Specific phobia among U.S. adolescents: phenomenology and typology. Depress Anxiety 29(12):1072–1082, 2012 23108894

Byock I: Dying Well: The Prospect for Growth at the End of Life. New York, Riverhead Books, 1997

Campbell-Sills L, Stein MB, Sherbourne CD, et al: Effects of medical comorbidity on anxiety treatment outcomes in primary care. Psychosom Med 75(8):713–720, 2013 23886736

Candy B, Jackson KC, Jones L, et al: Drug therapy for symptoms associated with anxiety in adult palliative care patients. Cochrane Database Syst Rev (10):CD004596, 2012 23076905

Cankurtaran ES, Ozalp E, Soygur H, et al: Mirtazapine improves sleep and lowers anxiety and depression in cancer patients: superiority over imipramine. Support Care Cancer 16(11):1291–1298, 2008 18299900

Celano CM, Daunis DJ, Lokko HN, et al: Anxiety Disorders and Cardiovascular Disease. Curr Psychiatry Rep 18(11):101, 2016 27671918

Crone CC, Gabriel GM, DiMartini A: An overview of psychiatric issues in liver disease for the consultation-liaison psychiatrist. Psychosomatics 47(3):188–205, 2006 16684936

Davydow DS, Gifford JM, Desai SV, et al: Posttraumatic stress disorder in general intensive care unit survivors: a systematic review. Gen Hosp Psychiatry 30(5):421–434, 2008 18774425

Davydow DS, Lease ED, Reyes JD: Posttraumatic stress disorder in organ transplant recipients: a systematic review. Gen Hosp Psychiatry 37(5):387–398, 2015 26073159

Dickerman AL, Barnhill JW: Abnormal thyroid function tests in psychiatric patients: a red herring? Am J Psychiatry 169(2):127–133, 2012 22318794

DiMatteo MR, Lepper HS, Croghan TW: Depression is a risk factor for noncompliance with medical treatment: meta-analysis of the effects of anxiety and depression on patient adherence. Arch Intern Med 160(14):2101–2107, 2000 10904452

Drugs that may cause psychiatric symptoms. Med Lett Drugs Ther 50(1301–1302):100–103, quiz 2, 104, 2008 19078866

Dulohery MM, Maldonado F, Limper AH: Drug-induced pulmonary disease, in Murray and Nadel's Textbook of Respiratory Medicine, 6th Edition. Edited by Broaddus VC, Mason RJ, Ernst JD. Philadelphia, PA, Elsevier Saunders, 2016, pp 1275–1294

Frankl V: Man's Search for Meaning. London, Hoddard-Stoughton, 1987

Fuller-Thomson E, Lacombe-Duncan A: Understanding the association between chronic obstructive pulmonary disease and current anxiety: a population-based study. COPD 13(5):622–631, 2016 26830204

Gander ML, von Känel R: Myocardial infarction and post-traumatic stress disorder: frequency, outcome, and atherosclerotic mechanisms. Eur J Cardiovasc Prev Rehabil 13(2):165–172, 2006 16575268

García-Llana H, Remor E, Del Peso G, et al: The role of depression, anxiety, stress and adherence to treatment in dialysis patients' health-related quality of life: a systematic review of the literature. Nefrologia 34(5):637–657, 2014 25259819

Generalized anxiety disorder: toxic worry. Harv Ment Health Lett 19(7):1–5, 2003 12543599

Generoso MB, Trevizol AP, Kasper S, et al: Pregabalin for generalized anxiety disorder: an updated systematic review and meta-analysis. Int Clin Psychopharmacol 32(1):49–55, 2017 27643884

Gotink RA, Chu P, Busschbach JJ, et al: Standardised mindfulness-based interventions in healthcare: an overview of systematic reviews and meta-analyses of RCTs (Electronic Resource). PLoS One 10(4):e0124344, 2015 25881019

Green BL, Epstein SA, Krupnick JL, et al: Trauma and medical illness: assessing trauma-related disorders in medical settings, in Assessing Psychological Trauma and PTSD. Edited by Wilson JP, Keane TM. New York, Guilford, 1997, pp 160–191

Greene T, Neria Y, Gross R: Prevalence, detection and correlates of PTSD in the primary care setting: a systematic review. J Clin Psychol Med Settings 23(2):160–180, 2016 26868222

Gregg RA, Rawls SM: Behavioral pharmacology of designer cathinones: a review of the preclinical literature. Life Sci 97(1):27–30, 2014 24231450

Guaiana G, Barbui C, Cipriani A: Hydroxyzine for generalised anxiety disorder. Cochrane Database Syst Rev (12):CD006815, 2010 21154375

Gulseren S, Gulseren L, Hekimsoy Z, et al: Depression, anxiety, health-related quality of life, and disability in patients with overt and subclinical thyroid dysfunction. Arch Med Res 37(1):133–139, 2006 16314199

Gunderson EW, Haughey HM, Ait-Daoud N, et al: "Spice" and "K2" herbal highs: a case series and systematic review of the clinical effects and biopsychosocial implications of synthetic cannabinoid use in humans. Am J Addict 21(4):320–326, 2012 22691010

Harman JS, Rollman BL, Hanusa BH, et al: Physician office visits of adults for anxiety disorders in the United States, 1985–1998. J Gen Intern Med 17(3):165–172, 2002 11929501

Hatch R, McKechnie S, Griffiths J: Psychological intervention to prevent ICU-related PTSD: who, when and for how long? Crit Care 15(2):141, 2011 21542870

Herr NR, Williams JW Jr, Benjamin S, et al: Does this patient have generalized anxiety or panic disorder? The Rational Clinical Examination systematic review. JAMA 312(1):78–84, 2014 25058220

House A, Stark D: Anxiety in medical patients. BMJ 325(7357):207–209, 2002 12142312

Iacovides A, Fountoulakis KN, Grammaticos P, et al: Difference in symptom profile between generalized anxiety disorder and anxiety secondary to hyperthyroidism. Int J Psychiatry Med 30(1):71–81, 2000 10900562

Jones GN, Ames SC, Jeffries SK, et al: Utilization of medical services and quality of life among low-income patients with generalized anxiety disorder attending primary care clinics. Int J Psychiatry Med 31(2):183–198, 2001 11760862

Kahana RJ, Bibring GL: Personality types in medical management, in Psychiatry and Medical Practice in a General Hospital. Edited by Zinberg N. New York, International Universities Press, 1964, pp 108–123

Kangas M: DSM-5 trauma and stress-related disorders: implications for screening for cancer-related stress. Front Psychiatry 4:122, 2013 24106482

Kaplan N: Systemic hypertension: therapy, in Braunwald's Heart Disease: A Textbook of Cardiovascular Medicine, 8th Edition. Edited by Libby P, Bonow RO, Mann DL, et al. Philadelphia, PA, WB Saunders, 2007, pp 1049–1068

Katon WJ, Roy-Byrne P, Russo J, et al: Cost-effectiveness and cost offset of a collaborative care intervention for primary care patients with panic disorder. Arch Gen Psychiatry 59(12):1098–1104, 2002 12470125

Katzman MA, Bleau P, Blier P, et al; Canadian Anxiety Guidelines Initiative Group on behalf of the Anxiety Disorders Association of Canada/Association Canadienne des troubles anxieux and McGill University: Canadian clinical practice guidelines for the management of anxiety, posttraumatic stress and obsessive-compulsive disorders. BMC Psychiatry 14 (suppl 1):S1, 2014 25081580

Kessler RC, Ormel J, Demler O, et al: Comorbid mental disorders account for the role impairment of commonly occurring chronic physical disorders: results from the National Comorbidity Survey. J Occup Environ Med 45(12):1257–1266, 2003 14665811

Kessler RC, Petukhova M, Sampson NA, et al: Twelve-month and lifetime prevalence and lifetime morbid risk of anxiety and mood disorders in the United States. Int J Methods Psychiatr Res 21(3):169–184, 2012 22865617

Ketterer MW, Knysz W, Khandelwal A, et al: Healthcare utilization and emotional distress in coronary artery disease patients. Psychosomatics 51(4):297–301, 2010 20587757

Kim HF, Yudofsky SC, Hales RE, et al: Neuropsychiatric aspects of seizure disorders, in The American Psychiatric Publishing Textbook of Neuropsychiatry and Behavioral Neurosciences. Edited by Yudofsky SC, Hales RE. Washington, DC, American Psychiatric Publishing, 2007, pp 649–676

Kreys TJ, Phan SV: A literature review of quetiapine for generalized anxiety disorder. Pharmacotherapy 35(2):175–188, 2015 25689246

Kroenke K, Spitzer RL, Williams JB, et al: Anxiety disorders in primary care: prevalence, impairment, comorbidity, and detection. Ann Intern Med 146(5):317–325, 2007 17339617

Kroenke K, Spitzer RL, Williams JB, et al: An ultra-brief screening scale for anxiety and depression: the PHQ-4. Psychosomatics 50(6):613–621, 2009 19996233

Kumano H, Kaiya H, Yoshiuchi K, et al: Comorbidity of irritable bowel syndrome, panic disorder, and agoraphobia in a Japanese representative sample. Am J Gastroenterol 99(2):370–376, 2004 15046231

Kwon OY, Park SP: Depression and anxiety in people with epilepsy. J Clin Neurol 10(3):175–188, 2014 25045369

Ladwig KH, Baumert J, Marten-Mittag B, et al: Posttraumatic stress symptoms and predicted mortality in patients with implantable cardioverter-defibrillators: results from the prospective living with an implanted cardioverter-defibrillator study. Arch Gen Psychiatry 65(11):1324–1330, 2008 18981344

Lavigne JE, Heckler C, Mathews JL, et al: A randomized, controlled, double-blinded clinical trial of gabapentin 300 versus 900 mg versus placebo for anxiety symptoms in breast cancer survivors. Breast Cancer Res Treat 136(2):479–486, 2012 23053645

Lee ST, Park JH, Kim M: Efficacy of the 5-HT1A agonist, buspirone hydrochloride, in migraineurs with anxiety: a randomized, prospective, parallel group, double-blind, placebo-controlled study. Headache 45(8):1004–1011, 2005 16109114

Lee YC, Lee CT, Lai YR, et al: Association of asthma and anxiety: a nationwide population-based study in Taiwan. J Affect Disord 189:98–105, 2016 26432033

Leibovici V, Koran LM, Murad S, et al: Excoriation (skin-picking) disorder in adults: a cross-cultural survey of Israeli Jewish and Arab samples. Compr Psychiatry 58:102–107, 2015 25682319

Maier W, Gänsicke M, Freyberger HJ, et al: Generalized anxiety disorder (ICD-10) in primary care from a cross-cultural perspective: a valid diagnostic entity? Acta Psychiatr Scand 101(1):29–36, 2000 10674948

Merikangas KR, Stevens DE: Comorbidity of migraine and psychiatric disorders. Neurol Clin 15(1):115–123, 1997 9058400

Micoulaud-Franchi JA, Lagarde S, Barkate G, et al: Rapid detection of generalized anxiety disorder and major depression in epilepsy: validation of the GAD-7 as a complementary tool to the NDDI-E in a French sample. Epilepsy Behav 57(Pt A):211–216, 2016 26694447

Montserrat-Capdevila J, Godoy P, Marsal JR, et al: Overview of the impact of depression and anxiety in chronic obstructive pulmonary disease. Lung 195(1):77–85, 2017 27900466

Munn Z, Jordan Z: The effectiveness of interventions to reduce anxiety, claustrophobia, sedation and non-completion rates of patients undergoing high technology medical imaging. JBI Library Syst Rev 10(19):1122–1185, 2012 27820328

Muskin PR: The medical hospital, in Psychodynamic Concepts in General Psychiatry. Edited by Schwartz HJ. Washington, DC, American Psychiatric Press, 1995, pp 69–88

Napp AE, Enders J, Roehle R, et al: Analysis and prediction of claustrophobia during MR imaging with the Claustrophobia Questionnaire: an observational prospective 18-month single-center study of 6500 patients. Radiology 283(1):148–157, 2017 27892781

Payne D, Massie MJ: Anxiety in palliative care, in Handbook of Psychiatry in Palliative Medicine. Edited by Chochinov HM, Breitbart W. New York, Oxford University Press, 2000, pp 63–74

Piet J, Würtzen H, Zachariae R: The effect of mindfulness-based therapy on symptoms of anxiety and depression in adult cancer patients and survivors: a systematic review and meta-analysis. J Consult Clin Psychol 80(6):1007–1020, 2012 22563637

Procyshyn RM, Bezchlibnyk-Butler KZ, Jeffries J: Benzodiazepines, in Clinical Handbook of Psychotropic Drugs, 21st Edition. Boston, MA, Hogrefe & Huber, 2015, pp 199–211

Rosenthal LJ, Kim V, Kim DR: Weaning from prolonged mechanical ventilation using an antipsychotic agent in a patient with acute stress disorder. Crit Care Med 35(10):2417–2419, 2007 17948335

Roy-Byrne PP, Stein MB, Russo J, et al: Panic disorder in the primary care setting: comorbidity, disability, service utilization, and treatment. J Clin Psychiatry 60(7):492–499, quiz 500, 1999 10453807

Roy-Byrne PP, Davidson KW, Kessler RC, et al: Anxiety disorders and comorbid medical illness. Gen Hosp Psychiatry 30(3):208–225, 2008 18433653

Sait Gönen M, Kisakol G, Savas Cilli A, et al: Assessment of anxiety in subclinical thyroid disorders. Endocr J 51(3):311–315, 2004 15256776

Sareen J, Jacobi F, Cox BJ, et al: Disability and poor quality of life associated with comorbid anxiety disorders and physical conditions. Arch Intern Med 166(19):2109–2116, 2006 17060541

Seng JS, Clark MK, McCarthy AM, et al: PTSD and physical comorbidity among women receiving Medicaid: results from service-use data. J Trauma Stress 19(1):45–56, 2006 16568470

Sherbourne CD, Wells KB, Meredith LS, et al: Comorbid anxiety disorder and the functioning and well-being of chronically ill patients of general medical providers. Arch Gen Psychiatry 53(10):889–895, 1996 8857865

Sherman AC, Pennington J, Latif U, et al: Patient preferences regarding cancer group psychotherapy interventions: a view from the inside. Psychosomatics 48(5):426–432, 2007 17878502

Simon GE, Ludman EJ, Tutty S, et al: Telephone psychotherapy and telephone care management for primary care patients starting antidepressant treatment: a randomized controlled trial. JAMA 292(8):935–942, 2004 15328325

Spiegel D, Bloom JR, Yalom I: Group support for patients with metastatic cancer. A randomized outcome study. Arch Gen Psychiatry 38(5):527–533, 1981 7235853

Stanley MA, Wilson NL, Novy DM, et al: Cognitive behavior therapy for generalized anxiety disorder among older adults in primary care: a randomized clinical trial. JAMA 301(14):1460–1467, 2009 19351943

Stark DP, House A: Anxiety in cancer patients. Br J Cancer 83(10):1261–1267, 2000 11044347

Strain JJ, Grossman S: Psychological Care of the Medically Ill. New York, Appleton-Century-Crofts, 1975

Stundner O, Kirksey M, Chiu YL, et al: Demographics and perioperative outcome in patients with depression and anxiety undergoing total joint arthroplasty: a population-based study. Psychosomatics 54(2):149–157, 2013 23194934

Sugaya N, Kaiya H, Kumano H, Nomura S: Relationship between subtypes of irritable bowel syndrome and severity of symptoms associated with panic disorder. Scand J Gastroenterol 43(6):675–681, 2008 18569984

Tapson VF: Pulmonary embolism, in Cecil Textbook of Medicine, 23rd Edition. Edited by Goldman L, Ausiello D. Philadelphia, PA, WB Saunders, 2007, pp 688–695

Thompson GN, Chochinov HM: Dignity-based approaches in the care of terminally ill patients. Curr Opin Support Palliat Care 2(1):49–53, 2008 18685395

Torelli P, D'Amico D: An updated review of migraine and co-morbid psychiatric disorders. Neurol Sci 25 (suppl 3):S234–S235, 2004 15549545

Trevor AJ, Way WL: Sedative-hypnotic drugs, in Basic and Clinical Pharmacology, 10th Edition. Edited by Katzung BG. New York, McGraw-Hill, 2007, pp 347–362

Tully PJ, Cosh SM: Generalized anxiety disorder prevalence and comorbidity with depression in coronary heart disease: a meta-analysis. J Health Psychol 18(12):1601–1616, 2013 23300050

Twomey C, O'Reilly G, Byrne M: Effectiveness of cognitive behavioural therapy for anxiety and depression in primary care: a meta-analysis. Fam Pract 32(1):3–15, 2015 25248976

U.S. Food and Drug Administration: FDA Drug Safety Communication: FDA warns about serious risks and death when combining opioid pain or cough medicines with benzodiazepines; requires its strongest warning. Safety Announcement 8/31/2016. Available at: https://www.fda.gov/Drugs/DrugSafety/ucm518473.htm. Accessed June 23, 2017.

van't Veer-Tazelaar PJ, van Marwijk HW, van Oppen P, et al: Stepped-care prevention of anxiety and depression in late life: a randomized controlled trial. Arch Gen Psychiatry 66(3):297–304, 2009 19255379

Verbeek DE, van Riezen J, de Boer RA, et al: A review on the putative association between beta-blockers and depression. Heart Fail Clin 7(1):89–99, 2011 21109212

Viederman M: The supportive relationship, the psychodynamic narrative, and the dying patient, in Handbook of Psychiatry in Palliative Medicine. Edited by Chochinov HM, Breitbart W. New York, Oxford University Press, 2000, pp 215–222

Volpato E, Banfi P, Rogers SM, et al: Relaxation techniques for people with chronic obstructive pulmonary disease: a systematic review and a meta-analysis. Evid Based Complement Alternat Med 2015:628365, 2015 26339268

Wen MC, Chan LL, Tan LC, et al: Depression, anxiety, and apathy in Parkinson's disease: insights from neuroimaging studies. Eur J Neurol 23(6):1001–1019, 2016 27141858

Wiltink J, Tschan R, Michal M, et al: Dizziness: anxiety, health care utilization and health behavior—results from a representative German community survey. J Psychosom Res 66(5):417–424, 2009 19379958

Wittchen HU, Kessler RC, Beesdo K, et al: Generalized anxiety and depression in primary care: prevalence, recognition, and management. J Clin Psychiatry 63 (suppl 8):24–34, 2002 12044105

Yalom I: Death and Dying. New York, Basic Books, 1980

Zaubler TS, Katon W: Panic disorder in the general medical setting. J Psychosom Res 44(1):25–42, 1998 9483462

CHAPTER 11

Somatic Symptom Disorder and Illness Anxiety Disorder

Peter Henningsen, M.D.

Somatic symptom disorder and *illness anxiety disorder* are diagnostic categories that were newly introduced in the fifth edition of the *Diagnostic and Statistical Manual of Mental Disorders* (DSM-5; American Psychiatric Association 2013). Although the categories are new, they refer to a well-known clinical profile with high relevance in all areas of medicine: patients who suffer from bodily distress over and beyond what would be expected from their documented organic disease and/or who express high health anxiety. Related disorders such as conversion disorder (functional neurological symptom disorder) and functional somatic syndromes are covered elsewhere in this book (see Chapter 25, "Chronic Fatigue and Fibromyalgia Syndromes," and Chapter 30, "Neurology and Neurosurgery"), but this chapter will also refer to classificatory overlap issues.

Clinical Description

Patients in all areas and at all levels of health care commonly report symptoms such as pain in different locations of the body; fatigue; or perceived disturbances of cardiovascular, gastrointestinal, or other organ functions in the form of palpitations, dizziness, diarrhea, limb weakness, or other manifestations. Some patients suffer from only one persisting symptom, but many complain of multiple symptoms concurrently and over time. Clinically, bodily distress and health anxiety occur across the life span, from adolescence (van Geelen et al. 2015) to old age. Suffering is not confined to the experience of bodily symptoms; it also entails psychological and behavioral aspects such as high health anxiety and checking behavior. In most patients, suffering is dominated by the experience of bodily distress itself, but in some, suffering is dominated by the anxiety aspect, and bodily symptoms are negligible. Patients with high health anxiety may be preoccupied with a particular diagnosis (e.g., cancer, AIDS), a bodily function (e.g., bowel movements), a normal variation in function (e.g., heart rate, blood pressure), or a vague somatic sensation (e.g., "tired heart"). The degree of patient insight varies; some patients recognize that their disease fears are excessive, while others firmly maintain the appropriateness of their convictions. However, these patients' beliefs are not of delusional intensity, and patients can acknowledge the possibility that their disease fears are exaggerated or that there may be no disease at all. Many patients continually check their bodies to reassure themselves; examples of illness anxiety behaviors include excessive breast self-examination or blood pressure and pulse monitoring.

The spectrum of severity in bodily distress and health anxiety is wide, reaching from mild symptoms with little functional impairment to severely disabling conditions (Creed et al. 2011). Diagnostic and therapeutic approaches to patients vary substantially across and within medical specialties, from biomedicine to psychiatry and psychology. Patients are often frustrated, doctors experience them as difficult to treat, and this type of health problem contributes, to a large and still-growing extent, to the global burden of disease (Rice et al. 2016).

In most patients with distressing bodily symptoms and high health anxiety, there is no well-defined structural organic pathology to be found that correlates with the symptoms, and hence the symptoms are typically said to be *functional* in nature. If organic pathology is present, it does not explain the extent of bodily symptoms and suffering, and even successful treatment and/or remission of the underlying pathology does not relieve the symptoms. Many medical specialists feel uncertain when having to decide about the relevance or nonrelevance of underlying organic disease. However, in diagnostic follow-up studies, only 0.5% of diagnoses of so-called functional symptoms and syndromes have to be revised, whereas an initial thorough evaluation of patients who are said to have functional symptoms reveals underlying organic pathology in up to 8% of cases (Eikelboom et al. 2016; Stone et al. 2009).

Importantly, the overall number of bodily symptoms is a more reliable predictor of disability and health care use—and hence, of overall severity—than is the severity of single symptoms or the specification of a subgroup of bodily symptoms as "medically unexplained" (Creed et al. 2013, Tomenson et al. 2013). High health anxiety independently adds to overall severity, especially in terms of use of specialist medical services (Bobevski et al. 2016; Tomenson et al. 2012). Functional limitations in this group of patients in terms of quality of life and work participation are at least as severe as those in well-defined medical diseases with comparable symptoms (Carson et al. 2011; Joustra et al. 2015). Long-term outcome is poor, with high rates of disability often persisting after many years (Rask et al. 2015).

Functional somatic symptoms and bodily distress in general are associated with higher rates of depression and anxiety than are diseases with comparable physical symptoms with well-defined organic pathology (i.e., irritable bowel syndrome vs. inflammatory bowel disease; fibromyalgia syndrome vs. rheumatoid arthritis). However, because many patients with enduring somatic symptoms do not have anxiety or depression, their symptoms cannot be explained as a nonspecific psychological reaction to the presence of bodily complaints or as a masked or somatized depression or anxiety alone (Henningsen et al. 2003). Wilhelm Stekel, who coined the term *somati-*

zation, saw it as being equivalent to the term *conversion*—it meant the expression of psychosocial conflicts via bodily symptoms. And there are at least two other meanings of the term *somatization:* 1) a mental disorder, such as depression or anxiety, manifesting as bodily symptoms; and 2) the most neutral meaning, presence of (multiple) bodily symptoms without reference to underlying conflicts or (other) mental disorders (Henningsen et al. 2005).

Classification in DSM-5

Tables 11–1 and 11–2 list the DSM-5 diagnostic criteria for somatic symptom disorder (SSD) and illness anxiety disorder (IAD), respectively.

The psychopathological features of the two disorders (SSD criterion B; IAD criteria A, C, and D) are essentially similar—that is, dysfunctional mental and behavioral aspects of health anxiety and health-related behavior. It is these features that turn the diagnoses into legitimately mental ones. The main distinction between the two diagnoses is that SSD requires the presence of distressing bodily symptoms, and IAD does not.

The two new diagnoses mark major changes in the diagnostic tradition in this field (Figure 11–1):

- Somatic Symptom and Related Disorders replaces the category of Somatoform Disorders, which had been part of the DSM classification since 1980, appearing in the third (DSM-III [American Psychiatric Association 1980]), revised third (DSM-III-R [American Psychiatric Association 1987]), and fourth editions (DSM-IV [American Psychiatric Association 1994]) and including the subcategories of somatization disorder, undifferentiated somatoform disorder, and pain disorder. Whereas a DSM-5 SSD diagnosis requires the presence of only one distressing bodily symptom, the prototypic somatization disorder diagnoses required the presence of multiple distressing bodily symptoms (DSM-III: 14 symptoms in men, 12 in women; DSM-III-R: 13 symptoms for both sexes; DSM-IV: four pain, two gastrointestinal, one sexual, and one neurological symptom)—a major reason why this category remained rare in research (see below).
- The diagnosis of somatoform disorder primarily rested on the determination that the bodily symptoms be medically unexplained, and this central requirement has been dropped in DSM-5 SSD criterion A. By contrast, the inclusion of positive psychobehavioral features in criterion B is new for SSD compared with the former somatoform disorder diagnoses.
- IAD is a follow-up category that replaces hypochondriasis in the older DSM editions. Whereas most patients previously diagnosed with hypochondriasis also reported distressing bodily symptoms and hence will in future qualify for SSD in DSM-5, a minority of these patients (about 25%) showed only the preoccupation with having a serious illness, without suffering from bodily distress; hence, this subgroup would now qualify for IAD in DSM-5 (Dimsdale et al. 2013; see also Figure 11–1).

Abandoning a strict criterion of "medical unexplainedness" in SSD has largely been welcomed, not least because of the problematic conceptual and pragmatic prob-

---

TABLE 11–1.   DSM-5 diagnostic criteria for somatic symptom disorder

---

A. One or more somatic symptoms that are distressing or result in significant disruption of daily life.

B. Excessive thoughts, feelings, or behaviors related to the somatic symptoms or associated health concerns as manifested by at least one of the following:

1. Disproportionate and persistent thoughts about the seriousness of one's symptoms.

2. Persistently high level of anxiety about health or symptoms.

3. Excessive time and energy devoted to these symptoms or health concerns.

C. Although any one somatic symptom may not be continuously present, the state of being symptomatic is persistent (typically more than 6 months).

Specify if:

With predominant pain (previously pain disorder): This specifier is for individuals whose somatic symptoms predominantly involve pain.

Specify if:

Persistent: A persistent course is characterized by severe symptoms, marked impairment, and long duration (more than 6 months).

Specify current severity:

Mild: Only one of the symptoms specified in Criterion B is fulfilled.

Moderate: Two or more of the symptoms specified in Criterion B are fulfilled.

Severe: Two or more of the symptoms specified in Criterion B are fulfilled, plus there are multiple somatic complaints (or one very severe somatic symptom).

Source.   Reprinted from American Psychiatric Association: *Diagnostic and Statistical Manual of Mental Disorders,* 5th Edition, Arlington, VA, American Psychiatric Association, 2013, p. 311. Copyright 2013, American Psychiatric Association. Used with permission.

---

lems of judging symptoms as medically unexplained (Creed et al. 2010). However, the potential overinclusiveness of the "one size fits all" category has raised fears about mislabeling patients with medical illness as having a mental disorder (Frances and Chapman 2013). Also, selection of positive psychobehavioral criteria has been criticized as being arbitrary and as not capturing the predictively most relevant psychobehavioral features, such as a self-concept of bodily weakness (Rief and Martin 2014).

The clinical relevance of the subdivision of "hypochondriasis" into two forms has been questioned on empirical grounds (Bailer et al. 2016), and further research on the clinical epidemiology of the two new categories is clearly needed.

Classification in ICD and Classificatory Overlap

In the 11th revision of the International Classification of Diseases (ICD-11), which is scheduled for publication in 2018, the category of somatoform disorder will also be replaced. ICD-11 will likely introduce a new category, bodily distress disorder (BDD), that very much resembles the central characteristics of SSD in DSM-5, with emphasis on distressing bodily symptoms and psychobehavioral features (Gureje and Reed 2016). The term *bodily distress* may better capture the fact that patients indeed suffer from their bodily symptoms, but for some, "distress" implies a psychological compo-

TABLE 11–2. DSM-5 diagnostic criteria for illness anxiety disorder

A. Preoccupation with having or acquiring a serious illness.

B. Somatic symptoms are not present or, if present, are only mild in intensity. If another medical condition is present or there is a high risk for developing a medical condition (e.g., strong family history is present), the preoccupation is clearly excessive or disproportionate.

C. There is a high level of anxiety about health, and the individual is easily alarmed about personal health status.

D. The individual performs excessive health-related behaviors (e.g., repeatedly checks his or her body for signs of illness) or exhibits maladaptive avoidance (e.g., avoids doctor appointments and hospitals).

E. Illness preoccupation has been present for at least 6 months, but the specific illness that is feared may change over that period of time.

F. The illness-related preoccupation is not better explained by another mental disorder, such as somatic symptom disorder, panic disorder, generalized anxiety disorder, body dysmorphic disorder, obsessive-compulsive disorder, or delusional disorder, somatic type.

Specify whether:

   Care-seeking type: Medical care, including physician visits or undergoing tests and procedures, is frequently used.

   Care-avoidant type: Medical care is rarely used.

Source. Reprinted from American Psychiatric Association: *Diagnostic and Statistical Manual of Mental Disorders,* 5th Edition, Arlington, VA, American Psychiatric Association, 2013, p. 315. Copyright 2013, American Psychiatric Association. Used with permission.

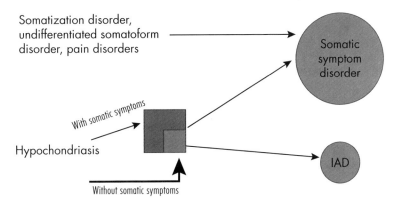

Coalescing and differentiating

FIGURE 11–1. Relationship of DSM-5 somatic symptom disorder and illness anxiety disorder (IAD) to DSM-IV predecessor disorders.

Source. Reprinted from Dimsdale JE, Creed F, Escobar J, Sharpe M, Wulsin L, Barsky A, Lee S, Irwin MR, Levenson J: "Somatic Symptom Disorder: An Important Change in DSM." *Journal of Psychosomatic Research* 75(3):223–228, 2013. Copyright 2013, Elsevier, Inc. Used with permission.

nent to this primarily bodily condition that patients, and some physicians, may find difficult to accept. In any case, similarity in content with difference in terminology between DSM and ICD must be considered as unfortunate.

Functional somatic syndromes usually are diagnosed in the relevant medical section of ICD (e.g., irritable bowel syndrome [IBS] in the chapter on gastroenterological diseases; fibromyalgia syndrome [FMS] in the chapter on rheumatological diseases). For a few functional somatic syndromes, research diagnostic criteria are available that help to define them more strictly (e.g., the Rome criteria for IBS; the Oxford criteria for chronic fatigue syndrome [CFS]). Most functional somatic syndrome diagnoses include no indication of severity.

Extensive overlap exists between the more specific, lead-symptom-oriented diagnostic perspective of functional somatic syndromes and the more general, symptom-pattern-oriented perspective of somatic symptom/bodily distress disorders. In one study based on diagnostic interviews, 95% of patients fulfilling criteria for at least one functional somatic syndrome also fulfilled criteria for bodily (dis)stress syndrome, as defined by Fink and Schröder (2010). First results with proxy measures for psychobehavioral criteria demonstrated significant overlap of SSD with somatoform and functional disorders. In a cohort of general practice patients diagnosed with "medically unexplained symptoms," more than 90% fulfilled criteria for DSM-IV somatoform disorder, but only 45% fulfilled criteria for SSD. Patients who met criteria for SSD were also more disabled than those who did not (van Dessel et al. 2016). In contrast, in a large tertiary care cohort of patients with one lead symptom—dizziness—irrespective of underlying functional or structural causes, diagnoses of SSD were much more frequent than were diagnoses of somatoform disorder (Limburg et al. 2016). In unselected samples of psychosomatic inpatients, SSD and somatoform disorders according to DSM-IV criteria appear to identify similar numbers of patients, with a degree of overlap of 60% or more, depending on the operationalization of the SSD criteria, in particular the psychobehavioral ones (Voigt et al. 2012; see also Dimsdale et al. 2013).

Epidemiology

Because there are as yet no epidemiological studies with the two new diagnostic categories of SSD and IAD, and especially no studies using gold standard diagnostic instruments such as the Structured Diagnostic Interview for DSM-5 (SCID-5; First et al. 2015), no reliable epidemiology on SSD and IAD is yet available. However, there is good reason to assume that rates of SSD will definitely be higher—in the population as well as in primary, specialist, and mental health care—than rates of the narrowly defined multisymptomatic somatoform subcategory of somatization disorder. The latter's very low prevalence rates of between 0.1% and 0.7% in the general population (Creed and Barsky 2004) were confounding, as they misleadingly contributed to underrecognition of the problem of patients with persistent physical symptoms in general. On the other hand, the requirement for positive psychobehavioral features in SSD will prevent the diagnosis from becoming as frequent and nonspecific as the somatoform subcategory of undifferentiated somatoform disorder.

Prevalence estimates for SSD based on a combination of proxy criteria for distressing symptoms and for the presence of at least one psychobehavioral aspect currently vary between approximately 4% in the general population and nearly 25% in a clinical sample of patients with fibromyalgia (Dimsdale et al. 2013; Häuser et al. 2015).

Health anxiety affects approximately 5.7% of the population across the life span and a 3.4% prevalence at the time of the interview (Sunderland et al. 2013). A U.K. study of 28,991 medical clinic patients found that almost 20% had high health anxiety (Tyrer et al. 2011). For IAD, the prevalence will probably be around 25% of the prevalence formerly found for hypochondriasis according to DSM-IV, which had variable rates in the population of up to 7% (Bailer et al. 2016; Creed and Barsky 2004). For epidemiological data on other diagnostic constructs, such as "medically unexplained symptoms" and "functional somatic syndromes," readers are referred to the review by Creed et al. (2011).

Etiology

Rather than using the specific terms SSD and IAD, this section will refer to bodily distress in general. Early (psychodynamic) models of bodily distress in general often implied a top-down process (i.e., psychogenic activations of peripheral physiology) as the major mechanism underlying the experience of enduring bodily symptoms. Models from past decades predominantly implied bottom-up mechanisms, wherein peripheral input from nociceptive and other sensors was conceptualized as being overly amplified by central or psychosocial factors (Van den Bergh et al. 2017). Empirical confirmation of these models has been mixed at best, with aspects such as the consistently worse accuracy of interoception in patients with bodily distress also speaking against the unchallenged validity of concepts such as "somatic amplification" (Van den Bergh et al. 2017). More recently, a model conceptualizing bodily distress as a disorder of perception is gaining ground, wherein perception is seen as being determined as much by the expectations or predictions that the brain continually constructs of its environment (including bodily states) as by peripheral sensory input. In this model, which is based on a view of the brain as a predictive coding machine, disorders of perception can arise from failures of inference due to overly precise predictions (Edwards et al. 2012; Van den Bergh et al. 2017; Wiech 2016). For example, for a patient with persistent somatic symptoms (e.g., chronic fatigue and pain) and B criterion behaviors, the top-down model might focus on unmet dependency needs creating autonomic arousal that leads to the symptoms; the bottom-up model might emphasize oversensitivity to perception of peripheral pain stimuli leading to chronic pain experience and exhaustion; and the perceptual model might focus on the patient's developed expectation that he or she will become exhausted if exertion is attempted, leading the patient to become deconditioned, with "confirmation" of the ill state when the patient is pushed to exert him- or herself. A perceptual model that integrates top-down and bottom-up processes not only has the virtue of being compatible with modern models of brain functioning but also provides targets for prevention and therapy, because it stresses the direct importance of communicative modifications of expectations and attention for the perception of bodily distress (Henningsen et al. 2018).

Genetic factors contribute to a predisposition to bodily distress as well as to chronic pain in general, but only to a limited extent, explaining up to 30% of the variance (Denk et al. 2014; Kato et al. 2010). Thus far, genome-wide and other studies attempting to identify single genes responsible for this predisposition have yielded inconsistent results; epigenetic mechanisms are increasingly seen as also being highly relevant (Denk et al. 2014). Such mechanisms offer a potential link to the well-established role played by childhood adversity as a predisposing factor for bodily distress, raising the odds of developing bodily distress up to fourfold (Afari et al. 2014).

Attachment patterns form another link between childhood adversity and somatization, with maternal insensitivity at 18 months predicting somatization in 5-year-old children, and attachment insecurity in adults predicting somatization, with the strongest links found between attachment anxiety and health anxiety (Maunder et al. 2017). Another developmentally grounded deficiency—in emotion recognition and regulation—has also long been linked to various facets of bodily distress, with alexithymic cultural patterns as the most prominent concept—*alexithymia* refers to an inability to "read" (i.e., perceive and name) one's own emotional states. Despite concerns about the nonspecificity of this concept, recent evidence supports the relevance of its link with bodily distress, and trials of psychotherapeutic interventions that specifically target deficiencies in emotion recognition and regulation in patients with bodily distress are under way (Kleinstäuber et al. 2016). On another level, cultural factors contribute to the predisposition to bodily distress, with culturally determined patterns of symptom expectation and interpretation clearly influencing rates of disability and health care use. For instance, chronic disabling back pain has been shown to be much more prevalent in Germany than in Great Britain, without clear differences in risk factors such as obesity or physical inactivity (Kirmayer and Sartorius 2007).

Organic illnesses, stressful work conditions, and adverse life events are important precipitating factors for bodily distress (Bonvanie et al. 2017; Halpin and Ford 2012; Hickie et al. 2006; Momsen et al. 2016; Tschan et al. 2011). If they are persisting, these factors and predisposing personality aspects obviously also contribute to the maintenance of the symptoms of bodily distress. Further maintaining factors arise from the often-difficult interactions of these patients with the health care system, leading to missed or delayed diagnosis, inappropriate treatments, and frustrations on all sides. Somatizing communication behavior and persistent beliefs about biomedical causations on the part of patients and doctors alike—but also systemic factors of the health care system—contribute to these significant barriers to improved diagnosis and treatment (Henningsen et al. 2011; Murray et al. 2016).

Diagnosis

Diagnosis of SSD and IAD can be difficult or relatively straightforward, depending on context. In mental health care settings and in psychosomatic and psychiatric consultation-liaison services, patients usually are referred with a suspected (differential) diagnosis of SSD or IAD in mind. In such a situation, it is not a complex task to ascertain whether the relevant diagnostic criteria are met, and the fact that there is no longer any necessity to ascertain bodily symptoms as being organically unexplained makes it easier to arrive at a diagnosis than was possible in diagnosing somatoform disorder. Valid self-report questionnaires exist for screening and for aiding in diagnosis; well-known examples are the Patient Health Questionnaire–15 for somatic symptom burden (Kroenke et al. 2002) and the Whiteley Index for health anxiety (Hedman et al. 2015). Self-report questionnaires for assessment of the psychobehavioral B criteria in SSD have also now been published (Toussaint et al. 2016).

Whereas diagnostic ascertainment is not a major difficulty in these contexts, forging a stable doctor–patient relationship as the basis for treatment often remains a difficult initial challenge, as discussed below (see "Treatment" section later in this chapter).

Diagnosis of SSD and IAD is more difficult in the context of primary and specialist somatic care, where the common initial assumption of patients and doctors usually is that an underlying organic cause will be found that explains the patient's bodily symptoms and heightened anxiety.

The following recommendations are aimed at primary care physicians and somatic specialists; they also form a basis for interventions by mental health care specialists (see also Academic Health Science Network for the North East and North Cumbria 2015; Schäfert et al. 2012).

- Consider the possibility of SSD in a patient with persistent physical symptoms as early as possible; do not equate such symptoms with malingering.
- Avoid repetitive, especially risky investigations undertaken solely to reassure and calm the patient or yourself; bear in mind that negative findings rarely provide lasting reassurance, and excessive evaluation introduces risk of additional complications and "incidentalomas" (Chidiac and Aron 1997).
- Be attentive to patient clues indicating bodily or emotional distress beyond the current main symptom and outside your specialist field. Screen for other physical symptoms, anxiety, and depression. Do not miss potential medication or alcohol misuse, or suicidal ideation.
- Assess the patient's experiences, expectations, functioning, beliefs, and illness behavior, especially in regard to catastrophizing, body checking, avoidance, and dysfunctional health care utilization.
- If psychobehavioral criteria of SSD/IAD are present, decide whether the patient has SSD or IAD—depending on actual presence, or absence, of distressing bodily symptoms.
- If SSD is diagnosed, determine whether it is mild, moderate, or severe, according to specifiers.

The diagnostic process in itself, if done well, has therapeutic potential—hence, the term *theragnostics* could be applied here as well.

Differential Diagnosis and Comorbidity

For SSD, the most relevant disorder in the differential diagnosis is persistent physical symptoms, be they organically well explained or not, with psychobehavioral features that are either not present or not pronounced enough to fulfill one of the B criteria. Obviously, the boundaries for this determination are not clear-cut, and views will differ, for example, on the point at which understandable fears of progression in a patient with fatigue and multiple sclerosis become disproportionate beliefs about symptom severity and persistently high anxiety (SSD criteria B1 and B2).

Rare conditions to consider in the differential diagnosis of SSD are factitious disorder (DSM-5 300.19), in which a patient intentionally produces, feigns, or exaggerates the symptoms of a disease with the aim of assuming the patient role, and malingering, which is not a disorder but rather a conscious attempt at deceiving others about the presence of symptoms. SSD with multiple symptoms that lead to multiple diagnostic and therapeutic activities can sometimes blend into factitious disorder—as, for example, when a patient with pain syndromes is repeatedly operated on or treated with intensive measures in emergency departments.

For IAD, the most relevant disorders in the differential diagnoses are generalized anxiety disorder (DSM-5 300.02), wherein excessive worry and anxiety are focused on several events and issues, not just on illness in particular, and delusional disorder, somatic type (DSM-5 297.1), wherein the belief of having or acquiring a disease is held with certainty and cannot be changed by either evidence to the contrary or reassurance.

As stated above, depressive and anxiety disorders are commonly present in patients with SSD; in fact, there appears to be a linear relationship between number of bodily symptoms and likelihood of depression or anxiety (Kisely et al. 1997). This relationship argues against the former psychodynamic notion that bodily symptoms are preferentially experienced when defense mechanisms do not allow mental symptoms to develop. In view of the high rates of depressive and anxiety disorders in patients with SSD, it is more appropriate to view the experience of somatic, depressive, and anxiety symptoms as related dimensions of distress rather than as independent comorbid conditions.

In more severe cases of SSD, personality disorders are frequently present and must be considered in assessment and treatment (Garcia-Campayo et al. 2007).

Treatment

Good management of patients with SSD or IAD should avoid the trap of entrenched dualistic "either mental or physical" thinking. The bodily complaints of patients need to be taken seriously even if no well-defined organic pathology is demonstrated and no clear-cut (other) mental disorder is present. Good communication with the patient is essential at all stages of disease and levels of care and should include reassurance, anticipation of likely outcomes of diagnostic tests, positive explanations of the disorder's "functional" character, and motivation of the patient to actively engage in coping with bodily distress. Encouraging a healthy lifestyle—physical, social, and other activities, such as good sleep hygiene, regular exercising, and fulfilling hobbies—is helpful.

In mild cases, these theragnostic principles can be sufficient, combined with a "watchful waiting" attitude and follow-up contacts. If these principles turn out not to be sufficient, some of the following techniques may be helpful:

• Frame context factors as amplifiers rather than causes of the patient's symptoms. Build an effective, blame-free narrative that is linked to physical as well as psychosocial mechanisms and that makes sense to the patient.
• Encourage—and monitor—more adaptive attitudes and behaviors, such as positive thinking, relaxation techniques, graded exercise, and self-help guides/groups. Set realistic goals with the patient.

- Provide symptomatic measures such as nonsteroidal pain relief, or laxatives; allow measures from complementary medicine according to the patient's wishes; explain that these measures are temporarily helpful but are less effective than self-management.
- Consider antidepressant medication if there is predominant pain or depression.
- Strictly avoid opioid pain medication and sedative-hypnotics.
- If appropriate, set appointments at regular intervals rather than waiting for the patient to initiate, so that the patient does not "need" symptom exacerbations as an entry ticket for a visit.

If these measures are still not sufficient, consider the following:

- Ensure that traumatic stressors and maintaining factors, such as domestic violence, medication misuse, factitious symptoms, or litigation, are assessed.
- If applicable, carefully frame referral to a psychotherapist for the patient as seeking additional expert advice in addition to the reappointment with you.
- If applicable, liaise with psychotherapist on diagnosis, possible difficulties, and further treatment planning.
- When outpatient care is not available or seems insufficient, consider integrated care with multidisciplinary treatment, including symptomatic measures, physiotherapy and occupational therapy requiring active patient participation, and psychotherapy.

Psychotherapy is an established treatment modality in patients with SSD/IAD, but it meets with specific challenges in the initial phases, when patients very often find it difficult to accept that a "talking cure" might help with their primarily bodily symptoms and concerns. The following recommendations for these initial phases of psychotherapy aim at building a sustainable therapeutic relationship independent of later differentiations according to the pattern of patient problems and school of psychotherapy (adapted and translated from Henningsen and Martin 2016):

- Clarify the patient's motivation for psychotherapeutic consultation. If applicable, confirm to him/her that you acknowledge his/her initial view that the symptoms have an as-yet-undetected organic basis and that he/she may "only" accept the consultation to please others.
- Use the measures described above as appropriate.
- Listen attentively to bodily complaints and relationship experiences connected to them (e.g., with doctors and other health professionals; with relatives and/or colleagues). Give feedback on the emotional aspects of these experiences (e.g., anger, disappointment, fear).
- In more chronic patients, give support in organizing the history of presenting complaints (and experiences) into a coherent narrative.
- Encourage the patient to extend his or her view of the possible influence of psychosocial as well as biological context factors (e.g., through time-limited use of a symptom-context diary [not recommended for patients with very high health anxiety]). Do not attempt to "reattribute" symptoms to a predominantly psychosocial cause.

- Negotiate realistic (i.e., modest) treatment goals. Advocate "better adaptation" and "coping"; avoid "cure" as a treatment goal.
- Resist the temptation to concentrate on psychosocial issues too early and too independently of lead complaints. If necessary, "somatize"—that is, inquire about current bodily symptoms.
- Liaise with others involved in the care of the patient to obtain relevant information, especially in regard to the necessity of further somatic diagnostic and therapeutic interventions, but also to send the message to the patient that constructive cooperation in caring for him or her is possible.

For severe cases of bodily distress, with long-term sickness and disability, integrated multimodal treatment in a day clinic or inpatient setting—with combinations of single and group psychotherapy, body-oriented psychotherapy, art therapy, physiotherapy, and somatic diagnostics and treatment (where needed)—is indicated but very often not available. In some countries (e.g., Germany), clinics and departments for psychosomatic medicine provide these treatments (Zipfel et al. 2016).

Evidence Base for Treatments

Recent years have seen considerable efforts to compile evidence-based recommendations for the management of patients with bodily distress and health anxiety. Such efforts have included several national guideline initiatives and Cochrane reviews focused on the overall pattern of symptoms, as well as many systematic and Cochrane reviews examining single functional somatic syndromes. These investigations have identified not only the (mostly moderate) effects of various treatments but also the unmet needs of this large group of patients and the barriers to better diagnosis and treatment (Creed et al. 2011; Fink and Rosendal 2015; Murray et al. 2016; Schäfert et al. 2012; van der Feltz-Cornelis et al. 2012).

As mentioned earlier, bodily distress in general is covered by diagnostic categories such as somatoform disorders and now SSD that are mostly used in mental health care settings. In trials conducted under this perspective, primary endpoints often relate to functioning (e.g., in measures of health-related quality of life) rather than to symptom intensity. By the very nature of this perspective and its underlying conceptualization, trials and reviews focusing on peripherally acting drugs and passive physical interventions do not exist.

Two Cochrane reviews on nonpharmacological and pharmacological interventions for somatoform disorders and medically unexplained physical symptoms (Kleinstäuber et al. 2014; Van Dessel et al. 2014) documented consistently low- to moderate-quality evidence for the efficacy of different forms of short-term psychotherapy and self-help interventions on follow-up—effect sizes usually were in the low to medium range (0.3–0.5). Most evidence refers to cognitive-behavioral interventions, but there is also evidence for psychodynamic and other psychosocial interventions. In view of the increasing relevance of online interventions, it is interesting to note that the first promising results have been published for exposure-based cognitive-behavioral therapy (CBT) delivered via the Internet to patients with SSD or IAD (Hedman et al. 2016).

In terms of pharmacotherapy, there is some very low-quality evidence for the efficacy of newer-generation and tricyclic antidepressants and of natural products such as St. John's wort in this group of patients. However, this evidence must be balanced against a relatively high rate of adverse effects, because these patients, as a result of their sensitivity to somatic sensations, are prone to unusual side effects of medications, including multiple types of "allergies" to drugs. It must also be borne in mind that none (!) of the pharmacological trials provided follow-up data. No evidence is yet available for the efficacy of training in enhanced care for primary care physicians (Rosendal et al. 2013).

For health anxiety/hypochondriasis, the evidence base is better, particularly for cognitive-behavioral interventions; a recent systematic review and meta-analysis documented effect sizes of around $d=1.0$ for CBT in comparison with control conditions (Cooper et al. 2017).

Most trials by far still refer to the treatment of single functional somatic syndromes, such as IBS or FMS, without stratification according to total number of bodily symptoms, psychobehavioral features, comorbidity, or other indicators of severity. There is consistent evidence that psychotherapy is effective under this more somatic perspective on bodily distress—an exemplary trial was conducted with patients with chronic fatigue syndrome (White et al. 2011). However, many trials involving patients with functional somatic syndromes report not only on mental health–type interventions but also on the effects of peripherally acting drugs and passive physical interventions (e.g., massage, spinal manipulation). For further details on the treatment of functional somatic syndromes such as fibromyalgia, irritable bowel syndrome, and chronic fatigue syndrome, readers are referred to other chapters in this textbook (see Chapter 19, "Gastrointestinal Disorders"; Chapter 25, "Chronic Fatigue and Fibromyalgia Syndromes"; and Chapter 30, "Neurology and Neurosurgery"), as well as papers by Henningsen et al. (2003, 2018).

Conclusion

The diagnoses SSD and IAD capture long-standing clinical problems of patients with enduring bodily distress and heightened health anxiety in a new way that will be evaluated empirically more thoroughly in the coming years. A biopsychosocial understanding of the factors contributing to vulnerability, triggering, and maintenance of these disorders is now commonplace—a new understanding of the brain as a predictive coding machine helps to integrate top-down and bottom-up aspects of symptom perception.

Stepped-care approaches are well suited to all levels of care in dealing with the wide spectrum of severity in this group of patients. Patients with early-stage SSD or IAD are usually seen in primary and specialist somatic care, and in these settings, aspects such as a validating attitude, good communication, and reflective use of somatic diagnostic and therapeutic measures are essential. In later and more severe stages, usually also seen in mental health care settings, these basic "theragnostic" essentials should be complemented by more specific measures, including disorder-oriented management of the therapeutic relationship and initial stages of psychotherapy. Psychopharmacotherapy has only a very limited role in managing this group of patients, primarily in those with comorbid mood or anxiety disorders. Multimodal treatments should be implemented for severe cases whenever possible.

In addition to these patient- and doctor-oriented measures, more systemic approaches—including undergraduate and postgraduate medical training and adaptations of health care systems to avoid mismanagement of these mostly chronic patients—are necessary.

References

Academic Health Science Network for the North East and North Cumbria: We need to talk about symptoms: an introduction. Information for health professionals on Persistent Physical Symptoms, Version 1. October 2015. Available at: http://www.ahsn-nenc.org.uk/wp-content/uploads/sites/3/2014/12/We-need-to-talk-about-symptons-an-introduction.pdf. Accessed April 24, 2017.
Afari N, Ahumada SM, Wright LJ, et al: Psychological trauma and functional somatic syndromes: a systematic review and meta-analysis. Psychosom Med 76(1):2–11, 2014 24336429
American Psychiatric Association: Diagnostic and Statistical Manual of Mental Disorders, 3rd Edition. Washington, DC, American Psychiatric Association, 1980
American Psychiatric Association: Diagnostic and Statistical Manual of Mental Disorders, 3rd Edition, Revised. Washington, DC, American Psychiatric Association, 1987
American Psychiatric Association: Diagnostic and Statistical Manual of Mental Disorders, 4th Edition. Washington, DC, American Psychiatric Association, 1994
American Psychiatric Association: Diagnostic and Statistical Manual of Mental Disorders, 5th Edition. Arlington, VA, American Psychiatric Association, 2013
Bailer J, Kerstner T, Witthöft M, et al: Health anxiety and hypochondriasis in the light of DSM-5. Anxiety Stress Coping 29(2):219–239, 2016 25846805
Bobevski I, Clarke DM, Meadows G: Health anxiety and its relationship to disability and service use: findings from a large epidemiological survey. Psychosom Med 78(1):13–25, 2016 26588821
Bonvanie IJ, Janssens KA, Rosmalen JG, Oldehinkel AJ: Life events and functional somatic symptoms: a population study in older adolescents. Br J Psychol 108(2):318–333, 2017 27221984
Carson A, Stone J, Hibberd C, et al: Disability, distress and unemployment in neurology outpatients with symptoms "unexplained by organic disease." J Neurol Neurosurg Psychiatry 82(7):810–813, 2011 21257981
Chidiac RM, Aron DC: Incidentalomas. A disease of modern technology. Endocrinol Metab Clin North Am 26(1):233–253, 1997 9074861
Cooper K, Gregory JD, Walker I, et al: Cognitive behaviour therapy for health anxiety: a systematic review and meta-analysis. Behav Cogn Psychother 45(2):110–123, 2017 28229805
Creed F, Barsky A: A systematic review of the epidemiology of somatisation disorder and hypochondriasis. J Psychosom Res 56(4):391–408, 2004 15094023
Creed F, Guthrie E, Fink P, et al: Is there a better term than "medically unexplained symptoms"? J Psychosom Res 68(1):5–8, 2010 20004295
Creed F, Henningsen P, Fink P (eds): Medically Unexplained Symptoms, Somatization and Bodily Distress: Developing Better Clinical Services. Cambridge, UK, Cambridge University Press, 2011
Creed FH, Tomenson B, Chew-Graham C, et al: Multiple somatic symptoms predict impaired health status in functional somatic syndromes. Int J Behav Med 20(2):194–205, 2013 22932928
Denk F, McMahon SB, Tracey I: Pain vulnerability: a neurobiological perspective. Nat Neurosci 17(2):192–200, 2014 24473267
Dimsdale JE, Creed F, Escobar J, et al: Somatic symptom disorder: an important change in DSM. J Psychosom Res 75(3):223–228, 2013 23972410
Edwards MJ, Adams RA, Brown H, et al: A Bayesian account of "hysteria". Brain 135(Pt 11):3495–3512, 2012 22641838

Eikelboom EM, Tak LM, Roest AM, Rosmalen JG: A systematic review and meta-analysis of the percentage of revised diagnoses in functional somatic symptoms. J Psychosom Res 88:60–67, 2016 27455914

Fink P, Rosendal M (eds): Functional Disorders and Medically Unexplained Symptoms: Assessment and Treatment. Aarhus, Denmark, Aarhus University Press, 2015

Fink P, Schröder A: One single diagnosis, bodily distress syndrome, succeeded to capture 10 diagnostic categories of functional somatic syndromes and somatoform disorders. J Psychosom Res 68(5):415–426, 2010 20403500

First MB, Williams JBW, Karg RS, Spitzer RL: Structured Clinical Interview for DSM-5—Research Version (SCID-5 for DSM-5, Research Version; SCID-5-RV). Arlington, VA, American Psychiatric Association, 2015

Frances A, Chapman S: DSM-5 somatic symptom disorder mislabels medical illness as mental disorder. Aust N Z J Psychiatry 47(5):483–484, 2013 23653063

Garcia-Campayo J, Alda M, Sobradiel N, et al: Personality disorders in somatization disorder patients: a controlled study in Spain. J Psychosom Res 62(6):675–680, 2007 17540225

Gureje O, Reed GM: Bodily distress disorder in ICD-11: problems and prospects. World Psychiatry 15(3):291–292, 2016 27717252

Halpin SJ, Ford AC: Prevalence of symptoms meeting criteria for irritable bowel syndrome in inflammatory bowel disease: systematic review and meta-analysis. Am J Gastroenterol 107(10):1474–1482, 2012 22929759

Häuser W, Bialas P, Welsch K, Wolfe F: Construct validity and clinical utility of current research criteria of DSM-5 somatic symptom disorder diagnosis in patients with fibromyalgia syndrome. J Psychosom Res 78(6):546–552, 2015 25864805

Hedman E, Lekander M, Ljótsson B, et al: Optimal cut-off points on the Health Anxiety Inventory, Illness Attitude Scales and Whiteley Index to identify severe health anxiety. PLoS One 10(4):e0123412, 2015 25849477

Hedman E, Axelsson E, Andersson E, et al: Exposure-based cognitive-behavioural therapy via the Internet and as bibliotherapy for somatic symptom disorder and illness anxiety disorder: randomised controlled trial. Br J Psychiatry 209(5):407–413, 2016 27491531

Henningsen P, Martin A: [Somatoform disorders/somatic symptom disorder], in [Psychotherapy: Function- and Disorder-Oriented approach] (in German). Edited by Herpertz S, Caspar F, Lieb K. Munich, Elsevier, 2016, pp 473–492

Henningsen P, Zimmermann T, Sattel H: Medically unexplained physical symptoms, anxiety, and depression: a meta-analytic review. Psychosom Med 65(4):528–533, 2003 12883101

Henningsen P, Jakobsen T, Schiltenwolf M, Weiss MG: Somatization revisited: diagnosis and perceived causes of common mental disorders. J Nerv Ment Dis 193(2):85–92, 2005 15684910

Henningsen P, Zipfel S, Herzog W: Management of functional somatic syndromes. Lancet 369(9565):946–955, 2007 17368156

Henningsen P, Fazekas C, Sharpe M: Barriers to improving treatment, in Medically Unexplained Symptoms, Somatization and Bodily Distress: Developing Better Clinical Services. Edited by Creed F, Henningsen P, Fink P. Cambridge, UK, Cambridge University Press, 2011, pp 124–131

Henningsen P, Zipfel S, Sattel H, Creed F: Management of functional somatic syndromes and bodily distress. Psychother Psychosom 87(1):12–31, 2018 29306954

Henningsen P, Gündel H, Kop W, et al; EURONET-SOMA Group: Persistent physical symptoms as perceptual dysregulation: a neuropsychobehavioral model and its clinical implications. Psychosom Med April 4, 2018 [Epub ahead of print] 29621046

Hickie I, Davenport T, Wakefield D, et al; Dubbo Infection Outcomes Study Group: Post-infective and chronic fatigue syndromes precipitated by viral and non-viral pathogens: prospective cohort study. BMJ 333(7568):575, 2006 16950834

Joustra ML, Janssens KA, Bültmann U, Rosmalen JG: Functional limitations in functional somatic syndromes and well-defined medical diseases. Results from the general population cohort LifeLines. J Psychosom Res 79(2):94–99, 2015 26026696

Kato K, Sullivan PF, Pedersen NL: Latent class analysis of functional somatic symptoms in a population-based sample of twins. J Psychosom Res 68(5):447–453, 2010 20403503

Kirmayer LJ, Sartorius N: Cultural models and somatic syndromes. Psychosom Med 69(9):832–840, 2007 18040090

Kisely S, Goldberg D, Simon G: A comparison between somatic symptoms with and without clear organic cause: results of an international study. Psychol Med 27(5):1011–1019, 1997 9300507

Kleinstäuber M, Witthöft M, Steffanowski A, et al: Pharmacological interventions for somatoform disorders in adults. Cochrane Database Syst Rev (11):CD010628, 2014 25379990

Kleinstäuber M, Gottschalk J, Berking M, et al: Enriching cognitive behavior therapy with emotion regulation training for patients with multiple medically unexplained symptoms (ENCERT): design and implementation of a multicenter, randomized, active-controlled trial. Contemp Clin Trials 47:54–63, 2016 26655432

Kroenke K, Spitzer RL, Williams JB: The PHQ-15: validity of a new measure for evaluating the severity of somatic symptoms. Psychosom Med 64(2):258–266, 2002 11914441

Limburg K, Sattel H, Radziej K, Lahmann C: DSM-5 somatic symptom disorder in patients with vertigo and dizziness symptoms. J Psychosom Res 91:26–32, 2016 27894459

Maunder RG, Hunter JJ, Atkinson L, et al: An attachment-based model of the relationship between childhood adversity and somatization in children and adults. Psychosom Med 79(5):506–513, 2017 27941580

Momsen AH, Nielsen CV, Nielsen MB, et al: Work participation and health-related characteristics of sickness absence beneficiaries with multiple somatic symptoms. Public Health 133:75–82, 2016 26715321

Murray AM, Toussaint A, Althaus A, Löwe B: The challenge of diagnosing non-specific, functional, and somatoform disorders: a systematic review of barriers to diagnosis in primary care. J Psychosom Res 80:1–10, 2016 26721541

Rask MT, Rosendal M, Fenger-Grøn M, et al: Sick leave and work disability in primary care patients with recent-onset multiple medically unexplained symptoms and persistent somatoform disorders: a 10-year follow-up of the FIP study. Gen Hosp Psychiatry 37(1):53–59, 2015 25456975

Rice AS, Smith BH, Blyth FM: Pain and the global burden of disease. Pain 157(4):791–796, 2016 26670465

Rief W, Martin A: How to use the new DSM-5 somatic symptom disorder diagnosis in research and practice: a critical evaluation and a proposal for modifications. Annu Rev Clin Psychol 10:339–367, 2014 24387234

Rosendal M, Blankenstein AH, Morriss R, et al: Enhanced care by generalists for functional somatic symptoms and disorders in primary care. Cochrane Database Syst Rev (10):CD008142, 2013 24142886

Schäfert R, Hausteiner-Wiehle C, Häuser W, et al: Non-specific, functional, and somatoform bodily complaints. Dtsch Arztebl Int 109(47):803–813, 2012 23248710

Stone J, Carson A, Duncan R, et al: Symptoms "unexplained by organic disease" in 1144 new neurology out-patients: how often does the diagnosis change at follow-up? Brain 132(Pt 10):2878–2888, 2009 19737842

Sunderland M, Newby JM, Andrews G: Health anxiety in Australia: prevalence, comorbidity, disability and service use. Br J Psychiatry 202(1):56–61, 2013 22500013

Tomenson B, McBeth J, Chew-Graham CA, et al: Somatization and health anxiety as predictors of health care use. Psychosom Med 74(6):656–664, 2012 22753632

Tomenson B, Essau C, Jacobi F, et al; EURASMUS Population Based Study Group: Total somatic symptom score as a predictor of health outcome in somatic symptom disorders. Br J Psychiatry 203(5):373–380, 2013 24072756

Toussaint A, Murray AM, Voigt K, et al: Development and validation of the Somatic Symptom Disorder-B Criteria Scale (SSD-12). Psychosom Med 78(1):5–12, 2016 26461855

Tschan R, Best C, Beutel ME, et al: Patients' psychological well-being and resilient coping protect from secondary somatoform vertigo and dizziness (SVD) 1 year after vestibular disease. J Neurol 258(1):104–112, 2011 20717689

Tyrer P, Cooper S, Crawford M, et al: Prevalence of health anxiety problems in medical clinics. J Psychosom Res 71(6):392–394, 2011 22118381

Van den Bergh O, Witthöft M, Petersen S, Brown RJ: Symptoms and the body: taking the inferential leap. Neurosci Biobehav Rev 74(Pt A):185–203, 2017 28108416

van der Feltz-Cornelis CM, Hoedeman R, Keuter EJ, Swinkels JA: Presentation of the multidisciplinary guideline medically unexplained physical symptoms (MUPS) and somatoform disorder in the Netherlands: disease management according to risk profiles. J Psychosom Res 72(2):168–169, 2012 22281461

Van Dessel N, den Boeft M, van der Wouden JC, et al: Non-pharmacological interventions for somatoform disorders and medically unexplained physical symptoms (MUPS) in adults. Cochrane Database Syst Rev (11):CD011142, 2014 25362239

van Dessel NC, van der Wouden JC, Dekker J, van der Horst HE: Clinical value of DSM IV and DSM 5 criteria for diagnosing the most prevalent somatoform disorders in patients with medically unexplained physical symptoms (MUPS). J Psychosom Res 82:4–10, 2016 26944392

van Geelen SM, Rydelius PA, Hagquist C: Somatic symptoms and psychological concerns in a general adolescent population: exploring the relevance of DSM-5 somatic symptom disorder. J Psychosom Res 79(4):251–258, 2015 26297569

Voigt K, Wollburg E, Weinmann N, et al: Predictive validity and clinical utility of DSM-5 somatic symptom disorder—comparison with DSM-IV somatoform disorders and additional criteria for consideration. J Psychosom Res 73(5):345–350, 2012 23062807

White PD, Goldsmith KA, Johnson AL, et al; PACE Trial Management Group: Comparison of adaptive pacing therapy, cognitive behaviour therapy, graded exercise therapy, and specialist medical care for chronic fatigue syndrome (PACE): a randomised trial. Lancet 377(9768):823–836, 2011 21334061

Wiech K: Deconstructing the sensation of pain: the influence of cognitive processes on pain perception. Science 354(6312):584–587, 2016 27811269

Zipfel S, Herzog W, Kruse J, Henningsen P: Psychosomatic medicine in Germany: more timely than ever. Psychother Psychosom 85(5):262–269, 2016 27509065

CHAPTER 12

Deception Syndromes

Factitious Disorders and Malingering

Charles V. Ford, M.D.

Loretta Sonnier, M.D.

Cheryl McCullumsmith, M.D., Ph.D.

> *Disease has been simulated in every age, and by all classes of society. The monarch, the mendicant, the unhappy slave, the proud warrior, the lofty statesman, even the minister of religion as well as the condemned malefactor and boy "creeping like a snail unwillingly to school," have sought to disguise their purposes, or obtain their desires, by feigning mental or bodily infirmities.*
>
> Gavin (1838), p. i

The above introductory paragraph to Hector Gavin's 1838 book *On the Feigned and Factitious Diseases of Soldiers and Seamen,* in which he described clinical features of factitious disorders and malingering, indicates the pervasiveness of simulated disease. Also noteworthy is that in the second century A.D., the Roman physician Galen devoted a chapter to simulated disease in one of his medical texts (Adams 1846).

In DSM-5 (American Psychiatric Association 2013) factitious disorders are placed into a new category, "Somatic Symptom and Related Disorders." Malingering continues to be classed as a "V" code. In real-life clinical situations, the boundaries of these and other syndromes (e.g., conversion disorder and "compensation neurosis") are often blurred (Hall and Hall 2012). Further, there are frequently elements of other nonmedical issues that contribute to symptom formation and presentation (Bass and Halligan 2007, 2014).

Interest in factitious disorders has increased markedly since the publication of Richard Asher's seminal paper in 1951 (Asher 1951). As of 2017, there are more than 3,000 publications in the medical literature focused on factitious disorders. In addition, there have been descriptions of several other syndromes related to factitious disorder, such as factitious allegations of sexual abuse (Feldman et al. 1994; Feldman-Schorrig 1996; Gibbon 1998), and even production of disease in one's pets (Munro and Thrusfield 2001). There are increasing reports of the use of the Internet to obtain medical information and even download medical reports to present as one's own (Levenson et al. 2007). Persons also may assume a false identity to enter chat rooms and support groups for chronic diseases (Pulman and Taylor 2012).

Frequently, patients with factitious disorders will exhibit *pseudologia fantastica*, a form of pathological lying characterized by a matrix of fact and fiction, although this is not a diagnostic criterion. These stories, told repetitively, usually present the storyteller in a grandiose manner and/or as a victim. Pseudologia fantastica is often associated with cognitive dysfunction, learning disabilities, or childhood traumatic experiences (King and Ford 1988). Neuropsychological testing is indicated for patients presenting with pseudologia fantastica or other forms of pathological lying. One middle-aged man with late-onset pathological lying was shown by neuropsychological testing to have developed behavior-variant frontotemporal dementia (Poletti et al. 2011).

Hardie and Reed (1998) described the overlaps in characteristics of persons who have pseudologia fantastica, those who create factitious illness, and those who engage in impostorship. They proposed the term *deception syndromes* to describe these syndromes—a concept that would provide more unity than does the current tendency to create increasing numbers of new syndromes and eponyms.

Factitious Disorders Imposed on Self

Clinical Description

Factitious Disorders With Physical Symptoms

Persons who have factitious disorders intentionally feign, exaggerate, aggravate, or self-induce symptoms or disease. They are conscious of their behaviors, although the underlying motivation may be unconscious. By convention, this diagnosis is also characterized by the surreptitious nature of the behavior. Patients who acknowledge that they have produced their own self-harm (e.g., self-mutilators) are not included in this diagnostic group. Inherent in factitious disorders is a paradox: the patient presents to a physician or other health care provider with the request for medical care but simultaneously conceals the known cause of the problem.

Self-induced factitious disorders fit into two major syndromes. Unfortunately, the terminology in the general medical literature is inconsistent, and the terms *Munchausen syndrome* and *factitious disorder* are often used interchangeably (Fink and Jensen 1989). In this chapter, *Munchausen syndrome* refers specifically to the subtype of factitious disorders originally described by Richard Asher in 1951. Risk factors for factitious disorder vary according to the subtype of the clinical syndrome. The most common subtype is *common factitious disorder* (or *nonperegrinating factitious disorder*), in which the person does not use aliases or travel from hospital to hospital. In this syndrome, female gender, unmarried status, age in the 30s, prior work or experience in the health care professions (e.g., nursing), and Cluster B personality disorders with borderline features are frequently found. For *full-blown Munchausen syndrome,* in which the patient uses aliases and travels from hospital to hospital (and often from state to state), risk factors include male gender, single marital status, age often in the 40s, and a personality disorder of the Cluster B type with at least some antisocial features. In their review of 93 cases of factitious disorder diagnosed at the Mayo Clinic, Krahn et al. (2003) found that 72% were women, of whom 65.7% had some association with health-related occupations. The mean age for women was 30.7 years, and the mean age for men was 40.0 years. A recent systematic review of 455 published cases reported 66% female, a mean age of 34.2 years, 27% in a healthcare or laboratory profession, and depression more common than personality disorder, with more patients self-inducing illness or injury (58.7%) than simulating or falsely reporting it (Yates and Feldman 2016). The psychological data in this study must be interpreted with caution in that the majority of cases were reported by nonpsychiatrists and only 37% of case reports described comorbid psychiatric disorders.

Few epidemiological data are available for factitious disorders. An Italian community study found a lifetime prevalence of 0.1% (Faravelli et al. 2004). Most investigators believe that factitious disorder is a relatively uncommon but not extremely rare disorder. A rough estimate is approximately 1 in 10,000 hospital admissions. Most hospital consultation services will see at least one inpatient with factitious disorder per year.

Classic Munchausen syndrome consists of three essential components: the simulation or self-induction of disease, pseudologia fantastica, and travel from hospital to hospital, often with the use of aliases to disguise identity. These patients frequently present in the emergency department with dramatic symptoms, such as hemoptysis, acute chest pain suggesting a myocardial infarction, or coma from self-induced hypoglycemia. Munchausen patients may make a career out of illness and hospitalizations; as many as 423 separate hospitalizations for an individual patient have been reported (Maur et al. 1973).

The types of symptoms and different diseases that have been simulated defy the imagination (Table 12–1). Essentially every subspecialty journal has published case reports of self-induced illness related to that particular subspecialty. Among the most common presentations have been chest pain, endocrine disorders such as hyperthyroidism or Cushing's syndrome, coagulopathies, infections, and neurological symptoms. The Munchausen patient often presents during evening or weekend hours, presumably in order to be evaluated by less senior or experienced clinicians. The patient is frequently admitted to an inpatient service, where he or she may become the "star patient" in view of the dramatic nature of the symptoms or the rarity of the presumed diagnosis. In addition, the patient may call attention to himself or herself by providing false information, such as claiming to be a former professional football player, a recipient of the Medal of Honor, or perhaps the president of a foreign university. Despite such reputed prominence, these patients and their physicians rarely receive telephone calls from concerned family members or friends. The Munchausen patient is usually willing to undergo multiple diagnostic studies. When inconsistencies in history, medical findings, or laboratory examinations create suspicions, caregivers often become more confrontational. At this point, the patient generally responds with irritation, new complaints, disruptive behavior, or threats to file a lawsuit. He or she may request discharge against medical advice or may simply disappear. Embarrassed and angry clinicians on the treatment team may console themselves by preparing a case presentation for grand rounds or perhaps for publication.

Munchausen syndrome is the most dramatic form of factitious behavior, and the eponym certainly has great popularity. Much more frequently seen, however, is what has been termed *common factitious disorder*. In this syndrome, the patient does not use aliases and tends to seek treatment repetitively with the same physician or within the same health system. She may carry a diagnosis—which, on careful reflection, was made with imprecise criteria—such as a bleeding coagulopathy or a collagen disease. In retrospect, when the true diagnosis is discovered, it can be determined that the history, both medical and personal, was inaccurate. These patients, while deceitful, are not as inclined to pseudologia fantastica as are patients with full-blown Munchausen syndrome.

Symptoms and signs for patients with common factitious disorder tend to be less dramatic, and their complaints are often more chronic or subjective. Some common symptoms include joint pain, recurrent abscesses, failure to heal following operations, hypoglycemic episodes, simulated renal colic, and blood dyscrasias. Factitious disorder as a cause for these patients' symptoms may not be suspected for months or even years. When the diagnosis is finally established, there may be disbelief among the medical care providers. "Splitting" behavior, in which the patient plays one group of providers against another group, is frequently seen.

Factitious Disorder With Psychological Symptoms

The large majority of published cases of factitious disorder describe physical symptoms alone. When factitious psychological symptoms are recognized, they are generally in association with either authentic or fabricated physical complaints. The reason for this may be that subspecialists in psychosomatic medicine are more likely to encounter patients with factitious psychological symptoms who are hospitalized on medical–surgical wards, or in the emergency department, than to see such patients on psychiatric units. One study of Spanish psychiatric inpatients found that 8% had factitious symptoms (Catalina et al. 2008). These were interpreted as largely being exaggeration or invention of symptoms to find support, social relationships, and safety in the hospital (and therefore may include malingering).

Patients with factitious psychological symptoms fabricate a wide range of symptoms. The most commonly reported include depression and suicidal thinking tied to claims of bereavement (Phillips et al. 1983; Snowdon et al. 1978). The patient reports that his or her emotional distress is due to the death of someone close such as a parent or child. Distress appears genuine, is often accompanied by tears, and characteristically elicits sympathy from medical personnel. Later, staff members may discover that the mourned person is very much alive, that the circumstances of the death were less dramatic than the patient reported, or that the death was many years in the past. Case reports of factitious psychological symptoms also describe feigned dissociative identity disorder (multiple personality disorder), substance use disorders, dissociative and conversion reactions, memory loss, and posttraumatic stress disorder. Multiple feigned psychological symptoms may be present in the same patient (Parker 1993). Some authors urge caution in diagnosing factitious disorder with predomi-

TABLE 12–1. Examples of factitious diseases

Symptom/disease	Method of production	Diagnostic clue
Infections	Injections of saliva or feces	Polymicrobial cultures
Hypoglycemic coma	Self-injection of insulin	Low C-peptide
	Oral hypoglycemic agents	Glyburide in urine
Fever of unexplained etiology[a]	Manipulation of thermometer	Dissociation of fever/pulse
Neurological disease	Anisocoria secondary to anticholinergic eye drops	Variable reactivity of pupils
Diarrhea	Laxative abuse	Laxative in stool
Pheochromocytoma	Epinephrine in urine	Low blood chromogranin A
Electrolyte imbalance	Diuretics	High urinary potassium
Vomiting	Ipecac	Increased urinary potassium with low chloride
Coagulopathies	Warfarin	Serum assay
Anemia	Self-bloodletting	No bleeding site or iron malabsorption
Pancytopenia	Methotrexate	Serum assay
Proteinuria	Egg white in urine	Large daily variations of urine protein
Purpura	Quinidine	Serum or urinary assay
Hyperthyroidism	Exogenous thyroid	Low serum thyroglobulin
Hematuria	Finger-prick blood to urine	No casts, few or no crenated red blood cells in urinalysis

[a]Now uncommon because of the use of instantaneous electronic thermometers.

Source. Adapted from Wallach 1994.

nantly psychological symptoms, especially factitious psychosis, because some patients with these symptoms eventually manifest clear-cut severe mental illness (Nicholson and Roberts 1994; Rogers et al. 1989).

Ganser's syndrome is closely related to factitious disorder with predominantly psychological symptoms (Wirtz et al. 2008). This syndrome is characterized by the provision of approximate answers *(Vorbeireden)* to questions (e.g., the examiner asks, "What is the color of snow?" and the patient answers, "Green"). Complaints of amnesia, disorientation, and perceptual disturbance are generally present as well. This syndrome was originally described by the nineteenth-century German psychiatrist Sigbert Ganser (1965) as a form of malingering seen in prisoners, but it also has been described in other settings, including general hospital units (Dalfen and Anthony 2000; Weiner and Braiman 1955). Ganser's syndrome was described in one patient who also had clear-cut factitious physical and psychological symptoms (Parker 1993). The etiology of this syndrome remains in question, and malingering, dissociation, and organic brain disease (Sigal et al. 1992) have been proposed as contributing factors.

Diagnosis and Assessment

The diagnosis of factitious disorder may be suggested by inconsistent laboratory results, physical findings that do not conform to reported symptoms, failure to respond as predicted to effective treatment for the disorder in question, and/or the accidental discovery of medical paraphernalia on the patient's person or in the room (see Table 12–1). Some potential diagnostic clues include polymicrobial cultures from a wound that does not heal or is recurrent, and inconsistent pupillary reactivity in a person with anisocoria who surreptitiously is using anticholinergic eye drops (Wallach 1994). Ultimately, the diagnosis of factitious disorder is made via detective work by health care providers who have a high index of suspicion. A review of past medical records from other institutions may be essential to establish the diagnosis (Krahn et al. 2003). On the surface the patient may appear normal, and a psychiatric interview per se cannot establish the diagnosis unless there is a "confession." The patient, even when confronted with irrefutable evidence of factitious behavior, typically denies that the illness was self-induced and rarely expresses any remorse.

The differential diagnosis of factitious disorder includes unusual, rare, or as-yet-undescribed and unknown diseases; somatic symptom and related disorders; and overt malingering.

Etiology

The reasons that a person might engage in factitious illness behavior are, to a large extent, speculative. Even when seen in long-term treatment, these patients are resistant to articulating their motivations; furthermore, the essential quality of the disorder—the need to deceive—creates a question of validity. Proposed motivations, both conscious and unconscious, include the need to be the center of attention, dependency issues, maladaptive reactions to loss or separation, anger at physicians, and/or the pleasure of deceiving others ("duping delight"). Before DSM-5, the diagnostic criteria included "the motivation for the behavior is to assume the sick role." In DSM-5 this was dropped, with emphasis instead on the centrality of deception.

The large majority of patients with factitious disorder have an underlying severe personality disorder, usually of the Cluster B type. Factitious behavior can be seen as a form of acting out, similar to other acting-out behaviors. Axis I comorbidity, including major depression and schizophrenia, has been described but is not common. However, it must be kept in mind that psychiatric symptoms also may be simulated.

Few patients have been extensively studied with regard to developmental history because very few will agree to see a psychotherapist, and even fewer open up honestly. In the very select few who have, a childhood history of parental illness, death, or abandonment, or personal illness or institutionalization, is common (Ford 1973). As a result of these childhood experiences, factitious behavior may be viewed, at least in some circumstances, as a learned coping mechanism.

The possible role of cerebral dysfunction for at least some patients has been proposed. Pankratz and Lezak (1987) reported that approximately one-third of the Munchausen patients in their series had deficits in conceptual organization. Abnormal findings on brain imaging also have been reported (Babe et al. 1992; Fénelon et al. 1991). Brain dysfunction also has been reported in approximately 20%–25% of persons with pseudologia fantastica and/or Munchausen syndrome (Ford 1996; King and Ford 1988).

Management and Treatment

Circulated "blacklists" that identify these patients have found disfavor in the United States, largely because of legal and ethical concerns, and would be considered a violation of the Health Insurance Portability and Accountability Act of 1996 (P.L. 104–191) (best known as HIPAA). However, identification of past factitious illness behavior is facilitated in systems with a common electronic medical record (e.g., U.S. Department of Veterans Affairs). Diagnosis of a factitious disorder by use of an electronic medical record (EMR) search was reported by Van Dinter and Welch (2009). These authors emphasized the importance of attention to legal and ethical issues in reviews of EMRs.

A major question in management is how to deal with a patient once a definitive diagnosis of factitious disorder has been established. No matter how understandable the anger at these deceptive patients might be, the temptation to "let them have it" must be resisted. To act out in an angry way plays into the patient's pathology by drawing the physician into a dramatized scene. A direct, accusative confrontation is likely to result in anger from the patient and in his or her subsequent departure from the hospital, often against medical advice, or with threats to bring a lawsuit for defamation. It has been suggested that the confrontation be more indirect, in a manner that allows face-saving for the patient or an opportunity for therapy. For example, a patient may be told, "When some patients are very upset, they often do something to themselves to create illness as a way of seeking help. We believe that something such as this must be going on, and we would like to help you focus on the true nature of your problem, which is emotional distress" (Eisendrath 2001). Unfortunately, such an approach, although logical and humane, does not usually result in the patient's acknowledgment of factitious illness behavior and acceptance of psychological treatment.

When present, comorbid psychiatric disorders such as depression (if not believed to be also factitious) should be appropriately treated; in at least one case in the literature, remission of factitious behavior with antidepressant medication was reported (Earle and Folks 1986). Psychotherapy with the patient who engages in factitious behavior is, at best, extremely difficult. Treatment should be conceptualized essentially as being for a severe underlying personality disorder manifested by acting-out defenses. Stone (1977) proposed vigorous persistent confrontation of the behavior, but most clinicians who have had experience with these patients find that such confrontation results in abandonment of treatment or increase in acting-out behaviors. Instead of direct confrontation, the patient may be provided with indirect confrontation or interpretation in ongoing supportive psychotherapy (Eisendrath 2001). This technique is based on the premise that if the patient can maintain a relationship with a physician that is not contingent on development of new physical symptoms, factitious behavior may be reduced. Such a treatment approach must be viewed as primarily symptomatic with no expectation of changes in the basic personality structure that predisposes a person to factitious illness behavior. Experience with this type of treatment indicates that there may be remissions that last a few months but that they are often followed by the patient leaving treatment without warning and reengaging in factitious illness behavior elsewhere. A systematic review of all known published reports of the management and outcome of patients with diagnosed factitious disorder found no evidence for any effective treatment (Eastwood and Bisson 2008).

In the medical care of patients with any somatizing disorder (including factitious illness and malingering), the physician should proceed with invasive diagnostic and treatment procedures only when objective evidence of medical disorder is available. Furthermore, physicians must be cautious when prescribing any potentially dangerous or habituating medication (Ford 1992).

Legal and ethical issues frequently arise in the assessment and treatment of patients with factitious disorder. In the past, the paternalistic model of medicine suggested that the physician was permitted to do essentially anything that would help establish the diagnosis. More recently, particularly in the United States, medical practice has emphasized patients' rights and informed consent. This creates a dilemma. On one hand, a failure to do all that is necessary to establish the diagnosis might be regarded as abdication of medical responsibility and ultimately harmful to the patient. On the other hand, even patients suspected of factitious behavior have rights to personal privacy, including privacy in one's belongings, confidentiality, and informed consent. One approach is to tell the patient that factitious illness behavior is suspected and request permission to rule this out. This has the risk of alienating a patient who does not have factitious illness. It may result in the patient with factitious disorder refusing permission, leaving the hospital, and perpetuating the same behavior at another medical facility.

Physicians may believe that the patient's outrageous behavior of factitious disease production would leave them free from the risk of malpractice suits. This is untrue, and there have been numerous reports of lawsuits initiated by these patients (Eisendrath and McNiel 2004; Janofsky 1994). The reasons for lawsuits may include overt greed, rage at a physician who was previously idealized (borderline behavior), or perhaps the opportunity to change one's highly dramatized role as a patient in a hospital to an equally dramatized role as a plaintiff in a courtroom.

Because patients with factitious disorder do create legal and ethical problems, it is prudent for the psychiatric consultant to suggest that the management plan require careful multidisciplinary collaboration and appropriate consultation with hospital administrators, hospital and personal attorneys, and the hospital ethics committee. It cannot be overemphasized that any decision to deviate from usual medical practice with such patients should not be made by a solitary individual. Such decisions should be carried out, and their rationale noted, with the patient's best interests at heart and should be documented in the chart. When factitious disorder is suspected, chart documentation in a factual, nonspeculative manner is highly recommended.

In view of these patients' self-destructive nature, many physicians, including psychiatrists, may question whether involuntary psychiatric hospitalization is indicated. Thresholds for involuntary commitment vary from state to state and from country to country. In the United States, because factitious disorder represents chronic behavior, which is not immediately suicidal, these patients usually do not meet the criteria for involuntary psychiatric hospitalization. It is also unclear what benefit would be achieved by acute psychiatric hospitalization in a patient who denies all psychiatric symptoms. In one case in Oregon, outpatient commitment resulted in lower medical costs and less iatrogenic morbidity for a patient with factitious disorder (McFarland et al. 1983).

The prognosis of patients with factitious symptoms is unclear. Some patients may, at some point in their lives, abandon their behavior (Bass and Taylor 2013). Death, probably as a result of the patient's miscalculations of the risk of the behavior, also has been reported (Eisendrath and McNiel 2004; Nichols et al. 1990).

Factitious Disorder Imposed on Another

The introduction of a new diagnosis in DSM-5 (American Psychiatric Association 2013), factitious disorder imposed on another (FDIA), clarified the previous ambiguous and often misleading diagnosis "factitious disorder by proxy," which was more frequently called "Munchausen by proxy" syndrome. The new diagnosis identifies, specifically, the perpetrator of factitious illness in others. This clarification is important and clinically useful but does provide, by way of an "official" psychiatric diagnosis, the potential of mitigation in the prosecution for behavior that is often criminal (Ford 2005). For purposes of clarity, this topic will be divided into two sections 1) factitious behaviors imposed on children, and 2) factitious behaviors imposed on adults.

Factitious Disorder Imposed on Children (Previously Known as Munchausen by Proxy Syndrome)

Factitious illness imposed on children has been described in the medical literature since the 1970s (Meadow 1977) and has been subsequently reported numerous times and in widely varying cultures (Bappal et al. 2001). The incidence of this phenomenon is sufficiently great that most large children's hospitals are likely to see at least one case per year. In numerous case reports and diagnoses, there has been some confusion as to diagnostic distinctions between the victims (children) and the perpetrators, identified as the need for further clarification in DSM-5. Other suggested terminology has included "medical child abuse" (Ali-Panzarella et al. 2017; Roesler and Jenny 2009); "caregiver fabricated illness" (CFI), recommended by the American Academy of Pediatrics (Flaherty and Macmillan 2013); and "fabricated or induced illness by carers" per the Royal College of Paediatrics and Child Health (2013). This plethora of terms has added to confusion among clinicians, who struggle to intervene with both the victims and the perpetrators of this invidious behavior.

Clinical features of FDIA constitute a broad spectrum of presentations including, but not limited to, fever, rash, bleeding, seizures, apnea, diarrhea, and vomiting (Ali-Panzarella et al. 2017). FDIA must be distinguished from exaggeration or misinterpretation of symptoms by anxious caregivers (see Table 12–2 for differential diagnosis). Given the wide range of abnormal illness behaviors seen in real-world practice, it is essential to identify deliberate deception as a key component of factitious illness (Bass and Halligan 2014). Males and females are victimized equally, and siblings are also frequently abused. Most victims are infants, while approximately 25% are older than 6 years. Mothers are the most common perpetrators, but fathers, grandparents and other caregivers have been reported (Flaherty and Macmillan 2013).

The diagnosis of FDIA in children is underrecognized, and accurate diagnosis often takes months to years. Failure to consider it in the differential diagnosis may result in unnecessary extensive testing and procedures. The diagnosis should be considered when signs, symptoms, and course of illnesses are repeatedly inconsistent with known illnesses and expected treatment responses. It must be kept in mind that the disease, even if surreptitiously induced, may be life-threatening. When FDIA is suspected, a consultation by a clinician who has expertise in factitious disorders is indicated. When such expertise is not available, it is advised that a detailed review of medical records, including those from other facilities, and, if legal procedures are met, a similar review of siblings be undertaken. Greiner et al. (2013) developed a screening instrument for early identification of medical child abuse in hospitalized children. The most important items were that the illness resolves when the child is separated from the caregiver and the caregiver a) has features of Munchausen syndrome; b) has a history of counseling/psychiatric care; c) has a history of child abuse; and d) signs the child out of hospital against medical advice or insists on transfer to another facility. Psychopathological features of perpetrators reported by Bass and Jones (2011) indicated a high incidence of current somatoform or factitious disorders either currently or in the past. More than half of the mothers exhibited pseudologia fantastica, in some cases dating from adolescence. A systematic review of 796 perpetrators found that most were mothers of the victim; in addition, perpetrators were frequently reported to work in health care–related professions and to have personal histories of childhood mistreatment (30%), personality disorder (18.6%), or depression (14.2%) (Yates and Bass 2017).

Management and treatment for these complex patients is rarely easy. The following recommendations are made with the caveat that both suspected victims and putative perpetrators of medical child abuse must be, unless ordered differently by the court, afforded all civil rights and protections consistent with state and federal law. There are reported cases in which overzealous clinicians or child protective agencies have made accusations that were later proven to be inaccurate (Rand and Feldman 1999).

When FDIA is strongly suspected, it is recommended that a multidisciplinary management team be established to assist in diagnosis and provide definitive data to outside parties, such as child protective services, law enforcement, and the courts. This multidisciplinary team (composed potentially of the hospital legal department, risk management, child advocacy physicians, hospital security, and social work and

TABLE 12–2. **Differential diagnosis of factitious disorder imposed on another/caregiver-facilitated illness in children**

Pediatric somatization syndromes

Somatic symptom disorder or illness anxiety disorder by proxy (parent's anxiety projected/displaced onto child)

Infanticide/murder

Psychosis in parent

Child abuse

Factitious behavior initiated by child

Malingering by child (e.g., school rejection)

Unrecognized physical disease

nursing services, in addition to the attending physician) may determine if measures such as video surveillance are indicated (Ali-Panzarella et al. 2017). The first responsibility of clinicians involved in these cases is to ensure the safety of the child. A review of 451 cases of medical child abuse (Sheridan 2003) indicated that the mortality rate was 6.0% and that 25% of the known siblings were deceased! Separation of the child from the caregiver not only might result in resolution of the child's illness but also may be lifesaving. It is obvious, however, that decisions as to whether a child should be separated from the caregiver and when he or she, if ever, should be returned home are to be made by the court, with input from involved clinicians and child protective services.

Children who are victims of FDIA, when returned home to the offending caregiver, are often, once again, the victims of further medical child abuse, although this is not inevitable. The following indicators of successful treatment of the perpetrator have been outlined by Schreier (2004): the abuser a) admits to the abuse and is able to describe specifically how he or she abused the child and has experienced the appropriate emotional response to harm caused to the child, b) has developed new strategies to identify and manage personal needs, and c) has demonstrated these skills, with monitoring, over a significant period of time. Many caregivers will require treatment for mood instability, personality disorders, and their own somatic symptom disorders. Success in reunification of the abused child with the caregiver depends on the degree and quality of acknowledgment of the abuse by the caretaker and associated family as well as the willingness and capacity to engage in treatment and management (Bass and Glaser 2014).

The child victim's medical care should be centralized to one treatment center and overseen by a primary physician or a specialist who can coordinate care. The child should be evaluated and monitored as to the presence of psychological symptoms and/or failure to meet developmental milestones. For those cases that required child protective services and/or court involvement, monitoring should continue indefinitely until all concern for abuse or relapse of abusing behavior has abated.

Factitious Disorder Imposed on Another: Adult Victims

Children have been the primary concern, but medical abuse of adults by caregivers has also been reported. A review of the relevant medical literature (Burton et al. 2015) found a wide range of victims, ages 21–82 years. Presenting symptoms varied from skin abscesses or rashes produced by injections of toxic substances to syncope and coma produced by means such as insulin injections. Many of the victims had medical problems that required a caretaker. The perpetrators were primarily caretakers, most were women, and many worked in health care. Most of the perpetrators continued to deny their complicity when confronted, although some confessed and were subject to criminal prosecution. Burton et al. (2015) recommend that FDIA in adults should be included in the differential diagnosis of patients presenting with a complex constellation of symptoms without a unifying etiology.

There have been multiple reports in which health care providers have been accused of causing epidemics of acute cardiac or pulmonary arrests and unusual patterns of deaths (Yorker 1996; Yorker et al. 2006), the so-called *angel of death syndrome* (Kalisch et al. 1980). Tragically, many of these epidemics have been shown to be caused by the very persons entrusted with the patients' care. In their detailed review of multiple hospital epidemics, Yorker et al. (2006) concluded that the perpetrators were usually nurses or nurse's aides and that the victims were physically compromised: critically ill, elderly, or very young. The epidemics tend to cluster on evening and night shifts and also involve numerous, often successful, resuscitations. Yorker et al. (2006) proposed that one motive of the perpetrators is the excitement and exhilaration derived from participating in "codes." This behavior constitutes serial murder, and prosecution has resulted in several convictions. Epidemiological techniques have been used to identify probable perpetrators, but such evidence is circumstantial and cannot be used alone to establish guilt (Sacks et al. 1988).

Malingering

Malingering is not a psychiatric diagnosis. DSM-5 describes malingering as "the intentional production of false or grossly exaggerated physical or psychological problems" (American Psychiatric Association 2013, p. 726). Motivation for malingering is usually external (e.g., to avoid military duty, imprisonment, or work; to obtain financial compensation; to evade criminal prosecution; to obtain drugs). Malingering often must be considered in a differential diagnosis, but caution must be exercised in making such a "diagnosis." First, feigning of symptoms is most often dimensional and continuous rather than an absolute condition; thus, malingering often coexists with real symptoms or illness (as summarized in Bass and Halligan 2014 and Berry and Nelson 2010). Second, malingering is less a diagnosis than a socially unacceptable behavior with legal ramifications (Szasz 1956). Third, clinicians are not trained or skilled in detecting feigned illness.

Malingering is most common in settings where there are external and tangible gains accrued by illness. Symptom exaggeration has been estimated at 46%–60% of Social Security disability claimants, 29%–30% of personal injury and disability claimants, 19% of criminal cases, and 8% of medical or psychiatric cases (Chafetz and Underhill 2013; Mittenberg et al. 2002). Several studies have demonstrated that financial incentives make a difference in expression of symptoms and disability. For example, patients with mild traumatic brain injury with financial incentives exhibited more abnormality and disability than those without such incentives (Binder and Rohling

1996; Paniak et al. 2002). Evidence suggest that malingering might not be as prevalent where financial incentives are lessened (Mayou 1995).

Clinical Features: Phenomenology, Course, and Prognosis

Malingering symptoms fall into four major categories: 1) production or simulation of an illness, 2) exacerbation of a previous illness, 3) exaggeration of symptoms, and 4) falsification of laboratory samples or laboratory reports. Embellishment of previous or concurrent illness is probably the form of malingering most frequently encountered by psychiatric consultants. Patients may intensify their complaints when they are asked directly about their symptoms or when they think they are being observed. When distracted, they become physically more relaxed and at times may be seen to engage in physical activities incompatible with their symptom reports.

The malingered symptom often disappears when the person either obtains the desired goal or is confronted with irrefutable evidence of malingering. However, it has been noted that some malingered symptoms persist even after the goal is attained. It may be that the person maintains symptoms as a face-saving mechanism, or perhaps the symptom has been incorporated as a habit into the individual's lifestyle.

Diagnosis and Assessment

While malingering is not a psychiatric diagnosis, the clinician should consider malingering when the following circumstances exist: symptom complaints incongruent with objective data, the presence of secondary gains, concurrent litigation, and/or the pursuit of disability. However, none of these considerations are evidence of malingering per se. Thus, there must be not only verification of an external motivation but also objective evidence to confirm the probability of malingering. For example, a patient who cannot walk independently in the consultation suite might later be seen walking normally on a sidewalk outside the hospital. Human or video monitoring can sometimes be used to detect symptom production.

Evaluation of malingering is a multimodal and longitudinal exercise. Symptom validity psychological tests establish that a patient is intentionally performing below chance expectations on simple memory or recognition tasks (Bush et al. 2005; Heilbronner et al. 2009). Symptom validity tests such as the Test of Memory Malingering, the Word Memory Test, and the Portland Digit Recognition Test can be used in combination with the validity subscales from the Minnesota Multiphasic Personality Inventory–II (MMPI-2) and the Psychological Assessment Inventory to help establish a pattern of symptom exaggeration (McCullumsmith and Ford 2011; McDermott and Feldman 2007). Preliminary evidence suggests some utility in functional neuroimaging to evaluate conscious symptom production (Jiang et al. 2015; Ofen et al. 2017); however, use of neuroimaging is fraught with legal implications (Moriarty 2008).

The differential diagnosis of malingering includes somatic symptom disorder, conversion disorder, and factitious disorder. These clinical syndromes have indistinct boundaries, and a person may meet criteria for different disorders at different times or present with a hybrid of them (Bass and Halligan 2016; Ford 1992; Hall and Hall 2012). Patients with a confirmed disorder (e.g., schizophrenia) may also malinger symptoms of that disorder (e.g., express suicidal command hallucinations in order to get admitted). Relevant factors that may play a role in assessment include evidence of past somatization as well as coexistence of anxiety, mood, substance use, or personality disorders. Patients with unconsciously determined somatic symptoms (e.g., conversion) are usually consistent in their symptom presentation irrespective of their audience or whether they believe they are being observed. An underrecognized variation is malingering imposed on another—that is, when caregivers misrepresent or embellish the symptoms of the identified patient for their own gain (Amlani et al. 2016; Dumitrascu et al. 2015).

Etiology

By definition, the etiology of malingering is to obtain external gain as a result of the symptoms. However, malingering does tend to be more common in persons who may have histrionic or antisocial personality features.

Management and Treatment

Malingering is more a management problem than a therapeutic issue. With this in mind, the primary physician and psychiatric consultant must be circumspect in their approach to the patient. Every note must be written with the awareness that it may be read by the patient or even become a courtroom exhibit. Malingering is often listed among diagnostic possibilities but is rarely proven conclusively in medical settings.

The person who is suspected of malingering, as a rule, should not be confronted with a direct accusation. Instead, subtle communication can indicate that the physician is "onto the game" (Kramer et al. 1979). One technique is to mention, almost in passing, that diagnostic tests indicate no "serious" basis for the symptoms. The person who is malingering may feel freer to discard the symptom if the physician suggests that patients with similar problems usually recover after a certain procedure is performed or a particular length of time has passed. Such suggestions are often followed by perceptible improvement, if not recovery. This technique provides face-saving mechanisms for the patient to discard the symptom. Still, some patients, particularly those seeking drugs, will leave and seek medical care elsewhere. Others, in an effort to prove the existence of their disease, may greatly intensify their symptoms. In doing so, they may create such a caricature of illness that their efforts to malinger become obvious to all.

Conclusion

Requests for psychiatric consultation on patients with suspected factitious disorder or malingering are relatively infrequent. However, when the psychiatric consultant does become involved with one of these cases, a disproportionate amount of time is typically required. Issues of diagnosis, legal and ethical considerations, and the need to provide liaison with the medical staff may make one of these patients the primary focus of one's clinical activities for several days. Nevertheless, they are fascinating patients who demonstrate the extreme end of the continuum of abnormal illness behavior. They are rarely forgotten.

Maur KV, Wasson KR, DeFord JW, Caranasos GJ: Munchausen's syndrome: a thirty-year history of peregrination par excellence. South Med J 66(6):629–632, 1973 4733204

Mayou R: Medico-legal aspects of road traffic accidents. J Psychosom Res 39(6):789–798, 1995 8568736

McCullumsmith CB, Ford CV: Simulated illness: the factitious disorders and malingering. Psychiatr Clin North Am 34(3):621–641, 2011 21889683

McDermott BE, Feldman MD: Malingering in the medical setting. Psychiatr Clin North Am 30(4):645–662, 2007 17938038

McFarland BH, Resnick M, Bloom JD: Ensuring continuity of care for a Munchausen patient through a public guardian. Hosp Community Psychiatry 34(1):65–67, 1983 6826153

Meadow R: Munchausen syndrome by proxy. The hinterland of child abuse. Lancet 2(8033):343–345, 1977 69945

Mittenberg W, Patton C, Canyock EM, et al: Base rates of malingering and symptom exaggeration. J Clin Exp Neuropsychol 24(8):1094–1102, 2002 12650234

Moriarty JC: Flickering admissibility: neuroimaging evidence in the U.S. courts. Behav Sci Law 26(1):29–49, 2008 18327830

Munro HM, Thrusfield MV: "Battered pets": Munchausen syndrome by proxy (factitious illness by proxy). J Small Anim Pract 42(8):385–389, 2001 11518417

Nichols GR 2nd, Davis GJ, Corey TS: In the shadow of the Baron: sudden death due to Munchausen syndrome. Am J Emerg Med 8(3):216–219, 1990 2184806

Nicholson SD, Roberts GA: Patients who (need to) tell stories. Br J Hosp Med 51(10):546–549, 1994 7921496

Ofen N, Whitfield-Gabrieli S, Chai XJ, et al: Neural correlates of deception: lying about past events and personal beliefs. Soc Cogn Affect Neurosci 12(1):116–127, 2017 27798254

Paniak C, Reynolds S, Toller-Lobe G, et al: A longitudinal study of the relationship between financial compensation and symptoms after treated mild traumatic brain injury. J Clin Exp Neuropsychol 24(2):187–193, 2002 11992201

Pankratz L, Lezak MD: Cerebral dysfunction in the Munchausen syndrome. Hillside J Clin Psychiatry 9(2):195–206, 1987 3428878

Parker PE: A case report of Munchausen syndrome with mixed psychological features. Psychosomatics 34(4):360–364, 1993 8351312

Phillips MR, Ward NG, Ries RK: Factitious mourning: painless patienthood. Am J Psychiatry 140(4):420–425, 1983 6837777

Poletti M, Borelli P, Bonuccelli U: The neuropsychological correlates of pathological lying: evidence from behavioral variant frontotemporal dementia. J Neurol 258(11):2009–2013, 2011 21512737

Pulman A, Taylor J: Munchausen by Internet: current research and future directions. J Med Internet Res 14(4):e115, 2012 22914203

Rand DC, Feldman MD: Misdiagnosis of Munchausen syndrome by proxy: a literature review and four new cases. Harv Rev Psychiatry 7(2):94–101, 1999 10471247

Roesler TA, Jenny C: Medical Child Abuse: Beyond Munchausen by Proxy Syndrome. Elk Grove Village, IL, American Academy of Pediatrics, 2009, pp 43–69

Rogers R, Bagby RM, Rector N: Diagnostic legitimacy of factitious disorder with psychological symptoms. Am J Psychiatry 146(10):1312–1314, 1989 2782477

Royal College of Paediatrics and Child Health: Fabricated or Induced Illness by Carers (FII): A Practical Guide for Paediatricians. London, Royal College of Paediatrics and Child Health, 2013

Sacks JJ, Herndon JL, Lieb SH, et al: A cluster of unexplained deaths in a nursing home in Florida. Am J Public Health 78(7):806–808, 1988 3381956

Schreier H: Munchausen by proxy. Curr Probl Pediatr Adolesc Health Care 34(3):126–143, 2004 15039661

Sheridan MS: The deceit continues: an updated literature review of Munchausen syndrome by proxy. Child Abuse Negl 27(4):431–451, 2003 12686328

Sigal M, Altmark D, Alfici S, Gelkopf M: Ganser syndrome: a review of 15 cases. Compr Psychiatry 33(2):134–138, 1992 1544298

Snowdon J, Solomons R, Druce H: Feigned bereavement: twelve cases. Br J Psychiatry 133:15–19, 1978 667502

Stone MH: Factitious illness. Psychological findings and treatment recommendations. Bull Menninger Clin 41(3):239–254, 1977 871556

Szasz TS: Malingering: diagnosis or social condemnation? Analysis of the meaning of diagnosis in the light of some interrelations of social structure, value judgment, and the physician's role. AMA Arch Neurol Psychiatry 76(4):432–443, 1956 13361605

Van Dinter TG Jr, Welch BJ: Diagnosis of Munchausen's syndrome by an electronic health record search. Am J Med 122(10):e3, 2009 19786149

Wallach J: Laboratory diagnosis of factitious disorders. Arch Intern Med 154(15):1690–1696, 1994 8042885

Weiner H, Braiman A: The Ganser syndrome: a review and addition of some unusual cases. Am J Psychiatry 111(10):767–773, 1955 14361763

Wirtz G, Baas U, Hofer H, et al: [Psychopathology of Ganser's syndrome. Literature review and case report] [in German]. Nervenarzt 79(5):543–557, 2008 18274720

Yates G, Bass C: The perpetrators of medical child abuse (Munchausen syndrome by proxy)—a systematic review of 796 cases. Child Abuse Negl 72:45–53, 2017 28750264

Yates GP, Feldman MD: Factitious disorder: a systematic review of 455 cases in the professional literature. Gen Hosp Psychiatry 41:20–28, 2016 27302720

Yorker BC: Hospital epidemics of factitious disorder by proxy, in The Spectrum of Factitious Disorders. Edited by Feldman MD, Eisendrath SJ. Washington, DC, American Psychiatric Press, 1996, pp 157–174

Yorker BC, Kizer KW, Lampe P, et al: Serial murder by healthcare professionals. J Forensic Sci 51(6):1362–1371, 2006 17199622

CHAPTER 13

Eating Disorders

Weronika Micula-Gondek, M.D.
Angela S. Guarda, M.D.

Eating disorders are associated with high use of clinical resources and frequent medical complications (Westmoreland et al. 2016), yet often go unrecognized in medical settings. Patients may present either emergently in crisis or seeking relief from chronic medical or psychiatric complications of the disorder. Symptom concealment and minimization are common, because patients are often anxious about changing their underlying eating and weight-control behaviors and may even explicitly deny having an eating disorder. Ambivalence toward behavior change is therefore the norm, and feelings of shame, embarrassment, and stigma further complicate patient engagement. Most cases respond to behavioral specialist treatment; however, the majority of persons with eating disorders remain untreated, and some are at risk of iatrogenic complications if the underlying behavioral condition is not recognized and addressed.

Anorexia nervosa (AN), bulimia nervosa (BN), binge-eating disorder (BED), and the newly defined avoidant/restrictive food intake disorder (ARFID) are the main diagnostic categories of eating disorders. These conditions are best thought of as motivated behavioral disorders with phenomenological parallels to addiction. Eating disorders are associated with a repertoire of increasingly driven behaviors that include restrained eating or dieting, binge eating, purging, and excessive exercise. With a cumulative population prevalence of more than 5% (Hoek 2016), these conditions are common and are likely to be encountered in any general practice or acute care setting. Familiarity with diagnostic screening questions, comorbid conditions, complications, medical stabilization, and effective treatment options is essential for the psychiatric consultant, given that medical morbidity and mortality rates are high, especially for AN (Arcelus et al. 2011; Fichter and Quadflieg 2016). When (as in the case of extreme AN) complications become life-threatening, ethical questions, including capacity to refuse treatment, become relevant to treatment planning.

We begin this chapter with a review of the main diagnostic categories of eating disorders in DSM-5 (American Psychiatric Association 2013), as well as the relevant comorbid psychiatric and medical diagnoses. We discuss assessment and differential diagnoses and outline what is known about the etiology and maintenance of eating disorders. This discussion is followed by a summary of medical complications and their management. We then review nutritional guidelines for refeeding in AN, as well as evidence-based treatments for each disorder. Finally, we address ethical issues that may be encountered by the psychiatric consultant, including capacity to refuse treatment, confidentiality, and involuntary treatment.

Diagnostic Categories

DSM-5 introduced several changes to the diagnostic classification of eating disorders to improve clinical utility and to reduce the size of the residual diagnostic category eating disorder not otherwise specified (EDNOS), which under DSM-IV (American Psychiatric Association 1994) was being applied in up to 50% of cases because the presenting symptoms did not fulfill criteria for a specific eating disorder. DSM-5 introduced binge-eating disorder as a separate diagnosis, broadened the criteria for AN and BN, and incorporated the DSM-IV section of Feeding and Eating Disorders of Infancy or Early Childhood into a revised and combined Feeding and Eating Disorders chapter. Six distinctive eating disorders are identified in DSM-5: pica, rumination disorder, ARFID, AN, BN, and BED. Clinically significant eating disorders that do not meet the criteria for any of the above are captured under two residual categories: other specified feeding or eating disorder (OSFED) and unspecified feeding or eating disorder (UFED) (Call et al. 2013; Keel et al. 2011).

Pica

Pica is characterized by developmentally inappropriate and culturally nonnormative consumption of nonnutritive substances (e.g., dirt, clay, soap, paper, paint chips) for at least 1 month. The prevalence of pica has not been established; however, the disorder is more common in children, patients with severe developmental disabilities, patients with medical comorbidities (especially iron deficiency), and patients requiring non-oral feeding methods. Anxiety, sense of loss of control or self-harm tendencies, and poor family functioning have been associated with pica (Kelly et al. 2014). Compulsive ice eating (pagophagia), a common form of pica, is associated with iron deficiency anemia and appears to have an elevated prevalence in pregnant women, malnourished children, and persons who have undergone gastric bypass surgery (Tabaac and Tabaac 2015). Extreme cases of pica have been associated with lead poisoning (from consuming paint chips) and with abdominal pain, constipation, and bezoar formation (when associated with trichotillomania).

Rumination Disorder

Rumination disorder is characterized by recurrent regurgitation of food, which may be re-chewed, re-swallowed, or spit out. To qualify for the diagnosis, these behaviors must be present for at least 1 month and must not be attributable to a gastrointestinal or other medical condition. Rumination disorder is common in patients with autism spectrum disorder and is highly comorbid with depression, anxiety, and obsessive-compulsive behaviors (Bryant-Waugh et al. 2010). When rumination occurs in the context of a neurodevelopmental disorder, the eating disturbance should be sufficiently severe to warrant additional clinical attention. Regurgitation and re-chewing of food can also be seen as eating disorder behaviors in some patients with binge–purge behavior and chronic AN or BN, and in these cases it should be differentiated from chewing and spitting behavior. Chewing and spitting behavior is also present in a significant proportion of patients with AN and BN and has been associated with higher severity of symptoms (Guarda et al. 2004).

Avoidant/Restrictive Food Intake Disorder

The diagnostic category of ARFID captures children, adolescents, and adults with severe food restriction or avoidance and significant weight loss or compromised growth and nutritional deficiencies who do not exhibit fear of weight gain, body image disturbance, or drive for thinness. Patients may rely on nutritional supplements to meet their caloric requirements, and the food intake disturbance often causes marked interference with psychosocial functioning (American Psychiatric Association 2013). Patients with ARFID may present with very complex medical and psychiatric histories and may cite multiple reasons for their decreased food intake. Some, including those with autism spectrum diagnoses, may reject foods with certain textures, consistencies, or tastes. Others may restrict their food repertoire or absolute caloric intake because of specific concerns, such as fears of choking, vomiting, food allergies, or abdominal pain with eating. They may react to stress or trauma by restricting food intake or develop idiosyncratic fears of certain additives or chemicals. The exact prevalence of ARFID in the general population is not well established. A recently published study reported a prevalence of 0.3% in the Australian population (Hay et al. 2017). It is estimated that about 5%–14% of inpatients in eating disorder programs have symptoms that meet criteria for ARFID. Children and adolescents with ARFID typically are male and younger and have significant psychiatric and medical comorbidity (Norris et al. 2016).

Anorexia Nervosa

The first medical description of AN was provided in 1874 by Sir William Gull in a report on two young female patients suffering from anorexia associated with extreme weight loss (Gull 1997). Gull also gave the disease its name. AN was described almost simultaneously by French physician Charles Lasègue, who focused on the hysterical nature of the illness. It was not until the mid-1960s, however, that Hilde Bruch introduced the notion of a body image disturbance involving overvaluation of thinness and morbid fear of fatness as core psychological features (Russell and Treasure 1989). Over the years, explanations for the etiology of AN have varied from the belief that self-starvation originates from pituitary insufficiency to psychoanalytic explanations attributing the cause of the disorder to a toxic, "anorexogenic family" or to patients' need to control their bodies (Dell'Osso et al. 2016).

DSM-5 has maintained the focus on AN as a syndrome of self-starvation but has shifted to emphasizing the behavioral nature of the disorder, because some patients deny fear of fatness or body dissatisfaction yet exhibit persistent dieting or exercise behaviors as well as lack of concern about the need to interrupt these behaviors despite escalating negative consequences. The three primary features of AN in DSM-5 are therefore 1) persistent food intake restriction and low body weight, 2) either intense fear of gaining weight *or* behavior that interferes with weight gain, and 3) either disturbance in self-perceived weight or shape *or* persistent lack of recognition of the seriousness of being in a starved state. *Low weight* is defined as less than minimally normal or less than minimally expected in children and adolescents based on their weight trajectory (Call et al. 2013). Additionally, DSM-5 eliminated the criterion of secondary amenorrhea, thereby broadening the diagnosis to include patients with AN who are premenarchal, who take exogenous hormones, or who are male (Attia and Roberto 2009). Two types of AN are distinguished: restricting type (AN-R), marked by severe dieting, fasting, and (in the majority) overexercising; and binge-eating/purging type (AN-BP), which additionally includes the regular use of bingeing and/or purging behaviors such as self-induced vomiting and misuse of laxatives and/or diuretics (American Psychiatric Association 2013).

Estimates for lifetime prevalence of AN are 0.9% for females and 0.3% for males (Hudson et al. 2007). AN is a very serious illness, with the highest mortality rate among all psychiatric disorders, primarily due to complications of starvation and suicide. The standardized mortality ratio has been reported to be as high as 5.35% (Fichter and Quadflieg 2016). Onset of AN is typically in adolescence or young adulthood, with peak incidence between 14 and 25 years (Smink et al. 2012). Although 25%–70% of patients with AN eventually recover, the process is often a protracted one, occurring over the course of 5–6 years and marked by multiple relapses and remissions (Keel and Brown 2010). There is a high degree of diagnostic crossover, in that about half of patients with restricting-type AN will progress to either AN-BP or BN over time (Eddy et al. 2002).

Bulimia Nervosa

Bulimia nervosa was first defined by Gerald Russell in 1979 in a report of 30 patients described as having a variant of AN involving normal weight or overweight and characterized by regular bingeing and purging symptoms, less menstrual irregularity than in AN, higher rates of depression, and a poor prognosis (Russell 1979). BN was formally recognized as a distinct eating disorder in DSM-III-R (American Psychiatric Association 1987; Castillo and Weiselberg 2017). The defining features are recurrent episodes of binge eating associated with a sense of loss of control over eating, use of compensatory behaviors to prevent weight gain or to promote weight loss, and self-evaluation that is unduly influenced by body weight and shape. As in AN, patients typically engage in dieting and restricting behavior. The distinction between BN and AN-BP is one of weight, with AN-BP taking precedence over the diagnosis of BN in individuals with a low body mass index (BMI) (typically defined as <18.5). The lifetime prevalence of BN is estimated as 1.5% in females and 0.1%–0.5% in males (Hoek 2014).In DSM-5, the diagnosis of BN was broadened by reducing the required frequency of bingeing from twice a week to once a week (Hoek 2014), because data indicated no clear difference in severity or prognosis associated with this criterion change (Attia et al. 2013). *Binge eating* is characterized by 1) recurrent episodes of eating, within a relatively brief period (less than 2 hours), a large amount of food (larger than most people would eat under similar circumstances and during the same time frame); and 2) a feeling of loss of control over eating during these episodes (American Psychiatric Association 2013). Patients with BN typically restrict their intake to low-calorie-density "safe" foods and skip meals but intermittently lose control and binge on high-calorie-density "forbidden" foods. Binges are typically followed by purging behavior to avoid weight gain.

The most commonly used inappropriate compensatory behavior in patients with BN is self-induced vomiting (56.6%–86.4%), followed by abuse of laxatives (8.3%) and abuse of diuretics (6.6%) (Forney et al. 2016). Up to 50% of patients with BN employ multiple methods of purging, and an increased repertoire of behaviors is associated with greater severity of illness and more extreme methods of weight control (Haedt et al. 2006). Although most patients initially stimulate the gag reflex with their fingers or an object in order to vomit, those who vomit frequently can often regurgitate food spontaneously in a controlled fashion without inducing a gag. Patients generally vomit within 30 to 60 minutes after eating, and vomit is nonbilious. Some patients may use less conventional purging methods. Syrup of ipecac was sometimes used as a purgative before its withdrawal from the U.S. market in 2010 following reports of cardiotoxicity and deaths (Silber 2005). Abuse of orlistat, a weight loss supplement that decreases fat absorption in the gut and causes fatty diarrhea, has also been described (Malhotra and McElroy 2002), and patients with comorbid type 1 diabetes mellitus may purge by intentionally skipping or reducing prescribed doses of insulin. Prompt identification of unusual purging behaviors is of primary importance to clinicians, because purging can result in severe electrolyte imbalances and other medical complications and has been associated with increased risk of death.

Binge-Eating Disorder

First described by Albert Stunkard in 1959 as a form of abnormal eating among obese patients, BED was included as a provisional diagnosis warranting further research in DSM-IV and was formally recognized as a distinct eating disorder in DSM-5. BED is the most common eating disorder diagnosis, with lifetime prevalence rates of 1.9%–2.6% in the U.S. population (Kessler et al. 2013). Whereas up to 90% of cases of AN and BN occur in females, BED is more equally distributed, with about one-third of patients being male (Hudson et al. 2007). Like BN, BED is characterized by recurrent weekly binge-eating episodes, accompanied by a sense of loss of control over eating, that extend over a period of 3 months or more. In contrast to BN, however, BED does not involve regular use of compensatory behaviors (Guerdjikova et al. 2017). Moreover, binge-eating episodes in BED must be associated with at least three of the following additional symptoms: eating alone, eating when not physically hungry, eating more rapidly than usual, eating until physically full and uncomfortable, and feeling disgusted with oneself, depressed, or guilty after a binge. Although preoccupation with shape and weight is not included in the diagnostic criteria, about 60% of patients with BED exhibit such preoccupations, a feature associated with more significant eating pathology, more psychological distress, and negative self-esteem, as well as worse treatment outcomes (Grilo et al. 2009). About 40% of patients with BED meet criteria for metabolic syndrome, and evidence suggests that BED represents an obesity-independent risk factor for hypertension, diabetes, and dyslipidemia (Barnes et al. 2011). Other medical conditions frequently comorbid with BED include sleep disorders, pain disorders, irritable bowel syndrome, and fibromyalgia. Even though BED is the most common eating disorder, it is often overlooked. Shame and embarrassment often keep patients from disclosing their symptoms to their treatment providers. Furthermore, in primary care or inpatient medical settings, clinicians have a tendency to focus on treatment of obesity and its complications and may fail to inquire about, recognize, or address underlying eating pathology (Wilfley et al. 2016). BED is one of the most common psychiatric diagnoses in morbidly obese individuals seeking weight-loss surgery, with rates estimated to be as high as 17% (Dawes et al. 2016). Although current literature does not demonstrate a direct association between BED and postsurgical outcomes, most experts recommend that individuals with BED pursue eating disorder treatment prior to surgery, because normalization of eating behavior is likely to favorably impact postsurgical weight and psychological outcomes (Sogg et al. 2016).

Other Specified Feeding or Eating Disorder and Unspecified Feeding or Eating Disorder

OSFED is a provisional diagnosis applied to presentations of clinically significant symptoms characteristic of an eating disorder that cause pronounced distress and functional impairment but do not meet full criteria for a specific eating disorder diagnosis. This heterogeneous category of eating disorder presentations (with an estimated lifetime prevalence of about 1.5%) encompasses purging disorder and night eating syndrome, as well as cases of atypical AN (see paragraph below) and cases of BN and BED with a low frequency of binge and/or purge episodes or a duration shorter than 3 months (Mustelin et al. 2016). Of these syndromes, atypical AN is the most likely to be encountered by inpatient consultation-liaison psychiatrists because it can be associated with significant acute medical morbidity.

Atypical anorexia nervosa is a syndrome that meets all of the criteria for AN except low weight. At baseline, individuals with atypical AN are commonly overweight or obese, and they may present at normal or above-normal weight, having sustained marked and often rapid weight loss. Atypical AN involves behaviors and cognitions similar to those seen in classic AN but is likely to be underrecognized, resulting in a delay in diagnosis. Patients with atypical AN are prone to the same potentially life-threatening medical complications seen in AN, including nutritional deficiency syndromes, refeeding syndrome, and dangerous electrolyte abnormalities. As in AN, patients have high levels of psychiatric comorbidity and distress over eating and body image (Sawyer et al. 2016). Atypical AN following massive weight loss has also been described in patients who have undergone bariatric surgery (Conceição et al. 2013).

Night eating syndrome, another example of OSFED, is defined as a circadian disturbance in both sleep–wake cycles and meal consumption, with excess calorie intake at night, often upon awakening from sleep, that is outside cultural norms and causes impairment of function. Patients may have a sense of loss of control over eating and may assume that they must eat to be able to go to sleep. The prevalence of night eating syndrome is highest in obese individuals, and, interestingly, weight loss interventions tend to improve night eating syndrome symptomatology (Gallant et al. 2012).

Finally, UFED is a residual category that does not require clarification as to why the criteria for a specific eating disorder are not met. This diagnosis may apply in situations in which there is not enough information to establish a more specific diagnosis (e.g., the emergency room) (American Psychiatric Association 2013).

Psychiatric Comorbidity in Patients With Eating Disorders

Patients with eating disorders have high rates of psychiatric comorbidity, with the likelihood of at least one comorbid psychiatric diagnosis estimated to be around 70% (Ulfvebrand et al. 2015). Anxiety disorders, followed by depressive disorders and substance use disorders (SUDs), are the most common comorbid conditions.

Major Depressive Disorder

Comorbid depression is common in both AN and BN, with lifetime prevalence estimates ranging from 20% to 98% (Ulfvebrand et al. 2015). The validity of depression rating scales in patients with eating disorders has been questioned, however, because of the overlap between physiological consequences of starvation and physical symptoms of depression, including fatigue, anhedonia, and weight or sleep changes. Furthermore, starvation is associated with a depressive syndrome that can be difficult to distinguish from major depressive disorder, although depression secondary to starvation generally reverses rapidly with refeeding, usually within days or a few weeks. Some have noted that the evidence base supporting a direct relationship between malnutrition in AN and depressive symptoms is not entirely consistent (Mattar et al. 2011), given that improvement in mood symptoms with refeeding is not closely correlated with BMI change (Mattar et al. 2012a, 2012b; Voderholzer et al. 2016). When truly comorbid, major depressive disorder may precede the onset of an eating disorder, and elevated rates of depression are found in relatives of patients with AN (Perdereau et al. 2008). Eating disorders, especially AN, are associated with an increased risk of suicidality, and suicide accounts for about 20%–30% of deaths in AN (Papadopoulos et al. 2009). Recent studies have documented shared genetic factors among AN, major depressive disorder, and suicide attempts (Thornton et al. 2016).

Anxiety Disorders and Obsessive-Compulsive Disorder

The lifetime prevalence of anxiety disorders (including DSM-IV obsessive-compulsive disorder [OCD][1]) is estimated at around 64% across the eating disorder diagnoses (Godart et al. 2002; Kaye et al. 2004). Social anxiety disorder and OCD are the most common comorbid disorders, with reported prevalence rates of 20% and 40%, respectively (Kaye et al. 2004). Methodological differences are implicated in inconsistencies between studies examining the impact of anxiety disorders on eating disorder outcomes, but evidence suggests that anxiety comorbidity may be associated with worse

[1] In DSM-5, OCD is now classified with the Obsessive-Compulsive and Related Disorders, but for the purposes of this discussion it remains grouped with the Anxiety Disorders.

prognosis, especially for AN (Godart et al. 2003). Anxiety disorders in AN are also positively associated with greater severity of illness, including lower BMI and higher levels of eating disorder psychopathology (Guarda et al. 2015). While in many cases anxiety disorders predate the onset of eating disorders (42% in clinical samples), food-related obsessive-compulsive symptomatology can also evolve during food restriction and can worsen with malnutrition. Common non-food/exercise-related or non-weight-related obsessional symptoms in patients with AN include concerns about symmetry and order and rituals involving checking and counting. It is difficult to distinguish state anxiety from trait anxiety in acutely ill patients, although multiple studies have shown that anxious traits—including perfectionism, harm avoidance, and obsessionality—tend to persist even after recovery from an eating disorder and are present in first-degree relatives of affected probands (Kaye et al. 2004). Importantly, and in contrast to classic OCD symptoms, preoccupations with food and weight or shape in AN are typically ego-syntonic and are not resisted (Swinbourne and Touyz 2007).

Substance Use Disorders

Patients with eating disorders have an elevated prevalence of SUDs, with rates as high as 37% among patients with BN, 27% among patients with AN, and 23% among patients with BED (Hudson et al. 2007). Comorbid SUDs contribute to increased mortality, medical complications, and psychopathology; poor functional outcomes; and high relapse rates (Munn-Chernoff and Baker 2016). Purging diagnoses, including both BN and AN-BP (the binge-eating/purging subtype of AN), are more strongly associated with SUDs than is AN-R (the restricting subtype of AN), with alcohol being the most frequent drug of choice. Caffeine and tobacco are commonly used as appetite suppressants by women with eating disorders, and amphetamines may be abused for their appetite-suppression effects. The high comorbidity between SUDs and eating disorders is not well understood, although some evidence supports a genetic association between bingeing/purging symptoms and SUDs (Munn-Chernoff et al. 2015). There are phenomenological similarities between SUDs and eating disorders, especially with respect to BN and BED. Shared components include cravings, lack of control over consumption, and minimization and denial of symptoms. Underlying personality vulnerabilities, including traits of impulsivity, novelty seeking, and affective dysregulation, are additionally characteristic of both eating disorders and SUDs (Harrop and Marlatt 2010). The treatment of patients with comorbid eating disorders and SUDs is challenging. Ideally, both disorders should be addressed at the same time, because improvement in one behavioral disorder may be paralleled by worsening symptomatology in the other behavioral disorder.

Other Psychiatric Comorbidity in Eating Disorders

A recent literature review and meta-analysis suggested high comorbidity between eating disorders and attention-deficit/hyperactivity disorder (ADHD) (Nazar et al. 2016). ADHD, which is characterized by impulse-control symptoms, has been most closely associated with overeating, emotional eating, and binge-eating behaviors (Kaisari et al. 2017).

Finally, somatic symptom disorders, particularly those involving predominant pain complaints, are often present in patients with eating disorders and are likely to be encountered in medical settings. Recurrent headaches and abdominal pain are common in patients with chronic AN, who may present with these symptoms as their chief complaint to medical specialists. Among hospitalized and emergency department patient populations, patients with eating disorders and somatic pain disorders may additionally have symptoms that meet criteria for dependence on opioids or benzodiazepines.

Diabetes and Eating Disorders

Perhaps the most significant comorbid medical condition with eating disorders is type 1 diabetes mellitus, because the co-occurrence of these two disorders is associated with elevated morbidity and mortality (Peveler et al. 2005) (see also Chapter 21, "Endocrine and Metabolic Disorders"). Adolescents with type 1 diabetes have a higher prevalence of BN compared with those without diabetes (7% vs. 2.8%), and the prevalence of disordered eating behaviors in patients with type 1 diabetes is close to 40% (Young et al. 2013). Individuals with type 1 diabetes mellitus may purge calories by intentionally skipping or reducing their prescribed doses of insulin, resulting in increased urinary excretion of glucose and weight loss. They are at increased risk of both acute and chronic complications of diabetes, including diabetic ketoacidosis (DKA), poor glycemic control, and elevated hemoglobin A1c levels, with microvascular sequelae, including retinopathy and nephropathy. Overdosing of insulin to induce hypoglycemia and justify binge eating and consumption of high-carbohydrate foods have also been described (Scheuing et al. 2014). Several factors associated with the development of disordered eating in patients with comorbid type 1 diabetes have been reported, including premorbid overweight or obesity, prepubertal onset of diabetes, and initial disease-related weight loss followed by weight gain after diagnosis and initiation of insulin therapy. Moreover, chronic management of diabetes depends on dietary restriction and carbohydrate counting, goals that may promote disordered eating behaviors in susceptible individuals. The diagnosis of disordered eating in patients with type 1 diabetes can be challenging. Unexplained weight loss, suboptimal glycemic control, and/or recurrent hypoglycemia or DKA, as well as missed appointments and reluctance to be weighed, should raise suspicion for an underlying eating disorder (Pinhas-Hamiel et al. 2015).

Assessment

The evaluation of patients with suspected eating disorders can be challenging. While patients often present to emergency rooms, primary care physicians, or medical specialists with nonspecific complaints, such as fatigue, anxiety, or dysthymia, or with physical complications of malnutrition or purging, such as gastrointestinal symptoms, secondary amenorrhea, stress fractures, hypotension, or syncope, they may not report, or may actively deny, that they have an eating disorder (Sangvai 2016). The Academy for Eating Disorders (2016) publishes an online medical guide to eating disorders that provides useful information on early recognition and medical risks of these disorders.

Initial assessment by consultation-liaison psychiatrists in the general medical setting can be complicated because of the similarities between patients with primary eating disorders and patients with underlying medical problems that lead to eating and weight disturbance. Whereas patients in the two groups may report similar frequencies of vomiting, patients with underlying eating disorder pathology are more likely than those whose eating and weight symptoms are solely related to their medical condition to also engage in restricting and/or bingeing behavior, laxative abuse, and excessive exercise (Carney and Yates 1998).

During the interview, clinicians should assume a nonjudgmental approach and inquire directly about disordered eating behaviors, because patients often minimize or deny symptoms. In addition to ambivalence toward treatment, patients struggle with feelings of shame about their behaviors and fear of being judged or not taken seriously by medical professionals. The latter concern may be especially pertinent when a patient is of normal or elevated body weight, as in atypical AN. Patients with BED or BN may be more forthcoming about their symptoms than those with AN because of distress related to binge eating or overweight. Women with BED often present with a combination of mild mood and anxiety symptoms, anhedonia, sleep disturbance, concentration problems, and a history of consistent weight gain or "yo-yo" dieting. Collateral information from a patient's family members is often critical to establishing a diagnosis. It may be useful to ask relatives whether they have noticed rapid weight changes or recent changes in the patient's behavior, including changes in the types and amounts of foods consumed, avoidance of family dinners or meals prepared by others, excessive exercising, or evidence of purging after meals or of binge eating, as well as general changes in mood or in social and academic functioning. In inpatients, nursing staff reports regarding unusual eating rituals, hiding of food, detailed food requests, or excessive fidgeting, exercising, or pacing in underweight patients can further clarify whether malnutrition may be related to an eating disorder.

Evaluation should include a detailed assessment of changes in body weight (maximum and minimum adult weights), current BMI, and weight trajectory in children and adolescents, as well as desired body weight. A desired BMI less than 18.5 in response to the question "What is the most you would feel comfortable weighing?" is suggestive of AN. Inquiring about a typical day's food intake and dietary variety may be helpful in assessing whether a patient's food choices are restricted to low-fat items and whether there is normal dietary variety, given that many patients with eating disorders maintain a monotonous and restricted food repertoire. Direct questions about binge eating—defined as an episodic sense of loss of control over eating associated with consumption of a large amount of palatable food, typically of high calorie density—should be asked. History taking should also address use of any purging behaviors, including self-induced vomiting and use of laxatives or diuretics. A question that may be helpful in distinguishing regular from excessive exercise is "How much exercise would you engage in if it did not burn calories?" Types of exercise and recent changes in exercise routines can also be informative. Most patients with AN prefer solitary exercise rather than (or in addition to) team sports, and aerobic exercise rather than strength training. Other relevant questions may address dieting behaviors, including calorie counting, label checking, frequent weighing, and preoccupations with body image; "feeling fat"; and new and/or expanding food intolerances. Most patients will endorse feeling overly preoccupied with thoughts of food, weight, and shape during much of their day.

A detailed medical review of systems and physical examination should be performed to assess for signs and symptoms of starvation and purging (Table 13–1). Current weight, height, body mass index, temperature, and vital signs should be recorded. Patients should be weighed in a hospital gown whenever possible, because some patients with AN will wear multiple layers of clothing or hide heavy objects in their pockets to conceal their true weight (Harrington et al. 2015).

Initial medical workup should include laboratory studies: complete blood count; comprehensive metabolic panel, to include electrolytes, blood urea nitrogen and serum creatinine, liver function tests, and serum phosphate; thyroid stimulating hormone; urinalysis; urine toxicology; and an electrocardiogram. Patients with amenorrhea of 6 or more months' duration should have a bone density evaluation (dual-energy x-ray absorptiometry [DXA] scan) to assess for osteoporosis.

Several quick-screening assessment tools may be helpful in establishing a diagnosis (Table 13–2). The SCOFF questionnaire is a five-question tool that is easy to administer and score. It has a sensitivity of about 92%–100% for both AN and BN and fairly high specificity (87.5%), and it has been tested and validated for routine screening in numerous settings across different countries (Morgan et al. 2000). The Eating Disorder Screen for Primary Care (ESP) is another simple-to-administer screener with sensitivity and specificity (100% and 71%, respectively) similar to those of the SCOFF (Cotton et al. 2003). For both tools, two or more abnormal responses represent a positive test score.

The Eating Disorder Examination Questionnaire (EDE-Q) is a longer, 36-item self-report measure that provides a more comprehensive assessment of specific eating disorder symptoms and behaviors and is frequently used to complement comprehensive clinical evaluation (Mond et al. 2008).

Differential Diagnosis

There is overlap between symptoms of eating disorders and symptoms of a variety of serious medical or psychiatric disorders that should be considered in the differential diagnosis. For example, cancer (e.g., hypothalamic tumors or other occult malignancies) and gastrointestinal disorders (e.g., peptic ulcer disease, celiac disease, inflammatory bowel disease) can be accompanied by weight loss associated with a variety of gastrointestinal symptoms, including abdominal pain, early satiety, vomiting, constipation, and diarrhea. Autoimmune and endocrine disorders, including hyperthyroidism and type 1 diabetes, can be associated with weight loss despite increased appetite. Patients with primary adrenal insufficiency can present with prominent weight loss, anorexia, fatigue, vomiting, and dehydration. Weight loss and nutritional deficiencies can also result from chronic infections (e.g., from HIV, tuberculosis, hepatitis C, parasites), as well as from advanced lung disease, kidney disease, or neurological disease (e.g., stroke, amyotrophic lateral sclerosis) that causes impairment in cognition, motor dysfunction, or dysphagia (Vanderschueren et al. 2005). An exhaustive workup to rule out all possible medical diagnoses is not indicated in the ma-

TABLE 13–1.   **Signs and symptoms of eating disorders**

Starvation related	Purging related
Dry skin, lanugo, hair loss	Parotid gland enlargement
Cold intolerance, hypothermia	Dental caries and erosion
Weakness, fatigue	Perioral acne
Low mood, poor concentration, insomnia	Low mood, poor concentration
Hot flashes, diaphoresis	Orthostatic tachycardia, dehydration
Sinus bradycardia, orthostasis	Heartburn/reflux/abdominal pain
Early satiety, bloating, constipation	Hematemesis
Primary or secondary amenorrhea	Amenorrhea/oligomenorrhea
Low libido	Muscle cramps, paresthesias
Decreased bone density, fractures	Palpitations, cardiac arrhythmias
Muscle wasting/cachexia	Diarrhea/constipation
Nose bleeds, bruising	Hemorrhoids/rectal prolapse
Stress fractures	Presyncope or syncope
Presyncope or syncope	

TABLE 13–2.   **Rapid screening assessment tools for eating disorders**

SCOFF	Eating Disorder Screen for Primary Care
Do you make yourself **Sick** because you feel uncomfortably full?	Are you satisfied with your eating patterns? (A "no" to this question is classified as an abnormal response.)
Do you worry you have lost **Control** over how much you eat?	Do you ever eat in secret? (A "yes" to this and all other questions is classified as an abnormal response.)
Have you recently lost more than **One** stone (14 lbs. or 7.7 kg) in a 3-month period?	Does your weight affect the way you feel about yourself?
Do you believe yourself to be **Fat** when others say you are thin?	Have any members of your family suffered with an eating disorder?
Would you say that **Food** dominates your life?	Do you currently suffer with or have you ever suffered in the past with an eating disorder?

jority of cases of AN or BN, in which the full behavioral and psychological profile of the disorder is met. However, in atypical cases, or in cases of ARFID, careful consideration should be given to the possibility of an underlying medical etiology for recent changes in eating behavior or weight. It is also possible for a secondary eating disorder to arise in the setting of a primary medical condition that initiated the weight loss or gastrointestinal symptoms.

Numerous psychiatric disorders, including depressive disorders, psychotic disorders with paranoid delusions related to food or poisoning, obsessive-compulsive and related disorders, and neurocognitive disorders, can be associated with appetite disturbance and weight loss. Patients with severe SUDs are at risk of weight loss and nutritional deficiencies, particularly patients with alcohol use disorder and patients who abuse stimulants (e.g., cocaine, amphetamines) that are known to cause anorexia and weight loss.

A thorough history, including assessment of preoccupations with weight and shape, eating disorder behaviors, collateral history from family members, and review of past medical records, is often helpful in clarifying the diagnosis when the medical evaluation is unrevealing. Admission to a behavioral eating disorders program for observation and nutritional rehabilitation can assist in providing additional useful information in complex cases. It is important to remember that an eating disorder diagnosis can be associated with a range of significant medical complications.

Etiology: Predisposing, Precipitating, and Sustaining Factors

The cause of eating disorders is multifactorial and includes biological, psychological, and sociocultural contributions. A useful conceptual etiological framework separates risk factors into those that predispose to the condition, those that precipitate its onset, and those that come to maintain the self-sustaining nature of the behaviors over time. The three major eating disorders—AN, BN and BED—are all heritable. Family studies have identified a number of inherited personality traits, including perfectionism, harm avoidance, cognitive rigidity, neuroticism, and low self-directedness, in individuals with eating disorders and in their first-degree relatives, suggesting that these may be predisposing traits. Evidence of a genetic predisposition is strongest for AN, for which twin studies have yielded heritability estimates of 0.48–0.74 (Bulik et al. 2016). A recent large study revealed a genomewide significant locus on chromosome 12 as well as significant correlations with several psychological (e.g., high neuroticism, high educational attainment) and metabolic traits (e.g., low BMI) (Duncan et al. 2017). Childhood anxiety has been associated with lower lifetime BMIs in AN (Dellava et al. 2010), and anxious personality traits may affect course and prognosis of the disorder (Guarda et al. 2015). Significant life stressors in the year of onset of an eating disorder are common precipitants (Degortes et al. 2014; Hay and Williams 2013; Horesh et al. 1995), and impaired stress-coping styles linked to the aforementioned personality traits or high anxiety may contribute to illness course or treatment response. Precipitating factors other than acute and chronic stressors in adolescents include dieting behavior (Evans et al. 2017); depressive symptoms and body dissatisfaction (Goldschmidt et al. 2015; Rohde et al. 2015); and excessive exercise, which is present in the majority of patients with AN and often precedes the onset of dieting behavior (Davis et al. 2005). Estrogen may play a facilitatory role, given the female preponderance in AN and its peripubertal age at onset. Once the diagnosis of an eating disorder is established, as in addiction, classical conditioning and habit are increasingly believed to play a role in maintaining the disorder as weight-control behaviors, including food restriction and exercise, become more compulsive, automatic, and habitual (Steinglass and Walsh 2006). Consistent with the motivated nature of eating disorders, alterations in reward processing have been implicated in these disorders (Kaye et al. 2013). In AN, for example, as the disorder progresses, the physiological consequences of starvation and purging behaviors lead to alterations in satiety and hunger signaling (Monteleone et al. 2008), neural reward circuitry (Bischoff-Grethe et al. 2013; Cha et al. 2016; Monteleone et al. 2017), and attention and decision-making processes (Foerde et al. 2015; Guillaume et al. 2015). Although these are consequences of the disorder, there is increasing evidence that some of these changes likely feed forward and come to sustain disordered eating and weight-control behaviors and eating disorder cognitions over time.

Medical Complications

Eating disorders are associated with high rates of medical complications and high morbidity. Multiple organ systems may be affected, resulting in organ failure or death. In general, medical complications, like the presenting signs and symptoms discussed earlier in this chapter, are best thought of as consequences of either starvation or binge-eating/purging behaviors. Patients who are underweight and who purge, or who have undergone rapid weight changes, are at the highest risk for medical complications. This group includes patients with atypical AN who may have been obese at baseline but have sustained rapid and extreme weight loss over several months with the onset of a clinical eating disorder; this group can also include some bariatric surgery patients who lose excessive weight very rapidly after their procedures. The vast majority of physiological complications reverse with refeeding and with normalization of eating behaviors; however, symptomatic treatment alone is rarely sufficient. Accurate and prompt diagnosis, along with referral for eating disorder–specific behavioral treatment, is of utmost importance, given that better outcomes have been associated with early treatment (Treasure and Russell 2011). In the subsections below, we review some of the major medical complications that bring patients with eating disorders to clinical attention in the hospital or emergency department setting, and that should alert clinicians to the possibility that an occult comorbid eating disorder may be present.

Metabolic and Fluid/Electrolyte Abnormalities

Electrolyte abnormalities and associated cardiac arrhythmia constitute one of the most common causes of death in patients with AN and BN (Williams et al. 2008; Winston 2008). Hypokalemia poses a major risk. Unexplained hypokalemia should raise suspicion for purging behaviors, as it can be the consequence of frequent vomiting and laxative or diuretic abuse. Hyponatremia may result from excessive water intake, a behavior often employed by patients with AN to suppress appetite, increase satiety, or artificially inflate weight. Over time, chronic polydipsia can lead to the syndrome of inappropriate antidiuretic hormone secretion attributable to a reset osmostat. Hypophosphatemia can be a presenting symptom associated with starvation in AN but is more commonly a complication of refeeding syndrome (as discussed in the section "Medical Stabilization, Behavioral and Nutritional Management, and Refeeding Syndrome" later in this chapter). Starvation-related hypoglycemia in patients with AN can present in the acute setting with altered mental status and/or coma. Recent rapid weight loss, or weight gain, may be the most obvious indicator of AN, or of onset of BED, respectively. Dehydration, secondary hypoaldosteronism, renal failure, and cardiac decompensation can all occur as consequences of severe purging behaviors.

Gastrointestinal Complications

In one study, more than 90% of patients presenting to a behavioral eating disorders program had symptoms that met criteria for a functional gastrointestinal disorder, most frequently irritable bowel syndrome, functional dyspepsia, and abdominal bloating (Boyd et al. 2005). Both starvation and purging are associated with delayed gastric emptying (Benini et al. 2004), and patients with AN have additionally been shown to have delayed intestinal and whole-gut transit times that contribute to symptoms of constipation, abdominal pain and bloating, or flatulence. Vomiting can lead to parotid gland hypertrophy, dental caries, gastrointestinal reflux disease and esophagitis, Mallory-Weiss tears and hematemesis, and (in extreme cases) Boerhaave's syndrome with esophageal rupture. Patients who vomit regularly have often lost their gag reflex and can regurgitate at will without inducing a gag. Both starvation and refeeding in AN can be associated with transaminitis and elevated amylase and lipase levels, which are generally asymptomatic. Acute gastric dilatation, a potentially life-threatening condition, can present with acute abdominal pain and bloating in a patient with AN following a large binge and may be associated with superior mesenteric artery syndrome, with risk of bowel necrosis or gastric perforation (Nakao et al. 2000). Chronic severe laxative abuse can lead to ileus and to hemorrhoids or rectal prolapse and impaired anorectal motility (Chiarioni et al. 2000). Gastrointestinal symptoms that develop as consequences of disordered eating behavior and malnutrition may in turn come to play a role in sustaining patterns of restricted food intake or purging behavior and complicate refeeding and weight restoration in AN (Hadley and Walsh 2003). In some cases, a gastrointestinal disorder may precede the onset of the eating disorder. It is not unusual, for example, for an eating disorder to develop following weight loss or vomiting related to a gastrointestinal viral illness that appeared not to resolve.

Gynecological and Obstetric Complications

Low BMI in AN is associated with the onset of secondary hypogonadotropic amenorrhea and infertility, with low serum levels of estrogen, follicle-stimulating hormone, and luteinizing hormone. Irregular menses and amenorrhea are also observed in a minority of patients with BN, as well as in some patients with BED, largely as a complication of morbid obesity. Although anovulatory patients with AN who desire fertility respond to hormonal interventions and assisted reproductive technologies, they are at risk of ovarian hyperstimulation and multiple pregnancies, intrauterine growth retardation, and (in those who purge by vomiting as part of their eating disorder behaviors) hyperemesis gravidarum (Franko and Walton 1993; Solmi et al. 2014). Most patients with an eating disorder who do become pregnant are able to control their eating disorder behaviors during pregnancy; however, postpartum they often struggle with relapse. Patients with eating disorders may also be at higher risk of postpartum depression in the setting of rapid weight loss resulting from the adoption of extreme weight loss strategies to return to their prepregnancy weight. Evidence suggests that the relative risks of unplanned pregnancies and abortions are higher in patients with AN than in matched control women, likely due to irregular menstruation being associated with lower contraceptive use and assumed lower risk of pregnancy in this population (Bulik et al. 2010).

Neurological Complications

Patients with eating disorders may present with either syncope or presyncopal symptoms related to fluid loss and dehydration. These symptoms typically result from fluid restriction or from excessive vomiting and diuretic or laxative abuse. Patients with hyponatremia due to excessive water intake or with hypoglycemia can present with a generalized seizure, and patients with profound hypoglycemia (in cases of extreme AN) can present with coma (Rich et al. 1990). Care should be taken not to correct severe hyponatremia too rapidly, because central pontine myelinolysis is a serious iatrogenic risk (Leroy et al. 2012; Patel et al. 2008). In patients who are chronically malnourished or who have lost weight rapidly, and especially in those with comorbid alcohol use disorders, thiamine must be administered prior to refeeding to avoid the risk of Wernicke's encephalopathy (Renthal et al. 2014). Neurological consequences of vitamin deficiencies, including Wernicke's, are also a concern in patients who have undergone bariatric surgery and are losing weight rapidly and/or vomiting excessively (Punchai et al. 2017).

Cardiovascular Complications

Cardiovascular complications of eating disorders may be related to cardiac structural changes, conduction or repolarization abnormalities, hemodynamic changes, or peripheral vascular problems (Sachs et al. 2016). Most, but not all, of these complications are reversible with nutritional rehabilitation, and some are life-threatening. The most common cardiovascular finding is bradycardia associated with starvation in patients with AN or following rapid weight loss in patients with atypical AN. Patients with a heart rate less than 40 beats per minute (bpm) should be admitted for cardiac monitoring and assessment. Asymptomatic resting heart rates may be as low as 25–30 bpm. Orthostatic hypotension or tachycardia may reflect dehydration from purging behaviors or fluid restriction or may result from impaired vagal tone and postural orthostatic hypotension. Pericardial effusions are relatively common in patients with AN. Bradycardia, pericardial effusions, and orthostatic hypotension all typically reverse with refeeding and weight restoration. Peripheral vascular changes can include Raynaud's syndrome and acrocyanosis in low-weight starved individuals. Severely underweight patients may also develop cardiac muscle atrophy and subsequent mitral valve prolapse. In chronic extreme AN, starvation cardiomyopathy may result in congestive heart failure. Echocardiographic assessment of cardiac and valvular function should be considered in individuals who show evidence of fluid overload on exam, in older chronically ill patients with AN, or in individuals with a history of using fenfluramine as a diet aid (before it was withdrawn from the market), or of abusing ipecac (no longer available in the United States), which is cardiotoxic in large doses.

Endocrine Complications

The most common endocrine complications in AN are hypogonadotropic amenorrhea and infertility. Amenorrhea is associated with rapid development of osteoporosis, which can be detected as early as 6 months following loss of regular menses and places patients at elevated risk for disabling hip and spinal compression fractures over the long term. Evidence to date does not support a significant effect of hormonal replacement therapy on bone density, perhaps because of activation of the hypothalamic-pituitary-adrenal (HPA) axis and hypercortisolemia as well as low insulin-like growth factor in AN, all of which likely contribute to bone loss. There is increasing evidence to suggest that bisphosphonates may help improve bone mineral density in chronically ill adult patients and that transdermal 17-β-estradiol increases spinal and hip bone mineral density in adolescents with AN (Misra and Klibanski 2011; Robinson et al. 2017). Weight restoration is the most effective intervention to prevent continued bone loss and is associated with increased bone density in adolescents who have not yet reached peak bone mass. A recent study supports the importance of ensuring normal vitamin D levels, given that spinal bone mineral density during weight restoration improved only for patients with normal vitamin D levels (Giollo et al. 2017). Laboratory findings indicative of sick euthyroid syndrome (i.e., low serum levels of thyroid hormones in clinically euthyroid patients with nonthyroidal systemic illness) are also commonly observed in individuals with AN; findings can include low triiodothyronine (T_3) and reverse T_3 (rT_3) with an elevated ratio of thyroxine (T_4) to rT_3 and in some cases suppression of thyroid-stimulating hormone, all of which normalize with refeeding.

Hematological and Immune Complications

Starvation in AN is associated with anemia, leukopenia, and thrombocytopenia, and histological changes reveal gelatinous marrow hypocellularity (Hütter et al. 2009; Sabel et al. 2013). The resultant immunocompromised state places patients with extreme AN and a BMI lower than 13 at risk of common and opportunistic infections, with case reports describing both mycobacterial and fungal infections (Hotta et al. 2004; Mogi et al. 2012).

Medical Stabilization, Behavioral and Nutritional Management, and Refeeding Syndrome

Consulting psychiatrists are most likely to encounter patients with eating disorders when a complication of their eating and weight-control behaviors brings them to medical attention. Additionally, some patients are admitted in the setting of self-injurious behaviors. Both nonsuicidal self-injury and suicide attempts are common in eating disorder patients, with suicide accounting for about 20%–30% of deaths from AN (Cucchi et al. 2016; Papadopoulos et al. 2009; Zerwas et al. 2015). The initial challenges in the acute setting are to medically and psychiatrically assess and stabilize these patients. Oral rather than intravenous replacement of electrolytes, including potassium, magnesium, and phosphate, is generally preferable; electrolytes and glucose should be monitored daily if unstable. Hypoglycemia and bradycardia are commonly present but usually asymptomatic.

When patients are malnourished and underweight, nutritional goals are focused on initiating refeeding and weight gain. For individuals who are normal weight or overweight, the priority is weight maintenance and normalization of eating behavior. Special attention should be paid to the risk of medical complications in patients who have undergone rapid and extensive weight loss, regardless of their presenting weight. Patients with atypical AN or with BN may appear healthy yet be medically and psychiatrically unstable.

All clinicians should be familiar with refeeding syndrome and its management, especially when treating severely malnourished patients with AN. *Refeeding syndrome* is a constellation of metabolic and clinical changes that may occur in malnourished patients during renourishment. The hallmark finding is hypophosphatemia resulting from depleted whole-body stores of phosphate in starvation coupled with intracellular movement of phosphate for anabolic processes as refeeding is initiated. Although hypophosphatemia can be a presenting feature in refeeding syndrome, it typically develops within 2–4 days of the initiation of refeeding and, if not recognized and treated, can result in cardiac arrhythmias, delirium, or death. Refeeding can also be associated with hypoglycemia, which is thought to be related to depleted glycogen stores and increased insulin release, resulting in unpredictable blood glucose fluctuations. Edema from third spacing due to low levels of serum albumin and other proteins and fragile tissues is common. Overzealous attempts to rapidly correct orthostatic hypotension can iatrogenically exacerbate edema, resulting in risk of congestive heart failure or anasarca. Low blood pressure and postural hypotension in AN are often due to autonomic instability and not simply to dehydration. Congestive heart failure following intravenous hydration is especially a risk in older patients with chronic AN, who may have an occult starvation-related cardiomyopathy. Echocardiography is indicated to assess cardiac function in these cases or those that progress to severe edema. Edema is also common in patients with a history of laxative or diuretic abuse and results from activation of the renin–aldosterone system due to persistent fluid losses leading to fluid retention and edema when diuretic or laxative use is abruptly interrupted following hospitalization (Roerig et al. 2010). In general, edema can be managed conservatively and will resolve during the first few weeks of refeeding. Rarely, use of a potassium-sparing diuretic may be indicated. Stimulant laxatives should be stopped, but a daily bowel regimen of a stool softener and fiber laxative or osmotic laxative can be helpful to normalize bowel function. Patients should be educated on the need for patience while renal and intestinal functions are allowed to return to normal and should be advised that some degree of temporary discomfort is to be expected. Conveying reassurance that edema and abdominal bloating will resolve is important, because these effects often contribute to body dissatisfaction and fear of normalizing eating and weight-control behaviors.

Historically, refeeding syndrome was believed to be caused by excessively rapid calorie advancement, and guidelines for refeeding in patients with AN recommended starting at low calorie levels and increasing levels gradually to prevent this complication. However, more recent data indicate that low BMI at admission, rather than a rapid rate of calorie escalation, is the strongest predictor of hypophosphatemia and refeeding risk (Garber et al. 2016; Redgrave et al. 2015; Society for Adolescent Health and Medicine 2014). Current recommendations for AN typically advocate starting with 1,500–2,000 calories per day and increasing these levels over a 1- to 2-week period to 3,000–3,500 calories per day to achieve a target rate of weight gain of 2–4 pounds per week. Finally, it is important to note that refeeding syndrome is most common with parenteral or enteral feeding. Meal-based oral refeeding should therefore be prioritized whenever possible, in order to both minimize the risk of refeeding complications and help patients overcome anxiety about consuming a variety of foods of differing calorie densities in regular meals. Competent inpatient or residential behavioral specialty programs for the treatment of eating disorders achieve average weekly rates of weight gain in this range. Use of short-term enteral feeding is advocated by some adolescent inpatient programs for medical stabilization and to prepare for transition to outpatient meal-based refeeding and family-based interventions (Garber et al. 2016) (as discussed below in the section "Psychopharmacological and Psychotherapeutic Treatments").

The treatment of patients with eating disorders in general medical settings can be challenging. The consultation psychiatrist can play an important role in providing guidance regarding behavioral management and in helping staff process countertransference reactions to ensure proper care. Patients with eating disorders will often continue to engage in disordered eating and weight-control behaviors on a general medical ward despite the life-threatening consequences of their disorders that led to hospitalization. Patients may refuse food or may deliberately hide it or throw it away. They may continue to exercise, or pace and stand constantly, and may vomit or surreptitiously abuse laxatives or diuretics. In addition to the use of daily weight checks, calorie counts, and tray checks to assess the amount of food consumed, a sitter may be helpful to observe the patient's behavior. Staff should instruct the patient to allow the sitter to check the toilet bowl before flushing for evidence of purging. Close nursing observation may additionally be indicated for patients with suicidal or self-injurious behaviors. The clinical team should firmly but supportively instruct the patient on the importance of refraining from engaging in disordered eating behaviors and review medical risks and complications (Wolfe et al. 2016). Caring for patients with eating disorders can evoke strong feelings in providers that range from negative countertransference to rescue fantasies. Patients are often bright and engaging and may be perceived as less sick or requiring of less attention on busy medical units. In extreme AN, a patient's severely cachectic appearance may be shocking or perplexing. In less severely underweight cases, some clinicians may overidentify with a patient's desire to diet and lose weight and unwittingly minimize the severity of pathological thoughts or behaviors. Caregivers may feel overwhelmed, frustrated, or annoyed by a patient's deceitful behavior and disengage, thereby jeopardizing the therapeutic relationship (King and de Sales 2000). Ideally, a psychiatric consultation should be obtained within 24 hours of admission, to help guide the treatment team in how to respond to the patient's behavior and support his or her treatment while being aware of their own emotional reactions. The consultant should evaluate patients for coexisting diagnoses and assist in coordinating transfer to a specialized behavioral eating disorder treatment program once medical issues are stabilized for continued nutritional rehabilitation and behavioral treatment (Sylvester and Forman 2008).

Psychopharmacological and Psychotherapeutic Treatments

Anorexia Nervosa

Psychological Treatments

Treatment of AN can be seen as comprising three phases: 1) medical stabilization and initiation of refeeding, 2) weight restoration and normalization of eating behavior, and 3) relapse prevention. Outpatient interventions for AN are more effective at achieving weight restoration and symptom remission in adolescents than in adults, and for acutely ill as opposed to chronic and severe cases. For adolescents, family-based therapy (FBT) is superior to individual therapy, and early weight gain with either therapy appears the strongest indicator of weight restoration and full remission at end of treatment (Le Grange et al. 2014). In FBT, the focus is on assisting parents to re-feed their child by regaining appropriate parental control over the adolescent's eating behavior and restoring his or her weight. Therapy is usually in weekly sessions, and responsibility for meals gradually shifts to the patient as weight is restored (Jones et al. 2012). Outcomes for FBT are favorable in most adolescents with a short duration of illness (i.e., 3 years or less) (Le Grange 1999), but inpatient treatment is indicated when patients are medically unstable or fail to gain weight. Medical stabilization and initiation of treatment for adolescents with severe AN who are at risk of medical complications is best achieved in a meal-based specialty behavioral program for eating disorders with proven capability in achieving average rates of weight gain of at least 2 pounds per week and in medically managing these patients. Access to such specialty programs is often limited, however, either geographically or by insurance coverage. If patients admitted to a general hospital refuse oral intake, nocturnal nasogastric feeding is often used to initiate weight gain before transitioning to oral feeding over the course of days or a few weeks (Golden et al. 2015; Kohn et al. 2011; Madden et al. 2015). Once completing meals and consuming a minimum of 1,500–2,000 calories per day by mouth, most adolescent patients can be discharged to outpatient FBT to complete treatment, although those with higher behavioral severity, poor compliance, and/or complex psychiatric comorbidity may require transfer to a more structured inpatient or residential behavioral eating disorders treatment program.

Although some adults with AN respond to outpatient treatment, no randomized controlled trial (RCT) of an outpatient psychotherapeutic intervention has been effective in achieving full weight restoration in a majority of adult patients. No one therapeutic approach has been shown to be consistently superior; however, cognitive-behavioral therapy (CBT) is the favored modality. A trial of an enhanced form of CBT for AN, CBT–Enhanced (CBT-E), reported that this intervention was effective in restoring weight in the majority of adolescent patients but only 36% of adults with AN (Calugi et al. 2015). A minimally acceptable rate of weight gain for outpatient treatment is 0.5–1.0 pound per week, which typically requires a daily intake of more than 3,000 calories, a goal best achieved with a regimen consisting of 2,000 calories in food consumed over three daily meals with the addition of three nutritional supplements of around 350 calories each. Recent research has focused on the potential utility of psychotherapy techniques known to be effective in treating anxiety disorders and OCD—namely, exposure and response prevention (ERP)—in addressing eating-related anxiety (i.e., fear of high-calorie-density foods) in AN (Steinglass et al. 2012). ERP-informed techniques are used in the majority of intensive treatment programs for AN that are meal-based, and evidence suggests that the variety of foods consumed and fat intake at program discharge by hospitalized patients predicts outcome at 1-year follow up (Schebendach et al. 2008). Nonetheless, there are no RCT data to support this approach.

Despite the relative ineffectiveness of outpatient treatment for adult AN, inpatient behavioral specialty programs are effective in restoring weight in the majority of patients with AN to a BMI greater than 19 and achieve average rates of weight gain of 2–4 pounds per week. Most programs are meal-based, although some prescribe supplemental nocturnal nasogastric feeding to boost lower average rates of weight gain closer to the 4 pounds per week achieved by more structured behavioral programs. Patient compliance with meals is achieved through implementation of a uniform behavioral protocol with explicit behavioral guidelines and expectations for completing meals. Patients earn increasing independence over choice of foods consumed as they successfully complete meals and achieve an adequate rate of weight gain. As they progress in treatment, patients become involved in therapeutic meal-based activities, including selecting, cooking, and eating in a variety of social settings. The goal of this approach is to practice normal eating behavior, challenge and reframe cognitive distortions that sustain unhealthy behaviors, regulate emotions, and reinforce and generalize skills needed to prevent relapse after discharge. Even in the best-established behavioral programs, however, rates of relapse following intensive treatment and weight restoration remain around 50%. Typically, relapse occurs within the first 6–9 months after discharge (Carter et al. 2004). Interventions aimed at relapse prevention following intensive treatment and weight restoration have been underdeveloped and understudied. The BMI at discharge from intensive treatment remains the strongest predictor of weight maintenance at follow-up, with compelling correlational data and clinical experience supporting the association of lower discharge BMIs with higher risk of rehospitalization (Guarda 2008; Rigaud et al. 2011). Higher discharge BMI is also predictive of improvement in eating disorder and comorbid psychiatric symptoms at follow-up (Makhzoumi et al. 2017).

Given this evidence, the consultation psychiatrist should aim to facilitate transfer of patients with eating disorders on the medical and surgical floors to an eating disorders behavioral treatment program with established weight gain outcomes when possible. Patients may be resistant to this recommendation, however, because behavior change and weight gain are anxiety provoking. Persuading patients to agree to intensive treatment is best achieved by taking a supportive and empathic stance, including use of motivational interviewing strategies and psychoeducation. Providing patients and their families with information about how physiological complications of starvation and/or purging contribute to maintenance of eating-disordered thoughts and behaviors is often key in helping patients commit to specialty treatment. Reassurance that ambivalence toward treatment is normal and that recovery is always possible is important in instilling hope. Many patients have tried to change and failed, and they may hold the overvalued idea that their illness is part of who they are (Tan et al. 2003). When patients with severe AN at high risk of morbidity or mortality refuse specialty care or deny the diagnosis, ethical issues relating to capacity to refuse treatment arise (see section "Ethical Issues" below).

Pharmacotherapy

Most classes of psychotropic medications have been tried in the treatment of AN without yielding convincing evidence that they promote weight gain, improve disordered cognitions, or treat comorbid psychopathology in the underweight state. Overall, RCTs of medications in the treatment of AN have been small and underpowered and plagued by methodological problems and high dropout rates. Most trials have examined the efficacy of appetite stimulants, antidepressants, anxiolytics, and atypical antipsychotics (Guarda 2008). Early clinical trials of clomipramine and amitriptyline did not show efficacy, and tricyclic antidepressants (TCAs) are often seen as risky in AN because of the increased risk of QTc interval prolongation in patients who are also at risk of electrolyte abnormalities (Frank and Shott 2016). Fluoxetine has been studied in the treatment of AN primarily because of its known benefit in the treatment of BN, but it has shown no advantage over placebo, even when administered with the serotonin precursor tryptophan (Attia et al. 1998; Barbarich et al. 2004b; Ferguson et al. 1999). Whereas a small open trial of fluoxetine in weight-restored patients with AN showed some promise in preventing relapse and helping to maintain restored weight (Kaye et al. 1991), subsequent RCTs have been inconclusive (Sebaaly et al. 2013). Chlorpromazine was the first antipsychotic to be studied in AN. Although patients showed initial weight gain and had shorter lengths of hospital stay, the side effect of seizures precluded its further use (Dally and Sargant 1960). Another typical antipsychotic, haloperidol, demonstrated some efficacy in a very small group of treatment-resistant patients with delusional body image disturbance (Mauri et al. 2013). Among atypical antipsychotics, olanzapine is the most studied, primarily because of its side effect of weight gain (likely related to antihistaminic properties). Two small open-label studies (Barbarich et al. 2004a; Powers et al. 2002) showed some improvement in weight and in mood and anxiety symptoms. Early studies comparing olanzapine with placebo initially reported promise in weight restoration and improvement in psychological symptoms (Attia et al. 2011; Bissada et al. 2008); however, a more recent meta-analysis concluded that current evidence does not support the use of antipsychotics in AN (de Vos et al. 2014).

Although benzodiazepines are frequently prescribed clinically for meal-related anxiety, a small RCT of alprazolam in inpatients with AN demonstrated no effect on anxiety, food intake, or weight (Steinglass et al. 2014). Both opioids and cannabinoids affect appetite and eating, but there is no evidence to support their use in AN. Additional negative medication trials have included cyproheptadine, lithium, zinc, estrogen, and human growth hormone. To date, no pharmacological agent is approved for the treatment of AN, which remains one of the most difficult-to-treat psychiatric conditions, especially when chronic in duration (Frank and Shott 2016).

Bulimia Nervosa

Psychological Treatments

Treatment of BN is focused on decreasing and eliminating binge-eating and purging behaviors, normalizing eating patterns, and addressing disordered cognitions and comorbid psychopathology (Mitchell et al. 2007). CBT is the treatment of choice for BN (Hay 2013; Kass et al. 2013; Murphy et al. 2010) and was first used by Fairburn in 1981. CBT for BN in both individual and group formats has been shown to be superior to placebo, medication alone, and other forms of therapy (Hay et al. 2009), including psychoanalytic therapy (Poulsen et al. 2014). CBT for BN additionally targets the overvaluation of shape and weight that drives extreme weight-control behaviors, including persistent dietary restraint and purging that in turn escalate binge eating and thereby maintain core psychopathology and intensify patients' concerns about their inability to control their food intake and weight (Fairburn et al. 2003). CBT-E is a modified version of CBT that addresses additional factors implicated in the maintenance of BN, including low self-esteem, emotional reactivity, perfectionism, and interpersonal difficulties (Cooper and Fairburn 2011). A recently published meta-analysis demonstrated that CBT-E for BN was effective in reducing both bulimic and depressive symptoms. In this study, greater improvement in binge eating and purging was associated with greater improvement in depressive symptoms (Linardon et al. 2017).

Interpersonal therapy (IPT) for BN focuses on interpersonal domains such as conflicts, inadequate social supports, and role transitions. It is the only psychological treatment that has outcomes comparable to those of CBT; however, the response to treatment is much slower (Agras et al. 2000; Fairburn et al. 1993). Dialectical behavioral therapy (DBT) has recently gained attention as a potential treatment for BN, given its focus on behavior change, self-acceptance, and emotional regulation, constructs believed to be of relevance to maintenance of BN. There is limited evidence that DBT may be an acceptable alternative to CBT or IPT, particularly for individuals with comorbid borderline personality disorder; however, its efficacy in reducing eating disorder symptoms has not been evaluated in RCTs (Bankoff et al. 2012). Integrative cognitive affective therapy (ICAT), a new form of therapy that emphasizes emotional dysregulation and its relationship with bulimic symptoms, is aimed at modifying factors that precipitate momentary negative emotions associated with disordered behaviors. ICAT was found to be as efficacious as enhanced CBT in reducing the frequency of binge eating and purging (Wonderlich et al. 2014).

Treatment retention and treatment completion are significant challenges in treatment studies, and dropouts are common in both individual and group therapy for BN (Fassino et al. 2009; Waller 1997). Access to specialty treatment is an additional challenge, although technology- and Internet-based interventions hold promise (Aardoom et al. 2013); a recent trial comparing traditionally delivered CBT and Internet-based CBT for BN showed no difference in dropout rates (Watson et al. 2017). Various forms of self-help interventions for BN are available, yet treatments that are more individualized and guided by mental health professionals have generally been found to be superior to unsupervised interventions (Beintner et al. 2014).

Pharmacotherapy

Fluoxetine is the only U.S. Food and Drug Administration (FDA)–approved medication for BN. In a large double-blind, placebo-controlled study of 387 participants with BN, high-dose fluoxetine (60 mg/day) was superior to placebo in reducing both binge-eating and purging episodes, as well as depressive symptoms, carbohydrate cravings, and eating disorder cognitions (Fluoxetine Bulimia Nervosa Collaborative Study Group 1992). A meta-analysis of 10 RCTs examining different antidepressants in patients with BN found these medications to be superior to placebo. There were no statistically significant differences between classes of medications, which included TCAs, monoamine oxidase inhibitors, fluoxetine, trazodone, and bupropion. However, patients in the medication arms were more likely than those in the placebo arms to discontinue treatment because of side effects (Bacaltchuk and Hay 2003). Although bupropion was found to be effective in reducing the frequency of bingeing and purging, it was associated with an increased risk of generalized tonic-clonic seizures, and its use is contraindicated in patients with BN (Horne et al. 1988). Antidepressants alone are less effective than psychological treatment (remission rates of 20% vs. 39%); however, the combination of antidepressants with psychotherapy is superior to therapy alone (remission rates of 49% vs. 36%) (Bacaltchuk et al. 2001). Among anticonvulsants studied in BN, topiramate seems to be the most effective in reducing the frequency of bingeing and purging and in decreasing food preoccupation and body weight. Similar efficacy for topiramate has been found in patients with BED (McElroy et al. 2009). In one RCT in patients with severe BN who had been engaging in binge/purge episodes at least seven times per week over a 6-month period, ondansetron, a selective antagonist of the type-3 serotonin receptor (5-HT$_3$), was associated with a significant decrease in binge eating and vomiting and with normalization of eating behaviors and satiety cues, likely through its pharmacological effect on vagal nerve neurotransmission (Faris et al. 2000).

Binge Eating Disorder: Psychological and Pharmacological Treatment

Treatment of BED is aimed at reducing disordered eating behaviors and cognitions, regulating mood, and improving health. Weight loss is generally not regarded as a primary treatment goal, because calorie-restrictive diets are thought to be associated with exacerbation of binge eating and perpetuation of disordered eating patterns. Despite this generally held belief, behavioral weight loss therapies have in controlled trials been shown to be only slightly less effective than CBT and IPT, which are considered the treatments of choice for BED (Grilo 2017). Typically delivered in 1-hour sessions over 12–24 weeks of treatment, CBT and IPT reduce binge eating over both the short and the longer term, although neither produces significant weight loss. However, both of these modalities are effective in preventing further weight gain in the majority of responders. IPT may be slightly more efficacious than CBT for patients with more severe eating disorder psychopathology and low self-esteem, but response to CBT tends to be faster than response to IPT in the majority of responders (Brownley et al. 2016). In terms of prognostic factors, undue influence of body weight or shape on self-evaluation in patients with BED has been associated with higher severity of symptoms and worse treatment outcomes across interventions (Grilo et al. 2013). Other psychological treatments, such as self-help approaches and mindfulness, are only slightly effective in decreasing binge eating and have no effect on weight loss. Behavioral weight loss therapies lack long-term benefits in reducing weight and bingeing symptoms (McElroy et al. 2015a). American Psychiatric Association guidelines recommend CBT as a first-line treatment with adjunctive pharmacotherapy, while the National Institute for Health and Care Excellence (NICE) guidelines support use of medication monotherapy for some patients with BED.

Various second-generation antidepressants, particularly selective serotonin re-uptake inhibitors such as citalopram, fluoxetine, and sertraline, appear to be effective in reducing the frequency of binges, although they do not contribute to weight loss. They may be a good choice for the large percentage of patients with BED with comor-bid depression. In the only RCT of bupropion for BED, patients in the active treatment arm demonstrated greater weight loss at 8 weeks but did not differ from those in the placebo arm in frequency of binges or food cravings (White and Grilo 2013). Topira-mate was effective in reducing binge-eating behaviors, obsessive-compulsive symp-toms, and impulsivity and produced significant and persistent weight loss in two short-term RCTs (McElroy et al. 2007). Whereas topiramate's use is limited by its ad-verse effects, especially nonspecific cognitive impairment, it may be a preferred agent for patients with BED and bipolar disorder (because it does not exacerbate mania as can antidepressants) and for patients with BED and alcohol use disorder (because it can reduce craving for alcohol). Lisdexamfetamine is the only medication approved by the FDA for treatment of moderate to severe BED in adults. However, its approval in January 2015 was based on two Phase II studies that excluded patients with comor-bid cardiac disease or comorbid psychiatric conditions, despite the high frequency of comorbid psychiatric diagnoses and metabolic syndrome in this condition (McElroy et al. 2015b). The higher dosage ranges of 50 mg/day and 70 mg/day, but not 30 mg/day, were superior to placebo in reducing binge-eating episodes. A recently pub-lished Phase III open-label 12-month extension study demonstrated safety and toler-ability consistent with that found in previous studies of lisdexamfetamine for the treatment of BED; however, this trial again was limited to patients without medical and psychiatric comorbidities (Gasior et al. 2017). It remains unclear whether the study's findings can be generalized to the majority of clinical populations with BED.

Ethical Issues

Eating disorders can be challenging to treat. A core feature of these conditions is am-bivalence toward behavior change. This ambivalence results from the motivated, ego-syntonic nature of at least some of the disordered eating and weight-control behav-iors patients engage in. Ambivalence toward treatment is especially characteristic of AN, a perplexing disorder in which patients may come to describe their illness as their identity and may ascribe positive valence to their ability to starve themselves, viewing it as a hidden strength, virtue, or coping skill, despite evidence that self-starvation is increasingly impairing their health and function. Patients may deny that they fear gaining weight or that they have a serious illness. They often rationalize their restricting or exercise behavior by adopting a series of seemingly rational expla-nations to disguise the motives for their limited food repertoire, low-calorie food choices, and excessive exercise routines from others and from themselves. Examples of such rationalizations include idiosyncratic food intolerances or allergies, ethical beliefs justifying a conversion to veganism, food preferences, or the decision to pur-sue a healthy lifestyle.

Although patients with AN may appear competent in all other spheres, they often demonstrate diminished capacity to consent to or to refuse treatment. Decisional ca-pacity is task-specific and includes the ability to express a choice about treatment, to understand risks and benefits of treatment, to appreciate how those risks and benefits apply to oneself, and to logically assess these options. A recent study (Elzakkers et al. 2017) found that up to one-third of hospitalized patients with severe AN showed impaired decisional capacity. Although their reasoning was relatively intact, they lacked the ability to appreciate the seriousness of their own situation, in that they were unable to fully weigh the downstream risks of treatment refusal or to grasp the potential benefits of treatment, and they lacked a normal sense of self-preservation. Furthermore, their decision-making performance was disturbed more globally, as evidenced by impaired performance on neurocognitive tasks, including the Iowa Gambling Task. Finally, impaired capacity was associated with worse outcomes at 2-year follow-up.

The majority of patients with AN seek treatment only when in crisis as a result of a medical or psychiatric complication or when under pressure or ultimatums from others, including family, friends, educators, or employers (Guarda 2008). A study of voluntary admissions to an inpatient behavioral eating disorders program found that one-third of patients with AN reported that they did not believe that they needed inpatient admission and felt coerced by others into entering the hospital. Within 2 weeks, however, nearly half (43%) of these patients reported that they now perceived their admission as appropriate and agreed that continued inpatient treatment was justified, supporting the idea that motivation for treatment is likely to improve with behavior change (Guarda et al. 2007).

Involuntary treatment of AN remains controversial, and questions regarding whether involuntary treatment is justified and whether individuals with life-threatening AN have the decisional capacity to refuse treatment have attracted increased attention, given the high lethality of this condition (Carney et al. 2007; Douzenis and Michopoulos 2015). Patients with AN appear to agree in theory that compulsory treatment is appropriate in life-threatening cases of the disorder, but they have difficulty applying the same logic to their own situation (Tan et al. 2010). Two reviews of involuntary treatment for AN found that in published comparisons of involuntary and voluntary patient groups, higher comorbidity, greater number of past admissions, longer duration of illness, and more frequent self-harm behaviors characterized the involuntary treatment group (Clausen and Jones 2014; Elzakkers et al. 2014). These findings suggested that case complexity and refractoriness to past treatment efforts—rather than severity of eating disorder symptoms or low BMI—are the primary drivers of involuntary treatment in most cases. Because involuntary treatment is coercive and infringes on patient autonomy, its use can be justified only if the likelihood of benefit outweighs the risk of harm, and it requires both access to appropriate expert treatment and expectation of benefit. These issues are case specific and are additionally limited by both insurance and geographic limitations regarding access to expert care. Many states lack behavioral eating disorder specialty programs that are capable of treating and restoring weight in a majority of patients with AN or that accept involuntary admissions. Because civil commitment laws are state specific, transfers across state lines of certified patients face both legal and logistical obstacles. This can also be the case if family members obtain legal guardianship, because some states do not allow psychiatric admissions under guardianship. Guardianship by a parent also places the guardian in a role often perceived as unsupportive by the patient, with the potential of further eroding a strained relationship and hindering the involvement of family as a therapeutic and supportive part of the treatment team.

For patients with severe and enduring AN who have failed multiple attempts at hospital-based behavioral weight restoration across several expert programs, evidence for effective interventions is lacking. Open trials have explored modified therapies such as intensive CBT-E for AN, cognitive remediation therapy with emotional skills training (CREST), and specialist supportive clinical management (Hay et al. 2012). For patients with severe and enduring AN, the strength of the therapeutic alliance has been shown to be a stronger predictor of outcome than treatment type, and instilling hope appears to be a key factor in this effect (Stiles-Shields et al. 2016).

Conclusion

Eating disorders affect approximately 5% of the population and are associated with some of the highest rates of morbidity and mortality among psychiatric diagnoses. They affect both males and females and patients of different ages, socioeconomic status, and ethnicity. Medical complications of these behavioral disorders are common and can involve all organs and systems. Management of patients with eating disorders in general medical settings is very challenging. Even though patients present with physical complications of malnutrition and/or purging, they may not be forthcoming about their eating or exercise behaviors. Thorough assessment and diagnostic screening include a collateral history from family members. Review of outside records is often essential in diagnosing these disorders. Disordered eating behaviors are driven and compelling, and patients may continue to engage in them in the inpatient setting, sabotaging their own care despite serious medical sequelae. These self-damaging behaviors can be difficult for caregivers to understand and can provoke strong emotions in clinical staff when patients appear to reject help. Consultation-liaison psychiatrists can play an important role in the multidisciplinary treatment team by assisting with prompt diagnosis, offering psychoeducation, and providing guidance in managing patient behavior and staff countertransference reactions so as to build a therapeutic alliance and ensure proper care, and can help with appropriate referral to an expert eating disorders behavioral program.

References

Aardoom JJ, Dingemans AE, Spinhoven P, et al: Treating eating disorders over the Internet: a systematic review and future research directions. Int J Eat Disord 46(6):539–552, 2013 23674367

Academy for Eating Disorders: Eating disorders: a guide to medical care—critical points for early recognition and medical risk management in the care of individuals with eating disorders, 3rd edition. 2016. Available at: http://www.aedweb.org/images/updatedmedicalcareguidelines/AED-Medical-Care-Guidelines_-English_02.28.17_NEW.pdf. Accessed September 23, 2017.

Agras WS, Walsh T, Fairburn CG, et al: A multicenter comparison of cognitive-behavioral therapy and interpersonal psychotherapy for bulimia nervosa. Arch Gen Psychiatry 57(5):459–466, 2000 10807486

American Psychiatric Association: Diagnostic and Statistical Manual of Mental Disorders, 3rd Edition, Revised. Washington, DC, American Psychiatric Association, 1987

American Psychiatric Association: Diagnostic and Statistical Manual of Mental Disorders, 4th Edition, Revised. Washington, DC, American Psychiatric Association, 1994

American Psychiatric Association: Diagnostic and Statistical Manual of Mental Disorders, 5th Edition. Arlington, VA, American Psychiatric Association, 2013

Arcelus J, Mitchell AJ, Wales J, et al: Mortality rates in patients with anorexia nervosa and other eating disorders. A meta-analysis of 36 studies. Arch Gen Psychiatry 68(7):724–731, 2011 21727255

Attia E, Roberto CA: Should amenorrhea be a diagnostic criterion for anorexia nervosa? Int J Eat Disord 42(7):581–589, 2009 19621464

Attia E, Haiman C, Walsh BT, et al: Does fluoxetine augment the inpatient treatment of anorexia nervosa? Am J Psychiatry 155(4):548–551, 1998 9546003

Attia E, Kaplan AS, Walsh BT, et al: Olanzapine versus placebo for out-patients with anorexia nervosa. Psychol Med 41(10):2177–2182, 2011 21426603

Attia E, Becker AE, Bryant-Waugh R, et al: Feeding and eating disorders in DSM-5. Am J Psychiatry 170(11):1237–1239, 2013 24185238

Bacaltchuk J, Hay P: Antidepressants versus placebo for people with bulimia nervosa. Cochrane Database Syst Rev (4):CD003391, 2003 14583971

Bacaltchuk J, Hay P, Trefiglio R: Antidepressants versus psychological treatments and their combination for bulimia nervosa. Cochrane Database Syst Rev (4):CD003385, 2001 11687197

Bankoff SM, Karpel MG, Forbes HE, et al: A systematic review of dialectical behavior therapy for the treatment of eating disorders. Eat Disord 20(3):196–215, 2012 22519897

Barbarich NC, McConaha CW, Gaskill J, et al: An open trial of olanzapine in anorexia nervosa. J Clin Psychiatry 65(11):1480–1482, 2004a 15554759

Barbarich NC, McConaha CW, Halmi KA, et al: Use of nutritional supplements to increase the efficacy of fluoxetine in the treatment of anorexia nervosa. Int J Eat Disord 35(1):10–15, 2004b 14705152

Barnes RD, Boeka AG, McKenzie KC, et al: Metabolic syndrome in obese patients with binge-eating disorder in primary care clinics: a cross-sectional study. Prim Care Companion CNS Disord 13(2):pii, 2011 21977358

Beintner I, Jacobi C, Schmidt UH: Participation and outcome in manualized self-help for bulimia nervosa and binge eating disorder—a systematic review and metaregression analysis. Clin Psychol Rev 34(2):158–176, 2014 24508686

Benini L, Todesco T, Dalle Grave R, et al: Gastric emptying in patients with restricting and binge/purging subtypes of anorexia nervosa. Am J Gastroenterol 99(8):1448–1454, 2004 15307858

Bischoff-Grethe A, McCurdy D, Grenesko-Stevens E, et al: Altered brain response to reward and punishment in adolescents with anorexia nervosa. Psychiatry Res 214(3):331–340, 2013 24148909

Bissada H, Tasca GA, Barber AM, et al: Olanzapine in the treatment of low body weight and obsessive thinking in women with anorexia nervosa: a randomized, double-blind, placebo-controlled trial. Am J Psychiatry 165(10):1281–1288, 2008 18558642

Boyd C, Abraham S, Kellow J: Psychological features are important predictors of functional gastrointestinal disorders in patients with eating disorders. Scand J Gastroenterol 40(8):929–935, 2005 16170899

Brownley KA, Berkman ND, Peat CM, et al: Binge-eating disorder in adults: a systematic review and meta-analysis. Ann Intern Med 165(6):409–420, 2016 27367316

Bryant-Waugh R, Markham L, Kreipe RE, et al: Feeding and eating disorders in childhood. Int J Eat Disord 43(2):98–111, 2010 20063374

Bulik CM, Hoffman ER, Von Holle A, et al: Unplanned pregnancy in women with anorexia nervosa. Obstet Gynecol 116(5):1136–1140, 2010 20966699

Bulik CM, Kleiman SC, Yilmaz Z: Genetic epidemiology of eating disorders. Curr Opin Psychiatry 29(6):383–388, 2016 27532941

Call C, Walsh BT, Attia E: From DSM-IV to DSM-5: changes to eating disorder diagnoses. Curr Opin Psychiatry 26(6):532–536, 2013 24064412

Calugi S, Dalle Grave R, Sartirana M, et al: Time to restore body weight in adults and adolescents receiving cognitive behaviour therapy for anorexia nervosa. J Eat Disord 3:21, 2015 26019868

Carney CP, Yates WR: The evaluation of eating and weight symptoms in the general hospital consultation setting. Psychosomatics 39(1):61–67, 1998 9538677

Carney T, Tait D, Touyz S: Coercion is coercion? Reflections on trends in the use of compulsion in treating anorexia nervosa. Australas Psychiatry 15(5):390–395, 2007 17828636

Carter JC, Blackmore E, Sutandar-Pinnock K, et al: Relapse in anorexia nervosa: a survival analysis. Psychol Med 34(4):671–679, 2004 15099421

Castillo M, Weiselberg E: Bulimia Nervosa/Purging Disorder. Curr Probl Pediatr Adolesc Health Care 47(4):85–94, 2017 28532966

Cha J, Ide JS, Bowman FD, et al: Abnormal reward circuitry in anorexia nervosa: a longitudinal, multimodal MRI study. Hum Brain Mapp 37(11):3835–3846, 2016 27273474

Chiarioni G, Bassotti G, Monsignori A, et al: Anorectal dysfunction in constipated women with anorexia nervosa. Mayo Clin Proc 75(10):1015–1019, 2000 11040849

Clausen L, Jones A: A systematic review of the frequency, duration, type and effect of involuntary treatment for people with anorexia nervosa, and an analysis of patient characteristics. J Eat Disord 2(1):29, 2014 25414793

Conceição E, Orcutt M, Mitchell J, et al: Eating disorders after bariatric surgery: a case series. Int J Eat Disord 46(3):274–279, 2013 23192683

Cooper Z, Fairburn CG: The evolution of "enhanced" cognitive behavior therapy for eating disorders: learning from treatment nonresponse. Cognit Behav Pract 18(3):394–402, 2011 23814455

Cotton MA, Ball C, Robinson P: Four simple questions can help screen for eating disorders. J Gen Intern Med 18(1):53–56, 2003 12534764

Cucchi A, Ryan D, Konstantakopoulos G, et al: Lifetime prevalence of non-suicidal self-injury in patients with eating disorders: a systematic review and meta-analysis. Psychol Med 46(7):1345–1358, 2016 26954514

Dally PJ, Sargant W: A new treatment of anorexia nervosa. BMJ 1(5188):1770–1773, 1960 13813846

Davis C, Blackmore E, Katzman DK, et al: Female adolescents with anorexia nervosa and their parents: a case-control study of exercise attitudes and behaviours. Psychol Med 35(3):377–386, 2005 15841873

Dawes AJ, Maggard-Gibbons M, Maher AR, et al: Mental health conditions among patients seeking and undergoing bariatric surgery: a meta-analysis. JAMA 315(2):150–163, 2016 26757464

Degortes D, Santonastaso P, Zanetti T, et al: Stressful life events and binge eating disorder. Eur Eat Disord Rev 22(5):378–382, 2014 25044613

Dellava JE, Thornton LM, Hamer RM, et al: Childhood anxiety associated with low BMI in women with anorexia nervosa. Behav Res Ther 48(1):60–67, 2010 19822312

Dell'Osso L, Abelli M, Carpita B, et al: Historical evolution of the concept of anorexia nervosa and relationships with orthorexia nervosa, autism, and obsessive-compulsive spectrum. Neuropsychiatr Dis Treat 12:1651–1660, 2016 27462158

de Vos J, Houtzager L, Katsaragaki G, et al: Meta analysis on the efficacy of pharmacotherapy versus placebo on anorexia nervosa. J Eat Disord 2(1):27, 2014 25379181

Douzenis A, Michopoulos I: Involuntary admission: the case of anorexia nervosa. Int J Law Psychiatry 39:31–35, 2015 25660351

Duncan L, Yilmaz Z, Gaspar H, et al: Significant locus and metabolic genetic correlations revealed in genome-wide association study of anorexia nervosa. Am J Psychiatry 174(9):850–858, 2017 28494655

Eddy KT, Keel PK, Dorer DJ, et al: Longitudinal comparison of anorexia nervosa subtypes. Int J Eat Disord 31(2):191–201, 2002 11920980

Elzakkers IF, Danner UN, Hoek HW, et al: Compulsory treatment in anorexia nervosa: a review. Int J Eat Disord 47(8):845–852, 2014 24990434

Elzakkers IFFM, Danner UN, Sternheim LC, et al: Mental capacity to consent to treatment and the association with outcome: a longitudinal study in patients with anorexia nervosa. BJPsych Open 3(3):147–153, 2017 28584660

Evans EH, Adamson AJ, Basterfield L, et al: Risk factors for eating disorder symptoms at 12 years of age: a 6-year longitudinal cohort study. Appetite 108:12–20, 2017 27612559

Fairburn C: A cognitive behavioural approach to the treatment of bulimia. Psychol Med 11(4):707–711, 1981 6948316

Fairburn CG, Jones R, Peveler RC, et al: Psychotherapy and bulimia nervosa. Longer-term effects of interpersonal psychotherapy, behavior therapy, and cognitive behavior therapy. Arch Gen Psychiatry 50(6):419–428, 1993 8498876

Fairburn CG, Cooper Z, Shafran R: Cognitive behaviour therapy for eating disorders: a "trans-diagnostic" theory and treatment. Behav Res Ther 41(5):509–528, 2003 12711261

Faris PL, Kim SW, Meller WH, et al: Effect of decreasing afferent vagal activity with ondansetron on symptoms of bulimia nervosa: a randomised, double-blind trial. Lancet 355(9206):792–797, 2000 10711927

Fassino S, Pierò A, Tomba E, et al: Factors associated with dropout from treatment for eating disorders: a comprehensive literature review. BMC Psychiatry 9:67, 2009 19818137

Ferguson CP, La Via MC, Crossan PJ, et al: Are serotonin selective reuptake inhibitors effective in underweight anorexia nervosa? Int J Eat Disord 25(1):11–17, 1999 9924648

Fichter MM, Quadflieg N: Mortality in eating disorders—results of a large prospective clinical longitudinal study. Int J Eat Disord 49(4):391–401, 2016 26767344

Fluoxetine Bulimia Nervosa Collaborative Study Group: Fluoxetine in the treatment of bulimia nervosa. A multicenter, placebo-controlled, double-blind trial. Arch Gen Psychiatry 49(2):139–147, 1992 1550466

Foerde K, Steinglass JE, Shohamy D, et al: Neural mechanisms supporting maladaptive food choices in anorexia nervosa. Nat Neurosci 18(11):1571–1573, 2015 26457555

Forney KJ, Buchman-Schmitt JM, Keel PK, et al: The medical complications associated with purging. Int J Eat Disord 49(3):249–259, 2016 26876429

Frank GK, Shott ME: The role of psychotropic medications in the management of anorexia nervosa: rationale, evidence and future prospects. CNS Drugs 30(5):419–442, 2016 27106297

Franko DL, Walton BE: Pregnancy and eating disorders: a review and clinical implications. Int J Eat Disord 13(1):41–47, 1993 8477276

Gallant AR, Lundgren J, Drapeau V: The night-eating syndrome and obesity. Obes Rev 13(6):528–536, 2012 22222118

Garber AK, Sawyer SM, Golden NH, et al: A systematic review of approaches to refeeding in patients with anorexia nervosa. Int J Eat Disord 49(3):293–310, 2016 26661289

Gasior M, Hudson J, Quintero J, et al: A phase 3, multicenter, open-label, 12-month extension safety and tolerability trial of lisdexamfetamine dimesylate in adults with binge eating disorder. J Clin Psychopharmacol 37(3):315–322, 2017 28383364

Giollo A, Idolazzi L, Caimmi C, et al: Vitamin D levels strongly influence bone mineral density and bone turnover markers during weight gain in female patients with anorexia nervosa. Int J Eat Disord 50(9):1041–1049, 2017 28593655

Godart NT, Flament MF, Perdereau F, et al: Comorbidity between eating disorders and anxiety disorders: a review. Int J Eat Disord 32(3):253–270, 2002 12210640

Godart NT, Flament MF, Curt F, et al: Anxiety disorders in subjects seeking treatment for eating disorders: a DSM-IV controlled study. Psychiatry Res 117(3):245–258, 2003 12686367

Golden NH, Katzman DK, Sawyer SM, et al; Society for Adolescent Health and Medicine: Position Paper of the Society for Adolescent Health and Medicine: medical management of restrictive eating disorders in adolescents and young adults. J Adolesc Health 56(1):121–125, 2015 25530605

Goldschmidt AB, Wall MM, Loth KA, et al: Risk factors for disordered eating in overweight adolescents and young adults. J Pediatr Psychol 40(10):1048–1055, 2015 26050243

Grilo CM: Psychological and behavioral treatments for binge-eating disorder. J Clin Psychiatry 78 (suppl 1):20–24, 2017 28125175

Grilo CM, Crosby RD, Masheb RM, et al: Overvaluation of shape and weight in binge eating disorder, bulimia nervosa, and sub-threshold bulimia nervosa. Behav Res Ther 47(8):692–696, 2009 19552897

Grilo CM, White MA, Gueorguieva R, et al: Predictive significance of the overvaluation of shape/weight in obese patients with binge eating disorder: findings from a randomized controlled trial with 12-month follow-up. Psychol Med 43(6):1335–1344, 2013 22967857

Guarda AS: Treatment of anorexia nervosa: insights and obstacles. Physiol Behav 94(1):113–120, 2008 18155737

Guarda AS, Coughlin JW, Cummings M, et al: Chewing and spitting in eating disorders and its relationship to binge eating. Eat Behav 5(3):231–239, 2004 15135335

Guarda AS, Pinto AM, Coughlin JW, et al: Perceived coercion and change in perceived need for admission in patients hospitalized for eating disorders. Am J Psychiatry 164(1):108–114, 2007 17202551

Guarda AS, Schreyer CC, Boersma GJ, et al: Anorexia nervosa as a motivated behavior: relevance of anxiety, stress, fear and learning. Physiol Behav 152(Pt B):466–472, 2015 25846837

Guerdjikova AI, Mori N, Casuto LS, et al: Binge eating disorder. Psychiatr Clin North Am 40(2):255–266, 2017 28477651

Guillaume S, Gorwood P, Jollant F, et al: Impaired decision-making in symptomatic anorexia and bulimia nervosa patients: a meta-analysis. Psychol Med 45(16):3377–3391, 2015 26497047

Gull WW: Anorexia nervosa (apepsia hysterica, anorexia hysterica). 1868. Obes Res 5(5):498–502, 1997 9385628

Hadley SJ, Walsh BT: Gastrointestinal disturbances in anorexia nervosa and bulimia nervosa. Curr Drug Targets CNS Neurol Disord 2(1):1–9, 2003 12769807

Haedt AA, Edler C, Heatherton TF, et al: Importance of multiple purging methods in the classification of eating disorder subtypes. Int J Eat Disord 39(8):648–654, 2006 16941627

Harrington BC, Jimerson M, Haxton C, et al: Initial evaluation, diagnosis, and treatment of anorexia nervosa and bulimia nervosa. Am Fam Physician 91(1):46–52, 2015 25591200

Harrop EN, Marlatt GA: The comorbidity of substance use disorders and eating disorders in women: prevalence, etiology, and treatment. Addict Behav 35(5):392–398, 2010 20074863

Hay P: A systematic review of evidence for psychological treatments in eating disorders: 2005–2012. Int J Eat Disord 46(5):462–469, 2013 23658093

Hay P, Williams SE: Exploring relationships over time between psychological distress, perceived stress, life events and immature defense style on disordered eating pathology. BMC Psychol 1(1):27, 2013 25566375

Hay P, Bacaltchuk J, Stefano S, Kashyap P: Psychological treatments for bulimia nervosa and binging. Cochrane Database Syst Rev (4):CD000562, 2009 19821271

Hay P, Touyz S, Sud R: Treatment for severe and enduring anorexia nervosa: a review. Aust N Z J Psychiatry 46(12):1136–1144, 2012 22696548

Hay P, Mitchison D, Collado AEL, et al: Burden and health-related quality of life of eating disorders, including Avoidant/Restrictive Food Intake Disorder (ARFID), in the Australian population. J Eat Disord 5:21, 2017 28680630

Hoek HW: Epidemiology of eating disorders in persons other than the high-risk group of young Western females. Curr Opin Psychiatry 27(6):423–425, 2014 25247454

Hoek HW: Review of the worldwide epidemiology of eating disorders. Curr Opin Psychiatry 29(6):336–339, 2016 27608181

Horesh N, Apter A, Lepkifker E, et al: Life events and severe anorexia nervosa in adolescence. Acta Psychiatr Scand 91(1):5–9, 1995 7754787

Horne RL, Ferguson JM, Pope HG Jr, et al: Treatment of bulimia with bupropion: a multicenter controlled trial. J Clin Psychiatry 49(7):262–266, 1988 3134343

Hotta M, Nagashima E, Takagi S, et al: Two young female patients with anorexia nervosa complicated by Mycobacterium tuberculosis infection. Intern Med 43(5):440–444, 2004 15206562

Hudson JI, Hiripi E, Pope HG Jr, et al: The prevalence and correlates of eating disorders in the National Comorbidity Survey Replication. Biol Psychiatry 61(3):348–358, 2007 16815322

Hütter G, Ganepola S, Hofmann WK: The hematology of anorexia nervosa. Int J Eat Disord 42(4):293–300, 2009 19040272

Jones M, Völker U, Lock J, et al: Family based early intervention for anorexia nervosa. Eur Eat Disord Rev 20(3):e137–e143, 2012 22438094

Kaisari P, Dourish CT, Higgs S: Attention Deficit Hyperactivity Disorder (ADHD) and disordered eating behaviour: a systematic review and a framework for future research. Clin Psychol Rev 53:109–121, 2017 28334570

Kass AE, Kolko RP, Wilfley DE: Psychological treatments for eating disorders. Curr Opin Psychiatry 26(6):549–555, 2013 24060917

Kaye WH, Weltzin TE, Hsu LK, et al: An open trial of fluoxetine in patients with anorexia nervosa. J Clin Psychiatry 52(11):464–471, 1991 1744064

Kaye WH, Bulik CM, Thornton L, et al: Comorbidity of anxiety disorders with anorexia and bulimia nervosa. Am J Psychiatry 161(12):2215–2221, 2004 15569892

Kaye WH, Wierenga CE, Bailer UF, et al: Nothing tastes as good as skinny feels: the neurobiology of anorexia nervosa. Trends Neurosci 36(2):110–120, 2013 23333342

Keel PK, Brown TA: Update on course and outcome in eating disorders. Int J Eat Disord 43(3):195–204, 2010 20186717

Keel PK, Brown TA, Holm-Denoma J, et al: Comparison of DSM-IV versus proposed DSM-5 diagnostic criteria for eating disorders: reduction of eating disorder not otherwise specified and validity. Int J Eat Disord 44(6):553–560, 2011 21321984

Kelly NR, Shank LM, Bakalar JL, et al: Pediatric feeding and eating disorders: current state of diagnosis and treatment. Curr Psychiatry Rep 16(5):446, 2014 24643374

Kessler RC, Berglund PA, Chiu WT, et al: The prevalence and correlates of binge eating disorder in the World Health Organization World Mental Health Surveys. Biol Psychiatry 73(9):904–914, 2013 23290497

King SJ, de Sales T: Caring for adolescent females with anorexia nervosa: registered nurses' perspective. J Adv Nurs 32(1):139–147, 2000 10886445

Kohn MR, Madden S, Clarke SD: Refeeding in anorexia nervosa: increased safety and efficiency through understanding the pathophysiology of protein calorie malnutrition. Curr Opin Pediatr 23(4):390–394, 2011 21670680

Le Grange D: Family therapy for adolescent anorexia nervosa. J Clin Psychol 55(6):727–739, 1999 10445863

Le Grange D, Accurso EC, Lock J, et al: Early weight gain predicts outcome in two treatments for adolescent anorexia nervosa. Int J Eat Disord 47(2):124–129, 2014 24190844

Leroy S, Gout A, Husson B, et al: Centropontine myelinolysis related to refeeding syndrome in an adolescent suffering from anorexia nervosa. Neuropediatrics 43(3):152–154, 2012 22473289

Linardon J, Wade T, de la Piedad Garcia X, et al: Psychotherapy for bulimia nervosa on symptoms of depression: a meta-analysis of randomized controlled trials. Int J Eat Disord 50(10):1124–1136, 2017 28804915

Madden S, Miskovic-Wheatley J, Wallis A, et al: A randomized controlled trial of in-patient treatment for anorexia nervosa in medically unstable adolescents. Psychol Med 45(2):415–427, 2015 25017941

Makhzoumi SH, Coughlin JW, Schreyer CC, et al: Weight gain trajectories in hospital-based treatment of anorexia nervosa. Int J Eat Disord 50(3):266–274, 2017 28186654

Malhotra S, McElroy SL: Orlistat misuse in bulimia nervosa. Am J Psychiatry 159(3):492–493, 2002 11870021

Mattar L, Huas C, Duclos J, et al: Relationship between malnutrition and depression or anxiety in anorexia nervosa: a critical review of the literature. J Affect Disord 132(3):311–318, 2011 20920829

Mattar L, Huas C, Godart N; EVHAN Group: Relationship between affective symptoms and malnutrition severity in severe anorexia nervosa. PLoS One 7(11):e49380, 2012a 23185320

Mattar L, Thiébaud MR, Huas C, et al: Depression, anxiety and obsessive-compulsive symptoms in relation to nutritional status and outcome in severe anorexia nervosa. Psychiatry Res 200(2–3):513–517, 2012b 22703719

Mauri M, Miniati M, Mariani MG, et al: Haloperidol for severe anorexia nervosa restricting type with delusional body image disturbance: a nine-case chart review. Eat Weight Disord 18(3):329–332, 2013 23907761

McElroy SL, Hudson JI, Capece JA, et al; Topiramate Binge Eating Disorder Research Group: Topiramate for the treatment of binge eating disorder associated with obesity: a placebo-controlled study. Biol Psychiatry 61(9):1039–1048, 2007 17258690

McElroy SL, Guerdjikova AI, Martens B, et al: Role of antiepileptic drugs in the management of eating disorders. CNS Drugs 23(2):139–156, 2009 19173373

McElroy SL, Guerdjikova AI, Mori N, et al: Overview of the treatment of binge eating disorder. CNS Spectr 20(6):546–556, 2015a 26594849

McElroy SL, Hudson JI, Mitchell JE, et al: Efficacy and safety of lisdexamfetamine for treatment of adults with moderate to severe binge-eating disorder: a randomized clinical trial. JAMA Psychiatry 72(3):235–246, 2015b 25587645

Misra M, Klibanski A: Bone health in anorexia nervosa. Curr Opin Endocrinol Diabetes Obes 18(6):376–382, 2011 21897220

Mitchell JE, Agras S, Wonderlich S: Treatment of bulimia nervosa: where are we and where are we going? Int J Eat Disord 40(2):95–101, 2007 17080448

Mogi A, Kosaka T, Yamaki E, et al: Pulmonary aspergilloma in patient with anorexia nervosa: case report. Ann Thorac Cardiovasc Surg 18(5):465–467, 2012 22374072

Mond JM, Myers TC, Crosby RD, et al: Screening for eating disorders in primary care: EDE-Q versus SCOFF. Behav Res Ther 46(5):612–622, 2008 18359005

Monteleone AM, Monteleone P, Esposito F, et al: Altered processing of rewarding and aversive basic taste stimuli in symptomatic women with anorexia nervosa and bulimia nervosa: an fMRI study. J Psychiatr Res 90:94–101, 2017 28249187

Monteleone P, Castaldo E, Maj M: Neuroendocrine dysregulation of food intake in eating disorders. Regul Pept 149(1–3):39–50, 2008 18582958

Morgan JF, Reid F, Lacey JH: The SCOFF questionnaire: a new screening tool for eating disorders. West J Med 172(3):164–165, 2000 18751246

Munn-Chernoff MA, Baker JH: A primer on the genetics of comorbid eating disorders and substance use disorders. Eur Eat Disord Rev 24(2):91–100, 2016 26663753

Munn-Chernoff MA, Grant JD, Agrawal A, et al: Genetic overlap between alcohol use disorder and bulimic behaviors in European American and African American women. Drug Alcohol Depend 153:335–340, 2015 26096536

Murphy R, Straebler S, Cooper Z, et al: Cognitive behavioral therapy for eating disorders. Psychiatr Clin North Am 33(3):611–627, 2010 20599136

Mustelin L, Lehtokari VL, Keski-Rahkonen A: Other specified and unspecified feeding or eating disorders among women in the community. Int J Eat Disord 49(11):1010–1017, 2016 27442991

Nakao A, Isozaki H, Iwagaki H, et al: Gastric perforation caused by a bulimic attack in an anorexia nervosa patient: report of a case. Surg Today 30(5):435–437, 2000 10819480

Nazar BP, Bernardes C, Peachey G, et al: The risk of eating disorders comorbid with attention-deficit/hyperactivity disorder: a systematic review and meta-analysis. Int J Eat Disord 49(12):1045–1057, 2016 27859581

Norris ML, Spettigue WJ, Katzman DK: Update on eating disorders: current perspectives on avoidant/restrictive food intake disorder in children and youth. Neuropsychiatr Dis Treat 12:213–218, 2016 26855577

Papadopoulos FC, Ekbom A, Brandt L, et al: Excess mortality, causes of death and prognostic factors in anorexia nervosa. Br J Psychiatry 194(1):10–17, 2009 19118319

Patel AS, Matthews L, Bruce-Jones W: Central pontine myelinolysis as a complication of refeeding syndrome in a patient with anorexia nervosa. J Neuropsychiatry Clin Neurosci 20(3):371–373, 2008 18806246

Perdereau F, Faucher S, Wallier J, et al: Family history of anxiety and mood disorders in anorexia nervosa: review of the literature. Eat Weight Disord 13(1):1–13, 2008 18319632

Peveler RC, Bryden KS, Neil HA, et al: The relationship of disordered eating habits and attitudes to clinical outcomes in young adult females with type 1 diabetes. Diabetes Care
28(1):84–88, 2005 15616238

Pinhas-Hamiel O, Hamiel U, Levy-Shraga Y: Eating disorders in adolescents with type 1 diabetes: challenges in diagnosis and treatment. World J Diabetes 6(3):517–526, 2015 25897361

Poulsen S, Lunn S, Daniel SI, et al: A randomized controlled trial of psychoanalytic psychotherapy or cognitive-behavioral therapy for bulimia nervosa. Am J Psychiatry 171(1):109–116,
2014 24275909

Powers PS, Santana CA, Bannon YS: Olanzapine in the treatment of anorexia nervosa: an open
label trial. Int J Eat Disord 32(2):146–154, 2002 12210656

Punchai S, Hanipah ZN, Meister KM, et al: Neurologic manifestations of vitamin B deficiency
after bariatric surgery. Obes Surg 27(8):2079–2082, 2017 28213665

Redgrave GW, Coughlin JW, Schreyer CC, et al: Refeeding and weight restoration outcomes in
anorexia nervosa: challenging current guidelines. Int J Eat Disord 48(7):866–873, 2015
25625572

Renthal W, Marin-Valencia I, Evans PA: Thiamine deficiency secondary to anorexia nervosa: an
uncommon cause of peripheral neuropathy and Wernicke encephalopathy in adolescence.
Pediatr Neurol 51(1):100–103, 2014 24938142

Rich LM, Caine MR, Findling JW, et al: Hypoglycemic coma in anorexia nervosa. Case report
and review of the literature. Arch Intern Med 150(4):894–895, 1990 2183736

Rigaud D, Pennacchio H, Bizeul C, et al: Outcome in AN adult patients: a 13-year follow-up in
484 patients. Diabetes Metab 37(4):305–311, 2011 21317006

Robinson L, Aldridge V, Clark EM, et al: Pharmacological treatment options for low bone mineral density and secondary osteoporosis in anorexia nervosa: a systematic review of the
literature. J Psychosom Res 98:87–97, 2017 28554377

Roerig JL, Steffen KJ, Mitchell JE, et al: Laxative abuse: epidemiology, diagnosis and management. Drugs 70(12):1487–1503, 2010 20687617

Rohde P, Stice E, Marti CN: Development and predictive effects of eating disorder risk factors
during adolescence: implications for prevention efforts. Int J Eat Disord 48(2):187–198,
2015 24599841

Russell G: Bulimia nervosa: an ominous variant of anorexia nervosa. Psychol Med 9(3):429–448,
1979 482466

Russell GF, Treasure J: The modern history of anorexia nervosa. An interpretation of why the
illness has changed. Ann N Y Acad Sci 575:13–27, discussion 27–30, 1989 2699184

Sabel AL, Gaudiani JL, Statland B, et al: Hematological abnormalities in severe anorexia nervosa. Ann Hematol 92(5):605–613, 2013 23392575

Sachs KV, Harnke B, Mehler PS, et al: Cardiovascular complications of anorexia nervosa: a systematic review. Int J Eat Disord 49(3):238–248, 2016 26710932

Sangvai D: Eating disorders in the primary care setting. Prim Care 43(2):301–312, 2016 27262009

Sawyer SM, Whitelaw M, Le Grange D, et al: Physical and psychological morbidity in adolescents with atypical anorexia nervosa. Pediatrics 137(4):e20154080, 2016 27025958

Schebendach JE, Mayer LE, Devlin MJ, et al: Dietary energy density and diet variety as predictors of outcome in anorexia nervosa. Am J Clin Nutr 87(4):810–816, 2008 18400701

Scheuing N, Bartus B, Berger G, et al; DPV Initiative; German BMBF Competence Network Diabetes Mellitus: Clinical characteristics and outcome of 467 patients with a clinically recognized eating disorder identified among 52,215 patients with type 1 diabetes: a multicenter
German/Austrian study. Diabetes Care 37(6):1581–1589, 2014 24623022

Sebaaly JC, Cox S, Hughes CM, et al: Use of fluoxetine in anorexia nervosa before and after
weight restoration. Ann Pharmacother 47(9):1201–1205, 2013 24259736

Silber TJ: Ipecac syrup abuse, morbidity, and mortality: isn't it time to repeal its over-the-
counter status? J Adolesc Health 37(3):256–260, 2005 16109351

Smink FR, van Hoeken D, Hoek HW: Epidemiology of eating disorders: incidence, prevalence
and mortality rates. Curr Psychiatry Rep 14(4):406–414, 2012 22644309

Society for Adolescent Health and Medicine: Refeeding hypophosphatemia in hospitalized adolescents with anorexia nervosa: a position statement of the Society for Adolescent Health and Medicine. J Adolesc Health 55(3):455–457, 2014 25151056

Sogg S, Lauretti J, West-Smith L: Recommendations for the presurgical psychosocial evaluation of bariatric surgery patients. Surg Obes Relat Dis 12(4):731–749, 2016 27179400

Solmi F, Sallis H, Stahl D, et al: Low birth weight in the offspring of women with anorexia nervosa. Epidemiol Rev 36(1):49–56, 2014 24025351

Steinglass J, Walsh BT: Habit learning and anorexia nervosa: a cognitive neuroscience hypothesis. Int J Eat Disord 39(4):267–275, 2006 16523472

Steinglass J, Albano AM, Simpson HB, et al: Fear of food as a treatment target: exposure and response prevention for anorexia nervosa in an open series. Int J Eat Disord 45(4):615–621, 2012 21541979

Steinglass JE, Kaplan SC, Liu Y, et al: The (lack of) effect of alprazolam on eating behavior in anorexia nervosa: a preliminary report. Int J Eat Disord 47(8):901–904, 2014 25139178

Stiles-Shields C, Bamford BH, Touyz S, et al: Predictors of therapeutic alliance in two treatments for adults with severe and enduring anorexia nervosa. J Eat Disord 4:13, 2016 27054037

Swinbourne JM, Touyz SW: The co-morbidity of eating disorders and anxiety disorders: a review. Eur Eat Disord Rev 15(4):253–274, 2007 17676696

Sylvester CJ, Forman SF: Clinical practice guidelines for treating restrictive eating disorder patients during medical hospitalization. Curr Opin Pediatr 20(4):390–397, 2008 18622192

Tabaac BJ, Tabaac V: Pica patient, status post gastric bypass, improves with change in medication regimen. Ther Adv Psychopharmacol 5(1):38–42, 2015 25653830

Tan JO, Hope T, Stewart A: Anorexia nervosa and personal identity: the accounts of patients and their parents. Int J Law Psychiatry 26(5):533–548, 2003 14522224

Tan JO, Stewart A, Fitzpatrick R, et al: Attitudes of patients with anorexia nervosa to compulsory treatment and coercion. Int J Law Psychiatry 33(1):13–19, 2010 19926134

Thornton LM, Welch E, Munn-Chernoff MA, et al: Anorexia nervosa, major depression, and suicide attempts: shared genetic factors. Suicide Life Threat Behav 46(5):525–534, 2016 26916469

Treasure J, Russell G: The case for early intervention in anorexia nervosa: theoretical exploration of maintaining factors. Br J Psychiatry 199(1):5–7, 2011 21719874

Ulfvebrand S, Birgegård A, Norring C, et al: Psychiatric comorbidity in women and men with eating disorders: results from a large clinical database. Psychiatry Res 230(2):294–299, 2015 26416590

Vanderschueren S, Geens E, Knockaert D, et al: The diagnostic spectrum of unintentional weight loss. Eur J Intern Med 16(3):160–164, 2005 15967329

Voderholzer U, Witte S, Schlegl S, et al: Association between depressive symptoms, weight and treatment outcome in a very large anorexia nervosa sample. Eat Weight Disord 21(1):127–131, 2016 26440611

Waller G: Drop-out and failure to engage in individual outpatient cognitive behavior therapy for bulimic disorders. Int J Eat Disord 22(1):35–41, 1997 9140733

Watson HJ, Levine MD, Zerwas SC, et al: Predictors of dropout in face-to-face and Internet-based cognitive-behavioral therapy for bulimia nervosa in a randomized controlled trial. Int J Eat Disord 50(5):569–577, 2017 27862108

Westmoreland P, Krantz MJ, Mehler PS: Medical complications of anorexia nervosa and bulimia. Am J Med 129(1):30–37, 2016 26169883

White MA, Grilo CM: Bupropion for overweight women with binge-eating disorder: a randomized, double-blind, placebo-controlled trial. J Clin Psychiatry 74(4):400–406, 2013 23656848

Wilfley DE, Citrome L, Herman BK: Characteristics of binge eating disorder in relation to diagnostic criteria. Neuropsychiatr Dis Treat 12:2213–2223, 2016 27621631

Williams PM, Goodie J, Motsinger CD: Treating eating disorders in primary care. Am Fam Physician 77(2):187–195, 2008 18246888

Winston AP: Management of physical aspects and complications of eating disorders. Psychiatry 7(4):174–178, 2008

Wolfe BE, Dunne JP, Kells MR: Nursing care considerations for the hospitalized patient with an eating disorder. Nurs Clin North Am 51(2):213–235, 2016 27229277

Wonderlich SA, Peterson CB, Crosby RD, et al: A randomized controlled comparison of integrative cognitive-affective therapy (ICAT) and enhanced cognitive-behavioral therapy (CBT-E) for bulimia nervosa. Psychol Med 44(3):543–553, 2014 23701891

Young V, Eiser C, Johnson B, et al: Eating problems in adolescents with type 1 diabetes: a systematic review with meta-analysis. Diabet Med 30(2):189–198, 2013 22913589

Zerwas S, Larsen JT, Petersen L, et al: The incidence of eating disorders in a Danish register study: associations with suicide risk and mortality. J Psychiatr Res 65:16–22, 2015 25958083

CHAPTER 14

Sleep Disorders

Lois E. Krahn, M.D.

Obtaining a sufficient quantity and quality of sleep is important for good health. Chronic partial sleep deprivation, also known as insufficient sleep, is common in our society. The consequences include depressed mood, interpersonal irritability, decreased daytime vigilance, weight gain, coronary artery disease, and cognitive impairment (Kecklund and Axelsson 2016). Determining what amount of sleep is sufficient for an individual is difficult for several reasons. Sleep duration gradually decreases from a starting length of 16 hours per 24-hour day as human beings transition from infancy to adulthood. Interindividual differences in the optimal amount of sleep range from 6 to 12 hours, with a mean of 7.5 hours for adults. When a primary sleep disorder, such as obstructive sleep apnea hypopnea (OSAH), is present, the continuity and depth of sleep may be compromised independently of sleep duration. Recognizing how much sleep any individual requires is complicated. Nonetheless, there is consensus that chronically inadequate sleep is detrimental to health.

Physiological Mechanisms of Normal Sleep

Sleep can be subdivided into two major components: rapid eye movement (REM) sleep, which is characterized by increased levels of cortical activation accompanied by reduced muscle tone to prevent corresponding movements, and non–rapid eye movement (NREM) sleep, which is separated into three distinct stages. The International Classification of Sleep Disorders was updated in 2014, with the most significant change relating to NREM sleep, which previously had four distinct phases (American Academy of Sleep Medicine 2014). Table 14–1 summarizes the characteristics and percentage of time spent in each sleep stage by healthy middle-aged adults.

Normal sleep progresses from wakefulness to stage N1 NREM sleep. From this stage of twilight sleep, a patient can be easily awakened by environmental stimuli. Stage N2 NREM sleep is deeper, and moderate environmental stimuli, such as a crack

TABLE 14–1.   Sleep stages in healthy adults

Stage	Percentage of total sleep	Polysomnographic characteristics	Physiological state
Stage N1 NREM	2–5	Slow eye movements	Easy to arouse
Stage N2 NREM	45–55	Spindles, K complexes	More difficult to arouse
Stage N3 NREM	13–23	Slow EEG frequency	Difficult to arouse
Stage R	20–25	Rapid eye movements Muscle atonia Increased EEG frequency	Variable arousal threshold Penile engorgement

Note.   EEG=electroencephalographic; NREM=non–rapid eye movement.

of thunder, no longer cause arousal but rather result in a distinctive electrophysiolog-ical event, the K complex. Sleep spindles and K complexes are used to identify stage N2 NREM sleep. When the electroencephalographic (EEG) tracing slows until at least 20% of the activity consists of higher-voltage slow waves, the sleep is rated stage N3 NREM. Previously subdivided into Stage III and IV sleep, stage N3 is also called *delta wave sleep, deep sleep,* or *slow-wave sleep.* A person awakens from this sleep stage only when environmental stimuli are marked, such as the prolonged loud noise of an alarm.

As the normal sleep cycle progresses, EEG activity gradually returns to the most common stage, N2 sleep. Stage N2 sleep evolves into the first REM sleep episode of the night. REM sleep, now called stage R, is characterized by high-frequency EEG ac-tivity, episodic bursts of vertical eye movements, muscle atonia, and penile tumes-cence. The first REM episode is often brief and typically occurs 70–100 minutes after the person falls asleep. The sleep cycle repeats four or five times during the night, subsequent REM episodes being of longer Center for Sleep Medicine duration. In general, slow-wave sleep is more common early in the night, and REM periods be-come longer toward morning. Because the last REM episode occurs at the very end of the major sleep period, people can recall their dreams, and men experience morning erections.

The data in Table 14–1 are useful as normative data because sleep study reports typically describe the percentage of the night spent in each complete stage, and thus subjects with normal sleep patterns can be compared with subjects with pathology. In healthy elderly subjects, the relative percentage of time spent in slow-wave sleep decreases, and sleep is generally more fragmented. Figure 14–1 is based on a meta-analysis of distribution of sleep stages over the life span and shows in the absence of pathology a progressive decrease in total sleep time plus stages N3 and R (Ohayon et al. 2004). Patients with disrupted sleep often spend most of the night in stages N1 and N2 and have little slow-wave or REM sleep. The exact roles of slow-wave sleep and REM sleep in a refreshing night's sleep are not well understood, but significant reduc-tions in either state can lead to undesirable results, including daytime sleepiness, de-pressed mood, and cognitive impairment. In animal studies, prolonged absolute sleep deprivation has resulted in death attributed to sepsis because of suspected un-derlying compromise of immune function (Everson and Toth 2000).

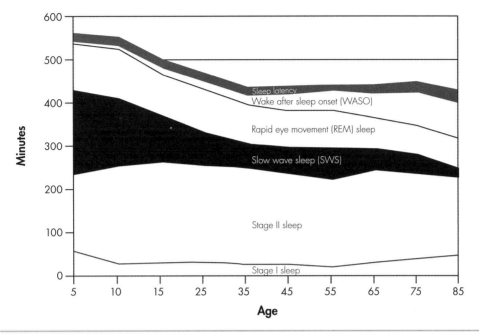

FIGURE 14–1. Changes in sleep architecture throughout the life cycle.

Source. Adapted from Ohayon MM, Carskadon MA, Guilleminault C, Vitiello MV: "Meta-Analysis of Quantitative Sleep Parameters From Childhood to Old Age in Healthy Individuals: Developing Normative Sleep Values Across the Human Lifespan." *Sleep* 27(7):1270, 2004. Copyright 2004, Oxford University Press. Used with permission.

Evaluation of Sleep

Office Evaluation

A diagnostic interview and physical examination remain the foundation of the sleep evaluation. Table 14–2 lists the many issues that require evaluation when assessing patients for a possible sleep disorder. The decision to refer a patient for a sleep medicine specialty evaluation and diagnostic testing is based on the history and physical examination. Sleep studies are not necessary for some disorders (e.g., restless legs syndrome) and can be avoided if the classic symptoms of the disorder are identified in the absence of any other factors. Clinicians need to obtain thorough medical and psychiatric histories, because many illnesses and disorders can alter sleep. As people age, sleep complaints become more common, not because of primary sleep disorders but rather because of comorbid conditions (Vitiello et al. 2002). Tables 14–3 and 14–4 list disorders that may lead to sleep problems. As a first step, treatment should be targeted to the underlying disease.

An interview with a bed partner is of great value, if feasible, especially in regard to snoring, respiratory pauses, and unusual behaviors. A validated questionnaire has been developed to collect data from family members concerning possible REM sleep behavior disorder and other common conditions (Figure 14–2). Presbycusis (age-related hearing loss) and/or sound sleep may limit the ability of a bed partner to pro-

TABLE 14–2.   **Essential issues in a sleep diagnostic interview of patients and bed partners**

Presenting complaint?

Sleep interruptions—Parenting issues? Caregiver issues?

Preferred sleep time—Early or late bedtime? Sleep position?

Sleep environment—Bed partner? Comfortable bedding? Bright light? Noise? Vibrations? Excessive heat/cold? Pets?

Sleep walking? Somnambulism? Sleep eating?

Nap schedule—Frequent or prolonged?

Excessive daytime somnolence?

Cataplexy? Sleep paralysis? Hallucinogenic experiences?

Nocturnal movements?

Gastrointestinal reflux—Diagnosed? Partially treated?

Erectile problems? Urinary frequency? Enuresis?

Depression, mania, or panic attacks?

Prescription drug use, abuse, or dependence?

Family sleep history?

Previous sleep evaluations?

Work schedule—Rotating shifts? On call?

Exercise schedule—Late in the evening?

Insomnia—Early? Middle? Late?

Motor vehicle accident due to sleepiness?

Alcohol, street drug, or caffeine use, abuse, or dependence?

Snoring? Observed pauses?

Pain—Chronic? Acute? Medications wear off?

Hangover effect? Amnesia?

Vivid dreams, nightmares?

Herbal preparations?

Childhood sleep history?

vide observations. Alternatively, a video or audio recording of the presenting complaint can yield valuable information (Koo et al. 2017).

Sometimes, even if the patient sleeps alone, a family member can provide useful information, particularly if the partner moved out of a shared bedroom because of the patient's intolerable snoring or unusual behaviors. Although the interview with the former bed partner may yield limited specific information about the patient's current symptoms, the partner's confirmation of the patient's sleep problems increases the likelihood that a pathological condition is present.

During the physical examination, the examiner should note the patient's level of alertness (in the waiting room and during the appointment), body mass index, neck circumference, nasopharyngeal abnormalities, protrusion of mandible, thyroid size, pulmonary findings, cardiac sounds, and cognition. Laboratory tests including thyroid-stimulating hormone, ferritin, B_{12}, and folate and a complete blood cell count are helpful in identifying medical disorders to include in the differential diagnosis of several sleep disorders.

TABLE 14–3.   **Selected causes of insomnia**

Primarily medical

Obstructive sleep apnea hypopnea

Chronic obstructive pulmonary disease

Asthma

Gastroesophageal reflux

Angina

Hypoglycemia

Congestive heart failure (orthopnea, paroxysmal nocturnal dyspnea)

Hyperthyroidism

Pain

Primarily neurological

Central sleep apnea

Dementia

Restless legs syndrome

Fatal familial insomnia

Primarily psychiatric

Medication-induced (e.g., xanthines, psychostimulants)

Insomnia disorder

Anxiety disorders

Circadian rhythm sleep–wake disorder, irregular sleep–wake type

Withdrawal-related (e.g., alcohol, benzodiazepines)

Paradoxical insomnia

Mood disorders (depression, mania)

Primarily environmental

Community noise (e.g., traffic, alarms, neighbors, gunshots)

Altered temperature (too hot, too cold)

Vibration (elevator, machinery)

Because of the cost and inconvenience of sleep studies, a clear need exists for cost-effective screening tools for determining which patients are good candidates for more definitive diagnostic testing. In children, careful visualization of tonsillar size has been found to be highly sensitive and specific as a screening test for obstructive sleep apnea (A.M. Li et al. 2002).

In one large-scale study with a community-based sample, investigators found that among adults, male sex, older age, higher body mass index, greater neck circumference, snoring, and repeated respiratory pauses were all independent correlates of moderate to severe breathing-related sleep disorder (Young et al. 2002).

Because many patients minimize excessive daytime sleepiness or slowly adapt to it, they may lose insight into the degree of their excessive daytime sleepiness. History from other sources, such as family members, may be necessary. Daytime symptoms related to excessive sleepiness can be evaluated with the brief and convenient Epworth Sleepiness Scale (Johns 1991) (Table 14–5).

TABLE 14–4.   Selected causes of excessive daytime sleepiness

Primarily neurological

Narcolepsy or hypersomnolence disorder

Delirium

Kleine-Levin syndrome

Narcolepsy secondary to another medical condition (tumor or trauma destroying the hypocretin neurons)

Central sleep apnea

Prader-Willi syndrome

Primarily medical

Obstructive sleep apnea hypopnea

Gastroesophageal reflux

Primarily psychiatric

Substance/medication-induced sleep disorder (e.g., alcohol, hypnotic, sedative) with onset during intoxication or with onset during discontinuation/withdrawal

Mood disorder

Altered sleep–wake schedule

Diagnostic Procedures

Techniques for measuring sleep and body functions during sleep have evolved since the initial description of REM sleep in 1953 (Aserinsky and Kleitman 1953). Until recently, most sleep studies were conducted in facilities using computerized equipment that monitor and store the multiple physiological measurements that comprise a polysomnographic study (Table 14–6). Trained technologists attend the patient during the study, making adjustments or intervening as needed. Today, a variety of portable devices are increasingly in use for patients suspected to be at high risk of OSAH (Claman and Sunwoo 2017; see section "Sleep-Related Breathing Disorders and Snoring" later in this chapter for more information on portable devices). Many patients welcome the availability of portable studies that can be conducted in the privacy and comfort of their homes. When the differential diagnosis includes sleep disorders other than obstructive sleep apnea, or when a patient sleeps poorly, portable studies have not been demonstrated to be as reliable. In these cases, the sleep study may need to be repeated in a laboratory setting.

Devices such as wrist actigraphs, an accelerometer that detects movement, have been studied in the hospital setting, but they are used mostly in ambulatory practice (Krahn et al. 1997). Precise determination of sleep–wake status is impossible with actigraphs, because the equipment measures limb acceleration and does not record EEG activity. One distinct advantage of actigraphy, however, is that the compact device can be worn 24 hours per day for up to 4 weeks. Longitudinal monitoring also allows identification of irregular sleep–wake patterns. Sleep diaries, completed by patients or caregivers, can be used but often are inaccurate due to the poor recall of sleep parameters, lack of adherence to daily documentation, or distorted perception (O'Brien et al. 2016).

The multiple sleep latency (MSL) test is used to identify disorders of excessive daytime sleepiness, including narcolepsy (Kretzschmar et al. 2016), though it has limita-

Mayo Sleep Questionnaire—*Informant*

Do you live with the patient? ☐ Yes ☐ No (If No, END FORM HERE)

Do you sleep in the same room as the patient? ☐ Yes ☐ No

If no, is it because of his/her sleep behaviors (i.e., snores too loud, acts out dreams, etc.)? ☐ Yes ☐ No

Please mark "Yes" if the described event has occurred *at least 3 times*.

1. Have you ever seen the patient appear to "act out his/her dreams" while sleeping (punched or flailed arms in the air, shouted or screamed)?
   ☐ No
   ☐ Yes
   - If Yes,
     a. How many months or years has this been going on?
        __ __ year(s)
        __ __ months
     b. Has the patient ever been injured from these behaviors (bruises, cuts, broken bones)?
        ☐ No
        ☐ Yes
     c. Has a bedpartner ever been injured from these behaviors (bruises, blows, pulled hair)?
        ☐ No
        ☐ Yes
        ☐ No bedpartner
     d. Has the patient told you about dreams of being chased, attacked or that involve defending himself/herself?
        ☐ No
        ☐ Yes
        ☐ Never told you about dreams
     e. If the patient woke up and told you about a dream, did the details of the dream match the movements made while sleeping?
        ☐ No
        ☐ Yes
        ☐ Never told you about dreams

2. Do the patient's legs repeatedly jerk or twitch during sleep (not just when falling asleep)?
   ☐ No
   ☐ Yes

3. Does the patient complain of a restless, nervous, tingly, or creepy-crawly feeling in his/her legs that disrupts his/her ability to fall or stay asleep?
   ☐ No
   ☐ Yes

- If Yes,
   a. Does the patient tell you that these leg sensations decrease when he/she moves them or walks around?
      ☐ No
      ☐ Yes
   b. When do these sensations seem to be the worst?
      ☐ before 6 pm
      ☐ after 6 pm

4. Has the patient ever walked around the bedroom or house while asleep?
   ☐ No
   ☐ Yes

5. Has the patient ever snorted or choked him/herself awake?
   ☐ No
   ☐ Yes

6. Does the patient ever seem to stop breathing during sleep?
   ☐ No
   ☐ Yes
   - If Yes,
     a. Is the patient currently being treated for this (e.g., CPAP)?
        ☐ No
        ☐ Yes

7. Does the patient have leg cramps at night (e.g., also called a "charley horse," with intense pain in certain muscles in the leg)?
   ☐ No
   ☐ Yes

8. Rate the patient's general level of alertness for the past 3 weeks on a scale from 0 to 10.

0	1	2	3	4	5	6	7	8	9	10
Sleep all day										Fully and normally awake

FIGURE 14–2. Mayo Sleep Questionnaire.

tions (Plante 2017). Patients must first undergo an overnight sleep study for exclusion of other sleep disorders caused by disrupted nocturnal sleep. If the patient has had, at minimum, 6 hours of sleep to preclude sleep deprivation, then a valid MSL test can be conducted the next day. Patients are asked to take four or five scheduled naps wearing a simplified set of leads—only EEG, electromyography (EMG), and electro-oculography (EOG). The MSL test is used to measure initial sleep latency and initial

TABLE 14–5.   **Epworth Sleepiness Scale**

How likely are you to doze off or fall asleep in the following situations, in contrast to feeling just tired? This refers to your usual way of life in recent times. Even if you have not done some of these things recently, try to work out how they would have affected you. Use the following scale to choose the most appropriate number for each situation:

0 = would never doze;
1 = slight chance of dozing;
2 = moderate chance of dozing;
3 = high chance of dozing.

Situation	Chance of dozing			
Sitting and reading	0	1	2	3
Sitting inactive in a public place	0	1	2	3
Passenger in a car (>60 minutes)	0	1	2	3
Lying down to rest in the afternoon	0	1	2	3
Sitting and talking	0	1	2	3
Sitting after lunch (without alcohol)	0	1	2	3
Sitting in traffic	0	1	2	3

TABLE 14–6.   **Components of polysomnography**

Essentials

Electroencephalography (EEG) (typically three channels)

Electromyography (EMG)—surface electrodes on chin and lower extremity

Electro-oculography (EOG) (two channels)

Electrocardiography (ECG)

Respiratory effort measurement

Airflow monitoring (nasal pressure or temperature)

Pulse oximetry

Options

Videotaping using infrared light source

Transcutaneous carbon dioxide monitoring

Esophageal pressure monitoring

Esophageal pH monitoring

Additional electromyography (upper extremities, intercostal muscles)

Additional electroencephalography (seizure detection)

REM latency, if present, for each nap. Patients are asked to stay awake between naps, to refrain from stimulants such as caffeine and prescribed medications, and to undergo drug screening for occult sedative use. The utility of MSL testing for patients with hypersomnolence due to a psychiatric disorder has not been as well studied and is suspected to be more limited (Plante 2017). The maintenance of wakefulness test (MWT) is a similar procedure with slight modifications. Instead of being asked to fall asleep, patients are asked to stay awake during four or five specified daytime sessions (Mitler et al. 1982). The data can be used to document that a patient with a treated sleep disorder such as OSAH or narcolepsy can maintain wakefulness sufficiently to drive or operate equipment requiring sustained vigilance. MWT results can be used as an outcome measure of effective treatment.

Sleep Disorders

Several disorders with signs and symptoms closely linked with sleep or the 24-hour sleep–wake schedule are generally classified as sleep disorders. Not all pathophysiological states that vary according to a 24-hour schedule—for example, tumor growth and abnormal cortisol production—are classified as sleep disorders, because circadian rhythmicity is not the defining feature (American Academy of Sleep Medicine 2014). The clearest example of this distinction would be restless legs syndrome, which is set apart from other neurological diseases by its periodicity and timing.

Narcolepsy and Other Disorders of Excessive Daytime Sleepiness

Narcolepsy is an excellent example of a disorder with dysfunction of a specific sleep state, in this case REM sleep. Isolated fragments of REM sleep intrude into wakefulness, and the result is the characteristic symptoms that invariably cause excessive daytime sleepiness. Narcolepsy in humans was first described in 1880 by the French neurologist Gelineau (Schenck et al. 2007). Since that time, narcolepsy has been observed in several dog breeds as well as in horses and sheep. These naturally occurring animal models have greatly facilitated investigations into the pathophysiology of narcolepsy.

Prevalence

Narcolepsy is a more common disorder than many recognize, with a prevalence similar to that of multiple sclerosis. For this reason, identification and treatment offer a valuable opportunity to prevent medical, occupational, and social complications. When patients present with sleepiness, many other conditions, including insufficient sleep and breathing-related sleep disorder, should be suspected before narcolepsy is diagnosed. Likely because of the broad differential diagnosis, the average delay between onset of symptoms and diagnosis is 10 years (Maski et al. 2017).

In a U.S. community sample, narcolepsy was observed to have a prevalence of 0.06% (Silber et al. 2002). All cases of narcolepsy met the diagnostic criteria on the basis of excessive daytime sleepiness and laboratory findings. In 64% of these cases, the patient had cataplexy. Incidence data from the same study confirmed the long-standing impression that narcolepsy is slightly more common in men (1.72 per 100,000) than women (1.05 per 100,000). The disease most commonly starts in the second decade of life and is a chronic condition.

Narcolepsy is no longer believed to be a familial disease, although rare cases of familial clusters have been identified (Taheri 2016). When narcolepsy is familial, the mode of inheritance is complex. Debate continues about whether narcolepsy is the result of an autoimmune or neurodegenerative process.

Clinical Features

Narcolepsy is characterized by chronic excessive daytime sleepiness with episodic sleep attacks (American Academy of Sleep Medicine 2014; American Psychiatric Association 2013). Approximately 65%–75% of patients with narcolepsy have cataplexy (also called narcolepsy type 1), in which an emotional trigger, most commonly laughter, provokes abrupt muscle atonia without loss of consciousness. Other associated symptoms include sleep paralysis (isolated loss of muscle tone associated with REM in normal sleep) and hypnagogic and hypnopompic hallucinations (vivid dreaming occurring at the time of sleep onset and awakening that can be difficult to distinguish from reality). When related to the dissociated components of REM sleep, such as muscle atonia (cataplexy and sleep paralysis) and vivid dreams (hypnagogic and hypnopompic hallucinations), these phenomena can intrude into wakefulness. Disturbed nocturnal sleep has been added as a fifth part of this constellation of symptoms.

Pathophysiological Mechanism

In 2000, patients with narcolepsy with cataplexy were reported to have undetectable levels of a newly identified neuropeptide, hypocretin (also known as orexin), in cerebrospinal fluid (CSF). Hypocretin is synthesized by a small number of neurons in the anterior hypothalamus that project widely throughout the central nervous system (CNS). After studies of other sleep and neurological disorders, the absence of this neuropeptide appears to be highly specific (99%) for narcolepsy (Mignot et al. 2002). Hypocretin influences sleep, appetite, and temperature. The genes for the ligands and receptors for hypocretin have been knocked out in mice, resulting in the development of excessive sleepiness, cataplexy, and obesity (Smart and Jerman 2002). An autoimmune mechanism has been suspected ever since the association between narcolepsy and a specific human leukocyte antigen (HLA) allele was recognized 25 years ago (Kornum et al. 2017).

Diagnostic Testing

The most important part of an evaluation for narcolepsy is a careful interview to screen for long-standing excessive daytime sleepiness and spells triggered by emotions. The definitive bedside test for cataplexy is demonstrating the transient absence of deep tendon reflexes during the episode (Krahn et al. 2000). This procedure also aids in differentiating cataplexy from pseudocataplexy (Krahn et al. 2001). However, cataplexy is difficult to provoke, and the episode is often too brief to allow for a physical examination.

   In most cases diagnostic testing in a sleep disorders center is necessary to supplement the clinical interview. The diagnosis must be as certain as possible before a life-long course of treatment is begun. A polysomnogram is important for ruling out other causes of excessive daytime sleepiness. This study is ideally preceded by wrist actigraphy to confirm adequate sleep in the weeks before testing in order to eliminate sleep deprivation as the cause. If polysomnography reveals that the patient has OSAH or another primary sleep disorder, these conditions must be stabilized before reliable daytime testing can be conducted. The MSL test quantifies the time required to fall asleep during daytime naps and confirms the presence of inappropriate daytime REM sleep. Hypocretin testing in the CSF is not yet clinically available.

Complications

Narcolepsy is associated with a poorer quality of life than is epilepsy (Maski et al. 2017). Without treatment, patients are at risk of motor vehicle accidents and occupational injuries related to sleepiness. Patients with narcolepsy have a higher-than-expected rate of OSAH, REM sleep behavior disorder, and periodic limb movements during sleep (Krahn et al. 2001). Patients with narcolepsy also have higher rates of obesity, which may be linked to the hypocretin deficiency.

Treatment

Patient education should emphasize the importance of a consistent sleep–wake schedule, the need for adequate sleep, the value of brief daytime naps, and refraining from driving a car when sleepy. Pharmacological options for narcolepsy include methylphenidate or amphetamines, which target excessive daytime sleepiness (Saini and Rye 2017). Extended-release preparations of methylphenidate and amphetamines have the advantage of continuous drug delivery, which reduces the daytime variability in alertness that may occur with the immediate-release forms (taken twice or three times a day). Tricyclic antidepressants and, to a lesser degree, selective serotonin reuptake inhibitors (SSRIs) historically have been used to treat cataplexy. Agents that increase the level of norepinephrine, and to a lesser degree serotonin, in the brain suppress REM sleep–related symptoms.

Modafinil and its R-enantiomer armodafinil are wake-promoting medications approved by the U.S. Food and Drug Administration (FDA) for the treatment of narcolepsy. Lacking sympathomimetic activity, these agents are not considered psychostimulants. Their mechanism of action is not completely understood (Thorpy 2016). Sodium oxybate (also known as gamma-hydroxybutyrate), a novel agent used for narcolepsy primarily in specialty settings, was approved by the FDA in 2002.

Hypersomnolence Disorder

Hypersomnolence disorder is a disorder of unknown etiology characterized by excessive daytime sleepiness in the absence of other specific symptoms (American Academy of Sleep Medicine 2014; American Psychiatric Association 2013). Patients typically have a prolonged duration of nocturnal sleep as well as unrefreshing daytime naps. The prevalence of hypersomnolence disorder is unknown, but the condition appears to develop at equal rates in both genders. As in narcolepsy, symptoms first appear in adolescence or young adulthood. This condition increases the risk of motor vehicle accidents and occupational or educational problems due to sleepiness. Depression may be another consequence (Saini and Rye 2017).

The clinical interview should concentrate on the duration of excessive daytime sleepiness, the sleep–wake schedule, and the presence of mood disorders. The presence of a mood disorder complicates the evaluation because both depression and antidepressant medications can alter sleep architecture. Because of the broad differential diagnosis, the evaluation for hypersomnolence disorder must be in-depth. Ideally the diagnostic testing consists of wrist actigraphy, polysomnography, MSL testing, and drug screening. The testing for respiratory arousals must be particularly rigorous, since any degree of upper airway resistance syndrome or subclinical sleep-related breathing disorder can produce persisting excessive daytime sleepiness. The diagnosis of hypersomnolence disorder is established on the basis of quantifiable excessive daytime sleepiness on the MSL test. Unlike patients with narcolepsy, those with hypersomnolence disorder have no sleep-onset REM episodes and have normal levels of hypocretin in the CSF.

There is less agreement regarding the treatment of hypersomnolence disorder than that of other sleep disorders. Patient education regarding adequate sleep is critical. A common strategy is initially to request patients to extend sleep time by at least an hour, with the intent to aid patients whose sleepiness may be related to inadequate nocturnal sleep. Long sleepers, who require an hour or more sleep than average to obtain adequate sleep, may be erroneously identified as having hypersomnolence disorder. Apart from sleep extension, treatment is otherwise similar to that for narcolepsy. In contrast to narcolepsy, however, daytime naps are not encouraged in hypersomnolence disorder because they are not refreshing. If the results after evaluation suggest the presence of a coexisting mood disorder, use of an antidepressant is appropriate and does not cause problems. More stimulating antidepressants are preferred.

Kleine-Levin syndrome, also known as recurrent hypersomnia, is an important part of the differential diagnosis of hypersomnolence. Patients with recurrent hypersomnia are generally male adolescents who engage in binge eating and have periodic hypersomnia that lasts several weeks (Miglis and Guilleminault 2016). The typical pattern is recurrent episodes, each lasting approximately a week, spanning 8 years. Depressed mood has been reported in 48% of affected patients (Arnulf et al. 2005). In the absence of any randomized controlled trials in Kleine-Levin syndrome, psychostimulants and lithium have been reported to prevent relapses (de Oliveira et al. 2016).

Parasomnias

Parasomnias are disorders in which patients have inappropriate motor behaviors during sleep. REM sleep behavior disorder is arguably of most interest because of the complex, distressing behaviors and the relationship with other neurological conditions.

REM Sleep Behavior Disorder

Patients with REM sleep behavior disorder appear to "act out their dreams" by yelling or gesturing during REM sleep (American Academy of Sleep Medicine 2014; American Psychiatric Association 2013). They lack the muscle atonia normally found in REM sleep and move in response to dream imagery. REM sleep behavior disorder appears to be more common than was originally suspected, although the prevalence has not been firmly established. Risk factors for this sleep disorder are male sex (90% of patients described in the literature) and advanced age (most patients have been age 50 years or older) (Schenck 2016). SSRIs and serotonin–norepinephrine reuptake inhibitors (SNRIs) have been suggested as possible triggers. Patients and their bed partners can be seriously injured by hitting, kicking, and other more complex behaviors. REM sleep behavior disorder is associated with several neurological disorders, including Parkinson's disease (15%–33% of patients), multiple system atrophy (69%–90%), and dementia with Lewy bodies (50%–80%) (Jacobs et al. 2016).

Polysomnography, optimally with extra EMG leads and videotaping, can be useful for documenting increased EMG tone during REM sleep. Patients can have increased muscle tone without reports of disruptive or inappropriate behaviors (REM sleep without atonia). These patients are not yet considered to have REM sleep behavior disorder, but the disease is expected to evolve. Polysomnography also helps identify complicating disorders, such as OSAH, which is of particular importance if benzodiazepine treatment is considered. Nocturnal seizures should be excluded. Treatment includes modifying the bedroom to reduce injury to the patient and bed partner. Bed partners often choose to sleep separately. Clonazepam has become the medication of choice because it reduces the muscle movement that occurs during REM sleep, reducing the risk of injury (S.X. Li et al. 2016), but there are no randomized controlled trials of treatment for REM sleep behavior disorder.

NREM Sleep Arousal Disorder

NREM parasomnias (DSM-5 NREM sleep arousal disorder), unlike REM sleep behavior disorder, are more common in children and adolescents than in adults. Patients, when not fully alert, act unusually, walk, or eat. Polysomnography is not always needed because the behaviors are often intermittent and therefore difficult to observe with a single night of monitoring. Sleep deprivation, nocturnal arousals, shifting bedtimes, and consumption of alcohol can precipitate episodes in susceptible individuals. Sleep deprivation has been used to trigger sleepwalking in studies of somnambulism (Dang-Vu et al. 2015).

Treatment of NREM sleep arousal disorders includes modifying the sleeping environment to promote safety, adhering to a consistent sleep schedule, reducing nocturnal awakenings, and, if warranted, using medications such as hypnotics to prevent arousal (Pilon et al. 2008).

Nocturnal panic disorder with episodes occurring exclusively during sleep is rare, while panic disorder with attacks occurring both during the day and at night is not uncommon. Treatment of this condition ideally includes a combination of medication and behavioral intervention. When panic or anxiety exists exclusively at night, most typically in NREM sleep, a broad differential diagnosis should include breathing-related sleep disorder, nightmares, and medical disorders (e.g., arrhythmia, angina, gastroesophageal reflux) triggering the anxiety. Whenever a patient presents with unusual behavior at night, the differential diagnosis must include epilepsy. In particular, seizures arising from a locus in the frontal lobe can result in stereotypical but bizarre events during slow-wave sleep (Dyken et al. 2001). Confirmed treatment of nocturnal panic disorder relies on medications, because behavioral measures are less feasible when an attack develops during sleep.

Nightmare Disorder

In DSM-5, the Parasomnia section includes nightmare disorder—repeated episodes of prolonged, highly distressing dreams that are subdivided into acute (duration <1 month), subacute (duration 1–6 months), and persistent (duration >6 months). These dreams can be accompanied by sweating, tachycardia, and tachypnea and can occur in the context of severe situational stress or posttraumatic stress disorder (PTSD). Nightmares can be associated with several medical conditions, including Parkinson's disease and congestive heart failure. Medications, notably beta-blockers, can provoke nightmares (American Psychiatric Association 2013). Treatment includes behavioral techniques such as exposure, relaxation, and rescripting therapy in which the upsetting content is reframed (Pruiksma et al. 2016). Medication options include tricyclic antidepressants (which suppress REM sleep) and benzodiazepines (which decrease arousals, thereby reducing dream recall). The alpha-adrenergic antagonist prazosin has been studied in nightmare disorder unaccompanied by PTSD, with unclear results to date (Kung et al. 2012).

Sleep-Related Breathing Disorders and Snoring

Sleep-related breathing disorder includes OSAH, central sleep apnea, and obesity hypoventilation syndrome (ICD-10 E66.2).

Obstructive Sleep Apnea Hypopnea

OSAH is the most notable of the sleep-related breathing disorders because of its high prevalence and its association with numerous medical complications if untreated (Chowdhuri et al. 2016). *Obstructive apnea* is defined as cessation of airflow lasting at least 10 seconds caused by impedance of respiratory effort as the result of airway obstruction. *Hypopnea* is defined as reduction in airflow resulting in at least a 4% decrease in oxygen saturation. Table 14–7 outlines the diagnostic criteria for OSAH. Both apneas and hypopneas are considered to be clinically significant markers of disease and as a result are reported together as the apnea–hypopnea index.

Prevalence

Patients with OSAH are the largest subgroup of patients referred to sleep disorders centers. Defined by an apnea–hypopnea index ≥5 in a recent systematic review, OSAH was reported to affect 9%–38% of the population (Senaratna et al. 2017). Advanced age, male gender, obesity, and postmenopausal status are all associated with a higher prevalence (Young et al. 2002). In subpopulations of patients with hypertension, heart disease, and adult-onset type 2 diabetes, 30%–40% of patients can have OSAH (Partinen 1995). Obstructive sleep apnea more commonly presents without marked obesity in several racial groups, including Asians, in whom craniofacial anatomic features can produce a narrower nasopharyngeal airway (K. Li et al. 2000).

Clinical Features

Most patients with OSAH snore. Obstructive events can lead to respiratory arousals and oxygen desaturation, resulting in nondipping nocturnal blood pressure (Crinion et al. 2017). Initially, blood pressure increases follow each obstructive event, but if apneic or hypopneic episodes are frequent, blood pressure can remain elevated throughout the night and day. In particular, pulmonary hypertension has been associated with severe OSAH.

The hemodynamic alterations of OSAH include systemic hypertension, increased right and left ventricular afterload, and increased cardiac output. Epidemiological data confirm an independent association between OSAH and these cardiovascular diseases. Possible mechanisms include a combination of intermittent hypoxia and hypercapnia, repeated arousals, increased renin-angiotensin-aldosterone activity, sustained increase in sympathetic tone, higher circulating levels of the inflammatory factor interleukin-2, and endothelial dysfunction (Crinion et al. 2017).

Pathophysiological Mechanism

Patients with OSAH experience intermittent collapse of the upper airway. The most common site of obstruction is the pharynx, a structure largely unsupported by carti-

---

TABLE 14–7.   DSM-5 diagnostic criteria for obstructive sleep apnea hypopnea

A.   Either (1) or (2):

    1.   Disproportionate and persistent thoughts about the seriousness of one's symptoms.

        a.   Nocturnal breathing disturbances: snoring, snorting/gasping, or breathing pauses during sleep.

        b.   Daytime sleepiness, fatigue, or unrefreshing sleep despite sufficient opportunities to sleep that is not better explained by another mental disorder (including a sleep disorder) and is not attributable to another medical condition.

    2.   Evidence by polysomnography of 15 or more obstructive apneas and/or hypopneas per hour of sleep regardless of accompanying symptoms.

Specify current severity:

   Mild: Apnea–hypopnea index is less than 15.

   Moderate: Apnea–hypopnea index is 15–30.

   Severe: Apnea–hypopnea index is greater than 30.

Source.   Reprinted from American Psychiatric Association: *Diagnostic and Statistical Manual of Mental Disorders,* 5th Edition, Arlington, VA, American Psychiatric Association, 2013, p. 378. Copyright 2013, American Psychiatric Association. Used with permission.

---

lage or bone that contorts during swallowing and speech. The pharyngeal musculature serves to keep the upper airway open and opposes the subatmospheric pressure in the pharynx itself. The genioglossus muscles also pull forward to keep the upper airway clear of obstruction. This balance is further influenced by anatomic structures (adipose tissue, tongue size, mandible, soft palate, and tonsils) and neuromuscular mechanisms (activity of the pharyngeal muscles affected by sleep state, degree of muscle relaxation, and hypnotic medications) (Rama et al. 2002). The obstructed upper airway leads to cessation or reduction of airflow resulting in a cortical arousal. The upper airway is more collapsible during REM sleep (because of muscle atonia) than during N3 NREM sleep (Carberry et al. 2016).

Diagnostic Testing

Polysomnographic data collected as part of a facility-based sleep study have been the standard for the diagnosis of breathing-related sleep disorder, with patients monitored in both NREM and REM sleep and in both supine and nonsupine positions (Kushida et al. 2005). In a split-night sleep study, once a diagnosis of breathing-related sleep disorder is established, a sleep technologist introduces an intervention that addresses the upper airway collapse. In the morning, the patient can be asked about tolerability of the therapy. A split-night study can confirm the diagnosis by comparing the symptomatic versus the newly treated state (Sands et al. 2016).

Increasingly, home apnea tests are being used to diagnose OSAH. The type of data produced by these tests depends on the specific technology employed. Measurements of peripheral arterial tone in the finger produce an apnea–hypopnea index that is not significantly different from measurements obtained by polysomnography (Camilon et al. 2014). Other types of home apnea monitors assess respiratory movement, body position, nasal airflow, heart rate, and oxygen saturation and can diagnose OSAH with acceptable agreement with polysomnography; however, they are less successful in assessing severity (Gjevre et al. 2011). Split-night studies, with treatment introduced partway through the night, cannot be done in the home environment. Other portable devices, with a limited array of measures, have been marketed and have clear limitations. Pulse oximetry monitors only oxygen saturation and heart rate. With this equipment, the clinician does not know heart rhythm, body position, or whether the patient is asleep or awake—or in NREM versus REM sleep (Jonas et al. 2017). False-negative results can be obtained from patients with OSAH so severe that they cannot fall asleep. Oxygen saturation can look deceptively normal in patients without pulmonary disease lying awake in bed at night. Only after patients fall asleep do they begin to experience significant oxygen desaturation.

Complications

The complications of OSAH lead to significant morbidity and mortality. Untreated OSAH has been associated with systemic hypertension, right-sided heart failure, cerebrovascular accidents, type 2 diabetes, cognitive impairment, and depression (Rakel 2009). The excessive daytime sleepiness that can result from untreated OSAH can put patients at risk of motor vehicle accidents, cognitive problems, irritability, and interpersonal difficulties. An association has been described between OSAH and gastroesophageal reflux.

Treatment

Since the early 1980s, the treatment of OSAH has been revolutionized by the use of nasal continuous positive airway pressure (CPAP). This treatment involves delivering pressurized air (typically 5–18 cm of water pressure) to sites of upper airway collapse (generally the oropharynx and less commonly the nasopharynx) to hold the airway open. Apnea and snoring are eliminated, allowing the patient to sleep continuously without being aroused to breathe. Self-titrating devices that modify the pressure setting breath by breath without requiring technologist involvement are now widely available (Nigam et al. 2016).

Patients with severe OSAH often report marked improvement, within days, in their mood and energy. This improvement provides positive reinforcement that leads to good compliance with nasal CPAP treatment (Singhal et al. 2016). Patients with milder OSAH have more adherence problems, with compliance estimated at 10%–50%. Optimizing compliance with CPAP is a challenge, but recent studies show that providing a safe hypnotic medication (zaleplon or zolpidem) short-term may be beneficial (Collen et al. 2009). Patients with OSAH who consume alcohol close to bedtime pose a challenge, because alcohol can increase collapse of the upper airway. These patients often need higher nasal CPAP settings to prevent apnea. In addition, if the sleep study is done when the patient has not been consuming alcohol, the selected pressure settings are insufficient on nights when the patient has ingested alcohol (Berry et al. 1991).

Another treatment of OSAH is bilevel positive airway pressure. This therapy represents a modification of CPAP whereby the positive pressure fluctuates depending on whether the airflow is inspiratory or expiratory. Bilevel pressure therapy is considerably more expensive than conventional CPAP and is reserved for patients who cannot tolerate CPAP. Supplemental oxygen alone is inadequate for OSAH because the oxygen cannot pass the obstruction to reach the lungs. Patients with both breathing-related sleep disorder and intrinsic lung disease who have persistent hypoxia despite using CPAP can benefit from supplemental oxygen delivered through the nasal CPAP mask. For patients who have apnea only in the supine position, effective treatment may include preventing them from lying on their backs. Inflatable devices resembling backpacks can serve the same purpose, but few data are available regarding long-term adherence. Some patients who refuse CPAP and have severe apnea during REM sleep have been offered a REM-suppressant medication such as a monoamine oxidase inhibitor. No published data are available regarding this practice. Abrupt discontinuation of the pharmacological agent should be avoided because of REM rebound, which can increase the risk of apnea.

Weight loss through diet and exercise is a critical component of the treatment plan for any overweight patient with breathing-related sleep disorder (Koo et al. 2017). Motivated patients can succeed. Gastric bypass surgery can be especially important for management of medically complicated obesity (see Chapter 28, "Surgery"). In general, a 20-pound weight loss can reduce the required CPAP pressure; however, many patients eventually seem to gain rather than lose weight, with the result that CPAP pressure needs to be increased.

Patients with abnormalities of the soft tissue or skeletal structures surrounding the upper airway may consider surgery. Surgical procedures include laser-assisted uvulo-palato-pharyngoplasty, tonsillectomy, mandibular advancement, tracheostomy, and neuromuscular electrical stimulation of the hypoglossal nerve. Patients must be carefully selected. They must have upper airway obstructions that are resectable (e.g., large tonsils) and have no other comorbid conditions (e.g., a high body mass index that compromises upper airway patency at multiple points). Oral appliances that pull the tongue or mandible forward are also a valuable option (Bartolucci et al. 2016).

Central Sleep Apnea and Obesity Hypoventilation Syndrome (DSM-5 Sleep-Related Hypoventilation)

Central sleep apnea, a condition in which patients have respiratory pauses without any airway collapse, is more likely to be asymptomatic than is OSAH. Because the patient's airway is not narrowed and vibrating, snoring is not a typical warning sign. Patients often present with insomnia rather than excessive daytime sleepiness. Patients with central sleep apnea are often older and have associated cardiac or cerebrovascular disease. Central sleep apnea can be differentiated from OSAH through the absence of snoring, this differentiation being confirmed by the presence of polysomnographic features of the apnea (Quaranta et al. 1997). Treatment can include a hypnotic agent to decrease arousals or supplemental oxygen to reduce hypoxia (Guilleminault and Robinson 1998). When central sleep apnea and OSAH coexist, treatment may include positive airway pressure therapy.

In some patients with marked obesity, OSAH with repetitive desaturation is absent, but patients still have a sleep-related breathing condition. Particularly during REM sleep, when muscle atonia affects all muscles but the diaphragm, patients may be unable to properly ventilate because of the difficulty in expanding their lungs due to their body mass. In obesity hypoventilation, polysomnography shows persisting oxygen desaturation without the fluctuating cessation of airflow and oxygen desaturation that occur in OSAH. Arterial blood gases or transcutaneous carbon dioxide data reveal hypercapnia (Egea-Santaolalla and Javaheri 2016). Obese patients commonly have both obesity hypoventilation and OSAH, in which case bilevel positive airway pressure is indicated. Other interventions include weight loss and avoiding any factor that may aggravate hypoventilation (e.g., discontinuing any sedating agents).

Restless Legs Syndrome and Periodic Limb Movements

Patients with restless legs syndrome (RLS) describe subjective discomfort of the lower extremities that worsens at night. Patients must have an irresistible need to move their legs in bed or during prolonged periods of sedentary activity, such as airplane flights. This condition was first described by Ekbom in 1945 (Ekbom 1945). As a result of these distressing symptoms, patients can experience insomnia or have unrefreshing sleep.

Prevalence

RLS is often unrecognized but far from rare. For years, all data about this condition were collected in clinical settings, and the prevalence in community samples was essentially unknown. A community-based survey showed a prevalence of RLS of 3% in respondents ages 18–29 years, 10% in those ages 30–79 years, and 19% in those ages 80 years and older. Risk factors for RLS were identified as greater age and high body mass index as well as nicotine dependence, diabetes mellitus, and lack of exercise (Phillips et al. 2000).

RLS sometimes occurs in association with anemia and iron deficiency, and can develop during the third trimester of pregnancy, likely because of functional anemia (Allen and Earley 2001). Case reports have shown that patients with RLS who donate blood may have an exacerbation of the condition (Silber and Richardson 2003).

RLS is known to occur secondary to diabetes, peripheral neuropathy, and uremia; 20%–30% of patients with renal failure experience RLS (Giannaki et al. 2014). Familial occurrence of RLS has been described, with an autosomal dominant mode of inheritance in several large families. In a large French Canadian kindred, RLS was mapped to chromosome 12q (Desautels et al. 2001). In familial RLS, the disorder can have a childhood onset.

Clinical Features

Clinical features of RLS are listed in Table 14–8. Periodic limb movement disorder is a condition that frequently overlaps with RLS. Approximately 90% of patients with RLS have intermittent muscle twitches called periodic limb movements (Trotti and Rye 2011). These movements are involuntary leg jerks that occur at night. They can cause insomnia and, as a result, excessive daytime sleepiness. Almost all patients with RLS have periodic limb movements, but many patients with periodic limb movements have no symptoms.

The periodic limb movements can affect a variety of muscles in the legs or arms. Periodic limb movements in the absence of subjective symptoms of restlessness are of uncertain clinical significance.

Periodic limb movements must be differentiated from nocturnal leg cramps, which are extremely painful sustained muscle contractions, particularly involving the gastrocnemius and soleus muscles. Predisposing factors include pregnancy, diabetes mellitus, electrolyte disturbances, and prior vigorous exercise. Nocturnal leg cramps

TABLE 14–8. **Clinical characteristics of restless legs syndrome**

Urge to move the limbs because of subjective discomfort

Motor restlessness

Symptoms worse or exclusively associated with sedentary activities

Symptoms at least partially relieved by activity

Symptoms worse in the evening or during the night

are not periodic and usually occur, at most, several times a night. The differential diagnosis of RLS and periodic limb movement disorder includes neuropathic pain, arthritis, restless insomnia, and drug-induced akathisia.

Complications

Patients with RLS experience irritability, depressed mood, or cognitive problems due to disturbed sleep; headache, especially on awakening; depressed mood; social isolation; and reduced libido (Becker and Novak 2014).

Pathophysiological Mechanism

RLS is believed to be a condition associated with decreased dopamine levels. Positron emission tomographic studies of RLS have shown decreased dopaminergic functioning in the caudate and putamen (Ruottinen et al. 2000). Treatment with dopaminergic agonists, even low dosages, leads to marked improvement. RLS has been strongly associated with anemia. It is not clear how CNS iron deficiency causes RLS, but it is thought to reduce dopaminergic activity (Dauvilliers and Winkelmann 2013).

Diagnostic Testing

Using a rating scale for RLS—for example, the scale from the International Restless Legs Syndrome Study Group (Walters et al. 2003)—has facilitated diagnosis. An overnight sleep study is not essential, because the diagnosis of RLS can be based on the patient's history. Polysomnography is valuable if a patient potentially has a coexisting sleep disorder, such as OSAH, or if the patient does not respond to treatment of RLS diagnosed on the basis of history alone. The most useful laboratory test is a complete blood count to assess for anemia and ferritin, especially when levels are 75 µg/L or less (Winkelman et al. 2016).

Treatment

Treatment of RLS primarily involves dopaminergic medications. Gabapentin has recently been recognized as the preferred agent for treatment of RLS because of its effectiveness and tolerability (Winkelman et al. 2016). Initiation of dopamine receptor direct agonists, such as pramipexole and ropinirole, should be considered with caution because of the risk of exacerbating restless legs by augmenting the symptoms as well as triggering behaviors such as compulsive gambling (Garcia-Borreguero et al. 2016). Long-acting benzodiazepines, such as clonazepam, and opioids, including codeine and methadone, also have been used but can lead to physical dependence. As a result, these drugs are not preferred treatment choices. Behavioral options include physical therapy and exercise—consisting of lower-body resistance training plus walking on a treadmill (Aukerman et al. 2006).

Insomnia Disorder

Insomnia is characterized by dissatisfaction with sleep quantity, sleep quality, sleep initiation, or sleep maintenance. The new DSM-5 insomnia disorder diagnosis no longer differentiates between insomnia as a primary condition and insomnia secondary to another psychiatric disorder. As outlined in Table 14–4, insomnia can be associated with a variety of medical, neurological, psychiatric, and environmental conditions. If possible, any factors that cause or exacerbate insomnia, such as gastroesophageal reflux, should be corrected (Ohayon and Roth 2003). However, for many patients, there are no specific triggers of insomnia, and insomnia is not a symptom of an underlying disorder.

Patients with the classic type of conditioned insomnia learn to associate sleeplessness with certain circumstances, such as their own bedrooms. These patients become progressively more tense as bedtime approaches.

Prevalence

With a prevalence of 10% in the U.S. population, insomnia is the most common sleep disorder, and it is more common in women than in men (American Academy of Sleep Medicine 2014). Insomnia is more often found in association with another psychiatric disorder or medical condition than as an isolated symptom or disorder.

Diagnosis

Polysomnography is not generally useful in establishing the diagnosis of insomnia disorder. Sometimes a patient's best sleep in years occurs in the unfamiliar setting of the sleep disorders center (Chesson et al. 2000). Home studies generally lack monitors that reliably measure actual sleep, having been developed to assess sleep-related breathing. Numerous rating scales that specifically address sleep—including the Pittsburgh Sleep Quality Index, the Insomnia Severity Index, the Dysfunctional Beliefs and Attitudes about Sleep Scale—have been developed to supplement the clinical interview and the more general assessment tools (e.g., Beck Depression Inventory) that might have an item or two addressing sleep.

Treatment

Treatment of insomnia includes improvements to optimize sleep habits and the sleep environment. The recommendations listed in Table 14–9 have been found to be particularly efficacious in the care of patients with chronic insomnia. Establishing a regular waking time 7 days a week optimizes biological rhythms. This is particularly helpful for patients who need to keep morning commitments but tend to naturally be "night owls" or have problems falling asleep at the desired bedtime. However, the clock tends to drift rapidly back to the old schedule as soon as there is variability in arising time (Brown et al. 2002).

Exercising in the late afternoon several hours before bedtime may improve sleep. One postulated mechanism is that a decrease in body temperature is associated with sleep, and body temperature decreases approximately 4 hours after exercise (Montgomery and Dennis 2002). Avoiding "clock watching" can help reduce the arousal effects of becoming annoyed as time passes. Most people recall only periods of wakefulness at night, so clock watching can reinforce the perception that no sleep has occurred. Patients should avoid alcohol and stimulants, including nicotine and caffeine, at any time during the day. Patients, particularly those prone to gastroesopha-

TABLE 14–9. **Lifestyle and environmental changes to optimize sleep**

Circadian issues

Avoid daytime naps.

Limit time in bed to 8 hours.

Get daily exercise, preferably finishing at least 4 hours before bedtime.

Keep regular sleep–wake cycle 7 days per week.

Avoid bright light in the evening or at night.

Seek bright light in the morning.

Reduction of sleep disruption

Avoid large quantities of fluids in the evening.

Minimize caffeine; a hot drink without caffeine may be beneficial.

Avoid alcoholic beverages.

Keep the bedroom quiet, dark, and at a comfortable temperature.

Develop a relaxing bedtime ritual.

Avoid worrying in bed by using tools such as list writing during the day.

Manage stress optimally during the day.

Turn off mobile devices.

Do not use the bed and bedroom except for sleep and for sexual activity.

Get assistance with pets and children.

Avoid large meals soon before bedtime.

Pursue medical intervention for problems such as gastroesophageal reflux, pain, and nausea.

geal reflux, should not eat near bedtime, and antacids and histamine$_2$-blocking medication before sleep can be beneficial. Introducing relaxing routines around bedtime also can be helpful.

Many studies have demonstrated the benefits of cognitive-behavioral therapy for insomnia (CBT-I) both in general and for patients with coexisting medical disorders (Wu et al. 2015). For example, CBT-I has been shown to be feasible and efficacious for insomnia in patients with cancer (Johnson et al. 2016), chronic obstructive pulmonary disease (Kapella et al. 2011), arthritis (Smith et al. 2015), heart failure (Redeker et al. 2015), and fibromyalgia (Martínez et al. 2014). CBT-I includes some extra components that specifically address sleep issues, including stimulus control techniques to help patients with psychophysiological, or conditioned, insomnia (Bootzin and Perlis 1992). These patients report that they are sleepy near bedtime, but as soon as they enter the sleeping environment, they become alert and unable to sleep. In order to interrupt this conditioned association between sleeplessness and the bedroom, clinicians instruct patients to refrain from "trying to sleep" when they find themselves lying in bed in a wakeful state. Instead, they should get up and go to a different setting and engage in a different activity (e.g., reading a book, watching relaxing television, listening to music) until they become sleepy again, and then return to bed. Patients are advised to repeat this process as often and as long as needed to extinguish the arousal state conditioned to the bedroom.

For patients with severe and persistent insomnia, sleep restriction—that is, instructing patients to spend no more hours in bed than they estimated they slept the previous night—may be helpful. Initially this period may be considerably shorter than 7.5 hours. When patients are able to sleep for essentially all of the time in bed for several nights, they are advised to increase their time in bed by half-hour increments until they achieve optimal sleep time and sleep efficiency. Although both pharmacological and behavioral treatments are effective for insomnia management over the initial weeks of treatment, the evidence for sustained improvement is stronger for behavioral treatment than for pharmacological therapy (Brasure et al. 2015). Research has successfully demonstrated that as few as one to two sessions of behavioral treatment may be beneficial (Morin and Espie 2004). However, the availability of medication may reduce patients' motivation and confidence in behavioral techniques.

Because access to providers with expertise in delivering CBT-I has been a barrier, considerable effort has been devoted to developing alternative approaches. Online CBT programs are now available, the best of which incorporate screening tools, sleep diaries, patient education, and demonstrations of behavioral techniques. "Sleep Healthy Using the Internet" (SHUTi) provides instruction on sleep hygiene, sleep restriction, stimulus control, cognitive restructuring, and relapse prevention. Outcome data from a trial of this program revealed improvement in sleep initiation and wakefulness after sleep onset at 9 weeks and 1 year (Ritterband et al. 2017).

Hypnotic medications have an important role in the management of short-term or intermittent insomnia, but most sleep specialists prefer a meaningful trial of nonpharmacological interventions in the care of patients with the chronic form of insomnia disorder. Efforts to avoid or minimize sedating medications are especially pertinent in the elderly. The benzodiazepine receptor agonists zaleplon, zolpidem, and eszopiclone have a relatively short half-life that minimizes the hangover effect (Table 14–10). Patients have been shown to maintain alertness adequate for driving and other activities that require sustained vigilance (Roth et al. 2001). Unusual sleep behaviors, including somnambulism and sleep eating, have been reported with these agents, especially with zolpidem, and especially when the dose is supratherapeutic or the drug is combined with another sedative such as alcohol. The prevalence of these phenomena is unknown (Tsai et al. 2009). Physical dependence has not been reported with the short-term use approved by the FDA. In 2013, in response to data showing lower clearance of zolpidem in women, the FDA issued a safety announcement recommending dosage reductions in women to reduce the risk of residual sleepiness in the morning (Krystal and Attarian 2016). Benzodiazepines, although less expensive than some nonbenzodiazepine hypnotics, can cause dependence and also are associated with impaired cognitive function the morning after use; as a consequence, these agents are less frequently used than in the past.

Several antidepressants with prominent sedative side effects, such as mirtazapine and trazodone, are valuable therapeutic options, especially if the patient has a coexisting mood or anxiety disorder. Mirtazapine has prominent antihistaminergic side effects at doses of 15 mg or less; however, undesirable weight gain can occur (Artigas et al. 2002). Tricyclic antidepressants such as doxepin (low-dose) have a role in insomnia treatment for selected patients, with careful consideration of their cardiac and anticholinergic side effects (Krystal et al. 2010). Antihistamines such as diphenhydramine are generally a poor choice because they quickly lose effectiveness and can exacerbate confusion in the medically ill or elderly. Ramelteon, a novel hypnotic that acts as a selective melatonin agonist, has been demonstrated to be well tolerated and free of morning residual effect (Devi and Shankar 2008). Another option is suvorexant, the

TABLE 14–10. Effects of half-lives of hypnotic drugs (including their active metabolites) on sleep

Drug	Half-life (h)	Rebound	Tolerance	Carryover sedation
Flurazepam	40+	Yes	Yes	Yes
Temazepam	10+	Yes	Yes	No
Trazodone (25–50 mg)	4–7	?	?	Yes
Triazolam	1–5	Yes	Yes	No
Ramelteon	1–3	No	?	No
Zaleplon	1	No	?	No
Zolpidem	1–2	Yes	Yes	Yes
Suvorexant	12	No	No	Yes
Doxepin	15	No	No	Yes

Note.   ? = No available data.

first FDA-approved dual orexin receptor antagonist. It should not be used in patients with narcolepsy because of its potential to exacerbate their symptoms (Dubey et al. 2015).

Paradoxical Insomnia

Paradoxical insomnia, previously known as sleep state misperception, is a rare and little-studied type of insomnia. Patients with this disorder describe subjective sleep disturbances that are not consistent with objective data. For the criteria for this diagnosis to be met, polysomnography must demonstrate normal duration and quality of sleep (American Academy of Sleep Medicine 2014). Treatment involves discussing with patients the discrepancy between subjective and objective data. Behavioral techniques and hypnotic medications have been used successfully in this group of patients. Paradoxical insomnia is of particular interest to psychiatrists because it is in many ways analogous to other amplified somatic complaints, except that patients focus on insufficient sleep as the source of their distress.

Conclusion

Sleep takes up one-third of a typical day. Obtaining an adequate quantity and quality of sleep is necessary for good health and the prevention of adverse outcomes. Many physiological processes and some medical conditions are altered by sleep. We have reviewed the clinical features, diagnostic testing, and treatment of the sleep disorders most commonly encountered by consultation-liaison psychiatrists. Interventions can prevent undesirable medical, psychiatric, and social consequences of sleep disorders. A growing menu of behavioral and pharmacological treatment options are available once the diagnosis of a specific sleep disorder has been established.

References

Allen RP, Earley CJ: Restless legs syndrome: a review of clinical and pathophysiologic features. J Clin Neurophysiol 18(2):128–147, 2001 11435804

American Academy of Sleep Medicine: International Classification of Sleep Disorders, 3rd Edition. Westchester, IL, American Academy of Sleep Medicine, 2014

American Psychiatric Association: Diagnostic and Statistical Manual of Mental Disorders, 5th Edition. Arlington, VA, American Psychiatric Association, 2013

Arnulf I, Zeitzer JM, File J, et al: Kleine-Levin syndrome: a systematic review of 186 cases in the literature. Brain 128(Pt 12):2763–2776, 2005 16230322

Artigas F, Nutt DJ, Shelton R: Mechanism of action of antidepressants. Psychopharmacol Bull 36 (suppl 2):123–132, 2002 12490828

Aserinsky E, Kleitman N: Regularly occurring periods of eye motility, and concomitant phenomena, during sleep. Science 118(3062):273–274, 1953 13089671

Aukerman MM, Aukerman D, Bayard M, et al: Exercise and restless legs syndrome: a randomized controlled trial. J Am Board Fam Med 19(5):487–493, 2006 16951298

Bartolucci ML, Bortolotti F, Raffaelli E, et al: The effectiveness of different mandibular advancement amounts in OSA patients: a systematic review and meta-regression analysis. Sleep Breath 20(3):911–919, 2016 26779903

Becker PM, Novak M: Diagnosis, comorbidities, and management of restless legs syndrome. Curr Med Res Opin 30(8):1441–1460, 2014 24805265

Berry RB, Desa MM, Light RW: Effect of ethanol on the efficacy of nasal continuous positive airway pressure as a treatment for obstructive sleep apnea. Chest 99(2):339–343, 1991 1989792

Bootzin RR, Perlis ML: Nonpharmacologic treatments of insomnia. J Clin Psychiatry 53 (suppl):37–41, 1992 1613018

Brasure M, MacDonald R, Fuchs E, et al: Management of Insomnia Disorder (AHRQ Publ No 15[16]-EHC027-EF). Rockville, MD, Agency for Healthcare Research and Quality, 2015 26844312

Brown FC, Buboltz WC Jr, Soper B: Relationship of sleep hygiene awareness, sleep hygiene practices, and sleep quality in university students. Behav Med 28(1):33–38, 2002 12244643

Camilon PR, Nguyen SA, Camilon MP, Gillespie MB: WatchPAT versus polysomnography: a meta-analysis (poster presentation). Otolaryngol Head Neck Surg 151 (1 suppl):P265, 2014

Carberry JC, Jordan AS, White DP, et al: Upper airway collapsibility (Pcrit) and pharyngeal dilator muscle activity are sleep stage dependent. Sleep 39(3):511–521, 2016 26612386

Chesson A Jr, Hartse K, Anderson WM, et al; Standards of Practice Committee of the American Academy of Sleep Medicine: Practice parameters for the evaluation of chronic insomnia. An American Academy of Sleep Medicine report. Sleep 23(2):237–241, 2000 10737341

Chowdhuri S, Quan SF, Almeida F, et al; ATS Ad Hoc Committee on Mild Obstructive Sleep Apnea: An official American Thoracic Society research statement: impact of mild obstructive sleep apnea in adults. Am J Respir Crit Care Med 193(9):e37–e54, 2016 27128710

Claman D, Sunwoo B: Improving accuracy of home sleep apnea testing. J Clin Sleep Med 13(1):9–10, 2017 27998372

Collen J, Lettieri C, Kelly W, et al: Clinical and polysomnographic predictors of short-term continuous positive airway pressure compliance. Chest 135(3):704–709, 2009 19017888

Crinion S, Silke R, McNicholas W: Obstructive sleep apnea as a cause of nocturnal nondipping blood pressure: recent evidence regarding clinical importance and underlying mechanisms. Eur Resp J 49(1):1601818, 2017 28077479

Dang-Vu TT, Zadra A, Labelle MA, et al: Sleep deprivation reveals altered brain perfusion patterns in somnambulism. PLoS One 10(8):e0133474, 2015 26241047

Dauvilliers Y, Winkelmann J: Restless legs syndrome: update on pathogenesis. Curr Opin Pulm Med 19(6):594–600, 2013 24048084

de Oliveira MM, Conti C, Prado GF: Pharmacological treatment for Kleine-Levin syndrome. Cochrane Database Syst Rev (5):CD006685, 2016 27153153

Desautels A, Turecki G, Montplaisir J, et al: Identification of a major susceptibility locus for restless legs syndrome on chromosome 12q. Am J Hum Genet 69(6):1266–1270, 2001 11704926

Devi V, Shankar PK: Ramelteon: a melatonin receptor agonist for the treatment of insomnia. J Postgrad Med 54(1):45–48, 2008 18296808

Dubey AK, Handu SS, Mediratta PK: Suvorexant: the first orexin receptor antagonist to treat insomnia. J Pharmacol Pharmacother 6(2):118–121, 2015 25969666

Dyken ME, Yamada T, Lin-Dyken DC: Polysomnographic assessment of spells in sleep: nocturnal seizures versus parasomnias. Semin Neurol 21(4):377–390, 2001 11774053

Egea-Santaolalla C, Javaheri S: Obesity hypoventilation syndrome. Current Sleep Medicine Reports 2(1):12–19, 2016

Ekbom K: Restless legs. Acta Med Scand Suppl 158:1–123, 1945

Everson CA, Toth LA: Systemic bacterial invasion induced by sleep deprivation. Am J Physiol Regul Integr Comp Physiol 278(4):R905–R916, 2000 10749778

Garcia-Borreguero D, Silber MH, Winkelman JW, et al: Guidelines for the first-line treatment of restless legs syndrome/Willis-Ekbom disease, prevention and treatment of dopaminergic augmentation: a combined task force of the IRLSSG, EURLSSG, and the RLS-F. Sleep Med 21:1–11, 2016 27448465

Gelineau J: De la narcolepsie. Lancette Francaise 53:626–628, 1880

Giannaki CD, Hadjigeorgiou GM, Karatzaferi C, et al: Epidemiology, impact, and treatment options of restless legs syndrome in end-stage renal disease patients: an evidence-based review. Kidney Int 85(6):1275–1282, 2014 24107848

Gjevre J, Taylor-Gjevre RM, Skomro R, et al: Comparison of polysomnographic and portable home monitoring assessments of obstructive sleep apnea in Saskatchewan women. Can Respir J 18(5):271–274, 2011 21969928

Guilleminault C, Robinson A: Central sleep apnea. Otolaryngol Clin North Am 31(6):1049–1065, 1998 9838017

Jacobs ML, Dauvilliers Y, St Louis EK, et al: Risk factor profile in Parkinson's disease subtype with REM sleep behavior disorder. J Parkinsons Dis 6(1):231–237, 2016 26889635

Johns MW: A new method for measuring daytime sleepiness: the Epworth sleepiness scale. Sleep 14(6):540–545, 1991 1798888

Johnson JA, Rash JA, Campbell TS, et al: A systematic review and meta-analysis of randomized controlled trials of cognitive behavior therapy for insomnia (CBT-I) in cancer survivors. Sleep Med Rev 27:20–28, 2016 26434673

Jonas DE, Amick HR, Feltner C, et al: Screening for obstructive sleep apnea in adults: evidence report and systematic review for the U.S. Preventative Services task force. JAMA 317(4):415–433, 2017 28118460

Kapella MC, Herdegen JJ, Perlis ML, et al: Cognitive behavioral therapy for insomnia comorbid with COPD is feasible with preliminary evidence of positive sleep and fatigue effects. Int J Chron Obstruct Pulmon Dis 6:625–635, 2011 22162648

Kecklund G, Axelsson J: Health consequences of shift work and insufficient sleep. BMJ 355:i5210, 2016 27803010

Koo SK, Kwon SB, Kim YJ, et al: Acoustic analysis of snoring sounds recorded with a smartphone according to obstruction site in OSAS patients. Eur Arch Otorhinolaryngol 274(3):1735–1740, 2017 27709292

Kornum B, Knudsen S, Ollila H, et al: Narcolepsy. Nat Rev Dis Primers 3:16100, 2017 28179647

Krahn LE, Lin SC, Wisbey J, et al: Assessing sleep in psychiatric inpatients: nurse and patient reports versus wrist actigraphy. Ann Clin Psychiatry 9(4):203–210, 1997 9511943

Krahn LE, Boeve BF, Olson EJ, et al: A standardized test for cataplexy. Sleep Med 1(2):125–130, 2000 10767653

Krahn LE, Hansen MR, Shepard JW: Pseudocataplexy. Psychosomatics 42(4):356–358, 2001 11496028

Kretzschmar U, Werth E, Sturzenegger C, et al: Which diagnostic findings in disorders with excessive daytime sleepiness are really helpful? A retrospective study. J Sleep Res 25(3):307–313, 2016 26864219

Krystal A, Attarian H: Sleep medications and women: a review of issues to consider for optimizing the care of women with sleep disorders. Current Sleep Medicine Reports 2(4):218–222, 2016

Krystal AD, Durrence HH, Scharf M, et al: Efficacy and safety of doxepin 1 mg and 3 mg in a 12-week sleep laboratory and outpatient trial of elderly subjects with chronic primary insomnia. Sleep 33(11):1553–1561, 2010 21102997

Kung S, Espinel Z, Lapid MI: Treatment of nightmares with prazosin: a systematic review. Mayo Clin Proc 87(9):890–900, 2012 22883741

Kushida CA, Littner MR, Morgenthaler T, et al: Practice parameters for the indications for polysomnography and related procedures: an update for 2005. Sleep 28(4):499–521, 2005 16171294

Li AM, Wong E, Kew J, et al: Use of tonsil size in the evaluation of obstructive sleep apnoea. Arch Dis Child 87(2):156–159, 2002 12138072

Li K, Kushida C, Powell N, et al: Obstructive sleep apnea syndrome: a comparison between Far-East Asian and white men. Laryngoscope 110(10 pt 1):1689–1693, 2000 11037826

Li SX, Lam SP, Zhang J, et al: A prospective, naturalistic follow-up study of treatment outcomes with clonazepam in rapid eye movement sleep behavior disorder. Sleep Med 21:114–120, 2016 27448481

Martínez MP, Miró E, Sánchez AI, et al: Cognitive-behavioral therapy for insomnia and sleep hygiene in fibromyalgia: a randomized controlled trial. J Behav Med 37(4):683–697, 2014 23744045

Maski K, Steinhart E, Williams D, et al: Listening to the patient voice in narcolepsy: diagnostic delay, disease burden and treatment efficacy. J Clin Sleep Medicine 13(3):419–425, 2017 27923434

Miglis MG, Guilleminault C: Kleine-Levin syndrome. Curr Neurol Neurosci Rep 16(6):60, 2016 27137943

Mignot E, Lammers GJ, Ripley B, et al: The role of cerebrospinal fluid hypocretin measurement in the diagnosis of narcolepsy and other hypersomnias. Arch Neurol 59(10):1553–1562, 2002 12374492

Mitler MM, Gujavarty KS, Sampson MG, et al: Multiple daytime nap approaches to evaluating the sleepy patient. Sleep 5 (suppl 2):S119–S127, 1982 7156647

Montgomery P, Dennis J: Physical exercise for sleep problems in adults aged 60+. Cochrane Database Syst Rev (4):CD003404, 2002 12519595

Morin C, Espie C: Insomnia: A Clinical Guide to Assessment and Treatment. New York, Springer, 2004

Nigam G, Riaz M, Pathak C, et al: Use of auto-titrating positive airway pressure devices for sleep-disordered breathing: the good, the bad and the ugly. Journal of Pulmonary & Respiratory Medicine 6:336, 2016

O'Brien E, Hart C, Wing RR: Discrepancies between self-reported usual sleep duration and objective measures of total sleep time in treatment-seeking overweight and obese individuals. Behav Sleep Med 14(5):539–549, 2016 26503348

Ohayon MM, Roth T: Place of chronic insomnia in the course of depressive and anxiety disorders. J Psychiatr Res 37(1):9–15, 2003 12482465

Ohayon MM, Carskadon MA, Guilleminault C, Vitiello MV: Meta-analysis of quantitative sleep parameters from childhood to old age in healthy individuals: developing normative sleep values across the human lifespan. Sleep 27(7):1255–1273, 2004 15586779

Partinen M: Epidemiology of obstructive sleep apnea syndrome. Curr Opin Pulm Med 1(6):482–487, 1995 9363086

Phillips B, Young T, Finn L, et al: Epidemiology of restless legs symptoms in adults. Arch Intern Med 160(14):2137–2141, 2000 10904456

Pilon M, Montplaisir J, Zadra A: Precipitating factors of somnambulism: impact of sleep deprivation and forced arousals. Neurology 70(24):2284–2290, 2008 18463368

Plante DT: Sleep propensity in psychiatric hypersomnolence: a systematic review and meta-analysis of multiple sleep latency test findings. Sleep Med Rev 31:48–57, 2017 26883161

Pruiksma KE, Cranston CC, Rhudy JL, et al: Randomized controlled trial to dismantle exposure, relaxation and rescripting therapy (ERRT) for trauma-related nightmares. Psychol Trauma 8:335–355, 2016 27977223

Quaranta AJ, D'Alonzo GE, Krachman SL: Cheyne-Stokes respiration during sleep in congestive heart failure. Chest 111(2):467–473, 1997 9041998

Rakel RE: Clinical and societal consequences of obstructive sleep apnea and excessive daytime sleepiness. Postgrad Med 121(1):86–95, 2009 19179816

Rama AN, Tekwani SH, Kushida CA: Sites of obstruction in obstructive sleep apnea. Chest 122(4):1139–1147, 2002 12377834

Redeker NS, Jeon S, Andrews L, et al: Feasibility and efficacy of a self-management intervention for insomnia in stable heart failure. J Clin Sleep Med 11(10):1109–1119, 2015 25979100

Ritterband LM, Thorndike FP, Ingersoll KS, et al: Effect of a web-case cognitive behavioral therapy for insomnia intervention with 1-year follow-up: a randomized clinical trial. JAMA Psychiatry 74(1):68–75, 2017 27902836

Roth T, Hajak G, Ustün TB: Consensus for the pharmacological management of insomnia in the new millennium. Int J Clin Pract 55(1):42–52, 2001 11219318

Roth T, Jaeger S, Jin R, et al: Sleep problems, comorbid mental disorders, and role functioning in the national comorbidity survey replication. Biol Psychiatry 60(12):1364–1371, 2006 16952333

Ruottinen H, Partinen M, Hublin C, et al: An FDOPA PET study in patients with periodic limb movement disorder and restless legs syndrome. Neurology 54(2):502–504, 2000 10668725

Saini P, Rye DB: Hypersomnia: evaluation, treatment, and social and economic aspects. Sleep Med Clin 12(1):47–60, 2017 28159097

Sands SA, Owens RL, Malhotra A: New approaches to diagnosing sleep-disordered breathing. Sleep Med Clin 11(2):143–152, 2016 27236052

Schenck CH: Expanded insights into idiopathic REM sleep behavior disorder. Sleep 39(1):7–9, 2016 26564130

Schenck CH, Bassetti CL, Arnulf I, et al: English translations of the first clinical reports on narcolepsy and cataplexy by Westphal and Gélineau in the late 19th century, with commentary. J Clin Sleep Med 3(3):301–311, 2007 17561602

Senaratna CV, Perret JL, Lodge CJ, et al: Prevalence of obstructive sleep apnea in the general population: a systematic review. Sleep Med Rev 34:70–81, 2017 27568340

Silber MH, Richardson JW: Multiple blood donations associated with iron deficiency in patients with restless legs syndrome. Mayo Clin Proc 78(1):52–54, 2003 12528877

Silber M, Krahn L, Olson E, et al: The epidemiology of narcolepsy in Olmsted County, Minnesota: a population-based study. Sleep 25(2):197–202, 2002 11902429

Singhal P, Joshi Y, Singh G, Kulkarni S: Study of factors affecting compliance of continuous positive airway pressure (CPAP) in obstructive sleep apnea-hypopnea syndrome (OSAHS) (abstract). Eur Respir J 48 (suppl 60):PA2362, 2016

Smart D, Jerman J: The physiology and pharmacology of the orexins. Pharmacol Ther 94(1–2):51–61, 2002 12191593

Smith MT, Finan PH, Buenaver LF, et al: Cognitive-behavioral therapy for insomnia in knee osteoarthritis: a randomized, double-blind, active placebo-controlled clinical trial. Arthritis Rheumatol 67(5):1221–1233, 2015 25623343

Taheri S: The genetics of narcolepsy, in Narcolepsy: A Clinical Guide. New York, Springer International Publishing, 2016, pp 3–10

Thorpy M: Modafinil/armodafinil in the treatment of narcolepsy, in Narcolepsy: A Clinical Guide. New York, Springer International Publishing, 2016, pp 331–339

Trotti LM, Rye DB: Restless legs syndrome. Handb Clin Neurol 100:661–673, 2011 21496614

Tsai JH, Yang P, Chen CC, et al: Zolpidem-induced amnesia and somnambulism: rare occurrences? Eur Neuropsychopharmacol 19(1):74–76, 2009 18819779

Vitiello MV, Moe KE, Prinz PN: Sleep complaints cosegregate with illness in older adults: clinical research informed by and informing epidemiological studies of sleep. J Psychosom Res 53(1):555–559, 2002 12127171

Walters AS, LeBrocq C, Dhar A, et al; International Restless Legs Syndrome Study Group: Validation of the International Restless Legs Syndrome Study Group rating scale for restless legs syndrome. Sleep Med 4(2):121–132, 2003 14592342

Winkelman JW, Armstrong MJ, Allen RP, et al: Practice guideline summary: Treatment of restless legs syndrome in adults: report of the Guideline Development, Dissemination, and Implementation Subcommittee of the American Academy of Neurology. Neurology 87(24):2585–2593, 2016 27856776

Wu JQ, Appleman ER, Salazar RD, et al: Cognitive behavioral therapy for insomnia comorbid with psychiatric and medical conditions: a meta-analysis. JAMA Intern Med 175(9):1461–1472, 2015 26147487

Young T, Peppard PE, Gottlieb DJ: Epidemiology of obstructive sleep apnea: a population health perspective. Am J Respir Crit Care Med 165(9):1217–1239, 2002 11991871

CHAPTER 15

Sexual Dysfunctions

Rosemary Basson, M.D.
Peter M. Rees, M.D., Ph.D.

Advances in surgical and medical treatment have greatly improved survival from a variety of chronic illnesses including many types of cancer. However, frequently, sexual function is negatively affected. Approximately 30% of the general population reports sexual difficulties, and about 10% reports long-lasting problems that cause distress, but in some medical conditions, such as end-stage renal disease (ESRD), sexual dysfunction seems almost inevitable: the prevalence of desire disorders in men and women may reach 100% (Peng et al. 2007).

The distress that accompanies sexual dysfunction in the context of illness also varies: a sizable proportion of individuals living with spinal cord injury—regardless of the segmental level of their injury—rate regaining sexual function as either the first or the second priority (Anderson 2004). Of 526 adults reporting chronic poor health, close to 40% confirmed that sexual health was still an important aspect of quality of life (Flynn et al. 2016). Psychiatrists should routinely address sexual health during their consultations; the attending physician may have avoided this subject entirely. Chronic illness may even increase the need for sexual intimacy (Owens and Tepper 2003), but when sexual activity was never particularly rewarding, being unable to engage may be acceptable.

Chronic medical illness can affect sexual function both directly and indirectly (Table 15–1). Disease-related interruption of the neurovascular pathways and the hormonal milieu may not be the major determinant of dissatisfaction. For instance, sexual function in both men and women with ESRD is mostly governed by the presence or absence of depression (Peng et al. 2005, 2007). Similarly, depression is the major factor influencing sexual function in men and women who have undergone bone marrow transplantation (Humphreys et al. 2007), in women with rheumatoid arthritis (Abda et al. 2016), in men and women with Parkinson's disease (Kummer et al. 2009), and in women with multiple sclerosis (Zivadinov et al. 1999) or diabetes (Bhasin et al. 2007).

TABLE 15–1.   Factors involved in sexual dysfunction associated with chronic disease

Type	Factor	Examples
Direct	Change in sexual desire from disease	Typically reduced (e.g., from high prolactin level and anemia of chronic renal failure)[a]; may be increased (e.g., from some brain injuries)[b]
	Disruption of genital response from disease	ED from multiple sclerosis,[c] hypertension,[c] orgasmic disorder from multiple sclerosis[e]
	Disruption of genital response from surgery	Radical prostatectomy and ED[f]; radical hysterectomy and reduced genital congestion, reduced lubrication[g]; orgasmic disorder after radical vulvectomy[h]
	Disruption of genital response from radiation	ED from vascular and neurological damage after radiotherapy for prostate cancer[i]; vaginal stenosis and friability from radiation for pelvic cancer[j]
	Dyspareunia and disruption of sexual desire and response from chemotherapy	Ovarian or testicular failure after chemotherapy for cancer[k] or after hematopoietic transplantation[l]
	Disruption of sexual desire and response from antiandrogen treatment	GnRH therapy for prostate cancer[m]
	Disruption of genital response from estrogen depletion by aromatase inhibitors	Dyspareunia and loss of sexual genital sensitivity from genito-urinary syndrome of menopause or from aromatase inhibition following breast cancer[n]
	Disruption of sexual desire and response from pain	Pain from any chronic condition is a potent sexual distraction
	Disruption of sexual desire and response from nonhormonal medications	Narcotics can depress desire through gonadotropin suppression[o]; SSRIs and SNRIs frequently reduce desire and response[p]
Indirect	Reduction of self-image	Reduced by disfiguring surgeries, stomas, incontinence, altered appearance (e.g., drooling and altered facies of Parkinson's disease; altered skin color and muscle wasting of renal failure)
	Depressed mood	Depression and mood lability commonly accompany chronic illness; depression is a major determinant of sexual function in men and women with renal failure[q] and women with multiple sclerosis[r] or diabetes[s]; strong link between ED and subsequent depression[t]

TABLE 15–1. Factors involved in sexual dysfunction associated with chronic disease (*continued*)

Type	Factor	Examples
Indirect (*cont'd*)	Impaired mobility	Reduced ability to caress, hug, and hold a partner; to sexually self-stimulate; to stimulate a partner; to move into positions for intercourse; to pelvically thrust after spinal cord injury, Parkinson's disease, brain injury, or amputation
	Reduced energy	Fatigue may take its toll on sexuality, especially desire (e.g., from renal failure or chemotherapy)
	Partnership difficulties	Difficulties in finding a partner; lack of privacy from institutionalization; dysfunction in the partner who assumes a caregiver role; fears of inability to satisfy partner; fear of becoming a burden to a partner; lack of independence; relationship discord from stressors of living with medicalized lives (e.g., three times weekly hemodialysis)
	Sense of loss of sexuality from imposed infertility	From surgery removing gonads or uterus, or from chemotherapy or radiotherapy causing gonadal failure
	Fear of sexual activity worsening medical condition	Avoiding sexual intercourse because of fear that a pregnancy would provoke cancer recurrence; fearing that a genital cancer could be contagious; fearing that sexual activity will cause another myocardial infarction

Note. ED=erectile dysfunction; GnRH=gonadotropin-releasing hormone; SNRIs=serotonin–norepinephrine reuptake inhibitors; SSRIs=selective serotonin reuptake inhibitors.

[a]Finkelstein et al. 2007; [b] Absher et al. 2000; [c]Rees et al. 2007; [d]Doumas and Douma 2006; [e]Tzortzis et al. 2008; [f]Penson et al. 2005; [g]Bergmark et al. 1999; [h]Likes et al. 2007; [i]Incrocci 2006; [j]Bruner et al. 1993; [k]Kornblith and Ligibel 2003; [l]Syrjala et al. 2008; [m]Basaria et al. 2002; [n]Fallowfield et al. 2004; [o]Hallinan et al. 2008; [p]Clayton et al. 2007; [q]Peng et al. 2005; [r]Zivadinov et al. 1999; [s]Bhasin et al. 2007; [t]Korfage et al. 2009.

Chronic illness commonly alters a person's sense of self (Anderson et al. 2007a, 2007b). Qualitative studies have shown that new issues in sexuality emerge as people live with a chronic illness (Kralik et al. 2001), including the need to adapt to and accept changes in the body. The realization that part of sexual intimacy involves meeting the needs of others is a further factor, as is the need to be able to communicate one's changed sexual needs.

Sexual dysfunction can be a harbinger of otherwise asymptomatic systemic disease. Of 32,616 healthy male participants in a U.S. study reporting erectile dysfunction (ED) in 1986, a fourfold higher risk of developing Parkinson's disease was found over the next 16 years of follow-up, suggesting that erectile difficulties can precede the onset of the classic motor features of parkinsonism by a substantial margin (Gao et al. 2007). ED is now accepted as an important risk factor for myocardial infarction (Abdelhamed et al. 2016).

Assessment

The details of assessment of sexual dysfunction are shown in Table 15–2. A psychosomatic approach is needed because sexual disorders in illness and in health reflect the interaction of mind and body. For instance, psychological stress alone can induce hypothalamic amenorrhea or male hypogonadotrophic hypogonadism, potentially causing dysfunction from reduced sex hormones. Alternatively, nerve damage from multiple sclerosis or radical pelvic surgery leads to orgasmic dysfunction or ED, which can undermine sexual self-confidence and mood, thereby compounding sexual dysfunction. Detailed and respectful inquiry is necessary, without assumptions about sexual orientation or gender, but with an acceptance of the range of sexual expression.

The assessment is guided by current models of human sexual response. Over the past 20 years, empirical and clinical studies have focused on the complexity, variability, flexibility, and circular nature of human sexual response (Figure 15–1). The traditional model of human sexual response stemming from the research of Masters, Johnson, and Kaplan was invariable and linear, progressing from desire to arousal to a plateau of high arousal, culminating in orgasm or ejaculation; a phase of resolution then followed. However, in both men and women, the relation between desire and arousal is variable and complex; women are mostly unable to separate the two (Brotto et al. 2009; Janssen et al. 2008). The motivations and incentives for sex are multiple and varied, with a wish to increase emotional intimacy between the partners being important for both men and women (Carpenter et al. 2009; Meston and Buss 2007). Sexual "desire"—as in "lust" or "drive"—is only one of many reasons that people engage in sexual activity. Thus, models have been constructed that reflect the multiple reasons to initiate or agree to sexual activity, the need for sexual stimuli in a context that is conducive to sexual arousal, and a variable order and overlap of the phases of desire and arousal (Bancroft 2008; Basson 2001; Basson and Schultz 2007; Janssen et al. 2000; Meuleman and van Lankveld 2005). The circular nature allows a building of arousal, inviting more intense stimulation, thereby triggering more powerful feelings of both arousal and desire.

TABLE 15–2.   **Assessment of sexual dysfunction associated with chronic illness**

Review medical and psychiatric history.

Review current medical status: consider respiratory, cardiac, mobility, and continence requirements for sexual activity, including intercourse, self-stimulation, and orgasm.

Review current medications.

List the sexual dysfunctions and their duration.

Clarify relationship status and quality.

Review the environment for sexual activity: home/institution/"medicalization" (e.g., hemodialysis machines, respirators, lack of independence in daily living).

Review any chronic pain.

Assess current mood.

Assess impact of illness on sexual self-image (concerns regarding attractiveness, physical appearance).

Review dysfunctions in detail; ask what the sexual difficulties are:

  For each complaint, clarify if the difficulty is the same with self-stimulation as with partnered sex; for ED, also check erections on waking from sleep.

  Clarify motivations for sexual activity, including desire or drive and desire to satisfy partner; identify reasons for avoiding sexual activity.

  Clarify subjective arousal or excitement and pleasure.

  Clarify genital congestion and lubrication or erection.

  Review variety and usefulness of sexual stimuli and sexual context.

  Assess couple's sexual communication.

  Inquire about distracting thoughts or negative emotions during sexual activity.

  Determine whether wanted orgasms are possible, very delayed, nonintense, or painful.

  Identify ejaculation difficulties: delayed, too early, painful, or absent.

  Determine whether intercourse is possible.

  Assess female dyspareunia: introital, deeper, how constant, exacerbation from partner's ejaculation fluid, postcoital burning, postcoital dysuria.

Clarify sexual response pre-illness: any dysfunction, how rewarding and how important sexual activity was, any desire discrepancy or paraphilia.

Review effect of medications on desire and response.

Review treatment of sexual dysfunction to date.

Complete a full physical examination, including a genital examination whenever this is necessary because of the medical condition (this is particularly important for neurological illness), as well as whenever generalized ED, dyspareunia, or pain with arousal occurs.

Perform laboratory investigations as necessary, especially when needed to monitor anemia, high prolactin level, thyroid replacement, or testosterone levels (in men). Estrogen levels usually are assessed by the history and the genital or pelvic examination.

Note.   ED=erectile dysfunction.

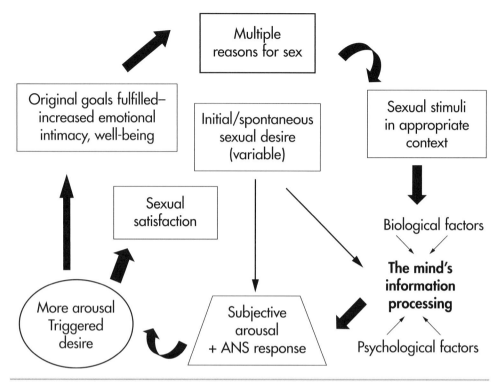

FIGURE 15–1.   Sexual response cycle.

A circular sexual response cycle of overlapping phases may be experienced many times during any one sexual encounter. Desire may or may not be present initially; it is triggered by the arousal to sexual stimuli. The sexual and nonsexual outcomes influence future sexual motivation. ANS=autonomic nervous system.

Source.   Reprinted with permission from Basson R: "Human Sex Response Cycles." *Journal of Sex and Marital Therapy* 27(1):33–43, 2001. Copyright 2001, Brunner Routledge. Used with permission.

Overview of Therapy for Sexual Dysfunction in the Medically Ill

In subsequent sections, we address specific therapies shown to benefit dysfunction precipitated by a particular illness or cancer. However, it is usually necessary first to explain the formulation—that is, the summary of the most important underlying causes of their difficulties—to the patient or couple. Reference to current models of human sexual response can be particularly helpful. Debility, fatigue, and pain frequently lessen innate or spontaneous desire, so that a sexual encounter beginning prior to sensing arousal or desire becomes the norm. This experience may be rather different from that before illness, especially for men (Katz and Dizon 2016); the type of sexual stimulation, context of the encounter, and ability to stay focused all may need to be modified, in addition to prescription of a needed medical adjunct (e.g., a phosphodiesterase type 5 [PDE-5] inhibitor or local estrogen therapy). In addition, if the interpersonal relationship is troubled, the chances that the couple will move on to enjoy a newly modified type of sexual interaction are slim. This may need to be explained and a necessary resource found. The knowledge that the partner of the less well person also may have developed major sexual dissatisfaction (Boller et al. 2015) encourages provision of therapy for both partners.

Standard therapies include psychoeducation, cognitive-behavioral therapy (CBT), mindfulness-based cognitive therapy (MBCT), and sex therapy. The latter usually involves sensate focus therapy, whereby each partner is encouraged to take turns giving or receiving sensual and later sexual touches, caresses, and kisses. Initially, genital areas and breasts are off limits. Past goals and expectations are put aside. Encouragement to stay in the moment is needed. Couples plan 15- to 20-minute sessions two to three times per week for 3–4 weeks. The clinician guides as to when breast and genital areas are included and when ultimately intercourse (if still possible) is also "on the menu."

Mindfulness, although practiced for some 3,500 years, is a new addition to therapy for sexual dysfunction (Mize 2015). Early studies show benefit for sexual dysfunction in health and after pelvic cancer (Brotto et al. 2008a, 2008b). Randomized wait-list-controlled studies show benefit for women with genito-pelvic pain and women with sexual interest/arousal disorder (Basson and Smith 2014; Brotto and Basson 2014; Brotto et al. 2015). Programs for men are also beginning (Kocsis and Newbury-Helps 2016). CBT can be very helpful in challenging a distorted self-view or catastrophic thinking from the changes imposed by the illness. Chronically unwell persons may view their sexual disability as so unattractive to their partner that they do not deserve care and attention. Some may even stay in a relationship in which they experience emotional, physical, or sexual abuse. Specific themes in therapy are shown in Table 15–3.

When sexual function deteriorates coincident with beginning a medication, the latter may be changeable (Table 15–4). When this is not possible, the patient is advised that at least part of the problem is the needed medication, and adjustments can be suggested. The context might be made more erotic, more intense sexual stimulation may be provided, and specific goals can be removed (e.g., that intercourse or orgasm must necessarily occur).

TABLE 15–3. **Themes in management of sexual dysfunction in the context of medical disorders**

Treat comorbid depression: consider using "sexually neutral" antidepressants, including mirtazapine, bupropion, or vortioxetine.

When current beneficial antidepressants appear to have compounded sexual dysfunction, consider use of PDE-5 inhibitors in men[a,b]; possible benefit from sildenafil for orgasmic dysfunction induced by SSRIs in women with multiple sclerosis.[c]

Address pain relief: suggest planning of sexual encounters at times of better pain control.

Share formulations of sexual dysfunctions with patients (and with partners when possible), referring to the human sexual response model.

Address logistics: privacy, safety from STI, pregnancy, need of assistance from health care providers, particularly when immobility is a problem.

Encourage openness between the sexual partners; fears of being physically unattractive, that scars are ugly, or that the stoma is upsetting to the "well" partner may not be accurate.

Encourage non-goal-oriented sexual activity. Acceptance that sexual activity will not be the same as pre-illness but need not be less satisfying is a realistic approach.

Note. PDE-5=phosphodiesterase type 5; SSRI=selective serotonin reuptake inhibitor; STI=sexually transmitted infection.
[a]Nurnberg et al. 2007; [b]Segraves et al. 2007; [c]Cordeau and Courtois 2014.

TABLE 15–4.   Frequently noted sexual side effects of commonly used medications

Medication	Sexual side effects	Comments
Antidepressants	SSRIs and SNRIs may cause low desire and delayed orgasm in 30%–50% of women and men[a] and new-onset ED in 22%–41% when patients are asked directly.[a] Trazodone may rarely cause priapism.	PDE-5 inhibitors[b,c] can reverse ED. Limited evidence of reversal of orgasmic delay in women with MS by sildenafil.[d] Limited evidence that bupropion can reverse SSRI-induced dysfunction.[e] Vortioxetine may be sexually neutral.[f]
Antipsychotics	Low desire in 50%–73%,[g] new-onset ED in up to 70% of patients taking traditional antipsychotics when patients are asked directly[g]; retrograde ejaculation.[h]	Second-generation antipsychotics, which do not raise prolactin level, may be preferable,[i] but other mechanisms may still cause dysfunction.[j]
Antihypertensives	*Low desire:* In comparison with ACE inhibitors[k] and angiotensin II antagonists,[l] beta-blockers reduce desire in men. Beta-blockers reduce desire in women in comparison with angiotensin II antagonists[m]; probably applies to agents with selective and nonselective beta-blockade. *ED:* Increased by centrally acting alpha-blockers; beta-blockers (conflicting data); little evidence from meta-analysis of 35,000 patients[n], probably only if nonselective and higher dose.[o] *Priapism:* Rarely from centrally acting alpha-blockers.	Use instead ACE inhibitors, angiotensin receptor antagonists, calcium channel blockers, or peripherally acting alpha-blockers.
Diuretics	ED from thiazides, chlorthalidone, spironolactone.[p]	Choose nonthiazide alternatives.
Antiandrogens	Agents such as GnRH agonists, flutamide, cyproterone acetate, and spironolactone in high doses will suppress GnRH, LH, and/or antagonism of androgen receptor, inhibiting sexual desire and response. Finasteride may lower desire, delay ejaculation, and cause ED.	Selective androgen receptor modulators not currently available.
Anabolic steroids (chronic use)	Low desire, ED, anejaculation, testicular atrophy.	

TABLE 15–4. Frequently noted sexual side effects of commonly used medications *(continued)*

Medication	Sexual side effects	Comments
Narcotics	Low desire in men via suppression of GnRH; limited evidence in women.	Testosterone supplementation for men, but minimal data are available.
Antiepileptic drugs	May increase SHBG and reduce free testosterone.[q]	Studies needed to confirm whether there is less sexual dysfunction from enzyme-neutral AEDs (e.g., oxcarbazepine, lamotrigine, levetiracetam).
Antiparkinsonian drugs	Compulsive sexual behavior from early use of dopamine agonists[r] with levodopa. Paraphilias from dopamine agonists plus levodopa.	Reversible side effects if dopamine agonist is discontinued.

Note. ACE=angiotensin-converting enzyme; AED=antiepileptic drug; ED=erectile dysfunction; GnRH=gonadotropin-releasing hormone; LH=luteinizing hormone; MS=multiple sclerosis; PDE-5=phosphodiesterase type 5; SHBG=sex hormone–binding globulin; SNRI=serotonin–norepinephrine reuptake inhibitor; SSRI=selective serotonin reuptake inhibitor.

[a]Kennedy et al. 1999; [b]Nurnberg et al. 2007; [c]Segraves et al. 2007; [d]Cordeau and Courtois 2014; [e]Clayton et al. 2004; [f]Sanchez et al. 2015; [g]Macdonald et al. 2003; [h]Dossenbach et al. 2005; [i]Knegtering et al. 2006; [j]Atmaca et al. 2005; [k]Fogari et al. 1998; [l]Fogari et al. 2002; [m]Fogari et al. 2004; [n]Ko et al. 2002; [o]Franzen et al. 2001; [p]Düsing 2005; [q]Rees et al. 2007; [r]Klos et al. 2005.

Sexual Function in Various Medical Conditions

Cardiac Disease

Factors known to strongly influence sexual function in patients with cardiac disease include the ease of treating any associated ED, concomitant depression, and personal or partner's fears that sexual activity is dangerous (Montorsi et al. 2003). Most patients report reduced frequency of sexual activity after myocardial infarction, and 10%–54% do not resume sexual activity at all (Drory et al. 2000). It is important to advise patients that risk of further cardiac damage is low and short-lasting. Energy requirements for sexual stimulation, intercourse, and orgasm are estimated to be 3–4 metabolic equivalents (METs)—similar to climbing a flight of stairs. For a 50-year-old patient with a previous myocardial infarction, the risk of a recurrence during the 2-hour period after sexual activity has been calculated to increase from 10 chances to 20 chances in a million per hour (Muller et al. 1996). The patient can be advised that risk is very low if no cardiac symptoms arise during exercise testing to 3–4 METs. Prescribing exercise will increase tolerance for sexual activity. Guidelines exist for the resumption of sexual activity in patients with cardiac disease according to degree of cardiovascular risk (DeBusk et al. 2000) (Table 15–5). U.S. and European cardiovascular society guidelines recommend that physicians counsel male and female patients about resuming sexual activity after acute myocardial infarction, but implementation of this advice is highly variable among clinicians (Lindau et al. 2014).

The PDE-5 inhibitors such as sildenafil can be used in men with cardiac disease provided that there is no risk of hypotension from concomitant prescription of nitrates or nonselective alpha-adrenergic blockers. Inhibitors of cytochrome P450 (CYP) 3A4 (e.g., cimetidine, efavirenz, erythromycin, ketoconazole, itraconazole, ritonavir) can significantly decrease metabolism of PDE-5 inhibitors to cause unwanted accumulation. All three available PDE-5 inhibitors (sildenafil, vardenafil, tadalafil) improve endothelial function. Sildenafil does not change the time to 1 mm ST segment depression during stress testing in men with chronic stable angina but can prolong the time to angina (Jackson 2002). In contrast, vardenafil may prolong the duration of ST depression in such men. The clinical significance of this is unclear. Vardenafil should not be prescribed to persons with the long QT syndrome, nor should it be prescribed to patients taking quinidine, procainamide, amiodarone, or sotalol because of further increase in the QT interval. The PDE-5 inhibitors should not be used in low-cardiac-output states (e.g., severe aortic stenosis). Intracavernosal injection of prostaglandin E_1 (PGE_1; alprostadil injection) by self or partner can be taught if PDE-5 inhibitors are contraindicated.

More than 50% of patients with coronary artery disease are depressed. The mutually reinforcing triad of depression, ischemic heart disease, and ED (Goldstein 2000) should encourage screening for the other two conditions if one is present. Sildenafil can improve sexual function and depression in men with heart failure (Freitas et al. 2006). Antidepressant-induced ED can be ameliorated with PDE-5 inhibitors (Nurnberg et al. 2007). Cardiac drugs rarely alter depression, although some (e.g., thiazides, spironolactone, digoxin) may reduce erectile function. Contrary to previous belief, a meta-analysis of 35,000 patients (Ko et al. 2002) suggested that beta-blockers cause only minimal ED—and only if nonselective and higher doses are used (Franzen et al. 2001).

TABLE 15–5. Management recommendations based on graded cardiovascular risk assessment

Grade of risk	Cardiovascular disease categories	Management recommendations
Low	Asymptomatic, <3 major risk factors for CAD, excluding age and gender	Primary care management
		Consider all first-line therapies
	Controlled hypertension	Reassess at regular intervals (6–12 months)
	Mild, stable angina	
	After successful coronary revascularization	
	Uncomplicated past MI (>6–8 weeks)	
	Mild valve disease	
	LVD/CHF (NYHA Class I)	
Intermediate	≥3 major risk factors for CAD, excluding gender	Evaluation by a cardiologist prior to initiation of any therapy for erectile dysfunction because of risk of myocardial ischemia during sexual activity and orgasm
	Moderate, stable angina	
	Recent MI (>2, <6 weeks)	
	LVD/CHF (NYHA Class II)	Specialized cardiovascular testing (e.g., ETT, echo)
	Noncardiac sequelae of atherosclerotic disease (e.g., CVA, peripheral vascular disease)	Restratification into high risk or low risk based on the results of cardiovascular assessment
High	Unstable or refractory angina	Priority referral for specialized cardiovascular management
	Uncontrolled hypertension	Treatment for sexual dysfunction to be deferred until cardiac condition stabilized and dependent on specialist recommendations
	LVD/CHF (NYHA Class III/IV)	
	Recent MI (<2 weeks), CVA	
	High-risk arrhythmias	
	Hypertrophic obstructive and other cardiomyopathies	
	Moderate or severe valve disease	

Note. CAD=coronary artery disease; CHF=congestive heart failure; CVA=cerebrovascular accident; echo=echocardiogram; ETT=exercise tolerance test; LVD=left ventricular dysfunction; MI=myocardial infarction; NYHA=New York Heart Association.

Chronic Obstructive Pulmonary Disease

Studies of sexual dysfunction in patients with chronic obstructive pulmonary disease (COPD) are limited. Most studies are in men and focus on ED, which is present in 70%–80% of men with COPD (whereas ED prevalence in age-matched men without COPD is closer to 60%) (Lauretti et al. 2016; Turan et al. 2016). One study showed that about one-third of patients with chronic respiratory failure who were using noninvasive mechanical ventilation were sexually active (Schönhofer et al. 2001). For some patients, noninvasive mechanical ventilation allowed intercourse, which had been impossible for several years. Ventilator settings for frequency and tidal volume had to be increased for the patients to reach orgasm. A Cochrane review (Levack et al. 2015) concluded that there were insufficient data in COPD to confirm benefit from either supplemental oxygen or testosterone in improving men's sexual function.

Rheumatic Disease

The sexual lives of men and women with rheumatic disease are frequently negatively affected by pain, debility, loss of mobility, comorbid depression, and genital tissue changes in some of the disorders. In a study examining 509 consecutive patients (men and women) with rheumatic disease, depression and anxiety were identified as the only predictors of sexual dysfunction, and this association remained even after adjustment for physical factors (Anyfanti et al. 2014). Because pain and depression are major determinants of sexual dysfunction in the context of many rheumatological conditions (Abda et al. 2016; Healey et al. 2009; van Nimwegen et al. 2015; Yilmaz et al. 2012), their control is a priority when addressing sexual dysfunction in these patients.

Impaired mobility can interfere with sexual caressing and specific sexual stimulation of the partner or the self. The movements needed to engage in intercourse may be too painful or impossible. Altered mobility can negatively affect self-image, particularly in adolescents, leading to difficulties forming relationships. Hip replacement in rheumatoid arthritis has a one in two chance of improving sexual function back to previous levels (Yoshino et al. 1984).

Aside from changes to the joints, other tissue changes may interfere with sexual function. Sjögren's syndrome is associated with vaginal dryness and dyspareunia, and patients report these symptoms more than twice as often as do healthy controls (Priori et al. 2015). In women with systemic sclerosis, loss of vaginal elasticity is common, as is vaginal dryness and ulcerations (Bhadauria et al. 1995). ED from associated vasculitis is common in systemic sclerosis, with a prevalence of up to 80% (Tristano 2009). PDE-5 inhibitors are shown to be effective in some but not all studies of men with systemic sclerosis.

Neurological Disease

Neurological disease can alter sexual motivation, sexual self-image, sexual desire, and ability to communicate sexual needs between partners. Its presence can increase vulnerability to sexual exploitation or coercion. Moreover, neurological disease frequently causes disruption of the sexual response system at brain, spinal cord, and peripheral nerve levels.

For the most part, neurological deficit leads to sexual deficit, but problematic increases can occur, such as hypersexuality from dopaminergic agonists given to treat Parkinson's disease or disinhibited hypersexuality from severe trauma to the prefrontal lobes or bilateral amygdaloid damage in the Klüver-Bucy syndrome, and also, albeit rarely, in strokes affecting the right temporal lobe. Ironically, the imposed anatomic changes and losses can sometimes lead to a more rewarding and more intimate sexuality than was experienced before the illness (e.g., radical pelvic surgery for gynecological cancer) (Corney et al. 1993).

Brain Injury

Whether from trauma or from stroke, brain injury is frequently associated with sexual problems, the prevalence of which can be difficult to estimate when the patient has extensive bodily injuries other than to the brain or when there are comorbidities such as depression or peripheral vascular disease. Depression, present in some 50% of patients (Kelly et al. 2006), is the most sensitive single predictor of sexual outcome after mechanical injury to the brain.

Damage to limbic structures or to their connections is the main cause of organic sexual dysfunction following stroke (Rees et al. 2007). Middle cerebral artery stroke causes injury to multiple limbic and paralimbic areas. Anterior cerebral artery ischemia damages the medial frontal cortex and adjoining cingulate gyrus receiving massive projections from limbic areas. Anterior choroidal artery strokes cause injury to the medial temporal limbic structures.

No clear relation has been found between the site of stroke or the duration of coma and the degree of sexual impairment (Boller et al. 2015). In some studies, close to 60% of stroke patients report sexual dysfunction. When their sexual partners are also assessed, a similar number report also having sexual dysfunction subsequent to all the changes in both of their lives, medical and psychological, since the partner's stroke (Boller et al. 2015). The most common dysfunctions are low desire, ED, premature or delayed ejaculation, and dyspareunia secondary to loss of lubrication. Antidepressant and antipsychotic medications can further add to the incidence of low desire and delayed/absent orgasm.

Severe head trauma can lead to pituitary injury with resultant secondary hypogonadism from impairment in LH and FSH production. This is suspected when a basal skull fracture involves the sphenoid bone that surrounds the pituitary gland or when diffuse cerebral edema compresses the third ventricle with pressure on the hypothalamus and the connecting portal veins alongside the pituitary stalk. Clinicians should screen for pituitary injury at 3 and 12 months following severe brain injury (Ghigo et al. 2005). If the patient has early diabetes insipidus, serious panhypopituitarism may already be present.

Brain trauma also may lead to impaired insight and cognition, causing difficulties in social interaction. Many survivors of brain trauma are young, and for these patients, engaging in the subtleties involved in forming and maintaining a sexual relationship may be particularly challenging. In response to growing recognition of health care providers' lack of attention to patients' sexual health after brain trauma (Moreno et al. 2015), rehabilitation centers are increasingly incorporating assessment and treatment of sexual dysfunction into their programs (Guo et al. 2015).

Parkinson's Disease

Given that Parkinson's disease involves the autonomic, limbic, and somatomotor systems, rates of sexual dysfunction are high. Further dysfunction from dopamine replacement therapy is possible. Traditionally, dopamine has been thought to play a major role in promoting sexual motivation, sexual arousal, and reward. Dopamine is important not only for motor function but also for general arousal, a circumstance that explains most of parkinsonism's effects on sexual behavior (Paredes and Agmo 2004). Prevalence rates of sexual dysfunction in Parkinson's disease vary from 40% to 68% in men and from 30% to 88% in women (Hand et al. 2010); symptoms include problems with erections and ejaculation (both premature and delayed) in men; difficulties with arousal, lubrication, and orgasm in women; and impaired sexual satisfaction and desire in both sexes—the latter being more common with left-side-predominant Parkinson's (Kummer et al. 2009). Distressing spontaneous orgasms and ejaculations are also reported (Kaut et al. 2012). Despite the involvement of dopaminergic pathways, it has been found that for men and women, depression (Kummer et al. 2009) and attitudes about sexuality and Parkinson's can be more important to their sexual functioning than are biomedical factors (DeLamater and Sill 2005). Healthy female partners of men with Parkinson's disease may experience more sexual dissatisfaction than women with Parkinson's disease (Brown et al. 1990).

Sexual dysfunction is almost invariably present in the parkinsonian variant of multiple system atrophy, for which ED may be an early sign. Some 50% of women with multiple system atrophy report reduced genital sensitivity, compared with only 4% of women with idiopathic Parkinson's disease (Oertel et al. 2003). Sexual dysfunction can occur at any stage of Parkinson's disease or can predate it, and ED may be considered a risk factor for developing Parkinson's disease (Gao et al. 2007).

Dopamine agonist drugs may increase sexual function and motivation through direct stimulation of the dopamine type 2 (D_2) receptors in the medial preoptic area and may also facilitate erections by inhibiting prolactin production and increasing oxytocin activity at the lumbosacral spinal cord. These effects help to explain why dopaminergic therapy may allow resumption of sexual activity in some patients with Parkinson's disease but may lead to hypersexuality in others. Dopamine agonist therapy is associated with compulsive sexual behavior in 2.0%–3.5% of Parkinson's patients, and with other impulse-control disorders in 13.6% (Weintraub et al. 2010). Individuals who develop pathological hypersexuality may compulsively use phone-sex lines or prostitution services and may make inappropriate advances to family members and acquaintances. A history of mood disorder, alcohol intake, personal traits of novelty seeking, early onset of Parkinson's disease, and early use of dopamine agonists are risk factors for pathological hypersexuality (Evans et al. 2005; Pezzella et al. 2005). It is currently thought that administration of dopamine agonists, especially in combination with L-dopa, may cause these symptoms through excessive stimulation of D_2 receptors, particularly the D_3 subclass (Klos et al. 2005). Sexual compulsions can be resolved by discontinuing dopamine agonist treatment while continuing L-dopa therapy (Klos et al. 2005). Use of deep brain stimulation may allow reduction of dopaminergic drugs, but it, too, can provoke hypersexuality (Bronner and Vodušek 2011).

This potential hypersexuality in Parkinson's disease is diametrically opposed to the disrupted genital function brought about by the neurodegenerative process; the combination of heightened desire with impaired genital function can be enormously problematic for a couple or patients in a nursing home environment.

Multiple Sclerosis

The prevalence of sexual dysfunction in men and women with multiple sclerosis is high, with the disease eventually affecting 75% of men (predominantly with ED and ejaculatory dysfunction) and up to 85% of women (with loss of genital sensation and impaired desire, arousal, lubrication, and orgasm) (Rees et al. 2007). Even at diagnosis, when duration of multiple sclerosis symptoms averaged 2.7 years, sexual dysfunction was present in 35% of women compared with 21% of healthy control subjects; furthermore, in 4 of 63 women with early disease, reduced genital sensation was a presenting symptom (Tzortzis et al. 2008). Fatigue, spasticity, pain, loss of self-esteem, depression, anxiety, and incontinence all contribute to sexual dysfunction in both men and women. Although bladder dysfunction generally correlates with sexual dysfunction in women, orgasm is typically preserved in women with urge incontinence (Cordeau and Courtois 2014). Nocturnal erections may be preserved in male patients with ED; however, this does not imply a psychogenic etiology as it would in men without neurological disease. PDE-5 inhibitors are effective for ED in men with multiple sclerosis, especially those with residual reflex erections and upper motor neuron lesions (Prévinaire et al. 2014). PDE-5 inhibitors may ameliorate orgasmic dysfunction from antidepressants in women (Cordeau and Courtois 2014). Genital vibratory stimulation can benefit orgasmic delay in men and women. Baclofen, tizanidine, botulin toxin, and sclerosing agents can lessen spasticity that interferes with sexual activity.

Amyotrophic Lateral Sclerosis

Published data on amyotrophic lateral sclerosis (ALS) are few. Patients with ALS have intact autonomic and sensory nerve supply to the genitalia. Consequently, the effect of ALS on sexuality is largely by way of motor incapacity through damaged efferent pathways of the brain stem and spinal cord.

Wasner et al. (2004) evaluated sexuality in 62 persons with ALS and found that 62% of the patients and 75% of their partners reported sexual difficulties, compared with 19% and 20%, respectively, before onset of the disease, yet sexual interest and activity remained. Fear of rejection and inhibition by physical limitation were important. The topic of sexuality was rarely discussed with medical personnel. Restricted pulmonary function made penetrative sexual intercourse difficult or impossible: however, five of the six ventilated patients in the study reported having intercourse at least once per month, which is consistent with an unexpectedly high importance of sexuality even in advanced disease.

Spinal Cord and Cauda Equina Injury

Data suggest that some 86% of patients with spinal cord injury retain sexual desire (Anderson et al. 2007a, 2007b), but such injuries are associated with the highest rate of sexual dysfunction from any neurological condition. Depending on the level and completeness of the spinal cord injury, sexual dysfunction is variable. Neurogenic bladder with incontinence appears to be a major influence on sexuality for women with spinal cord injury (Cramp et al. 2015)—the sensations preceding orgasm can be confused with urination, leading to avoidance of orgasm.

Very low lesions involving the S2, S3, and S4 vertebrae allow mental excitement to cause a degree of erection and vaginal lubrication and vulvar swelling, but reflexive erection of the penis and vulvar swelling are lost. The T10–L2 sympathetic outflow from the spinal cord is thought to provide the erections/lubrication that accompany mental sexual excitement.

With strong stimulation (vibrator), many men with lesions above the lumbosacral level can ejaculate. This may occur extremely quickly, and the ability to delay ejaculation, if desired, may not be present (Courtois and Charvier 2015). Reflex ejaculation is accompanied by cardiac, muscle, and autonomic sensations similar to orgasm and similar to autonomic hyperreflexia. This hyperreflexia generally affects patients with lesions above T6, because signals to inhibit sympathetic outflow are interrupted. Sustained genital stimulation, whether sexual or painful, travels through the somatic and visceral afferents to the thoracic segments of the spinal cord and can reflexively trigger sudden generalized vasoconstriction, thereby increasing blood pressure. There may be a pounding headache, flushing of the neck and face, increased skin temperature, and even blurred vision. Hypotensive treatment may be necessary; nifedipine is the usual choice, although it is not ideal (Courtois et al. 2012). Reflex orgasms from a vibrator placed on or near the clitoris, or even from manual stimulation, can also occur in women despite complete lesions. With time, neuroplasticity may allow stimulation to body areas—including the torso, shoulders, and neck—to be highly sexually arousing (Anderson et al. 2007a, 2007b; Duggal et al. 2010). Women with complete lesions at any level of the spinal cord may still experience orgasm from cervical vibrostimulation, possibly mediated through an intact neural supply to the cervix traveling separately in the vagus nerve outside the spinal neuraxis (Komisaruk et al. 2004).

Injuries to the medullary cone or to the cauda equina will interrupt the innervation to the genitalia from the autonomic and somatic nerves, causing variable loss of genital sensation and genital congestion as well as loss of voluntary control of the bladder and bowel.

PDE-5 inhibitors and intracavernosal PGE_1 are effective in augmenting reflex and psychogenic erections. A recent large international study confirmed sildenafil's safety and efficacy in treating sexual dysfunction in spinal cord injury (Ohl et al. 2017). Benefits extended to men with complete lesions, and the ability to ejaculate was often restored with the return of firmer erections, thereby avoiding medical intervention for desired sperm retrieval. Ejaculation is also facilitated by midodrine combined with penile vibratory stimulation, which is more effective than penile vibratory stimulation alone (Soler et al. 2007); however, injuries below the T10 vertebra show less improvement.

Epilepsy

Hyposexuality commonly follows but does not predate the onset of epilepsy and is particularly common in temporal lobe epilepsy (Rees et al. 2007). Epilepsy also can provoke involuntary sexual gestures during a seizure. This occurs when the seizure arises in the mesolimbic temporal structures or the interhemispheric parietal cortex subserving genital sensation. Also, an erotic aura can precede a seizure. Given that automatisms typically occur during the amnestic phase of the seizure, their frequency is probably underreported; video-electroencephalography detected sexual automatisms in 11% of 200 selected patients having medically refractive seizures (Dobesberger et al. 2004). Characteristically, women who have reflex orgasms with their seizures are profoundly hyposexual.

Enzyme-inducing antiepileptic drugs, including phenytoin, barbiturates, and carbamazepine (but not oxcarbazepine), increase the level of sex hormone–binding globulin by an unknown mechanism. Although the total (free plus bound) serum concentration of testosterone is generally unchanged by these anticonvulsants, the increase in sex hormone–binding globulin raises the proportion of bound testosterone and reduces the level of free or bioavailable testosterone. These older antiepileptic drugs impair male sexuality, but data on women are inconclusive. The CYP enzyme-*inhibiting* antiepileptic drug valproic acid may increase serum androgen levels and estradiol level in both men and women. At least in theory, enzyme-*neutral* antiepileptic drugs are less likely to cause sexual side effects. The latter include oxcarbazepine, gabapentin, pregabalin, levetiracetam, and lamotrigine. Some evidence indicates that lamotrigine has the lowest profile of sexual side effects (Devinsky 2005).

Dementia

Up to 25% of patients with dementia may lose normal inhibitory control of sexual behavior (Verdelho and Gonçalves-Pereira 2017). Inappropriate sexual gestures with caregivers—or with other patients when institutionalized—or public self-stimulation may occur. Inappropriate sexual behavior is more common in men. Anxiety may be a risk factor (Canevelli et al. 2017). These difficulties can be compounded by frustration with inability to experience sexual release when self-stimulation is ineffective in producing orgasm because of ED. Although such behavior is not usually dangerous, it can cause immense distress to all concerned. It is important to confirm that what appears to be inappropriate or disinhibited sexual behavior is not simply a result of frustration over lack of privacy (e.g., inability to be alone to self-stimulate or to be with the intimate partner). Still, in some health care facilities, there is no recognition and acceptance of the sexual needs of institutionalized patients. Psychiatric consultants should not only assess the problematic sexual behavior but also negotiate an appropriate environment for—and willingness of hospital staff to allow—patient sexual expression. An underlying medical condition (e.g., urinary tract infection) should be sought at the onset of such behaviors (Verdelho and Gonçalves-Pereira 2017).

When medical treatment is necessary to prevent harm to the patient or others, serotonergic antidepressants may be better tolerated than antipsychotics (Verdelho and Gonçalves-Pereira 2017). Antiandrogen therapy is sometimes considered. Scientific study is very limited, but spironolactone, medroxyprogesterone acetate (MPA), and gonadotropin-releasing hormone agonists are of some benefit. There is also anecdotal evidence of benefit from anticonvulsants such as carbamazepine, cholinesterase inhibitors such as rivastigmine, and nonselective beta-blockers (De Giorgi and Series 2016). When decisions concerning the use of pharmacological therapy are made, the inclusion of health care team members, the family, and possibly legal advice is recommended.

Diabetes

Diabetes poses risk for sexual dysfunction in both men and women. In men only, diabetic control and length of disease correlate with the incidence of dysfunction—notably ED and ejaculatory dysfunction. In women with diabetes, sexual dysfunction has been strongly linked to comorbid depression in the vast majority of studies (Bhasin et al. 2007). In men, insulin resistance and increased adiposity are associated with low levels of testosterone; in women, insulin resistance is associated with high testosterone levels (Sarkar et al. 2017).

Some studies suggest that ED may affect up to 85% of men with diabetes (Peak et al. 2016); both type 1 and type 2 are present in many sampled cohorts. In uncomplicated type 2 diabetes without other risk factors for coronary artery disease, ED can signal silent cardiac ischemia (Gazzaruso et al. 2004), yet some 63% of diabetic patients report never having been questioned about sexual dysfunction (Peak et al. 2016). Etiologies of diabetes-induced ED are multifactorial and can include endothelial and smooth muscle dysfunction, autonomic and somatic neuropathy, and interpersonal or psychological issues. Men with both diabetes and ED tend to have a history of poor metabolic control, untreated hypertension, peripheral neuropathy, micro- and macroalbuminuria, retinopathy, cardiovascular disease, diuretic treatment, obesity-related testosterone decline, and psychological vulnerability (Bhasin et al. 2007). Along with improving glycemic control, PDE-5 inhibitors are the first-line treatment for ED in diabetes; however, these drugs are less effective in some men with diabetes than in others (Bhasin et al. 2007). Vacuum devices or intracavernosal injections of PGE_1 are second-line options. Ejaculatory problems are common. Sympathetic neuropathy causes anejaculation from lack of vas deferens peristalsis or retrograde ejaculation from malfunction of the internal urethral sphincter. Sometimes emission occurs, but not expulsion; semen seeps out of the penis, and orgasmic intensity may be less.

Improving glycemic control may reverse ejaculatory dysfunction. Sympathomimetics have limited success, but recently using both imipramine and pseudoephedrine benefited 61% of men (Peak et al. 2016). When infertility is an issue, sperm can be retrieved by bladder washing after either sexual stimulation, penile vibrator stimulation, or electrostimulation of the prostatic nerve plexus per rectum, prior to intrauterine insemination.

In men with abdominal obesity and hyperlipidemia, low testosterone is common. The pathogenesis of low testosterone is complex and includes higher levels of estrogen and leptin, inflammation, and direct testicular damage. Testosterone replacement improves insulin resistance, lipid profiles, and sexual function but will inhibit fertility, so off-label clomiphene can be used to stimulate endogenous testosterone production.

A meta-analysis of 26 studies found an increased risk of sexual dysfunction in women with diabetes (odds ratios [ORs]=2.27 and 2.49 for type 1 and 2, respectively) compared with healthy control women (Pontiroli et al. 2013). Meta-regression indicated that sexual dysfunction may be related to increased body weight. In some but not all series, reduced lubrication from hyperglycemia-induced vaginal mucosal dehydration, dyspareunia, orgasmic difficulty, and sexual dissatisfaction were about twice as common in women with diabetes compared with control subjects. Of note, both in studies limited to type 1 or to type 2 and in prospective studies (Enzlin et al. 2009), the only predictors of sexual dysfunction were having depression and being married. This finding is in marked contrast to findings in men, in whom poor glycemic control and diabetic complications are the main predictors of sexual dysfunction.

Because of cardiovascular risk, systemic estrogen is generally avoided in diabetes. Topical estrogen can be prescribed via a vaginal ring, tablet, or cream for genito-urinary syndrome of menopause (American College of Obstetricians and Gynecologists 2014). There are no specific treatments for diabetes-associated female sexual dysfunction, but care is needed to optimally treat urinary and vaginal infections and associated sexual pain with subsequent loss of sexual motivation. In addition, screening for treatable comorbid depression is strongly recommended.

Male Hypogonadism

Investigating and treating the primary pathology in secondary hypogonadism is vital. The underlying disease may be life-threatening, as in hemochromatosis or a prolactinoma, and the presenting symptoms are typically sexual. Once the underlying disorder leading to secondary hypogonadism is addressed, including cases of primary testicular failure, testosterone replacement usually improves sexual desire and alleviates the delayed ejaculation, diminished ejaculate, low sperm count, and variable ED. Transdermal, as opposed to parenteral, preparations are recommended to avoid peaks and troughs in testosterone levels, which tend to cause both erythrocytosis and mood changes. The concept of "late-onset hypogonadism" in older men is controversial, with recent research noting little benefit from testosterone supplementation and increased cardiovascular risk (Budoff et al. 2017; Busnelli et al. 2017).

End-Stage Renal Disease

Sexual dysfunction is extremely common in men and women with ESRD. The etiology is complex because of comorbidities, including diabetes, hypertension, coronary artery disease, and depression (Peng et al. 2005, 2007). Associated symptoms relevant to sexual activity include pain in bones and joints from osteodystrophy, fatigue, anorexia, nausea, stomatitis, pruritus, and malnutrition. Reported prevalence of ED is as high as 85%, with anemia, endothelial dysfunction, uremia, and autonomic nerve dysfunction all contributing (Basson et al. 2010). PDE-5 inhibitors can be used if no contraindications are identified; the dose is reduced in renal insufficiency but not during dialysis. Transplantation may improve ED, and sildenafil is both effective and safe posttransplant (Basson et al. 2010). Recombinant human erythropoietin therapy is guided by hemoglobin levels and can improve ED in men who are receiving dialysis, but not when uremia is present. Low desire is present in up to 100% of men with ESRD; low testosterone, high prolactin, anemia, depression, chronic pain, and psychosexual factors, including altered self-image and medicalization of the bedroom in home hemodialysis, all contribute. Testosterone therapy has been of limited benefit, in part because of the anemia and high prolactin level. Erythropoietin partially corrects low testosterone levels (Basson et al. 2010).

Low sexual desire is present in up to 100% of women with ESRD and those undergoing hemodialysis and is as high as 80% posttransplantation (Basson et al. 2010). Multiple factors are involved, including anemia, negative outcomes to sexual interactions, high prolactin level, depression, chronic pain, and psychosexual and interpersonal issues. Forty percent of women with ESRD are totally amenorrheic, fewer than 10% have regular menstrual periods, and premature menopause is common—all predisposing to dyspareunia from estrogen deficiency.

Children with ESRD will face many obstacles when it comes time to form sexual relationships. Their lives have been medicalized, which limits social interaction. Puberty may have been delayed, reducing sexual self-confidence. Their situation is compounded by the negative effects of medical interventions on sexual responsiveness.

Cancer

Advances in the management of malignant disease have allowed more lives to be saved, so now the emphasis is also on the quality of those lives. Negative sexual sequelae are present in most cancer patients, 50% of whom would definitely seek treatment for sexual dysfunction were it available (Huyghe et al. 2009). The most pertinent causes of sexual dysfunction in cancer are shown in Tables 15–6 and 15–7.

Nerve-damage surgery or radiation can damage the pelvic autonomic nerves in the inferior hypogastric plexus and cavernous nerves and interrupt genital congestion, leading to ED or dyspareunia from decreased lubrication, all indirectly delaying or preventing orgasm. Experience of orgasm is possible (e.g., with a vibrator) because sympathetic fibers to the genital structures take multiple routes.

Surgeries to allow both oncological cure and preservation of function are evolving. Mesorectal incision for rectal cancer leads to better sexual and cancer outcomes. Here, the superior hypogastric plexus, both hypogastric nerves, pelvic plexus, and neurovascular bundles are spared (Kim et al. 2016). Robotic-assisted cavernosal nerve-sparing laparoscopic radical prostatectomy may allow better erectile function than either open or other laparoscopic approaches, but outcome mostly depends on age and presurgical erectile function (Kadıoğlu et al. 2015). Brachytherapy may preserve function better than external beam radiation (Chung and Gillman 2014). "Penile rehabilitation" with intermittent or, preferably, daily PDE-5 inhibitors is also advocated, beginning even several days before surgery (Moskovic et al. 2010). A meta-analysis of nerve-sparing radical surgery for cervical cancer identified no worsening of prognosis and improved sexual function as compared with non-nerve-sparing surgery (Kim et al. 2016). Nerve-sparing cystectomy with penile rehabilitation benefits erectile function, and similarly, sparing the anterior vaginal wall, with its neurovascular bundles, may preserve function in women (Bennett et al. 2016).

Abrupt Loss of Gonadal Hormones

Although premature ovarian failure from chemotherapy is a major factor influencing sexual outcome, it has not yet been shown that hormonal changes per se are responsible. A pilot study of women with past breast cancer and complex endocrine status as a result of ongoing antiestrogen therapy used multiple regression analysis to determine what influenced the sexual outcome (Alder et al. 2008). The study found that relationship factors predicted desire, but a history of chemotherapy predicted problematic arousal, lubrication, orgasm, and pain. However, no relation was seen between sexual function and androgen levels, including androgen metabolites. The researchers concluded that the chemotherapy-associated decline in sexual function was mediated by androgen-independent pathways. It may be the sudden, often severe menopausal symptoms of poor sleep, hot flashes, mood swings, and vaginal dryness that most severely reduce sexual motivation. Local (vaginal) estrogen to benefit dryness and dyspareunia is generally considered safe, even with a history of estrogen-dependent cancer (American College of Obstetricians and Gynecologists and Farrell 2016).

Androgen deprivation therapy for prostate cancer may be continuous or intermittent. In the latter group, desire improves when patients are in the "off" phase of therapy (Tunn 2007); ED can be treated with PDE-5 inhibitors. However, the insults to body image from weight gain, loss of muscle mass, gynecomastia, and genital shrink-

TABLE 15–6. **Possible direct effects of malignant disease and its treatment on sexual function**

Insult	Dysfunction
Loss of sexual organs: breast, vulva, penis	Reduced desire and response; intercourse possibly precluded
Chemotherapy-induced gonadal failure	Reduced desire and response
Surgical section of pelvic autonomic nerves causing failure of erection, vulvar and vaginal congestion	Reduced desire and arousal, ED, dyspareunia
Retroperitoneal lymph node dissection for testicular cancer or lymphoma	Failure of emission
Pelvic radiation damage to tissues, including vagina, to autonomic nerve and vascular supply of penis, vagina, vulva; higher doses causing neurogenic orgasmic disorder	Reduced desire and arousal, ED, dyspareunia or inability to accommodate penis or dildo, orgasmic disorder
Hormonal manipulation depleting testosterone, as in androgen deprivation therapy, and estrogen, as with aromatase inhibitors, bilateral oophorectomy, withdrawal of estrogen therapy	Reduced desire and arousal, ED, orgasmic and ejaculatory disorder, dyspareunia

Note. ED=erectile dysfunction.

TABLE 15–7. **Indirect effects of malignant disease on sexual function[a]**

Knowledge of potentially terminal disease

Pain and depression

Fear of inability to satisfy partner, especially when vagina is stenosed from radiation or when ED from radical pelvic surgery or radiation is not improved by PDE-5 inhibitors or intracavernosal PGE_1

Fear of transmitting cancer through intercourse

Fear that sexual intercourse was causative of the cancer (e.g., anal or cervical cancer)

Feeling "neutered" from loss of sexual organs

Feeling asexual due to loss of fertility after chemotherapy

Perception of premature aging with premature menopause

Feeling unattractive from presence of stoma, ileal conduit, surgical disfigurement

Note. ED=erectile dysfunction; PDE-5=phosphodiesterase type 5; PGE_1=prostaglandin E_1.
[a]All may lower sexual motivation and response.

age can be severe. With the loss of seemingly "innate" libido, beginning a sexual experience can feel so foreign that without clinician advice, men may never attempt any kind of sexual activity (Katz and Dizon 2016).

Preservation of fertility in patients with cancer is now sometimes possible (Chiles and Schlegel 2016; Flyckt and Falcone 2016; Kim et al. 2016). Sperm banking for men is relatively straightforward but may be precluded for men unwilling to self-stimulate or unable to ejaculate due to stress of diagnosis. Vibrostimulation may be an option, but many men still regret that their future fertility was not addressed. For women, delaying cancer treatment to allow one cycle of hormone stimulation followed by cryopreservation of either a mature oocyte or an embryo may be a very difficult decision. Moreover, in some situations (e.g., after hormone receptor–positive breast cancer), pregnancy may increase the risk of recurrence. The more established option of using embryos can prove difficult, as the embryo becomes shared property with the current partner unless donor sperm are used. When time is insufficient for these two approved options, ovarian tissue cryopreservation can be considered. It is helpful for psychiatrists to have some understanding of the current and emerging options to preserve fertility for their patients as they prepare for definitive cancer treatment.

Positive Sexual Sequelae in Cancer Survivors

Positive effects on sexuality also can be seen. For example, when therapy for the cancer has been extreme, as in bone marrow transplantation, survivors have described the experience of treasuring life and focusing on each moment, including the sexually intimate moments. Sexual "performance" is no longer a goal—indeed, sexual dysfunction may remain some 5 years after marrow transplantation, especially in women (Syrjala et al. 2008)—but closeness and sharing erotic touches is reported as being more rewarding than sexual intercourse was before cancer. Excellent reviews describe clinical management of sexuality in women (Carr 2015; Huffman et al. 2016) and men (Kadıoğlu et al. 2015; Katz and Dizon 2016).

Surgeries Resulting in Ostomies

Sexual difficulties associated with stomas range from hesitancy to even begin a relationship to fear that a current partner will now be offended by odor, leakage, or noise from passing flatus. Sexual self-image is vulnerable, particularly in adolescents, who already may be feeling unattractive. However, limited study suggests that by young adulthood, marked adaptation may occur such that sexual confidence nevertheless emerges (Erwin-Toth 1999). For older patients, one case–control study suggested that male veterans with stomas had a higher prevalence of ED and were less sexually active compared with those requiring major intestinal surgery that did not involve stoma creation (Symms et al. 2008). A study of 141 patients consecutively recruited from one clinic indicated widespread sexual dysfunction in men and women. More severe dysfunction was present in patients who currently or previously had stomas compared with patients who had never required a stoma (Reese et al. 2014). Of men with stomas, those discontinuing sexual activity adapted less well generally, reporting more isolation and interference with social activities.

Lower Urinary Tract Symptoms in Men and Women

Various urinary symptoms are common and are associated with an increased prevalence of sexual dysfunction in both men and women.

In men, symptoms include urgency, frequency, and nocturia; benign prostatic hyperplasia is often present. ED and lower urinary tract symptoms co-occur and likely share the same etiology. Surgery for benign prostatic hyperplasia precipitates ED in some 10% of cases, and the risk of delayed ejaculation is approximately 20% (Miner et al. 2006).

Pharmacological therapy for lower urinary tract symptoms (traditionally, alpha-adrenergic antagonists and 5-alpha-reductase inhibitors, and more recently, antimuscarinics and PDE-5 inhibitors) may negatively or positively affect sexual function. Combination treatment with alpha-adrenergic receptor antagonists and 5-alpha-reductase inhibitors produces cumulative risks of sexual side effects (Roehrborn et al. 2008). By contrast, treatment of sexual dysfunction with PDE-5 inhibitors can improve lower urinary tract symptoms.

In women, symptoms of lower urinary tract infection include frequency, urgency, nocturia, urinary incontinence, hesitancy, and postvoiding dribbling. When infection is absent, the combination of urinary urgency, frequency, and nocturia, with or without incontinence, constitutes the overactive bladder syndrome. Urinary urgency, frequency, nocturia, pelvic pain, and dyspareunia constitute painful bladder syndrome or interstitial cystitis. Dyspareunia may accompany both of these syndromes—the pain is usually located at the introitus (vaginal entrance). Well-designed studies are lacking, and the pathophysiology of sexual dysfunction is unclear. Data are sparse on the effects of medications (oxybutynin, tolterodine, solifenacin) for lower urinary tract symptoms on women's sexual function. Pelvic floor muscle training is effective for lower urinary tract symptoms and can benefit sexual function including dyspareunia (Giuseppe et al. 2007). The effect of urogynecological surgical therapy, including suburethral slings and prolapse surgeries for lower urinary tract symptoms, on women's sexual function is variable.

Simple Hysterectomy for Benign Disease

Prospective studies have now confirmed that most women report improved sexual function after hysterectomy for benign disease, regardless of operative method (Thakar 2015). The autonomic nerves traveling to the vulva in the cardinal and uterosacral ligaments are spared in a simple hysterectomy because the incisions in those ligaments are near the midline, whereas the autonomic nerves are in the more lateral portions of the ligaments. Probably underlying the postoperative improvement in sexual function is the lessening of dyspareunia and better sexual self-image resulting from the relief of prolapse or chronic menorrhagia.

Bilateral Salpingo-Oophorectomy

Three prospective studies have shown that perimenopausal women receiving bilateral salpingo-oophorectomy along with a simple hysterectomy for benign disease did not develop negative sexual effects when followed up over the next 1–3 years (Aziz et al. 2005; Farquhar et al. 2006; Teplin et al. 2007). A large national survey of 2,207 American women found an increased prevalence of *distress* about low sexual desire in women with a relatively recent bilateral salpingo-oophorectomy, but not an increased prevalence of low desire per se (West et al. 2008). The indications for undertaking bilateral salpingo-oophorectomy in this large survey were not given; almost certainly, some would have been for malignant disease.

Conclusion

Neither the debility nor the interruption of sexual response caused by disease or iatrogenesis removes the sexual needs of most persons with chronic illness. When physicians treating the disease or cancer avoid the subject of sexual health, patients may be reluctant to initiate this discussion, an all-too-common situation. By routinely addressing sexual health, psychiatrists are well suited to assess, diagnose, and direct the management of sexual disorders while treating comorbid depression or other psychiatric disorders (Stevenson 2004).

References

Abda E, Selim Z, Teleb S, et al: Sexual function in females with rheumatoid arthritis: relationship with physical and psychosocial states. Arch Rheumatol 31(3):239–247, 2016. Available at: http://www.archivesofrheumatology.org/full-text/804. Accessed May 28, 2017.

Abdelhamed A, Hisasue S, Nada EA, et al: Relation between erectile dysfunction and silent myocardial ischemia in diabetic patients: a multidetector computed tomographic coronary angiographic study. Sex Med 4(3):e127–e134, 2016 27375006

Absher JR, Vogt BA, Clark DG, et al: Hypersexuality and hemiballism due to subthalamic infarction. Neuropsychiatry Neuropsychol Behav Neurol 13(3):220–229, 2000 10910094

Alder J, Zanetti R, Wight E, et al: Sexual dysfunction after premenopausal stage I and II breast cancer: do androgens play a role? J Sex Med 5(8):1898–1906, 2008 18554258

American College of Obstetricians and Gynecologists: ACOG Practice Bulletin No. 141: management of menopausal symptoms. Obstet Gynecol 123(1):202–216, 2014 24463691

American College of Obstetricians and Gynecologists' Committee on Gynecologic Practice, Farrell R: ACOG Committee Opinion No. 659 Summary: the use of vaginal estrogen in women with a history of estrogen-dependent breast cancer. Obstet Gynecol 127(3):618–619, 2016 26901332

Anderson KD: Targeting recovery: priorities of the spinal cord-injured population. J Neurotrauma 21(10):1371–1383, 2004 15672628

Anderson KD, Borisoff JF, Johnson RD, et al: Long-term effects of spinal cord injury on sexual function in men: implications for neuroplasticity. Spinal Cord 45(5):338–348, 2007a 17016492

Anderson KD, Borisoff JF, Johnson RD, et al: Spinal cord injury influences psychogenic as well as physical components of female sexual ability. Spinal Cord 45(5):349–359, 2007b 17033619

Anyfanti P, Pyrpasopoulou A, Triantafyllou A, et al: Association between mental health disorders and sexual dysfunction in patients suffering from rheumatic diseases. J Sex Med 11(11):2653–2660, 2014 25124339

Atmaca M, Kuloglu M, Tezcan E: A new atypical antipsychotic: quetiapine-induced sexual dysfunctions. Int J Impot Res 17(2):201–203, 2005 15284834

Aziz A, Brännström M, Bergquist C, Silfverstolpe G: Perimenopausal androgen decline after oophorectomy does not influence sexuality or psychological well-being. Fertil Steril 83(4):1021–1028, 2005 15820815

Bancroft J: Sexual arousal and response: the psychosomatic circle, in Human Sexuality and Its Problems, 3rd Edition. Edited by Bancroft JHJ. Edinburgh, UK, Churchill, Livingstone, Elsevier, 2008, pp 96–106

Basaria S, Lieb J 2nd, Tang AM, et al: Long-term effects of androgen deprivation therapy in prostate cancer patients. Clin Endocrinol (Oxf) 56(6):779–786, 2002 12072048

Basson R: Human sex-response cycles. J Sex Marital Ther 27(1):33–43, 2001 11224952

Basson R, Schultz WW: Sexual sequelae of general medical disorders. Lancet 369(9559):409–424, 2007 17276781

Basson R, Smith KB: Incorporating mindfulness meditation into the treatment of provoked vestibulodynia. Current Sexual Health Reports 6(1):20–29, 2014. Available at: https://link.springer.com/article/10.1007/s11930-013-0008-0. Accessed May 28, 2017.

Basson R, Rees P, Wang R, et al: Sexual function in chronic illness. J Sex Med 7(1 Pt 2):374–388, 2010 20092445

Bennett N, Incrocci L, Baldwin D, et al: Cancer, benign gynecology, and sexual function—issues and answers. J Sex Med 13(4):519–537, 2016 27045256

Bergmark K, Avall-Lundqvist E, Dickman PW, et al: Vaginal changes and sexuality in women with a history of cervical cancer. N Engl J Med 340(18):1383–1389, 1999 10228188

Bhadauria S, Moser DK, Clements PJ, et al: Genital tract abnormalities and female sexual function impairment in systemic sclerosis. Am J Obstet Gynecol 172(2 Pt 1):580–587, 1995 7856689

Bhasin S, Enzlin P, Coviello A, et al: Sexual dysfunction in men and women with endocrine disorders. Lancet 369(9561):597–611, 2007 17307107

Boller F, Agrawal K, Romano A: Sexual function after strokes. Handb Clin Neurol 130:289–295, 2015 26003250

Bronner G, Vodušek DB: Management of sexual dysfunction in Parkinson's disease. Ther Adv Neurol Disord 4(6):375–383, 2011 22164191

Brotto LA, Basson R: Group mindfulness-based therapy significantly improves sexual desire in women. Behav Res Ther 57:43–54, 2014 24814472

Brotto LA, Basson R, Luria M: A mindfulness-based group psychoeducational intervention targeting sexual arousal disorder in women. J Sex Med 5(7):1646–1659, 2008a 18507718

Brotto LA, Heiman JR, Goff B, et al: A psychoeducational intervention for sexual dysfunction in women with gynecologic cancer. Arch Sex Behav 37(2):317–329, 2008b 17680353

Brotto LA, Heiman JR, Tolman DL: Narratives of desire in mid-age women with and without arousal difficulties. J Sex Res 46(5):387–398, 2009 19291528

Brotto LA, Basson R, Smith KB, et al: Mindfulness-based group therapy for women with provoked vestibulodynia. Mindfulness 6(3):417–432, 2015. Available at: https://link.springer.com/article/10.1007/s12671-013-0273-z. Accessed January 13, 2018.

Brown RG, Jahanshahi M, Quinn N, Marsden CD: Sexual function in patients with Parkinson's disease and their partners. J Neurol Neurosurg Psychiatry 53(6):480–486, 1990 2380728

Bruner DW, Lanciano R, Keegan M, et al: Vaginal stenosis and sexual function following intracavitary radiation for the treatment of cervical and endometrial carcinoma. Int J Radiat Oncol Biol Phys 27(4):825–830, 1993 8244811

Budoff MJ, Ellenberg SS, Lewis CE, et al: Testosterone treatment and coronary artery plaque volume in older men with low testosterone. JAMA 317(7):708–716, 2017 28241355

Busnelli A, Somigliana E, Vercellini P: "Forever Young"—testosterone replacement therapy: a blockbuster drug despite flabby evidence and broken promises. Hum Reprod 32(4):719–724, 2017 28333214

Canevelli M, Lucchini F, Garofalo C, et al: Inappropriate sexual behaviors among community-dwelling patients with dementia. Am J Geriatr Psychiatry 25(4):365–371, 2017 28017516

Carpenter LM, Nathanson CA, Kim YJ: Physical women, emotional men: gender and sexual satisfaction in midlife. Arch Sex Behav 38(1):87–107, 2009 17851747

Carr SV: Psychosexual health in gynecological cancer. Int J Gynaecol Obstet 131 (suppl 2):S159–S163, 2015 26433674

Chiles KA, Schlegel PN: Role for male reconstruction in the era of assisted reproductive technology. Fertil Steril 105(4):891–892, 2016 26945097

Chung E, Gillman M: Prostate cancer survivorship: a review of erectile dysfunction and penile rehabilitation after prostate cancer therapy. Med J Aust 200(10):582–585, 2014 24882489

Clayton AH, Warnock JK, Kornstein SG, et al: A placebo-controlled trial of bupropion SR as an antidote for selective serotonin reuptake inhibitor-induced sexual dysfunction. J Clin Psychiatry 65(1):62–67, 2004 14744170

Clayton A, Kornstein S, Prakash A, et al: Changes in sexual functioning associated with dulox-etine, escitalopram, and placebo in the treatment of patients with major depressive disorder. J Sex Med 4(4 Pt 1):917–929, 2007 17627739

Cordeau D, Courtois F: Sexual disorders in women with MS: assessment and management. Ann Phys Rehabil Med 57(5):337–347, 2014 24930089

Corney RH, Crowther ME, Everett H, et al: Psychosexual dysfunction in women with gynae-cological cancer following radical pelvic surgery. Br J Obstet Gynaecol 100(1):73–78, 1993 8427843

Courtois F, Charvier K: Sexual dysfunction in patients with spinal cord lesions. Handb Clin Neurol 130:225–245, 2015 26003247

Courtois F, Rodrigue X, Côté I, et al: Sexual function and autonomic dysreflexia in men with spinal cord injuries: how should we treat? Spinal Cord 50(12):869–877, 2012 22869221

Cramp JD, Courtois FJ, Ditor DS: Sexuality for women with spinal cord injury. J Sex Marital Ther 41(3):238–253, 2015 24325679

DeBusk R, Drory Y, Goldstein I, et al: Management of sexual dysfunction in patients with cardiovascular disease: recommendations of The Princeton Consensus Panel. Am J Cardiol 86(2):175–181, 2000 10913479

DeLamater JD, Sill M: Sexual desire in later life. J Sex Res 42(2):138–149, 2005 16123844

Devinsky O: Neurologist-induced sexual dysfunction: enzyme-inducing antiepileptic drugs. Neurology 65(7):980–981, 2005 16217046

De Giorgi R, Series H: Treatment of inappropriate sexual behavior in dementia. Curr Treat Options Neurol 18(9):41, 2016 27511056

Dobesberger J, Walser G, Unterberger I, et al: Genital automatisms: a video-EEG study in patients with medically refractory seizures. Epilepsia 45(7):777–780, 2004 15230701

Dossenbach M, Hodge A, Anders M, et al: Prevalence of sexual dysfunction in patients with schizophrenia: international variation and underestimation. Int J Neuropsychopharmacol 8(2):195–201, 2005 15631645

Doumas M, Douma S: Sexual dysfunction in essential hypertension: myth or reality? J Clin Hypertens (Greenwich) 8(4):269–274, 2006 16596030

Drory Y, Kravetz S, Weingarten M: Comparison of sexual activity of women and men after a first acute myocardial infarction. Am J Cardiol 85(11):1283–1287, 2000 10831940

Duggal N, Rabin D, Bartha R, et al: Brain reorganization in patients with spinal cord compression evaluated using fMRI. Neurology 74(13):1048–1054, 2010 20200344

Düsing R: Sexual dysfunction in male patients with hypertension: influence of antihypertensive drugs. Drugs 65(6):773–786, 2005 15819590

Enzlin P, Rosen R, Wiegel M, et al; DCCT/EDIC Research Group: Sexual dysfunction in women with type 1 diabetes: long-term findings from the DCCT/EDIC study cohort. Diabetes Care 32(5):780–785, 2009 19407075

Erwin-Toth P: The effect of ostomy surgery between the ages of 6 and 12 years on psychosocial development during childhood, adolescence, and young adulthood. J Wound Ostomy Continence Nurs 26(2):77–85, 1999 10373863

Evans AH, Lawrence AD, Potts J, et al: Factors influencing susceptibility to compulsive dopaminergic drug use in Parkinson disease. Neurology 65(10):1570–1574, 2005 16301483

Fallowfield L, Cella D, Cuzick J, et al: Quality of life of postmenopausal women in the Arimidex, Tamoxifen, Alone or in Combination (ATAC) Adjuvant Breast Cancer Trial. J Clin Oncol 22(21):4261–4271, 2004 15514369

Farquhar CM, Harvey SA, Yu Y, et al: A prospective study of 3 years of outcomes after hysterectomy with and without oophorectomy. Am J Obstet Gynecol 194(3):711–717, 2006 16522402

Finkelstein FO, Shirani S, Wuerth D, Finkelstein SH: Therapy Insight: sexual dysfunction in patients with chronic kidney disease. Nat Clin Pract Nephrol 3(4):200–207, 2007 17389889

Flyckt R, Falcone T: Fertility preservation in the female cancer patient, in Cancer and Fertility (Current Clinical Urology). Edited by Sabanegh ES. Basel, Switzerland, Springer International Publishing, 2016, pp 143–154

Flynn KE, Lin L, Bruner DW, et al: Sexual satisfaction and the importance of sexual health to quality of life throughout the life course of U.S. adults. J Sex Med 13(11):1642–1650, 2016 27671968

Fogari R, Zoppi A, Corradi L, et al: Sexual function in hypertensive males treated with lisinopril or atenolol: a cross-over study. Am J Hypertens 11(10):1244–1247, 1998 9799042

Fogari R, Preti P, Derosa G, et al: Effect of antihypertensive treatment with valsartan or atenolol on sexual activity and plasma testosterone in hypertensive men. Eur J Clin Pharmacol 58(3):177–180, 2002 12107602

Fogari R, Preti P, Zoppi A, et al: Effect of valsartan and atenolol on sexual behavior in hypertensive postmenopausal women. Am J Hypertens 17(1):77–81, 2004 14700518

Franzen D, Metha A, Seifert N, et al: Effects of beta-blockers on sexual performance in men with coronary heart disease. A prospective, randomized and double blinded study. Int J Impot Res 13(6):348–351, 2001 11918251

Freitas D, Athanazio R, Almeida D, et al: Sildenafil improves quality of life in men with heart failure and erectile dysfunction. Int J Impot Res 18(2):210–212, 2006 16121207

Gao X, Chen H, Schwarzschild MA, et al: Erectile function and risk of Parkinson's disease. Am J Epidemiol 166(12):1446–1450, 2007 17875583

Gazzaruso C, Giordanetti S, De Amici E, et al: Relationship between erectile dysfunction and silent myocardial ischemia in apparently uncomplicated type 2 diabetic patients. Circulation 110(1):22–26, 2004 15210604

Ghigo E, Masel B, Aimaretti G, et al: Consensus guidelines on screening for hypopituitarism following traumatic brain injury. Brain Inj 19(9):711–724, 2005 16195185

Giuseppe PG, Pace G, Vicentini C: Sexual function in women with urinary incontinence treated by pelvic floor transvaginal electrical stimulation. J Sex Med 4(3):702–707, 2007 17034409

Goldstein I: The mutually reinforcing triad of depressive symptoms, cardiovascular disease, and erectile dysfunction. Am J Cardiol 86(2A)(suppl):41F–45F, 2000 10899278

Guo M, Bosnyak S, Bontempo T, et al: Let's talk about sex!—improving sexual health for patients in stroke rehabilitation. BMJ Qual Improv Rep 4(1):ii, 2015 26734449

Hallinan R, Byrne A, Agho K, et al: Erectile dysfunction in men receiving methadone and buprenorphine maintenance treatment. J Sex Med 5(3):684–692, 2008 18093096

Hand A, Gray WK, Chandler BJ, Walker RW: Sexual and relationship dysfunction in people with Parkinson's disease. Parkinsonism Relat Disord 16(3):172–176, 2010 19892579

Healey EL, Haywood KL, Jordan KP, et al: Ankylosing spondylitis and its impact on sexual relationships. Rheumatology (Oxford) 48(11):1378–1381, 2009 19535610

Huffman LB, Hartenbach EM, Carter J, et al: Maintaining sexual health throughout gynecologic cancer survivorship: a comprehensive review and clinical guide. Gynecol Oncol 140(2):359–368, 2016 26556768

Humphreys CT, Tallman B, Altmaier EM, Barnette V: Sexual functioning in patients undergoing bone marrow transplantation: a longitudinal study. Bone Marrow Transplant 39(8):491–496, 2007 17322932

Huyghe E, Sui D, Odensky E, Schover LR: Needs assessment survey to justify establishing a reproductive health clinic at a comprehensive cancer center. J Sex Med 6(1):149–163, 2009 18823323

Incrocci L: Sexual function after external-beam radiotherapy for prostate cancer: what do we know? Crit Rev Oncol Hematol 57(2):165–173, 2006 16325413

Jackson G: Phosphodiesterase type-5 inhibitors in cardiovascular disease: experimental models and potential clinical applications. Eur Heart J Suppl 4 (suppl H):H19–H23, 2002

Janssen E, Everaerd W, Spiering M, Janssen J: Automatic processes and the appraisal of sexual stimuli: toward an information processing model of sexual arousal. J Sex Res 37(1):8–23, 2000

Janssen E, McBride KR, Yarber W, et al: Factors that influence sexual arousal in men: a focus group study. Arch Sex Behav 37(2):252–265, 2008 18040768

Kadıoğlu A, Ortaç M, Brock G: Pharmacologic and surgical therapies for sexual dysfunction in male cancer survivors. Transl Androl Urol 4(2):148–159, 2015 26816821

Katz A, Dizon DS: Sexuality after cancer: a model for male survivors. J Sex Med 13(1):70–78, 2016 2675508

Kaut O, Asmus F, Paus S: Spontaneous unwelcome orgasms due to pramipexole and ropini-role. Mov Disord 27(10):1327–1328, 2012 22903628

Kelly DF, McArthur DL, Levin H, et al: Neurobehavioral and quality of life changes associated with growth hormone insufficiency after complicated mild, moderate, or severe traumatic brain injury. J Neurotrauma 23(6):928–942, 2006 16774477

Kennedy SH, Dickens SE, Eisfeld BS, Bagby RM: Sexual dysfunction before antidepressant therapy in major depression. J Affect Disord 56(2–3):201–208, 1999 10701478

Kim SY, Kim SK, Lee JR, Woodruff TK: Toward precision medicine for preserving fertility in cancer patients: existing and emerging fertility preservation options for women. J Gynecol Oncol 27(2):e22, 2016 26768785

Klos KJ, Bower JH, Josephs KA, et al: Pathological hypersexuality predominantly linked to adjuvant dopamine agonist therapy in Parkinson's disease and multiple system atrophy. Parkinsonism Relat Disord 11(6):381–386, 2005 16109498

Knegtering H, Boks M, Blijd C, et al: A randomized open-label comparison of the impact of olanzapine versus risperidone on sexual functioning. J Sex Marital Ther 32(4):315–326, 2006 16709552

Ko DT, Hebert PR, Coffey CS, et al: Beta-blocker therapy and symptoms of depression, fatigue, and sexual dysfunction. JAMA 288(3):351–357, 2002 12117400

Kocsis A, Newbury-Helps J: Mindfulness in sex therapy and intimate relationships (MSIR): clinical protocol and theory development. Mindfulness 7(3):690–699, 2016. Available at: https://link.springer.com/article/10.1007/s12671-016-0506-z. Accessed May 28, 2017.

Komisaruk BR, Whipple B, Crawford A, et al: Brain activation during vaginocervical self-stimulation and orgasm in women with complete spinal cord injury: fMRI evidence of mediation by the vagus nerves. Brain Res 1024(1–2):77–88, 2004 15451368

Korfage IJ, Pluijm S, Roobol M, et al: Erectile dysfunction and mental health in a general population of older men. J Sex Med 6(2):505–512, 2009 19067789

Kornblith AB, Ligibel J: Psychosocial and sexual functioning of survivors of breast cancer. Semin Oncol 30(6):799–813, 2003 14663780

Kralik D, Koch T, Telford K: Constructions of sexuality for midlife women living with chronic illness. J Adv Nurs 35(2):180–187, 2001 11442697

Kummer A, Cardoso F, Teixeira AL: Loss of libido in Parkinson's disease. J Sex Med 6(4):1024–1031, 2009 19040621

Lauretti S, Cardaci V, Barrese F, Calzetta L: Chronic obstructive pulmonary disease (COPD) and erectile dysfunction (ED): results of the BRED observational study. Arch Ital Urol Androl 88(3):165–170, 2016 27711087

Levack WM, Weatherall M, Hay-Smith EJ, et al: Goal setting and strategies to enhance goal pursuit for adults with acquired disability participating in rehabilitation. Cochrane Database Syst Rev (7):CD009727, 2015 26189709

Likes WM, Stegbauer C, Tillmanns T, Pruett J: Pilot study of sexual function and quality of life after excision for vulvar intraepithelial neoplasia. J Reprod Med 52(1):23–27, 2007 17286063

Lindau ST, Abramsohn EM, Bueno H, et al: Sexual activity and counseling in the first month after acute myocardial infarction among younger adults in the United States and Spain: a prospective, observational study. Circulation 130(25):2302–2309, 2014 25512442

Macdonald S, Halliday J, MacEwan T, et al: Nithsdale Schizophrenia Surveys 24: sexual dysfunction. Case-control study. Br J Psychiatry 182:50–56, 2003 12509318

Meston CM, Buss DM: Why humans have sex. Arch Sex Behav 36(4):477–507, 2007 17610060

Meuleman EJ, van Lankveld JJ: Hypoactive sexual desire disorder: an underestimated condition in men. BJU Int 95(3):291–296, 2005 15679780

Miner M, Rosenberg MT, Perelman MA: Treatment of lower urinary tract symptoms in benign prostatic hyperplasia and its impact on sexual function. Clin Ther 28(1):13–25, 2006 16490576

Mize SJS: A review of mindfulness-based sex therapy interventions for sexual desire and arousal difficulties: from research to practice. Current Sexual Health Reports 7(2):89–97, 2015. Available at: https://link.springer.com/article/10.1007/s11930-015-0048-8. Accessed May 28, 2017.

Montorsi F, Briganti A, Salonia A, et al: Erectile dysfunction prevalence, time of onset and association with risk factors in 300 consecutive patients with acute chest pain and angiographically documented coronary artery disease. Eur Urol 44(3):360–364, discussion 364–365, 2003 12932937

Moreno A, Gan C, Zasler N, McKerral M: Experiences, attitudes, and needs related to sexuality and service delivery in individuals with traumatic brain injury. NeuroRehabilitation 37(1):99–116, 2015 26409696

Moskovic DJ, Mohamed O, Sathyamoorthy K, et al: The female factor: predicting compliance with a post-prostatectomy erectile preservation program. J Sex Med 7(11):3659–3665, 2010 20819141

Muller JE, Mittleman MA, Maclure M, et al; Determinants of Myocardial Infarction Onset Study Investigators: Triggering myocardial infarction by sexual activity. Low absolute risk and prevention by regular physical exertion. JAMA 275(18):1405–1409, 1996 8618365

Nurnberg HG, Fava M, Gelenberg AJ, et al: Open-label sildenafil treatment of partial and nonresponders to double-blind treatment in men with antidepressant-associated sexual dysfunction. Int J Impot Res 19(2):167–175, 2007 16871270

Oertel WH, Wächter T, Quinn NP, et al: Reduced genital sensitivity in female patients with multiple system atrophy of parkinsonian type. Mov Disord 18(4):430–432, 2003 12671951

Ohl DA, Carlsson M, Stecher VJ, Rippon GA: Efficacy and safety of sildenafil in men with sexual dysfunction and spinal cord injury. Sex Med Rev 5(4):521–528, 2017 28341580

Owens AF, Tepper MS: Chronic illnesses and disabilities affecting women's sexuality. Female Patient (Parsippany) 28(1):45–50, 2003

Paredes RG, Agmo A: Has dopamine a physiological role in the control of sexual behavior? A critical review of the evidence. Prog Neurobiol 73(3):179–226, 2004 15236835

Peak TC, Gur S, Hellstrom WJG: Diabetes and sexual function. Current Sexual Health Reports 8(1):9–18, 2016. Available at: https://link.springer.com/article/10.1007/s11930-016-0065-2. Accessed May 28, 2017.

Peng YS, Chiang CK, Kao TW, et al: Sexual dysfunction in female hemodialysis patients: a multicenter study. Kidney Int 68(2):760–765, 2005 16014053

Peng YS, Chiang CK, Hung KY, et al: The association of higher depressive symptoms and sexual dysfunction in male haemodialysis patients. Nephrol Dial Transplant 22(3):857–861, 2007 17121784

Penson DF, McLerran D, Feng Z, et al: 5-year urinary and sexual outcomes after radical prostatectomy: results from the prostate cancer outcomes study. J Urol 173(5):1701–1705, 2005 15821561

Pezzella FR, Colosimo C, Vanacore N, et al: Prevalence and clinical features of hedonistic homeostatic dysregulation in Parkinson's disease. Mov Disord 20(1):77–81, 2005 15390130

Pontiroli AE, Cortelazzi D, Morabito A: Female sexual dysfunction and diabetes: a systematic review and meta-analysis. J Sex Med 10(4):1044–1051, 2013 23347454

Prévinaire JG, Lecourt G, Soler JM, Denys P: Sexual disorders in men with multiple sclerosis: evaluation and management. Ann Phys Rehabil Med 57(5):329–336, 2014 24958443

Priori R, Minniti A, Derme M, et al: Quality of sexual life in women with primary Sjögren syndrome. J Rheumatol 42(8):1427–1431, 2015 26136488

Rees PM, Fowler CJ, Maas CP: Sexual function in men and women with neurological disorders. Lancet 369(9560):512–525, 2007 17292771

Reese JB, Finan PH, Haythornthwaite JA, et al: Gastrointestinal ostomies and sexual outcomes: a comparison of colorectal cancer patients by ostomy status. Support Care Cancer 22(2):461–468, 2014 24091721

Roehrborn CG, Siami P, Barkin J, et al; CombAT Study Group: The effects of dutasteride, tamsulosin and combination therapy on lower urinary tract symptoms in men with benign prostatic hyperplasia and prostatic enlargement: 2-year results from the CombAT study. J Urol 179(2):616–621, discussion 621, 2008 18082216

Sanchez C, Asin KE, Artigas F: Vortioxetine, a novel antidepressant with multimodal activity: review of preclinical and clinical data. Pharmacol Ther 145:43–57, 2015 25016186

Sarkar M, Wellons M, Cedars MI, et al: Testosterone levels in pre-menopausal women are associated with nonalcoholic fatty liver disease in midlife. Am J Gastroenterol 112(5):755–762, 2017 28291240

Schönhofer B, Von Sydow K, Bucher T, et al: Sexuality in patients with noninvasive mechanical ventilation due to chronic respiratory failure. Am J Respir Crit Care Med 164(9):1612–1617, 2001 11719298

Segraves RT, Lee J, Stevenson R, et al: Tadalafil for treatment of erectile dysfunction in men on antidepressants. J Clin Psychopharmacol 27(1):62–66, 2007 17224715

Soler JM, Previnaire JG, Plante P, et al: Midodrine improves ejaculation in spinal cord injured men. J Urol 178(5):2082–2086, 2007 17869290

Stevenson RW: Sexual medicine: why psychiatrists must talk to their patients about sex. Can J Psychiatry 49(10):673–677, 2004 15560313

Symms MR, Rawl SM, Grant M, et al: Sexual health and quality of life among male veterans with intestinal ostomies. Clin Nurse Spec 22(1):30–40, 2008 18091126

Syrjala KL, Kurland BF, Abrams JR, et al: Sexual function changes during the 5 years after high-dose treatment and hematopoietic cell transplantation for malignancy, with case-matched controls at 5 years. Blood 111(3):989–996, 2008 17878404

Teplin V, Vittinghoff E, Lin F, et al: Oophorectomy in premenopausal women: health-related quality of life and sexual functioning. Obstet Gynecol 109(2 Pt 1):347–354, 2007 17267835

Thakar R: Is the uterus a sexual organ? Sexual function following hysterectomy. Sex Med Rev 3(4):264–278, 2015 27784599

Tristano AG: The impact of rheumatic diseases on sexual function. Rheumatol Int 29(8):853–860, 2009 19152092

Tunn U: The current status of intermittent androgen deprivation (IAD) therapy for prostate cancer: putting IAD under the spotlight. BJU Int 99 (suppl 1):19–22, discussion 23–24, 2007 17229164

Turan O, Ure I, Turan PA: Erectile dysfunction in COPD patients. Chron Respir Dis 13(1):5–12, 2016 26647416

Tzortzis V, Skriapas K, Hadjigeorgiou G, et al: Sexual dysfunction in newly diagnosed multiple sclerosis women. Mult Scler 14(4):561–563, 2008 18710825

van Nimwegen JF, Arends S, van Zuiden GS, et al: The impact of primary Sjögren's syndrome on female sexual function. Rheumatology (Oxford) 54(7):1286–1293, 2015 25652072

Verdelho A, Gonçalves-Pereira M: Inappropriate sexual behaviors in dementia, in Neuropsychiatric Symptoms of Cognitive Impairment and Dementia. Cham, Switzerland, Springer International Publishing, 2017, pp 251–262

Wasner M, Bold U, Vollmer TC, Borasio GD: Sexuality in patients with amyotrophic lateral sclerosis and their partners. J Neurol 251(4):445–448, 2004 15083290

Weintraub D, Koester J, Potenza MN, et al: Impulse control disorders in Parkinson disease: a cross-sectional study of 3090 patients. Arch Neurol 67(5):589–595, 2010 20457959

West SL, D'Aloisio AA, Agans RP, et al: Prevalence of low sexual desire and hypoactive sexual desire disorder in a nationally representative sample of US women. Arch Intern Med 168(13):1441–1449, 2008 18625925

Yilmaz H, Yilmaz SD, Polat HA, et al: The effects of fibromyalgia syndrome on female sexuality: a controlled study. J Sex Med 9(3):779–785, 2012 22240036

Yoshino S, Fujimori J, Morishige T, Uchida S: Bilateral joint replacement of hip and knee joints in patients with rheumatoid arthritis. Arch Orthop Trauma Surg 103(1):1–4, 1984 6466058

Zivadinov R, Zorzon M, Bosco A, et al: Sexual dysfunction in multiple sclerosis, II: correlation analysis. Mult Scler 5(6):428–431, 1999 10618700

CHAPTER 16

Substance-Related Disorders

Michael Weaver, M.D., DFASAM

Psychiatric consultants in hospital settings often encounter patients with substance use disorders (SUDs). Patients who are intoxicated are more likely to be injured in traumatic accidents, and there is a significant association between having a SUD and injury from physical trauma. Risk-taking behavior associated with drug use can lead to sexually transmitted diseases and other infections, including those acquired through injection drug use (e.g., cellulitis, endocarditis, HIV, hepatitis C virus [HCV]). SUDs are more prevalent in patients who have depression or anxiety disorders or other psychiatric comorbidities (including personality disorders) and in those who use tobacco or alcohol. Patients with a dual diagnosis (i.e., both SUD and another major psychiatric disorder) may present with complex clinical histories and symptoms that make diagnosis challenging. Intoxication and withdrawal symptoms may be mistaken for other psychiatric or medical symptoms. Hospitalization may be prolonged by delirium due to intoxication or withdrawal.

Assessment

Prevalence rates for SUDs among hospitalized patients are 15%–30% (Katz et al. 2008), and rates are even higher among trauma patients or psychiatric inpatients. With rates this high, it is important to be alert for SUDs in inpatients. However, even careful assessment by clinicians looking for SUDs may not identify all current users. A combination of universal questionnaire screening and urine toxicology for those at high risk is more effective than either alone. Findings from physical examination and laboratory studies can provide important clues to SUDs (Tables 16–1 and 16–2). Although many of these findings can be caused by other diseases, the differential diagnosis should include SUD, and additional information can help verify this.

TABLE 16–1.   Physical examination indications of substance use disorders

Body system	Examination finding	Medical indication	Substance(s)
Eyes	Scleral icterus	Cirrhosis (alcoholic or viral)	Alcohol, any injected drug
	Conjunctival injection	Recent ingestion	Marijuana
	Pinpoint pupils	Opioid intoxication	Opioids
	Horizontal nystagmus	Acute intoxication	Alcohol
	Vertical nystagmus	Acute phencyclidine intoxication	Hallucinogen
Head and neck	Smell of alcohol on breath	Recent ingestion	Alcohol
	Nasal septal perforation	Snorting drugs	Stimulants
	Poor dentition	Inadequate oral hygiene	Stimulants, opioids
Cardiac	Irregular heart rhythm	Atrial fibrillation ("holiday heart")	Alcohol
	New murmur	Endocarditis from injection drug use	Opioids, stimulants, other injected drugs
	Tachycardia	Intoxication	Stimulants, marijuana
		Acute withdrawal	Alcohol
Abdomen	Enlarged, tender liver	Acute hepatitis (alcoholic or viral)	Alcohol, any injected drug
	Shrunken, hard, or nodular liver	Cirrhosis (alcoholic or viral)	Alcohol, any injected drug
	Caput medusae	Cirrhosis (alcoholic or viral)	Alcohol, any injected drug
	Epigastric tenderness	Pancreatitis, gastritis	Alcohol
	Enlarged colon	Constipation	Opioids
Extremities	Tremulousness, hyperreflexia	Acute withdrawal	Alcohol
	Ataxia	Acute intoxication	Alcohol
		Wernicke's encephalopathy	Alcohol
	Reduced light touch sensation	Peripheral neuropathy	Alcohol
	Reduced strength	Muscle atrophy	Alcohol
Skin	Jaundice	Cirrhosis (alcoholic or viral)	Alcohol, any injected drug
	Spider angiomas	Cirrhosis (alcoholic or viral)	Alcohol, any injected drug
	Track marks, fresh needle marks	Injection drug use	Opioids, stimulants, other injected drugs

TABLE 16–2. Laboratory indications of substance use disorders			
Laboratory test	**Change in result**	**Medical indication**	**Substance(s)**
Albumin	Reduced	Malnutrition, cirrhosis	Any
Blood alcohol level	Alcohol present	Recent alcohol ingestion	Alcohol
Folate	Reduced	Malnutrition	Alcohol
International normalized ratio, prothrombin time	Increased	Cirrhosis (alcoholic or viral)	Alcohol, any injected drug
Mean corpuscular volume	Increased	Bone marrow suppression, B_{12} deficiency	Alcohol
Thiamine	Reduced	Wernicke-Korsakoff syndrome	Alcohol
Transaminases (alanine aminotransferase, aspartate aminotransferase)	Increased	Acute hepatitis (alcoholic or viral)	Alcohol, any injected drug
Urine drug test	Positive	Recent drug use	Any
White blood cell count	Reduced	Bone marrow suppression, human immunodeficiency virus	Alcohol, any injected drug

A good general health history can elicit risk factors for SUDs. Erratic occupational history, relational problems with partners and children, accidents, burns and fractured bones, and charges for driving under the influence may be clues to probe further into possible SUD. A simple screening tool for problems with alcohol use is the CAGE questionnaire (questions about Cutting down, Annoyance with criticism, Guilty feelings, and Eye-openers), which has been modified for screening for drug use and is known as the CAGE-AID (Adapted to Include Drugs) questionnaire (Brown and Rounds 1995). The more responses that are affirmative, the more likely that the person answering has an SUD warranting further investigation by the clinician.

Asking directly about alcohol and drug use is important and even therapeutic for the patient. Often, the clinician should ask first about socially accepted substances, such as nicotine and caffeine (coffee, tea, soda, and energy drinks). This will establish an initial level of comfort for the patient in addressing questions about use of substances. The clinician should inquire next about alcohol use. Specifically, the clinician should ask about beer, wine, and whiskey, because many patients do not consider beer to be "alcohol," which they equate with hard liquor. The clinician should then ask about misuse of over-the-counter and prescription medications. Finally, the clinician should ask about illicit drugs. By this time, the patient will have a sense that the practitioner is soliciting information in a nonjudgmental fashion for the purpose of helping. The clinician should ask about cannabis (marijuana) first, because its use is prevalent, carries less social stigma, and is legal in some states. Inquiries should then be made about cocaine and heroin use, as well as other illicit substances. The amount of money spent on a daily, weekly, or monthly basis for drugs also may be used to quantify drug use. It is important to ask whether the patient has ever injected drugs in the past or shared needles.

In the United States, many states require hospitals to report pregnant women suspected of heavy alcohol or other drug use to local public health authorities when the women present for delivery. Two states (Illinois and Minnesota) require reporting before delivery for referral to treatment; the other states and federal law require only reporting at birth (the newborn is not legally an independent citizen until birth) (Child Welfare Information Gateway 2016). This reporting requirement may cause women to be even more wary of acknowledging that they have a problem (Weaver et al. 2014b). In many cases across the nation, legislators and the courts have ruled that SUD in pregnancy is not a criminal matter, and there is no evidence that punitive approaches work. The federal Child Abuse Prevention and Treatment Act requires states to have policies and procedures to notify Child Protective Services of substance-exposed newborns (Child Welfare Information Gateway 2016). The mandate to report varies significantly, so clinicians should be familiar with legislation in their state and community.

Some patients are able to use illicit substances while hospitalized. They may bring in drugs and paraphernalia at admission in clothing, or visitors may bring drugs to a patient during the inpatient stay. Occasionally, a patient may obtain drugs from another patient or from hospital personnel. Substance intoxication may present with altered mental status, unexpected resolution of withdrawal symptoms, or a change in patient behavior. Drug use while in the hospital may be verified by urine drug testing, especially confirmatory testing for specific substances not prescribed. Hospital security personnel may be able to search the room and possibly the patient's belongings.

The hospital's risk management department should be notified of any illicit drug use on the premises by a patient. Depending on circumstances, this need not result in a drastic response such as immediate discharge of the patient but may be used as an opportunity for brief intervention to address the seriousness of the patient's addiction (Jewell et al. 2011).

Substance-Related Disorders

Alcohol and Sedatives

In the United States, 90% of men and 70% of women consume alcohol (Johnston et al. 2002) in the form of beer, wine, or liquor. Alcohol use disorders (AUDs) result in 25,000 deaths per year from accidents and 175,000 deaths annually from heart disease, cancer, and suicide (Schuckit and Tapert 2004).

In addition to alcohol, sedative drugs include benzodiazepines, barbiturates, and other sleeping pills. The newer medications zolpidem, zaleplon, and eszopiclone act on the benzodiazepine subtype 1 receptor (Richardson and Roth 2001) and thus are similar to typical benzodiazepines (e.g., diazepam, alprazolam). Zolpidem and eszopiclone abuse is relatively rare in comparison with benzodiazepine abuse, but patients with a history of SUD or psychiatric comorbidity are at higher risk for abuse of these medications (Hajak et al. 2003).

Intoxication

The clinical features of acute sedative (including alcohol) intoxication are slurred speech, incoordination, unsteady gait, and impaired attention or memory; severe overdose may lead to stupor or coma. Psychiatric manifestations include inappropriate behavior, labile mood, and impaired judgment. Physical signs include nystagmus and decreased reflexes.

A benzodiazepine antagonist, flumazenil, is available for the treatment of acute benzodiazepine intoxication. Nausea and vomiting are its most common side effects. It may not completely reverse respiratory depression and may provoke withdrawal seizures in patients with benzodiazepine dependence (Penninga et al. 2016). Flumazenil should be withheld in patients with a history of or current seizures and in patients who have overdosed on drugs that lower the seizure threshold. Flumazenil should not routinely be administered to comatose patients when the identity of the ingested drug(s) is not certain. Repeat doses should be administered slowly in patients who are physically dependent on benzodiazepines. Flumazenil is short acting, and sedation may recur after an initial awakening. This can be treated by repeating doses at 20-minute intervals as needed.

Withdrawal

Patients may develop an acute alcohol withdrawal syndrome when chronic alcohol use is interrupted by hospital admission. An identical syndrome occurs in patients chronically taking benzodiazepines or other sedatives if the medication is discontinued during admission. Acute withdrawal is most safely managed in an inpatient setting if the patient has been using high doses of sedatives, has a history of seizures or delirium tremens, or has unstable comorbid medical or psychiatric problems (Saitz

1998). The severity of the withdrawal syndrome is affected by concurrent medical illness. Up to 20% of patients develop delirium tremens if left untreated (Cross and Hennessey 1993). Recognition and effective treatment of alcohol withdrawal are important to prevent mortality or prolonged hospitalization resulting from complications.

Even when patients acknowledge heavy drinking, they often underestimate the amount, which may be because of minimization or because alcohol is an amnestic agent, and drinkers quickly lose count of how much they have had to drink. It is simplest to ask all patients admitted to the hospital in a nonjudgmental manner about drinking and to be alert for signs of acute alcohol withdrawal. Individual variability in the threshold at which a patient may develop withdrawal is significant, and those who drink most days of the week are more likely to develop withdrawal as a result of tolerance. Not all daily drinkers will develop withdrawal, but it is difficult to predict who will. The best predictor of whether a patient will develop acute withdrawal while hospitalized is a history of acute alcohol withdrawal.

The alcohol withdrawal syndrome has two phases: early withdrawal and late withdrawal (Table 16–3). The signs and symptoms of early withdrawal usually develop within 48 hours of the last drink. This time frame may be prolonged if the patient has taken long-acting sedatives or accelerated in extremely heavy users. The initial indication of withdrawal is an elevation of vital signs (heart rate, blood pressure, temperature). Tremors develop next: first, a fine tremor of the hands and fasciculation of the tongue, sometimes followed by gross tremors of the extremities. Disorientation and mild hallucinations (often auditory, occasionally visual) may develop as the syndrome progresses, accompanied by diaphoresis.

Late alcohol withdrawal is also known as *delirium tremens* ("the DTs") and consists of worsening autonomic dysregulation that is responsible for much of the morbidity and mortality attributed to alcohol withdrawal. It begins after early withdrawal, usually 72 hours or more after the last drink, and peaks around 5 days (Schuckit 2014).

Some patients do not progress from early to late withdrawal, and the symptoms simply subside after a few days with or without treatment, but it is impossible to predict which patients will progress. The signs of late withdrawal consist of worsening diaphoresis; nausea and vomiting (which may result in aspiration pneumonia); delirium with frank hallucinations; and rapid, severe fluctuation in vital signs. Sudden changes in blood pressure and heart rate may result in complications such as myocardial infarction or a cerebrovascular event, and increased QT variability elevates the risk for serious cardiac arrhythmias (Bär et al. 2007). Hyperthermia is also associated with higher mortality. Progression to late withdrawal results in significant morbidity and even death, but adequate treatment of early withdrawal helps prevent progression to late withdrawal (Schuckit 2014).

The revised Clinical Institute Withdrawal Assessment for Alcohol (CIWA-Ar) is commonly used to assess severity of withdrawal (Sullivan et al. 1989). It can be used to determine an appropriate pharmacotherapy dose for patients in withdrawal who also have other medical illnesses (Weaver et al. 2006). Regular assessments should continue until the withdrawal syndrome has been under control (CIWA-Ar score <6) for at least 24 hours. If no withdrawal signs have manifested after 48 hours, then it is usually safe to discontinue monitoring for withdrawal. Standardized algorithms with frequent assessment for signs of withdrawal also facilitate efficient treatment of postoperative patients at risk for withdrawal (Lansford et al. 2008).

TABLE 16–3. **Alcohol withdrawal signs**

Sign	Early withdrawal	Late withdrawal (delirium tremens)
Onset	<48 hours after last drink	After onset of early withdrawal
Heart rate	80–110 beats/minute	>120 beats/minute
Temperature	<101.5°F	>101.5°F
Blood pressure	Slight increase (especially systolic)	Significant hypotension or hypertension
Respiratory rate	12–20 breaths/minute	>20 breaths/minute
Tremors	Fine tremor of hands and tongue	Gross tremors, all extremities
Consciousness	Agitated	Delirious
Orientation	Mildly disoriented	Completely disoriented
Hallucinations	Mild auditory and/or visual	Visual, auditory, tactile
Seizures	Possible	Unusual

Pharmacotherapy is indicated for management of moderate to severe withdrawal, and any cross-tolerant medication may be used. It is inappropriate to give beverage alcohol to prevent or treat alcohol withdrawal. Use of intravenous alcohol infusion is reserved for poisoning with methanol, isopropanol, or ethylene glycol and should not be given for treatment of acute alcohol withdrawal because of complications such as intoxication with delirium or development of gastritis (Weaver 2007). Both benzodiazepines and barbiturates effectively treat alcohol withdrawal (Mayo-Smith and American Society of Addiction Medicine Working Group on Pharmacological Management of Alcohol Withdrawal 1997). In the United States, alcohol withdrawal is most often managed with benzodiazepines, but barbiturates also have been used successfully to treat acute alcohol withdrawal syndrome in general medical inpatients, with phenobarbital the most common choice. Its long half-life provides some protection if the patient leaves the hospital prematurely (Mo et al. 2016; Weaver et al. 2009). Several alternative non-sedative-hypnotic medications are available for the treatment of acute alcohol withdrawal. Beta-adrenergic blockers (atenolol, propranolol), clonidine, and anticonvulsant agents (carbamazepine, valproate) decrease alcohol withdrawal symptoms and have been used successfully in treatment of mild withdrawal. However, they are not cross-tolerant with alcohol and may result in progression of the withdrawal syndrome. These alternative medications are not appropriate as single agents to treat moderate or severe withdrawal.

In addition to pharmacotherapy for alcohol withdrawal, some patients need intravenous glucose, because many individuals with AUD are hypoglycemic as a result of poor diet and hepatic dysfunction. It is essential to administer thiamine and folate (see discussion below), as well as magnesium and phosphate, before or concurrently with glucose.

Severe withdrawal (delirium tremens), manifested by abnormal and fluctuating vital signs with delirium, should be treated aggressively in an intensive care environment with sufficiently large doses of medication to suppress the withdrawal (Weaver 2007). Medications with a rapid onset of action should be used intravenously for immediate effect. Lorazepam and diazepam have a rapid onset of action when given intravenously, although the duration of action is shorter than when given orally. For example, lorazepam (1–4 mg every 10–30 minutes) should be given until the patient is calm but awake and the heart rate is less than 120 beats/minute (Weaver 2007). A continuous intravenous infusion may be warranted to control withdrawal symptoms, and the infusion rate can be titrated to the desired level of consciousness. After the patient is stabilized, the clinician can substitute an equivalent dose of a long-acting sedative-hypnotic that will be tapered.

Up to 40% of patients admitted to intensive care units (ICUs) have an AUD, and withdrawal is associated with prolonged lengths of stay (Moss and Burnham 2006). Prevention strategies include screening of ICU patients for SUDs and assessment for development of acute withdrawal syndromes (de Wit et al. 2008). The key to treating withdrawal syndromes in the ICU is to anticipate that they may occur and treat them vigorously to prevent new problems in critically ill patients (Weaver and Schnoll 1996). No specific benzodiazepine is superior to any other for alcohol withdrawal treatment in the ICU, although longer-acting benzodiazepines may allow for a smoother withdrawal course. Severe alcohol withdrawal that is refractory to high-dose benzodiazepines has been treated successfully with the addition of phenobarbital (Gold et al. 2007), propofol (Brotherton et al. 2016), dexmedetomidine (Linn and Loeser 2015), baclofen (Liu and Wang 2015), and even ketamine (Wong et al. 2015).

Patients who abuse alcohol often have some degree of liver dysfunction when admitted to the hospital, either from acute alcohol-induced hepatitis or from cirrhosis due to long-term consumption. Hepatically metabolized sedatives such as benzodiazepines and barbiturates may worsen hepatic encephalopathy in patients with cirrhosis. These medications should be used with caution to avoid adverse outcomes from accumulation of metabolites requiring liver metabolism. Lorazepam, temazepam, and oxazepam are intermediate-acting benzodiazepines that have no active metabolites (hepatic metabolism of these involves only glucuronidation for excretion), unlike other benzodiazepines, which makes them safer in severe liver disease. Despite the long half-life and metabolism by the liver, phenobarbital is still safe to use for patients with liver disease who are not at risk for hepatic encephalopathy because approximately 30% is excreted unchanged in the urine (Hadama et al. 2001). This is an advantage over most long-acting benzodiazepines (e.g., chlordiazepoxide and diazepam), which undergo extensive liver metabolism to additional active metabolites (Olkkola and Ahonen 2008).

Effects on Medical Disorders

An individual with AUD reduces his or her life span by 10–15 years. Chronic alcohol use causes many potential medical problems, including cardiovascular disease, liver damage, and cancer (alcohol is a known teratogen). AUDs are independent risk factors for the development of community-acquired pneumonia (de Roux et al. 2006). Magnesium excretion is increased by alcohol intake, so magnesium repletion is important to prevent hypokalemia, which can lead to acute cardiac arrhythmias and muscle weakness (Elisaf et al. 2002). AUD is also associated with persistent vascular endothelial damage leading to atherosclerosis, with complications such as hypertension and other cardiovascular diseases; this heightened cardiovascular and metabolic risk persists even after 2 years of abstinence (Di Gennaro et al. 2007). Behavior problems may occur in hospitalized patients with AUD, including surgical patients. These may include agitation, sleep disturbances, and verbal abuse (Williams et al. 2008). Alcohol also interacts with many different medications in many ways (Table 16–4).

Patients with AUD have longer surgical ICU lengths of stay, higher rates of ICU readmission, and increased risk of death (Clark et al. 2013). A history of alcohol use is an important independent risk factor for delirium and other neurocognitive complications in an ICU setting (Dubois et al. 2001). Acute intoxication or withdrawal from other substances may result in delirium and can be easily missed by failing to obtain a full history of substance use from the patient or family members or by failing to use urine or blood toxicology testing on admission. Even patients admitted with minor injuries have higher morbidity, with significantly longer hospital lengths of stay, including ICU stays with days on mechanical ventilation (Bard et al. 2006), when they have AUD. Alcohol use results in postoperative complications, especially from development of alcohol withdrawal syndrome (Salottolo et al. 2017), so patients at risk for alcohol withdrawal should have elective surgical procedures postponed until they have achieved 7–10 days of abstinence (Bard et al. 2006); if this is not feasible, adequate prophylaxis for alcohol withdrawal should be provided.

AUD leads to vitamin deficiency states as a result of reduced transport across the intestinal lining, reduced capacity of the liver to store vitamins, and poor nutrition (Thomson 2000). Vitamin repletion, especially thiamine and folate, is important for all patients with AUD. Wernicke's encephalopathy results from thiamine deficiency and consists of ophthalmoplegia, ataxia, and altered mental status; this may be difficult to differentiate from acute alcohol intoxication. It is a medical emergency requiring immediate treatment with parenteral thiamine to prevent development of Korsakoff's syndrome, the irreversible form of thiamine deficiency consisting of chronic loss of working memory accompanied by confabulation (Sechi and Serra 2007). Thiamine must be given before or concurrently with intravenous glucose because giving glucose alone to a thiamine-deficient patient can precipitate Wernicke's encephalopathy due to thalamic neuronal damage (Thomson et al. 2002). High-dose thiamine (≥ 500 mg)—given intravenously three times a day for 2–3 days initially—is safe and effective, and additional doses are based on clinical response (Nishimoto et al. 2017).

Pharmacological Treatment

Three medications have been approved by the U.S. Food and Drug Administration (FDA) for treatment of alcohol dependence. Disulfiram acts as an aversive agent by inhibition of aldehyde dehydrogenase, which prevents metabolism of alcohol to acetaldehyde. Ingestion of alcohol results in accumulation of acetaldehyde in the blood, leading to nausea and vomiting, flushing, palpitations, dyspnea, hypotension, headache, and sympathetic overactivity. This reaction to alcohol consumption discourages further drinking. Metronidazole has been reported to cause a disulfiram-like effect when alcohol is consumed while taking it, but this has been disputed; however, it is recommended that patients avoid alcohol while taking metronidazole and for at least 48 hours after stopping it (Williams and Woodcock 2000).

Naltrexone affects alcohol consumption through blockade of opioid receptors because some reinforcing effects of alcohol are mediated through the endogenous opioid system. Naltrexone reduces the pleasurable effects of alcohol, which reduces the risk of relapse, especially among those with a family history of alcoholism and those with strong cravings (Jarosz et al. 2013). Naltrexone is available as a daily pill or as a

TABLE 16–4.   Interactions between alcohol and medications

Medication	Clinical interaction
Warfarin, oral anticoagulants	Acute: increased anticoagulant effect Chronic: decreased anticoagulant effect
Chlorpropamide Disulfiram Griseofulvin Metronidazole Quinacrine	Nausea and vomiting, flushing, palpitations, dyspnea, hypotension, headache, and sympathetic overactivity
Diazepam	Increased sedation (increased absorption)
Antihistamines Benzodiazepines Opioids	Increased sedation
Chloral hydrate Chlorpromazine Cimetidine	Increased intoxication (decreased alcohol metabolism)

monthly intramuscular depot injection given in a physician's office. Because naltrexone is an opioid blocker, treatment of acute or postoperative pain can be challenging in a patient who is using naltrexone for treatment of AUD. For unexpected severe pain such as trauma, nonopioid analgesics should be considered, including nonsteroidal anti-inflammatory agents, or local anesthesia with a nerve block or epidural catheter can be used (Vickers and Jolly 2006). It also may be feasible to titrate typical opioid analgesics upward to patient comfort under medical observation without causing oversedation or respiratory depression.

Acamprosate antagonizes N-methyl-D-aspartate glutamate receptors, restoring balance between excitatory and inhibitory neurotransmission that was deregulated by chronic alcohol consumption, which reduces negative affect and craving during abstinence (Plosker 2015). Acamprosate has no known drug interactions. Compared with disulfiram and naltrexone, which have multiple drug interactions and potential complications (hepatotoxicity), acamprosate may be a good choice for patients with medical and/or psychiatric comorbidities, especially those taking other medications.

Timely follow-up after hospitalization is essential to monitor effectiveness and adverse effects of medications for abstinence. For patients who are motivated to remain abstinent, one of these medications may be started in the inpatient setting, but only if a practitioner is identified to continue it in the outpatient setting.

Opioids

In 2014, more than 10 million people in the United States used prescription opioids for nonmedical purposes (Center for Behavioral Health Statistics and Quality 2016). From 2000 to 2014, opioid overdose deaths quadrupled. In 2014, for the first time, opioid overdose exceeded automobile crashes as a cause of death (Compton et al. 2016), and more than 33,000 people died from opioid overdoses in the United States in 2015. Eighty percent of new heroin users report previous misuse of prescription opioids (Jones 2013).

Intoxication

Acute opioid intoxication is characterized by decreased level of consciousness, substantially decreased respiration, miotic pupils, and absent bowel sounds. Prescription opioid analgesics can lead to intoxication or overdose. Oral controlled-release oxycodone is ingested by crushing the tablets and then snorting the powder; when taken in this way by people who have no tolerance to the drug, a single 80-mg dose (the highest strength available in a single tablet) can be fatal. Illicit fentanyl is 100 times more potent than morphine, and the recent practice of adding it to heroin, often without the knowledge of the user, has resulted in overdose or death (Frank and Pollack 2017). Meperidine or tramadol can cause seizures in overdose. Meperidine, in particular, can cause an agitated delirium due to accumulation of normeperidine, which is a neuroexcitatory toxic metabolite; this is most prevalent in patients with acute or chronic renal impairment and results in reduced clearance of normeperidine (Adunsky et al. 2002).

Opioid overdose is treated with naloxone, given intravenously at an initial dose of 0.4 mg, but if no response is seen in 3–5 minutes, additional doses can be given up to a total of 1–2 mg. The duration of action of naloxone is 20–40 minutes, so repeated doses or a continuous infusion may be necessary for patients who have taken long-acting opioids such as methadone.

Withdrawal

The physical signs of opioid withdrawal are very distinctive and include nausea, vomiting, abdominal pain, diarrhea, myalgias, piloerection, restlessness, lacrimation, rhinorrhea, and yawning. The time of onset after last use is fairly consistent (about 8 hours for short-acting opioids such as heroin or oxycodone), which is a prominent factor in repeated administration after development of tolerance. This is in contrast to delirium tremens from alcohol and sedatives, in which minor signs of acute withdrawal often do not progress to severe withdrawal; onset and severity of opioid withdrawal are consistent and predictable for the vast majority of daily users. Opioid withdrawal is treated with substitution of a long-acting opioid (methadone or buprenorphine) for detoxification over several days.

Hospitalization is usually unnecessary for opioid withdrawal alone unless the patient has concurrent medical or psychiatric illness that warrants hospitalization (e.g., unstable angina, brittle diabetes mellitus, suicidality). Methadone is frequently used to treat acute withdrawal from opioids, but current U.S. federal regulations restrict the use of methadone for treatment of opioid use disorder (OUD). Methadone may be used by a physician for temporary maintenance or detoxification when a patient with OUD is admitted to a hospital for an illness other than OUD. A method of titrating the amount of methadone based on symptoms has been used extensively to titrate methadone for opioid withdrawal, without causing oversedation or severe patient discomfort (Weaver et al. 1999). The patient should be evaluated and the symptom score reassessed every 6 hours for the first 24 hours. After 24 hours, the total dose of methadone administered is calculated; this dose is approximately equivalent to the dose of opioid the individual was taking. After being stabilized on this dose of methadone for 24 hours, the patient can be tapered off by approximately 10%–20% per day. The duration of action of methadone allows it to be given once daily as a single dose (when treating opioid withdrawal in contrast to pain treatment). Most patients do not experience euphoria with methadone administration.

Buprenorphine is also used to treat opioid withdrawal. It is classified as a Schedule III controlled substance and may only be prescribed in the United States by certified and specially trained physicians who have registered with the Center for Substance Abuse Treatment (1993) of the Substance Abuse and Mental Health Services Administration (SAMHSA; information on the training and registration process is available at www.buprenorphine.samhsa.gov). As is done with methadone, buprenorphine may be prescribed for temporary maintenance or detoxification when a patient with OUD is admitted to a hospital for an illness other than OUD. When a patient develops opioid withdrawal symptoms (at least 5 points on the Clinical Opiate Withdrawal Scale [Wesson and Ling 2003]), a small dose of buprenorphine (2–4 mg) is given sublingually and the patient is monitored closely for improvement in symptoms. Additional small doses are given every 1–2 hours until withdrawal signs have subsided. After stabilization, buprenorphine can be given sublingually once daily and tapered off by approximately 10%–20% per day.

Clonidine is not approved by the FDA for the treatment of opioid withdrawal, although it is commonly used for this purpose. A transdermal clonidine patch is effective for mild withdrawal symptoms and can be left on the skin for 7 days. Typical oral clonidine protocols use 0.1–0.3 mg of clonidine every 2–4 hours for the first 24 hours, usually 0.8–1.2 mg/day. Subsequently, clonidine is given three to four times a day, with the total daily dose reduced by 0.1 or 0.2 mg on each subsequent day. The total duration for this regimen is 10–14 days. It is important to monitor for hypotension during clonidine therapy and then to taper clonidine gradually to avoid hypertensive rebound (Gowing et al. 2004). Clonidine should be avoided in hypotensive patients (systolic blood pressure <100 mm Hg). In addition to orthostatic hypotension, side effects of clonidine include sedation, dry mouth, and constipation; these are more likely at higher doses.

Other medications may provide relief of other symptoms of opioid withdrawal: muscle relaxants for spasms and twitching, nonsteroidal anti-inflammatory drugs for aches, antiemetics for nausea, loperamide or bismuth subsalicylate for diarrhea, and a sleeping medication with low abuse potential (e.g., trazodone) for insomnia.

Opioid withdrawal syndrome during pregnancy can lead to fetal distress and premature labor as a result of increased oxygen consumption by both the mother and the fetus (Cooper et al. 1983). Even minimal symptoms in the mother may indicate fetal distress, because the fetus may be more susceptible to withdrawal symptoms. Buprenorphine has now emerged as a first-line medication alongside methadone (World Health Organization 2014). Naloxone should not be administered to a pregnant woman except as a last resort for severe opioid overdose, because withdrawal precipitated by an opioid antagonist can result in spontaneous abortion, premature labor, or stillbirth.

Effects on Medical Disorders

Even infrequent heroin use is associated with a 3.5-fold excess risk of mortality, with the cause of death most commonly infections or injury (Lopez-Quintero et al. 2015). Chronic infection with HCV can lead to cirrhosis, and the rate of HCV infection among methadone maintenance (MM) patients is 70% (Weaver et al. 2005). Accurate data about drug and alcohol use among patients with liver disease or liver transplant candidates are difficult to obtain because patients underreport because they believe that divulging this information will harm their chances of receiving further care, especially access to a liver transplant (Weinrieb et al. 2000). It is inappropriate to require patients who are stable on methadone or buprenorphine to discontinue this treatment before any surgical procedure or other intervention.

Individuals admitted to the hospital with opioid dependence may have pain from various sources, including trauma or infection. Acute opioid withdrawal syndrome also may be painful because of myalgias and intestinal cramping. Adequate treatment of pain with opioid analgesics will also ameliorate opioid withdrawal signs. It may be difficult to distinguish pain due to opioid withdrawal from pain due to other causes; the best course of action is to give the patient the benefit of the doubt and provide appropriate amounts of opioid analgesics to treat complaints of pain adequately (Weaver and Schnoll 2002). Sedation and mild reduction in respiratory rate are indicators that the pain and withdrawal are adequately being treated; additional requests for opioids despite these signs may indicate that the patient is seeking higher doses in an attempt to achieve euphoria beyond relief of pain and withdrawal symptoms. Narcotic bowel syndrome is a form of bowel hyperalgesia with chronic or recurring abdominal pain that is worsened with continued or escalating dosages of opioids (Drossman and Szigethy 2014); improvement in symptoms is observed after gradual tapering and discontinuation of opioids (see Chapter 19, "Gastrointestinal Disorders," for discussion of narcotic bowel syndrome).

Some opioids, including tramadol, meperidine, dextromethorphan, and methadone, are weak serotonin reuptake inhibitors (Gillman 2005). When given—especially at high doses—with monoamine oxidase inhibitors or other serotonergic drugs, they can cause serotonin syndrome (see Chapter 36, "Psychopharmacology"). Opioids that do not have serotonin activity are morphine, oxycodone, and buprenorphine; these would be better choices for patients taking other serotonergic medications.

Pharmacological Treatment

Prescribing methadone for withdrawal or long-term treatment of OUD requires a special state and federal license; however, methadone can be prescribed in the United States for treatment of acute or chronic pain by any physician with a Drug Enforcement Administration (DEA) license, similar to laws for other Schedule II medications. If an MM client is hospitalized, such as for a traumatic injury or medical illness, the maintenance dose should be continued throughout hospitalization. The hospital physician should contact the MM program to verify the client's current dose and arrange for dosing to resume after discharge.

Acutely ill or injured MM patients experience the same pain despite receiving methadone because methadone reaches steady-state levels in the body and does not provide additional analgesia. Patients receiving MM with acute pain should be treated for pain with opioid or nonopioid medications, as would be appropriate if they were not receiving MM. The patient's usual MM dose should be continued and additional short-acting opioid analgesics administered. Higher-than-usual opioid analgesic doses may be required because of opioid cross-tolerance (Alford et al. 2006). If the patient cannot take oral medication, methadone can be given by the intramuscular or subcutaneous route. The parenteral dose should be given as one-half to two-thirds of the maintenance dose, divided into two to four equal doses per day. Mixed agonist and antagonist opioid analgesics, such as pentazocine, nalbuphine, and butorphanol, should not be administered because they precipitate acute withdrawal and block the analgesic effects of agonist opioids.

Many different medications affect methadone metabolism, primarily because it is metabolized by cytochrome P450 3A4. Risperidone, carbamazepine, rifampicin, and many antiretrovirals can lower serum methadone levels, resulting in opioid withdrawal symptoms. These interactions usually do not have life-threatening consequences for patients, other than acute discomfort and risk of relapse to OUD (Ferrari et al. 2004). Diazepam, fluoxetine, and erythromycin can elevate methadone serum levels and increase the risk of opioid intoxication. Methadone can prolong the QTc interval. A dose relation has been observed between methadone and QTc interval, with most problems occurring at dosages greater than 100 mg/day (Stallvik et al. 2013). Torsades de pointes has been reported with very high doses of methadone in outpatient settings, occurring in a few patients who had risk factors for arrhythmias. The risk of QTc prolongation is increased when methadone is given intravenously; is used in conjunction with other QTc-prolonging drugs (e.g., antipsychotics, amiodarone, erythromycin) or drugs that inhibit cytochrome P450 3A4; and is administered to patients with hypokalemia, hypocalcemia, hypomagnesemia, or impaired liver function (Vieweg et al. 2013).

Buprenorphine reduces illicit opioid use with long-term therapy (Kakko et al. 2003) and is taken sublingually. It is available alone or in a combination preparation with naloxone, an opioid antagonist that has poor oral absorption. Buprenorphine has a lower potential for causing respiratory depression than methadone. It does not appear to prolong the QTc interval (Stallvik et al. 2013), unlike methadone. Buprenorphine does have the potential to be misused as an injectable agent. Administration of buprenorphine or buprenorphine/naloxone may precipitate an acute opioid withdrawal syndrome in patients with physical dependence on opioids (Walsh and Eissenberg 2003).

Buprenorphine is well suited for outpatient maintenance treatment of OUD; however, treatment of acute pain is challenging in patients on buprenorphine maintenance because of the drug's high opioid receptor affinity, long half-life, and partial agonism of opioid receptors (which may inhibit the action of other opioid analgesics) (Anderson et al. 2017). For patients undergoing surgery in which only mild postoperative pain is expected or in which postoperative pain can be adequately controlled with continuous regional anesthesia, buprenorphine can be continued; it can also be continued for patients who are at high risk of relapse to opioid misuse. For elective surgery in which postoperative pain is expected to be difficult to manage, buprenorphine can be discontinued prior to surgery in consultation with the prescriber. Postoperative pain management planning involves multimodal analgesia with nonpharmacological as well as pharmacological modalities, regional analgesia, and local anesthetic infiltration. If supplemental opioid analgesics are required for patients on buprenorphine, patient-controlled analgesia is recommended, and oral dosing is preferred over intravenous administration where possible; basal infusion of opioids should be avoided. Due to established opioid tolerance, large opioid doses may be required for some patients, so it is appropriate to have the patient in a monitored setting, including ICU admission to monitor respiratory status.

Buprenorphine has fewer drug interactions than methadone does, so it is safer when used for patients with medical comorbidities such as HIV who are taking antiretroviral medications. However, buprenorphine may cause elevation of liver trans-aminase levels in patients with chronic HCV infection (Petry et al. 2000), which has a very high prevalence among patients who have injected opioids and are receiving maintenance treatment, and monitoring of liver enzymes may be necessary. Buprenorphine toxicity has been linked to use of benzodiazepines (Tracqui et al. 1998), so patients who require chronic benzodiazepine therapy for anxiety disorders or who have a history of sedative dependence may not be appropriate candidates for buprenorphine maintenance. Illicitly bought heroin is adulterated with other compounds that may be harmful to the fetus, so elimination of heroin use and provision of adequate doses of methadone or buprenorphine are needed to prevent harm to the fetus from exposure to these other compounds. Pregnant women who use opioids should be referred for prenatal care as well as for maintenance treatment from a local MM or buprenorphine program, if available. Newborns of mothers maintained on buprenorphine and of mothers maintained on methadone have a similar incidence of neonatal abstinence syndrome (Jones et al. 2005). Women can breast-feed while receiving MM or buprenorphine as long as they are not using any illicit drugs (McCarthy and Posey 2000) and are not HIV positive.

Naltrexone is also used as a medication to assist with maintaining abstinence in patients with OUD. Daily oral dosing or monthly intramuscular injections result in blockade of opioid effects if opioids are used. Naltrexone causes immediate withdrawal symptoms if administered prior to detoxification. Patients who discontinue antagonist therapy and resume opioid use should be made aware of the risk of serious overdose. This risk may be a result of loss of tolerance to opioids and a resulting misjudgment of dose at the time of relapse (Strang et al. 2003).

Stimulants

Amphetamines, including methamphetamine, and cocaine are the most prevalent abused stimulants, but this class also includes prescription stimulants such as methylphenidate and dextroamphetamine, as well as "designer drugs" such as methylenedioxymethamphetamine (MDMA; Ecstasy). In 2015, 1.7 million people age 12 years or older (0.6% of the U.S. population) were current misusers of prescription stimulants, 1.9 million (0.7% of the population) were current users of cocaine, and approximately 900,000 (0.3% of the population) were current users of methamphetamine (Center for Behavioral Health Statistics and Quality 2016).

Caffeine is a mild stimulant found in coffee, tea, soda, and energy drinks. Reports of caffeine intoxication have been rising because of the availability of energy drinks with high caffeine content, and this can mimic symptoms of anxiety disorders. Compelling evidence indicates that caffeine can produce a SUD in some individuals (Juliano et al. 2012). Energy drink consumption is associated with progression to nonmedical use of prescription stimulants, and caffeine increases the reinforcing effects of nicotine and may increase the rate of alcohol-related injuries. It is important to ask all patients about consumption of caffeine and use of other drugs.

Khat is a plant with psychostimulant properties that has been long used socially and in religious rituals in some African and Middle Eastern countries. The primary psychoactive compound in khat leaves is cathinone, which is chemically altered into much more potent stimulant designer drugs known collectively as "bath salts." Synthetic cathinone compound availability has evolved rapidly to evade legal regulation and detection by routine drug testing. Young adults are the primary users (Paillet-Loilier et al. 2014; Weaver et al. 2015).

Intoxication

Stimulant intoxication includes behavior changes such as hypervigilance, psychomotor agitation, grandiosity, and impaired judgment. People should approach acutely intoxicated stimulant users in a subdued manner, avoid speaking in a loud voice or moving quickly, not approach the patient from behind, and avoid touching the patient unless absolutely sure that it is safe to do so (Weaver et al. 1999). Treatment of acute toxicity includes acute stabilization of airway, breathing, and circulation; administration of activated charcoal; seizure control with benzodiazepines; aggressive management of hypertension; and management of hyperthermia.

Many experts advise that beta-blockers should not be considered first-line agents for controlling chest pain or hypertension in patients using cocaine because that would leave alpha-adrenergic stimulation unopposed, but this remains controversial (Dattilo et al. 2008). Phentolamine (an alpha-adrenergic antagonist) or nitroglycerin can be used for treatment of cocaine-related hypertension, coronary artery vasoconstriction, or tachycardia (Chan et al. 2006).

Effects on Medical and Psychiatric Disorders

Use of stimulants may result in many serious health consequences (Table 16–5). Known psychiatric disorders may be exacerbated by stimulant use. Use of stimulants can make schizophrenia more susceptible to relapse and can cause panic attacks to increase in intensity and frequency. Chronic stimulant use can lead to paranoid psychosis that is clinically indistinguishable from schizophrenia, but this effect usually abates after a prolonged period of abstinence. Several studies suggest that use of MDMA can lead to cognitive decline in otherwise healthy young people (Gouzoulis-Mayfrank et al. 2000); this neurotoxicity occurs at typical recreational doses. Patients presenting with psychosis or cognitive decline should be suspected of stimulant abuse and screened carefully.

Stimulants are used therapeutically for multiple conditions and are prescribed appropriately for attention-deficit/hyperactivity disorder, narcolepsy, fatigue in multiple sclerosis, refractory depression, and palliative care. When prescribed stimulants such as methylphenidate or dextroamphetamine are also used nonmedically by patients who have valid prescriptions for them, clinicians may see unintended side effects such as elevation in resting heart rate or other cardiovascular complications; these effects may be a clue to the prescriber that unauthorized dosage escalation is occurring. Patients prescribed stimulants who also have cardiovascular disease are at higher risk for complications. When used at therapeutic dosages in healthy adults, stimulants present little or no cardiac risk (Habel et al. 2011). Chest pain is the most common reason that cocaine users seek emergency care. Stimulant use disorder is a major cause of cerebrovascular and cardiovascular disease in young adults (O'Connor et al. 2005). In numerous case reports, MDMA (Ecstasy) use resulted in rhabdomyolysis, hyperthermia, serotonin syndrome, hyponatremia with cerebral edema, fulminant hepatic failure, or stroke (Hall and Henry 2006). Synthetic cathinone use can also lead to similar complications (Weaver et al. 2015). Acute toxicity is common

TABLE 16–5. **Effects of stimulant use**

Psychological	Central nervous system
Emotional lability	Headache
Irritability	Transient focal neurological deficits
Insomnia	Tremor
Exaggerated startle reactions	Myoclonus
Paranoia	Bradykinesia
Aggressive behavior	Dyskinesia
Anxiety	Cerebral vasculitis
Depression	Cerebral edema
Hallucinations	Cerebral hemorrhage
Psychosis	Cerebral infarction
Delirium	Cerebral atrophy
	Toxic encephalopathy
Obstetric	
Placenta previa	**Cardiovascular**
Premature rupture of membranes	Hypertension
Placental abruption	Arrhythmias
Spontaneous abortion	Cardiomyopathy
	Myocardial ischemia/infarction
Fetal	
Intrauterine growth retardation	**Head and neck**
Fetal hypertension	Dental enamel erosion
Congenital malformations	Gingival ulceration
	Mydriasis
Pulmonary	Chronic rhinitis
Chronic productive cough	Nasal septal perforation
Asthma exacerbation	
Pulmonary edema	**Other**
Pulmonary hemorrhage	Hyperthermia
Pneumothorax	Rhabdomyolysis
Pneumomediastinum	Acute renal failure
Bronchiolitis obliterans	

and often manifests with a constellation of psychiatric and medical effects, which may be severe (e.g., anxiety, agitation, psychosis, tachycardia). Treatment of acute intoxication involves supportive care targeting the signs and symptoms (Weaver et al. 2015). Both prescribed and illicit stimulants interact with other medications, potentially leading to serious adverse reactions, often cardiovascular in nature (Table 16–6).

Pharmacological Treatment

Abrupt discontinuation of stimulants does not cause gross physiological sequelae, so they are not tapered off or replaced with a cross-tolerant drug during medically supervised withdrawal. Most pharmacological agents have not proven significantly

TABLE 16–6. **Clinical interactions between stimulants and other substances or medications**

Clinical interaction effect	Drug
Increased blood pressure, increased heart rate	Alcohol
	Beta-blockers
	Caffeine
	Carbamazepine
	Monoamine oxidase inhibitors
	Nonsteroidal anti-inflammatory medications
Arrhythmias	Anticholinergics
	Bromocriptine
	Digoxin
	Halothane anesthetics
	Calcium channel blockers
Reduced blood pressure	Haloperidol

better than placebo for long-term management of abstinence for stimulant-dependent patients (Brensilver et al. 2013).

Nicotine

In the United States, 15% of the adult population smokes cigarettes and more than 16 million Americans live with a smoking-related disease (Jamal et al. 2016). Cigarette smoking can interact with medications to produce clinically significant reductions in levels of drugs such as estradiol, haloperidol, imipramine, pentazocine, propranolol, and theophylline (Smith 2009).

Electronic cigarettes, also referred to as "e-cigarettes," consist of a battery and a heating element that vaporizes a solution ("e-liquid"), which the user inhales (known as "vaping"). E-liquids contain nicotine, flavorings, and propylene glycol or vegetable glycerin (Weaver et al. 2014a). E-cigarettes are now the most commonly used tobacco product among youth, having surpassed conventional cigarettes in 2014; in 2015, current use of e-cigarettes was reported by 16% of high school students (U.S. Department of Health and Human Services 2016).

Withdrawal

Symptoms of nicotine withdrawal are similar with all tobacco products, whether cigarettes, e-cigarettes, chewing tobacco, or snuff. Withdrawal symptoms include irritability, difficulty concentrating, restlessness, anxiety, depression, and increased appetite (Karan et al. 2003). Reaction time and attention are also impaired. Withdrawal symptoms peak around 48 hours after the last use, then gradually diminish over several weeks. Symptoms of dysphoria, anhedonia, and depression may continue for several months after cessation. The withdrawal syndrome from nicotine is similar to that of other stimulants.

Nicotine replacement therapy (NRT) is used in hospitalized smokers to treat acute nicotine withdrawal symptoms and to promote smoking cessation (Rigotti et al.

2008). Research supports the inclusion of NRT in interventions for hospitalized smokers, along with counseling, because pharmacotherapy and counseling may be synergistic. Nicotine replacement products include a patch, gum, lozenge, nasal spray, and inhaler; all provide similar relief from withdrawal symptoms and efficacy for smoking cessation (Stead et al. 2012). No significant adverse effects have been reported for NRT (Lee and Fariss 2017). Even patients with hypertension and/or cardiovascular disease benefit from NRT, including those in an inpatient hospital setting (Joseph and Fu 2003). However, NRT is not routinely recommended for smokers with acute coronary syndromes because safety has not been established, and most of these patients have minimal nicotine withdrawal symptoms when they are hospitalized in a tobacco-free environment (Joseph and Fu 2003). Counseling for smoking cessation is appropriate for smokers hospitalized with acute cardiovascular complications. Clinically significant drug interactions of NRT include reduced analgesia from opioids and reduced sedation from benzodiazepines (Kroon 2006).

Pharmacological Treatment

Varenicline is a nicotinic receptor partial agonist that is without significant drug interactions. Because it is renally excreted, dosage reductions are recommended in patients with renal insufficiency. Varenicline's side effects of nausea and vomiting may be problematic in some medically ill patients. Sustained-release bupropion increases smoking cessation rates by inhibiting dopamine uptake. Both varenicline and bupropion exert their beneficial effects on smoking cessation over time and are usually started around 10 days prior to quitting smoking, so they may not be appropriate to start in hospitalized patients who are only beginning to consider smoking cessation.

Cannabis

In 2015, more than 22 million people in the United States age 12 years or older reported use of cannabis within the past 30 days, and between 2002 and 2015, the percentage of past-month cannabis users increased steadily, from 6.2% to 8.3% (Center for Behavioral Health Statistics and Quality 2016). Currently, 28 states and the District of Columbia have legalized the use of cannabis for treatment of medical conditions, and 8 of these states and the District of Columbia have also legalized cannabis for recreational use (National Conference of State Legislatures 2017). These changes in state policy have markedly altered cannabis use patterns as well as perceived levels of risk. The primary use of cannabis in the United States remains recreational, with only 10% reporting use solely for medical purposes, and 36% reporting mixed medical/recreational use (Schauer et al. 2016).

Synthetic cannabinoids were originally formulated for research purposes. Products used recreationally include synthetic cannabinoids (either single agents or mixtures) sprayed on psychoactively inert pulverized plant matter of virtually unknown content to resemble potpourri or incense (Uchiyama et al. 2010). The term "Spice" is now generally applied to all products containing synthetic cannabinoids, regardless of branding (Johnson et al. 2013).

Intoxication

The onset of acute intoxication occurs within minutes when cannabis is smoked, and the effects last for 3–4 hours (American Psychiatric Association 2013). With regular use, impairment of concentration and motor performance lasts for 12–24 hours as a result of accumulation of cannabis in adipose tissue, with slow release of tetrahydrocannabinol from fatty tissue stores and enterohepatic recirculation. Compared with tetrahydrocannabinol in cannabis, synthetic cannabinoids are often more potent and may have a longer half-life, which may lead to greater toxicity (Harris and Brown 2013). Acute effects of synthetic formulations are similar to those of cannabis.

Acute intoxication with cannabis alone rarely requires medical treatment, although dysphoria may result in distress that causes the user to seek help. Placing the distraught user in a quiet environment and maintaining gentle support is often sufficient until the acute effects subside; more severe paranoia or psychosis may require close observation with possible administration of a benzodiazepine or haloperidol for sedation.

Withdrawal

Heavy cannabis use for more than 3 weeks results in a withdrawal syndrome after abrupt cessation (American Psychiatric Association 2013). Cannabis withdrawal begins within 10 hours of the last dose and consists of irritability, agitation, depression, insomnia, nausea, anorexia, and tremor. Most symptoms peak in 48 hours and last for 5–7 days. Some symptoms, such as unusual dreams and irritability, can persist for weeks (Budney et al. 2004). Cannabis withdrawal is uncomfortable but not life-threatening. Thus, treatment is entirely supportive and nearly always accomplished without the need for adjunctive medications.

Effects on Medical and Psychiatric Disorders

Chronic cannabis use can have multiple psychiatric and medical repercussions. It can cause cognitive deficits that persist for at least hours after acute intoxication. Very heavy use is associated with persistent decrements in neurocognitive performance, even after 28 days of abstinence (Bolla et al. 2002). Cannabis use is associated with measurable health consequences as well as increases in health care costs (Pacula et al. 2008). The recent report of the National Academies of Sciences, Engineering, and Medicine (2017) concluded that oral cannabinoids have modest therapeutic benefits for pain relief, control of nausea and vomiting, and multiple sclerosis–related spasticity, but smoking it is a poor delivery system. Better alternatives are available for nausea and vomiting caused by cancer chemotherapy. Data do not support the use of cannabis for glaucoma. No statistically significant association has been found between cannabis use and the incidence of lung or head and neck cancer, and there is limited evidence for a statistically significant association between cannabis use and the incidence of nonseminomatous testicular germ cell tumors (National Academies of Sciences, Engineering, and Medicine 2017).

Cannabinoid hyperemesis syndrome, a disorder originally characterized in chronic cannabis users, involves cycles of vomiting and abdominal pain that are relieved by bathing or showering with hot water, an unusual feature that helps to confirm the diagnosis (Sorensen et al. 2017). Although previously rare, this syndrome has become more common in recent years with the increased availability and use of synthetic cannabinoids (see also Chapter 19, "Gastrointestinal Disorders," for a discussion of cannabis hyperemesis syndrome).

Adverse psychological effects are common with synthetic cannabinoids and are more severe than with cannabis, especially acute psychosis, which may persist for a significant period (up to several months). Consequences of severe toxicity have included seizures, acute renal failure, and myocardial infarction. Two deaths have been reported, one from a cardiac ischemic event and the other from extreme anxiety leading to suicide (Fattore and Fratta 2011).

Hallucinogens

Drugs considered hallucinogens are a diverse group and include lysergic acid diethylamide (LSD), certain designer drugs (e.g., NBOMe ["N-bomb"]), and many other compounds (e.g., mescaline, psilocybin, phencyclidine [PCP], ketamine). Hallucinogens produce perceptual distortions and cognitive changes with a clear sensorium, without impairment in level of consciousness or attention (Abraham et al. 1996).

Intoxication

In general, acute physiological complications of hallucinogen intoxication rarely require medical treatment. However, malignant hyperthermia and seizures may occur with hallucinogen intoxication. Warning signs for hallucinogen hyperthermia are agitation, dry skin, and increased muscle tension. Intoxication with PCP causes a characteristic vertical nystagmus (it can also cause horizontal or rotatory nystagmus), which helps to identify it as the cause when a patient presents with intoxication by an unknown drug (Weaver and Schnoll 2007).

Effects on Medical and Psychiatric Disorders

Hallucinogen use may result in long-term psychiatric consequences, such as anxiety, depression, or psychosis. Patients may present with apathy, hypomania, paranoia, delusions, hallucinations, formal thought disorder, or dissociative states. Treatment of prolonged anxiety, depression, or psychosis is the same as when not associated with hallucinogen use. Hallucinogen use also may result in medical consequences. Up to a third of frequent ketamine users experience severe gastrointestinal cramping known as "k-cramps," but the cause is unknown, and no treatment exists currently (Muetzelfeldt et al. 2008). PCP may cause hypertensive encephalopathy or life-threatening hyperthermia (Weaver and Schnoll 2008). No pharmacological treatment is available for hallucinogen use disorder.

Gamma-Hydroxybutyrate

Gamma-hydroxybutyrate (GHB) is a sedative that is both a precursor and a metabolite of gamma-aminobutyric acid (GABA). It has been used as a sleep aid and for treatment of narcolepsy; it also increases episodic secretion of growth hormone, so some bodybuilders use it to promote muscle growth.

Intoxication

GHB's effects have been likened to those of alcohol, with mild euphoria, mild numbing, and pleasant disinhibition. GHB is not detectable by routine drug screening. The dose–response curve for GHB is exceedingly steep, so small increases in the amount ingested may lead to significant intensification of effects and onset of central nervous system depression. Concurrent use of sedatives or alcohol may increase the risk of vomiting, aspiration, or respiratory depression; use with stimulants may increase the risk of seizure. In cases of acute GHB intoxication, physicians should provide physiological support and maintain a high index of suspicion for intoxication with other drugs. Most patients who overdose on GHB or related compounds recover completely if they receive proper medical attention, but there have been deaths (Zvosec et al. 2001). Management of GHB ingestion in a spontaneously breathing patient includes oxygen supplementation, intravenous access, and comprehensive physiological and cardiac monitoring. Atropine can be used for persistent symptomatic bradycardia.

Withdrawal

The symptoms of GHB withdrawal include anxiety, tremor, insomnia, and "feelings of doom," which may persist for several weeks after stopping the drug (Galloway et al. 1997). Severe withdrawal involves agitation, delirium, and psychosis (McDaniel and Miotto 2001). The treatment of GHB withdrawal is with benzodiazepines, which may require very high doses (Dyer et al. 2001). Antipsychotics or pentobarbital (Sivilotti et al. 2001) may have some utility in treatment of severe GHB withdrawal.

Inhalants

Examples of illicitly used inhalants include glue, dry-cleaning fluids (carbon tetrachloride), gasoline, aerosol propellants from whipped cream cans or deodorant sprays, amyl nitrite, butyl nitrite, nitrous oxide ("laughing gas"), and some industrial solvents. Inhalants are used by 9% of adolescents in the United States, and about 20% who try them will go on to develop a use disorder (Nguyen et al. 2016).

Many of the inhalants are similar to general anesthetics and sensitize the myocardium to catecholamines; fatal arrhythmias have been reported resulting from inhalant abuse (Shepherd 1989). Antiarrhythmic medications can be given as needed, and supplemental oxygen is administered for hypoxia and to enhance clearance of the inhalant. Cases of methemoglobinemia have been reported secondary to butyl nitrite abuse (Bogart et al. 1986). Chronic complications from abuse usually clear if the patient remains abstinent, but impairment of working memory and executive cognitive function may persist (see also Chapter 35, "Medical Toxicology").

Linkage to Addiction Treatment

A psychiatric consultant can address acute issues of intoxication and withdrawal in the inpatient setting. Hospitalization affords an excellent opportunity ("teachable moment") for addressing patients' substance use and engaging them in treatment (Martins et al. 2007). Brief interventions with trauma patients who have a positive blood alcohol concentration at the time of injury can reduce their future alcohol intake and risk of trauma recidivism (Gentilello et al. 1999). Several inpatient substance abuse consultation services have been described in the literature, but there has been little formal assessment of their efficacy (Murphy et al. 2009).

Acute and long-term treatments are necessary once the diagnosis of SUD is made. Recovery from SUD is possible, and individuals who receive treatment have less disability than do those who do not receive treatment (Hasin et al. 2007). Hospitalized patients identified to have a SUD should be provided with information linking them to local community treatment resources. In the United States, physicians certified in treatment of addictive disorders can be found through the American Society of Addiction Medicine (www.asam.org) or the American Academy of Addiction Psychiatry (www.aaap.org). At times, it may be appropriate to refer the patient to a nonphysician counselor, which can be found through the Association for Addiction Professionals (www.naadac.org).

Conclusion

The hospital setting is a good place to identify a SUD and initiate a brief intervention. SUD treatment is cost-effective, and even multiple episodes of treatment are worthwhile. It can be very rewarding for any health care practitioner to assist a patient who was impaired by substance use to return to normal functioning in society.

References

Abraham HD, Aldridge AM, Gogia P: The psychopharmacology of hallucinogens. Neuropsychopharmacology 14(4):285–298, 1996 8924196

Adunsky A, Levy R, Heim M, et al: Meperidine analgesia and delirium in aged hip fracture patients. Arch Gerontol Geriatr 35(3):253–259, 2002 14764364

Alford DP, Compton P, Samet JH: Acute pain management for patients receiving maintenance methadone or buprenorphine therapy. Ann Intern Med 144(2):127–134, 2006 16418412

American Psychiatric Association: Diagnostic and Statistical Manual of Mental Disorders, 5th Edition. Arlington, VA, American Psychiatric Association, 2013

Anderson TA, Quaye ANA, Ward EN, et al: To stop or not, that is the question: acute pain management for the patient on chronic buprenorphine. Anesthesiology 126(6):1180–1186, 2017 28511196

Bär KJ, Boettger MK, Koschke M, et al: Increased QT interval variability index in acute alcohol withdrawal. Drug Alcohol Depend 89(2–3):259–266, 2007 17350180

Bard MR, Goettler CE, Toschlog EA, et al: Alcohol withdrawal syndrome: turning minor injuries into a major problem. J Trauma 61(6):1441–1445, discussion 1445–1446, 2006 17159688

Bogart L, Bonsignore J, Carvalho A: Massive hemolysis following inhalation of volatile nitrites. Am J Hematol 22(3):327–329, 1986 3717148

Bolla KI, Brown K, Eldreth D, et al: Dose-related neurocognitive effects of marijuana use. Neurology 59(9):1337–1343, 2002 12427880

Brensilver M, Heinzerling KG, Shoptaw S: Pharmacotherapy of amphetamine-type stimulant dependence: an update. Drug Alcohol Rev 32(5):449–460, 2013 23617468

Brotherton AL, Hamilton EP, Kloss HG, et al: Propofol for treatment of refractory alcohol withdrawal syndrome: a review of the literature. Pharmacotherapy 36(4):433–442, 2016 26893017

Brown RL, Rounds LA: Conjoint screening questionnaires for alcohol and other drug abuse: criterion validity in a primary care practice. Wis Med J 94(3):135–140, 1995 7778330

Budney AJ, Hughes JR, Moore BA, et al: Review of the validity and significance of cannabis withdrawal syndrome. Am J Psychiatry 161(11):1967–1977, 2004 15514394

Center for Behavioral Health Statistics and Quality: Key substance use and mental health indicators in the United States: results from the 2015 National Survey on Drug Use and Health (HHS Publication No. SMA 16-4984, NSDUH Series H-51), September 2016. Available at: https://www.samhsa.gov/data/sites/default/files/NSDUH-FFR1-2015/NSDUH-FFR1-2015/NSDUH-FFR1-2015.pdf. Accessed February 2, 2018.

Center for Substance Abuse Treatment: Treatment Improvement Protocol 2: Pregnant Substance-Abusing Women. Rockville, MD, Center for Substance Abuse Treatment, 1993

Chan GM, Sharma R, Price D, et al: Phentolamine therapy for cocaine-association acute coronary syndrome (CAACS). J Med Toxicol 2(3):108–111, 2006 18072128

Child Welfare Information Gateway: Parental Drug Use as Child Abuse. Washington, DC, U.S. Department of Health and Human Services, Children's Bureau, 2016

Clark BJ, Keniston A, Douglas IS, et al: Healthcare utilization in medical intensive care unit survivors with alcohol withdrawal. Alcohol Clin Exp Res 37(9):1536–1543, 2013 23647435

Compton WM, Jones CM, Baldwin GT: Relationship between nonmedical prescription-opioid use and heroin use. N Engl J Med 374(2):154–163, 2016 26760086

Cooper JR, Altman F, Brown BS, et al: Research on the Treatment of Narcotic Addiction—State of the Art (NIDA Treatment Research Monograph Series). Rockville, MD, U.S. Department of Health and Human Services, 1983

Cross GM, Hennessey PT: Principles and practice of detoxification. Prim Care 20(1):81–93, 1993 8464950

Dattilo PB, Hailpern SM, Fearon K, et al: Beta-blockers are associated with reduced risk of myocardial infarction after cocaine use. Ann Emerg Med 51(2):117–125, 2008 17583376

de Roux A, Cavalcanti M, Marcos MA, et al: Impact of alcohol abuse in the etiology and severity of community-acquired pneumonia. Chest 129(5):1219–1225, 2006 16685012

de Wit M, Gennings C, Zilberberg M, et al: Drug withdrawal, cocaine and sedative use disorders increase the need for mechanical ventilation in medical patients. Addiction 103(9):1500–1508, 2008 18636996

Di Gennaro C, Biggi A, Barilli AL, et al: Endothelial dysfunction and cardiovascular risk profile in long-term withdrawing alcoholics. J Hypertens 25(2):367–373, 2007 17211243

Drossman D, Szigethy E: The narcotic bowel syndrome: a recent update. Am J Gastroenterol Suppl 2(1):22–30, 2014 25207609

Dubois MJ, Bergeron N, Dumont M, et al: Delirium in an intensive care unit: a study of risk factors. Intensive Care Med 27(8):1297–1304, 2001 11511942

Dyer JE, Roth B, Hyma BA: Gamma-hydroxybutyrate withdrawal syndrome. Ann Emerg Med 37(2):147–153, 2001 11174231

Elisaf M, Liberopoulos E, Bairaktari E, et al: Hypokalaemia in alcoholic patients. Drug Alcohol Rev 21(1):73–76, 2002 12189007

Fattore L, Fratta W: Beyond THC: the new generation of cannabinoid designer drugs. Front Behav Neurosci 5:60, 2011 22007163

Ferrari A, Coccia CP, Bertolini A, et al: Methadone—metabolism, pharmacokinetics and interactions. Pharmacol Res 50(6):551–559, 2004 15501692

Frank RG, Pollack HA: Addressing the fentanyl threat to public health. N Engl J Med 376(7):605–607, 2017 28199808

Galloway GP, Frederick SL, Staggers FE Jr, et al: Gamma-hydroxybutyrate: an emerging drug of abuse that causes physical dependence. Addiction 92(1):89–96, 1997 9060200

Gentilello LM, Rivara FP, Donovan DM, et al: Alcohol interventions in a trauma center as a means of reducing the risk of injury recurrence. Ann Surg 230(4):473–480, discussion 480–483, 1999 10522717

Gillman PK: Monoamine oxidase inhibitors, opioid analgesics and serotonin toxicity. Br J Anaesth 95(4):434–441, 2005 16051647

Gold JA, Rimal B, Nolan A, et al: A strategy of escalating doses of benzodiazepines and phenobarbital administration reduces the need for mechanical ventilation in delirium tremens. Crit Care Med 35(3):724–730, 2007 17255852

Gouzoulis-Mayfrank E, Daumann J, Tuchtenhagen F, et al: Impaired cognitive performance in drug free users of recreational ecstasy (MDMA). J Neurol Neurosurg Psychiatry 68(6):719–725, 2000 10811694

Gowing L, Farrell M, Ali R, et al: Alpha2 adrenergic agonists for the management of opioid withdrawal. Cochrane Database Syst Rev (4):CD002024, 2004 15495025

Habel LA, Cooper WO, Sox CM, et al: ADHD medications and risk of serious cardiovascular events in young and middle-aged adults. JAMA 306(24):2673–2683, 2011 22161946

Hadama A, Ieiri I, Morita T, et al: P-hydroxylation of phenobarbital: relationship to (S)-mephenytoin hydroxylation (CYP2C19) polymorphism. Ther Drug Monit 23(2):115–118, 2001 11294510

Hajak G, Müller WE, Wittchen HU, et al: Abuse and dependence potential for the non-benzo-diazepine hypnotics zolpidem and zopiclone: a review of case reports and epidemiological data. Addiction 98(10):1371–1378, 2003 14519173

Hall AP, Henry JA: Acute toxic effects of "Ecstasy" (MDMA) and related compounds: over-view of pathophysiology and clinical management. Br J Anaesth 96(6):678–685, 2006 16595612

Harris CR, Brown A: Synthetic cannabinoid intoxication: a case series and review. J Emerg Med 44(2):360–366, 2013 22989695

Hasin DS, Stinson FS, Ogburn E, et al: Prevalence, correlates, disability, and comorbidity of DSM-IV alcohol abuse and dependence in the United States: results from the National Epi-demiologic Survey on Alcohol and Related Conditions. Arch Gen Psychiatry 64(7):830–842, 2007 17606817

Jamal A, King BA, Neff LJ, et al; Centers for Disease Control and Prevention: Current cigarette smoking among adults—United States, 2005–2015. MMWR Morb Mortal Wkly Rep 65(44):1205–1211, 2016 27832052

Jarosz J, Miernik K, Wąchal M, et al: Naltrexone (50 mg) plus psychotherapy in alcohol-depen-dent patients: a meta-analysis of randomized controlled trials. Am J Drug Alcohol Abuse 39(3):144–160, 2013 23721530

Jewell C, Tomlinson J, Weaver MF: Identification and management of prescription opioid abuse in hospitalized patients. J Addict Nurs 22(1–2):32–38, 2011

Johnson LA, Johnson RL, Portier RB: Current "legal highs." J Emerg Med 44(6):1108–1115, 2013 23528960

Johnston LD, O'Malley PM, Bachman JG: Monitoring the Future: National Survey Results on Drug Use, 1975–2001, Vol 1: Secondary School Students. Rockville, MD, National Institute on Drug Abuse, 2002

Jones CM: Heroin use and heroin use risk behaviors among nonmedical users of prescription opioid pain relievers—United States, 2002–2004 and 2008–2010. Drug Alcohol Depend 132(1–2):95–100, 2013 23410617

Jones HE, Johnson RE, Jasinski DR, et al: Randomized controlled study transitioning opioid-dependent pregnant women from short-acting morphine to buprenorphine or methadone. Drug Alcohol Depend 78(1):33–38, 2005 15769555

Joseph AM, Fu SS: Smoking cessation for patients with cardiovascular disease: what is the best approach? Am J Cardiovasc Drugs 3(5):339–349, 2003 14728068

Juliano LM, Evatt DP, Richards BD, et al: Characterization of individuals seeking treatment for caffeine dependence. Psychol Addict Behav 26(4):948–954, 2012 22369218

Kakko J, Svanborg KD, Kreek MJ, et al: 1-year retention and social function after buprenor-phine-assisted relapse prevention treatment for heroin dependence in Sweden: a ran-domised, placebo-controlled trial. Lancet 361(9358):662–668, 2003 12606177

Karan LD, Dani JA, Benowitz N: The pharmacology of nicotine and tobacco, in Principles of Addiction Medicine, 3rd Edition. Edited by Graham AW, Shultz TK. Chevy Chase, MD, American Society of Addiction Medicine, 2003, pp 225–248

Katz A, Goldberg D, Smith J, et al: Tobacco, alcohol, and drug use among hospital patients: con-current use and willingness to change. J Hosp Med 3(5):369–375, 2008 18951399

Kroon LA: Drug interactions and smoking: raising awareness for acute and critical care provid-ers. Crit Care Nurs Clin North Am 18(1):53–62, xii, 2006 16546008

Lansford CD, Guerriero CH, Kocan MJ, et al: Improved outcomes in patients with head and neck cancer using a standardized care protocol for postoperative alcohol withdrawal. Arch Otolaryngol Head Neck Surg 134(8):865–872, 2008 18711062

Lee PN, Fariss MW: A systematic review of possible serious adverse health effects of nicotine replacement therapy. Arch Toxicol 91(4):1565–1594, 2017 27699443

Linn DD, Loeser KC: Dexmedetomidine for Alcohol Withdrawal Syndrome. Ann Pharmaco-ther 49(12):1336–1342, 2015 26400008

Liu J, Wang LN: Baclofen for alcohol withdrawal. Cochrane Database Syst Rev (4):CD008502, 2015 25836263

Lopez-Quintero C, Roth KB, Eaton WW, et al: Mortality among heroin users and users of other internationally regulated drugs: a 27-year follow-up of users in the Epidemiologic Catchment Area Program household samples. Drug Alcohol Depend 156:104–111, 2015 26386826

Martins SS, Copersino ML, Soderstrom CA, et al: Sociodemographic characteristics associated with substance use status in a trauma inpatient population. J Addict Dis 26(2):53–62, 2007 17594998

Mayo-Smith MF; American Society of Addiction Medicine Working Group on Pharmacological Management of Alcohol Withdrawal: Pharmacological management of alcohol withdrawal. A meta-analysis and evidence-based practice guideline. JAMA 278(2):144–151, 1997 9214531

McCarthy JJ, Posey BL: Methadone levels in human milk. J Hum Lact 16(2):115–120, 2000 11153342

McDaniel CH, Miotto KA: Gamma hydroxybutyrate (GHB) and gamma butyrolactone (GBL) withdrawal: five case studies. J Psychoactive Drugs 33(2):143–149, 2001 11476261

Mo Y, Thomas MC, Karras GE Jr: Barbiturates for the treatment of alcohol withdrawal syndrome: a systematic review of clinical trials. J Crit Care 32:101–107, 2016 26795441

Moss M, Burnham EL: Alcohol abuse in the critically ill patient. Lancet 368(9554):2231–2242, 2006 17189035

Muetzelfeldt L, Kamboj SK, Rees H, et al: Journey through the K-hole: phenomenological aspects of ketamine use. Drug Alcohol Depend 95(3):219–229, 2008 18355990

Murphy MK, Chabon B, Delgado A, et al: Development of a substance abuse consultation and referral service in an academic medical center: challenges, achievements and dissemination. J Clin Psychol Med Settings 16(1):77–86, 2009 19219627

National Academies of Sciences, Engineering, and Medicine: The health effects of cannabis and cannabinoids: current state of evidence and recommendations for research. Washington, DC, National Academies Press, January 12, 2017

National Conference of State Legislatures: State medical marijuana laws, 2017. Available at: http://www.ncsl.org/research/health/state-medical-marijuana-laws.aspx. Accessed May 28, 2017.

Nguyen J, O'Brien C, Schapp S: Adolescent inhalant use prevention, assessment, and treatment: a literature synthesis. Int J Drug Policy 31:15–24, 2016 26969125

Nishimoto A, Usery J, Winton JC, et al: High-dose parenteral thiamine in treatment of Wernicke's encephalopathy: case series and review of the literature. In Vivo 31(1):121–124, 2017 28064230

O'Connor AD, Rusyniak DE, Bruno A: Cerebrovascular and cardiovascular complications of alcohol and sympathomimetic drug abuse. Med Clin North Am 89(6):1343–1358, 2005 16227066

Olkkola KT, Ahonen J: Midazolam and other benzodiazepines. Handb Exp Pharmacol 182(182):335–360, 2008 18175099

Pacula RL, Ringel J, Dobkin C, et al: The incremental inpatient costs associated with marijuana comorbidity. Drug Alcohol Depend 92(1–3):248–257, 2008 17928166

Paillet-Loilier M, Cesbron A, Le Boisselier R, et al: Emerging drugs of abuse: current perspectives on substituted cathinones. Subst Abuse Rehabil 5:37–52, 2014 24966713

Penninga EI, Graudal N, Ladekarl MB, et al: Adverse events associated with flumazenil treatment for the management of suspected benzodiazepine intoxication—a systematic review with meta-analyses of randomised trials. Basic Clin Pharmacol Toxicol 118(1):37–44, 2016 26096314

Petry NM, Bickel WK, Piasecki D, et al: Elevated liver enzyme levels in opioid-dependent patients with hepatitis treated with buprenorphine. Am J Addict 9(3):265–269, 2000 11000922

Plosker GL: Acamprosate: a review of its use in alcohol dependence. Drugs 75(11):1255–1268, 2015 26084940

Richardson GS, Roth T: Future directions in the management of insomnia. J Clin Psychiatry 62 (suppl 10):39–45, 2001 11388590

PART III

Specialties and Subspecialties

Rigotti NA, Munafo MR, Stead LF: Smoking cessation interventions for hospitalized smokers: a systematic review. Arch Intern Med 168(18):1950–1960, 2008 18852395

Saitz R: Introduction to alcohol withdrawal. Alcohol Health Res World 22(1):5–12, 1998 15706727

Salottolo K, McGuire E, Mains CW, et al: Occurrence, predictors, and prognosis of alcohol withdrawal syndrome and delirium tremens following traumatic injury. Crit Care Med 45(5):867–874, 2017 28266937

Schauer GL, King BA, Bunnell RE, et al: Toking, vaping, and eating for health or fun: marijuana use patterns in adults, U.S., 2014. Am J Prev Med 50(1):1–8, 2016 26277652

Schuckit MA: Recognition and management of withdrawal delirium (delirium tremens). N Engl J Med 371(22):2109–2113, 2014 25427113

Schuckit MA, Tapert S: Alcohol, in The American Psychiatric Publishing Textbook of Substance Abuse Treatment, 3rd Edition. Edited by Galanter M, Kleber HD. Washington, DC, American Psychiatric Publishing, 2004, pp 151–166

Sechi G, Serra A: Wernicke's encephalopathy: new clinical settings and recent advances in diagnosis and management. Lancet Neurol 6(5):442–455, 2007 17434099

Shepherd RT: Mechanism of sudden death associated with volatile substance abuse. Hum Toxicol 8(4):287–291, 1989 2777268

Sivilotti ML, Burns MJ, Aaron CK, et al: Pentobarbital for severe gamma-butyrolactone withdrawal. Ann Emerg Med 38(6):660–665, 2001 11719746

Smith RG: An appraisal of potential drug interactions in cigarette smokers and alcohol drinkers. J Am Podiatr Med Assoc 99(1):81–88, 2009 19141727

Sorensen CJ, DeSanto K, Borgelt L, et al: Cannabinoid hyperemesis syndrome: diagnosis, pathophysiology, and treatment—a systematic review. J Med Toxicol 13(1):71–87, 2017 28000146

Stallvik M, Nordstrand B, Kristensen Ø, et al: Corrected QT interval during treatment with methadone and buprenorphine—relation to doses and serum concentrations. Drug Alcohol Depend 129(1–2):88–93, 2013 23084592

Stead LF, Perera R, Bullen C, et al: Nicotine replacement therapy for smoking cessation. Cochrane Database Syst Rev (11):CD000146, 2012 23152200

Strang J, McCambridge J, Best D, et al: Loss of tolerance and overdose mortality after inpatient opiate detoxification: follow up study. BMJ 326(7396):959–960, 2003 12727768

Sullivan JT, Sykora K, Schneiderman J, et al: Assessment of alcohol withdrawal: the revised clinical institute withdrawal assessment for alcohol scale (CIWA-Ar). Br J Addict 84(11):1353–1357, 1989 2597811

Thomson AD: Mechanisms of vitamin deficiency in chronic alcohol misusers and the development of the Wernicke-Korsakoff syndrome. Alcohol Alcohol Suppl 35 (1 suppl):2–7, 2000 11304071

Thomson AD, Cook CCH, Touquet R, et al; Royal College of Physicians, London: The Royal College of Physicians report on alcohol: guidelines for managing Wernicke's encephalopathy in the accident and Emergency Department. Alcohol Alcohol 37 (6 suppl):513–521, 2002 12414541

Tracqui A, Kintz P, Ludes B: Buprenorphine-related deaths among drug addicts in France: a report on 20 fatalities. J Anal Toxicol 22(6):430–434, 1998 9788517

Uchiyama N, Kikura-Hanajiri R, Ogata J, et al: Chemical analysis of synthetic cannabinoids as designer drugs in herbal products. Forensic Sci Int 198(1–3):31–38, 2010 20117892

U.S. Department of Health and Human Services: E-Cigarette Use Among Youth and Young Adults. A Report of the Surgeon General. Atlanta, GA, U.S. Department of Health and Human Services, Centers for Disease Control and Prevention, National Center for Chronic Disease Prevention and Health Promotion, Office on Smoking and Health, 2016

Vickers AP, Jolly A: Naltrexone and problems in pain management. BMJ 332(7534):132–133, 2006 16424470

Vieweg WV, Hasnain M, Howland RH, et al: Methadone, QTc interval prolongation and torsade de pointes: case reports offer the best understanding of this problem. Ther Adv Psychopharmacol 3(4):219–232, 2013 24167694

Walsh SL, Eissenberg T: The clinical pharmacology of buprenorphine: extrapolating from the laboratory to the clinic. Drug Alcohol Depend 70 (2 suppl):S13–S27, 2003 12738347

Weaver MF: Dealing with the DTs: managing alcohol withdrawal in hospitalized patients. The Hospitalist 11:22–25, 2007

Weaver MF, Schnoll SH: Drug overdose and withdrawal syndromes. Curr Opin Crit Care 2(3):242–247, 1996

Weaver M, Schnoll S: Abuse liability in opioid therapy for pain treatment in patients with an addiction history. Clin J Pain 18 (4 suppl):S61–S69, 2002 12479255

Weaver MF, Schnoll SH: Phencyclidine and ketamine, in Gabbard's Treatments of Psychiatric Disorders, 4th Edition. Glen O. Gabbard, M.D., Editor in Chief. Washington, DC, American Psychiatric Publishing, 2007, pp 271–280

Weaver MF, Schnoll SH: Hallucinogens and club drugs, in The American Psychiatric Publishing Textbook of Substance Abuse Treatment, 4th Edition. Edited by Galanter M, Kleber HD. Washington, DC, American Psychiatric Publishing, 2008, pp 191–200

Weaver MF, Jarvis MAE, Schnoll SH: Role of the primary care physician in problems of substance abuse. Arch Intern Med 159(9):913–924, 1999 10326934

Weaver MF, Cropsey KL, Fox SA: HCV prevalence in methadone maintenance: self-report versus serum test. Am J Health Behav 29(5):387–394, 2005 16201855

Weaver MF, Hoffman HJ, Johnson RE, et al: Alcohol withdrawal pharmacotherapy for inpatients with medical comorbidity. J Addict Dis 25(2):17–24, 2006 16785215

Weaver MF, Jewell C, Tomlinson J: Phenobarbital for treatment of alcohol withdrawal. J Addict Nurs 20(1):1–5, 2009

Weaver M, Breland A, Spindle T, et al: Electronic cigarettes: a review of safety and clinical issues. J Addict Med 8(4):234–240, 2014a 25089953

Weaver MF, Jones HE, Wunsch MJ: Alcohol and other drug use during pregnancy: management of the mother and child, in Principles of Addiction Medicine, 5th Edition. Edited by Ries R, Fiellin D, Miller S, Saitz R. Chevy Chase, MD, American Society of Addiction Medicine, 2014b, pp 1254–1271

Weaver MF, Hopper JA, Gunderson EW: Designer drugs 2015: assessment and management. Addict Sci Clin Pract 10:8, 2015 25928069

Weinrieb RM, Van Horn DH, McLellan AT, et al: Interpreting the significance of drinking by alcohol-dependent liver transplant patients: fostering candor is the key to recovery. Liver Transpl 6(6):769–776, 2000 11084066

Wesson DR, Ling W: The Clinical Opiate Withdrawal Scale (COWS). J Psychoactive Drugs 35(2):253–259, 2003 12924748

Williams CS, Woodcock KR: Do ethanol and metronidazole interact to produce a disulfiram-like reaction? Ann Pharmacother 34(2):255–257, 2000 10676835

Williams G, Daly M, Proude EM, et al: The influence of alcohol and tobacco use in orthopaedic inpatients on complications of surgery. Drug Alcohol Rev 27(1):55–64, 2008 18034382

Wong A, Benedict NJ, Armahizer MJ, et al: Evaluation of adjunctive ketamine to benzodiazepines for management of alcohol withdrawal syndrome. Ann Pharmacother 49(1):14–19, 2015 25325907

World Health Organization: Guidelines for the identification and management of substance use and substance use disorders in pregnancy. Geneva, Switzerland, WHO Press, 2014, pp 10–14. Available at: http://apps.who.int/iris/bitstream/10665/107130/1/9789241548731_eng.pdf. Accessed June 7, 2017.

Zvosec DL, Smith SW, McCutcheon JR, et al: Adverse events, including death, associated with the use of 1,4-butanediol. N Engl J Med 344(2):87–94, 2001 11150358

CHAPTER 17

Heart Disease

Peter A. Shapiro, M.D.

Cardiovascular disease is the cause of death for one-third of American adults and the leading cause of death and disease burden in the developed world (Mozaffarian et al. 2016). Some patients experience sudden fatal illness; others have a chronic course with a marked impact on their life experience. The interface between psychiatry and cardiovascular disease includes both the effects of psychosocial factors on the cardiovascular system and the effects of cardiovascular disease on the brain, psychological function, and psychopathology. Many psychological states and traits have been identified as contributing to risk for the development or exacerbation of heart disease. Treatments for psychiatric disorders may also increase cardiovascular disease risk. Unhealthy behaviors (which can be associated with psychiatric illness), such as sedentary lifestyle, overeating, smoking, and heavy alcohol use, also add to the risk of heart disease, especially coronary disease. Conversely, heart disease seems to contribute to risk for numerous psychiatric problems, especially depression, anxiety, and cognitive disorders. Medications and other treatments for heart diseases often have psychiatric effects. Because heart disease is so common, psychiatrists must deal with the effects of cardiovascular comorbidity in the care of their patients, evaluating the role of medical factors in their mental health and recognizing the potential impact of psychiatric interventions on the cardiovascular system. Unfortunately, patients with serious mental disorders tend to receive insufficient screening and treatment for heart disease (Laursen et al. 2009).

Coronary Artery Disease

Coronary artery disease (CAD) risk factors include hypertension, smoking, dyslipidemia, diabetes mellitus, male sex, and family history. Increased public awareness about modifiable CAD risk factors and dissemination of effective treatments have resulted in reductions in the prevalence of some of these factors. Nevertheless, the incidence of first acute myocardial infarction (MI) in the United States is about 635,000 cases per year, and of recurrent MI about 300,000 per year (Mozaffarian et al. 2016). One-third of patients die within the first hour after the onset of symptoms, before receiving any treatment. Aggressive use of thrombolysis, revascularization and stenting procedures, beta-adrenergic blockers, angiotensin-converting enzyme (ACE) inhibitors and angiotensin II receptor blockers, statins, and aspirin and other antiplatelet agents has reduced mortality in those who survive long enough to receive acute care. Estimated 28-day survival after acute MI for patients who survive to hospital admission is greater than 90% (Eisen et al. 2016). Depression is the most prominent of the many psychiatric conditions and psychological factors associated with CAD.

Congestive Heart Failure

The prevalence of congestive heart failure (CHF) in the United States is over 2%. In individuals older than 65 years, the annual incidence of CHF approaches 1%. By and large, heart failure is characterized by a progressive downhill course; the 5-year mortality rate in CHF is 50%, with death generally occurring within 1 year after the onset of advanced symptoms, although rescue therapies such as ventricular assist devices may alter this trajectory (Mozaffarian et al. 2016). Risk factors for CHF include CAD, valvular disease, sleep apnea, congenital defects, alcohol overuse, obesity, and tobacco use. The primary modes of death are pump failure and cardiac arrhythmias. Treatment with beta-adrenergic blockers, ACE inhibitors, angiotensin II receptor blockers, spironolactone, or implantable cardiac defibrillators reduces the risk of death, whereas treatment with inotropic agents does not, although these agents improve functional status in severely ill patients. Biventricular pacing, cardiac resynchronization therapies, long-term ventricular assist devices, heart transplantation, and sacubitril/valsartan (a new drug combining angiotensin receptor blockade and neprilysin inhibition) may improve both survival and quality of life (QoL) (McMurray et al. 2014; Slaughter et al. 2009; Yancy et al. 2013). Depression and other psychiatric illnesses are associated with incidence and an adverse prognosis of CHF. Depressed patients are prone to treatment nonadherence and delay in seeking hospitalization after onset of worsening symptoms (Riegel et al. 2011). Takotsubo cardiomyopathy is an acute, reversible form of heart failure associated specifically with intense emotional excitement (see discussion in "Acute Mental Stress" subsection under "Effects of Psychological Factors on the Heart and on Heart Disease Risk").

Heart Transplantation

Heart transplantation is a treatment option for some patients with severe heart failure, and occasionally for patients with intractable recurrent myocardial ischemia or ventricular arrhythmias, but its use is limited by donor scarcity. Patients eligible for heart transplantation typically have an expected survival of less than 2 years unless they receive a transplant. With transplantation, expected 5-year survival is now around 75%–80% (Organ Procurement and Transplant Network 2017). In view of the limited donor supply and the demands placed on the patient by immunosuppression and the care regimen, transplant programs generally screen patients and exclude from candidacy those with significant contraindications, which may include some behavioral and psychiatric issues. Patients entering the transplant process may experience anxiety about "passing" the evaluation, anxiety and depression while on the waiting list, and delirium and a variety of emotional and psychological reactions after transplantation, including elevated mood, depression, anxiety, acute and posttraumatic stress disorders, sexual dysfunction, and difficulty negotiating the social role transitions that occur over the course of recovery (Shapiro 1990). For a detailed discussion, see Chapter 29, "Organ Transplantation."

Left Ventricular Assist Devices

The mismatch between the shortage of available donors of hearts for transplantation and the large number of patients dying of CHF provided impetus for the development of artificial heart technology (D.J. Goldstein and Oz 2000). Early experience with use of left ventricular assist devices (LVADs) designed to be used for periods of weeks to months as a bridge to transplantation indicated that they improved hemodynamics, renal and liver function, cerebral perfusion, and functional status, but neuropsychiatric issues were common, including delirium, stroke, cognitive impairment, pain, and depressed mood. Subsequent design improvements and randomized trials have demonstrated survival and QoL benefits for LVAD, both as a long-term ("destination") therapy and as a "bridge to recovery" (Mehra et al. 2017; Rogers et al. 2017; Slaughter et al. 2009). Neuropsychiatric complications of LVAD treatment include delirium, stroke, and depression. Prior cerebrovascular disease increases the risk of neuropsychiatric complications after LVAD placement (Petrucci et al. 2009). LVAD treatment may be construed as a form of extended cardiac life support, and patients (or their health care agents) sometimes request withdrawal of this support (i.e., LVAD deactivation). Counseling before device implantation, as well as psychiatry, palliative care, and ethics consultations, may be helpful and necessary to address this issue (Nakagawa et al. 2017).

Cardiac Arrhythmias

Causes of cardiac arrhythmias include primary disorders of the cardiac conduction system, ischemia, heart failure, valvular disease, drugs, thyroid disease, genetic abnormalities, infection, metabolic derangement, and psychological stress. Many arrhythmias are idiopathic. Common arrhythmias include atrial fibrillation, sinus node dysfunction, and ventricular tachyarrhythmias.

Atrial fibrillation can cause decreased cardiac output and intra-atrial thrombus formation with risk for subsequent embolic stroke. Beta-blockers, calcium channel blockers, amiodarone, ablation procedures, and cardioversion are used to achieve heart rate or rhythm control. Warfarin and other anticoagulants decrease stroke risk but increase bleeding risk. Emotional factors such as anxiety, anger, acute stress, and panic are associated with episodes of atrial fibrillation; conversely, awareness of symptoms and diagnosis may lead to increased anxiety. Sinus node dysfunction may lead to symptomatic bradycardia, with lightheadedness and syncope, or to sick sinus syndrome, with episodes of both tachycardia and bradycardia. Lithium may contribute to sinus node dysfunction. Ventricular tachyarrhythmias may degenerate to ventricular fibrillation, with cardiac arrest and sudden cardiac death. There are more than 300,000 cases of sudden cardiac death in the United States yearly, and about half of these occur in patients with no history of heart disease. These arrhythmia events may be idiopathic or associated with myocardial ischemia or heart failure; emotional stress increases the risk of ventricular tachyarrhythmias and sudden death, especially in individuals with predisposing heart disease. Implanted defibrillator therapy has become the standard of care for secondary prevention of sudden cardiac death and for primary prevention in patients with reduced left ventricular ejection fraction.

Hypertension

High blood pressure affects about one-third of adults in the United States and is associated with increased risk of stroke, MI, CHF, and renal failure. Most hypertension is "essential," or idiopathic. Typical treatments include diet (reducing sodium intake), weight loss, exercise, diuretics, beta-blockers, angiotensin receptor blockers, and ACE inhibitors. The relationship of psychological factors to the development of hypertension has been a subject of controversy, with mixed findings in large-scale observational studies.

Several large-scale prospective studies with longitudinal follow-up ranging from 11 to 22 years have identified associations between psychological factors and hypotension. A 15-year prospective study found that two components of Type A behavior—namely, "time urgency–impatience" and "hostility"—were each associated with almost double the rate of developing hypertension. In contrast, anxiety symptoms, depression symptoms, and "achievement-striving-competitiveness" (another Type A component) did not predict hypertension (Yan et al. 2003). In a Norwegian epidemiological study, high baseline depression and anxiety symptoms were both associated with *low* systolic blood pressure at 11-year follow-up, and the magnitude and direction of anxiety or depression symptom changes over time were inversely associated with the magnitude of the change in systolic blood pressure. These effects were not accounted for by use of antihypertensive and antidepressant medication (Hildrum et al. 2008). However, a 22-year follow-up of a population-based cohort of 3,310 normotensive persons without chronic diseases from the National Health and Nutrition Examination Survey I (NHANES I) Epidemiologic Follow-up Study found that combined symptoms of depression and anxiety ("negative affect") were associated with an increased risk of developing hypertension. The risk of hypertension was increased in both men and women and was most pronounced (more than threefold) in black women (Jonas and Lando 2000).

A review (Rutledge and Hogan 2002) of 15 prospective studies of psychological traits affecting the development of hypertension, with sample sizes varying from 78 to 4,650 subjects and follow-up for 2.5–21 years, found small but significant effects for anger, anxiety, depression, and other variables, with an overall magnitude of effect suggesting an 8% increase in prospective hypertension risk associated with a high level of one or more of the psychological variables. Anxiety was associated with modest increased risk (hazard ratio, 1.55) of hypertension in a 2015 meta-analysis of 8 prospective studies (Pan et al. 2015), but some studies have found an association of hypertension with depression but not with anxiety (Maatouk et al. 2016).

The main psychiatric consequence of hypertension seems to be long-term neuro-cognitive impairment and increased risk of dementia (Iadecola et al. 2016). Treatment that successfully controls blood pressure reduces this risk (Forette et al. 2002; Vinyoles et al. 2008). Among patients older than 60 years, adherence to antihypertensive therapy is associated with better blood pressure control and better cognitive function (Vinyoles et al. 2008). "White-coat hypertension," defined as persistently high blood pressure at visits to the doctor's office but normal ambulatory and self-measured blood pressure, is associated with increased long-term risk of stroke but not of heart disease (Angeli et al. 2005). Behavioral treatments appear to have a modest effect at best on hypertension (Linden and Moseley 2006; Perez et al. 2009); however, combined treatments may be helpful in paroxysmal hypertension, especially if paroxysmal episodes of high blood pressure are linked to panic or anxiety (Pickering and Clemow 2008).

Congenital Heart Disease

Psychological maladjustment is common in children after surgery for congenital heart disease (Latal et al. 2009), and lifetime rates of mood and anxiety disorders in survivors of congenital heart disease may be as high as 50% (Kovacs et al. 2009); the association of congenital disease with later psychological difficulties may depend on residual somatic symptoms (Eslami et al. 2013). Elevated posttraumatic stress disorder (PTSD) symptoms are present in 10%–20% of patients and are associated with depression symptoms (Deng et al. 2016). Elevated depression symptoms are associated with poorer prognosis (Kourkoveli et al. 2015).

Overall IQ scores are typically in the normal range in persons with congenital heart disease but lower than those of healthy control subjects, and subtle neuropsychological deficits are common (Forbess et al. 2002; Miatton et al. 2007). For cyanotic conditions, delayed repair appears to exacerbate intellectual impairment (Newburger et al. 1984). Other common psychological problems among children and young adults with congenital heart disease include concerns about exclusion from participation in peer group activities such as sports and gym class, problems with appearance (e.g., short stature, cyanosis, drug side effects on appearance), concerns about attractiveness, capacity to develop intimate relationships, exclusion from work, and fears about mortality (Kendall et al. 2001). Sexual dysfunction is common in men who have had surgery for congenital heart disease (Vigl et al. 2009).

Parents of children with critical congenital heart disease frequently have anxiety and depression symptoms as well as high rates of PTSD and psychological distress. The period after cardiac surgery is a time of heightened risk (Woolf-King et al. 2017). Parental anxiety and overprotectiveness may play a role in the development of anxiety in congenital heart disease patients (Ong et al. 2011)

Psychiatric Disorders in Heart Disease

The development of cardiac disease in a previously healthy individual is associated with a variety of psychological reactions. Perhaps most fundamentally, it is difficult to maintain denial about one's mortality after a cardiac event. Viewing oneself as having heart disease has effects at every level of psychological development: increasing concerns about dependency, autonomy, control, and ability to provide for others; provoking loss of self-esteem and concern about loss of love; and inciting fears about vitality, sexuality, and mortality. The maintenance of denial has been associated with mental well-being and may manifest as minimizing the severity of the event or attributing symptoms to a noncardiac source; excessive denial can be detrimental if it leads to delay in seeking treatment or failure to accept the need to maintain a treatment regimen. By contrast, inadequate denial or exaggeration of the illness can lead to invalidism or mental disorder in cardiac patients.

Attention to one's heartbeat, conscious experience of twinges of chest pain or palpitations, and preoccupation with minor physical symptoms may result in hypochondriacal avoidance of activity and increased visits to the doctor and emergency room. Research with hypochondriacal, somatizing, and panic disorder patients, who make up a large portion of patients presenting to emergency rooms with noncardiac chest pain, has demonstrated their high level of somatic awareness (Barsky et al. 1994b, 1996; Campbell et al. 2017).

Depression

Depression in Coronary Artery Disease

Depression appears to be the most common psychiatric disorder in CAD patients (Barth et al. 2004; Glassman and Shapiro 1998; Rugulies 2002; van Melle et al. 2004; Wulsin and Singal 2003). Numerous surveys of patients with established coronary disease, acute MI, and unstable angina consistently indicate a point prevalence of depression in the range of 15%–20% (Barth et al. 2004; van Melle et al. 2004). Depression can be persistent, and subsyndromal depression in CAD patients often evolves into major depressive disorder (MDD) (Hance et al. 1996), belying the notion that depression is a "normal" reaction to illness that does not deserve attention. The point prevalence of depression in the months following coronary artery bypass graft (CABG) surgery is also in the range of 20%–30% (Blumenthal et al. 2003; Connerney et al. 2001). Elevated symptom scores on depression rating scales such as the Beck Depression Inventory are even more common and may predict subsequent MDD (Frasure-Smith et al. 1995a, 1995b). The availability of good social support reduces the likelihood of persistent depression after an acute coronary event (Frasure-Smith et al. 2000). Guidelines (Davidson et al. 2006; Lichtman et al. 2008) recommend screening for depression in patients with CAD, but the added value of screening is not established (Thombs et al. 2013).

Depression in Congestive Heart Failure

As in patients with coronary disease, the prevalence of MDD in patients with congestive heart failure is about 20% (Jiang et al. 2001; Rutledge et al. 2006; Westlake et al. 2005). An additional 30%–35% of patients have subsyndromal or mild depression symptoms (Jiang et al. 2001; Westlake et al. 2005). Patients with more severe depression symptoms tend to have worse functional status and poorer exercise tolerance (Westlake et al. 2005).

Anxiety and Trauma- and Stressor-Related Disorders

Anxiety in Coronary Artery Disease

High levels of anxiety are common in patients with acute coronary disease, and anxiety prevalence rates in patients with chronic heart disease range from 5% to 40% (Frasure-Smith and Lespérance 2008; Sullivan et al. 2000). Structured interviews yield a prevalence of generalized anxiety and other anxiety disorders of 5%–7% in patients with CAD (Bunevicius et al. 2013; Frasure-Smith and Lespérance 2008). Screening tools are sensitive but have low specificity in this population.

Intense subjective distress and fear of dying in the immediate aftermath of an acute coronary event are associated with an increased risk of developing clinically significant anxiety 1 week to several weeks after the event (Whitehead et al. 2005). Some patients with CAD have a family history of death in the parent of the same sex as a result of the same illness. This history is often associated with the conscious fantasy that the patient's death at the age at which the parent died is inevitable, leading to considerable vigilance, avoidance, and other anxiety behaviors.

Anxiety in Congestive Heart Failure

Among individuals with CHF, about 13% have anxiety disorders, and 30% have elevated symptoms of anxiety (Easton et al. 2016; Yohannes et al. 2010). One study reported a 10% prevalence of panic disorder in CHF patients treated in a cardiology clinical practice (Müller-Tasch et al. 2008). Predictors of an anxiety disorder in CHF patients were previous history of mental illness, diabetes, angina, and worse functional status. Both anxiety symptoms (Tsuchihashi-Makaya et al. 2009) and diagnosed anxiety disorders (Cully et al. 2009) have been associated with increased health care utilization in CHF patients.

Panic Disorder and Mitral Valve Prolapse

Depending on the echocardiographic criteria employed, 5%–20% or more of patients with panic disorder have mitral valve prolapse (Margraf et al. 1988). Individuals with mitral valve prolapse may be asymptomatic or may experience occasional palpitations or "fluttering" sensations in the precordium, and it has been proposed that these sensations give rise to catastrophic cognitions that stimulate panic attacks in predisposed individuals (Barlow 1988). However, the link between panic disorder and mitral valve prolapse has been questioned, and a 2008 systematic review found the evidence for an association inconclusive at best (Filho et al. 2008).

Anxiety Associated With Automatic Implantable Cardioverter Defibrillators

Malignant ventricular arrhythmias account for a substantial fraction of fatal events among individuals with CAD and CHF. Although the use of automatic implantable cardioverter defibrillators (AICDs) reduces mortality (Epstein et al. 2008), the experience of defibrillation is unpleasant for patients and has been likened to being "kicked in the chest." AICD discharges are associated with iatrogenic anxiety, particularly in patients who experience repetitive, frequent, or early discharges after device implantation. Significant anxiety and depression symptoms were still present more than

12 months after implantation in 15%–30% of AICD patients (Lang et al. 2014; Magyar-Russell et al. 2011).

Although anxiety symptoms, anxiety disorders, and impaired QoL are more common in patients who have received shocks (Jacq et al. 2009), the likelihood of developing anxiety is also associated with predisposing personality traits such as social inhibition, negative affectivity, and sensitivity to anxiety (Bostwick and Sola 2011; Van den Broek et al. 2008). In one study, individual psychological trait factors such as optimism, past history of depression, trait anxiety, and perceived social support accounted for 25%–40% of the variance in self-reported QoL in patients 9–18 months following AICD implantation, while the experience of having been shocked accounted for only 1%–7% of the variance (Sears et al. 2005). Although full-fledged PTSD appears to occur in fewer than 5% of AICD patients, symptoms of the disorder, such as avoidance, hypervigilance, and re-experiencing, are common, especially in patients experiencing multiple sequential shocks. A variety of other reactions to implanted defibrillators have been described, including feelings of invulnerability, dependency, and withdrawal (Fricchione et al. 1989; Morris et al. 1991). Despite the potential for unpleasant experiences, most patients with implanted defibrillators report satisfaction with their experience with the device (Bostwick and Sola 2011).

Anxiety and Supraventricular Tachycardia

Patients with supraventricular tachycardia often experience anxiety, especially with paroxysmal arrhythmias (e.g., paroxysmal supraventricular tachycardia; see section "Diagnostic Issues" later in this chapter).

Posttraumatic Stress Disorder in Cardiac Disease

PTSD rates averaging 12%–15% (range, 0%–38%) have been reported in patients with cardiac disease (Edmondson and von Känel 2017; Vilchinsky et al. 2017). Proposed risk factors include personality traits such as repressive coping, alexithymia, and neuroticism; history of depression or of previous trauma; younger age; female gender; limited social support; dissociative symptoms during, and acute stress reactions immediately following, index cardiac events; and subjective factors related to the experience of the event.

A circular association of PTSD with incident acute coronary events and defibrillator discharges, and of these medical events with the development of acute stress disorder and PTSD, has been established, wherein preexisting PTSD increases the risk of coronary events and of cardiac event–related mortality by 25%–50%, coronary events are associated with subsequent incident PTSD, and PTSD after a coronary event is associated with an increased risk of further coronary events and higher mortality. The mechanisms by which PTSD leads to cardiac events are probably both behavioral (e.g., smoking, nonadherence, substance use) and physiological (e.g., altered hypothalamic-pituitary-adrenal [HPA] axis, altered autonomic cardiovascular regulation) (Edmondson and von Känel 2017; Edmondson et al. 2013).

Anxiety and Cardiac Surgery

Heart-focused anxiety increases before cardiac surgery but tends to return to normal levels within 1–6 months after surgery. About 20% of patients continue to experience clinically significant heart-focused anxiety 6 months after surgery (Hoyer et al. 2008).

The presence of high anxiety symptoms before surgery has been associated with increased mortality risk, after adjustment for other known mortality risk factors (Tully et al. 2008; Williams et al. 2014).

Delirium and Neurocognitive Dysfunction After Cardiac Surgery

After CABG surgery and open-heart procedures, many patients experience altered mental status with an impaired level of consciousness for some days. Whether these patients are identified as experiencing delirium appears to depend on the sensitivity of the observer and on the degree to which the patient's obtundation or agitation interferes with postoperative management. Even with use of structured diagnostic criteria (e.g., ICD-10, DSM-5) and validated rating scales, reported incidence rates for delirium in post–cardiac surgery patients range from 6% to more than 50% (Detroyer et al. 2008; Kazmierski et al. 2008; Koster et al. 2009; Rudolph et al. 2009). Emboli from valvular structures, intracardiac thrombus, and the cardiopulmonary bypass circuit contribute to subsequent cognitive impairment. Adverse cerebral effects that may persist after surgery include focal deficits, persistent cognitive impairment, diminished level of consciousness, and seizures. Strong risk factors for delirium include older age, previous cerebrovascular disease, previous psychiatric illness, postoperative atrial fibrillation, pre- or perioperative blood product transfusions, and longer time on ventilator support. Prolonged sedation with opiates, renal failure, and metabolic derangement have also been identified as delirium risk factors. In patients older than 70 years, diabetes, hyponatremia, fever, and fluid overload during surgery are additional risk factors (Gosselt et al. 2015; Kazmierski et al. 2008; Smulter et al. 2013). Delirium after cardiac surgery is associated with other negative outcomes, including long-term cognitive impairment and increased mortality (Crocker et al. 2016). There is little evidence that avoidance of heart–lung bypass (i.e., "off-pump" surgery) improves neuropsychological outcomes (Afilalo et al. 2012; van Dijk et al. 2007). There is limited and conflicting evidence supporting postoperative use of agents such as risperidone or dexmedetomidine for prevention or treatment of delirium after cardiac surgery (Gosselt et al. 2015; Maldonado et al. 2009; Mu et al. 2015; Pandharipande et al. 2007). Current guidelines emphasize early mobilization, adequate nonnarcotic pain management, and avoidance of prolonged sedation to reduce the incidence of delirium after cardiac surgery (Barr et al. 2013).

Psychiatric Side Effects of Cardiac Drugs

A few cardiac medications can have neuropsychiatric side effects (Table 17–1). Beta-adrenergic blockers and carvedilol can exacerbate fatigue. Profound hypothyroidism caused by amiodarone can present as progressive cognitive decline, depression, or fatigue.

Psychogenic Cardiac Disability Syndromes

A psychogenic disability syndrome with overvalued ideas or convictions about the severity of one's cardiac illness sometimes occurs after a patient experiences symptoms attributed to heart disease, regardless of whether actual heart disease exists. For

TABLE 17–1.   Selected psychiatric side effects of cardiac drugs

Drug/class	Effects
Digoxin	Visual hallucinations (classically, yellow rings around objects), delirium, depression
Beta-blockers	Fatigue, sexual dysfunction
Alpha-blockers	Depression, sexual dysfunction
Lidocaine	Agitation, delirium, psychosis
Carvedilol	Fatigue, insomnia
Methyldopa	Depression, confusion, insomnia
Reserpine	Depression
Clonidine	Depression
ACE inhibitors	Mood elevation or depression (rare)
Amiodarone	Mood disorders secondary to thyroid effects
Diuretics	Hypokalemia/hyponatremia resulting in anorexia, weakness, apathy

Note.   ACE=angiotensin-converting enzyme.

some patients, apparent clinging to symptoms of disease and the resulting disability may serve a defensive function. Most such patients have symptoms that meet diagnostic criteria for somatic symptom disorder. Illness anxiety and panic may also increase focus on somatic symptoms, and factitious disorder and malingering must also be considered in the differential diagnosis of patients who appear to cling to cardiac disability (Rief et al. 2004).

Sexual Dysfunction

Sexual dysfunction after the onset of heart disease occurs as a consequence of both physical and psychological factors. Physical factors include medications; comorbid medical conditions such as peripheral vascular disease and diabetes mellitus; endothelial dysfunction; and low cardiac output (Kapur and Schwarz 2007). Psychological factors include depression, anxiety, and fear of provoking a heart attack. Coital angina accounts for 5% of angina attacks, but it is rare in patients who do not experience angina during strenuous physical exertion. The metabolic demand of coitus is about equal to the demand of walking 2–3 miles/hour (DeBusk 2003) (see Chapter 15, "Sexual Dysfunctions"). Erectile dysfunction in men with CHF can often be treated with phosphodiesterase type 5 (PDE-5) inhibitors, which may result in concomitant improvement in mood, with appropriate precautions about contraindicated concurrent treatment with nitrates and alpha-adrenergic blockers (Mandras et al. 2007; Webster et al. 2004). Avoidance of intercourse out of fear is associated with greater anxiety and depression in CAD patients, but not with the degree of stenosis due to atherosclerotic plaque or the number of affected arteries (Kazemi-Saleh et al. 2007).

Effects of Psychological Factors on the Heart and on Heart Disease Risk

Depression

Depression and Coronary Artery Disease

A history of depressive disorder or elevated symptoms of depression is associated with a near doubling of risk for subsequent development of ischemic heart disease and for coronary disease death (Goldstein et al. 2015; Herbst et al. 2007; Rugulies 2002; Wulsin and Singal 2003). The risk is probably higher in individuals with MDD (Surtees et al. 2008). Depression also heightens the risk of ventricular arrhythmias (ventricular tachycardia/ventricular fibrillation) resulting in discharge of AICDs and of cardiac arrest, independent of other established CAD risk factors (Whang et al. 2009). In patients with preexisting CAD, those with depression had a mortality risk three- to fourfold higher than that in nondepressed coronary patients (Lichtman et al. 2014). The association between depression and adverse outcomes cannot be explained by confounding of depression with severity of heart disease (Kronish et al. 2009), although in some studies, somatic symptoms associated with depression had a stronger effect on CAD prognosis than did cognitive–affective symptoms (Linke et al. 2009; Martens et al. 2010). Onset of depression after an acute event, severity of depression measured shortly after the acute coronary event, and persistence of depression (with or without active treatment) all increased the long-term risk of all-cause mortality after acute coronary events (Lichtman et al. 2014).

Depression following CABG surgery predicts recurrent cardiac events at 12 months and over many years of follow-up (Connerney et al. 2001, 2010), and both moderate and severe depression symptoms before surgery, and even mild depression persisting from baseline to 6-month follow-up after surgery, are predictors of increased long-term mortality (Blumenthal et al. 2003).

Vital exhaustion—defined as a mental state of unusual fatigue, feelings of dejection or defeat, and increased irritability—is associated with increased risk of incident coronary disease. A psychotherapeutic intervention to reduce exhaustion was reported to reduce angina complaints, but not recurrent cardiac events, after angioplasty (Appels et al. 2005, 2006; Frestad and Prescott 2017). Although vital exhaustion has been conceptualized as being distinct from depression (e.g., it does not include self-critical thoughts, and HPA axis activity is diminished rather than increased) (Appels et al. 2005), its overlap with depression is substantial, and the independent effect of nondepression components of vital exhaustion on CAD risk is uncertain (McGowan et al. 2004).

In contrast to depression, positive emotional characteristics such as optimism and "emotional vitality" have been associated with reduced incidence of CAD, and absence of positive emotion has been identified as a risk factor for CAD events (Davidson et al. 2010a, 2010b; Giltay et al. 2004; Lundgren et al. 2015). Investigators have tended to view these positive characteristics as independent of depression, rather than simply an absence of depression (Kubzansky and Thurston 2007).

Depression clearly adversely affects patients' perceptions of their heart disease status and QoL. Ruo et al. (2003) examined 1,024 patients with stable CAD to evaluate the contributions of depressive symptoms and objective measures of cardiac function to patient-perceived health status. The patients who had depressive symptoms (20%) were more likely to report coronary disease symptom burden, physical limitations, diminished QoL, and impaired health. In multivariate analyses, depression symptoms showed significant independent associations with these health status outcomes, whereas exercise capacity, left ventricular ejection fraction, and myocardial ischemia did not. These findings suggest that efforts to improve subjective health and functional status in patients with coronary disease should address depression symptoms. A subsequent study (Ruo et al. 2006) in 2,675 postmenopausal women found that depression (new-onset or persistent) had as powerful an impact on patients' self-ratings of their health as recent acute coronary events, heart failure, or coronary bypass surgery.

Mechanisms linking depression and CAD.   Candidate psychophysiological mechanisms linking depression to adverse CAD outcomes include platelet dysfunction, autonomic dysfunction, and abnormalities of inflammation (York et al. 2009). However, the literature is inconclusive (Poole et al. 2011). Inflammation contributes to the development of atherosclerosis and acute coronary events (Libby et al. 2002). Inflammatory cytokines are elevated in CAD patients, and the magnitude of elevation of interleukin-6 (IL-6), tumor necrosis factor-alpha, and C reactive protein (CRP) predicts coronary and cerebrovascular disease events and progression of heart failure (Cesari et al. 2003; Fisman et al. 2006). Depression has been shown to be associated with increased circulating levels of IL-6, CRP, and intercellular adhesion molecule 1 (ICAM-1) (Empana et al. 2005; Liukkonen et al. 2006; Miller et al. 2002; Vaccarino et al. 2007), but depression increases the risk of CAD incidence and events even after controlling for inflammation (Empana et al. 2005; Vaccarino et al. 2007). Platelet dysfunction in depression is complex, with abnormal increases in platelet activation and enhancement of platelet aggregation in response to serotonin, but not to other agonists (Williams 2012). Increased platelet activation may contribute to increased risk of coronary thrombus formation. A synergistic effect of increased inflammatory cytokines co-occurring with platelet activation has been proposed to contribute to risk of CAD events (Williams 2012; Williams et al. 2014). Selective serotonin reuptake inhibitor (SSRI) antidepressants that inhibit serotonin storage in platelets have been found to reduce CAD event risk in some (e.g., Sauer et al. 2003) but not all (e.g., Kimmel et al. 2011) studies. SSRIs that have the highest binding affinity for the serotonin transporter, such as fluoxetine, paroxetine, and sertraline, have the strongest effect (Sauer et al. 2003).

Several measures of cardiac autonomic control—indexed by heart rate variability (HRV) or heart period variability (HPV)—are also deranged in depression, indicating elevated sympathetic activation, suppression of vagal tone, and increased propensity to cardiac arrhythmias (R.M. Carney et al. 2001). Some studies have attributed the association between depression and reduced HRV primarily to antidepressant drug use (Licht et al. 2008). However, HRV measures were no different in depressed and nondepressed patients with stable CAD in a large patient cohort in the Heart and Soul Study, raising doubt about the importance of the autonomic derangements seen in depression in explaining subsequent events (Gehi et al. 2005b). Other HRV measures less specifically linked to sympathetic nervous system activation may account for a part of the mortality risk attributable to depression after MI (R.M. Carney et al. 2005).

Some studies (e.g., Konttinen et al. 2016; Stenman et al. 2013) have suggested that antidepressants, especially tricyclic antidepressants (TCAs), might be responsible for excess cardiovascular events and deaths in patients with depression. None of these studies were randomized trials, however, and they could not exclude the confounding effect of depression itself on outcomes (O'Connor et al. 2008). No prospective randomized study of SSRIs in CAD or heart failure patients has found an association of SSRI use with increased mortality risk.

Depression's negative effect on cardiovascular outcomes may be most importantly mediated by negative effects on behavior and adherence to treatment recommendations (Whooley et al. 2008). Depression reduces the likelihood that patients will maintain ideal cardiovascular health behaviors (España-Romero et al. 2013). Poor adherence to the medical regimen in CAD patients is associated with increased recurrent cardiac events and mortality (Gehi et al. 2007; Rasmussen et al. 2007), and demonstrated effects of depression in coronary disease patients include lower rates of smoking cessation, exercise, dietary modification, and adherence to medication regimen (Dempe et al. 2013; Gehi et al. 2005a; Glassman 1993; Kronish et al. 2006; Ziegelstein et al. 2000). Depressed CHF patients are prone to nonadherence and delay in seeking hospitalization after onset of worsening symptoms (Riegel et al. 2011). Improvement in depression symptoms is followed by improved adherence to the medical regimen in heart disease patients (Rieckmann et al. 2006). However, it remains to be demonstrated in an intervention trial that depression treatment changes any of these candidate mechanisms in a way that accounts for any part of the variance in any cardiovascular outcome.

Numerous clinical trials in CAD patients have investigated depression treatment outcomes; some have also addressed cardiovascular outcomes (Shapiro 2015). Randomized, placebo-controlled, double-blind trials have demonstrated at least modest antidepressant efficacy for fluoxetine (Strik et al. 2000), sertraline (Glassman et al. 2002), citalopram (Lespérance et al. 2007), and escitalopram (J.M. Kim et al. 2015), and equivocal benefit for mirtazapine (Honig et al. 2007). In general, these antidepressants were well tolerated, with low rates of discontinuation due to adverse effects. Older trials demonstrated efficacy for TCAs, but their unfavorable adverse-effect profile renders them unsuitable for first- or second-line treatment of depression in patients with CAD (Glassman et al. 1993). Other medications with some evidence of efficacy and tolerability in treatment of depression in CAD patients include bupropion (Roose et al. 1991) and nefazodone (Lespérance et al. 2003). Intensive aerobic exercise training has also demonstrated beneficial effects on depression in patients with CAD and CHF (Blumenthal et al. 2012a, 2012b). Collaborative care trials with stepped interventions, including brief education, counseling, problem-solving therapy, and antidepressants, have demonstrated substantial benefit for patients with depression after acute coronary events (Davidson et al. 2010c, 2013; Huffman et al. 2014) and after coronary bypass surgery (Rollman et al. 2009).

Two trials have examined the effects of depression intervention on cardiovascular outcomes and mortality in CAD patients. In the Enhancing Recovery in Coronary Heart Disease (ENRICHD) trial, patients with depression or low social support received cognitive-behavioral therapy (CBT) or usual care for 6 months; some patients also received open (nonrandomized) treatment with antidepressants (Berkman et al. 2003). Recurrent cardiac events and mortality were ascertained through 30 months of follow-up. In the Myocardial INfarction and Depression-Invention Trial (MIND-IT), patients received a variety of interventions, with an 18-month follow-up (van Melle et al. 2007). Neither study showed a significant effect of the intervention on cardiac outcomes and mortality.

It is notable that in all of these post-MI depression intervention trials, persistence of depression was associated with higher cardiac morbidity and mortality over long-term follow-up (R.M. Carney et al. 2004, 2009; de Jonge et al. 2007; Glassman et al. 2009). Recovery from depression was associated with better long-term cardiac prognosis, but treatment per se was not. A congruent effect was found in an observational study of patients after CABG surgery, in which patients whose depression improved in the 6 months after surgery had a better cardiac prognosis than patients whose depression persisted or worsened (Blumenthal et al. 2003). Conversely, patients with new onset or worsening of depression in the months following MI appear to have a worse cardiac prognosis (Dickens et al. 2008; Parker et al. 2008). These findings suggest two possibilities: First, depression may be driving cardiac outcomes, in which case stronger antidepression effects, or treatments that directly target mediating mechanisms, may be needed to mitigate adverse medical outcome risks associated with depression (Rutledge et al. 2013; Shapiro 2013, 2015; Teply et al. 2016). Alternatively, short-term deterioration in cardiac status may be driving new onset or persistence of depression, and the apparent effect of depression on cardiac outcomes is confounded by worsening health status, in which case depression treatment is unlikely to have an effect on cardiac outcomes (Shapiro 2013; Ziegelstein 2013).

Depression and Congestive Heart Failure

Depression arising de novo in patients after the diagnosis of coronary disease is associated with a 1.5-fold increased risk of subsequent development of CHF, even after adjustment for confounding factors (May et al. 2009). Depression in CHF patients is associated with about a 1.5- to 3-fold increased risk of new cardiac events or death (Gathright et al. 2017; Sokoreli et al. 2016). Depressed CHF patients in the hospital tend to receive a lower intensity of invasive interventions and referral to outpatient disease management programs, which may contribute to their risk of death (Albert et al. 2009).

A multicenter study of 460 outpatients with CHF showed that compared with non-depressed patients, patients with significant depression symptoms had both worse subjective health status at baseline (even after adjustment for objective measures of illness) and more deterioration in health status over short-term follow-up. Depression predicted worsening of heart failure symptoms, physical and social functioning, and QoL. Depression symptoms were the strongest predictor of decline in health status (Rumsfeld et al. 2003).

Mechanisms such as those postulated to underlie the relationship of depression and coronary disease have been proposed to account for the effect of depression on CHF outcomes (Joynt et al. 2004), but little pathophysiological research has been performed specifically in depressed patients with heart failure.

Clinical trials of escitalopram and sertraline have failed to demonstrate substantial effects on mood or beneficial effects on cardiovascular morbidity and mortality in patients with depression and CHF (Angermann et al. 2016; O'Connor et al. 2010). CBT was shown in one study to improve mood in depressed patients with heart failure but not to improve patient engagement with CHF self-care (Freedland et al. 2015).

Anxiety and Trauma- and Stressor-Related Disorders

Anxiety and Coronary Disease

The relationship of anxiety symptoms and disorders to CAD remains unsettled. Several studies have found that anxiety symptoms increase the risk of incident CAD (Eaker et al. 2005; Shen et al. 2008; Thurston et al. 2013), and in middle-aged and older men without heart disease, anxiety is associated with incident MI even after controlling for other predictors (Shen et al. 2008). However, lifetime anxiety *disorders* were not associated with risk of CAD in a large epidemiological survey of older adults (Herbst et al. 2007). Anxiety symptoms and tension also modestly increase the risk of incident atrial fibrillation (Eaker et al. 2005).

Epidemiological studies do demonstrate an association of anxiety with sudden cardiac death (Kawachi et al. 1994a, 1994b). In patients with CAD, phobic anxiety is also associated with increased risk of ventricular arrhythmias, and the co-occurrence of anxiety and depression symptoms elevates this risk further (Watkins et al. 2006). For patients with preexisting CAD, studies of the effect of anxiety on prognosis have reported mixed findings. A meta-analysis found a weak association of anxiety with mortality in CAD patients in unadjusted analyses, but not after adjustment for relevant covariates (Celano et al. 2015).

A very large prospective epidemiological cohort study found a nearly twofold increased incidence of CAD in panic disorder patients, after controlling for tobacco use, comorbid depression, medications, and obesity (Gomez-Caminero et al. 2005). In the Women's Health Initiative, panic attacks were common in healthy postmenopausal women and were associated with increased risk of subsequent CAD, stroke, and all-cause mortality (Smoller et al. 2007).

Posttraumatic Stress Disorder and Coronary Disease

Increased coronary disease incidence also occurs in association with elevated PTSD symptom severity (Edmondson and von Känel 2017; Edmondson et al. 2013; Kubzansky et al. 2007; Vilchinsky et al. 2017). PTSD in patients with established coronary disease is associated with physical symptom burden and impaired QoL and has a stronger association with self-reported cardiovascular health status than do objective measures of cardiac function (Cohen et al. 2009). Anxiety in acute coronary syndrome patients is associated with reduced adherence to smoking cessation and exercise recommendations (Kuhl et al. 2009).

Anger, Type A Behavior, and Hostility

Type A behavior pattern—characterized by anger, impatience, aggravation, and irritability—was linked in influential studies in the 1970s (Rosenman et al. 1975) to an approximately twofold increased risk of incident coronary disease and fatal coronary events in men, although many subsequent studies had mixed findings or negative findings. Anger and hostility, considered as "toxic components" within the Type A concept, have also been studied as risk factors for coronary disease, with a majority of (but not all) studies finding that high anger and high hostility are linked to increased cardiovascular risk (Chida and Steptoe 2009; Krantz et al. 2006). In two studies, group counseling to reduce anger and type A behavior patterns substantially reduced mortality and recurrent infarction (Friedman et al. 1986; Gulliksson et al. 2011).

Type D Personality

The combined tendency to experience negative affects (anxiety or depression) and to inhibit expression of negative emotions in social interactions has been termed Type D (for "distressed") personality (Denollet 2005) and has been linked in European studies to increased risk of coronary events and arrhythmias (Denollet et al. 1995; van den Broek et al. 2009). However, more recent methodologically sound studies suggest that early Type D studies overestimated the prognostic relevance (Grande et al. 2012).

Acute Mental Stress

George Engel, who championed the biopsychosocial model in medicine, provided vivid examples from the news media of acute mental stress preceding acute coronary events (Engel 1976), and epidemiological studies of disasters have helped to demonstrate the relationship between acute stressful life events and risk of sudden cardiac death (Dimsdale 2008; Nakagawa et al. 2009). Even sports events, such as World Cup soccer matches, can have an epidemiologically significant stress effect on the incidence of coronary events (Wilbert-Lampen et al. 2008). In the aftermath of the destruction of the World Trade Center in New York City in September 2001, patients with implanted defibrillators had an increased frequency of ventricular tachycardia and ventricular fibrillation episodes, even if they were geographically distant and at no risk of physical harm (Shedd et al. 2004; Steinberg et al. 2004). Acute emotional stress can provoke a variety of supraventricular arrhythmias, as well as ventricular tachycardia and fibrillation (Ziegelstein 2007). Animal models demonstrate that the combination of acute stress and underlying myocardial ischemia can provoke ventricular tachyarrhythmias, an effect mediated by stress-induced sympathetic nervous system activation (DeSilva 1993).

In laboratory settings, provocation of acute mental stress results in elevations in heart rate and blood pressure and alterations in indices of cardiac autonomic regulation, with diminished parasympathetic and elevated sympathetic activation, in both healthy volunteers and patients with CAD (Sheps et al. 2002). Coronary vasospasm and mental stress–induced platelet activation are additional mechanisms of mental stress–induced ischemia in at least some cases (Reid et al. 2009; Yeung et al. 1991). Patients with CAD may experience ischemia during mental stress. Ischemia occurs at lower levels of rate–pressure product elevation during mental stress than during exercise stress, and may be asymptomatic (Rozanski et al. 1988). Emotional arousal in the course of everyday life, especially anger, has similar hemodynamic and autonomic effects; acute emotional stress can be identified as a trigger in up to 20%–30% of acute coronary events (Jiang 2015). In patients with coronary disease, mental stress–induced ischemia is associated with more than a doubling of the risk of death, even after adjustment for other prognostic variables (Jiang 2015). Mental stress–induced myocardial ischemia in CAD patients is also associated with heightened QT interval variability, increasing proarrhythmic risk (Hassan et al. 2009). A placebo-controlled trial of escitalopram demonstrated substantial reductions in mental stress–induced ischemia but not in exercise-induced ischemia (Jiang et al. 2013), but to date no study has demonstrated an effect of any antidepressant on clinical cardiac outcomes for patients with mental stress–induced ischemia.

Acute stress cardiomyopathy, sometimes referred to as Takotsubo cardiomyopathy or "broken heart syndrome," is an uncommon illness occurring in the setting of sudden emotional stress or surprise (Auzel et al. 2016). Affected individuals, who are predominantly female, experience abrupt onset of ventricular dysfunction, with characteristic ventricular apical ballooning seen on echocardiography, with chest pain and/or hypotension, in the absence of atherosclerosis or CAD (Tsai et al. 2009; Wittstein 2007). Prior history of anxiety disorders is associated with increased risk (Nayeri et al. 2017; Salmoirago-Blotcher et al. 2016). Most patients recover, with improvement in ventricular function occurring over several days to weeks (Bielecka-Dabrowa et al. 2010; Wittstein 2007). An abrupt surge in sympathetic nervous system activation is believed to cause the ventricular dysfunction (Wittstein 2016).

Chronic Mental Stress

The cumulative effect of chronic or recurring emotional stressors on risk of MI was strikingly demonstrated in the INTERHEART study (Rosengren et al. 2004), a 52-country investigation evaluating chronic stress in more than 11,000 MI patients and more than 13,000 matched control subjects. Work stress, family stress, and general stress over the past year were each associated with significantly increased risk of MI (odds ratios>2). The total number of stressors reported also correlated with MI risk. Chronic job strain is associated with a doubling of risk for recurrent CAD events (see, e.g., Aboa-Eboulé et al. 2007).

Low Social Support

Although social support is an omnibus term covering a variety of quantitative (i.e., How many relationships?) and qualitative (i.e., What kinds of relationships?) aspects of social relationships, most studies in this area have shown an association between low levels of social support and increased risk of coronary disease development and progression. The effect of social support is moderated by socioeconomic status, depression, and cultural factors (Lett et al. 2005; Wang et al. 2006). In two trials, efforts to improve social support for post-MI patients with low social support did not improve cardiac outcomes (Burg et al. 2005; Frasure-Smith et al. 1997).

Other Psychiatric Disorders

Increased cardiovascular mortality risk is also associated with schizophrenia and bipolar disorder (Correll et al. 2017; Sowden and Huffman 2009). Adults with bipolar I disorder have increased rates and earlier age at onset of hypertension and CAD compared with the general population, even after other predictive variables are controlled (Goldstein et al. 2009). The extent to which cardiovascular risk is influenced by the pathophysiological effects of these psychiatric illnesses—as opposed to the effects of lifestyle and associated behaviors (e.g., smoking) and treatments (e.g., antipsychotic drugs, lithium, anticonvulsants)—is uncertain. Most atypical antipsychotic agents increase the risk of metabolic syndrome (Mitchell et al. 2013; Ringen et al. 2014). Schizophrenia and bipolar disorder are each associated with high rates of other medical comorbidities (C.P. Carney and Jones 2006; R.M. Carney et al. 2006).

Diagnostic Issues

Most psychiatric diagnoses are reached in a straightforward fashion in patients with heart disease; however, confusion may arise because of the overlap of symptoms of heart disease with symptoms of psychiatric disorders, and because treatments for heart disease may cause psychiatric side effects. A depression diagnosis should never be based solely on a positive score on a depression screening measure (Thombs et al. 2013). The most frequent problem in psychiatric diagnosis is attribution of symptoms of depression to the underlying cardiac disease or to a "normal" reaction to the illness, with a resultant underdiagnosis of depression. Generally in practice, however, an inclusive approach is appropriate, with symptoms such as fatigue and poor sleep counted toward a diagnosis of depression even if those symptoms might also be attributable to the patient's cardiac condition (see Chapter 7, "Depression"). Patients who report somatic symptoms of depression should be evaluated for the presence of the cardinal mood and interest symptoms, and they should be considered to be depressed if these symptoms are present. Patients with advanced heart failure often develop appetite loss and cachexia, but in the absence of loss of self-esteem, loss of interest in ordinarily enjoyable events, or depressed mood, these patients should not be diagnosed with a depressive disorder.

Paroxysmal Supraventricular Tachycardia

Paroxysmal supraventricular tachycardia (PSVT) occurs in young and middle-aged adults and may manifest as symptoms of shortness of breath, chest discomfort, and apprehension. Because these features may overlap with those of generalized anxiety disorder and panic attacks, there is a significant risk of misdiagnosis. A retrospective study of 107 patients with PSVT found that criteria for panic disorder were met by 59 patients (67%); PSVT had been unrecognized after initial medical evaluation in 55% and remained unrecognized for a median of 3.3 years. Prior to the eventual identification of PSVT, nonpsychiatric physicians attributed patient symptoms to panic, anxiety, or stress for 32 (54%) of the 59 patients (Lessmeier et al. 1997). Of course, some patients may have both PSVT and an anxiety disorder, with symptomatic attacks including elements of each.

Atypical Chest Pain and Palpitations

Typical anginal chest pain in CAD occurs with exertion or after eating; is not exacerbated by palpation of the chest or by inspiration; is described as dull, pressure-like, or burning rather than sharp or stabbing; and is experienced across the precordium rather than in a pinpoint area of the left side of the chest. Many patients present for evaluation of atypical chest pain (Campbell et al. 2017). Although atypical features do not conclusively rule out a diagnosis of CAD, 40%–70% of patients with no history of documented CAD and few CAD risk factors ultimately receive a diagnosis of panic disorder, somatic symptom disorder, or depression (Campbell et al. 2017). Patients with noncardiac chest pain demonstrate a high prevalence of anxiety disorders (approximately 40%–60%), including panic and social phobia; depression (approximately 5%–25%); and somatoform disorders (2%–15%), as well as subsyndromal symptoms of these disorders (Hocaoglu et al. 2008; Jonsbu et al. 2009; White et al. 2008). More than half of children with noncardiac chest pain have an anxiety disorder, usually panic disorder (Achiam-Montal et al. 2013). A small randomized trial reported that an 8-week course of paroxetine treatment was beneficial in noncardiac chest pain patients who did not meet criteria for panic disorder or depression (Doraiswamy et al. 2006); some of these patients might have "non-fearful" panic attacks (Foldes-Busque et al. 2015). Factitious disorder and deception (malingering) can also present with noncardiac chest pain.

In the absence of CAD, characteristics of chest pain patients predicting panic disorder include female sex, atypical chest pain quality, younger age, lower education and income, and high self-reported anxiety (Dammen et al. 1999; Huffman and Pollack 2003).

CBT, breath retraining–relaxation exercises, and hypnosis have shown promise in controlled trials as treatments to reduce noncardiac chest pain. However, specific psychotherapy and pharmacotherapy for associated psychiatric diagnoses have not been demonstrated to reduce noncardiac chest pain (Kisely et al. 2015; van Beek et al. 2013).

Psychiatric disorders are also common in patients complaining of palpitations, especially panic disorder, MDD, and somatic symptom disorders (Barsky et al. 1994a; Jonsbu et al. 2009). Even when a patient with palpitations has a history of panic disorder, clinical examination alone may not be sufficient to exclude significant arrhythmias. Ambulatory electrocardiographic monitoring with loop recording is the most sensitive method for identifying the presence of a specific arrhythmia in patients with palpitations (Thavendiranathan et al. 2009).

Treatment Issues

Stress Management and Health Education Interventions in Coronary Artery Disease

Psychoeducational and stress management interventions for patients with CAD may encompass a variety of components, including diet and nutrition advice, anger reduction, relaxation exercises and meditation, smoking cessation assistance, counseling on sexual activity, and supervised exercise training. These interventions have been found to reduce MI recurrence and mortality (Dusseldorp et al. 1999). Longer intervention programs with more hours of intervention and more tailoring of program content to individual needs appear to have greater long-term effects on cardiac outcomes (Linden 2000). Meta-analyses have been critical of the quality of individual trials and guarded in their assessment of the benefits of psychological interventions in CAD patients, suggesting effects ranging from modest benefits for anxiety and depression symptoms only (Rees et al. 2004) to reductions in cardiac and all-cause mortality and nonfatal MI associated with interventions with behavioral components, especially supervised exercise (Janssen et al. 2013; Rutledge et al. 2013; Welton et al. 2009; Whalley et al. 2014). Sexual counseling can reduce anxiety and improve sexual function and satisfaction in CAD patients (Steinke et al. 2013). Specialized counseling is also recommended before AICD implantation (Dunbar et al. 2012).

Psychotherapy

Psychological reactions to the experience of heart disease may include feelings of anxiety and sadness, as well as concerns about survival and well-being, the effects of illness on social roles and relationships, and the impact on loved ones. Denial is nearly universal as an initial reaction to illness and can be either helpful (by staving off depressed and anxious mood) or hurtful (by leading to treatment nonadherence). Conversely, preoccupation with disease can lead to abnormal illness behavior, unnecessary disability, and impaired QoL. Psychotherapy for patients with heart disease might be aimed at reducing psychological distress or at improving functional status and medical outcomes, or some combination of both (Whalley et al. 2014).

The ENRICHD trial tested the effects of a CBT intervention versus usual care in patients with a recent MI and either low social support or depression. Most patients in the intervention arm received 6–10 individual or group therapy sessions. The trial demonstrated a small but statistically significant benefit of the CBT intervention on measures of social support and depression (Berkman et al. 2003). Innovative collaborative care models employing stepped care with brief counseling, problem-solving therapy, and CBT, sometimes along with medication, have been successful in reducing depression symptoms and improving health-related QoL in patients following CABG and after acute coronary events (Davidson et al. 2010c, 2013; Huffman et al. 2014; Rollman et al. 2009) but have not been shown to improve cardiac outcomes (Herrmann-Lingen et al. 2016). Attention to patient preferences for psychotherapy versus medication as first-line therapy appears to improve patient satisfaction (Davidson et al. 2013).

Role transition problems linked to changes in social roles, including changes caused by development of illness, are a prototypical focus of interpersonal psychotherapy (IPT) of depression. Therefore, IPT would seem to be readily applicable to the treatment of patients who experience depression after the onset or exacerbation of heart disease. However, the only published controlled trial of IPT for depression in patients with CAD, the CREATE trial (Lespérance et al. 2007), found no added benefit of IPT compared with clinical management alone.

Focused counseling and psychoeducation have been recommended to improve understanding and reduce stress and anxiety for heart disease patients who are preparing to have implanted defibrillators or LVADs, and to improve sexual functioning in cardiac patients (Dunbar et al. 2012; Nakagawa et al. 2017; Steinke et al. 2013).

Psychopharmacological Treatment

Common adverse cardiac effects of psychiatric drugs are listed in Table 17–2 (see also Chapter 36, "Psychopharmacology").

TABLE 17–2. **Selected cardiac side effects of psychotropic drugs**

Drug/class	Cardiac effects
Lithium	Sinus node dysfunction and arrest
SSRIs	Slowing of heart rate; occasional sinus bradycardia or sinus arrest
TCAs	Orthostatic hypotension; atrioventricular conduction disturbance; class IA antiarrhythmic effect; proarrhythmia in overdose and in setting of ischemia
MAOIs	Orthostatic hypotension
First-generation antipsychotics	Orthostatic hypotension (especially low-potency drugs); QT interval prolongation; torsade de pointes
Second-generation antipsychotics	Variable; QT interval prolongation; ventricular arrhythmias; metabolic syndrome
Clozapine	Effects listed above plus orthostatic hypotension; myocarditis
Carbamazepine	Class IA antiarrhythmic effects; atrioventricular block; hyponatremia
Cholinesterase inhibitors	Decreased heart rate

Note.   MAOIs=monoamine oxidase inhibitors; SSRIs=selective serotonin reuptake inhibitors; TCAs=tricyclic antidepressants.

Antidepressants

Antidepressants must be used at therapeutically effective dosages in cardiac patients with depression; it is counterproductive to use inadequate dosages out of fear of side effects or prolongation of metabolism. Unless the patient has severe right-sided heart failure resulting in hepatic congestion, ascites, and jaundice, it is unlikely that metabolism of oral psychotropic medication (except for lithium) will be substantially impaired because of heart disease.

TCAs.   TCAs cause orthostatic hypotension, cardiac conduction delay (bundle branch block or complete atrioventricular nodal block), and, in overdose, ventricular arrhythmias (including potentially lethal ventricular tachycardia and ventricular fibrillation). QRS interval prolongation results from interference with phase 1 (depolarization across the cell membrane) of the action potential in the specialized cardiac conduction system. Prolongation of the QT interval is predominantly caused by prolongation of the QRS interval, and ventricular tachycardia or fibrillation can occur with marked prolongation of the QT interval (typically >500 msec). Cardiac pacemakers can obviate the risk of heart block associated with TCAs. More commonly problematic, however, is orthostatic hypotension, which can lead to syncope and falls. Nortriptyline and desipramine tend to cause less orthostatic hypotension than tertiary-amine TCAs and are better tolerated by patients with cardiac disease (Roose and Glassman 1989).

TCAs have quinidine-like effects on cardiac conduction and are classified as type IA antiarrhythmics. Drugs of this class have been shown to increase mortality in post-MI patients with premature ventricular contractions (Morganroth and Goin 1991), an effect believed to be moderated by episodic myocardial ischemia. Consequently,

TCAs should generally not be used as first-line agents for treatment of depression in ischemic heart disease patients, although their efficacy may occasionally offset the risk in selected patients. Consideration should be given to the totality of the clinical situation, including depression severity, past treatment responses, concomitant medications, and electrocardiogram (ECG) findings (Glassman et al. 1993).

SSRIs.   SSRIs have little to no cardiac effect in healthy subjects. The most commonly observed effect is slowing of the heart rate, generally by a clinically insignificant 1–2 beats per minute. Occasional cases of sinus bradycardia or sinus arrest, with light-headedness or syncope, have been reported (Roose et al. 1998a, 1998b). The combination of beta-adrenergic blockade and SSRIs may result in additive slowing of the heart rate with increased risk of symptoms. In addition, some SSRIs (fluoxetine, paroxetine, fluvoxamine) inhibit the metabolism of beta-blockers through the cytochrome P450 (CYP) 2D6 pathway (responsible for the metabolism of most beta-blockers), potentially causing the blood levels and effects of beta-adrenergic blockers to be increased.

In patients with preexisting heart disease, the effects of SSRIs on heart rate are similar to those seen in disease-free patients, and no blood pressure, cardiac conduction, or arrhythmia effects have been noted (Roose et al. 1994, 1998a, 1998b). The SAD-HART study was a double-blind, placebo-controlled, randomized trial examining the effect of sertraline in patients with MDD immediately after an acute coronary event. Sertraline had no effect on heart rate, blood pressure, arrhythmias, ejection fraction, or cardiac conduction, and adverse events were rare. All patients in the SADHART study began medication within 30 days of the index acute coronary event (Glassman et al. 2002). Sertraline was more effective than placebo in treating depression in patients with a prior history of depression, but it did not differ from placebo in patients without a prior history (Glassman et al. 2006).

The CREATE trial (Lespérance et al. 2007) was a 12-week randomized controlled study utilizing a two-by-two factorial design to compare citalopram (20–40 mg/day) with placebo treatment, while simultaneously comparing clinical management with and without interpersonal psychotherapy, for treatment of depression in patients with stable coronary disease. Citalopram was significantly superior to placebo both in improving depression symptoms and with respect to remission rates.

Mirtazapine treatment (30–45 mg/day) of depression in patients who had had an acute coronary event was evaluated in the MIND-IT randomized placebo-controlled trial (Honig et al. 2007). This study employed several measures of depression at 8 and 24 weeks. Findings were mixed, but mirtazapine was superior to placebo on some measures at both follow-up assessments. Mirtazapine was well tolerated by the patients in this trial, with no effects on heart rate, blood pressure, or electrocardiographic parameters, and no difference from placebo in the rate of major adverse cardiac events.

Randomized placebo-controlled studies of citalopram, escitalopram (the MOOD-HF trial), and sertraline (the SADHART-CHF trial) in depressed CHF patients found the drugs to be well tolerated but failed to find a beneficial effect on mood or medical outcomes (Angermann et al. 2016; Fraguas et al. 2009; O'Connor et al. 2010). A very small ($N=28$) randomized double-blind, placebo-controlled trial in patients with chronic heart failure found paroxetine superior to placebo in reducing depressive symptoms (Gottlieb et al. 2007).

Dose-dependent QT interval prolongation occurs with citalopram treatment, and to a lesser degree with other SSRIs (Castro et al. 2013). Although the U.S. Food and Drug Administration (FDA) has imposed a boxed warning against use of citalopram dosages greater than 40 mg/day because of concerns about ventricular arrhythmias, there is little evidence that higher dosages of citalopram are associated with an increased risk of sudden cardiac death (Zivin et al. 2013).

Other antidepressants. The cardiovascular effects of other antidepressants have been less fully studied than those of TCAs and SSRIs, especially in patients with cardiac disease. Bupropion appears to have few cardiovascular effects but may increase blood pressure occasionally (Roose et al. 1991). The serotonin–norepinephrine reuptake inhibitor venlafaxine behaves like an SSRI at low dosages and displays noradrenergic effects at higher dosages. The main cardiovascular effect of this dual action is a tendency to increase blood pressure in a dose-dependent fashion at dosages of 150 mg/day or higher. There may be a diminution of this hypertensive effect of venlafaxine with its extended-release formulation. Venlafaxine's effects in patients with preexisting heart disease or hypertension have not been evaluated.

Clinical experience with mirtazapine in patients with hypertension has also demonstrated instances of worsening hypertension, although the frequency of this adverse effect is unknown. In a study using Swedish national registry data, mirtazapine was the antidepressant most associated with sudden cardiac death (Danielsson et al. 2016); however, no other study to date has corroborated this risk.

Monoamine oxidase inhibitors (MAOIs) cause hypotension and orthostatic hypotension; dietary indiscretions leading to high circulating levels of tyramine can cause hypertensive crises. Sympathomimetic agents can increase blood pressure in patients on MAOIs, although hypertensive crises are infrequent. The use of intravenous pressors (epinephrine, isoproterenol, norepinephrine, dopamine, dobutamine) in patients receiving MAOIs requires caution (Krishnan 1995).

Antipsychotics

Antipsychotics are used in cardiac disease patients with comorbid schizophrenia, schizoaffective disorder, bipolar disorder, or other psychotic disorders, as well as in the (off-label) management of delirium in acute cardiac care settings. First-generation antipsychotics continue to play a role in the management of acute psychotic symptoms in cardiac patients, in part because of the availability of parenteral formulations for haloperidol, few cardiovascular effects, and extensive experience with the use of intravenous haloperidol in the critically ill.

For chronically psychotic patients with heart disease, the choice of antipsychotic is based on side-effect profile. The principal cardiovascular effects of antipsychotics are orthostatic hypotension and QT interval prolongation. Orthostatic hypotension secondary to antipsychotic drugs is related to these drugs' alpha-adrenergic receptor–blocking effects (seen especially with clozapine and low-potency antipsychotics such as chlorpromazine) and is often accompanied by sedative effects. Few data are available on the frequency or clinical significance of orthostatic effects of antipsychotic drugs in patients with heart disease. More attention has been paid to the less common but much more dramatic and dangerous side effect of cardiac arrest secondary to ventricular tachyarrhythmias in patients on antipsychotics (Beach et al. 2013). The characteristic tachyarrhythmia is torsade de pointes (TdP), a polymorphic tachycardia with the appearance of "twisting of the points" of the QRS complex. QT prolongation caused by antipsychotics, unlike that caused by TCAs, is related to impaired repolarization of the ventricular conduction tissue at the end of systole. Aripiprazole carries little risk of QT interval prolongation, although there have been isolated case reports of prolonged QT interval and sudden death (Polcwiartek et al. 2015). The QT interval normally is less than 450 msec in men and 460 msec in women. Because the normal QT interval is dependent on heart rate, evaluation customarily adjusts for heart rate, by one of several formulas, to yield a corrected QT interval (QTc). The risk of TdP increases gradually with increasing QTc interval, such that risk is approximately doubled when the QTc reaches 500 msec, compared with the risk associated with a QTc of 400 msec. Intravenous haloperidol is frequently employed in delirious open-heart surgery patients, and although it does have the potential to prolong the QT interval, its use at dosages of up to 1,000 mg/24 hours has been reported without complications (Tesar et al. 1985). Clearly, electrocardiographic monitoring is important in intensive care settings and is recommended during antipsychotic treatment when the QTc is greater than 450 msec in men or 470 msec in women, although in the absence of structural heart disease there is little risk of TdP as long as the QTc remains lower than 500 msec. A QTc interval over 500 msec is generally considered a contraindication to the use of haloperidol and other QT-prolonging agents.

Before prescribing drugs that prolong the QT interval, risk factors for TdP should be reviewed. These include female sex; familial long QT syndrome; family or personal history of sudden cardiac death, syncope, or unexplained seizure; arrhythmias; personal history of hypertension; other medications that prolong the QT interval or that may interfere with metabolism of other QT-prolonging agents; valvular heart disease; and bradycardia. Laboratory values of particular importance are magnesium, calcium, and potassium levels. Class IA and III antiarrhythmic drugs, dolasetron, droperidol, tacrolimus, levomethadyl acetate, other antipsychotics, many antibiotics ("floxacins"), and antifungals may increase the risk of TdP (Beach et al. 2013).

A large cohort study taking advantage of statewide Medicaid prescription data found that antipsychotic use was associated with a doubling of the risk of sudden cardiac death; the increase in the absolute risk of sudden cardiac death was about 0.15%, meaning that 1 extra death would occur for every 666 persons treated for 1 year with antipsychotics (Ray et al. 2009). It seems clear that this risk would be higher in patients with preexisting cardiac disease maintained on antipsychotics. A recent Swedish registry study identified haloperidol, risperidone, olanzapine, and quetiapine as the antipsychotics associated with the highest risk of sudden cardiac death (Danielsson et al. 2016). For elderly patients receiving antipsychotics for agitation or behavioral disturbance (e.g., psychotic symptoms in dementia), the risk of death associated with antipsychotics is substantially higher, due mostly to cardiac events and infections (Schneider et al. 2005), a circumstance that led the FDA to require a boxed warning against the use of antipsychotics in elderly patients with dementia.

Polymorphic ventricular tachycardia can also occur in the absence of a long QT interval. Brugada syndrome is a rare disorder characterized by a history of syncope and risk of sudden death due to polymorphic ventricular tachyarrhythmias. Lithium has been reported to provoke Brugada syndrome, and drugs that interfere with the sodium channel and prolong the depolarization phase of the action potential, including phenothiazines, TCAs, and carbamazepine, might also increase risk (Laske et al. 2007).

Second-generation antipsychotics also increase cardiovascular disease risk indirectly through promotion of the metabolic syndrome (i.e, dyslipidemia, obesity, hypertension, and impaired glycemic control). Olanzapine and clozapine appear most likely, and aripiprazole and ziprasidone least likely, to induce metabolic syndrome. In the Clinical Antipsychotic Trials of Intervention Effectiveness (CATIE) study, olanzapine and quetiapine were associated with a slight increase, and risperidone, ziprasidone, and perphenazine with a slight decrease, in the 10-year risk of heart disease (Bobes et al. 2007; Correll et al. 2006, 2009; Daumit et al. 2008; Newcomer and Hennekens 2007).

Myocarditis has been estimated to occur in 0.01%–1.0% of patients treated with clozapine, generally within the first few weeks of treatment. Cardiomyopathy has also been reported, with onset up to a few years after starting clozapine, even without prior acute myocarditis (Alawami et al. 2014; Mackin 2008).

Anxiolytics

Benzodiazepines have no specific cardiac effects. Reduction of anxiety tends to reduce sympathetic nervous system activation and, therefore, to slow heart rate, decrease myocardial workload, and reduce myocardial irritability. Before the introduction of beta-blockers into acute coronary care, benzodiazepines were widely used for prophylaxis of infarct extension and arrhythmias in patients with acute coronary syndrome, but this practice has largely been abandoned. Oxazepam, lorazepam, and temazepam do not undergo phase I hepatic metabolism and may be better tolerated by patients with heart failure with hepatic congestion. Buspirone has no cardiovascular effects.

Stimulants

Stimulants are often used for treatment of depressed medically ill patients, particularly those with pronounced apathy, fatigue, or psychomotor slowing. Stimulant treatment of attention-deficit/hyperactivity disorder (ADHD) in adults increases systolic and diastolic blood pressure by about 5 mm Hg (Wilens et al. 2005), but the dosages used in ADHD treatment are typically higher than those that would be used in cardiac patients. At dosages of 5–30 mg/day, dextroamphetamine and methylphenidate are generally well tolerated by heart disease patients, including patients with a history of cardiac arrhythmias and angina (Masand and Tesar 1996), and have little effect on heart rate and blood pressure. Clinical response generally occurs within days rather than weeks. The safety of a long-term treatment that raises blood pressure by 5 mm Hg has been questioned (Nissen 2006), but several large-scale studies have found no evidence of increased risk of cardiovascular adverse events in children, adolescents, or adults receiving stimulant treatment (Cooper et al. 2011; Olfson et al. 2012; Peyre et al. 2014; Winterstein et al. 2012). Nevertheless, a cardiology consultation may be prudent before prescribing stimulants for patients with heart disease.

Lithium

Lithium occasionally causes sinus node dysfunction and even sinus arrest. There are no studies of the use of lithium in patients with heart disease. Generally, even in patients with reduced cardiac output, lithium can be safely used by adjusting the dosage downward. Because renal function is sometimes impaired in advanced heart failure, lithium dosing requires further reduction. Caution is necessary for patients taking ACE inhibitors, angiotensin II receptor blockers, and/or diuretics, especially thiazides, and for those on salt-restricted diets. In patients with acute CHF exacerbations and acute coronary syndromes, rapid electrolyte and fluid balance shifts can occur; lithium is best avoided during such episodes because of the difficulty managing fluctuations in lithium levels as cardiac therapy (especially diuretics) is adjusted.

Other Mood Stabilizers

Valproic acid and lamotrigine have no cardiovascular effects. Carbamazepine resembles TCAs in having quinidine-like class IA antiarrhythmic effects and may cause atrioventricular conduction disturbances.

Cholinesterase Inhibitors and *N*-Methyl-D-Aspartate Receptor Antagonists

The procholinergic effect of cholinesterase inhibitors may cause vagotonic effects, including bradycardia or heart block. For the *N*-methyl-D-aspartate (NMDA) receptor antagonist memantine, hypertension is the only cardiac effect described by the manufacturer on the basis of premarketing controlled trials.

Electroconvulsive Therapy

Electroconvulsive therapy (ECT) leads to an initial sympathetic discharge, with tachycardia and hypertension, followed by a parasympathetic reflex response, with instances of bradycardia and arrhythmia. Excessive bradycardia can be prevented by premedication with atropine. Excessive sympathetic response may induce myocardial ischemia; for elderly patients or those with known coronary disease, monitoring the ECG is essential, and treatment with intravenous beta-blockers is sometimes required. ECT has been used safely in patients with ischemic heart disease, heart failure, and heart transplants. Acute MI or recent malignant tachyarrhythmias are relatively strong contraindications. Takotsubo cardiomyopathy has been reported after ECT; a case of successful reintroduction of ECT after prior Takotsubo cardiomyopathy response to ECT has also been reported (Kent et al. 2009; O'Reardon et al. 2008). Cardiac effects of ECT are discussed in greater detail in Chapter 38, "Electroconvulsive Therapy and Other Brain Stimulation Therapies."

Cardiac–Psychiatric Drug Interactions

A few drug interactions between psychotropic and cardiovascular drugs are worth noting (Table 17–3). Many psychotropic drugs lower blood pressure; their interaction with antihypertensives, vasodilators, and diuretics may potentiate hypotension. TCAs and antipsychotics that prolong the QT interval may interact with antiarrhythmics such as quinidine, procainamide, moricizine, and amiodarone and result in further QT prolongation or atrioventricular block. Although SSRIs may increase the risk of bleeding, most do not appear to have a clinically significant effect on the international normalized ratio (INR) in patients treated with warfarin. The largest INR effects occur with fluoxetine and fluvoxamine (Holbrook et al. 2005). In patients under-

TABLE 17–3. **Selected psychotropic drug interactions with cardiovascular drugs**

Psychotropic agent	Cardiovascular agent	Effect
SSRIs	Beta-blockers	Additive bradycardic effects
	Warfarin	Increased bleeding risk, especially with paroxetine and fluoxetine, despite little effect on INR
MAOIs	Epinephrine, dopamine	Hypertension
TCAs	Class IA antiarrhythmics, amiodarone	Prolonged QT interval, increased AV block
Lithium	ACE inhibitors, angiotensin II receptor blockers	Increased lithium level
	Thiazide diuretics	Increased lithium level
Phenothiazines	Beta-blockers	Hypotension

Note. ACE=angiotensin-converting enzyme; AV=atrioventricular; INR=international normalized ratio; MAOIs=monoamine oxidase inhibitors; SSRIs=selective serotonin reuptake inhibitors; TCAs= tricyclic antidepressants.

going CABG, SSRIs do not increase bleeding risk or hospital mortality, even when administered with warfarin, antiplatelet therapies, and/or nonsteroidal anti-inflammatory drugs (D.H. Kim et al. 2009). Over the long term, however, concomitant SSRI use approximately doubles the risk of bleeding associated with antiplatelet agents and warfarin alone (Cochran et al. 2011; Labos et al. 2011).

Drug Interactions: Cytochrome P450 Issues

CYP2D6 is responsible for the metabolism of many beta-blockers, carvedilol, and anti-arrhythmics; this metabolic pathway is inhibited by haloperidol, fluoxetine, and paroxetine, with resulting elevation of blood levels of CYP2D6 substrates. Conversely, amiodarone is a 2D6 inhibitor and can elevate blood levels of TCAs, fluoxetine, and risperidone. CYP3A4 is responsible for metabolism of alprazolam, midazolam, triazolam, zolpidem, buspirone, carbamazepine, and haloperidol, and of calcium channel blockers, many statins, cyclosporine, and tacrolimus. The 3A4 system is inhibited by amiodarone, diltiazem, verapamil, grapefruit juice, and nefazodone—and, to a lesser degree, by fluoxetine and sertraline. Thus, for example, the combination of nefazodone and haloperidol might increase the risk of ventricular arrhythmias, because increased haloperidol levels may result in greater QT prolongation. Carbamazepine and St. John's wort are inducers of CYP3A4 activity. Many Web-based resources for review of cytochrome P450 interactions are available; further discussion of this topic is provided in Chapter 36, "Psychopharmacology."

Conclusion

Because heart disease is so common, psychiatrists have ample opportunity to consider the many issues it raises in the course of mental health care. The meaning and psychological impact of heart disease for the patient, the threat of death, the effects and interactions of cardiac and psychiatric medications, and the wide range of emotional responses and psychiatric disorders that affect and are affected by cardiovascular disease and its treatment—all of these issues require the psychiatrist's thoughtful vigilance and an integrated, biopsychosocial treatment perspective. The continuing rapid introduction of new technologies and treatments in cardiology and cardiac surgery, and in psychiatry, will alter some of what psychiatrists need to know, but not the fundamental human condition and the experience of crisis posed by life-threatening illness.

References

Aboa-Eboulé C, Brisson C, Maunsell E, et al: Job strain and risk of acute recurrent coronary heart disease events. JAMA 298(14):1652–1660, 2007 17925517

Achiam-Montal M, Tibi L, Lipsitz JD: Panic disorder in children and adolescents with noncardiac chest pain. Child Psychiatry Hum Dev 44(6):742–750, 2013 23378228

Afilalo J, Rasti M, Ohayon SM, et al: Off-pump vs. on-pump coronary artery bypass surgery: an updated meta-analysis and meta-regression of randomized trials. Eur Heart J 33(10):1257–1267, 2012 21987177

Alawami M, Wasywich C, Cicovic A, et al: A systematic review of clozapine induced cardiomyopathy. Int J Cardiol 176(2):315–320, 2014 25131906

Albert NM, Fonarow GC, Abraham WT, et al: Depression and clinical outcomes in heart failure: an OPTIMIZE-HF analysis. Am J Med 122(4):366–373, 2009 19332232

American Psychiatric Association: Diagnostic and Statistical Manual of Mental Disorders, 4th Edition. Washington, DC, American Psychiatric Association, 1994

Angeli F, Verdecchia P, Gattobigio R, et al: White-coat hypertension in adults. Blood Press Monit 10(6):301–305, 2005 16496443

Angermann CE, Gelbrich G, Störk S, et al; MOOD-HF Study Investigators and Committee Members: Effect of escitalopram on all-cause mortality and hospitalization in patients with heart failure and depression: the MOOD-HF randomized clinical trial. JAMA 315(24):2683–2693, 2016 27367876

Appels A, Bär F, van der Pol G, et al: Effects of treating exhaustion in angioplasty patients on new coronary events: results of the randomized Exhaustion Intervention Trial (EXIT). Psychosom Med 67(2):217–223, 2005 15784786

Appels A, van Elderen T, Bär F, et al: Effects of a behavioural intervention on quality of life and related variables in angioplasty patients: results of the EXhaustion Intervention Trial. J Psychosom Res 61(1):1–7, discussion 9–10, 2006 16813838

Auzel O, Mustafic H, Pillière R, et al: Incidence, Characteristics, Risk Factors, and Outcomes of Takotsubo Cardiomyopathy With and Without Ventricular Arrhythmia. Am J Cardiol 117(8):1242–1247, 2016 26874546

Barlow DH: Anxiety and Its Disorders. New York, Guilford, 1988

Barr J, Fraser GL, Puntillo K, et al; American College of Critical Care Medicine: Clinical practice guidelines for the management of pain, agitation, and delirium in adult patients in the intensive care unit. Crit Care Med 41(1):263–306, 2013 23269131

Barsky AJ, Cleary PD, Coeytaux RR, et al: Psychiatric disorders in medical outpatients complaining of palpitations. J Gen Intern Med 9(6):306–313, 1994a 8077994

Barsky AJ, Cleary PD, Sarnie MK, et al: Panic disorder, palpitations, and the awareness of cardiac activity. J Nerv Ment Dis 182(2):63–71, 1994b 8308534

Barsky AJ, Delamater BA, Clancy SA, et al: Somatized psychiatric disorder presenting as palpitations. Arch Intern Med 156(10):1102–1108, 1996 8638998

Barth J, Schumacher M, Herrmann-Lingen C: Depression as a risk factor for mortality in patients with coronary heart disease: a meta-analysis. Psychosom Med 66(6):802–813, 2004 15564343

Beach SR, Celano CM, Noseworthy PA, et al: QTc prolongation, torsades de pointes, and psychotropic medications. Psychosomatics 54(1):1–13, 2013 23295003

Berkman LF, Blumenthal J, Burg M, et al; Enhancing Recovery in Coronary Heart Disease Patients Investigators (ENRICHD): Effects of treating depression and low perceived social support on clinical events after myocardial infarction: the Enhancing Recovery in Coronary Heart Disease Patients (ENRICHD) Randomized Trial. JAMA 289(23):3106–3116, 2003 12813116

Bielecka-Dabrowa A, Mikhailidis DP, Hannam S, et al: Takotsubo cardiomyopathy—the current state of knowledge. Int J Cardiol 142(2):120–125, 2010 20051293

Blumenthal JA, Lett HS, Babyak MA, et al; NORG Investigators: Depression as a risk factor for mortality after coronary artery bypass surgery. Lancet 362(9384):604–609, 2003 12944059

Blumenthal JA, Babyak MA, O'Connor C, et al: Effects of exercise training on depressive symptoms in patients with chronic heart failure: the HF-ACTION randomized trial. JAMA 308(5):465–474, 2012a 22851113

Blumenthal JA, Sherwood A, Babyak MA, et al: Exercise and pharmacological treatment of depressive symptoms in patients with coronary heart disease: results from the UPBEAT (Understanding the Prognostic Benefits of Exercise and Antidepressant Therapy) study. J Am Coll Cardiol 60(12):1053–1063, 2012b 22858387

Bobes J, Arango C, Aranda P, et al; CLAMORS Study Collaborative Group: Cardiovascular and metabolic risk in outpatients with schizophrenia treated with antipsychotics: results of the CLAMORS Study. Schizophr Res 90(1–3):162–173, 2007 17123783

Bostwick JM, Sola CL: An updated review of implantable cardioverter/defibrillators, induced anxiety, and quality of life. Heart Fail Clin 7(1):101–108, 2011 21109213

Bunevicius A, Staniute M, Brozaitiene J, et al: Screening for anxiety disorders in patients with coronary artery disease. Health Qual Life Outcomes 11:37, 2013 23497087

Burg MM, Barefoot J, Berkman L, et al; ENRICHD Investigators: Low perceived social support and post-myocardial infarction prognosis in the enhancing recovery in coronary heart disease clinical trial: the effects of treatment. Psychosom Med 67(6):879–888, 2005 16314592

Campbell KA, Madva EN, Villegas AC, et al: Non-cardiac chest pain: a review for the consultation-liaison psychiatrist. Psychosomatics 58(3):252–265, 2017 28196622

Carney CP, Jones LE: Medical comorbidity in women and men with bipolar disorders: a population-based controlled study. Psychosom Med 68(5):684–691, 2006 17012521

Carney CP, Jones L, Woolson RF: Medical comorbidity in women and men with schizophrenia: a population-based controlled study. J Gen Intern Med 21(11):1133–1137, 2006 17026726

Carney RM, Blumenthal JA, Stein PK, et al: Depression, heart rate variability, and acute myocardial infarction. Circulation 104(17):2024–2028, 2001 11673340

Carney RM, Blumenthal JA, Freedland KE, et al; ENRICHD Investigators: Depression and late mortality after myocardial infarction in the Enhancing Recovery in Coronary Heart Disease (ENRICHD) study. Psychosom Med 66(4):466–474, 2004 15272090

Carney RM, Blumenthal JA, Freedland KE, et al: Low heart rate variability and the effect of depression on post-myocardial infarction mortality. Arch Intern Med 165(13):1486–1491, 2005 16009863

Carney RM, Freedland KE, Steinmeyer B, et al: History of depression and survival after acute myocardial infarction. Psychosom Med 71(3):253–259, 2009 19251868

Castro VM, Clements CC, Murphy SN, et al: QT interval and antidepressant use: a cross sectional study of electronic health records. BMJ 346:f288, 2013 23360890

Celano CM, Millstein RA, Bedoya CA, et al: Association between anxiety and mortality in patients with coronary artery disease: a meta-analysis. Am Heart J 170(6):1105–1115, 2015 26678632

Cesari M, Penninx BW, Newman AB, et al: Inflammatory markers and onset of cardiovascular events: results from the Health ABC study. Circulation 108(19):2317–2322, 2003 14568895

Chida Y, Steptoe A: The association of anger and hostility with future coronary heart disease: a meta-analytic review of prospective evidence. J Am Coll Cardiol 53(11):936–946, 2009 19281923

Cochran KA, Cavallari LH, Shapiro NL, et al: Bleeding incidence with concomitant use of antidepressants and warfarin. Ther Drug Monit 33(4):433–438, 2011 21743381

Cohen BE, Marmar CR, Neylan TC, et al: Posttraumatic stress disorder and health-related quality of life in patients with coronary heart disease: findings from the Heart and Soul Study. Arch Gen Psychiatry 66(11):1214–1220, 2009 19884609

Connerney I, Shapiro PA, McLaughlin JS, et al: Relation between depression after coronary artery bypass surgery and 12-month outcome: a prospective study. Lancet 358(9295):1766–1771, 2001 11734233

Connerney I, Sloan RP, Shapiro PA, et al: Depression is associated with increased mortality 10 years after coronary artery bypass surgery. Psychosom Med 72(9):874–881, 2010 20841558

Cooper WO, Habel LA, Sox CM, et al: ADHD drugs and serious cardiovascular events in children and young adults. N Engl J Med 365(20):1896–1904, 2011 22043968

Correll CU, Frederickson AM, Kane JM, et al: Metabolic syndrome and the risk of coronary heart disease in 367 patients treated with second-generation antipsychotic drugs. J Clin Psychiatry 67(4):575–583, 2006 16669722

Correll CU, Manu P, Olshanskiy V, et al: Cardiometabolic risk of second-generation antipsychotic medications during first-time use in children and adolescents. JAMA 302(16):1765–1773, 2009 19861668

Correll CU, Solmi M, Veronese N, et al: Prevalence, incidence and mortality from cardiovascular disease in patients with pooled and specific severe mental illness: a large-scale meta-analysis of 3,211,768 patients and 113,383,368 controls. World Psychiatry 16(2):163–180, 2017 28498599

Crocker E, Beggs T, Hassan A, et al: Long-term effects of postoperative delirium in patients undergoing cardiac operation: a systematic review. Ann Thorac Surg 102(4):1391–1399, 2016 27344279

Cully JA, Johnson M, Moffett ML, et al: Depression and anxiety in ambulatory patients with heart failure. Psychosomatics 50(6):592–598, 2009 19996230

Dammen T, Ekeberg O, Arnesen H, et al: The detection of panic disorder in chest pain patients. Gen Hosp Psychiatry 21(5):323–332, 1999 10572773

Danielsson B, Collin J, Jonasdottir Bergman G, et al: Antidepressants and antipsychotics classified with torsades de pointes arrhythmia risk and mortality in older adults—a Swedish nationwide study. Br J Clin Pharmacol 81(4):773–783, 2016 26574175

Daumit GL, Goff DC, Meyer JM, et al: Antipsychotic effects on estimated 10-year coronary heart disease risk in the CATIE schizophrenia study. Schizophr Res 105(1–3):175–187, 2008 18775645

Davidson KW, Kupfer DJ, Bigger JT, et al; National Heart, Lung, and Blood Institute Working Group: Assessment and treatment of depression in patients with cardiovascular disease: National Heart, Lung, and Blood Institute Working Group Report. Psychosom Med 68(5):645–650, 2006 17012516

Davidson KW, Burg MM, Kronish IM, et al: Association of anhedonia with recurrent major adverse cardiac events and mortality 1 year after acute coronary syndrome. Arch Gen Psychiatry 67(5):480–488, 2010a 20439829

Davidson KW, Mostofsky E, Whang W: Don't worry, be happy: positive affect and reduced 10-year incident coronary heart disease: the Canadian Nova Scotia Health Survey. Eur Heart J 31(9):1065–1070, 2010b 20164244

Davidson KW, Rieckmann N, Clemow L, et al: Enhanced depression care for patients with acute coronary syndrome and persistent depressive symptoms: coronary psychosocial evaluation studies randomized controlled trial. Arch Intern Med 170(7):600–608, 2010c 20386003

Davidson KW, Bigger JT, Burg MM, et al: Centralized, stepped, patient preference-based treatment for patients with post-acute coronary syndrome depression: CODIACS vanguard randomized controlled trial. JAMA Intern Med 173(11):997–1004, 2013 23471421

DeBusk RF: Sexual activity in patients with angina. JAMA 290(23):3129–3132, 2003 14679276

de Jonge P, Honig A, van Melle JP, et al; MIND-IT Investigators: Nonresponse to treatment for depression following myocardial infarction: association with subsequent cardiac events. Am J Psychiatry 164(9):1371–1378, 2007 17728422

Dempe C, Jünger J, Hoppe S, et al: Association of anxious and depressive symptoms with medication nonadherence in patients with stable coronary artery disease. J Psychosom Res 74(2):122–127, 2013 23332526

Deng LX, Khan AM, Drajpuch D, et al: Prevalence and correlates of post-traumatic stress disorder in adults with congenital heart disease. Am J Cardiol 117(5):853–857, 2016 26803381

Denollet J: DS14: standard assessment of negative affectivity, social inhibition, and Type D personality. Psychosom Med 67(1):89–97, 2005 15673629

Denollet J, Sys SU, Brutsaert DL: Personality and mortality after myocardial infarction. Psychosom Med 57(6):582–591, 1995 8600485

DeSilva RA: Cardiac arrhythmias and sudden cardiac death, in Medical-Psychiatric Practice. Edited by Stoudemire A, Fogel BS. Washington, DC, American Psychiatric Press, 1993, pp 199–236

Detroyer E, Dobbels F, Verfaillie E, et al: Is preoperative anxiety and depression associated with onset of delirium after cardiac surgery in older patients? A prospective cohort study. J Am Geriatr Soc 56(12):2278–2284, 2008 19112653

Dickens C, McGowan L, Percival C, et al: New onset depression following myocardial infarction predicts cardiac mortality. Psychosom Med 70(4):450–455, 2008 18434496

Dimsdale JE: Psychological stress and cardiovascular disease. J Am Coll Cardiol 51(13):1237–1246, 2008 18371552

Doraiswamy PM, Varia I, Hellegers C, et al: A randomized controlled trial of paroxetine for noncardiac chest pain. Psychopharmacol Bull 39(1):15–24, 2006 17065971

Dunbar SB, Dougherty CM, Sears SF, et al; American Heart Association Council on Cardiovascular Nursing, Council on Clinical Cardiology, and Council on Cardiovascular Disease in the Young: Educational and psychological interventions to improve outcomes for recipients of implantable cardioverter defibrillators and their families: a scientific statement from the American Heart Association. Circulation 126(17):2146–2172, 2012 23008437

Dusseldorp E, van Elderen T, Maes S, et al: A meta-analysis of psychoeducational programs for coronary heart disease patients. Health Psychol 18(5):506–519, 1999 10519467

Eaker ED, Sullivan LM, Kelly Hayes M, et al: Tension and anxiety and the prediction of the 10-year incidence of coronary heart disease, atrial fibrillation, and total mortality: the Framingham Offspring Study. Psychosom Med 67(5):692–696, 2005 16204425

Easton K, Coventry P, Lovell K, et al: Prevalence and measurement of anxiety in samples of patients with heart failure: meta-analysis. J Cardiovasc Nurs 31(4):367–379, 2016 25930162

Edmondson D, von Känel R: Post-traumatic stress disorder and cardiovascular disease. Lancet Psychiatry 4(4):320–329, 2017 28109646

Edmondson D, Kronish IM, Shaffer JA, et al: Posttraumatic stress disorder and risk for coronary heart disease: a meta-analytic review. Am Heart J 166(5):806–814, 2013 24176435

Eisen A, Giugliano RP, Braunwald E: Updates on acute coronary syndrome: a review. JAMA Cardiol 1(6):718–730, 2016 27438381

Empana JP, Sykes DH, Luc G, et al; PRIME Study Group: Contributions of depressive mood and circulating inflammatory markers to coronary heart disease in healthy European men: the Prospective Epidemiological Study of Myocardial Infarction (PRIME). Circulation 111(18):2299–2305, 2005 15867179

Engel GL: Editorial: Psychologic factors in instantaneous cardiac death. N Engl J Med 294(12):664–665, 1976 1246260

Epstein AE, DiMarco JP, Ellenbogen KA, et al: ACC/AHA/HRS 2008 guidelines for device-based therapy of cardiac rhythm abnormalities: a report of the American College of Cardiology/American Heart Association Task Force on Practice Guidelines (Writing Committee to Revise the ACC/AHA/NASPE 2002 Guideline Update for Implantation of Cardiac Pacemakers and Antiarrhythmia Devices) developed in collaboration with the American Association for Thoracic Surgery and Society of Thoracic Surgeons. J Am Coll Cardiol 51(21):e1–e62, 2008 18498951

Eslami B, Sundin O, Macassa G, et al: Anxiety, depressive and somatic symptoms in adults with congenital heart disease. J Psychosom Res 74(1):49–56, 2013 23272988

España-Romero V, Artero EG, Lee DC, et al: A prospective study of ideal cardiovascular health and depressive symptoms. Psychosomatics 54(6):525–535, 2013 24012292

Filho AS, Maciel BC, Martín-Santos R, et al: Does the association between mitral valve prolapse and panic disorder really exist? Prim Care Companion J Clin Psychiatry 10(1):38–47, 2008 18311420

Fisman EZ, Benderly M, Esper RJ, et al: Interleukin-6 and the risk of future cardiovascular events in patients with angina pectoris and/or healed myocardial infarction. Am J Cardiol 98(1):14–18, 2006 16784912

Foldes-Busque G, Fleet RP, Denis I, et al: Nonfearful panic attacks in patients with noncardiac chest pain. Psychosomatics 56(5):513–520, 2015 25583556

Forbess JM, Visconti KJ, Hancock-Friesen C, et al: Neurodevelopmental outcome after congenital heart surgery: results from an institutional registry. Circulation 106(12) (suppl 1):I95–I102, 2002 12354716

Forette F, Seux ML, Staessen JA, et al; Systolic Hypertension in Europe Investigators: The prevention of dementia with antihypertensive treatment: new evidence from the Systolic Hypertension in Europe (Syst-Eur) study. Arch Intern Med 162(18):2046–2052, 2002 12374512

Fraguas R, da Silva Telles RM, Alves TC, et al: A double-blind, placebo-controlled treatment trial of citalopram for major depressive disorder in older patients with heart failure: the relevance of the placebo effect and psychological symptoms. Contemp Clin Trials 30(3):205–211, 2009 19470312

Frasure-Smith N, Lespérance F: Depression and anxiety as predictors of 2-year cardiac events in patients with stable coronary artery disease. Arch Gen Psychiatry 65(1):62–71, 2008 [Erratum (incorrect information in abstract and table) in JAMA Psychiatry 72(8):851, 2015] 18180430

Frasure-Smith N, Lespérance F, Talajic M: Depression and 18-month prognosis after myocardial infarction. Circulation 91(4):999–1005, 1995a 7531624

Frasure-Smith N, Lespérance F, Talajic M: The impact of negative emotions on prognosis following myocardial infarction: is it more than depression? Health Psychol 14(5):388–398, 1995b 7498109

Frasure-Smith N, Lespérance F, Prince RH, et al: Randomised trial of home-based psychosocial nursing intervention for patients recovering from myocardial infarction. Lancet 350(9076):473–479, 1997 9274583

Frasure-Smith N, Lespérance F, Gravel G, et al: Social support, depression, and mortality during the first year after myocardial infarction. Circulation 101(16):1919–1924, 2000 10779457

Freedland KE, Carney RM, Rich MW, et al: Cognitive behavior therapy for depression and self-care in heart failure patients: a randomized clinical trial. JAMA Intern Med 175(11):1773–1782, 2015 26414759

Frestad D, Prescott E: Vital exhaustion and coronary heart disease risk: a systematic review and meta-analysis. Psychosom Med 79(3):260–272, 2017 27902666

Fricchione GL, Olson LC, Vlay SC: Psychiatric syndromes in patients with the automatic internal cardioverter defibrillator: anxiety, psychological dependence, abuse, and withdrawal. Am Heart J 117(6):1411–1414, 1989 2729084

Friedman M, Thoresen CE, Gill JJ, et al: Alteration of type A behavior and its effect on cardiac recurrences in post myocardial infarction patients: summary results of the recurrent coronary prevention project. Am Heart J 112(4):653–665, 1986 3766365

Gathright EC, Goldstein CM, Josephson RA, et al: Depression increases the risk of mortality in patients with heart failure: a meta-analysis. J Psychosom Res 94:82–89, 2017 28183407

Gehi A, Haas D, Pipkin S, et al: Depression and medication adherence in outpatients with coronary heart disease: findings from the Heart and Soul Study. Arch Intern Med 165(21):2508–2513, 2005a 16314548

Gehi A, Mangano D, Pipkin S, et al: Depression and heart rate variability in patients with stable coronary heart disease: findings from the Heart and Soul Study. Arch Gen Psychiatry 62(6):661–666, 2005b 15939843

Gehi AK, Ali S, Na B, et al: Self-reported medication adherence and cardiovascular events in patients with stable coronary heart disease: the heart and soul study. Arch Intern Med 167(16):1798–1803, 2007 17846400

Giltay EJ, Geleijnse JM, Zitman FG, et al: Dispositional optimism and all-cause and cardiovascular mortality in a prospective cohort of elderly Dutch men and women. Arch Gen Psychiatry 61(11):1126–1135, 2004 15520360

Glassman AH: Cigarette smoking: implications for psychiatric illness. Am J Psychiatry 150(4):546–553, 1993 8465868

Glassman AH, Shapiro PA: Depression and the course of coronary artery disease. Am J Psychiatry 155(1):4–11, 1998 9433332

Glassman AH, Roose SP, Bigger JT Jr: The safety of tricyclic antidepressants in cardiac patients. Risk-benefit reconsidered. JAMA 269(20):2673–2675, 1993 8487453

Glassman AH, O'Connor CM, Califf RM, et al; Sertraline Antidepressant Heart Attack Randomized Trial (SADHEART) Group: Sertraline treatment of major depression in patients with acute MI or unstable angina. JAMA 288(6):701–709, 2002 12169073

Glassman AH, Bigger JT, Gaffney M, et al: Onset of major depression associated with acute coronary syndromes: relationship of onset, major depressive disorder history, and episode severity to sertraline benefit. Arch Gen Psychiatry 63(3):283–288, 2006 16520433

Glassman AH, Bigger JT Jr, Gaffney M: Psychiatric characteristics associated with long-term mortality among 361 patients having an acute coronary syndrome and major depression: seven-year follow-up of SADHART participants. Arch Gen Psychiatry 66(9):1022–1029, 2009 19736359

Goldstein BI, Fagiolini A, Houck P, et al: Cardiovascular disease and hypertension among adults with bipolar I disorder in the United States. Bipolar Disord 11(6):657–662, 2009 19689508

Goldstein BI, Carnethon MR, Matthews KA, et al; American Heart Association Atherosclerosis; Hypertension and Obesity in Youth Committee of the Council on Cardiovascular Disease in the Young: Major depressive disorder and bipolar disorder predispose youth to accelerated atherosclerosis and early cardiovascular disease: a scientific statement from the American Heart Association. Circulation 132(10):965–986, 2015 26260736

Goldstein DJ, Oz MC: Cardiac Assist Devices. Armonk, NY, Futura, 2000

Gomez-Caminero A, Blumentals WA, Russo LJ, et al: Does panic disorder increase the risk of coronary heart disease? A cohort study of a national managed care database. Psychosom Med 67(5):688–691, 2005 16204424

Gosselt AN, Slooter AJ, Boere PR, et al: Risk factors for delirium after on-pump cardiac surgery: a systematic review. Crit Care 19:346, 2015 26395253

Gottlieb SS, Kop WJ, Thomas SA, et al: A double-blind placebo-controlled pilot study of controlled-release paroxetine on depression and quality of life in chronic heart failure. Am Heart J 153(5):868–873, 2007 17452166

Grande G, Romppel M, Barth J: Association between type D personality and prognosis in patients with cardiovascular diseases: a systematic review and meta-analysis. Ann Behav Med 43(3):299–310, 2012 22237826

Gulliksson M, Burell G, Vessby B, et al: Randomized controlled trial of cognitive behavioral therapy vs standard treatment to prevent recurrent cardiovascular events in patients with coronary heart disease: Secondary Prevention in Uppsala Primary Health Care project (SUPRIM). Arch Intern Med 171(2):134–140, 2011 21263103

Hance M, Carney RM, Freedland KE, et al: Depression in patients with coronary heart disease. A 12-month follow-up. Gen Hosp Psychiatry 18(1):61–65, 1996 8666215

Hassan M, Mela A, Li Q, et al: The effect of acute psychological stress on QT dispersion in patients with coronary artery disease. Pacing Clin Electrophysiol 32(9):1178–1183, 2009 19719496

Herbst S, Pietrzak RH, Wagner J, et al: Lifetime major depression is associated with coronary heart disease in older adults: results from the National Epidemiologic Survey on Alcohol and Related Conditions. Psychosom Med 69(8):729–734, 2007 17942842

Herrmann-Lingen C, Beutel ME, Bosbach A, et al; SPIRR-CAD Study Group: A Stepwise Psychotherapy Intervention for Reducing Risk in Coronary Artery Disease (SPIRR-CAD): results of an observer-blinded, multicenter, randomized trial in depressed patients with coronary artery disease. Psychosom Med 78(6):704–715, 2016 27187851

Hildrum B, Mykletun A, Holmen J, et al: Effect of anxiety and depression on blood pressure: 11-year longitudinal population study. Br J Psychiatry 193(2):108–113, 2008 18669991

Hocaoglu C, Gulec MY, Durmus I: Psychiatric comorbidity in patients with chest pain without a cardiac etiology. Isr J Psychiatry Relat Sci 45(1):49–54, 2008 18587169

Holbrook AM, Pereira JA, Labiris R, et al: Systematic overview of warfarin and its drug and food interactions. Arch Intern Med 165(10):1095–1106, 2005 15911722

Honig A, Kuyper AM, Schene AH, et al; MIND-IT Investigators: Treatment of post-myocardial infarction depressive disorder: a randomized, placebo-controlled trial with mirtazapine. Psychosom Med 69(7):606–613, 2007 17846258

Hoyer J, Eifert GH, Einsle F, et al: Heart-focused anxiety before and after cardiac surgery. J Psychosom Res 64(3):291–297, 2008 18291244

Huffman JC, Pollack MH: Predicting panic disorder among patients with chest pain: an analysis of the literature. Psychosomatics 44(3):222–236, 2003 12724504

Huffman JC, Mastromauro CA, Beach SR, et al: Collaborative care for depression and anxiety disorders in patients with recent cardiac events: the Management of Sadness and Anxiety in Cardiology (MOSAIC) randomized clinical trial. JAMA Intern Med 174(6):927–935, 2014 24733277

Iadecola C, Yaffe K, Biller J, et al; American Heart Association Council on Hypertension; Council on Clinical Cardiology; Council on Cardiovascular Disease in the Young; Council on Cardiovascular and Stroke Nursing; Council on Quality of Care and Outcomes Research; and Stroke Council: Impact of hypertension on cognitive function: a scientific statement from the American Heart Association. Hypertension 68(6):e67–e94, 2016 27977393

Jacq F, Foulldrin G, Savouré A, et al: A comparison of anxiety, depression and quality of life between device shock and nonshock groups in implantable cardioverter defibrillator recipients. Gen Hosp Psychiatry 31(3):266–273, 2009 19410106

Janssen V, De Gucht V, Dusseldorp E, et al: Lifestyle modification programmes for patients with coronary heart disease: a systematic review and meta-analysis of randomized controlled trials. Eur J Prev Cardiol 20(4):620–640, 2013 23022703

Jiang W: Emotional triggering of cardiac dysfunction: the present and future. Curr Cardiol Rep 17(10):91, 2015 26298307

Jiang W, Alexander J, Christopher E, et al: Relationship of depression to increased risk of mortality and rehospitalization in patients with congestive heart failure. Arch Intern Med 161(15):1849–1856, 2001 11493126

Jiang W, Velazquez EJ, Kuchibhatla M, et al: Effect of escitalopram on mental stress-induced myocardial ischemia: results of the REMIT trial. JAMA 309(20):2139–2149, 2013 23695483

Jonas BS, Lando JF: Negative affect as a prospective risk factor for hypertension. Psychosom Med 62(2):188–196, 2000 10772396

Jonsbu E, Dammen T, Morken G, et al: Cardiac and psychiatric diagnoses among patients referred for chest pain and palpitations. Scand Cardiovasc J 43(4):256–259, 2009 19431049

Joynt KE, Whellan DJ, O'connor CM: Why is depression bad for the failing heart? A review of the mechanistic relationship between depression and heart failure. J Card Fail 10(3):258–271, 2004 15190537

Kapur V, Schwarz ER: The relationship between erectile dysfunction and cardiovascular disease, part I: pathophysiology and mechanisms. Rev Cardiovasc Med 8(4):214–219, 2007 18192944

Kawachi I, Colditz GA, Ascherio A, et al: Prospective study of phobic anxiety and risk of coronary heart disease in men. Circulation 89(5):1992–1997, 1994a 8181122

Kawachi I, Sparrow D, Vokonas PS, et al: Symptoms of anxiety and risk of coronary heart disease. The Normative Aging Study. Circulation 90(5):2225–2229, 1994b 7955177

Kazemi-Saleh D, Pishgou B, Assari S, et al: Fear of sexual intercourse in patients with coronary artery disease: a pilot study of associated morbidity. J Sex Med 4(6):1619–1625, 2007 17970974

Kazmierski J, Kowman M, Banach M, et al: Clinical utility and use of DSM-IV and ICD-10 criteria and the Memorial Delirium Assessment Scale in establishing a diagnosis of delirium after cardiac surgery. Psychosomatics 49(1):73–76, 2008 18212180

Kendall L, Lewin RJ, Parsons JM, et al: Factors associated with self-perceived state of health in adolescents with congenital cardiac disease attending paediatric cardiologic clinics. Cardiol Young 11(4):431–438, 2001 11558953

Kent LK, Weston CA, Heyer EJ, et al: Successful retrial of ECT two months after ECT-induced Takotsubo cardiomyopathy. Am J Psychiatry 166(8):857–862, 2009 19651751

Kim DH, Daskalakis C, Whellan DJ, et al: Safety of selective serotonin reuptake inhibitor in adults undergoing coronary artery bypass grafting. Am J Cardiol 103(10):1391–1395, 2009 19427434

Kim JM, Bae KY, Stewart R, et al: Escitalopram treatment for depressive disorder following acute coronary syndrome: a 24-week double-blind, placebo-controlled trial. J Clin Psychiatry 76(1):62–68, 2015 25375836

Kimmel SE, Schelleman H, Berlin JA, et al: The effect of selective serotonin re-uptake inhibitors on the risk of myocardial infarction in a cohort of patients with depression. Br J Clin Pharmacol 72(3):514–517, 2011 21557758

Kisely SR, Campbell LA, Yelland MJ, et al: Psychological interventions for symptomatic management of non-specific chest pain in patients with normal coronary anatomy. Cochrane Database Syst Rev (6):CD004101, 2015 26123045

Konttinen H, Kilpi F, Moustgaard H, et al: Socioeconomic position and antidepressant use as predictors of coronary heart disease mortality: a population-based registry study of 362,271 Finns. Psychosom Med 78(2):144–152, 2016 26780300

Koster S, Hensens AG, van der Palen J: The long-term cognitive and functional outcomes of postoperative delirium after cardiac surgery. Ann Thorac Surg 87(5):1469–1474, 2009 19379886

Kourkoveli P, Rammos S, Parissis J, et al: Depressive symptoms in patients with congenital heart disease: incidence and prognostic value of self-rating depression scales. Congenit Heart Dis 10(3):240–247, 2015 24975053

Kovacs AH, Saidi AS, Kuhl EA, et al: Depression and anxiety in adult congenital heart disease: predictors and prevalence. Int J Cardiol 137(2):158–164, 2009 18707776

Krantz DS, Olson MB, Francis JL, et al: Anger, hostility, and cardiac symptoms in women with suspected coronary artery disease: the Women's Ischemia Syndrome Evaluation (WISE) Study. J Womens Health (Larchmt) 15(10):1214–1223, 2006 17199462

Krishnan KRR: Monoamine oxidase inhibitors, in American Psychiatric Press Textbook of Psychopharmacology. Edited by Schatzberg AF, Nemeroff CB. Washington, DC, American Psychiatric Press, 1995, pp 183–193

Kronish IM, Rieckmann N, Halm EA, et al: Persistent depression affects adherence to secondary prevention behaviors after acute coronary syndromes. J Gen Intern Med 21(11):1178–1183, 2006 16899061

Kronish IM, Rieckmann N, Schwartz JE, et al: Is depression after an acute coronary syndrome simply a marker of known prognostic factors for mortality? Psychosom Med 71(7):697–703, 2009 19592517

Kubzansky LD, Thurston RC: Emotional vitality and incident coronary heart disease: benefits of healthy psychological functioning. Arch Gen Psychiatry 64(12):1393–1401, 2007 18056547

Kubzansky LD, Koenen KC, Spiro A 3rd, et al: Prospective study of posttraumatic stress disorder symptoms and coronary heart disease in the Normative Aging Study. Arch Gen Psychiatry 64(1):109–116, 2007 17199060

Kuhl EA, Fauerbach JA, Bush DE, et al: Relation of anxiety and adherence to risk-reducing recommendations following myocardial infarction. Am J Cardiol 103(12):1629–1634, 2009 19539067

Labos C, Dasgupta K, Nedjar H, et al: Risk of bleeding associated with combined use of selective serotonin reuptake inhibitors and antiplatelet therapy following acute myocardial infarction. CMAJ 183(16):1835–1843, 2011 21948719

Lang S, Becker R, Wilke S, et al: Anxiety disorders in patients with implantable cardioverter defibrillators: frequency, course, predictors, and patients' requests for treatment. Pacing Clin Electrophysiol 37(1):35–47, 2014 24102228

Laske C, Soekadar SR, Laszlo R, et al: Brugada syndrome in a patient treated with lithium. Am J Psychiatry 164(9):1440–1441, 2007 17728436

Latal B, Helfricht S, Fischer JE, et al: Psychological adjustment and quality of life in children and adolescents following open-heart surgery for congenital heart disease: a systematic review. BMC Pediatr 9:6, 2009 19161602

Laursen TM, Munk-Olsen T, Agerbo E, et al: Somatic hospital contacts, invasive cardiac procedures, and mortality from heart disease in patients with severe mental disorder. Arch Gen Psychiatry 66(7):713–720, 2009 19581562

Lespérance F, Frasure-Smith N, Laliberté MA, et al: An open-label study of nefazodone treatment of major depression in patients with congestive heart failure. Can J Psychiatry 48(10):695–701, 2003 14674053

Lespérance F, Frasure-Smith N, Koszycki D, et al; CREATE Investigators: Effects of citalopram and interpersonal psychotherapy on depression in patients with coronary artery disease: the Canadian Cardiac Randomized Evaluation of Antidepressant and Psychotherapy Efficacy (CREATE) trial. JAMA 297(4):367–379, 2007 17244833

Lessmeier TJ, Gamperling D, Johnson-Liddon V, et al: Unrecognized paroxysmal supraventricular tachycardia. Potential for misdiagnosis as panic disorder. Arch Intern Med 157(5):537–543, 1997 9066458

Lett HS, Blumenthal JA, Babyak MA, et al: Social support and coronary heart disease: epidemiologic evidence and implications for treatment. Psychosom Med 67(6):869–878, 2005 16314591

Libby P, Ridker PM, Maseri A: Inflammation and atherosclerosis. Circulation 105(9):1135–1143, 2002 11877368

Licht CM, de Geus EJ, Zitman FG, et al: Association between major depressive disorder and heart rate variability in the Netherlands Study of Depression and Anxiety (NESDA). Arch Gen Psychiatry 65(12):1358–1367, 2008 19047522

Lichtman JH, Bigger JT Jr, Blumenthal JA, et al; American Heart Association Prevention Committee of the Council on Cardiovascular Nursing; American Heart Association Council on Clinical Cardiology; American Heart Association Council on Epidemiology and Prevention; American Heart Association Interdisciplinary Council on Quality of Care and Outcomes Research; American Psychiatric Association: Depression and coronary heart disease: recommendations for screening, referral, and treatment: a science advisory from the American Heart Association Prevention Committee of the Council on Cardiovascular Nursing, Council on Clinical Cardiology, Council on Epidemiology and Prevention, and Interdisciplinary Council on Quality of Care and Outcomes Research: endorsed by the American Psychiatric Association. Circulation 118(17):1768–1775, 2008 18824640

Lichtman JH, Froelicher ES, Blumenthal JA, et al; American Heart Association Statistics Committee of the Council on Epidemiology and Prevention and the Council on Cardiovascular and Stroke Nursing: Depression as a risk factor for poor prognosis among patients with acute coronary syndrome: systematic review and recommendations: a scientific statement from the American Heart Association. Circulation 129(12):1350–1369, 2014 24566200

Linden W: Psychological treatments in cardiac rehabilitation: review of rationales and outcomes. J Psychosom Res 48(4–5):443–454, 2000 10880665

Linden W, Moseley JV: The efficacy of behavioral treatments for hypertension. Appl Psychophysiol Biofeedback 31(1):51–63, 2006 16565886

Linke SE, Rutledge T, Johnson BD, et al: Depressive symptom dimensions and cardiovascular prognosis among women with suspected myocardial ischemia: a report from the National Heart, Lung, and Blood Institute-sponsored Women's Ischemia Syndrome Evaluation. Arch Gen Psychiatry 66(5):499–507, 2009 19414709

Liukkonen T, Silvennoinen-Kassinen S, Jokelainen J, et al: The association between C-reactive protein levels and depression: results from the northern Finland 1966 birth cohort study. Biol Psychiatry 60(8):825–830, 2006 16616729

Lundgren O, Garvin P, Jonasson L, et al: Psychological resources are associated with reduced incidence of coronary heart disease. An 8-year follow-up of a community-based Swedish sample. Int J Behav Med 22(1):77–84, 2015 24430130

Maatouk I, Herzog W, Böhlen F, et al: Association of hypertension with depression and generalized anxiety symptoms in a large population-based sample of older adults. J Hypertens 34(9):1711–1720, 2016 27341438

Mackin P: Cardiac side effects of psychiatric drugs. Hum Psychopharmacol 23 (suppl 1):3–14, 2008 18098218

Magyar-Russell G, Thombs BD, Cai JX, et al: The prevalence of anxiety and depression in adults with implantable cardioverter defibrillators: a systematic review. J Psychosom Res 71(4):223–231, 2011 21911099

Maldonado JR, Wysong A, van der Starre PJ, et al: Dexmedetomidine and the reduction of postoperative delirium after cardiac surgery. Psychosomatics 50(3):206–217, 2009 19567759

Mandras SA, Uber PA, Mehra MR: Sexual activity and chronic heart failure. Mayo Clin Proc 82(10):1203–1210, 2007 17908527

Margraf J, Ehlers A, Roth WT: Mitral valve prolapse and panic disorder: a review of their relationship. Psychosom Med 50(2):93–113, 1988 3287421

Martens EJ, Hoen PW, Mittelhaeuser M, et al: Symptom dimensions of post-myocardial infarction depression, disease severity and cardiac prognosis. Psychol Med 40(5):807–814, 2010 19691872

Masand PS, Tesar GE: Use of stimulants in the medically ill. Psychiatr Clin North Am 19(3):515–547, 1996 8856815

May HT, Horne BD, Carlquist JF, et al: Depression after coronary artery disease is associated with heart failure. J Am Coll Cardiol 53(16):1440–1447, 2009 19371828

McGowan L, Dickens C, Percival C, et al: The relationship between vital exhaustion, depression and comorbid illnesses in patients following first myocardial infarction. J Psychosom Res 57(2):183–188, 2004 15465074

McMurray JJV, Packer M, Desai AS, et al; PARADIGM-HF Investigators and Committees: Angiotensin-neprilysin inhibition versus enalapril in heart failure. N Engl J Med 371(11):993–1004, 2014 25176015

Mehra MR, Naka Y, Uriel N, et al; MOMENTUM 3 Investigators: A fully magnetically levitated circulatory pump for advanced heart failure. N Engl J Med 376(5):440–450, 2017 27959709

Miatton M, De Wolf D, François K, et al: Neuropsychological performance in school-aged children with surgically corrected congenital heart disease. J Pediatr 151(1):73–78, 78.e1, 2007 17586194

Miller GE, Stetler CA, Carney RM, et al: Clinical depression and inflammatory risk markers for coronary heart disease. Am J Cardiol 90(12):1279–1283, 2002 12480034

Mitchell AJ, Vancampfort D, Sweers K, et al: Prevalence of metabolic syndrome and metabolic abnormalities in schizophrenia and related disorders—a systematic review and meta-analysis. Schizophr Bull 39(2):306–318, 2013 22207632

Morganroth J, Goin JE: Quinidine-related mortality in the short-to-medium-term treatment of ventricular arrhythmias. A meta-analysis. Circulation 84(5):1977–1983, 1991 1834365

Morris PL, Badger J, Chmielewski C, et al: Psychiatric morbidity following implantation of the automatic implantable cardioverter defibrillator. Psychosomatics 32(1):58–64, 1991 2003140

Mozaffarian D, Benjamin EJ, Go AS, et al; Writing Group Members; American Heart Association Statistics Committee; Stroke Statistics Subcommittee: Heart disease and stroke statistics—2016 update: a report from the American Heart Association. Circulation 133(4):e38–e360, 2016 26673558

Mu JL, Lee A, Joynt GM: Pharmacologic agents for the prevention and treatment of delirium in patients undergoing cardiac surgery: systematic review and meta-analysis. Crit Care Med 43(1):194–204, 2015 25289932

Müller-Tasch T, Frankenstein L, Holzapfel N, et al: Panic disorder in patients with chronic heart failure. J Psychosom Res 64(3):299–303, 2008 18291245

Nakagawa I, Nakamura K, Oyama M, et al: Long-term effects of the Niigata-Chuetsu earthquake in Japan on acute myocardial infarction mortality: an analysis of death certificate data. Heart 95(24):2009–2013, 2009 19541690

Nakagawa S, Yuzefpolskaya M, Colombo PC, et al: Palliative care interventions before left ventricular assist device implantation in both bridge to transplant and destination therapy. J Palliat Med 20(9):977–983, 2017 28504892

Nayeri A, Rafla-Yuan E, Farber-Eger E, et al: Pre-existing psychiatric illness is associated with increased risk of recurrent Takotsubo cardiomyopathy. Psychosomatics 58(5):527–532, 2017 28602445

Newburger JW, Silbert AR, Buckley LP, et al: Cognitive function and age at repair of transposition of the great arteries in children. N Engl J Med 310(23):1495–1499, 1984 6717539

Newcomer JW, Hennekens CH: Severe mental illness and risk of cardiovascular disease. JAMA 298(15):1794–1796, 2007 17940236

Nissen SE: ADHD drugs and cardiovascular risk. N Engl J Med 354(14):1445–1448, 2006 16549404

O'Connor CM, Jiang W, Kuchibhatla M, et al: Antidepressant use, depression, and survival in patients with heart failure. Arch Intern Med 168(20):2232–2237, 2008 19001200

O'Connor CM, Jiang W, Kuchibhatla M, et al; SADHART-CHF Investigators: Safety and efficacy of sertraline for depression in patients with heart failure: results of the SADHART-CHF (Sertraline Against Depression and Heart Disease in Chronic Heart Failure) trial. J Am Coll Cardiol 56(9):692–699, 2010 20723799

Olfson M, Huang C, Gerhard T, et al: Stimulants and cardiovascular events in youth with attention-deficit/hyperactivity disorder. J Am Acad Child Adolesc Psychiatry 51(2):147–156, 2012 22265361

Ong L, Nolan RP, Irvine J, et al: Parental overprotection and heart-focused anxiety in adults with congenital heart disease. Int J Behav Med 18(3):260–267, 2011 20842471

O'Reardon JP, Lott JP, Akhtar UW, et al: Acute coronary syndrome (Takotsubo cardiomyopathy) following electroconvulsive therapy in the absence of significant coronary artery disease: case report and review of the literature. J ECT 24(4):277–280, 2008 18955900

Organ Procurement and Transplant Network: National data. 2017. Available at: https://optn.transplant.hrsa.gov/data/view-data-reports/national-data/#. Accessed September 24, 2017.

Pan Y, Cai W, Cheng Q, et al: Association between anxiety and hypertension: a systematic review and meta-analysis of epidemiological studies. Neuropsychiatr Dis Treat 11:1121–1130, 2015 25960656

Pandharipande PP, Pun BT, Herr DL, et al: Effect of sedation with dexmedetomidine vs lorazepam on acute brain dysfunction in mechanically ventilated patients: the MENDS randomized controlled trial. JAMA 298(22):2644–2653, 2007 18073360

Parker GB, Hilton TM, Walsh WF, et al: Timing is everything: the onset of depression and acute coronary syndrome outcome. Biol Psychiatry 64(8):660–666, 2008 18602090

Perez MI, Linden W, Perry T Jr, et al: Failure of psychological interventions to lower blood pressure: a randomized controlled trial. Open Med 3(2):e92–e100, 2009 19946397

Petrucci RJ, Wright S, Naka Y, et al; HeartMate II Clinical Investigators: Neurocognitive assessments in advanced heart failure patients receiving continuous-flow left ventricular assist devices. J Heart Lung Transplant 28(6):542–549, 2009 19481013

Peyre H, Hoertel N, Hatteea H, et al: Adulthood self-reported cardiovascular risk and ADHD medications: results from the 2004–2005 National Epidemiologic Survey on Alcohol and Related Conditions. J Clin Psychiatry 75(2):181–182, 2014 24602253

Pickering TG, Clemow L: Paroxysmal hypertension: the role of stress and psychological factors. J Clin Hypertens (Greenwich) 10(7):575–581, 2008 18607143

Polcwiartek C, Sneider B, Graff C, et al: The cardiac safety of aripiprazole treatment in patients at high risk for torsade: a systematic review with a meta-analytic approach. Psychopharmacology (Berl) 232(18):3297–3308, 2015 26231497

Poole L, Dickens C, Steptoe A: The puzzle of depression and acute coronary syndrome: reviewing the role of acute inflammation. J Psychosom Res 71(2):61–68, 2011 21767684

Rasmussen JN, Chong A, Alter DA: Relationship between adherence to evidence-based pharmacotherapy and long-term mortality after acute myocardial infarction. JAMA 297(2):177–186, 2007 17213401

Ray WA, Chung CP, Murray KT, et al: Atypical antipsychotic drugs and the risk of sudden cardiac death. N Engl J Med 360(3):225–235, 2009 19144938

Rees K, Bennett P, West R, et al: Psychological interventions for coronary heart disease. Cochrane Database Syst Rev (2):CD002902, 2004 15106183

Reid GJ, Seidelin PH, Kop WJ, et al: Mental-stress-induced platelet activation among patients with coronary artery disease. Psychosom Med 71(4):438–445, 2009 19251865

Rieckmann N, Gerin W, Kronish IM, et al: Course of depressive symptoms and medication adherence after acute coronary syndromes: an electronic medication monitoring study. J Am Coll Cardiol 48(11):2218–2222, 2006 17161249

Rief W, Nanke A, Emmerich J, et al: Causal illness attributions in somatoform disorders: associations with comorbidity and illness behavior. J Psychosom Res 57(4):367–371, 2004 15518672

Riegel B, Lee CS, Dickson VV; Medscape: Self care in patients with chronic heart failure. Nat Rev Cardiol 8(11):644–654, 2011 21769111

Ringen PA, Engh JA, Birkenaes AB, et al: Increased mortality in schizophrenia due to cardiovascular disease—-a non-systematic review of epidemiology, possible causes, and interventions. Front Psychiatry 5:137, 2014 25309466

Rogers JG, Pagani FD, Tatooles AJ, et al: Intrapericardial left ventricular assist device for advanced heart failure. N Engl J Med 376(5):451–460, 2017 28146651

Rollman BL, Belnap BH, LeMenager MS, et al: Telephone-delivered collaborative care for treating post-CABG depression: a randomized controlled trial. JAMA 302(19):2095–2103, 2009 19918088

Roose SP, Glassman AH: Cardiovascular effects of tricyclic antidepressants in depressed patients with and without heart disease. J Clin Psychiatry 50:S1–S18, 1989

Roose SP, Dalack GW, Glassman AH, et al: Cardiovascular effects of bupropion in depressed patients with heart disease. Am J Psychiatry 148(4):512–516, 1991 1900980

Roose SP, Glassman AH, Attia E, et al: Comparative efficacy of selective serotonin reuptake inhibitors and tricyclics in the treatment of melancholia. Am J Psychiatry 151(12):1735–1739, 1994 7977878

Roose SP, Glassman AH, Attia E, et al: Cardiovascular effects of fluoxetine in depressed patients with heart disease. Am J Psychiatry 155(5):660–665, 1998a 9585718

Roose SP, Laghrissi-Thode F, Kennedy JS, et al: Comparison of paroxetine and nortriptyline in depressed patients with ischemic heart disease. JAMA 279(4):287–291, 1998b 9450712

Rosengren A, Hawken S, Ôunpuu S, et al; INTERHEART Investigators: Association of psychosocial risk factors with risk of acute myocardial infarction in 11119 cases and 13648 controls from 52 countries (the INTERHEART study): case-control study. Lancet 364(9438):953–962, 2004 15364186

Rosenman RH, Brand RJ, Jenkins D, et al: Coronary heart disease in Western Collaborative Group Study. Final follow-up experience of 8 1/2 years. JAMA 233(8):872–877, 1975 1173896

Rozanski A, Bairey CN, Krantz DS, et al: Mental stress and the induction of silent myocardial ischemia in patients with coronary artery disease. N Engl J Med 318(16):1005–1012, 1988 3352695

Rudolph JL, Jones RN, Levkoff SE, et al: Derivation and validation of a preoperative prediction rule for delirium after cardiac surgery. Circulation 119(2):229–236, 2009 19118253

Rugulies R: Depression as a predictor for coronary heart disease. a review and meta-analysis. Am J Prev Med 23(1):51–61, 2002 12093424

Rumsfeld JS, Havranek E, Masoudi FA, et al; Cardiovascular Outcomes Research Consortium: Depressive symptoms are the strongest predictors of short-term declines in health status in patients with heart failure. J Am Coll Cardiol 42(10):1811–1817, 2003 14642693

Ruo B, Rumsfeld JS, Hlatky MA, et al: Depressive symptoms and health-related quality of life: the Heart and Soul Study. JAMA 290(2):215–221, 2003 12851276

Ruo B, Bertenthal D, Sen S, et al: Self-rated health among women with coronary disease: depression is as important as recent cardiovascular events. Am Heart J 152(5):921.e1–921.e7, 2006 17070159

Rutledge T, Hogan BE: A quantitative review of prospective evidence linking psychological factors with hypertension development. Psychosom Med 64(5):758–766, 2002 12271106

Rutledge T, Reis VA, Linke SE, et al: Depression in heart failure a meta-analytic review of prevalence, intervention effects, and associations with clinical outcomes. J Am Coll Cardiol 48(8):1527–1537, 2006 17045884

Rutledge T, Redwine LS, Linke SE, et al: A meta-analysis of mental health treatments and cardiac rehabilitation for improving clinical outcomes and depression among patients with coronary heart disease. Psychosom Med 75(4):335–349, 2013 23630306

Salmoirago-Blotcher E, Rosman L, Wittstein IS, et al: Psychiatric history, post-discharge distress, and personality characteristics among incident female cases of Takotsubo cardiomyopathy: a case-control study. Heart Lung 45(6):503–509, 2016 27553636

Sauer WH, Berlin JA, Kimmel SE: Effect of antidepressants and their relative affinity for the serotonin transporter on the risk of myocardial infarction. Circulation 108(1):32–36, 2003 12821544

Schneider LS, Dagerman KS, Insel P: Risk of death with atypical antipsychotic drug treatment for dementia: meta-analysis of randomized placebo-controlled trials. JAMA 294(15):1934–1943, 2005 16234500

Sears SF, Lewis TS, Kuhl EA, et al: Predictors of quality of life in patients with implantable cardioverter defibrillators. Psychosomatics 46(5):451–457, 2005 16145190

Shapiro PA: Life after heart transplantation. Prog Cardiovasc Dis 32(6):405–418, 1990 2159649

Shapiro PA: Depression treatment and coronary artery disease outcomes: time for reflection. J Psychosom Res 74(1):4–5, 2013 23272981

Shapiro PA: Management of depression after myocardial infarction. Curr Cardiol Rep 17(10):80, 2015 26277362

Shedd OL, Sears SF Jr, Harvill JL, et al: The World Trade Center attack: increased frequency of defibrillator shocks for ventricular arrhythmias in patients living remotely from New York City. J Am Coll Cardiol 44(6):1265–1267, 2004 15364330

Shen BJ, Avivi YE, Todaro JF, et al: Anxiety characteristics independently and prospectively predict myocardial infarction in men the unique contribution of anxiety among psychologic factors. J Am Coll Cardiol 51(2):113–119, 2008 18191733

Sheps DS, McMahon RP, Becker L, et al: Mental stress-induced ischemia and all-cause mortality in patients with coronary artery disease: results from the Psychophysiological Investigations of Myocardial Ischemia study. Circulation 105(15):1780–1784, 2002 11956119

Slaughter MS, Rogers JG, Milano CA, et al; HeartMate II Investigators: Advanced heart failure treated with continuous-flow left ventricular assist device. N Engl J Med 361(23):2241–2251, 2009 19920051

Smoller JW, Pollack MH, Wassertheil-Smoller S, et al: Panic attacks and risk of incident cardiovascular events among postmenopausal women in the Women's Health Initiative Observational Study. Arch Gen Psychiatry 64(10):1153–1160, 2007 17909127

Smulter N, Lingehall HC, Gustafson Y, et al: Delirium after cardiac surgery: incidence and risk factors. Interact Cardiovasc Thorac Surg 17(5):790–796, 2013 23887126

Sokoreli I, de Vries JJ, Pauws SC, et al: Depression and anxiety as predictors of mortality among heart failure patients: systematic review and meta-analysis. Heart Fail Rev 21(1):49–63, 2016 26572543

Sowden GL, Huffman JC: The impact of mental illness on cardiac outcomes: a review for the cardiologist. Int J Cardiol 132(1):30–37, 2009 19004512

Steinberg JS, Arshad A, Kowalski M, et al: Increased incidence of life-threatening ventricular arrhythmias in implantable defibrillator patients after the World Trade Center attack. J Am Coll Cardiol 44(6):1261–1264, 2004 15364329

Steinke EE, Jaarsma T, Barnason SA, et al; Council on Cardiovascular and Stroke Nursing of the American Heart Association and the ESC Council on Cardiovascular Nursing and Allied Professions (CCNAP): Sexual counseling for individuals with cardiovascular disease and their partners: a consensus document from the American Heart Association and the ESC Council on Cardiovascular Nursing and Allied Professions (CCNAP). Circulation 128(18):2075–2096, 2013 23897867

Stenman M, Holzmann MJ, Sartipy U: Antidepressant use before coronary artery bypass surgery is associated with long-term mortality. Int J Cardiol 167(6):2958–2962, 2013 22959870

Strik JJ, Honig A, Lousberg R, et al: Efficacy and safety of fluoxetine in the treatment of patients with major depression after first myocardial infarction: findings from a double-blind, placebo-controlled trial. Psychosom Med 62(6):783–789, 2000 11138997

Sullivan MD, LaCroix AZ, Spertus JA, Hecht J: Five-year prospective study of the effects of anxiety and depression in patients with coronary artery disease. Am J Cardiol 86(10):1135–1138, A6, A9, 2000 11074214

Surtees PG, Wainwright NW, Luben RN, et al: Depression and ischemic heart disease mortality: evidence from the EPIC-Norfolk United Kingdom prospective cohort study. Am J Psychiatry 165(4):515–523, 2008 18245176

Teply RM, Packard KA, White ND, et al: Treatment of depression in patients with concomitant cardiac disease. Prog Cardiovasc Dis 58(5):514–528, 2016 26562328

Tesar GE, Murray GB, Cassem NH: Use of high-dose intravenous haloperidol in the treatment of agitated cardiac patients. J Clin Psychopharmacol 5(6):344–347, 1985 4067002

Thavendiranathan P, Bagai A, Khoo C, et al: Does this patient with palpitations have a cardiac arrhythmia? JAMA 302(19):2135–2143, 2009 19920238

Thombs BD, Roseman M, Coyne JC, et al: Does evidence support the American Heart Association's recommendation to screen patients for depression in cardiovascular care? An updated systematic review. PLoS One 8(1):e52654, 2013 23308116

Thurston RC, Rewak M, Kubzansky LD: An anxious heart: anxiety and the onset of cardiovascular diseases. Prog Cardiovasc Dis 55(6):524–537, 2013 23621962

Tsai TT, Nallamothu BK, Prasad A, et al: Clinical problem-solving. A change of heart. N Engl J Med 361(10):1010–1016, 2009 19726776

Tsuchihashi-Makaya M, Kato N, Chishaki A, et al: Anxiety and poor social support are independently associated with adverse outcomes in patients with mild heart failure. Circ J 73(2):280–287, 2009 19096191

Tully PJ, Baker RA, Knight JL: Anxiety and depression as risk factors for mortality after coronary artery bypass surgery. J Psychosom Res 64(3):285–290, 2008 18291243

Vaccarino V, Johnson BD, Sheps DS, et al; National Heart, Lung, and Blood Institute: Depression, inflammation, and incident cardiovascular disease in women with suspected coronary ischemia: the National Heart, Lung, and Blood Institute-sponsored WISE study. J Am Coll Cardiol 50(21):2044–2050, 2007 18021871

van Beek MH, Oude Voshaar RC, Beek AM, et al: A brief cognitive-behavioral intervention for treating depression and panic disorder in patients with noncardiac chest pain: a 24-week randomized controlled trial. Depress Anxiety 30(7):670–678, 2013 23625592

Van den Broek KC, Nyklíček I, Van der Voort PH, et al: Shocks, personality, and anxiety in patients with an implantable defibrillator. Pacing Clin Electrophysiol 31(7):850–857, 2008 18684282 van den Broek KC, Nyklícek I, van der Voort PH, et al: Risk of ventricular arrhythmia after implantable defibrillator treatment in anxious type D patients. J Am Coll Cardiol 54(6):531–537, 2009 19643315

van Dijk D, Spoor M, Hijman R, et al; Octopus Study Group: Cognitive and cardiac outcomes 5 years after off-pump vs on-pump coronary artery bypass graft surgery. JAMA 297(7):701–708, 2007 17312289

van Melle JP, de Jonge P, Spijkerman TA, et al: Prognostic association of depression following myocardial infarction with mortality and cardiovascular events: a meta-analysis. Psychosom Med 66(6):814–822, 2004 15564344

van Melle JP, de Jonge P, Honig A, et al; MIND-IT Investigators: Effects of antidepressant treatment following myocardial infarction. Br J Psychiatry 190:460–466, 2007 17541103

Vigl M, Hager A, Bauer U, et al: Sexuality and subjective wellbeing in male patients with congenital heart disease. Heart 95(14):1179–1183, 2009 19364753

Vilchinsky N, Ginzburg K, Fait K, et al: Cardiac-disease-induced PTSD (CDI-PTSD): a systematic review. Clin Psychol Rev 55:92–106, 2017 28575815

Vinyoles E, De la Figuera M, Gonzalez-Segura D: Cognitive function and blood pressure control in hypertensive patients over 60 years of age: COGNIPRES study. Curr Med Res Opin 24(12):3331–3339, 2008 18954496

Wang HX, Mittleman MA, Leineweber C, et al: Depressive symptoms, social isolation, and progression of coronary artery atherosclerosis: the Stockholm Female Coronary Angiography Study. Psychother Psychosom 75(2):96–102, 2006 16508344

Watkins LL, Blumenthal JA, Davidson JRT, et al: Phobic anxiety, depression, and risk of ventricular arrhythmias in patients with coronary heart disease. Psychosom Med 68(5):651–656, 2006 17012517

Webster LJ, Michelakis ED, Davis T, et al: Use of sildenafil for safe improvement of erectile function and quality of life in men with New York Heart Association classes II and III congestive heart failure: a prospective, placebo-controlled, double-blind crossover trial. Arch Intern Med 164(5):514–520, 2004 15006828

Welton NJ, Caldwell DM, Adamopoulos E, et al: Mixed treatment comparison meta-analysis of complex interventions: psychological interventions in coronary heart disease. Am J Epidemiol 169(9):1158–1165, 2009 19258485

Westlake C, Dracup K, Fonarow G, et al: Depression in patients with heart failure. J Card Fail 11(1):30–35, 2005 15704061

Whalley B, Thompson DR, Taylor RS: Psychological interventions for coronary heart disease: Cochrane systematic review and meta-analysis. Int J Behav Med 21(1):109–121, 2014 23179678

Whang W, Kubzansky LD, Kawachi I, et al: Depression and risk of sudden cardiac death and coronary heart disease in women: results from the Nurses' Health Study. J Am Coll Cardiol 53(11):950–958, 2009 19281925

White KS, Raffa SD, Jakle KR, et al: Morbidity of DSM-IV Axis I disorders in patients with noncardiac chest pain: psychiatric morbidity linked with increased pain and health care utilization. J Consult Clin Psychol 76(3):422–430, 2008 18540735

Whitehead DL, Strike P, Perkins-Porras L, et al: Frequency of distress and fear of dying during acute coronary syndromes and consequences for adaptation. Am J Cardiol 96(11):1512–1516, 2005 16310432

Whooley MA, de Jonge P, Vittinghoff E, et al: Depressive symptoms, health behaviors, and risk of cardiovascular events in patients with coronary heart disease. JAMA 300(20):2379–2388, 2008 19033588

Wilbert-Lampen U, Leistner D, Greven S, et al: Cardiovascular events during World Cup soccer. N Engl J Med 358(5):475–483, 2008 18234752

Wilens TE, Hammerness PG, Biederman J, et al: Blood pressure changes associated with medication treatment of adults with attention-deficit/hyperactivity disorder. J Clin Psychiatry 66(2):253–259, 2005 15705013

Williams MS: Platelets and depression in cardiovascular disease: a brief review of the current literature. World J Psychiatry 2(6):114–123, 2012 24175177

Williams MS, Rogers HL, Wang N-Y, et al: Do platelet-derived microparticles play a role in depression, inflammation, and acute coronary syndrome? Psychosomatics 55(3):252–260, 2014 24374086

Winterstein AG, Gerhard T, Kubilis P, et al: Cardiovascular safety of central nervous system stimulants in children and adolescents: population based cohort study. BMJ 345:e4627, 2012 22809800

Wittstein IS: The broken heart syndrome. Cleve Clin J Med 74 (suppl 1):S17–S22, 2007 17455537

Wittstein IS: The sympathetic nervous system in the pathogenesis of Takotsubo syndrome. Heart Fail Clin 12(4):485–498, 2016 27638019

Woolf-King SE, Anger A, Arnold EA, et al: Mental health among parents of children with critical congenital heart defects: a systematic review. J Am Heart Assoc 6(2):e004862, 2017 28151402

Wulsin LR, Singal BM: Do depressive symptoms increase the risk for the onset of coronary disease? A systematic quantitative review. Psychosom Med 65(2):201–210, 2003 12651987

Yan LL, Liu K, Matthews KA, et al: Psychosocial factors and risk of hypertension: the Coronary Artery Risk Development in Young Adults (CARDIA) study. JAMA 290(16):2138–2148, 2003 14570949

Yancy CW, Jessup M, Bozkurt B, et al: 2013 ACCF/AHA guideline for the management of heart failure: executive summary: a report of the American College of Cardiology Foundation/American Heart Association Task Force on practice guidelines. Circulation 128(16):1810–1852, 2013 23741057

Yeung AC, Vekshtein VI, Krantz DS, et al: The effect of atherosclerosis on the vasomotor response of coronary arteries to mental stress. N Engl J Med 325(22):1551–1556, 1991 1944439

Yohannes AM, Willgoss TG, Baldwin RC, et al: Depression and anxiety in chronic heart failure and chronic obstructive pulmonary disease: prevalence, relevance, clinical implications and management principles. Int J Geriatr Psychiatry 25(12):1209–1221, 2010 20033905

York KM, Hassan M, Sheps DS: Psychobiology of depression/distress in congestive heart failure. Heart Fail Rev 14(1):35–50, 2009 18368481

Ziegelstein RC: Acute emotional stress and cardiac arrhythmias. JAMA 298(3):324–329, 2007 17635893

Ziegelstein RC: Improving depression and reducing cardiac events: which is the chicken and which is the egg? J Psychosom Res 74(5):454–457, 2013 23597336

Ziegelstein RC, Fauerbach JA, Stevens SS, et al: Patients with depression are less likely to follow recommendations to reduce cardiac risk during recovery from a myocardial infarction. Arch Intern Med 160(12):1818–1823, 2000 10871976

Zivin K, Pfeiffer PN, Bohnert AS, et al: Evaluation of the FDA warning against prescribing citalopram at doses exceeding 40 mg. Am J Psychiatry 170(6):642–650, 2013 23640689

CHAPTER 18

Lung Disease

Thomas Ritz, Ph.D.

Juliet Kroll, M.A.

Alexandra Kulikova, M.S.

Chelsey Werchan, M.A.

E. Sherwood Brown, M.D., Ph.D.

In this chapter we review psychiatric aspects of the common pulmonary disorders, as well as the use of psychiatric medications in patients with these disorders. Some lung diseases are discussed elsewhere in this book, including tuberculosis in Chapter 26 ("Infectious Diseases"), cystic fibrosis and childhood asthma in Chapter 32 ("Pediatrics"), sleep-related breathing disorders in Chapter 14 ("Sleep Disorders"), lung cancer in Chapter 22 ("Oncology"), lung transplant in Chapter 29 ("Organ Transplantation"), and ventilator issues in Chapter 28 ("Surgery").

Asthma

Asthma is a chronic inflammatory disorder of the airways that is characterized by variable airway obstruction and airway hyperresponsiveness to various trigger factors. Symptoms of asthma include shortness of breath, chest tightness, cough, and wheezing, as well as restrictions in physical, social, and occupational functioning (see Chapter 32 for a discussion of asthma in children). The prevalence of asthma has increased significantly in past decades. Worldwide, an estimated 300 million people have asthma, and deaths from asthma have been estimated at 250,000 cases annually (Global Initiative for Asthma 2012). Prevalence rates vary internationally from 1% to 18%. In children, asthma is the most common chronic disease. In the United States, racial and ethnic minorities, in particular Puerto Ricans, African Americans, and American Indians/Alaskan Natives, are disproportionately affected (Leong et al. 2012). In addition to substantial personal suffering, the economic costs of asthma are considerable, with estimated costs of $56 billion in 2007 in the United States alone, and are increasing (Centers for Disease Control and Prevention 2013).

Emotions and Stress as Asthma Triggers

Historically, asthma has been viewed as one of the seven prototypical psychosomatic illnesses. Earlier psychoanalytic theory of psychosomatic medicine advanced the notion that asthma was the outcome of a conflictual constellation in the mother–child relationship (Alexander 1950). With advances of the biomedical model of asthma, which emphasizes cellular and molecular processes, the focus of the field has shifted to empirical research more compatible with a biopsychosocial view of asthma etiology and its course (Ritz et al. 2013). Earlier clinical and epidemiological findings indicated that many asthma patients viewed psychological factors as primary or secondary triggers of their asthma exacerbations, although study findings pertaining to this perception have varied considerably (Weiner 1977). Systematic questionnaire surveys indicate that up to one-fourth of people with asthma believe that emotions and stress are among their top asthma triggers, and these perceptions are associated with diminished illness control and more emergency treatments, independent of possible mood disorder comorbidity (Ritz et al. 2016).

Stress and Comorbid Psychiatric Disorders: Cross-Sectional and Longitudinal Associations With Asthma

Ample research points to an elevated comorbidity of asthma and psychiatric illness, in particular anxiety (Katon et al. 2004; Roy-Byrne et al. 2008) and depression (Trojan et al. 2014). Comorbid panic disorder has been found in 6.5%–24% of adults and 0.6%–4.7% of children and adolescents (Katon et al. 2004). In a large-scale cross-national study, adults with self-reported asthma had significantly elevated odds of also being diagnosed with panic disorder/agoraphobia, generalized anxiety disorder, posttraumatic stress disorder, social phobia, dysthymia/major depressive disorder (MDD), or alcohol use disorder (Scott et al. 2007). For a similar range of disorders in adult patients, including bipolar disorder and binge-eating disorder, the likelihood of a subsequent diagnosis of asthma was also elevated (Alonso et al. 2014). Comorbidities appear to depend on race or ethnicity, with particularly high comorbidity of panic disorder among urban patients with asthma who were from Puerto Rico and the Dominican Republic (21.1%) compared with asthma patients who were African American (6.7%) (Feldman et al. 2010). Suicidality (Kuo et al. 2010) and schizophrenia (Pedersen et al. 2012) are also more common in asthma patients. Common underlying risk factors, such as a genetic predisposition to both types of disorders or perinatal factors, may explain these findings (Meuret et al. 2017). Psychological disorders may produce some of the distress that triggers asthma symptoms, and such disorders are associated prospectively with problems in asthma control, emergency room visits, and hospitalizations (Favreau et al. 2014; Schneider et al. 2008).

Longitudinal studies have additionally demonstrated associations among stress, psychiatric disorders, and asthma onset. Panic disorder in early adulthood was related to a greater likelihood of developing asthma 20 years later (Hasler et al. 2005), while early adulthood asthma was predictive of later onset of panic disorder. A meta-analysis of longitudinal studies confirmed the bidirectional nature of the association between distress and atopic disorders (allergic disorders, characterized by type I hypersensitivity reactions, in that sample mostly asthma), with a stronger role of atopic disease in predicting subsequent psychological distress than the reverse (Chida et al. 2008). Perinatal factors may account for some of these associations. Stress during pregnancy, such as negative life events, anxiety, and depression, has been linked to childhood asthma and atopic illness in a number of studies (Andersson et al. 2016). Blood cord mononuclear cells of mothers with higher prenatal stress show signs of elevated inflammatory cytokine responses when challenged with antigens, a characteristic that could affect early-life programming of lung structure and function (Wright 2010). A variety of early-life challenges, such as parental mental illness, parenting problems, and exposure to domestic or neighborhood violence, have also been found to predict childhood asthma prospectively, sometimes in interaction with other environmental exposures (Exley et al. 2015). Recent research suggests that alterations of the lung or intestinal microbiome through psychological stress may also constitute a common risk factor for both affective disorders and asthma (Trueba et al. 2016). Overall, these findings indicate that psychosocial factors and mental health–related factors are critical players in asthma etiology, manifestation, and management and are important in the early stages of asthma development.

Psychosocial Factors: Influence on Asthma Through Biological and Illness Management Pathways

Influences of psychosocial factors on asthma unfold directly through their impact on pathophysiological processes or affect the illness indirectly through health behaviors and illness management. Airway and immune system function are susceptible to direct psychological influences, through nervous system and endocrine pathways. Vagal excitation and hyperventilation-associated negative affect lead to bronchoconstriction that is clinically significant in approximately one-fourth of patients (Isenberg et al. 1992; Ritz 2012) and can produce asthma symptoms. Stressful life episodes have been demonstrated to exacerbate asthma in children within a few days of stressor onset (Sandberg et al. 2004), and studies with sensitized mice show differential upregulation of allergy-relevant cytokine production depending on the acute versus chronic character of stressors (Kang and Weaver 2010). Immune cells of asthmatic children from low socioeconomic status (SES) families exposed to chronic stress respond to antigen stimulation with an elevated production of inflammatory cytokines (Marin et al. 2009). Downregulation of messenger RNA of beta-adrenergic and glucocorticoid receptors that are potentially relevant for lung health has been shown in children with chronic stress and low SES (Miller and Chen 2006). Sputum analysis of asthma patients during stressful periods (e.g., exams) demonstrated that allergy-relevant cytokine production is also elevated in the airways upon allergen challenge (Liu et al. 2002). Some of the allergic inflammatory processes correlate with overactivation in distinct areas of the limbic system (Rosenkranz et al. 2012). The well-documented facilitation of respiratory infections through stress could also mediate asthma exacerbations, given the importance of infections as asthma triggers (Trueba and Ritz 2013).

Interaction with comorbidity or underlying risk factors may worsen the impact of stress in asthma, as has been shown for depression (Miller et al. 2009) and for polymorphisms of glucocorticoid and beta$_2$-receptor genes (Rehm et al. 2012). Influences of stress on asthma can be counterbalanced by resilience factors, such as positive life experiences (Sandberg et al. 2002). Because psychobiological processes are superimposed on specific developmental trajectories of lung mechanics and immune system development and are embedded in a multitude of physical and social environmental disease mediators and moderators, the multilevel framework of a biopsychosocial asthma analysis is required (Wright and Subramanian 2007).

Whereas some psychosocial factors may affect biological pathways directly, others may affect asthma indirectly through adverse health behaviors or compromised management (Chen et al. 2007). Stress can influence dietary behaviors and substance use, giving rise to adverse influences on asthma through obesity (Sivapalan et al. 2015) or smoking (Bakakos et al. 2016). Seminal studies of "psychomaintenance" of asthma conducted in the early 1970s at the National Jewish Hospital in Denver, Colorado, demonstrated that aspects of anxiety indirectly influence asthma control through their effect on management variables (Kinsman et al. 1973). Thus, patients' asthma-related fears were associated with physicians' corticosteroid prescriptions. Patients' beliefs about their illness and its treatment motivate and guide self-management behaviors and therefore influence asthma outcomes (Kaptein et al. 2010). As shown for Latino cultures (McQuaid et al. 2009), specific beliefs and concerns about medication can interfere with adequate asthma management. Patients' perceptions of asthma symptoms are of great importance. A substantial proportion of patients inaccurately assess their dyspnea (Janssens et al. 2009); imaging studies examining cortical processing of the perception of dyspnea have identified neurophysiological pathways involving areas relevant to interoception (i.e., the perception of bodily responses such as respiration) and emotion, such as the insular cortex and amygdala (von Leupoldt et al. 2008). The close association between interoception and emotion is also reflected in the association of anxiety with enhanced processing of respiratory symptoms (von Leupoldt et al. 2011).

Asthma Management: Behavioral Interventions and Psychotherapy

Beyond the first-line treatments of anti-inflammatory and bronchodilatory medication, multidisciplinary behavioral medicine team efforts should ideally address the need for education in asthma self-management and for adjunctive behavioral treatments (Ritz et al. 2013).

Asthma education is recognized as essential and effective in improving asthma control (Global Initiative for Asthma 2012; National Heart, Lung, and Blood Institute/National Asthma Education and Prevention Program 2007). Patients need training in the proper use of inhalers, self-monitoring of asthma symptoms or lung function, avoidance and management of triggering factors, and self-adjustment of medication using asthma action plans devised by their treating physician. Regular physical activity and exercise are also recommended, because they are safe for patients and improve fitness and asthma outcomes (Eichenberger et al. 2013). In daily life, physical activity is associated with bronchodilation; nevertheless, patients complain about symptoms, possibly because in stronger exercise, hyperreactive airways of asthma patients can also constrict, a response that can be controlled by bronchodilators or warm-up protocols (Ritz et al. 2010).

Because adherence to maintenance medication is often low, interventions have been devised to improve outcomes (Bårnes and Ulrik 2015). However, intervention effects on overall adherence levels and asthma outcomes have remained disappointing, and new intervention modes utilizing electronic monitoring, smartphone applications, and the Internet are now being explored. Training in accurate perception of airway obstruction using feedback from self-measurements of lung function has shown promise for improving medication adherence and reducing underperception of airway status in minority children with asthma (Feldman et al. 2012).

A range of behavioral interventions with varying support by psychophysiological rationales have also been tested. Studies of relaxation training, yoga, and meditation have produced mixed results (Lahmann et al. 2009; Pbert et al. 2012; Posadzki and Ernst 2011), which is not surprising, given that physical activation, rather than deactivation, dilates the airways. By contrast, various forms of breathing training show more promise, with clinical trial evidence supporting slow abdominal breathing (Thomas et al. 2009), slow breathing with heart rate variability feedback (Lehrer et al. 2004), and hypoventilation training with (Ritz et al. 2014) or without (Bruton and Lewith 2005) feedback of end-tidal carbon dioxide levels. Although some of these techniques also yield effects on lung function, benefits are seen mostly for asthma symptoms, quality of life, and bronchodilator or maintenance medication needs.

More comprehensive programs of psychotherapy have been tested to address common psychiatric asthma comorbidities, such as panic or depression, and the negative effect of these symptoms on asthma outcomes. These interventions typically target both general concerns of patients and asthma-specific concerns, such as hyperventilation (Lehrer et al. 2008). For example, Parry et al. (2012) randomly assigned 94 high-anxiety asthma patients to either intervention or control groups to compare the effectiveness of anxiety self-management education in reducing asthma-specific fear. The patients who received the cognitive-behavioral therapy (CBT) intervention showed lower levels of asthma-specific panic fear at the end of the treatment, as well as at the 6-month follow-up, suggesting the efficacy of CBT in managing comorbid asthma and anxiety. However, no asthma-specific illness outcomes were reported. In another study, adults with persistent asthma showed improvements in quality of life and asthma control following a six-session self-regulation intervention that focused on identifying goals, problems, and barriers to asthma management (Baptist et al. 2013). Thus, CBT is associated with positive effects on anxiety, asthma control, and quality of life for patients with asthma (Kew et al. 2016).

Chronic Obstructive Pulmonary Disease

Chronic obstructive pulmonary disease (COPD) is a chronic respiratory disease based on an inflammatory response of the lung to noxious particles or gases, often due to tobacco smoking or environmental exposures, such as smoke from open fireplaces or biomass fuel stoves in developing countries (Global Initiative for Chronic Obstructive Lung Disease 2017). The resulting airflow limitation is progressive and, in contrast to asthma, only partially reversible. Patients experience symptoms of persistent cough and dyspnea (an uncomfortable sensation of breathlessness). These symptoms are associated with limitations in daily activities and can generate considerable fear and distress, reducing quality of life considerably (von Leupoldt et al. 2012). Systemic inflammation may additionally contribute to COPD severity and the comorbidity commonly observed with other somatic diseases, including lung cancer, cardiovascular diseases, respiratory tract infections, skeletal muscle dysfunction, and diabetes. Late stages of COPD are characterized by insufficient gas exchange, hyperinflation of the lungs, respiratory muscle weakening, and emphysema, requiring long-term oxygen therapy, mechanical ventilation, or surgical procedures. In 2010, the worldwide prevalence of COPD was estimated at 11.7%, although rates vary widely across countries (Adeloye et al. 2015). The highest rates are found in older segments of the population, especially in individuals older than 60 years. COPD is a leading cause of morbidity and mortality, with rates increasing due to changes in world population demographics.

Comorbidity of COPD With Psychiatric Illness and Special Psychological Considerations

The prevalence of comorbid psychiatric symptoms, in particular mood and anxiety disorders, is generally high in COPD (Rapsey et al. 2015). Although prevalence rates vary considerably across studies, recent reviews estimate that approximately one-fourth of COPD patients experience clinically significant depression (Panagioti et al. 2014). Clinically significant anxiety is estimated to be two times more prevalent in patients with COPD than in the general population, with panic-related symptoms or panic disorder being up to 10 times more prevalent. These psychiatric comorbidities impact COPD management, with increased frequency of exacerbations, hospitalizations, and hospital readmissions due to anxiety and depression (Coventry et al. 2011; Laurin et al. 2012). Physical activity is also hampered by COPD (Spruit et al. 2010), further reducing both psychological and physical functioning. Consequently, quality of life of COPD patients with comorbid psychiatric diagnoses is impaired considerably (Blakemore et al. 2014). Psychiatric comorbidities often remain undetected (Kunik et al. 2005), further complicating patient management. Reasons for these comorbidities are likely multifactorial but include concerns about functional and social limitations, life-threatening states of dyspnea and suffocation, and end-of-life questions. Inflammatory mechanisms in COPD could constitute a psychobiological link to anxiety and depression (Barnes and Celli 2009), but research remains in its infancy. That retrospectively reported psychiatric diagnoses (in particular, depression, generalized anxiety disorder, and alcohol use disorder) are more common among individuals who subsequently develop COPD than among those who do not supports a potential etiological role of clinically significant emotional distress (Rapsey et al. 2015).

Qualitative research points to the importance of additional psychological considerations in COPD. Lindqvist and Hallberg (2010) identified six core areas of concern from patient interviews: "feelings of guilt due to self-inflicted disease," "making sense of existence," "adjusting to bodily restrictions," "surrendering to fate," "making excuses for smoking-related causes," and "creating compliance with daily medication." Feelings of guilt about one's smoking habit and its effects on one's health appear to be central, hindering acceptance of the chronic condition with its functional

delirium, seizures, dementia, mania, and psychosis. Psychotic symptoms generally remit rapidly with steroids.

Sarcoidosis rarely has been investigated from a psychological standpoint. A large study of members of the Dutch Sarcoidosis Society found that perceived stress was high and was related to depressive symptoms (De Vries and Drent 2004). In addition, psychiatric comorbidity was reported in 44% of Italian sarcoidosis patients, with MDD in 25%, panic disorder in 6.3%, bipolar disorder in 6.3%, generalized anxiety disorder in 5%, and obsessive-compulsive disorder in 1.3% (Goracci et al. 2008). Depression is associated with poorer quality of life in sarcoidosis (Yeager et al. 2005).

Other Respiratory Conditions

Many individuals experience symptom patterns that mimic asthma or COPD. Such symptoms include the experience of disabling breathlessness, chronic cough, "air hunger," and suffocation. Consideration of alternative diagnoses that may present in a manner similar to asthma is essential for correct diagnosis and treatment. Inappropriate treatment with medications such as systemic corticosteroids can result in deleterious side effects, ineffective treatment, and even morbidity (Benninger et al. 2011; Idrees and FitzGerald 2015).

Somatic Cough Disorder (Psychogenic Cough) and Tic Cough (Habit Cough)

In many respiratory conditions, chronic cough—defined as cough that is present for at least 4 weeks in children and 8 weeks in adults—is often the only symptom. However, chronic cough may also be present in the absence of any pulmonary or extrapulmonary (e.g., gastroesophageal reflux disease) etiology. In these cases, chronic cough, when unresponsive to medical management, is categorized as somatic cough disorder (previously psychogenic cough) or tic cough (previously known as habit cough) (Haydour et al. 2014; Vertigan et al. 2015). The American College of Chest Physicians (CHEST) Guideline and Expert Panel Report concluded that only low-quality evidence exists to support the definition or diagnosis of somatic cough disorder or tic cough (Vertigan et al. 2015). *Somatic cough disorder* is broadly indicated by core features, including chronic persistence, nonresponsiveness to medical treatment, daytime occurrence, absence at night, and the potential of a barking or honking sound. *Tic cough* is further classified as a psychogenic cough with single dry coughs (tics) that are suppressible, distractible, suggestible, and variable (Vertigan 2017). Despite low-quality evidence and lack of control groups, CHEST guidelines recommend nonpharmacological trials of hypnosis, suggestion therapy, combinations of reassurance and counseling, or referral to a psychologist or psychiatrist for treatment (Haydour et al. 2014; Vertigan et al. 2015).

Hyperventilation

The term *hyperventilation syndrome* was first introduced by Kerr et al. in 1937 and has since garnered both attention and controversy, with little consensus among definitions of symptomatology or diagnostic criteria (Bass 1997; Kerr et al. 1938). Hyperventilation arises when breathing occurs in excess of metabolic demand, which acutely leads to dyspnea and anxiety, and reduction of the partial pressure of carbon dioxide (pCO_2) (Wilhelm et al. 2001). Symptoms of hyperventilation include breathlessness out of proportion to actual physical effort, chest pain that is usually atypical in angina, dizziness, paresthesias, fatigue, and palpitations (Tavel 1990). Terms used to describe this collection of symptoms have included *dysfunctional breathing, behavioral breathlessness, neurocirculatory asthenia,* and *psychogenic dyspnea* (Howell 1990; Jones et al. 2013). Problematic hyperventilation is estimated to occur in up to 10% of the general population, more commonly in children and adolescents, and even more commonly in those who also have asthma (D'Alba et al. 2015; Gridina et al. 2013).

There is no clearly elucidated pathophysiology underlying hyperventilation, which can occur in both acute and chronic forms (Gardner 1996). Acute hyperventilation is easily diagnosed due to rapid breathing (tachypnea) or frequent deep breaths; chronic hyperventilation is more problematic, requiring more nuanced diagnosis to identify the subtleties of a modest increase in respiratory rate or tidal volume. Affected individuals frequently seek medical care and undergo extensive and expensive testing in attempts to identify an organic cause of symptoms (Decuyper et al. 2012).

Many physicians regard hyperventilation as a manifestation of anxiety, but a more complex interaction may be involved among organic respiratory, physiological, and psychiatric disturbances that induce symptomatic hypocapnia (i.e., deficiency of carbon dioxide in arterial blood) (Gardner 1996). Chronic hyperventilation is often observed in anxiety disorders, particularly panic disorder, where it generates several characteristic physical symptoms, including shortness of breath and dizziness (Meuret and Ritz 2010). Anxious patients with complaints of air hunger often take large "sigh" breaths, which results in overbreathing and induces hypocapnia. Additionally, neuroticism is viewed as a risk factor for the development of hyperventilation because it is strongly associated with self-reported hyperventilation symptoms (Decuyper et al. 2012).

Hyperventilation and anxiety can function in both a bidirectional and progressive manner, with symptoms of anxiety influencing breathing patterns, and hyperventilation symptoms generating psychological distress. Primary treatment for hyperventilation includes psychoeducation and interventions targeted at reducing hyperventilation. These interventions include diaphragmatic breathing, cognitive training, and hypoventilation training (Jones et al. 2013; Meuret et al. 2010).

Vocal Cord Dysfunction

Vocal cord dysfunction (VCD) was first described in the 1840s and occurs when abnormal adduction of the vocal cords during the inspiratory phase of the respiratory cycle produces airflow obstruction at the larynx (Dunn et al. 2015). VCD can mimic persistent asthma in up to 10% of patients seeking evaluation; if not diagnosed appropriately, VCD is often treated with asthma medications, with significant resulting morbidity and costs (Traister et al. 2016). Symptoms of VCD include wheezing, coughing, shortness of breath, chest tightness, and dyspnea. VCD can also be comorbid with asthma, with some studies showing that more than 50% of patients with VCD have an additional asthma diagnosis (Newman et al. 1995). The exact cause of VCD is not established but is likely multifactorial (Goldberg and Kaplan 2000). Factors predictive of VCD include younger age, female sex, high body mass index, history of childhood sexual trauma, and presence of anxiety or depression (Goldberg and Kaplan 2000; Idrees and FitzGerald 2015; Li et al. 2016). The condition is largely treated with breathing strategies aimed at reducing laryngeal muscle tone, and psychological interventions may also be useful in management of both adult and pediatric patients; however, continued research with longitudinal study designs is needed (Guglani et al. 2014).

Psychiatric Effects of Pulmonary Drugs

Systemic corticosteroids are frequently prescribed for patients with pulmonary diseases. Long-term corticosteroid use is associated with side effects, such as suppression of the hypothalamic-pituitary-adrenal (HPA) axis and immune system, glaucoma, cataracts, truncal obesity, thinning and bruising of the skin, and loss of bone mineral density.

Corticosteroids are also associated with an increased risk of depression, mania, and mixed episodes (Judd et al. 2014) Acute, high-dose corticosteroid therapy appears to be more strongly associated with mania or hypomania, while chronic, lower-dose therapy may be more associated with depression. Psychotic symptoms, including delusions, hallucinations, and disorganized thought processes, also can occur. The most common neuropsychiatric effects of corticosteroids may be cognitive changes. The hippocampus, a brain region involved in memory, appears to be particularly sensitive to corticosteroid effects, with some studies showing volume decreases (Brown 2009; Brown et al. 2004). Diffuse cognitive changes, including delirium, are also reported during corticosteroid therapy (Fardet et al. 2012). Dose is the most definitively established risk factor for psychiatric side effects of corticosteroids. Even inhaled corticosteroids can cause HPA axis suppression at higher doses, as well as psychiatric side effects. Corticosteroid-induced psychiatric symptoms and their treatment are discussed in detail in Chapter 24 ("Rheumatology").

Other medications used for pulmonary diseases also have psychiatric side effects. Theophylline and beta$_2$-adrenergic agonists are sometimes associated with anxiety, insomnia, restlessness, agitation, and depression. Theophylline may even be associated with an increased risk of suicidal ideation (Favreau et al. 2012). Initial reports suggested that leukotriene inhibitors may cause psychiatric symptoms, such as agitation, insomnia, anxiety, depression, and suicidal ideation, although more recent analyses do not suggest a link with completed suicide (Gibbons and Mann 2011). Other than dose reduction or discontinuation, no known treatments have been established for psychiatric side effects of these medications.

Psychopharmacology in Pulmonary Disease

Psychiatric disorders are common among people with pulmonary diseases. The symptoms may be influenced by disability, activity limitations, and changes in quality of life, as well as breathlessness and medication side effects. In general, pharmacological treatment of psychiatric disorders such as depression, anxiety, and psychosis in this population is similar to that in other patient populations. However, the likelihood that patients with chronic respiratory diseases are already taking several medications increases the risk of additive side effects (e.g., QTc prolongation) and drug–drug interactions, particularly for drugs metabolized by the cytochrome P450 system. When possible, clinicians should avoid prescribing psychiatric medications that depress the respiratory system (e.g., benzodiazepines); if used, these agents should be prescribed at the lowest dosage that provides symptom relief. Sedating medications are contraindicated in hypercapnic patients (i.e., those with chronically elevated pCO_2) because they can suppress hypoxic respiratory drive.

Although limited, there is also evidence suggesting potential benefits of pharmacotherapy in managing adult respiratory asthma and its psychiatric comorbidities. A randomized 12-week clinical trial of citalopram in 82 adults with both asthma and MDD showed reductions in oral corticosteroid use and depression symptom scores in patients receiving citalopram vs. placebo (Brown et al. 2005). Additionally, trends toward reductions in depression scores, as well as a correlation between changes in asthma (based on the Asthma Control Questionnaire and pulmonary function [FEV_1% of predicted]) and changes in depressive symptoms, have been observed in small proof-of-concept randomized trials of escitalopram and bupropion in outpatients with asthma and MDD (Brown et al. 2007, 2012). These studies may have meaningful clinical implications for the management of both asthma and MDD with antidepressant medications; however, physiological mechanisms that drive the relationship between both conditions and the medication response remain unclear.

A recent meta-analysis concluded that benzodiazepines are safe and effective as hypnotics in less severe COPD (Lu et al. 2016); however, they also have a higher rate of adverse respiratory events (Chung et al. 2015; Ekström et al. 2014). Benzodiazepines have not been shown to be effective in relieving breathlessness in advanced COPD (Simon et al. 2016); low-dose opioids are suggested as a safer and more effective alternative (Ekström et al. 2014). Antipsychotic use has been associated with an acute and dose-dependent increased risk of acute respiratory failure in patients with COPD (Wang et al. 2017). Chronic antipsychotic use uncommonly causes laryngeal and other respiratory dyskinesias. Additional research, including larger-scale clinical studies that incorporate integrative approaches to pulmonary disease management, is needed to improve our understanding of the interaction between respiratory disease and psychiatric illness and to create better-targeted treatment approaches.

Conclusion

In this chapter, we discussed the nature, prevalence, and treatment of psychiatric disorders frequently observed in patients with pulmonary diseases. The symptoms and treatment outcomes of many pulmonary diseases are strongly influenced by mood, emotions, and the presence of psychiatric comorbidities and are mediated by biological factors, as well as through treatment adherence and overall functioning and quality of life. The management of psychiatric disorders in this population can include both psychosocial approaches and pharmacotherapy. When psychiatric medications are given, an appreciation of the potential for side effects and drug–drug interactions is essential.

References

Adeloye D, Chua S, Lee C, et al; Global Health Epidemiology Reference Group (GHERG): Global and regional estimates of COPD prevalence: systematic review and meta-analysis. J Glob Health 5(2):020415, 2015 26755942

Alexander F: Psychosomatic Medicine: Its Principles and Applications. New York, WW Norton, 1950

Alonso J, de Jonge P, Lim CC, et al: Association between mental disorders and subsequent adult onset asthma. J Psychiatr Res 59:179–188, 2014 25263276

Andersson NW, Hansen MV, Larsen AD, et al: Prenatal maternal stress and atopic diseases in the child: a systematic review of observational human studies. Allergy 71(1):15–26, 2016 26395995

Bakakos P, Kostikas K, Loukides S: Smoking asthma phenotype: diagnostic and management challenges. Curr Opin Pulm Med 22(1):53–58, 2016 26606078

Baptist AP, Ross JA, Yang Y, et al: A randomized controlled trial of a self-regulation intervention for older adults with asthma. J Am Geriatr Soc 61(5):747–753, 2013 23617712

Bårnes CB, Ulrik CS: Asthma and adherence to inhaled corticosteroids: current status and future perspectives. Respir Care 60(3):455–468, 2015 25118311

Barnes PJ, Celli BR: Systemic manifestations and comorbidities of COPD. Eur Respir J 33(5):1165–1185, 2009 19407051

Bass C: Hyperventilation syndrome: a chimera? J Psychosom Res 42(5):421–426, 1997 91944014

Benninger C, Parsons JP, Mastronarde JG: Vocal cord dysfunction and asthma. Curr Opin Pulm Med 17(1):45–49, 2011 21330824

Blakemore A, Dickens C, Guthrie E, et al: Depression and anxiety predict health-related quality of life in chronic obstructive pulmonary disease: systematic review and meta-analysis. Int J Chron Obstruct Pulmon Dis 9:501–512, 2014 24876770

Brown ES: Effects of glucocorticoids on mood, memory, and the hippocampus. Treatment and preventive therapy. Ann N Y Acad Sci 1179:41–55, 2009 19906231

Brown ES, Varghese FP, McEwen BS: Association of depression with medical illness: does cortisol play a role? Biol Psychiatry 55(1):1–9, 2004 14706419

Brown ES, Vigil L, Khan DA, et al: A randomized trial of citalopram versus placebo in outpatients with asthma and major depressive disorder: a proof of concept study. Biol Psychiatry 58(11):865–870, 2005 15993860

Brown ES, Vornik LA, Khan DA, et al: Bupropion in the treatment of outpatients with asthma and major depressive disorder. Int J Psychiatry Med 37(1):23–28, 2007 17645195

Brown ES, Howard C, Khan DA, et al: Escitalopram for severe asthma and major depressive disorder: a randomized, double-blind, placebo-controlled proof-of-concept study. Psychosomatics 53(1):75–80, 2012 22221724

Bruton A, Lewith GT: The Buteyko breathing technique for asthma: a review. Complement Ther Med 13(1):41–46, 2005 15907677

Centers for Disease Control and Prevention: Asthma facts: CDC's National Asthma Control Program grantees. July 2013. Available at: https://www.cdc.gov/asthma/pdfs/asthma_facts_program_grantees.pdf. Accessed June 8, 2017.

Chen E, Chim LS, Strunk RC, et al: The role of the social environment in children and adolescents with asthma. Am J Respir Crit Care Med 176(7):644–649, 2007 17556714

Chida Y, Hamer M, Steptoe A: A bidirectional relationship between psychosocial factors and atopic disorders: a systematic review and meta-analysis. Psychosom Med 70(1):102–116, 2008 18158379

Chung WS, Lai CY, Lin CL, et al: Adverse respiratory events associated with hypnotics use in patients of chronic obstructive pulmonary disease: a population-based case-control study. Medicine (Baltimore) 94(27):e1110, 2015 26166105

Coventry PA, Gemmell I, Todd CJ: Psychosocial risk factors for hospital readmission in COPD patients on early discharge services: a cohort study. BMC Pulm Med 11:49, 2011 22054636

Coventry PA, Bower P, Keyworth C, et al: The effect of complex interventions on depression and anxiety in chronic obstructive pulmonary disease: systematic review and meta-analysis. PLoS One 8(4):e60532, 2013 23585837

D'Alba I, Carloni I, Ferrante AL, et al: Hyperventilation syndrome in adolescents with and without asthma. Pediatr Pulmonol 50(12):1184–1190, 2015 25470247

Decuyper M, De Bolle M, Boone E, et al: The relevance of personality assessment in patients with hyperventilation symptoms. Health Psychol 31(3):316–322, 2012 22149121

De Vries J, Drent M: Relationship between perceived stress and sarcoidosis in a Dutch patient population. Sarcoidosis Vasc Diffuse Lung Dis 21(1):57–63, 2004 15127976

Dunn NM, Katial RK, Hoyte FCL: Vocal cord dysfunction: a review. Asthma Res Pract 1:9, 2015 27965763

Eichenberger PA, Diener SN, Kofmehl R, et al: Effects of exercise training on airway hyperreactivity in asthma: a systematic review and meta-analysis. Sports Med 43(11):1157–1170, 2013 23846823

Ekström MP, Bornefalk-Hermansson A, Abernethy AP, et al: Safety of benzodiazepines and opioids in very severe respiratory disease: national prospective study. BMJ 348:g445, 2014 24482539

Exley D, Norman A, Hyland M: Adverse childhood experience and asthma onset: a systematic review. Eur Respir Rev 24(136):299–305, 2015 26028641

Fardet L, Petersen I, Nazareth I: Suicidal behavior and severe neuropsychiatric disorders following glucocorticoid therapy in primary care. Am J Psychiatry 169(5):491–497, 2012 22764363

Farver-Vestergaard I, Jacobsen D, Zachariae R: Efficacy of psychosocial interventions on psychological and physical health outcomes in chronic obstructive pulmonary disease: a systematic review and meta-analysis. Psychother Psychosom 84(1):37–50, 2015 25547641

Favreau H, Bacon SL, Joseph M, et al: Association between asthma medications and suicidal ideation in adult asthmatics. Respir Med 106(7):933–941, 2012 22495109

Favreau H, Bacon SL, Labrecque M, et al: Prospective impact of panic disorder and panic-anxiety on asthma control, health service use, and quality of life in adult patients with asthma over a 4-year follow-up. Psychosom Med 76(2):147–155, 2014 24470131

Feldman JM, Mayefsky L, Beckmann L, et al: Ethnic differences in asthma-panic disorder comorbidity. J Allergy Clin Immunol 125(3):760–762, 2010 20132974

Feldman JM, Kutner H, Matte L, et al: Prediction of peak flow values followed by feedback improves perception of lung function and adherence to inhaled corticosteroids in children with asthma. Thorax 67(12):1040–1045, 2012 23154987

Gardner WN: The pathophysiology of hyperventilation disorders. Chest 109(2):516–534, 1996 8620731

Gibbons RD, Mann JJ: Strategies for quantifying the relationship between medications and suicidal behaviour: what has been learned? Drug Saf 34(5):375–395, 2011 21513361

Global Initiative for Asthma (GINA): Global Strategy for Asthma Management and Prevention: 2012 update. 2012. Available at: http://www.ginasthma.org/local/uploads/files/GINA_Report_March13.pdf. Accessed March 5, 2014.

Global Initiative for Chronic Obstructive Lung Disease (GOLD): Global Strategy for the Diagnosis, Management and Prevention of COPD. 2017. Available at: http://goldcopd.org/gold-2017-global-strategy-diagnosis-management-prevention-copd/. Accessed June 8, 2017.

Goldberg BJ, Kaplan MS: Non-asthmatic respiratory symptomatology. Curr Opin Pulm Med 6(1):26–30, 2000 10608422

Goracci A, Fagiolini A, Martinucci M, et al: Quality of life, anxiety and depression in sarcoidosis. Gen Hosp Psychiatry 30(5):441–445, 2008 18774427

Gosselink R, De Vos J, van den Heuvel SP, et al: Impact of inspiratory muscle training in patients with COPD: what is the evidence? Eur Respir J 37(2):416–425, 2011 21282809

Gridina I, Bidat E, Chevallier B, et al: [Prevalence of chronic hyperventilation syndrome in children and teenagers] [in French]. Arch Pediatr 20(3):265–268, 2013 23375424

Guglani L, Atkinson S, Hosanagar A, et al: A systematic review of psychological interventions for adult and pediatric patients with vocal cord dysfunction. Front Pediatr 2:82, 2014 25152871

Hasler G, Gergen PJ, Kleinbaum DG, et al: Asthma and panic in young adults: a 20-year prospective community study. Am J Respir Crit Care Med 171(11):1224–1230, 2005 15764721

Haydour Q, Alahdab F, Farah M, et al: Management and diagnosis of psychogenic cough, habit cough, and tic cough: a systematic review. Chest 146(2):355–372, 2014 24833061

Holland AE, Hill CJ, Jones AY, et al: Breathing exercises for chronic obstructive pulmonary disease. Cochrane Database Syst Rev (10):CD008250, 2012 23076942

Howcroft M, Walters EH, Wood-Baker R, et al: Action plans with brief patient education for exacerbations in chronic obstructive pulmonary disease. Cochrane Database Syst Rev (12):CD005074, 2016 27990628

Howell JBL: Behavioural breathlessness. Thorax 45(4):287–292, 1990 2278552

Idrees M, FitzGerald JM: Vocal cord dysfunction in bronchial asthma. A review article. J Asthma 52(4):327–335, 2015 25365113

Isenberg SA, Lehrer PM, Hochron S: The effects of suggestion and emotional arousal on pulmonary function in asthma: a review and a hypothesis regarding vagal mediation. Psychosom Med 54(2):192–216, 1992 1565756

Janssens T, Verleden G, De Peuter S, et al: Inaccurate perception of asthma symptoms: a cognitive-affective framework and implications for asthma treatment. Clin Psychol Rev 29(4):317–327, 2009 19285771

Jones M, Harvey A, Marston L, et al: Breathing exercises for dysfunctional breathing/hyperventilation syndrome in adults. Cochrane Database Syst Rev (5):CD009041, 2013 23728685

Judd LL, Schettler PJ, Brown ES, et al: Adverse consequences of glucocorticoid medication: psychological, cognitive, and behavioral effects. Am J Psychiatry 171(10):1045–1051, 2014 25272344

Kang DH, Weaver MT: Airway cytokine responses to acute and repeated stress in a murine model of allergic asthma. Biol Psychol 84(1):66–73, 2010 19879322

Kaptein AA, Scharloo M, Fischer MJ, et al: Illness perceptions and COPD: an emerging field for COPD patient management. J Asthma 45(8):625–629, 2008 18951252

Kaptein AA, Klok T, Moss-Morris R, et al: Illness perceptions: impact on self-management and control in asthma. Curr Opin Allergy Clin Immunol 10(3):194–199, 2010 20386435

Katon WJ, Richardson L, Lozano P, et al: The relationship of asthma and anxiety disorders. Psychosom Med 66(3):349–355, 2004 15184694

Kerr WJ, Dalton JW, Gliebe PA: Some physical phenomena associated with anxiety states and their relation to hyperventilation. Annals of Internal Medicine 11(6):961–992, 1937

Kerr WJ, Gliebe PA, Dalton JW: Physical phenomena associated with anxiety states: the hyperventilation syndrome. California and Western Medicine 48(1):12–16, 1938 18744341

Kessler R, Ståhl E, Vogelmeier C, et al: Patient understanding, detection, and experience of COPD exacerbations: an observational, interview-based study. Chest 130(1):133–142, 2006 16840393

Kew KM, Nashed M, Dulay V, et al: Cognitive behavioural therapy (CBT) for adults and adolescents with asthma. Cochrane Database Syst Rev (9):CD011818, 2016 27649894

Kinsman RA, Luparello T, O'Banion K, et al: Multidimensional analysis of the subjective symptomatology of asthma. Psychosom Med 35(3):250–267, 1973 4710144

Krumholz A, Stern BJ: Neurologic manifestations of sarcoidosis. Handb Clin Neurol 119:305–333, 2014 24365304

Kunik ME, Roundy K, Veazey C, et al: Surprisingly high prevalence of anxiety and depression in chronic breathing disorders. Chest 127(4):1205–1211, 2005 15821196

Kuo CJ, Chen VC, Lee WC, et al: Asthma and suicide mortality in young people: a 12-year follow-up study. Am J Psychiatry 167(9):1092–1099, 2010 20634368

Lahham A, McDonald CF, Holland AE: Exercise training alone or with the addition of activity counseling improves physical activity levels in COPD: a systematic review and meta-analysis of randomized controlled trials. Int J Chron Obstruct Pulmon Dis 11:3121–3136, 2016 27994451

Lahmann C, Nickel M, Schuster T, et al: Functional relaxation and guided imagery as complementary therapy in asthma: a randomized controlled clinical trial. Psychother Psychosom 78(4):233–239, 2009 19401624

Laurin C, Moullec G, Bacon SL, et al: Impact of anxiety and depression on chronic obstructive pulmonary disease exacerbation risk. Am J Respir Crit Care Med 185(9):918–923, 2012 22246177

Lehrer PM, Vaschillo E, Vaschillo B, et al: Biofeedback treatment for asthma. Chest 126(2):352–361, 2004 15302717

Lehrer PM, Karavidas MK, Lu SE, et al: Psychological treatment of comorbid asthma and panic disorder: a pilot study. J Anxiety Disord 22(4):671–683, 2008 17693054

Leong AB, Ramsey CD, Celedón JC: The challenge of asthma in minority populations. Clin Rev Allergy Immunol 43(1–2):156–183, 2012 21538075

Li RC, Singh U, Windom HP, et al: Clinical associations in the diagnosis of vocal cord dysfunction. Ann Allergy Asthma Immunol 117(4):354–358, 2016 27590638

Lindqvist G, Hallberg LR: "Feelings of guilt due to self-inflicted disease": a grounded theory of suffering from chronic obstructive pulmonary disease (COPD). J Health Psychol 15(3):456–466, 2010 20348366

Liu LY, Coe CL, Swenson CA, et al: School examinations enhance airway inflammation to antigen challenge. Am J Respir Crit Care Med 165(8):1062–1067, 2002 11956045

Livermore N, Sharpe L, McKenzie D: Prevention of panic attacks and panic disorder in COPD. Eur Respir J 35(3):557–563, 2010 19741029

Lu XM, Zhu JP, Zhou XM: The effect of benzodiazepines on insomnia in patients with chronic obstructive pulmonary disease: a meta-analysis of treatment efficacy and safety. Int J Chron Obstruct Pulmon Dis 11:675–685, 2016 27110106

Marin TJ, Chen E, Munch JA, et al: Double-exposure to acute stress and chronic family stress is associated with immune changes in children with asthma. Psychosom Med 71(4):378–384, 2009 19196805

McQuaid EL, Vasquez J, Canino G, et al: Beliefs and barriers to medication use in parents of Latino children with asthma. Pediatr Pulmonol 44(9):892–898, 2009 19672958

Meuret AE, Ritz T: Hyperventilation in panic disorder and asthma: empirical evidence and clinical strategies. Int J Psychophysiol 78(1):68–79, 2010 20685222

Meuret AE, Rosenfield D, Seidel A, et al: Respiratory and cognitive mediators of treatment change in panic disorder: evidence for intervention specificity. J Consult Clin Psychol 78(5):691–704, 2010 20873904

Meuret AE, Kroll J, Ritz T: Panic disorder comorbidity with medical conditions and treatment implications. Annu Rev Clin Psychol 13:209–240, 2017 28375724

Miller BD, Wood BL, Lim J, et al: Depressed children with asthma evidence increased airway resistance: "vagal bias" as a mechanism? J Allergy Clin Immunol 124(1):66–73.e1, 10, 2009 19523670

Miller GE, Chen E: Life stress and diminished expression of genes encoding glucocorticoid receptor and beta2-adrenergic receptor in children with asthma. Proc Natl Acad Sci U S A 103(14):5496–5501, 2006 16567656

National Heart, Lung, and Blood Institute/National Asthma Education and Prevention Program: Expert Panel Report: Guidelines for the Diagnosis and Management of Asthma (NIH Publ No 07-4051). Bethesda, MD, National Institutes of Health, 2007

Newman KB, Mason UG 3rd, Schmaling KB: Clinical features of vocal cord dysfunction. Am J Respir Crit Care Med 152(4 Pt 1):1382–1386, 1995 7551399

Ngai SP, Jones AY, Tam WW: Tai Chi for chronic obstructive pulmonary disease (COPD). Cochrane Database Syst Rev (6):CD009953, 2016 27272131

Panagioti M, Scott C, Blakemore A, et al: Overview of the prevalence, impact, and management of depression and anxiety in chronic obstructive pulmonary disease. Int J Chron Obstruct Pulmon Dis 9:1289–1306, 2014 25419126

Parry GD, Cooper CL, Moore JM, et al: Cognitive behavioural intervention for adults with anxiety complications of asthma: prospective randomised trial. Respir Med 106(6):802–810, 2012 22398158

Pbert L, Madison JM, Druker S, et al: Effect of mindfulness training on asthma quality of life and lung function: a randomised controlled trial. Thorax 67(9):769–776, 2012 22544892

Pedersen MS, Benros ME, Agerbo E, et al: Schizophrenia in patients with atopic disorders with particular emphasis on asthma: a Danish population-based study. Schizophr Res 138(1):58–62, 2012 22391212

Posadzki P, Ernst E: Yoga for asthma? A systematic review of randomized clinical trials. J Asthma 48(6):632–639, 2011 21627405

Puhan MA, Gimeno-Santos E, Cates CJ, et al: Pulmonary rehabilitation following exacerbations of chronic obstructive pulmonary disease. Cochrane Database Syst Rev (12):CD005305, 2016 27930803

Rapsey CM, Lim CC, Al-Hamzawi A, et al: Associations between DSM-IV mental disorders and subsequent COPD diagnosis. J Psychosom Res 79(5):333–339, 2015 26526305

Rehm KE, Xiang L, Elci OU, et al: Variability in laboratory immune parameters is associated with stress hormone receptor polymorphisms. Neuroimmunomodulation 19(4):220–228, 2012 22441538

Ritz T: Airway responsiveness to psychological processes in asthma and health. Front Physiol 3:343, 2012 22973233

Ritz T, Rosenfield D, Steptoe A: Physical activity, lung function, and shortness of breath in the daily life of individuals with asthma. Chest 138(4):913–918, 2010 20472861

Ritz T, Meuret AE, Trueba AF, et al: Psychosocial factors and behavioral medicine interventions in asthma. J Consult Clin Psychol 81(2):231–250, 2013 23025250

Ritz T, Rosenfield D, Steele AM, et al: Controlling Asthma by Training of Capnometry-assisted Hypoventilation (CATCH) vs slow breathing: a randomized controlled trial. Chest 146(5):1237–1247, 2014 25122497

Ritz T, Wittchen HU, Klotsche J, et al; sap-NEEDs study group: Asthma trigger reports are associated with low quality of life, exacerbations, and emergency treatments. Ann Am Thorac Soc 13(2):204–211, 2016 26599372

Rosenkranz MA, Busse WW, Sheridan JF, et al: Are there neurophenotypes for asthma? Functional brain imaging of the interaction between emotion and inflammation in asthma. PLoS One 7(8):e40921, 2012 22870208

Roy-Byrne PP, Davidson KW, Kessler RC, et al: Anxiety disorders and comorbid medical illness. Gen Hosp Psychiatry 30(3):208–225, 2008 18433653

Sandberg S, McCann DC, Ahola S, et al: Positive experiences and the relationship between stress and asthma in children. Acta Paediatr 91(2):152–158, 2002 11952001

Sandberg S, Järvenpää S, Penttinen A, et al: Asthma exacerbations in children immediately following stressful life events: a Cox's hierarchical regression. Thorax 59(12):1046–1051, 2004 15563703

Schneider A, Löwe B, Meyer FJ, et al: Depression and panic disorder as predictors of health outcomes for patients with asthma in primary care. Respir Med 102(3):359–366, 2008 18061424

Scott KM, Von Korff M, Ormel J, et al: Mental disorders among adults with asthma: results from the World Mental Health Survey. Gen Hosp Psychiatry 29(2):123–133, 2007 17336661

Simon ST, Higginson IJ, Booth S, et al: Benzodiazepines for the relief of breathlessness in advanced malignant and non-malignant diseases in adults. Cochrane Database Syst Rev (10):CD007354, 2016 27764523

Sivapalan P, Diamant Z, Ulrik CS: Obesity and asthma: current knowledge and future needs. Curr Opin Pulm Med 21(1):80–85, 2015 25405670

Spruit MA, Watkins ML, Edwards LD, et al; Evaluation of COPD Longitudinally to Identify Predictive Surrogate Endpoints (ECLIPSE) study investigators: Determinants of poor 6-min walking distance in patients with COPD: the ECLIPSE cohort. Respir Med 104(6):849–857, 2010 20471236

Tavel ME: Hyperventilation syndrome—hiding behind pseudonyms? Chest 97(6):1285–1288, 1990 2189694

Thomas M, McKinley RK, Mellor S, et al: Breathing exercises for asthma: a randomised controlled trial. Thorax 64(1):55–61, 2009 19052047

Traister RS, Fajt ML, Petrov AA: The morbidity and cost of vocal cord dysfunction misdiagnosed as asthma. Allergy Asthma Proc 37(2):25–31, 2016 26932166

Trojan TD, Khan DA, Defina LF, et al: Asthma and depression: the Cooper Center Longitudinal Study. Ann Allergy Asthma Immunol 112(5):432–436, 2014 24650441

Trueba AF, Ritz T: Stress, asthma, and respiratory infections: pathways involving airway immunology and microbial endocrinology. Brain Behav Immun 29:11–27, 2013 23041248

Trueba AF, Ritz T, Trueba G: The role of the microbiome in the relationship of asthma and affective disorders. Adv Exp Med Biol 874:263–288, 2016 26589224

Vertigan AE: Somatic cough syndrome or psychogenic cough—what is the difference? J Thorac Dis 9(3):831–838, 2017 28449492

Vertigan AE, Murad MH, Pringsheim T, et al; CHEST Expert Cough Panel: Somatic cough syndrome (previously referred to as psychogenic cough) and tic cough (previously referred to as habit cough) in adults and children: CHEST guideline and expert panel report. Chest 148(1):24–31, 2015 25856777

Volpato E, Banfi P, Rogers SM, et al: Relaxation techniques for people with chronic obstructive pulmonary disease: a systematic review and a meta-analysis. Evid Based Complement Alternat Med 2015:628365, 2015 26339268

von Leupoldt A, Sommer T, Kegat S, et al: The unpleasantness of perceived dyspnea is processed in the anterior insula and amygdala. Am J Respir Crit Care Med 177(9):1026–1032, 2008 18263796

von Leupoldt A, Chan PY, Bradley MM, et al: The impact of anxiety on the neural processing of respiratory sensations. Neuroimage 55(1):247–252, 2011 21111831

von Leupoldt A, Fritzsche A, Trueba AF, et al: Behavioral medicine approaches to chronic obstructive pulmonary disease. Ann Behav Med 44(1):52–65, 2012 22351032

Wang MT, Tsai CL, Lin CW, et al: Association between antipsychotic agents and risk of acute respiratory failure in patients with chronic obstructive pulmonary disease. JAMA Psychiatry 74(3):252–260, 2017 28055066

Weiner H: Psychobiology and Human Disease. New York, Elsevier, 1977

Wiles L, Cafarella P, Williams MT: Exercise training combined with psychological interventions for people with chronic obstructive pulmonary disease. Respirology 20(1):46–55, 2015 25339508

Wilhelm FH, Gerlach AL, Roth WT: Slow recovery from voluntary hyperventilation in panic disorder. Psychosom Med 63(4):638–649, 2001 11485118

Wright RJ: Perinatal stress and early life programming of lung structure and function. Biol Psychol 84(1):46–56, 2010 20080145

Wright RJ, Subramanian SV: Advancing a multilevel framework for epidemiologic research on asthma disparities. Chest 132 (5 suppl):757S–769S, 2007 17998340

Yeager H, Rossman MD, Baughman RP, et al; ACCESS Research Group: Pulmonary and psychosocial findings at enrollment in the ACCESS study. Sarcoidosis Vasc Diffuse Lung Dis 22(2):147–153, 2005 16053031

Yohannes AM, Alexopoulos GS: Pharmacological treatment of depression in older patients with chronic obstructive pulmonary disease: impact on the course of the disease and health outcomes. Drugs Aging 31(7):483–492, 2014 24902934

CHAPTER 19

Gastrointestinal Disorders

Catherine C. Crone, M.D.

Jeanne M. Lackamp, M.D.

Andrew R. Alkis, M.D.

Gastrointestinal (GI) disorders cover a wide range of illnesses that span from mouth to anus and include the liver, pancreas, and gall bladder. While some disorders are uncommon, others—such as gastroesophageal reflux disease, peptic ulcer, and irritable bowel syndrome—are commonplace. Physical and psychological distress caused by GI disorders results in high rates of health care utilization, billions of dollars in annual health care costs, lost productivity, and reduced quality of life (QoL). Additionally, there is an interrelationship between the brain and the gut that adds to the complexity of care. Psychiatrists will often encounter patients with concurrent GI disorders, and the presence of these disorders may need to be factored into clinical evaluation and subsequent care. This chapter covers a number of GI disorders, both structural and functional in origin, and is organized according to organ/GI region.

Functional Gastrointestinal Disorders

Patients often present to health care providers with various forms of GI distress that are found to lack specific structural or physiological etiologies. These represent functional gastrointestinal disorders (FGIDs), a broad spectrum of symptom-defined diagnoses (e.g., functional heartburn, functional dyspepsia, cyclic vomiting syndrome) that may consist of any combination of motility disturbance, visceral hypersensitivity, altered gut microbiota, and altered central nervous system (CNS) processing (Drossman 2016). The unifying construct behind FGIDs is the influence of the *brain–gut axis*, which refers to the bidirectional communication pathways between the CNS and the enteric nervous system (Carabotti et al. 2015). Disturbances along these pathways can result in functional GI problems. The existence of the brain–gut axis is thought to help explain how psychosocial factors, personality styles, and comorbid psychiatric disorders can influence the onset and course of various FGIDs, such as irritable bowel syndrome, functional dyspepsia, and functional nausea and vomiting. Among patients with FGIDs, a premorbid history of traumatic events, particularly sexual and physical abuse, is often present. Neuroticism, hostility, maladaptive coping, and emotional hypersensitivity are personality traits that are commonly observed. Comorbid psychiatric syndromes, particularly depression, anxiety, and somatization, are also frequently noted. Psychotropic medications and psychotherapy have a role in the treatment of many FGIDs, although their mechanism of action is not clearly understood. For example, antidepressants can provide analgesic and autonomic effects in addition to their anxiolytic and antidepressant activity. To meet the need for consistency in diagnosis of FGIDs, the Rome criteria were developed and refined through an iterative consensus process. The most recent edition, the Rome IV criteria, involved the work of clinicians and researchers from more than 20 countries (Drossman 2016).

Oropharyngeal Disorders

Rumination Syndrome

Rumination syndrome is an FGID involving effortless and repetitive regurgitation of recently ingested food, which is subsequently re-swallowed or spit out (Absah et al. 2017). Compared with vomiting, regurgitation is not typically preceded by nausea or retching, and unlike reflux, regurgitated material is not acidic and consists of recently ingested food. The behavior normally occurs while eating or a short time afterward. Although originally described in children and adults with intellectual disabilities, regurgitation syndrome is now recognized to also occur in adolescents and adults of normal intelligence (Kessing et al. 2014). Considered an uncommon diagnosis, the actual prevalence is unknown, as the syndrome is often misdiagnosed (as, e.g., gastroesophageal reflux disease, bulimia, gastroparesis) because patients often complain of "vomiting" or "reflux" (Absah et al. 2017). Postprandial dyspepsia, nausea, heartburn, or chest pain may accompany rumination syndrome, and weight loss has been reported in up to 40% of patients. Limited case series have suggested that up to 20%–30% of patients may have comorbid psychiatric disorders, including eating disorders (Olden 2001). Rumination can also develop following a stressful life event (Hejazi and McCallum 2014). Diagnosis is primarily clinical, but high-resolution and gastroduodenal manometry can be confirmatory. Treatment is focused on patient education and diaphragmatic breathing; the latter restores the gastroesophageal pressure gradient and impedes rumination. Biofeedback and relaxation techniques may be incorporated as well (Barba et al. 2015, 2016; see also Chapter 32, "Pediatrics," and Chapter 13, "Eating Disorders").

Burning Mouth Syndrome

Primary burning mouth syndrome (BMS) is characterized by chronic persistent intraoral pain unaccompanied by evidence of oral mucosal changes (Ducasse et al. 2013). BMS typically involves the tongue, lips, and/or hard palate and primarily occurs in perimenopausal and postmenopausal women, in whom its prevalence may be 18%–33%. In comparison, reported prevalence in general populations ranges from 1% to

15% (Zakrzewska and Buchanan 2016). Pain is usually sudden in onset and described as burning, tingling, or numbness (Charleston 2013). Dysgeusia and xerostomia often accompany BMS, which may be triggered by dental work, physical illness, or stress (Zakrzewska and Buchanan 2016). Primary BMS is considered to be a neuropathic pain disorder whose underlying pathophysiology is not fully understood; it is a diagnosis of exclusion (Ducasse et al. 2013). Secondary BMS arises from a variety of causative factors, including autoimmune disorders (e.g., Sjögren's syndrome), diabetes, nutritional deficiencies, and medications (e.g., selective serotonin reuptake inhibitors [SSRIs], antiretrovirals, angiotensin II receptor blockers) (Charleston 2013; Ducasse et al. 2013). Psychiatric comorbidity—particularly major depressive disorder, generalized anxiety disorder, and illness anxiety disorder—is common among BMS patients (de Souza et al. 2012).

Treatment of BMS is challenging because of limited evidence. However, double-blind randomized controlled trials (RCTs) have demonstrated beneficial effects from clonazepam in addition to other agents (Heckmann et al. 2012; Rodríguez de Rivera Campillo et al. 2010). Cognitive-behavioral therapy (CBT) has also shown benefits in randomized clinical trials (Kisely et al. 2016; Komiyama et al. 2013).

Xerostomia

Xerostomia is a subjective complaint of dry mouth, which may be accompanied by decreased saliva production (Villa et al. 2014). When present, xerostomia can contribute to dental caries and thrush, along with complaints of dysgeusia or dysphagia (Wolff et al. 2017). Xerostomia is more common among women than among men and may be caused by a number of conditions, including connective tissue disorders, radiation therapy, anxiety, and depression (Han et al. 2015; Villa et al. 2014). Psychotropic agents are a major contributor to xerostomia. All antidepressants, benzodiazepines, typical and atypical antipsychotics, lithium, and carbamazepine can cause xerostomia (Fratto and Manzon 2014). Psychotropic side effects may be particularly problematic for patients who are also taking other medications that produce xerostomia (e.g., antihypertensives, diuretics, opioids, anticholinergics). Management of symptoms may require medication changes or dosage reductions, avoidance of caffeine and/or alcohol, or use of cholinergic agents such as pilocarpine or cevimeline; measures such as sips of water, ice chips, sugarless gum or candies, xylitol-containing lozenges, saliva substitutes, or topical fluoride may also provide relief (Han et al. 2015; Villa et al. 2014).

Dysphagia

Dysphagia results when conditions or circumstances interfere with the coordinated neuromuscular contractions necessary for swallowing (Clavé and Shaker 2015; Roden and Altman 2013). Neurological, autoimmune, oncological, and GI disorders are common causes of dysphagia (Roden and Altman 2013). Medications often contribute to dysphagia by producing xerostomia, sedation, pharyngeal weakness, dystonia, or reflux. Drugs with anticholinergic activity may interfere with the pharyngeal and esophageal phases of swallowing, which are controlled by the parasympathetic nervous system (Visser et al. 2014). Case reports frequently cite antipsychotic medications as a cause of dysphagia, particularly secondary to acute dystonia, parkinsonism, or tardive dyskinesia/dystonia (Dziewas et al. 2007; Nieves et al. 2007; O'Neill and Remington 2003). Whereas acute dystonia responds to intravenous diphenhy-dramine or benztropine, dysphagia from drug-induced parkinsonism requires reduction of antipsychotic dosing, switching of agents, or discontinuation of therapy (Dziewas et al. 2007; Nieves et al. 2007; O'Neill and Remington 2003). Tardive dyskinesia/dystonia–associated dysphagia may respond to similar measures, with additional benefits from clonazepam (Nieves et al. 2007; O'Neill and Remington 2003). Dysphagia may also be caused by muscular rigidity in neuroleptic malignant syndrome or, rarely, serotonin syndrome (Passmore et al. 2004; Shamash et al. 1994).

Upper Gastrointestinal Disorders

In this section, we address several of the most common upper-GI entities—both organic and nonorganic (previously functional). Not all Rome IV clinical entities are covered in the following section, and some entities not included in Rome IV are discussed here. The reader is encouraged to not get tripped up by specific diagnostic labels, but rather to recognize the similarities in diagnostic criteria, symptomatology, and treatments across these syndromes. The critical elements to consider in upper-GI disorders are 1) How do patients present and describe their conditions? and 2) What can we do to minimize harm and improve symptoms?

Esophagitis and Related Syndromes

Symptomatic reflux continues to be a significant health issue in Western countries, where upward of 20%–40% of people report reflux symptoms (Bashashati et al. 2014; Weijenborg et al. 2015). The prevalence of reflux seems to be on the rise, perhaps as related to increasing obesity and associated issues (diets high in fat, alcohol use, and sedentary lifestyles), psychosocial stressors, anatomic issues (e.g., hiatal hernia), and medications (Brahm and Kelly-Rehm 2011; Nwokediuko 2012). It is important to consider these clinical entities carefully, because, as noted by some authors, "heartburn is the GI symptom most commonly encountered in clinical practice" (Miwa et al. 2016).

In addition to reflux proper, there are multiple functional esophageal disorders defined as "disorders presenting with symptoms assumed to originate from the esophagus without a structural or anatomic explanation" (Weijenborg et al. 2015). According to the Rome IV diagnostic criteria, there are several such gut/brain–mediated esophageal disorders: functional heartburn, functional chest pain, reflux hypersensitivity syndrome, globus, and functional dysphagia (Drossman and Hasler 2016). The myriad labels for upper-GI disorders can cause confusion for clinicians. Here we will review gastroesophageal reflux disease, non-erosive reflux disease, functional heartburn, noncardiac chest pain, globus, and functional dysphagia.

Gastroesophageal Reflux Disease, Non-Erosive Reflux Disease, and Functional Heartburn

Gastroesophageal reflux disease (GERD) refers to the "heartburn" sensation that is experienced when gastric contents and gastric acid reenter the esophagus from the stomach. It has been commonly believed that problematic acid exposure in the esophagus, by virtue of increased gastric acid production and/or increasing transient lower esophageal sphincter relaxations (TLESRs), causes discomfort. Furthermore, gastric acid was felt to directly affect the tissue integrity of the esophagus by causing increased permeability and dilation of intracellular spaces, and thus painful tissue damage. Reflux is a normal occurrence, so decreased lower esophageal sphincter pressure and/or increased numbers of TLESRs have been implicated in bothersome symptoms (Nwokediuko 2012; van Soest et al. 2007).

The relationship of GERD to psychiatric syndromes such as major depressive disorder is complex. Possible mechanisms underlying this relationship may include reflux leading to depression; psychological issues leading to increased perception of GERD symptoms; stress leading to decreased lower esophageal sphincter pressure, altered esophageal motility, increased gastric acid secretion, and/or delayed gastric acid clearance from the esophagus; depression that is comorbid with unhealthy behaviors (e.g., smoking, overeating, alcohol consumption, sedentary lifestyle); and *psychiatric medications themselves* contributing to GERD symptoms (Chou et al. 2014; Martín-Merino et al. 2010). Medication effects can include benzodiazepines leading to decreased lower esophageal sphincter pressure, and anticholinergic medications, such as tricyclic antidepressants (TCAs), leading to decreased gastric transit, impaired GI peristalsis, and/or decreased salivary secretions. SSRIs also may contribute to GERD by increasing gastric acidity via increased vagal tone (Andrade and Sharma 2016; Anglin et al. 2014; Bahuva et al. 2015).

Updated theories regarding esophagitis suggest that inflammatory cytokines triggered by acid exposure, rather than gastric acid exposure itself, may be responsible for causing heartburn symptoms ("GERD"). On the other hand, the presence of a high-acidity "acid pocket" in the proximal stomach (separated from meal contents and general gastric acid) may be the source of discomfort due to acid exposure. The presence of this pocket also might help to explain complaints of postprandial heartburn occurring when general gastric acidity is normally at its lowest (Miwa et al. 2016).

Patients with endoscopically identified cellular changes in the esophagus are labeled as having "GERD," whereas patients without such cellular changes (more than 70% of patients with reflux symptoms) are labeled as having "NERD" (non-erosive reflux disease) (Quigley and Lacy 2013). NERD patients may have esophageal hypersensitivity in addition to esophageal acid exposure (de Bortoli et al. 2016b; Miwa et al. 2016). Although psychological symptoms such as anxiety, depression, and "neurosis" are common in GERD patients (affecting more than one-third), and psychological stress may worsen symptom perception in more than half of all cases, patients with NERD may have a higher likelihood of psychiatric comorbidities as compared with GERD patients (Ciovica et al. 2009; Ostovaneh et al. 2014).

To further complicate matters, in "functional heartburn"—a clinical entity currently defined as "retrosternal burning discomfort or pain refractory to optimal antisecretory therapy in the absence of GERD, histopathological mucosal abnormalities, major motor disorders, or structural explanations" (Aziz et al. 2016, p. 1371)—no structural, motoric, or chemical cause of patients' reported discomfort can be found, and investigations into organic causes of discomfort are fruitless. Rather, these symptoms may be related to altered pain perception (Aziz et al. 2016; Weijenborg et al. 2016). Compared with GERD and NERD, functional heartburn may be more strongly correlated with psychological symptoms (Bilgi et al. 2017; Miwa et al. 2016). Patients with functional heartburn may bear the closest resemblance to patients with irritable bowel syndrome (IBS), a population identified as having high levels of anxiety and neuroticism, heightened perception of physical symptoms, and decreased QoL (de

Bortoli et al. 2016a). de Bortoli et al. (2016a) found that IBS and anxiety occurred in two-thirds of patients with functional heartburn, possibly identifying a connection to hypersensitivity and altered pain modulation.

Reflux disorders are among the most costly chronic GI disorders, with estimated direct and indirect costs of $10 billion annually in the United States alone (Bashashati et al. 2014). GERD-related discomfort is commonly treated with histamine-2 receptor antagonists (e.g., H_2 blockers such as ranitidine) and proton pump inhibitors (e.g., PPIs such as omeprazole) (Hershcovici et al. 2012). Some psychiatric medications increase the risk of GERD. Thus, whereas antidepressants are used in the treatment of many of the functional upper-GI disorders discussed in this chapter, antidepressants are not considered first-line treatment for symptoms related to *endoscopically identified cellular changes* in the esophagus. While some authors have opined that buspirone (with combined serotonin agonism and dopamine antagonism) might be helpful in patients with "ineffective esophageal motility," evidence to support this suggestion is limited (Scheerens et al. 2015). If patients have both psychiatric (e.g., depression, anxiety) and GERD symptoms, it is prudent to treat all symptoms aggressively and to change or adjust dosages of psychiatric medication if GI symptoms emerge or notably worsen after medication initiation.

Patients with NERD respond less well to PPI medications (Ostovaneh et al. 2014). Functional heartburn patients do not merit treatment with GI-specific medications, because they do not have organic pathology, but they may respond to psychiatric medications found to modulate pain perception, such as TCAs, as well as to other behavioral therapies (Aziz et al. 2016).

Noncardiac Chest Pain

Roughly 6 million patients present annually to U.S. emergency departments with chest pain symptoms, and up to 90% of these symptoms are noncardiac in origin (Burgstaller et al. 2014). Noncardiac chest pain (NCCP) may be attributed to esophageal symptoms in 30%–50% of cases (Coss-Adame et al. 2014; Nguyen and Eslick 2012). In any initial presentation with chest pain, patients merit a thorough and sensitive workup, including cardiac and GI evaluations, to rule out significant organic pathology.

Many cases of NCCP may be classified as functional esophageal disorders. Some authors postulate that up to 80% of patients with "unexplained noncardiac chest pain" have lower thresholds for pain perception in the esophagus relative to healthy control subjects (Bashashati et al. 2014; Remes-Troche 2010). Esophageal hypersensitivity is a symptom with various components, causes, and (depending on the patient) proposed treatments. Clinicians should bear in mind that the symptom of esophageal hypersensitivity may be related to sensory and/or motoric dysfunction and is found in a variety of esophageal disorders, including functional heartburn, functional chest pain, reflux hypersensitivity, globus, and functional dysphagia (Coss-Adame and Rao 2015; Farmer et al. 2017b).

Various antidepressants have shown benefit in reducing patients' perceptions of the frequency and intensity of NCCP (Coss-Adame et al. 2014; Nguyen and Eslick 2012; Nwokediuko 2012; Remes-Troche 2010; Viazis et al. 2012; Weijenborg et al. 2015). Whereas SSRIs for NCCP have shown mixed results, TCAs have been used to treat NCCP for many years. Positive effects of antidepressants in GERD/NCCP patients have been noted even in the absence of improvement in anxiety or depression scores, thus implying that a mechanism other than amelioration of underlying psychiatric disorders is responsible for improvement (Bashashati et al. 2014; Nguyen and Eslick 2012; Weijenborg et al. 2015).

Esophageal NCCP patients have responded well to CBT in several RCTs (Jonsbu et al. 2011; Marchand et al. 2012; van Beek et al. 2013), with reduction of pain severity, depression, and anxiety (and commensurate improvement in QoL). However, GERD patients were not excluded from these trials, thus making the results difficult to interpret. Other modalities, including hypnotherapy and biofeedback, have been tested, but results have been inconclusive, largely because of mixed patient populations (Coss-Adame and Rao 2015; Coss-Adame et al. 2014; Nwokediuko 2012).

Globus

Globus is the nonpainful sensation of a lump or mass in the throat without clear evidence of a structural lesion, reflux, or an esophageal motor disorder (Drossman 2016). The sensation may be persistent or intermittent, occurs between meals, is relieved by ingestion of solids or liquids, and does not interfere with actual swallowing. Chronic cough, hoarseness, catarrh, and a persistent clearing of the throat may accompany globus (Kortequee et al. 2013). The sensation is common, acknowledged by up to half of healthy individuals, and is responsible for up to 4% of otolaryngology referrals (Drossman 2016; Lee and Kim 2012). Symptoms tend to be chronic in nature. Although the etiology of globus is unknown, it is thought to be multifactorial, arising from conditions such as laryngeal and pharyngeal dysfunction, esophageal dysmotility, visceral hypersensitivity, elevated upper-esophageal sphincter pressure, anatomic abnormalities, gastroesophageal reflux, medication side effects, and/or psychological factors (Haft et al. 2016; Lee and Kim 2012; Selleslagh et al. 2014). The contribution of psychological factors is suggested by studies demonstrating increased numbers of stressful life events preceding the onset of globus and symptom exacerbation with emotional duress (Deary et al. 1992; Harris et al. 1996). Diagnosis is based on history and an examination to rule out clear pathology, followed by reassurance. Two recent RCTs suggested added benefits from low-dose amitriptyline or paroxetine (Chen et al. 2016; You et al. 2013), and a case series supported hypnotically assisted relaxation therapy (Kiebles et al. 2010).

Functional Dysphagia

Oropharyngeal dysphagia is a symptom defined as difficulty in effectively moving an alimentary bolus from the mouth to the esophagus (Wirth et al. 2016)—basically, the inability to chew and swallow food successfully. Dysphagia can be caused by medical disorders (e.g., esophageal diseases, head/neck cancer or treatment, stroke) (Smithard 2016; Tanrivermis Sayit et al. 2016; Uppal and Wang 2016); iatrogenesis (e.g., prolonged intubation, botulinum toxin injections, antipsychotics); and the aging process itself (Wirth et al. 2016). Sequelae can include choking, aspiration, and malnutrition (Wirth et al. 2016).

Functional dysphagia is defined as "a sensation of abnormal bolus transit through the esophageal body in the absence of structural, mucosal, or motor abnormalities to explain the symptom" (Aziz et al. 2016, p. 1376), and is diagnosed only after a thorough evaluation to rule out organic issues (Farmer et al. 2017b). It differs from *globus*, which involves the sensation of "a lump in the throat" in the absence of food boluses—and, in fact, globus can improve when swallowing and eating (Aziz et al. 2016). Functional dysphagia can be challenging to diagnose, because even so-called normal patients (i.e., without esophageal pathology) may have trouble with food bolus transit at times. Although acute stress can trigger acute peristaltic dysfunction, it is difficult to draw parallels between this experience and functional dysphagia's chronic symptoms (Aziz et al. 2016).

Treatment for functional dysphagia can include reassurance; guidance for meals (e.g., sit upright, chew thoroughly, follow solids with liquids); and a trial of a PPI to rule out GERD spectrum symptoms (Aziz et al. 2016). In addition, esophageal dilation may be helpful in some patients (Colon et al. 2000; Naini et al. 2007). There is no clear evidence supporting the use of psychiatric medications in this population (Aziz et al. 2016).

Nausea and Vomiting

Functional nausea and vomiting disorders reviewed here include cyclic vomiting syndrome and cannabinoid hyperemesis syndrome (CHS) (both in Rome IV; Drossman and Hasler 2016), as well as anticipatory nausea/vomiting. In patients with frequent vomiting, disordered eating behaviors (with purging) and intracranial pathology (with increased intracranial pressure) should not be overlooked. Hyperemesis gravidarum is discussed in Chapter 31, "Obstetrics and Gynecology," and cancer-related nausea/vomiting is discussed in Chapter 22, "Oncology."

Cyclic vomiting syndrome.   Cyclic vomiting syndrome is characterized by intense episodes of vomiting, separated by periods without vomiting. Previously largely identified in children, with a pediatric prevalence ranging from 1% to 15%, there has been increased recognition of this syndrome in adults (Bhandari and Venkatesan 2016; Hermus et al. 2016; Sezer and Sezer 2016). In both children and adults, QoL can be significantly affected by this diagnosis (Hermus et al. 2016; Kumar et al. 2012; Levinthal 2016).

The four phases of cyclic vomiting syndrome are the prodromal phase, the emetic phase, the recovery phase, and the interepisode (asymptomatic) phase (Bhandari and Venkatesan 2016). Vomiting episodes may have triggers (e.g., migraine headaches, seizures, menstrual cycles, stressors, foods, sleep deprivation) or may be unrelated to any stimuli or environmental cues (Bhandari and Venkatesan 2016; Kumar et al. 2012; Levinthal 2016). The pathogenesis of cyclic vomiting syndrome remains unknown, although genetic factors, mitochondrial dysfunction, brain–gut axis neurocircuitry, and other etiologies may be involved (Bhandari and Venkatesan 2016; Levinthal 2016; Millichap 2016). Both in pediatric and in adult populations, migraine, anxiety, depression, and IBS are common personal and family comorbidities (Kumar et al. 2012), although it is unknown whether the psychiatric comorbidities are contributors to, or the results of, cyclic vomiting syndrome. Indeed, the stress of having episodic nausea and vomiting can unfortunately trigger additional episodes (Bhandari and Venkatesan 2016).

During acute episodes of nausea and vomiting, patients may require intravenous fluids, antiemetics, anxiolytics, and analgesics (Sezer and Sezer 2016). Several case reports have noted successful use of chlorpromazine (Hermus et al. 2016; Özdemir et al. 2014). Prophylactic medications may include amitriptyline, anticonvulsants, and supplements/cofactors such as coenzyme Q10 and L-carnitine (Bhandari and Venkatesan 2016). Abortive medications, used at the start of an episode to prevent further decompensation, may include sumatriptan, ondansetron, benzodiazepines, and diphenhydramine (Bhandari and Venkatesan 2016; Kumar et al. 2012).

Cannabinoid hyperemesis syndrome. Cannabinoid hyperemesis syndrome is sometimes mistaken for idiopathic cyclic vomiting syndrome, delaying appropriate treatment. Although cannabinoids have commonly been considered beneficial for nausea, heavy and/or prolonged cannabis use can result in extreme nausea/vomiting and abdominal pain (Hermes-Laufer et al. 2016). Unlike individuals with idiopathic cyclic vomiting syndrome, persons with cannabinoid hyperemesis syndrome compulsively take hot showers or baths (Jones and Abernathy 2016; Sorensen et al. 2017).

The presumed mechanism for cannabinoid hyperemesis syndrome involves dysregulation of the endogenous cannabinoid system (Hermes-Laufer et al. 2016). In cases of heavy cannabis use, GI-slowing effects appear to overtake central antiemetic effects (Inayat et al. 2017). The mechanism may also involve re-calibration of the thermoregulatory system (via the hypothalamic-pituitary-adrenal [HPA] axis) by excessive cannabinoid exposure, causing hypothermia that in turn triggers compulsive bathing in hot water (Hermes-Laufer et al. 2016; Simonetto et al. 2012).

Complications of cannabinoid hyperemesis syndrome include hospitalizations for dehydration and electrolyte shifts. Symptoms resolve with cessation of cannabis use, and although case reports have noted symptomatic improvement with haloperidol, many providers do not endorse prescribing antipsychotics in patients who continue to use cannabis (Inayat et al. 2017; Jones and Abernathy 2016; Sorensen et al. 2017). Patients can be resistant to the suggestion of cannabinoid abstinence, but referral to appropriate chemical dependency services should be considered.

Anticipatory nausea and vomiting. Anticipatory nausea (sometimes accompanied by vomiting) is a classically conditioned response to repeated episodes of nausea and vomiting caused by chemotherapy, structural abnormalities (e.g., gastric outflow stricture), or gastric bypass surgery (Ahrari et al. 2017). *Expectations* that nausea and vomiting will occur also can influence the likelihood of developing anticipatory nausea and vomiting (Kamen et al. 2014). A multisite study revealed that the presence of anticipatory nausea was significantly associated with increased likelihood of suffering chemotherapy-induced nausea and vomiting during subsequent treatment cycles (Molassiotis et al. 2016).

Risk factors for anticipatory nausea and vomiting include female gender, age younger than 50 years, history of depression or anxiety, predilection to motion sickness, and history of morning sickness during pregnancy (Ahrari et al. 2017; Kamen et al. 2014; Qureshi et al. 2016). There appears to be a bidirectional relationship between anticipatory nausea and chemotherapy-induced nausea/vomiting, wherein each can trigger the other (Ahrari et al. 2017).

Improvements in the management of nausea and vomiting have resulted in decreased rates of anticipatory nausea and vomiting. Prophylaxis is "the cornerstone of (anticipatory nausea) prevention" (Ahrari et al. 2017; Kamen et al. 2014). Compared with other types of nausea and vomiting, anticipatory nausea and vomiting do not respond well to standard antiemetics (Kamen et al. 2014; Qureshi et al. 2016), which have been found to paradoxically worsen symptoms, perhaps because in certain patients these drugs come to be experienced as a conditioned stimulus in themselves (Qureshi et al. 2016). Behavioral interventions are the most effective treatment (Kamen et al. 2014). Progressive muscle relaxation, systemic desensitization, hypnosis, and cognitive distraction have each been found helpful (Figueroa-Moseley et al. 2007; Kamen et al. 2014; Kravits 2015; Redd et al. 2001). Benzodiazepines may reduce the anxiety associated with anticipatory nausea and vomiting; however, they do not modify the response, nor is their use advisable in patients at risk of falls or confusion (Ahrari et al. 2017; Kravits 2015).

Gastroparesis

GI motility and functional disorders may account for roughly 40% of referrals to gastroenterologists (Camilleri 2016). Gastroparesis is characterized by delayed gastric emptying in the absence of identifiable mechanical obstruction (Camilleri 2016; Malamood et al. 2017). The most common cause is diabetic autonomic neuropathy; other causes include postsurgical, postvagotomy, idiopathic, iatrogenic (e.g., medications), and postinfectious syndromes (Camilleri 2016; Malamood et al. 2017; Oh and Pasricha 2013; Pan et al. 2017). Symptoms of gastroparesis include abdominal pain, early satiety (postprandial fullness), nausea, vomiting, and bloating (Camilleri 2016; Malamood et al. 2017; Woodhouse et al. 2017). Anxiety, depression, and somatization are common comorbidities, although it is not known whether these conditions are precursors or sequelae of gastroparesis. In patients with anxiety and depression, higher anxiety/depression scores are associated with greater gastroparesis symptom severity (Hasler et al. 2010).

One study identified several predictors of symptom improvement—including male sex, prodromal infection, and antidepressant use—as well as several predictors of no improvement—including obesity, history of smoking, abdominal pain, severe GERD, and moderate to severe depression (Pasricha et al. 2015).

Eating multiple low-fat small meals, consuming more liquids than solids, and ensuring optimal glucose control in patients with diabetes are dietary changes that may be helpful (Bielefeldt 2012; Enweluzo and Aziz 2013; Patrick and Epstein 2008). Commonly used pharmacological treatments include prokinetic medications (e.g., metoclopramide, erythromycin) and antiemetic medications (Camilleri 2016). Often prescribed for gastroparesis, metoclopramide has dopamine D_2 receptor–blocking properties that can cause extrapyramidal symptoms and tardive dyskinesia, in addition to somnolence, anxiety, depression, and decreased mental acuity (Enweluzo and Aziz 2013).

Antidepressants may be another treatment option and may act by prokinetic effects, by reducing pain or nausea/vomiting, or by simply alleviating distress associated with gastroparesis (Bielefeldt 2012). Mirtazapine has become a popular agent for gastroparesis, largely related to its enhancement of receptive relaxation of the gastric fundus and provision of nausea relief (Malamood et al. 2017; Song et al. 2014), and has been beneficial for patients whose gastroparesis is resistant to conventional therapies (Oh and Pasricha 2013; Yin et al. 2014). Although phenothiazines, benzodiazepines, and TCAs were previously used in gastroparesis, these drugs have since fallen out of favor.

Peptic Ulcer Disease and Dyspepsia

Current lifetime prevalence of peptic ulcer disease (PUD) ranges from 5% to 10%, with 4 million people affected by PUD worldwide each year (Chung and Shelat 2017; Lanas and Chan 2017). Peptic ulcers traditionally were linked to infection with *Helicobacter pylori* and chronic use of nonsteroidal anti-inflammatory drugs (NSAIDs), with an estimated 50% of peptic ulcers attributable to *H. pylori,* 25% to NSAIDs, and 25% to other sources. Additional causes include other infections and substance use (e.g., potassium chloride, bisphosphonates, crack cocaine, amphetamine, heavy alcohol use) (Jones 2006; Levenstein 2000). The contribution of tobacco smoking to PUD incidence remains unclear, although tobacco is believed to impair duodenal ulcer healing (Chung and Shelat 2017).

In duodenal peptic ulcers, patients report a gnawing sensation in the abdomen that often improves with food—as opposed to gastric peptic ulcers, which can be associated with postprandial pain and weight loss (Lanas and Chan 2017). The risk of ulcer bleeding is heightened in patients who take NSAIDs or other antiplatelet agents, and in those who take SSRI medications.

As one of the classic "psychosomatic disorders," peptic ulcers have been studied by gastroenterologists and psychiatrists for decades. The physician and psychoanalyst Franz Alexander studied psychological influences on GI disorders in the 1930s and included PUD in his 1950 book *Psychosomatic Medicine: Its Principles and Applications* (Alexander 1950). In a study in a large cohort of army draftees, Mirsky et al. (1957) successfully predicted which men would develop duodenal ulcers by evaluating psychological criteria along with the biological criterion of high baseline pepsinogen secretion. A significant body of research has demonstrated that stressful life events, and perhaps personality characteristics, play a role in PUD. One recent study noted that a high "stress index" more than doubled the chances of developing an ulcer (Levenstein et al. 2015); other researchers have noted increased ulcer incidence in people experiencing intense stressors, natural disasters, and refugee status (Lanas and Chan 2017).

Evidence suggests an association between psychiatric disorders and increased risk of PUD. Epidemiological data on more than 43,000 subjects showed that all mood and anxiety disorders were significantly associated with PUD (especially generalized anxiety disorder and panic disorder); alcohol and nicotine dependence attenuated some, but not all, of this association (Goodwin et al. 2009). As in other upper-GI disorders, patient with PUD symptoms also often have comorbid psychiatric symptoms. One recent study of more than 900 patients found that anxiety symptoms were independently associated with GI ulcers (Niles et al. 2015). However, correlation does not imply causation.

Patients with PUD are often started on multiple medications, including antibiotics, PPIs, and/or H_2 blockers. Despite these treatments, there is recent evidence of antibiotic resistance contributing to decreased eradication of *H. pylori* over time, and an increase in the popularity of incorporating probiotics as augmenting agents (Hołubiuk and Imiela 2016; Lau et al. 2016). Several small RCTs in the 1980s (Andersen et al. 1984; Ries et al. 1984) demonstrated benefits from TCAs (doxepin, trimipramine)—perhaps via these agents' antihistaminic and anticholinergic effects—in the treatment and prevention of duodenal ulcers. However, because of their side effects (e.g., weight gain, constipation, dry mouth), TCAs are no longer used for PUD.

Nonulcer Dyspepsia (Functional Dyspepsia)

According to Rome IV criteria, *functional dyspepsia* is defined as symptomatic distress—involving one or more of four core features—that is not associated with any structural disease (Stanghellini et al. 2016). The four bothersome core symptoms of functional dyspepsia are postprandial fullness, early satiety, epigastric pain, and epigastric burning (Camilleri and Stanghellini 2013; Oustamanolakis and Tack 2012). The Rome IV criteria maintained two subcategories of functional dyspepsia (initially proposed in Rome III): *postprandial distress syndrome* (PDS; meal-induced dyspepsia) and *epigastric pain syndrome* (EPS; epigastric discomfort that is not associated with postprandial state and that actually may improve with eating) (Camilleri and Stanghellini 2013; Quigley and Lacy 2013; Schmulson and Drossman 2017).

Functional dyspepsia has a presentation similar to that of gastroparesis, and the boundary between the two conditions is blurred (Camilleri 2016). Overlapping features include delayed gastric emptying, impaired fundal accommodation, visceral hypersensitivity, and abnormal pain processing (Camilleri 2016; Ford et al. 2017). Functional dyspepsia may have a relapsing and remitting course, with up to 80% of patients reporting symptoms associated with meals (Ford et al. 2017).

Patients with functional dyspepsia report higher levels of psychological symptoms in comparison with healthy (non–functional dyspepsia) individuals (Ford et al. 2017). Functional dyspepsia patients have high rates of neuroticism, anxiety, depression, hostility, tension, posttraumatic stress disorder, and somatization (Faramarzi et al. 2015; Ford et al. 2017; Levy et al. 2006; North et al. 2007; Oustamanolakis and Tack 2012; Piacentino et al. 2011). However, these symptoms may reflect the influence of psychological factors on the experience and expression of functional dyspepsia symptoms, rather than constituting causes of the condition (Piacentino et al. 2011).

Psychotropic medications are often used to treat functional dyspepsia; commonly prescribed agents include antidepressants, acotiamide (an acetylcholinesterase inhibitor), and buspirone (Camilleri 2016; Ford et al. 2017; Scheerens et al. 2015; Talley et al. 2015). A recent review concluded that symptomatic benefit was most notable with TCAs and antipsychotics (Ford et al. 2017). In a multisite RCT comparing amitriptyline and escitalopram in 292 patients with functional dyspepsia, the TCA produced significantly more improvement in functional dyspepsia symptoms compared with the SSRI, with the difference largely attributable to pain relief (Talley et al. 2015). Buspirone also seems to benefit functional dyspepsia patients by enhancing gastric fundus relaxation and improving gastric accommodation (Camilleri 2016). In patients in whom functional dyspepsia is accompanied by weight loss, mirtazapine may be helpful (Tack et al. 2016). Therapies such as relaxation training, cognitive therapy, and hypnotherapy have also been used in patients with functional dyspepsia and have led to symptomatic improvement (Camilleri and Stanghellini 2013; Oustamanolakis and Tack 2012).

Upper-Gastrointestinal Bleeding and Selective Serotonin Reuptake Inhibitors

Despite their relatively robust tolerability and safe side-effect profiles, SSRIs have been associated with an increased risk of upper-GI bleeding (Wee 2017). Normally, serotonin is released from platelets, promoting platelet aggregation and hemostasis.

However, because serotonin is not synthesized by platelets de novo, adequate platelet serotonin requires receptor reuptake of serotonin from plasma. This process is blocked by SSRIs, and platelet aggregation is thereby impaired (Anglin et al. 2014; Cheng et al. 2015; Patel et al. 2015; Wee 2017).

Despite differences in research design and antidepressants investigated, most studies suggest that there is about double the risk of GI hemorrhage in patients who are taking SSRIs (odds ratio=2.36; Anglin et al. 2014) compared with controls (Cheng et al. 2015; Dalton et al. 2006; Laporte et al. 2017; Loke et al. 2008). Furthermore, patients taking a combination of SSRIs and NSAIDs have more than two times the risk of upper-GI bleeding compared with patients taking SSRIs alone (Oka et al. 2014). Serotonin–norepinephrine reuptake inhibitors (SNRIs) do not appear to carry this risk (Cheng et al. 2015).

Whereas the absolute effect of SSRIs in increasing upper-GI bleeding in healthy adults is considered to be small (comparable to the risk associated with low-dose NSAIDs), the odds of upper-GI bleeding are greater for patients who have additional upper-GI hemorrhage risk factors, such as concurrent use of NSAIDs and other antiplatelet drugs (e.g., clopidogrel); who are elderly; who have thrombocytopenia or platelet dysfunction (e.g., von Willebrand's disease); or who have a history of upper-GI bleeding (Andrade and Sharma 2016; Bahuva et al. 2015; Kuo et al. 2014; Oka et al. 2014). For such patients, great care is recommended when selecting an antidepressant.

Lower Gastrointestinal Disorders

Inflammatory Bowel Disease: Crohn's Disease and Ulcerative Colitis

Inflammatory bowel disease (IBD) is a chronic, relapsing and remitting bowel disorder that involves inflammation of the intestinal mucosa. Common symptoms include diarrhea, fever, and abdominal cramps/pain, as well as bleeding, anorexia, weight loss, and fatigue. Ulcerative colitis and Crohn's disease are the two forms of IBD, which differ according to the extent of mucosal damage and GI tract involvement. For ulcerative colitis, the mucosal layer from rectum to colon may be affected, whereas Crohn's disease involves transmural inflammation of any portion of the GI tract. Complications of IBD can lead to bowel obstruction or perforation, malnutrition, fistulas, and ulcerations, along with increased risk of colon cancer. The peak incidence of IBD occurs between the ages of 15 and 30 years, with a smaller peak occurring at ages 60 years and older. Extraintestinal manifestations of IBD are common and may predate the diagnosis of IBD; these manifestations include musculoskeletal, skin, or eye involvement and (more rarely) cardiac, pulmonary, neurological, hepatobiliary (e.g., primary sclerosing cholangitis), pancreatic, or renal involvement (Vavricka et al. 2015). Abdominal pain without evidence of mucosal inflammation is present in more than one-third of IBD patients and is referred to as *comorbid irritable bowel syndrome* (IBS-IBD). IBS-IBD is more prevalent among patients with Crohn's disease patients than among those with ulcerative colitis (Regueiro et al. 2017).

Epidemiology of IBD.   The overall incidence and prevalence of IBD have continued to rise across the globe but remain greatest in developed countries (Ye et al. 2015). This trend is thought to be at least partly due to changes brought by modernization and development (e.g., diet, hygiene, exposure to pathogens). The annual incidence ranges from 0 to 20.2 per 100,000 for Crohn's disease and from 0 to 24.3 per 100,000 for ulcerative colitis across North America and Europe (Ananthakrishnan 2015), whereas recent data from the National Health Interview Study reported that an estimated 3.1 million adults in the United States had ever received a diagnosis of IBD (Dahlhamer et al. 2016).

Pathophysiology of IBD.   The underlying pathophysiology of IBD is not completely understood but appears to involve complex interactions between the gut microbiome and immune system, genetic, and environmental factors, resulting in a dysregulated immune response and inflammation (de Souza and Fiocchi 2016). Smoking increases the risk of developing Crohn's disease and worsens its course, but serves a protective function in ulcerative colitis (Ananthakrishnan 2015). Sleep deprivation appears to increase the risk of ulcerative colitis onset and contributes to IBD flares (Ananthakrishnan et al. 2014).

Stress and IBD.   The relationship between stress and IBD is thought to be due to interactions involving the HPA axis, autonomic nervous system, mast cell activation, and inflammatory cytokine production, as well as changes in intestinal permeability and gut microbiota (Bonaz and Bernstein 2013). Although experimentally induced psychological stress in healthy humans and animal models of colitis results in increased intestinal permeability, examination of the impact of stress on IBD patients has yielded inconsistent results (Triantafillidis et al. 2013; Vanuytsel et al. 2014). A cross-sectional study of 478 IBD patients showed a strong relationship between perceived stress and IBD symptoms but no—or a only modest—relationship between perceived stress and intestinal inflammation in ulcerative colitis and Crohn's disease (Targownik et al. 2015). Subsequent data obtained over a 6-month period by this same group continued to show no relationship between perceived stress and presence of intestinal inflammation (Sexton et al. 2017). A Swedish prospective cohort study found that men who had shown low stress resilience as adolescents were at increased risk of IBD (Melinder et al. 2017).

Anxiety/depression and IBD.   Given that IBD is a chronic disorder often involving significant morbidity, impaired functioning, and reduced QoL, the presence of anxiety and depression is not surprising. A recent systematic review reported pooled incidence rates of 19% and 21% for anxiety and depressive symptoms, respectively. In the face of active IBD, these rates rise to 28% and 66% (Mikocka-Walus et al. 2016a). Anxiety and/or depressive symptoms among IBD patients are associated with lower health-related QoL, medication nonadherence, increased risk of hospital readmission and surgery, greater perceived stress, increased disease activity, and poor response to IBD treatment across most, but not all studies (Allegretti et al. 2015; Luo et al. 2016; Mikocka-Walus et al. 2016b). For example, a large prospective cohort study using clinical and treatment data from more than 2,000 IBD patients found significant relationships between the presence of depressive and anxiety symptoms and risk for clinical recurrences (Mikocka-Walus et al. 2016b). Similarly, an Internet cohort study of more than 2,000 Crohn's disease patients, which examined whether affective-cognitive depressive symptoms were linked to disease exacerbation, focused on symptoms that would not overlap with physical symptoms of IBD (Gaines et al. 2016). A significant association between depressive symptoms and elevated Crohn's disease activity was noted at 12 months (Gaines et al. 2016). While anxiety and depressive symptoms impact the course of established IBD, there is less evidence about their influence on IBD onset. The Nurses' Health Study, which followed a large population of women, noted that recent depressive symptoms were associated with an increased risk of Crohn's disease (Ananthakrishnan et al. 2013). Studies focused on anxiety have been fewer, though a Canadian study using a nationally representative sample reported a greater than twofold odds of generalized anxiety disorder among IBD patients compared with those without IBD (Fuller-Thomson et al. 2015).

IBD and quality of life. Compared with the general population, IBD patients have a significantly reduced health-related QoL, both during remission and during active disease (Iglesias et al. 2010). Disease activity/severity—as measured by work disability, number of relapses, corticosteroid use, and hospitalization rate—is the strongest predictor of health-related QoL across studies (Hoivik et al. 2012; Huppertz-Hauss et al. 2015, 2016; van der Have et al. 2014; Yoon et al. 2017). Psychological distress (anxiety, depression), perceived stress, fatigue, and personality styles such as alexithymia also appear to influence health-related QoL (Iglesias-Rey et al. 2014). Active treatment of IBD with medication and surgery (including ostomies) improves perceptions of health-related QoL (Abdalla et al. 2016; Burisch et al. 2014; Herrera-deGuise et al. 2015). The presence of comorbid IBS symptoms significantly affects health-related QoL, as noted in a cross-sectional study of 378 IBD patients (Gracie et al. 2017). The subgroup with true IBS symptoms and no active IBD had significantly worse QoL, with QoL levels comparable to those of patients with active IBD with intestinal mucosal inflammation. Levels of anxiety, depression, and somatization were also greater among the IBS-IBD patients. Several disease-specific measures of health-related QoL have been developed for IBD patient populations; the Inflammatory Bowel Disease Questionnaire (IBDQ) remains the most established and well-validated and is available in several languages (Alrubaiy et al. 2015).

Psychological and pharmacological interventions in IBD. Due to recognition of elevated rates of anxiety and depressive symptoms, reduced QoL, overlapping IBS symptomatology and the possible interaction between stress and IBD, psychotherapeutic approaches have been tested in IBD including CBT, gut-directed hypnotherapy, mindfulness-based treatment, stress management, and multi-convergent therapy (Knowles et al. 2013). The majority of these have yielded mixed results, although there is some indication of improved QoL and psychological well-being. In an RCT of 199 patients using a computerized CBT program, those who completed the program showed significant improvements in IBDQ and 12-item Short Form Health Survey (SF-12) mental health scores, but these did not persist at 6-month follow-up (McCombie et al. 2016). A study of 60 patients comparing group mindfulness-based therapy with treatment as usual yielded significant improvements in anxiety, depression, mindfulness, and QoL; some improvement persisted after 6 months (Neilson et al. 2016). Small studies of gut-directed hypnotherapy in active ulcerative colitis have shown reductions in inflammatory markers (e.g., IL-6, TNF-α) and steroid usage (Mawdsley et al. 2008; Miller and Whorwell 2008). A subsequent RCT of 54 UC patients with quiescent disease demonstrated significantly longer periods of disease remission (Keefer et al. 2013).

Limited data are available on the role of psychopharmacological agents in IBD, despite the fact that nearly one-third of patients either are taking or have taken antidepressants (Mikocka-Walus et al. 2012). IBD patients are usually prescribed antidepressants to treat anxiety and/or depression rather than functional symptoms. Most patients report improvement in psychological well-being, and a small portion report improvements in IBD disease activity (Mikocka-Walus and Andrews 2014). Evidence from clinical studies is relatively weak, but the majority report some benefits on IBD course, such as improvements related to QoL, clinical disease activity, and steroid usage (Goodhand et al. 2012; Macer et al. 2017; Yanartas et al. 2016). Although studies utilizing specific agents are few, one study reported mild to moderate improvement in residual bowel symptoms with low-dose TCAs (Iskandar et al. 2014), and another reported improvement in mean physical, psychological, and social QoL scores with duloxetine 60 mg/day (Daghaghzadeh et al. 2015).

Irritable Bowel Syndrome

IBS is characterized by abdominal pain related to defecation and associated with changes in stool appearance or frequency. The updated Rome IV diagnostic criteria for IBS include chronicity of symptoms along with abdominal pain and change in bowel habits (Drossman 2016). Additional symptoms may include flatulence, bloating, distention, stool urgency or straining, a persistent sensation of incomplete bowel evacuation, and presence of mucus in the feces. Active symptoms must have been present over the past 3 months, and symptom onset must have occurred at least 6 months before diagnosis. During the 3 months of active symptoms, abdominal pain must have been present at least once weekly (Drossman 2016). IBS can be subdivided according to predominant bowel pattern: diarrhea (IBS-D), constipation (IBS-C), or mixed. Diagnosis is based on symptomatic history without the presence of accompanying alarm symptoms (e.g., fever, weight loss, rectal bleeding) that suggest a more serious underlying GI condition. Comorbid conditions are common and include GERD, nausea, functional dyspepsia, chronic pelvic pain, chronic fatigue syndrome, temporomandibular joint dysfunction, interstitial cystitis, fibromyalgia, headache, backache, anxiety, depression, and/or sleep disturbance (Drossman 2016; Riedl et al. 2008; Talley 2006).

Epidemiology of IBS.   Global prevalence pf IBS is estimated at between 10% and 15%, according to the International Foundation for Functional Gastrointestinal Disorders (2016), with prevalence highest in South America (21%) and lowest in South Asia (7%) (Lovell and Ford 2012). Globally, there is a predominance of females with IBS, with rates in women 1.5–3 times higher than those in men, but this is not seen in South Asia, South America, and Africa (Lovell and Ford 2012). The prevalence of IBS is higher in individuals younger than 50 years, suggesting that IBS symptoms may remit over time (Canavan et al. 2014a; Lovell and Ford 2012). Despite the frequency of IBS, only 30% of individuals with the disorder seek medical treatment in the United States; 80% of these individuals have IBS-D (Canavan et al. 2014b; Hungin et al. 2005). IBS is the most commonly diagnosed GI disorder by gastroenterologists in the outpatient setting, accounting for 2.4–3.5 million annual physician visits in the United States (International Foundation for Functional Gastrointestinal Disorders 2016). In the United States, the cost per patient per year ranges from $742 to $7,547 (Ricci et al. 2000; Talley et al. 1995).

Pathophysiology of IBS. Despite extensive investigation, the pathophysiology of IBS remains unknown, but it is thought to involve multiple factors, including abnormal GI motility, visceral hypersensitivity, intestinal permeability, altered gut microbiota, inflammatory processes, altered stress responses, changes in serotonin signaling, genetic factors, and psychological dysfunction. A large contributor to the proposed pathophysiology of IBS involves the brain–gut axis, which allows bidirectional communication between the CNS and the enteric nervous system (Bohórquez and Liddle 2015; Furness 2012; Goyal and Hirano 1996; Savidge et al. 2007). At present, no pathophysiological abnormalities are considered specific to all IBS patients.

Altered colonic motility has been observed among IBS patients. Other contributors to the pathophysiology of IBS include autonomic dysfunction and visceral hypersensitivity. A recent evaluation of five cohort studies conducted by Simrén et al. (2018) underscored the continued relevance of visceral hypersensitivity by showing a gradual increase in GI symptom severity with increasing visceral hypersensitivity to balloon distention. This increase was independent of anxiety, depression, and somatization scores (Simrén et al. 2018). Functional magnetic resonance imaging (fMRI) has shown a link between defective processing of visceral pain and dysfunctional fear and anticipation of pain in individuals with IBS (Hong et al. 2016; Icenhour et al. 2015).

Serotonin signaling in the gut is important for motility, secretion, vasodilatation, and visceral sensation. Release and transport of serotonin in the colonic mucosa have been reported to be disturbed in IBS (Mawe et al. 2006). Studies have shown that an increase in plasma serotonin is associated with IBS-D, whereas a reduction in plasma serotonin is associated with IBS-C (Atkinson et al. 2006).

Diet has been extensively researched as a contributing factor in IBS, with a focus on fermentable oligo-, di-, and monosaccharides and polyols (FODMAPs), which are short-chain carbohydrates that are poorly absorbed by the intestine. FODMAPs not only are osmotically active but also are fermentable by enteric bacteria, producing excess amounts of H_2 and methane, which leads to bloating and abdominal pain (Ong et al. 2010). Several RCTs have shown reductions in IBS symptoms with a low-FODMAP diet, although the long-term safety and tolerability of this diet are not known (Böhn et al. 2015; Halmos et al. 2014; Rao et al. 2015; Shepherd et al. 2008).

Psychological factors are known to affect the perception of GI symptoms and pain. In the past, psychological factors were viewed as influencing symptom distress and help-seeking behavior in IBS patients. A history of sexual, emotional, or physical trauma was present in 26%–44% of individuals referred to specialty clinics with functional GI disorders (Drossman et al. 1995). Recent studies suggest that psychological factors also may contribute to the development of IBS. A recent meta-analysis and systematic review pooling 11 studies noted that depression and anxiety were each associated with an approximately twofold increase in risk of developing IBS (Sibelli et al. 2016). A larger prospective population-based study reported that after results were adjusted for age, gender, and baseline abdominal pain, high levels of illness behavior, sleep problems, and somatic symptoms remained independent predictors of IBS onset (Nicholl et al. 2008). A greater number of stressful life events and higher hypochondriasis scores were highly predictive of postinfectious IBS in another group of patients (Gwee et al. 1999). fMRI has demonstrated reduced intrinsic brain activity in the prefrontal cortex, posterior cingulate cortex, and bilateral inferior parietal cortex in individuals with IBS and comorbid anxiety and depression (Qi et al. 2016).

IBS and quality of life.   QoL in IBS patients has consistently been shown to be worse than that in the general population and comparable to that in patients with other chronic disorders, such as asthma, migraine, IBD, and GERD (Ballou and Keefer 2017), as well as those with even more serious conditions, such as diabetes mellitus and end-stage renal failure (Gralnek et al. 2000). Individuals with IBS miss 3–4 days of additional work annually in comparison with healthy control subjects (Dean et al. 2005; Hungin et al. 2003). In a recent study examining the burden of IBS on daily functioning, commonly reported areas of impairment included job and social functioning, as well as eating habits (e.g., eating alone) (Ballou and Keefer 2017). Patients who did not seek medical care or who were followed only by primary care providers reported better QoL compared with patients seen by specialists (Simrén et al. 2004). This is consistent with findings that IBS symptom severity plays a significant role in QoL (Coffin et al. 2004; Sabate et al. 2008). The presence of extraintestinal symptoms (e.g., fatigue, sleep disturbance, sexual dysfunction) and psychological distress (e.g., health anxiety) also contributes to reduced QoL (Rey et al. 2008; Sabate et al. 2008). In one study, patients referred to a gastroenterologist reported a moderate but not statistically significant improvement in QoL for 3 months following the visit, but this improvement was no longer present after 1 year (Canavan et al. 2015).

Psychiatric comorbidity in IBS.   Approximately 50% of people with IBS report psychiatric symptoms of clinical relevance (Creed et al. 2013; Hillilä et al. 2007). The lifetime prevalence of a comorbid psychiatric disorder is estimated to range from 38% to 100% among IBS patients (Woodman et al. 1998). In most studies that do not exclude persons with a psychiatric diagnosis, prevalence rates of comorbid psychiatric disorders exceed 90% (Hausteiner-Wiehle and Henningsen 2014). Depression is the most common comorbid disorder (prevalence of 6%–70%), followed by anxiety (5%–50%), DSM-IV (American Psychiatric Association 1994) somatization disorders (15%–47%), panic disorder (0%–41%), and trauma-related disorders (8%–36%) (Hausteiner-Wiehle and Henningsen 2014). With the changes in DSM-5 (American Psychiatric Association 2013), the frequency with which individuals with IBS present with symptoms that meet the criteria for somatic symptom disorder requires further investigation (Hausteiner-Wiehle and Henningsen 2014). A recent meta-analysis pooling six retrospective cohort studies found an increased prevalence of bipolar disorder in persons with IBS (Tseng et al. 2016). Bidirectional comorbidity exists between anxiety or depression and IBS, as elevated rates of IBS have been found among patients with panic attacks (17%–47%), generalized anxiety disorder (17%–37%), and depressive disorders (17%–59%) (Hausteiner-Wiehle and Henningsen 2014). Frequently, however, psychiatric disorders predate the onset of IBS symptoms. The presence of psychiatric comorbidity is associated with more severe GI symptoms, greater functional impairment, greater psychological distress, lower QoL, and worse prognosis (Karling et al. 2007; Lee et al. 2009). The greater the number of psychiatric diagnoses, the greater the physical role limitations and number of days of restricted activity (Laird et al. 2017). Differences in coping mechanisms or personality styles also have been noted in individuals with IBS, with elevated levels of catastrophizing and neuroticism (Palsson and Drossman 2005). Psychological factors (e.g., somatization, trait anxiety, maladaptive coping, catastrophizing) rather than somatic factors more closely correlate with severity of IBS and worse outcomes (Hausteiner-Wiehle and Henningsen 2014).

Psychological interventions in IBS.   Recognition of the interactions among stress, psychopathology, and IBS has spurred studies examining the effects of psychological interventions on IBS symptoms and QoL. CBT, hypnotherapy, mindfulness, psychodynamic psychotherapy, and stress management and relaxation therapy all have been studied in clinical trials. CBT is the most commonly utilized and most well studied. There is strong evidence supporting its use as a first-line approach, with a number needed to treat of 3 (Ford et al. 2014). Currently there is no single streamlined cognitive-behavioral approach to IBS, and most clinical data were obtained from CBT performed face-to-face. Despite study heterogeneity, common components in CBT for IBS include providing patients with psychoeducation on the stress response and its relation to GI symptoms, teaching patients to develop insight into cognitive and behavioral responses to IBS symptoms and fear of symptoms, and helping patients to learn methods based on these responses for reducing psychological and physical distress (Ford et al. 2014). A recent meta-analysis comparing CBT with other medical treatments showed a reduction in bowel symptoms and improvements in QoL and psychological distress that persisted beyond the treatment phase into long-term follow-up (Ballou and Keefer 2017). Findings from a positron emission tomography (PET) study of how CBT benefits IBS patients were interpreted as showing reductions in hypervigilance to visceral stimuli (Lackner et al. 2006).

Hypnotherapy utilizing one of two standardized approaches (the North Carolina protocol or the Manchester approach) has been shown to have long-term benefits equal in effectiveness to a low-FODMAP diet. The number needed to treat for hypnotherapy is 4 (Ford et al. 2014). One study comparing psychodynamic therapy with antidepressant treatment showed that the two were equally efficacious, and both were superior to treatment as usual (Creed et al. 2003). Psychodynamic psychotherapy may be an effective approach in IBS patients with a trauma history (Creed et al. 2005). The number needed to treat for psychodynamic psychotherapy is 3.5 (Ford et al. 2014).

Psychopharmacological interventions in IBS.   A recent systematic review and meta-analysis of psychological interventions and antidepressants in IBS concluded that both approaches are effective (Ford et al. 2014). Antidepressants, specifically TCAs and SSRIs, have been used in many clinical trials in IBS. The estimated number needed to treat to prevent persistent IBS symptoms was 4 for both TCAs and SSRIs; however, significant heterogeneity among SSRI studies was noted (Ford et al. 2014). Another meta-analysis (Xie et al. 2015) concluded that patients receiving SSRIs showed no statistically significant differences in symptoms compared with the control groups. A third meta-analysis concluded that insufficient evidence exists to support use of SSRIs to treat individuals with IBS who do not have a comorbid psychiatric condition (Bundeff and Woodis 2014). The rationale for trying antidepressants in IBS patients is threefold: the frequent psychiatric comorbidity in these patients, the central effects of antidepressants on pain modulation, and the central or peripheral effects of these agents on visceral sensitivity and motor activity (Harris and Chang 2006). From their side-effect profiles, it would seem that TCAs would be more appropriate for IBS-D (IBS with diarrhea), whereas SSRIs would be a better choice for IBS-C (IBS with constipation). However, at present there are few clinical data to support this theory, because most studies do not distinguish between IBS-C and IBS-D (Ford et al. 2014). Finally, it is important to note that research to date has not established whether improvement in mood or anxiety underlies the improvement in IBS symptoms in those who respond to antidepressants (Ford et al. 2014).

Most clinical trials investigating TCAs have used low dosages of several different TCAs (i.e., imipramine, amitriptyline, desipramine, doxepin, trimipramine). Even though pooled results involving more than 740 patients in placebo-controlled trials showed significant benefits for IBS, dropout rates were sometimes high (Abdul-Baki et al. 2009; Ford et al. 2009). A recent meta-analysis of antidepressant studies found a statistically significant incidence of adverse effects with antidepressants compared with placebo (number needed to harm of 9). The most common side effects were drowsiness and dry mouth (more pronounced with TCAs) (Ford et al. 2014). An fMRI study suggested that TCAs work in the CNS to blunt pain and other symptoms exacerbated by stress in IBS patients (Morgan et al. 2005). The effectiveness of low-dose TCAs for functional bowel disorders was supported in a post hoc analysis of an RCT of desipramine (Halpert et al. 2005). Clinical response to treatment was associated with detectable desipramine blood levels; however, no relation was established between clinical response and total desipramine dosage or plasma drug level.

Given that serotonin plays a significant role in control of gut function and pain pathways in the peripheral and enteric nervous systems, along with the presence of abnormal serotonin signaling and release in IBS, the choice of SSRIs is not surprising. Several randomized clinical trials have investigated SSRIs such as paroxetine, fluoxetine, or citalopram. A double-blind RCT in IBS that added paroxetine 10–40 mg to a high-fiber diet noted significant improvement in overall well-being but no statistically significant benefit in abdominal pain, bloating, or social functioning (Tabas et al. 2004). An RCT using extended-release paroxetine (12.5–50 mg/day) showed statistically significant reductions in Clinical Global Impression—Improvement (CGI-I) scores but not in the composite pain score (the primary outcome) (Masand et al. 2009). An RCT in patients with constipation-predominant IBS (i.e., IBS-C) found that fluoxetine (20 mg/day) significantly reduced abdominal discomfort and bloating in comparison with placebo and resulted in improvements in stool consistency and bowel movement frequency; these benefits were independent of presence of depression (Vahedi et al. 2005). In contrast, another RCT comparing fluoxetine 20 mg/day with placebo showed no statistically significant benefit in reduction of visceral sensitivity, bloating, flatulence, or incomplete evacuation or in global symptom relief (Kuiken et al. 2003). Regarding citalopram, one double-blind RCT demonstrated that intravenous citalopram was superior to placebo in improving overall well-being and in reducing number of days of abdominal pain, severity of bloating, and IBS symptom impact on daily life (Tack et al. 2006). An additional study comparing citalopram with imipramine and placebo found no statistical improvement in primary or secondary outcomes from either antidepressant (Talley et al. 2008). Finally, Ladabaum et al. (2010) found no statistical difference between oral citalopram 20–40 milligrams and placebo in achieving "adequate relief" reports from patients. Although the evidence for SSRIs is less positive and less consistent than the evidence for TCAs, SSRIs do offer greater tolerability than TCAs and can be used if other treatment has not proven efficacious. Small open-label studies of SNRIs have shown encouraging but not conclusive evidence of benefit in IBS (Brennan et al. 2009; Kaplan et al. 2014; Lewis-Fernández et al. 2016).

Centrally Mediated Gastrointestinal Disorders

The Rome IV criteria added a new category of centrally mediated disorders of GI pain, in which the primary clinical focus is abdominal pain out of proportion to structural or physiological abnormalities (Keefer et al. 2016). This category is further subdivided into centrally mediated abdominal pain syndrome (CAPS) and narcotic bowel syndrome (NBS).

Centrally Mediated Abdominal Pain Syndrome

CAPS is characterized as severe, continuous or near-continuous abdominal pain that causes significant disruption in daily functioning. The pain is chronic and is often described as burning or colicky and as diffuse in nature versus localized (Whorwell et al. 2016). Compared with other visceral pain disorders such as IBS, functional dyspepsia, or chronic pelvic pain, CAPS pain is not linked to food intake, defecation, or menses. Accompanying complaints of non-GI pain, such as musculoskeletal pain, are often present, as are comorbid disorders such as fibromyalgia or chronic fatigue syndrome (Keefer et al. 2016). Increased health care utilization, work absenteeism, and disability have been noted. The prevalence of CAPS is reported to be 0.5%–2%, peaking between the ages of 35 and 44 years, and CAPS may be twice as common in women (Drossman 2016). The pathophysiology is suspected to be similar to that of other FGIDs in which there is an alteration in central sensory processing of pain signals (Keefer et al. 2016). This mechanism is also thought to explain the influence of certain psychosocial factors—such as depression, unresolved losses, and both physical and sexual abuse—on the clinical presentation of CAPS. Diagnosis involves a careful history to discern whether organic causes of pain are present, with testing reserved for cases in which evidence from the physical exam suggests the latter (Keefer et al. 2016). Treatment is focused on fostering adaptation to chronic pain and should include patient education, a collaborative treatment plan, and psychological interventions (e.g., CBT, hypnotherapy, mindfulness training, acceptance and commitment therapy), along with antidepressants (i.e., TCAs, SNRIs) to help provide analgesic relief (Keefer and Mandal 2015; Törnblom and Drossman 2015) while avoiding narcotics.

Narcotic Bowel Syndrome (Opioid-Induced Gastrointestinal Hyperalgesia)

NBS is characterized by chronic or recurrent abdominal pain of ongoing or worsening severity despite escalating dosages of opioids to relieve pain. Similar in quality to the pain reported in CAPS, NBS occurs in approximately 4%–6% of patients who take opioids long-term and is not attributable to opioid-related GI side effects such as reflux, nausea, abdominal bloating/distension, or constipation, or to underlying structural disease (Kurlander and Drossman 2014). NBS patients experience pain relief from opioids for increasingly shorter periods of time, and unlike in opioid tolerance, increases in dosage worsen pain (Farmer et al. 2017a). Because NBS can occur alongside structural disease, it should be considered when pain complaints seem out of proportion to what can be explained structurally (Whorwell et al. 2016). Management is focused on reduction of pain through gradual tapering and discontinuation of opioids. Early incorporation of an antidepressant (i.e. TCA, SNRI, SSRI) is recommended, along with clonidine to manage withdrawal symptoms, benzodiazepines for marked anxiety, and behavioral techniques to foster coping skills and reduce catastrophizing, hypervigilance to pain, and cognitive inflexibility (Drossman and Szigethy 2014; Keefer and Mandal 2015). Despite reports of successful detoxification and significant reductions in pain, resumption of narcotic use is common (Drossman et al. 2012; Farmer et al. 2013).

Hepatic Disorders

Hepatitis C

Epidemiology

The hepatitis C virus (HCV) remains one of the most common blood-borne pathogens, affecting 2%–3% of the world's population (Hauser and Kern 2015). In the United States, an estimated 3.5 million individuals are chronically infected, and a large proportion of persons are unaware of being infected (Spach 2016). Approximately one-third of infected individuals eventually develop cirrhosis or hepatocellular carcinoma, and HCV infection continues to be the leading indication for orthotopic liver transplantation. Intravenous drug use is the route of transmission for more than 50% of infections; perinatal exposure and sexual contact are less common causes (Spach 2016). The prevalence of HCV infection is significantly higher among individuals with serious mental illness, with a pooled prevalence of 17.4% compared with 1% in the general population in North America (Hughes et al. 2016). Comorbidity with HIV infection is frequent.

Clinical Presentation and CNS Effects

Acute infection with HCV is often asymptomatic, which is one of the reasons that patients are unaware of being infected until long-term consequences such as cirrhosis arise. Symptoms of chronic HCV infection include fatigue and cognitive difficulties (Monaco et al. 2015; Yarlott et al. 2017). Fatigue is reported by more than 50% of patients (Negro et al. 2015). Studies of cognitive impairment in HCV infection have generally shown disturbances—in executive function, sustained attention, working memory, verbal learning, and verbal recall—that are similar to disturbances found in HIV-associated mild neurocognitive disorder (Negro et al. 2015; Yarlott et al. 2017). Because such impairment has also been reported in individuals with absent or mild liver disease, it is not attributable to hepatic encephalopathy. Neuroimaging studies suggest the presence of neuroinflammation due to HCV (Bokemeyer et al. 2011; Grover et al. 2012). Improvements in cognitive functioning, fatigue, and cerebral metabolism have been noted after successful antiviral treatment and sustained virological response in some, but not all, studies (Kraus et al. 2013; Pattullo et al. 2011).

Treatment of Hepatitis C

Prior to 2011, treatment of HCV was based on a regimen of interferon (IFN) and ribavirin. Treatment tolerability was hampered by side effects, including flu-like symptoms, anemia, fatigue, depression, insomnia, and irritability, as well as by the length of treatment required (24–48 weeks). IFN-induced depression, often with suicidal ideation, arose in approximately 25%–30% of patients, significantly impairing QoL and prompting premature treatment discontinuation (Sockalingam et al. 2013, 2015). Concerns about IFN-induced depression contributed to reluctance to prescribe IFN regimens in patients with comorbid psychiatric and substance use disorders, although successful treatment was possible with multidisciplinary collaboration. Clinical trials demonstrated that prophylactic antidepressant therapy could reduce the incidence and severity of IFN-induced depression in patients with and without a preexisting history of mood disorder (de Knegt et al. 2011; Hou et al. 2013; Schaefer et al. 2012). Rarely, IFN-induced mania, delirium, and psychosis were reported. In most but not all cases, IFN-induced psychiatric disorders resolved after treatment was discontinued or completed (Cheng et al. 2009).

Currently, IFN-based therapy has fallen out of favor with the introduction of direct-acting antiviral agents (DAAs) (e.g., protease inhibitors, nonstructural protein 5B [NS5B] and 5A [NS5A] inhibitors), which offer marked advancements in treatment tolerability, length of therapy, and sustained virological response. DAAs have not been found to cause significant psychiatric side effects, and treatment discontinuation rates have been minimal. Studies including "high-risk" patients receiving opioid substitution therapy (i.e., methadone, buprenorphine) have also shown optimal treatment adherence and clinical responsiveness, even among subjects who continued to use illicit drugs (Dore et al. 2016; Grebely et al. 2016; Rowan and Bhulani 2015). Side effects of DAAs are usually mild and consist of fatigue, headache, insomnia, and nausea. Compared with IFN-based regimens, DAAs impose a greater need for caution because of the risk of clinically relevant drug–drug interactions (Dick et al. 2016; Menon et al. 2015; Smolders et al. 2016; Soriano et al. 2015). This risk is primarily an issue with the 3D regimen (paritaprevir/ritonavir, ombitasvir, and dasabuvir) due to the presence of ritonavir.

Hepatic Encephalopathy

Background and Pathogenesis

Hepatic encephalopathy (HE)—defined as "brain dysfunction caused by liver insufficiency or portosystemic shunting" (American Association for the Study of Liver Diseases and European Association for the Study of the Liver 2014)—affects 30%–45% of patients with cirrhosis, and its presence is associated with poorer prognosis independent of the severity of liver disease (Kandiah and Kumar 2016). HE is classified on the basis of four factors: underlying cause, severity of manifestations (grades 0–4), time course, and existence of precipitating factors (American Association for the Study of Liver Diseases and European Association for the Study of the Liver 2014). Clinically, HE manifests in a myriad of ways, from grossly asymptomatic to significant disturbances in consciousness, cognition, mood, and behavior, culminating in coma. HE can be mistaken for a primary psychiatric disorder but symptomatically worsens following addition of psychotropic medications. Motor disturbances, including incoordination, asterixis, ataxia, and extrapyramidal symptoms, may accompany cognitive and behavioral changes (Basu and Shah 2015; Suraweera et al. 2016). The pathogenesis of HE remains unclear, but one component appears to involve the liver's reduced capacity to detoxify ammonia, a by-product derived from the intestinal breakdown of protein. Excess ammonia reaches the systemic circulation and brain, resulting in a number of adverse functional and anatomical effects (Butterworth 2015; Grover et al. 2015; Nardone et al. 2016; Wijdicks 2016). Other suggested contributors to HE include increased production of neurosteroids (γ-aminobutyric acid [GABA] receptor agonists), excess manganese, elevated levels of short-chain fatty acids, and amino acid disturbances, as well as activation of microglia and genes coding for pro-inflammatory cytokines (Butterworth 2016; Grover et al. 2015; Wijdicks 2016).

Diagnosis of Hepatic Encephalopathy

Clinical diagnosis of HE is by exclusion of other causes of altered mental status (e.g., substance use, intracranial hemorrhage) in patients with cirrhosis. Because of the lack of a consistent correlation between serum ammonia levels and severity of HE, levels are not routinely recommended for diagnosis (Edula and Pyrsopoulos 2015; Sussman 2015; Vilstrup et al. 2014). Psychometric testing, however, may be helpful, particularly in the presence of covert HE (grades 0–1). Initial electroencephalography (EEG) findings demonstrate posterior dominant alpha rhythm slowing followed by theta and high-amplitude delta waves as HE progresses (Edula and Pyrsopoulos 2015; Nabi et al. 2014). Triphasic waves, which are not specific to HE, tend to appear with background slowing in HE of grade 2–3 severity (Wijdicks 2016). Digital analysis and spectral EEG offer greater sensitivity than routine EEG in detecting early HE (Nabi et al. 2014). Critical flicker frequency, a nonverbal neurophysiological test, can be utilized for both covert and overt HE (Suraweera et al. 2016). There is no established role for brain imaging in the clinical diagnosis of HE, except to rule out other causes of altered mental status.

Management of Hepatic Encephalopathy

Treatment of HE is focused on identification and correction of precipitating factors, which are thought to affect 80% of patients (Kandiah and Kumar 2016; Sussman 2015). Infection, dehydration, GI bleeding, constipation, and medications (e.g., sedative-hypnotics) may aggravate HE, and metabolic derangements are common. Beyond addressing these precipitating factors, treatment of overt HE is focused on reducing ammonia levels, primarily through use of the nonabsorbable disaccharides (lactulose and lactitol; the latter is not available in the United States). Use of these agents appears to benefit patient survival and reduce the frequency of serious complications (e.g., liver failure, spontaneous bacterial peritonitis) (Morgan 2016). Nonabsorbable disaccharides reduce ammonia formation and absorption by decreasing colonic transit time, reducing ionization of ammonia, and altering the gut microbiome (Morgan 2016). Rifaximin, a nonabsorbable antibiotic, may be added to or used in place of lactulose to alter gut flora (Jawaro et al. 2016; Vilstrup et al. 2014). L-Ornithine-L-aspartate may also be considered in HE patients who do not respond to or tolerate lactulose, and is able to stimulate the removal of ammonia by remaining hepatocytes (Suraweera et al. 2016; Sussman 2015). Evidence suggests potential benefits from probiotics and branched-chain amino acids (Jawaro et al. 2016; Viramontes Hörner et al. 2017). Flumazenil, a short-acting benzodiazepine antagonist, improves HE but does not produce long-term benefits or improved outcomes (Kandiah and Kumar 2016). Low-protein diets should be avoided to prevent muscle wasting, with consequent negative effects on ammonia load and metabolism. Large portosystemic shunts may be considered in patients who are unresponsive to standard therapy (Wijdicks 2016). Liver transplantation is considered the definitive treatment for HE, although some cognitive deficits may persist afterward (Bajaj et al. 2010; Umapathy et al. 2014).

Minimal Hepatic Encephalopathy

The term *minimal hepatic encephalopathy* (MHE) refers to clinically undetectable HE that is discernible only with psychometric testing. Present among a majority of patients with cirrhosis, MHE has a negative impact on QoL, work abilities, and driving skills and is predictive of subsequent onset of overt HE (Weissenborn 2015). Patients exhibit impairments in selective attention, psychomotor speed, visuospatial functioning, response inhibition, and delayed information processing (Basu and Shah 2015; Nardone et al. 2016). The Psychometric Hepatic Encephalopathy Scale (PHES), composed of five subtests, is considered the "gold standard" for diagnosing MHE but reportedly lacks U.S. norms (Nabi et al. 2014; Nardone et al. 2016). The Repeatable Battery for the Assessment of Neuropsychological Status (RBANS) is an alternative option, and a modified version specific for HE has been developed (Nabi et al. 2014). Some have recommended using a combination of Number Connection A and B, Digit Symbol, and Block Design tests for diagnosis (Grover et al. 2015). Computerized tests such as inhibitory control testing offer good sensitivity and specificity (Nabi et al. 2014; Nardone et al. 2016; Vilstrup et al. 2014). EncephalApp_Stroop is a smartphone application that is considered to be a valid and reliable screening tool (Bajaj et al. 2013). Management of MHE involves lifestyle alterations, with use of agents such as lactulose and rifaximin on a case-by-case basis (Nardone et al. 2016; Vilstrup et al. 2014).

Psychopharmacology in Liver Disease

When prescribing psychotropic medications for patients with liver disease, clinicians should take into account the severity of the disease, the medication being considered, the margin between therapeutic and toxic plasma levels, and whether the patient has or is at high risk of hepatic encephalopathy. Therapeutic drug monitoring may be helpful, but results should be interpreted with caution in the face of altered protein binding (Crone et al. 2016). Generally, drugs with a narrow therapeutic window (e.g., lithium) should be avoided when possible. Hepatic dysfunction alters the absorption, distribution, metabolism, and elimination of most psychotropic medications. Although no specific biochemical test directly conveys the degree of pharmacokinetic disturbance present, the Child–Pugh Scale (CPS) provides a rough estimate to guide dosing in liver disease (Albers et al. 1989; Table 19–1). Among patients rated as having CPS-A (mild) liver failure, most can tolerate 75%–100% of a standard initial dose. Patients with CPS-B (moderate) disease require more cautious dosing; a 50%–75% reduction in the normal starting dose is prudent. Prolongation of the elimination half-life will delay the time required for drug levels to reach steady state; thus, smaller incremental dosing increases are recommended. Patients with CPS-B cirrhosis can often be successfully treated with 50% of a typical psychotropic dose. Patients with CPS-C (severe) cirrhosis will usually have some degree of HE, and medications must be carefully monitored to avoid toxicity or worsening mental status (Crone et al. 2016). Benzodiazepines should be avoided in patients at risk of HE, but when these agents are

TABLE 19–1.   **Child–Pugh Scale**

Factor	1 Point	2 Points	3 Points
Serum bilirubin (mmol/L)	≤34	35–50	≥51
Serum albumin (g/dL)	>3.5	3.0–3.5	<3.0
Prothrombin time (s)	<4	4–6	>6
International normalized ratio (INR)	<1.7	1.7–2.3	>2.3
Ascites	None	Slight, medically controlled	Moderate–severe, poorly controlled
Encephalopathy	None	Stage 1–2	Stage 3–4
Total score[a]	5–6	7–9	10–15
Child–Pugh Scale score	A	B	C

[a]Combine scores together from all five factors.

needed (e.g., for delirium tremens), a benzodiazepine requiring only phase II glucu-ronidation, and not oxidative metabolism, should be prescribed—specifically, loraz-epam, temazepam, or oxazepam. Glucuronidation is generally preserved in cirrhosis. Even when drugs do not depend on hepatic metabolism, some (e.g., gabapentin, lith-ium) should be used cautiously because impaired renal function and fluctuations in fluid balance may be present (e.g., as a result of diuretics prescribed for ascites).

Psychotropic Drug–Induced Hepatitis, Hepatic Dysfunction, and Hepatic Failure

Drug-induced liver injury (DILI) ranges from mild asymptomatic transaminase ele-vations to rare cases of fulminant hepatic failure. Most reactions are idiosyncratic (and are therefore unpredictable), are not dose dependent, and develop after a vari-able time taking the drug in question. Fortunately, liver injury usually resolves after the drug is discontinued, although full recovery may take up to a year. Epidemiolog-ical data suggest that approximately 20 new cases per 100,000 persons occur annually (Leise et al. 2014). Identification of patient risk factors for idiosyncratic DILI has proven difficult, with conflicting findings regarding age, sex, alcohol use, and pres-ence of liver disease (Björnsson 2014; Leise et al. 2014). Some evidence suggests that women may be more susceptible to severe DILI (Andrade et al. 2005; Reuben et al. 2010). Although it is unclear whether patients with chronic liver disease are at greater risk of DILI, having less hepatic reserve could prove problematic if injury occurs (Björnsson 2014, Sarges et al. 2016). U.S. Food and Drug Administration guidelines advise against prescribing valproate or duloxetine in patients with liver disease.

There are three classes of DILI: hepatocellular, cholestatic, and mixed. Hepatocel-lular damage causes significant elevation in alanine aminotransferase (ALT) relative to alkaline phosphatase (AP), whereas AP is increased more with cholestatic injury. Although most psychotropic medications carry some risk of hepatotoxicity, overall risks are very low (Au and Pockros 2013; Marwick et al. 2012; Sarges et al. 2016; Sedky et al. 2012; Voican et al. 2014). For most patients, evidence does not support ordering of repeated liver function tests during treatment with a particular drug (except for valproate) because of the idiosyncratic nature of DILI (Crone et al. 2016; Senior 2009).

However, because it is unclear which patients who develop DILI may progress to severe hepatic injury, suspected medications should be discontinued in patients who develop ALT elevations greater than 3 times the upper limit of normal, total bilirubin elevations greater than 2 times the upper limit of normal, or symptoms of hepatic dysfunction (e.g., right upper quadrant pain, dark urine, pruritus, jaundice, nausea, anorexia) (Crone et al. 2016; Voican et al. 2014).

Pancreatic Disorders

Drug-Induced Pancreatitis

Drug-induced pancreatitis is an infrequent cause of acute pancreatitis, accounting for approximately 5% of cases (Vinklerová et al. 2010). Although most cases are mild, prompt recognition is necessary to reduce the risk of serious complications (e.g., chronic pancreatitis, multiorgan failure) (Kaurich 2008). Accurate diagnosis is difficult because clinical presentations often are not readily distinguishable from other causes of acute pancreatitis (Nitsche et al. 2010). Most cases develop within a few weeks to months of starting a particular drug and are not dose-dependent. Certain populations—women, children, elderly persons, and persons with advanced HIV infection or IBD—are at greater risk of drug-induced pancreatitis (Nitsche et al. 2010). Valproic acid is the most common cause of psychotropic-induced pancreatitis, with the majority of cases involving children (Gerstner et al. 2007). The true incidence of drug-induced pancreatitis is considered to be 1 in 40,000, and presenting symptoms typically include abdominal pain, nausea, vomiting, diarrhea, and anorexia. Transient asymptomatic hyperamylasemia occurs in about 20% of adults who are taking valproic acid, but this effect does not correlate with a greater risk of pancreatitis (Zaccara et al. 2007). Infrequent case reports have linked pancreatitis with other anticonvulsants, including carbamazepine, lamotrigine, topiramate, levetiracetam, gabapentin, and vigabatrin (Zaccara et al. 2007). Among antipsychotics, clozapine, olanzapine, quetiapine, and risperidone have been associated with the greatest number of cases, and haloperidol, ziprasidone, and aripiprazole with the fewest (Silva et al. 2016). However, population-based studies have yielded conflicting results as to whether antipsychotics cause pancreatitis (Bodén et al. 2012; Gasse et al. 2008). Mirtazapine has been linked to cases, whereas cases associated with bupropion, venlafaxine, and SSRIs have been infrequently reported (Hussain and Burke 2008). For SSRIs, the actual risk has been called into question (Ljung et al. 2012). Rechallenge with the offending drug after an episode of pancreatitis is not advised, even when a lower dosage or a different route of administration is used, because of the risk of recurrence. However, substitution of the offending agent with another drug of the same class is considered an acceptable option.

Pancreatic Cancer

Pancreatic cancer is the fourth leading cause of cancer-related deaths in the United States (Fernandez-del Castillo and Jimenez 2017). Most cases are diagnosed at an advanced stage, with older age at diagnosis contributing to a poor prognosis and a

5-year survival rate of approximately 5%. Symptoms are nonspecific and often include anorexia, weight loss, fatigue, abdominal pain, and jaundice. Since the early 1930s, there have been reports of a higher-than-expected incidence of depression in pancreatic cancer compared with other GI malignancies (Fras et al. 1967; Holland et al. 1986; Jia et al. 2010; Mayr and Schmid 2010), with onset of depressive symptoms often occurring prior to the diagnosis of pancreatic cancer (Olson et al. 2016; Sebti et al. 2015). Recent work has attempted to discern the underlying physiological connection between pancreatic cancer and depression. Breitbart et al. (2014) reported that higher levels of interleukin-6 in patients with pancreatic cancer correlated with greater severity of depressive symptoms. Early identification of depression is important, given that depression has been linked to reduced survival due to less likelihood of receiving appropriate cancer treatment (Boyd et al. 2012).

Conclusion

The GI system's functions include oral intake, digestion, absorption, and metabolism. Disorders affecting the GI tract produce considerable disruption in daily function, productivity, overall health, long-term survival, and QoL. Psychological distress secondary to GI disorders is common, but psychological distress also may precede the onset of a GI disorder and contribute to its development, clinical course, and subsequent treatment response. The effect of psychological factors is particularly notable in functional GI disorders, which lack clear evidence of physiological or structural abnormalities. Increasing evidence indicates a strong link between the brain and the gut that helps to explain the interactions between psychological factors and GI disorders. Psychotherapeutic and psychopharmacological approaches can be beneficial for GI patients, even in the absence of clear psychopathology, with the benefit resulting from the effect on central brain–gut mechanisms.

References

Abdalla MI, Sandler RS, Kappelman MD, et al: The impact of ostomy on quality of life and functional status of Crohn's disease patients. Inflamm Bowel Dis 22(11):2658–2664, 2016 27661669

Abdul-Baki H, El Hajj II, Elzahabi L, et al: A randomized controlled trial of imipramine in patients with irritable bowel syndrome. World J Gastroenterol 15(29):3636–3642, 2009 19653341

Absah I, Rishi A, Talley NJ, et al: Rumination syndrome: pathophysiology, diagnosis, and treatment. Neurogastroenterol Motil 29(4), 2017 27766723

Ahrari S, Chow R, Goodall S, DeAngelis C: Anticipatory nausea: current landscape and future directions. Ann Palliat Med 6(1):1–2, 2017 28061530

Albers I, Hartmann H, Bircher J, Creutzfeldt W: Superiority of the Child-Pugh classification to quantitative liver function tests for assessing prognosis of liver cirrhosis. Scand J Gastroenterol 24(3):269–276, 1989 2734585

Alexander F: Psychosomatic Medicine: Its Principles and Applications. New York, Norton, 1950

Allegretti JR, Borges L, Lucci M, et al: Risk factors for rehospitalization within 90 days in patients with inflammatory bowel disease. Inflamm Bowel Dis 21(11):2583–2589, 2015 26244647

Alrubaiy L, Rikaby I, Dodds P, et al: Systematic review of health-related quality of life measures for inflammatory bowel disease. J Crohn's Colitis 9(3):284–292, 2015 25576752

American Association for the Study of Liver Diseases, European Association for the Study of the Liver: Hepatic encephalopathy in chronic liver disease: 2014 practice guideline by the European Association for the Study of the Liver and the American Association for the Study of Liver Diseases. J Hepatol 61(3):642–659, 2014 25015420

American Psychiatric Association: Diagnostic and Statistical Manual of Mental Disorders, 4th Edition. Washington, DC, American Psychiatric Association, 1994

American Psychiatric Association: Diagnostic and Statistical Manual of Mental Disorders, 5th Edition. Arlington, VA, American Psychiatric Association, 2013

Ananthakrishnan AN: Epidemiology and risk factors for IBD. Nat Rev Gastroenterol Hepatol 12(4):205–217, 2015 25732745

Ananthakrishnan AN, Khalili H, Pan A, et al: Association between depressive symptoms and incidence of Crohn's disease and ulcerative colitis: results from the Nurses' Health Study. Clin Gastroenterol Hepatol 11(1):57–62, 2013 22944733

Ananthakrishnan AN, Khalili H, Konijeti GG, et al: Sleep duration affects risk for ulcerative colitis: a prospective cohort study. Clin Gastroenterol Hepatol 12(11):1879–1886, 2014 24780288

Andersen OK, Bergsåker-Aspøy J, Halvorsen L, Giercksky KE: Doxepin in the treatment of duodenal ulcer. A double-blind clinical study comparing doxepin and placebo. Scand J Gastroenterol 19(7):923–925, 1984 6397849

Andrade C, Sharma E: Serotonin reuptake inhibitors and risk of abnormal bleeding. Psychiatr Clin North Am 39(3):413–426, 2016 27514297

Andrade RJ, Lucena MI, Fernández MC, et al; Spanish Group for the Study of Drug-Induced Liver Disease: Drug-induced liver injury: an analysis of 461 incidences submitted to the Spanish registry over a 10-year period. Gastroenterology 129(2):512–521, 2005 [Erratum in: Gastroenterology 129(5):1808, 2005] 16083708

Anglin R, Yuan Y, Moayyedi P, et al: Risk of upper gastrointestinal bleeding with selective serotonin reuptake inhibitors with or without concurrent nonsteroidal anti-inflammatory use: a systematic review and meta-analysis. Am J Gastroenterol 109(6):811–819, 2014 24777151

Atkinson W, Lockhart S, Whorwell PJ, et al: Altered 5-hydroxytryptamine signaling in patients with constipation- and diarrhea-predominant irritable bowel syndrome. Gastroenterology 130(1):34–43, 2006 16401466

Au JS, Pockros PJ: Drug-induced liver injury from antiepileptic drugs. Clin Liver Dis 17(4):687–697, x, 2013 24099025

Aziz Q, Fass R, Gyawali CP, et al: Functional esophageal disorders. Gastroenterology 150:1368–1379, 2016 27144625

Bahuva R, Yee J, Gupta S, Atreja A: SSRI and the risk of gastrointestinal bleed: more than what meets the eye. Am J Gastroenterol 110(2):346, 2015 25646912

Bajaj JS, Schubert CM, Heuman DM, et al: Persistence of cognitive impairment after resolution of overt hepatic encephalopathy. Gastroenterology 138(7):2332–2340, 2010 20178797

Bajaj JS, Thacker LR, Heuman DM, et al: The Stroop smartphone application is a short and valid method to screen for minimal hepatic encephalopathy. Hepatology 58(3):1122–1132, 2013 23389962

Ballou S, Keefer L: The impact of irritable bowel syndrome on daily functioning: characterizing and understanding daily consequences of IBS. Neurogastroenterol Motil 29(4), 2017 27781332

Barba E, Burri E, Accarino A, et al: Biofeedback-guided control of abdominothoracic muscular activity reduces regurgitation episodes in patients with rumination. Clin Gastroenterol Hepatol 13(1):100.e1–106.e1, 2015 24768808

Barba E, Accarino A, Soldevilla A, et al: Randomized, placebo-controlled trial of biofeedback for the treatment of rumination. Am J Gastroenterol 111(7):1007–1013, 2016 27185077

Bashashati M, Hejazi RA, Andrews CN, Storr MA: Gastroesophageal reflux symptoms not responding to proton pump inhibitor: GERD, NERD, NARD, esophageal hypersensitivity or dyspepsia? Can J Gastroenterol Hepatol 28(6):335–341, 2014 24719900

Basu PP, Shah NJ: Clinical and neurologic manifestations of minimal hepatic encephalopathy and overt hepatic encephalopathy. Clin Liver Dis 19(3):461–472, 2015 26195201

Bhandari S, Venkatesan T: Novel treatments for cyclic vomiting syndrome: beyond ondansetron and amitriptyline. Curr Treat Options Gastroenterol 14(4):495–506, 2016 27757817

Bielefeldt K: Gastroparesis: concepts, controversies, and challenges. Scientifica (Cairo) 2012:424802, 2012 24278691

Bilgi MM, Vardar R, Yıldırım E, et al: Prevalence of psychiatric comorbidity in symptomatic gastroesophageal reflux subgroups. Dig Dis Sci 62(4):984–993, 2017 27565506

Björnsson ES: Epidemiology and risk factors for idiosyncratic drug-induced liver injury. Semin Liver Dis 34(2):115–122, 2014 24879977

Bodén R, Bexelius TS, Mattsson F, et al: Antidopaminergic drugs and acute pancreatitis: a population-based study. BMJ Open 2(3), 2012 22581796

Böhn L, Störsrud S, Liljebo T, et al: Diet low in FODMAPs reduces symptoms of irritable bowel syndrome as well as traditional dietary advice: a randomized controlled trial. Gastroenterology 149(6):1399–1407, 2015 26255043

Bohórquez DV, Liddle RA: The gut connectome: making sense of what you eat. J Clin Invest 125(3):888–890, 2015 25729849

Bokemeyer M, Ding XQ, Goldbecker A, et al: Evidence for neuroinflammation and neuroprotection in HCV infection-associated encephalopathy. Gut 60(3):370–377, 2011 20926642

Bonaz BL, Bernstein CN: Brain-gut interactions in inflammatory bowel disease. Gastroenterology 144(1):36–49, 2013 23063970

Boyd CA, Benarroch-Gampel J, Sheffield KM, et al: The effect of depression on stage at diagnosis, treatment, and survival in pancreatic adenocarcinoma. Surgery 152(3):403–413, 2012 22938900

Brahm NC, Kelly-Rehm MC: Antidepressant-mediated gastroesophageal reflux disease. Consult Pharm 26(4):274–278, 2011 21486738

Breitbart W, Rosenfeld B, Tobias K, et al: Depression, cytokines, and pancreatic cancer. Psychooncology 23(3):339–345, 2014 24136882

Brennan BP, Fogarty KV, Roberts JL, et al: Duloxetine in the treatment of irritable bowel syndrome: an open-label pilot study. Hum Psychopharmacol 24(5):423–428, 2009 19548294

Bundeff AW, Woodis CB: Selective serotonin reuptake inhibitors for the treatment of irritable bowel syndrome. Ann Pharmacother 48(6):777–784, 2014 24651166

Burgstaller JM, Jenni BF, Steurer J, et al: Treatment efficacy for non-cardiovascular chest pain: a systematic review and meta-analysis. PLoS One 9(8):e104722, 2014 25111147

Burisch J, Weimers P, Pedersen N, et al; EpiCom-Group: Health-related quality of life improves during one year of medical and surgical treatment in a European population-based inception cohort of patients with inflammatory bowel disease—an ECCO-EpiCom study. J Crohn's Colitis 8(9):1030–1042, 2014 24560877

Butterworth RF: Pathogenesis of hepatic encephalopathy and brain edema in acute liver failure. J Clin Exp Hepatol 5 (suppl 1):S96–S103, 2015 26041966

Butterworth RF: Pathogenesis of hepatic encephalopathy in cirrhosis: the concept of synergism revisited. Metab Brain Dis 31(6):1211–1215, 2016 26521983

Camilleri M: Pharmacological agents currently in clinical trials for disorders in neurogastroenterology. J Clin Invest 123(10):4111–4120, 2013 24084743

Camilleri M: Functional dyspepsia and gastroparesis. Dig Dis 34(5):491–499, 2016 27332558

Camilleri M, Stanghellini V: Current management strategies and emerging treatments for functional dyspepsia. Nat Rev Gastroenterol Hepatol 10(3):187–194, 2013 23381190

Canavan C, West J, Card T: The epidemiology of irritable bowel syndrome. Clin Epidemiol 6:71–80, 2014a 24523597

Canavan C, West J, Card T: Review article: the economic impact of the irritable bowel syndrome. Aliment Pharmacol Ther 40(9):1023–1034, 2014b 25199904

Canavan C, West J, Card T: Change in quality of life for patients with irritable bowel syndrome following referral to a gastroenterologist: a cohort study. PLoS One 10(10):e0139389, 2015 26431458

Carabotti M, Scirocco A, Maselli MA, Severi C: The gut-brain axis: interactions between enteric microbiota, central and enteric nervous systems. Ann Gastroenterol 28(2):203–209, 2015 25830558

Charleston L 4th: Burning mouth syndrome: a review of recent literature. Curr Pain Headache Rep 17(6):336, 2013 23645183

Chen DY, Jia L, Gu X, et al: Comparison of paroxetine and amitriptyline in the treatment of refractory globus pharyngeus. Dig Liver Dis 48(9):1012–1017, 2016 27378704

Cheng YC, Chen CC, Ho AS, Chiu NY: Prolonged psychosis associated with interferon therapy in a patient with hepatitis C: case study and literature review. Psychosomatics 50(5):538–542, 2009 19855041

Cheng YL, Hu HY, Lin XH, et al: Use of SSRI, but not SNRI, increased upper and lower gastrointestinal bleeding: a nationwide population-based cohort study in Taiwan. Medicine (Baltimore) 94(46):e2022, 2015 26579809

Chou PH, Lin CC, Lin CH, et al: Prevalence of gastroesophageal reflux disease in major depressive disorder: a population-based study. Psychosomatics 55(2):155–162, 2014 23953172

Chung KT, Shelat VG: Perforated peptic ulcer—an update. World J Gastrointest Surg 9(1):1–12, 2017 28138363

Ciovica R, Riedl O, Neumayer C, et al: The use of medication after laparoscopic antireflux surgery. Surg Endosc 23(9):1938–1946, 2009 19169748

Clavé P, Shaker R: Dysphagia: current reality and scope of the problem. Nat Rev Gastroenterol Hepatol 12(5):259–270, 2015 25850008

Coffin B, Dapoigny M, Cloarec D, et al: Relationship between severity of symptoms and quality of life in 858 patients with irritable bowel syndrome. Gastroenterol Clin Biol 28(1):11–15, 2004 15041804

Colon VJ, Young MA, Ramirez FC: The short- and long-term efficacy of empirical esophageal dilation in patients with nonobstructive dysphagia: a prospective, randomized study. Am J Gastroenterol 95(4):910–913, 2000 10763936

Coss-Adame E, Rao SS: A review of esophageal chest pain. Gastroenterol Hepatol (N Y) 11(11):759–766, 2015 27134590

Coss-Adame E, Erdogan A, Rao SS: Treatment of esophageal (noncardiac) chest pain: an expert review. Clin Gastroenterol Hepatol 12(8):1224–1245, 2014 23994670

Creed F, Fernandes L, Guthrie E, et al; North of England IBS Research Group: The cost-effectiveness of psychotherapy and paroxetine for severe irritable bowel syndrome. Gastroenterology 124(2):303–317, 2003 12557136

Creed F, Guthrie E, Ratcliffe J, et al: Reported sexual abuse predicts impaired functioning but a good response to psychological treatments in patients with severe irritable bowel syndrome. Psychosom Med 67(3):490–499, 2005 15911915

Creed FH, Tomenson B, Chew-Graham C, et al: Multiple somatic symptoms predict impaired health status in functional somatic syndromes. Int J Behav Med 20(2):194–205, 2013 22932928

Crone CC, Marcangelo M, Lackamp J, et al: Gastrointestinal disorders, in Clinical Manual of Psychopharmacology in the Medically Ill, 2nd Edition. Edited by Levenson JL, Ferrando SJ. Washington, DC, American Psychiatric Association Publishing, 2016, pp 129–193

Daghaghzadeh H, Naji F, Afshar H, et al: Efficacy of duloxetine add on in treatment of inflammatory bowel disease patients: a double-blind controlled study. J Res Med Sci 20(6):595–601, 2015 26600836

Dahlhamer JM, Zammitti EP, Ward BW, et al: Prevalence of inflammatory bowel disease among adults aged > 18 years—United States, 2015. MMWR Morb Mortal Wkly Rep 65(42):1166–1169, 2016 27787492

Dalton SO, Sørensen HT, Johansen C: SSRIs and upper gastrointestinal bleeding: what is known and how should it influence prescribing? CNS Drugs 20(2):143–151, 2006 16478289

Dean BB, Aguilar D, Barghout V, et al: Impairment in work productivity and health-related quality of life in patients with IBS. Am J Manag Care 11 (1 suppl):S17–S26, 2005 15926760

Deary IJ, Smart A, Wilson JA: Depression and "hassles" in globus pharyngis. Br J Psychiatry 161:115–117, 1992 1638307 de Bortoli N, Frazzoni L, Savarino EV, et al: Functional heartburn overlaps with irritable bowel syndrome more often than GERD. Am J Gastroenterol 111(12):1711–1717, 2016a 27644732

de Bortoli N, Ottonello A, Zerbib F, et al: Between GERD and NERD: the relevance of weakly acidic reflux. Ann N Y Acad Sci 1380(1):218–229, 2016b 27472432

de Knegt RJ, Bezemer G, Van Gool AR, et al: Randomised clinical trial: escitalopram for the prevention of psychiatric adverse events during treatment with peginterferon-alfa-2a and ribavirin for chronic hepatitis C. Aliment Pharmacol Ther 34(11–12):1306–1317, 2011 21999489

de Souza FTA, Teixeira AL, Amaral TMP, et al: Psychiatric disorders in burning mouth syndrome. J Psychosom Res 72(2):142–146, 2012 22281456

de Souza HSP, Fiocchi C: Immunopathogenesis of IBD: current state of the art. Nat Rev Gastroenterol Hepatol 13(1):13–27, 2016 26627550

Dick TB, Lindberg LS, Ramirez DD, Charlton MR: A clinician's guide to drug-drug interactions with direct-acting antiviral agents for the treatment of hepatitis C viral infection. Hepatology 63(2):634–643, 2016 26033675

Dore GJ, Altice F, Litwin AH, et al; C-EDGE CO-STAR Study Group: Elbasvir-grazoprevir to treat hepatitis C virus infection in persons receiving opioid agonist therapy: a randomized trial. Ann Intern Med 165(9):625–634, 2016 27537841

Drossman DA: Functional gastrointestinal disorders and the Rome IV process, in Rome IV Functional Gastrointestinal Disorders: Disorders of Gut–Brain Interaction, 4th Edition. Edited by Drossman DA, Chang L, Chey WD, et al. Raleigh, NC, Rome Foundation, 2016, pp 2–32

Drossman DA, Hasler WL: Rome IV—Functional GI disorders: disorders of gut-brain interaction. Gastroenterology 150(6):1257–1261, 2016 27147121

Drossman D, Szigethy E. The narcotic bowel syndrome: a recent update. Am J Gastroenterol Suppl 2(1):22–30, 2014 25207609

Drossman DA, Talley NJ, Leserman J, et al: Sexual and physical abuse and gastrointestinal illness. Review and recommendations. Ann Intern Med 123(10):782–794, 1995 7574197

Drossman DA, Morris CB, Edwards H, et al: Diagnosis, characterization, and 3-month outcome after detoxification of 39 patients with narcotic bowel syndrome. Am J Gastroenterol 107(9):1426–1440, 2012 22710577

Ducasse D, Courtet P, Olie E: Burning mouth syndrome: current clinical, physiopathologic, and therapeutic data. Reg Anesth Pain Med 38(5):380–390, 2013 23970045

Dziewas R, Warnecke T, Schnabel M, et al: Neuroleptic-induced dysphagia: case report and literature review. Dysphagia 22(1):63–67, 2007 17024549

Edula RGR, Pyrsopoulos NT: New methods of testing and brain imaging in hepatic encephalopathy: a review. Clin Liver Dis 19(3):449–459, 2015 26195200

Enweluzo C, Aziz F: Gastroparesis: a review of current and emerging treatment options. Clin Exp Gastroenterol 6:161–165, 2013 24039443

Faramarzi M, Azadfallah P, Book HE, et al: The effect of psychotherapy in improving physical and psychiatric symptoms in patients with functional dyspepsia. Iran J Psychiatry 10(1):43–49, 2015 26005480

Farmer AD, Ferdinand E, Aziz Q: Opioids and the gastrointestinal tract—a case of narcotic bowel syndrome and literature review. J Neurogastroenterol Motil 19(1):94–98, 2013 23350054

Farmer AD, Gallagher J, Bruckner-Holt C, Aziz Q: Narcotic bowel syndrome. Lancet Gastroenterol Hepatol 2(5):361–368, 2017a 28397700

Farmer AD, Ruffle JK, Aziz Q: The role of esophageal hypersensitivity in functional esophageal disorders. J Clin Gastroenterol 51(2):91–99, 2017b 28005634

Fernandez-del Castillo C, Jimenez RE: Epidemiology and non-familial risk factors for exocrine pancreatic cancer. March 23, 2017. Available at: https://www.uptodate.com/contents/epidemiology-and-nonfamilial-risk-factors-for-exocrine-pancreatic-cancer. Accessed April 19, 2017.

Figueroa-Moseley C, Jean-Pierre P, Roscoe JA, et al: Behavioral interventions in treating anticipatory nausea and vomiting. J Natl Compr Canc Netw 5(1):44–50, 2007 17239325

Ford AC, Talley NJ, Schoenfeld PS, et al: Efficacy of antidepressants and psychological therapies in irritable bowel syndrome: systematic review and meta-analysis. Gut 58(3):367–378, 2009 19001059

Ford AC, Quigley EM, Lacy BE, et al: Effect of antidepressants and psychological therapies, including hypnotherapy, in irritable bowel syndrome: systematic review and meta-analysis. Am J Gastroenterol 109(9):1350–1365, quiz 1366, 2014 24935275

Ford AC, Luthra P, Tack J, et al: Efficacy of psychotropic drugs in functional dyspepsia: systematic review and meta-analysis. Gut 66(3):411–420, 2017 26567029

Fras I, Litin EM, Pearson JS: Comparison of psychiatric symptoms in carcinoma of the pancreas with those in some other intra-abdominal neoplasms. Am J Psychiatry 123(12):1553–1562, 1967 4381627

Fratto G, Manzon L: Use of psychotropic drugs and associated dental diseases. Int J Psychiatry Med 48(3):185–197, 2014 25492713

Fuller-Thomson E, Lateef R, Sulman J: Robust association between inflammatory bowel disease and generalized anxiety disorder: findings from a nationally representative Canadian study. Inflamm Bowel Dis 21(10):2341–2348, 2015 26218145

Furness JB: The enteric nervous system and neurogastroenterology. Nat Rev Gastroenterol Hepatol 9(5):286–294, 2012 22392290

Gaines LS, Slaughter JC, Horst SN, et al: Association between affective-cognitive symptoms of depression and exacerbation of Crohn's disease. Am J Gastroenterol 111(6):864–870, 2016 27045927

Gasse C, Jacobsen J, Pedersen L, et al: Risk of hospitalization for acute pancreatitis associated with conventional and atypical antipsychotics: a population-based case-control study. Pharmacotherapy 28(1):27–34, 2008 18154471

Gerstner T, Büsing D, Bell N, et al: Valproic acid-induced pancreatitis: 16 new cases and a review of the literature. J Gastroenterol 42(1):39–48, 2007 17322992

Goodhand JR, Greig FIS, Koodun Y, et al: Do antidepressants influence the disease course in inflammatory bowel disease? A retrospective case-matched observational study. Inflamm Bowel Dis 18(7):1232–1239, 2012 22234954

Goodwin RD, Keyes KM, Stein MB, Talley NJ: Peptic ulcer and mental disorders among adults in the community: the role of nicotine and alcohol use disorders. Psychosom Med 71(4):463–468, 2009 19443694

Goyal RK, Hirano I: The enteric nervous system. N Engl J Med 334(17):1106–1115, 1996 8598871

Gracie DJ, Williams CJ, Sood R, et al: Negative effects on psychological health and quality of life of genuine irritable bowel syndrome-type symptoms in patients with inflammatory bowel disease. Clin Gastroenterol Hepatol 15(3):376–384.e5, 2017 27189912

Gralnek IM, Hays RD, Kilbourne A, et al: The impact of irritable bowel syndrome on health-related quality of life. Gastroenterology 119(3):654–660, 2000 10982758

Grebely J, Mauss S, Brown A, et al: Efficacy and safety of ledipasvir/sofosbuvir with and without ribavirin in patients with chronic HCV genotype 1 infection receiving opioid substitution therapy: analysis of phase 3 ION trials. Clin Infect Dis 63(11):1405–1411, 2016 27553375

Grover VPB, Pavese N, Koh SB, et al: Cerebral microglial activation in patients with hepatitis C: in vivo evidence of neuroinflammation. J Viral Hepat 19(2):e89–e96, 2012 22239531

Grover VPB, Tognarelli JM, Massie N, et al: The why and wherefore of hepatic encephalopathy. Int J Gen Med 8:381–390, 2015 26719720

Gwee KA, Leong YL, Graham C, et al: The role of psychological and biological factors in postinfective gut dysfunction. Gut 44(3):400–406, 1999 10026328

Haft S, Carey RM, Farquhar D, Mirza N: Anticholinergic medication use is associated with globus pharyngeus. J Laryngol Otol 130(12):1125–1129, 2016 27786147

Halmos EP, Power VA, Shepherd SJ, et al: A diet low in FODMAPs reduces symptoms of irritable bowel syndrome. Gastroenterology 146(1):67–75.e5, 2014 24076059

Halpert A, Dalton CB, Diamant NE, et al: Clinical response to tricyclic antidepressants in functional bowel disorders is not related to dosage. Am J Gastroenterol 100(3):664–671, 2005 15743366

Han P, Suarez-Durall P, Mulligan R: Dry mouth: a critical topic for older adult patients. J Prosthodont Res 59(1):6–19, 2015 25498205

Harris LA, Chang L: Irritable bowel syndrome: new and emerging therapies. Curr Opin Gastroenterol 22(2):128–135, 2006 16462168

Harris MB, Deary IJ, Wilson JA: Life events and difficulties in relation to the onset of globus pharyngis. J Psychosom Res 40(6):603–615, 1996 8843039

Hasler WL, Parkman HP, Wilson LA, et al; NIDDK Gastroparesis Clinical Research Consortium: Psychological dysfunction is associated with symptom severity but not disease etiology or degree of gastric retention in patients with gastroparesis. Am J Gastroenterol 105(11):2357–2367, 2010 20588262

Hauser P, Kern S: Psychiatric and substance use disorders co-morbidities and hepatitis C: diagnostic and treatment implications. World J Hepatol 7(15):1921–1935, 2015 26244067

Hausteiner-Wiehle C, Henningsen P: Irritable bowel syndrome: relations with functional, mental, and somatoform disorders. World J Gastroenterol 20(20):6024–6030, 2014 24876725

Heckmann SM, Kirchner E, Grushka M, et al: A double-blind study on clonazepam in patients with burning mouth syndrome. Laryngoscope 122(4):813–816, 2012 22344742

Hejazi RA, McCallum RW: Rumination syndrome: a review of current concepts and treatments. Am J Med Sci 348(4):324–329, 2014 24642653

Hermes-Laufer J, Del Puppo L, Inan I, et al: Cannabinoid hyperemesis syndrome: a case report of Cyclic severe hyperemesis and abdominal pain with long-term cannabis use. Case Rep Gastrointest Med 2016:2815901, 2016 27980870

Hermus IP, Willems SJ, Bogman AC, et al: Cyclic vomiting syndrome: an update illustrated by a case report. Prim Care Companion CNS Disord 18(3), 2016 27733950

Herrera-deGuise C, Casellas F, Robles V, et al: Predictive value of early restoration of quality of life in Crohn's disease patients receiving antitumor necrosis factor agents. J Gastroenterol Hepatol 30(2):286–291, 2015 25302652

Hershcovici T, Achem SR, Jha LK, Fass R: Systematic review: the treatment of noncardiac chest pain. Aliment Pharmacol Ther 35(1):5–14, 2012 22077344

Hillilä MT, Siivola MT, Färkkilä MA: Comorbidity and use of health-care services among irritable bowel syndrome sufferers. Scand J Gastroenterol 42(7):799–806, 2007 17558902

Hoivik ML, Moum B, Solberg IC, et al; IBSEN Study Group: Health-related quality of life in patients with ulcerative colitis after a 10-year disease course: results from the IBSEN study. Inflamm Bowel Dis 18(8):1540–1549, 2012 21936030

Holland JC, Korzun AH, Tross S, et al: Comparative psychological disturbance in patients with pancreatic and gastric cancer. Am J Psychiatry 143(8):982–986, 1986 3524279

Hołubiuk Ł, Imiela J: Diet and Helicobacter pylori infection. Prz Gastroenterol 11(3):150–154, 2016 27713775

Hong JY, Naliboff B, Labus JS, et al: Altered brain responses in subjects with irritable bowel syndrome during cued and uncued pain expectation. Neurogastroenterol Motil 28(1):127–138, 2016 26526698

Hou XJ, Xu JH, Wang J, Yu YY: Can antidepressants prevent pegylated interferon-α/ribavirin-associated depression in patients with chronic hepatitis C: meta-analysis of randomized, double-blind, placebo-controlled trials? PLoS One 8(10):e76799, 2013 24204676

Hughes E, Bassi S, Gilbody S, et al: Prevalence of HIV, hepatitis B, and hepatitis C in people with severe mental illness: a systematic review and meta-analysis. Lancet Psychiatry 3(1):40–48, 2016 26620388

Hungin AP, Whorwell PJ, Tack J, Mearin F: The prevalence, patterns and impact of irritable bowel syndrome: an international survey of 40,000 subjects. Aliment Pharmacol Ther 17(5):643–650, 2003 12641512

Hungin APS, Chang L, Locke GR, et al: Irritable bowel syndrome in the United States: prevalence, symptom patterns and impact. Aliment Pharmacol Ther 21(11):1365–1375, 2005 15932367

Huppertz-Hauss G, Høivik ML, Langholz E, et al: Health-related quality of life in inflammatory bowel disease in a European-wide population-based cohort 10 years after diagnosis. Inflamm Bowel Dis 21(2):337–344, 2015 25569735

Huppertz-Hauss G, Lie Høivik M, Jelsness-Jørgensen LP, et al: Health-related quality of life in patients with inflammatory bowel disease 20 years after diagnosis: results from the IBSEN study. Inflamm Bowel Dis 22(7):1679–1687, 2016 27206016

Hussain A, Burke J: Mirtazapine associated with recurrent pancreatitis—a case report. J Psychopharmacol 22(3):336–337, 2008 18208920

Icenhour A, Langhorst J, Benson S, et al: Neural circuitry of abdominal pain-related fear learning and reinstatement in irritable bowel syndrome. Neurogastroenterol Motil 27(1):114–127, 2015 25557224

Iglesias M, Vázquez I, Barreiro-de Acosta M, et al: Health related quality of life in patients with Crohn's disease in remission. Rev Esp Enferm Dig 102(11):624–630, 2010 21142382

Iglesias-Rey M, Barreiro-de Acosta M, Caamaño-Isorna F, et al: Psychological factors are associated with changes in the health-related quality of life in inflammatory bowel disease. Inflamm Bowel Dis 20(1):92–102, 2014 24193152

Inayat F, Virk HU, Ullah W, Hussain Q: Is haloperidol the wonder drug for cannabinoid hyperemesis syndrome? BMJ Case Rep 2017 28052951

International Foundation for Functional Gastrointestinal Disorders: About IBS: Statistics. May 10, 2016. Available at: https://aboutibs.org/facts-about-ibs/statistics.html. Accessed July 21, 2017.

Iskandar HN, Cassell B, Kanuri N, et al: Tricyclic antidepressants for management of residual symptoms in inflammatory bowel disease. J Clin Gastroenterol 48(5):423–429, 2014 24406434

Jawaro T, Yang A, Dixit D, Bridgeman MB: Management of hepatic encephalopathy: a primer. Ann Pharmacother 50(7):569–577, 2016 27126547

Jia L, Jiang SM, Shang YY, et al: Investigation of the incidence of pancreatic cancer-related depression and its relationship with the quality of life of patients. Digestion 82(1):4–9, 2010 20145402

Jones MP: The role of psychosocial factors in peptic ulcer disease: beyond Helicobacter pylori and NSAIDs. J Psychosom Res 60(4):407–412, 2006 16581366

Jones JL, Abernathy KE: Successful treatment of suspected cannabinoid hyperemesis syndrome using haloperidol in the outpatient setting. Case Rep Psychiatry 2016:3614053, 2016 27597918

Jonsbu E, Dammen T, Morken G, et al: Short-term cognitive behavioral therapy for non-cardiac chest pain and benign palpitations: a randomized controlled trial. J Psychosom Res 70(2):117–123, 2011 21262413

Kamen C, Tejani MA, Chandwani K, et al: Anticipatory nausea and vomiting due to chemotherapy. Eur J Pharmacol 722:172–179, 2014 24157982

Kandiah PA, Kumar G: Hepatic encephalopathy: the old and the new. Crit Care Clin 32(3):311–329, 2016 27339673

Kaplan A, Franzen MD, Nickell PV, et al: An open-label trial of duloxetine in patients with irritable bowel syndrome and comorbid generalized anxiety disorder. Int J Psychiatry Clin Pract 18(1):11–15, 2014 23980534

Karling P, Danielsson A, Adolfsson R, Norrback KF: No difference in symptoms of irritable bowel syndrome between healthy subjects and patients with recurrent depression in remission. Neurogastroenterol Motil 19(11):896–904, 2007 17973640

Kaurich T: Drug-induced acute pancreatitis. Proc Bayl Univ Med Cent 21(1):77–81, 2008 18209761

Keefer L, Mandal S: The potential role of behavioral therapies in the management of centrally mediated abdominal pain. Neurogastroenterol Motil 27(3):313–323, 2015 25428520

Keefer L, Taft TH, Kiebles JL, et al: Gut-directed hypnotherapy significantly augments clinical remission in quiescent ulcerative colitis. Aliment Pharmacol Ther 38(7):761–771, 2013 23957526

Keefer L, Drossman DA, Guthrie E, et al: Centrally mediated disorders of gastrointestinal pain. Gastroenterology 150:1408–1419, 2016 27144628

Kessing BF, Smout AJ, Bredenoord AJ: Current diagnosis and management of the rumination syndrome. J Clin Gastroenterol 48(6):478–483, 2014 24921208

Kiebles JL, Kwiatek MA, Pandolfino JE, et al: Do patients with globus sensation respond to hypnotically assisted relaxation therapy? A case series report. Dis Esophagus 23(7):545–553, 2010 20459447

Kisely S, Forbes M, Sawyer E, et al: A systematic review of randomized trials for the treatment of burning mouth syndrome. J Psychosom Res 86:39–46, 2016 27302545

Knowles SR, Monshat K, Castle DJ: The efficacy and methodological challenges of psychotherapy for adults with inflammatory bowel disease: a review. Inflamm Bowel Dis 19(12):2704–2715, 2013 23846488

Komiyama O, Nishimura H, Makiyama Y, et al: Group cognitive-behavioral intervention for patients with burning mouth syndrome. J Oral Sci 55(1):17–22, 2013 23485596

Kortequee S, Karkos PD, Atkinson H, et al: Management of globus pharyngeus. Int J Otolaryngol 2013:946780, 2013 23935629

Kraus MR, Schäfer A, Teuber G, et al: Improvement of neurocognitive function in responders to an antiviral therapy for chronic hepatitis C. Hepatology 58(2):497–504, 2013 23300053

Kravits KG: Hypnosis for the management of anticipatory nausea and vomiting. J Adv Pract Oncol 6(3):225–229, 2015 26557409

Kuiken SD, Tytgat GN, Boeckxstaens GE: The selective serotonin reuptake inhibitor fluoxetine does not change rectal sensitivity and symptoms in patients with irritable bowel syndrome: a double blind, randomized, placebo-controlled study. Clin Gastroenterol Hepatol 1(3):219–228, 2003 15017494

Kumar N, Bashar Q, Reddy N, et al: Cyclic vomiting syndrome (CVS): is there a difference based on onset of symptoms—pediatric versus adult? BMC Gastroenterol 12:52, 2012 22639867

Kuo CY, Liao YT, Chen VC: Risk of upper gastrointestinal bleeding when taking SSRIs with NSAIDs or aspirin. Am J Psychiatry 171(5):582, 2014 24788285

Kurlander JE, Drossman DA: Diagnosis and treatment of narcotic bowel syndrome. Nat Rev Gastroenterol Hepatol 11(7):410–418, 2014 24751914

Lackner JM, Lou Coad M, Mertz HR, et al: Cognitive therapy for irritable bowel syndrome is associated with reduced limbic activity, GI symptoms, and anxiety. Behav Res Ther 44(5):621–638, 2006 16039604

Ladabaum U, Sharabidze A, Levin TR, et al: Citalopram provides little or no benefit in nondepressed patients with irritable bowel syndrome. Clin Gastroenterol Hepatol 8(1):42–48.e1, 2010 19765674

Laird KT, Tanner-Smith EE, Russell AC, et al: Comparative efficacy of psychological therapies for improving mental health and daily functioning in irritable bowel syndrome: a systematic review and meta-analysis. Clin Psychol Rev 51:142–152, 2017 27870997

Lanas A, Chan FK: Peptic ulcer disease. Lancet 390(10094):613–624, 2017 28242110

Laporte S, Chapelle C, Caillet P, et al: Bleeding risk under selective serotonin reuptake inhibitor (SSRI) antidepressants: a meta-analysis of observational studies. Pharmacol Res 118:19–32, 2017 27521835

Lau CS, Ward A, Chamberlain RS: Probiotics improve the efficacy of standard triple therapy in the eradication of Helicobacter pylori: a meta-analysis. Infect Drug Resist 9:275–289, 2016 27994474

Lee BE, Kim GH: Globus pharyngeus: a review of its etiology, diagnosis and treatment. World J Gastroenterol 18(20):2462–2471, 2012 22654443

Lee S, Wu J, Ma YL, et al: Irritable bowel syndrome is strongly associated with generalized anxiety disorder: a community study. Aliment Pharmacol Ther 30(6):643–651, 2009 19552631

Leise MD, Poterucha JJ, Talwalkar JA: Drug-induced liver injury. Mayo Clin Proc 89(1):95–106, 2014 24388027

Levenstein S: The very model of a modern etiology: a biopsychosocial view of peptic ulcer. Psychosom Med 62(2):176–185, 2000 10772394

Levenstein S, Rosenstock S, Jacobsen RK, Jorgensen T: Psychological stress increases risk for peptic ulcer, regardless of Helicobacter pylori infection or use of nonsteroidal anti-inflammatory drugs. Clin Gastroenterol Hepatol 13(3):498–506, 2015 25111233

Levinthal DJ: The cyclic vomiting syndrome threshold: a framework for understanding pathogenesis and predicting successful treatments. Clin Transl Gastroenterol 7(10):e198, 2016 27787513

Levy RL, Olden KW, Naliboff BD, et al: Psychosocial aspects of the functional gastrointestinal disorders. Gastroenterology 130(5):1447–1458, 2006 16678558

Lewis-Fernández R, Lam P, Lucak S, et al: An open-label pilot study of duloxetine in patients with irritable bowel syndrome and comorbid major depressive disorder. J Clin Psychopharmacol 36(6):710–715, 2016 27755218

Ljung R, Rück C, Mattsson F, et al: Selective serotonin reuptake inhibitors and the risk of acute pancreatitis: a Swedish population-based case-control study. J Clin Psychopharmacol 32(3):336–340, 2012 22544014

Loke YK, Trivedi AN, Singh S: Meta-analysis: gastrointestinal bleeding due to interaction between selective serotonin uptake inhibitors and non-steroidal anti-inflammatory drugs. Aliment Pharmacol Ther 27(1):31–40, 2008 17919277

Lovell RM, Ford AC: Global prevalence of and risk factors for irritable bowel syndrome: a meta-analysis. Clin Gastroenterol Hepatol 10(7):712–721.e4, 2012 22426087

Luo XP, Mao R, Chen BL, et al: Over-reaching beyond disease activity: the influence of anxiety and medical economic burden on health-related quality of life in patients with inflammatory bowel disease. Patient Prefer Adherence 11:23–31, 2016 28053510

Macer BJD, Prady SL, Mikocka-Walus A: Antidepressants in inflammatory bowel disease: a systematic review. Inflamm Bowel Dis 23(4):534–550, 2017 28267046

Malamood M, Roberts A, Kataria R, et al: Mirtazapine for symptom control in refractory gastroparesis. Drug Des Devel Ther 11:1035–1041, 2017 28408802

Marchand A, Belleville G, Fleet R, et al: Treatment of panic in chest pain patients from emergency departments: efficacy of different interventions focusing on panic management. Gen Hosp Psychiatry 34(6):671–680, 2012 22840563

Martín-Merino E, Ruigómez A, García Rodríguez LA, et al: Depression and treatment with antidepressants are associated with the development of gastro-oesophageal reflux disease. Aliment Pharmacol Ther 31(10):1132–1140, 2010 20199498

Marwick KFM, Taylor M, Walker SW: Antipsychotics and abnormal liver function tests: systematic review. Clin Neuropharmacol 35(5):244–253, 2012 22986798

Masand PS, Pae CU, Krulewicz S, et al: A double-blind, randomized, placebo-controlled trial of paroxetine controlled-release in irritable bowel syndrome. Psychosomatics 50(1):78–86, 2009 19213976

Mawdsley JE, Jenkins DG, Macey MG, et al: The effect of hypnosis on systemic and rectal mucosal measures of inflammation in ulcerative colitis. Am J Gastroenterol 103(6):1460–1469, 2008 18510607

Mawe GM, Coates MD, Moses PL: Review article: intestinal serotonin signalling in irritable bowel syndrome. Aliment Pharmacol Ther 23(8):1067–1076, 2006 16611266

Mayr M, Schmid RM: Pancreatic cancer and depression: myth and truth. BMC Cancer 10:569, 2010 20961421

McCombie A, Gearry R, Andrews J, et al: Does computerized cognitive behavioral therapy help people with inflammatory bowel disease? A randomized controlled trial. Inflamm Bowel Dis 22(1):171–181, 2016 26360545

Melinder C, Hiyoshi A, Fall K, et al: Stress resilience and the risk of inflammatory bowel disease: a cohort study of men living in Sweden. BMJ Open 7(1):e014315, 2017 28130207

Menon RM, Badri PS, Wang T, et al: Drug-drug interaction profile of the all-oral anti-hepatitis C virus regimen of paritaprevir/ritonavir, ombitasvir, and dasabuvir. J Hepatol 63(1):20–29, 2015 25646891

Mikocka-Walus A, Andrews JM: Attitudes towards antidepressants among people living with inflammatory bowel disease: an online Australia-wide survey. J Crohns Colitis 8(4):296–303, 2014 24074632

Mikocka-Walus AA, Gordon AL, Stewart BJ, Andrews JM: The role of antidepressants in the management of inflammatory bowel disease (IBD): a short report on a clinical case-note audit. J Psychosom Res 72(2):165–167, 2012 22281460

Mikocka-Walus A, Knowles SR, Keefer L, Graff L: Controversies revisited: a systematic review of the comorbidity of depression and anxiety with inflammatory bowel diseases. Inflamm Bowel Dis 22(3):752–762, 2016a 26841224

Mikocka-Walus A, Pittet V, Rossel JB, von Känel R; Swiss IBD Cohort Study Group: Symptoms of depression and anxiety are independently associated with clinical recurrence of inflammatory bowel disease. Clin Gastroenterol Hepatol 14(6):829.e1–835.e1, 2016b 26820402

Miller V, Whorwell PJ: Treatment of inflammatory bowel disease: a role for hypnotherapy? Int J Clin Exp Hypn 56(3):306–317, 2008 18569141

Millichap JG: Prognosis of cyclic vomiting syndrome. Pediatr Neurol Briefs 30(1):6, 2016 27004140

Mirsky IA, Reiser MF, Thaler M, Weiner H: Etiology of duodenal ulcer, I: relation of specific psychological characteristics to rate of gastric secretion (serum pepsinogen). Psychosom Med 19(1):1–10, 1957 13400987

Miwa H, Kondo T, Oshima T: Gastroesophageal reflux disease-related and functional heartburn: pathophysiology and treatment. Curr Opin Gastroenterol 32(4):344–352, 2016 27206157

Molassiotis A, Lee PH, Burke TA, et al: Anticipatory nausea, risk factors, and its impact on chemotherapy-induced nausea and vomiting: results from the Pan European Emesis Registry Study. J Pain Symptom Manage 51(6):987–993, 2016 26891606

Monaco S, Mariotto S, Ferrari S, et al: Hepatitis C virus-associated neurocognitive and neuropsychiatric disorders: advances in 2015. World J Gastroenterol 21(42):11974–11983, 2015 26576086

Morgan MY: Current state of knowledge of hepatic encephalopathy (part III): non-absorbable disaccharides. Metab Brain Dis 31(6):1361–1364, 2016 27638474

Morgan V, Pickens D, Gautam S, et al: Amitriptyline reduces rectal pain related activation of the anterior cingulate cortex in patients with irritable bowel syndrome. Gut 54(5):601–607, 2005 15831901

Nabi E, Bajaj JS, Gautam S, et al: Useful tests for hepatic encephalopathy in clinical practice. Curr Gastroenterol Rep 16(1):362, 2014 24357348

Naini P, Dutta SK, Karhadkar AS, et al: Critical evaluation of esophageal dilation in nonobstructive dysphagia with and without esophageal rings. J Clin Gastroenterol 41(4):362–365, 2007 17413602

Nardone R, Taylor AC, Höller Y, et al: Minimal hepatic encephalopathy: a review. Neurosci Res 111:1–12, 2016 27153746

Negro F, Forton D, Craxì A, et al: Extrahepatic morbidity and mortality of chronic hepatitis C. Gastroenterology 149(6):1345–1360, 2015 26319013

Neilson K, Ftanou M, Monshat K, et al: A controlled study of a group mindfulness intervention for individuals living with inflammatory bowel disease. Inflamm Bowel Dis 22(3):694–701, 2016 26529560

Nguyen TM, Eslick GD: Systematic review: the treatment of noncardiac chest pain with antidepressants. Aliment Pharmacol Ther 35(5):493–500, 2012 22239853

Nicholl BI, Halder SL, Macfarlane GJ, et al: Psychosocial risk markers for new onset irritable bowel syndrome—results of a large prospective population-based study. Pain 137(1):147–155, 2008 17928145

Nieves JE, Stack KM, Harrison ME, Gorman JM: Dysphagia: a rare form of dyskinesia? J Psychiatr Pract 13(3):199–201, 2007 17522565

Niles AN, Dour HJ, Stanton AL, et al: Anxiety and depressive symptoms and medical illness among adults with anxiety disorders. J Psychosom Res 78(2):109–115, 2015 25510186

Nitsche CJ, Jamieson N, Lerch MM, Mayerle JV: Drug induced pancreatitis. Best Pract Res Clin Gastroenterol 24(2):143–155, 2010 20227028

North CS, Hong BA, Alpers DH: Relationship of functional gastrointestinal disorders and psychiatric disorders: implications for treatment. World J Gastroenterol 13(14):2020–2027, 2007 17465442

Nwokediuko SC: Current trends in the management of gastroesophageal reflux disease: a review. ISRN Gastroenterol 2012:391631, 2012 22844607

Oh JH, Pasricha PJ: Recent advances in the pathophysiology and treatment of gastroparesis. J Neurogastroenterol Motil 19(1):18–24, 2013 23350043

Oka Y, Okamoto K, Kawashita N, et al: Meta-analysis of the risk of upper gastrointestinal hemorrhage with combination therapy of selective serotonin reuptake inhibitors and nonsteroidal anti-inflammatory drugs. Biol Pharm Bull 37(6):947–953, 2014 24681541

Olden KW: Rumination. Curr Treat Options Gastroenterol 4(4):351–358, 2001 11469994

Olson SH, Xu Y, Herzog K, et al: Weight loss, diabetes, fatigue, and depression preceding pancreatic cancer. Pancreas 45(7):986–991, 2016 26692445

O'Neill JL, Remington TL: Drug-induced esophageal injuries and dysphagia. Ann Pharmacother 37(11):1675–1684, 2003 14565800

Ong DK, Mitchell SB, Barrett JS, et al: Manipulation of dietary short chain carbohydrates alters the pattern of gas production and genesis of symptoms in irritable bowel syndrome. J Gastroenterol Hepatol 25(8):1366–1373, 2010 20659225

Ostovaneh MR, Saeidi B, Hajifathalian K, et al: Comparing omeprazole with fluoxetine for treatment of patients with heartburn and normal endoscopy who failed once daily proton pump inhibitors: double-blind placebo-controlled trial. Neurogastroenterol Motil 26(5):670–678, 2014 24533896

Oustamanolakis P, Tack J: Dyspepsia: organic versus functional. J Clin Gastroenterol 46(3):175–190, 2012 22327302

Özdemir HH, Bulut S, Berilgen MS, et al: Resistant cyclic vomiting syndrome successfully responding to chlorpromazine. Acta Med (Hradec Kralove) 57(1):28–29, 2014 25006660

Palsson OS, Drossman DA: Psychiatric and psychological dysfunction in irritable bowel syndrome and the role of psychological treatments. Gastroenterol Clin North Am 34(2):281–303, 2005 15862936

Pan W, Wang Z, Tian F, et al: Electroacupuncture combined with mosapride alleviates symptoms in diabetic patients with gastroparesis. Exp Ther Med 13(4):1637–1643, 2017 28413522

Pasricha PJ, Yates KP, Nguyen L, et al: Outcomes and factors associated with reduced symptoms in patients with gastroparesis. Gastroenterology 149(7):1762–1774, 2015 26299414

Passmore MJ, Devarajan S, Ghatavi K, et al: Serotonin syndrome with prolonged dysphagia. Can J Psychiatry 49:79–80, 2004 14763689

Patel H, Gaduputi V, Sakam S, et al: Serotonin reuptake inhibitors and post-gastrostomy bleeding: reevaluating the link. Ther Clin Risk Manag 11:1283–1289, 2015 26346885

Patrick A, Epstein O: Review article: gastroparesis. Aliment Pharmacol Ther 27(9):724–740, 2008 18248660

Pattullo V, McAndrews MP, Damyanovich A, Heathcote EJ: Influence of hepatitis C virus on neurocognitive function in patients free from other risk factors: validation from therapeutic outcomes. Liver Int 31(7):1028–1038, 2011 21733093

Piacentino D, Cantarini R, Alfonsi M, et al: Psychopathological features of irritable bowel syndrome patients with and without functional dyspepsia: a cross sectional study. BMC Gastroenterol 11:94, 2011 21871075

Qi R, Liu C, Weng Y, et al: Disturbed interhemispheric functional connectivity rather than structural connectivity in irritable bowel syndrome. Front Mol Neurosci 9:141, 2016 27999530

Quigley EM, Lacy BE: Overlap of functional dyspepsia and GERD—diagnostic and treatment implications. Nat Rev Gastroenterol Hepatol 10(3):175–186, 2013 23296247

Qureshi F, Shafi A, Ali S, Siddiqui N: Clinical predictors of anticipatory emesis in patients treated with chemotherapy at a tertiary care cancer hospital. Pak J Med Sci 32(2):337–340, 2016 27182235

Rao SS, Yu S, Fedewa A: Systematic review: dietary fibre and FODMAP-restricted diet in the management of constipation and irritable bowel syndrome. Aliment Pharmacol Ther 41(12):1256–1270, 2015 25903636

Redd WH, Montgomery GH, DuHamel KN: Behavioral intervention for cancer treatment side effects. J Natl Cancer Inst 93(11):810–823, 2001 11390531

Regueiro M, Greer JB, Szigethy E: Etiology and treatment of pain and psychosocial issues in patients with inflammatory bowel diseases. Gastroenterology 152(2):430–439, 2017 27816599

Remes-Troche JM: The hypersensitive esophagus: pathophysiology, evaluation, and treatment options. Curr Gastroenterol Rep 12(5):417–426, 2010 20669058

Reuben A, Koch DG, Lee WM; Acute Liver Failure Study Group: Drug-induced acute liver failure: results of a U.S. multicenter, prospective study. Hepatology 52(6):2065–2076, 2010 20949552

Rey E, García-Alonso MO, Moreno-Ortega M, et al: Determinants of quality of life in irritable bowel syndrome. J Clin Gastroenterol 42(9):1003–1009, 2008 18719505

Ricci JF, Jhingran P, McLaughlin T, Carter EG: Costs of care for irritable bowel syndrome in managed care. Journal of Clinical Outcomes Management 7(6):23–28, 2000

Riedl A, Schmidtmann M, Stengel A, et al: Somatic comorbidities of irritable bowel syndrome: a systematic analysis. J Psychosom Res 64(6):573–582, 2008 18501257

Ries RK, Gilbert DA, Katon W: Tricyclic antidepressant therapy for peptic ulcer disease. Arch Intern Med 144(3):566–569, 1984 6367680

Roden DF, Altman KW: Causes of dysphagia among different age groups: a systematic review of the literature. Otolaryngol Clin North Am 46(6):965–987, 2013 24262954

Rodríguez de Rivera Campillo E, López-López J, Chimenos-Küstner E: Response to topical clonazepam in patients with burning mouth syndrome: a clinical study. Bull Group Int Rech Sci Stomatol Odontol 49(1):19–29, 2010 22750263

Rowan PJ, Bhulani N: Psychosocial assessment and monitoring in the new era of non-interferon-alpha hepatitis C virus treatments. World J Hepatol 7(19):2209–2213, 2015 26380046

Sabate JM, Veyrac M, Mion F, et al: Relationship between rectal sensitivity, symptoms intensity and quality of life in patients with irritable bowel syndrome. Aliment Pharmacol Ther 28(4):484–490, 2008 18544074

Sarges P, Steinberg JM, Lewis JH: Drug-induced liver injury: highlights from a review of the 2015 literature. Drug Saf 39(9):801–821, 2016 27142208

Savidge TC, Newman P, Pothoulakis C, et al: Enteric glia regulate intestinal barrier function and inflammation via release of S-nitrosoglutathione. Gastroenterology 132(4):1344–1358, 2007 17408650

Schaefer M, Sarkar R, Knop V, et al: Escitalopram for the prevention of peginterferon-α2a-associated depression in hepatitis C virus-infected patients without previous psychiatric disease: a randomized trial. Ann Intern Med 157(2):94–103, 2012 22801672

Scheerens C, Tack J, Rommel N: Buspirone, a new drug for the management of patients with ineffective esophageal motility? United European Gastroenterol J 3(3):261–265, 2015 26137300

Schmulson MJ, Drossman DA: What is new in Rome IV. J Neurogastroenterol Motil 23(2):151–163, 2017 28274109

Sebti J, Desseigne F, Saltel P: Prodromal depression in pancreatic cancer: retrospective evaluation on ten patients. Palliat Support Care 13(3):801–807, 2015 24959882

Sedky K, Nazir R, Joshi A, et al: Which psychotropic medications induce hepatotoxicity? Gen Hosp Psychiatry 34(1):53–61, 2012 22133982

Selleslagh M, van Oudenhove L, Pauwels A, et al: The complexity of globus: a multidisciplinary perspective. Nat Rev Gastroenterol Hepatol 11(4):220–233, 2014 24296583

Senior JR: Monitoring for hepatotoxicity: what is the predictive value of liver "function" tests? Clin Pharmacol Ther 85(3):331–334, 2009 19129750

Sexton KA, Walker JR, Graff LA, et al: Evidence of bidirectional associations between perceived stress and symptoms activity: a prospective longitudinal investigation in inflammatory bowel disease. Inflamm Bowel Dis 23(3):473–483, 2017 28221251

Sezer OB, Sezer T: A new approach to the prophylaxis of cyclic vomiting: topiramate. J Neurogastroenterol Motil 22(4):656–660, 2016 27302967

Shamash J, Miall L, Williams F, et al: Dysphagia in the neuroleptic malignant syndrome. Br J Psychiatry 164(6):849–850, 1994 7953002

Shepherd SJ, Parker FC, Muir JG, Gibson PR: Dietary triggers of abdominal symptoms in patients with irritable bowel syndrome: randomized placebo-controlled evidence. Clin Gastroenterol Hepatol 6(7):765–771, 2008 18456565

Sibelli A, Chalder T, Everitt H, et al: A systematic review with meta-analysis of the role of anxiety and depression in irritable bowel syndrome onset. Psychol Med 46(15):3065–3080, 2016 27605134

Silva MA, Key S, Han E, Malloy MJ: Acute pancreatitis associated with antipsychotic medication: evaluation of clinical features, treatment, and polypharmacy in a series of cases. J Clin Psychopharmacol 36(2):169–172, 2016 26859276

Simonetto DA, Oxentenko AS, Herman ML, Szostek JH: Cannabinoid hyperemesis: a case series of 98 patients. Mayo Clin Proc 87(2):114–119, 2012 22305024

Simrén M, Brazier J, Coremans G, et al: Quality of life and illness costs in irritable bowel syndrome. Digestion 69(4):254–261, 2004 15256832

Simrén M, Törnblom H, Palsson OS, et al: Visceral hypersensitivity is associated with GI symptom severity in functional GI disorders: consistent findings from five different patient cohorts. Gut 67(2):255–262, 2018 28104632

Smithard DG: Dysphagia management and stroke units. Curr Phys Med Rehabil Rep 4(4):287–294, 2016 28018754

Smolders EJ, de Kanter CTMM, de Knegt RJ, et al: Drug-drug interactions between direct-acting antivirals and psychoactive medications. Clin Pharmacokinet 55(12):1471–1494, 2016 27317413

Sockalingam S, Tseng A, Giguere P, Wong D: Psychiatric treatment considerations with direct acting antivirals in hepatitis C. BMC Gastroenterol 13:86, 2013 23672254

Sockalingam S, Sheehan K, Feld JJ, Shah H: Psychiatric care during hepatitis C treatment: the changing role of psychiatrists in the era of direct-acting antivirals. Am J Psychiatry 172(6):512–516, 2015 26029803

Song J, Lin N, Tian F, et al: Successful treatment of gastroparesis with the antidepressant mirtazapine: a case report. J Nippon Med Sch 81(6):392–394, 2014 25744484

Sorensen CJ, DeSanto K, Borgelt L, et al: Cannabinoid hyperemesis syndrome: diagnosis, pathophysiology, and treatment—a systematic review. J Med Toxicol 13(1):71–87, 2017 28000146

Soriano V, Labarga P, Barreiro P, et al: Drug interactions with new hepatitis C oral drugs. Expert Opin Drug Metab Toxicol 11(3):333–341, 2015 25553890

Spach DH: HCV epidemiology in the United States (Hepatitis C Online Web site). September 5, 2016. Available at: http://www.hepatitisc.uw.edu/go/screening-diagnosis/epidemiology-us/core-concept/all. Accessed March 16, 2017.

Stanghellini V, Chan FK, Hasler WL, et al: Gastroduodenal disorders. Gastroenterology 150(6):1380–1392, 2016 27147122

Suraweera D, Sundaram V, Saab S: Evaluation and management of hepatic encephalopathy: current status and future directions. Gut Liver 10(4):509–519, 2016 27377741

Sussman NL: Treatment of overt hepatic encephalopathy. Clin Liver Dis 19(3):551–563, 2015 26195208

Tabas G, Beaves M, Wang J, et al: Paroxetine to treat irritable bowel syndrome not responding to high-fiber diet: a double-blind, placebo-controlled trial. Am J Gastroenterol 99(5):914–920, 2004 15128360

Tack J, Broekaert D, Fischler B, et al: A controlled crossover study of the selective serotonin reuptake inhibitor citalopram in irritable bowel syndrome. Gut 55(8):1095–1103, 2006 16401691

Tack J, Ly HG, Carbone F, et al: Efficacy of mirtazapine in patients with functional dyspepsia and weight loss. Clin Gastroenterol Hepatol 14(3):385–392.e4, 2016 26538208

Talley NJ: Irritable bowel syndrome. Intern Med J 36(11):724–728, 2006 17040359

Talley NJ, Gabriel SE, Harmsen WS, et al: Medical costs in community subjects with irritable bowel syndrome. Gastroenterology 109(6):1736–1741, 1995 7498636

Talley NJ, Kellow JE, Boyce P, et al: Antidepressant therapy (imipramine and citalopram) for irritable bowel syndrome: a double-blind, randomized, placebo-controlled trial. Dig Dis Sci 53(1):108–115, 2008 17503182

Talley NJ, Locke GR, Saito YA, et al: Effect of amitriptyline and escitalopram on functional dyspepsia: a multicenter, randomized controlled study. Gastroenterology 149(2):340–349, 2015 25921377

Tanrivermis Sayit A, Elmali M, Saglam D, Celenk C: The diseases of airway-tracheal diverticu-lum: a review of the literature. J Thorac Dis 8(10):E1163–E1167, 2016 27867581

Targownik LE, Sexton KA, Bernstein MT, et al: The relationship among perceived stress, symp-toms, and inflammation in persons with inflammatory bowel disease. Am J Gastroenterol 110(7):1001–1012, quiz 1013, 2015 26077178

Törnblom H, Drossman DA: Centrally targeted pharmacotherapy for chronic abdominal pain. Neurogastroenterol Motil 27(4):455–467, 2015 25651186

Triantafillidis JK, Merikas E, Gikas A: Psychological factors and stress in inflammatory bowel disease. Expert Rev Gastroenterol Hepatol 7(3):225–238, 2013 23445232

Tseng PT, Zeng BS, Chen YW, et al: A meta-analysis and systematic review of the comorbidity between irritable bowel syndrome and bipolar disorder. Medicine (Baltimore) 95(33):e4617, 2016 27537599

Umapathy S, Dhiman RK, Grover S, et al: Persistence of cognitive impairment after resolution of overt hepatic encephalopathy. Am J Gastroenterol 109(7):1011–1019, 2014 24777152

Uppal DS, Wang AY: Update on the endoscopic treatments for achalasia. World J Gastroenterol 22(39):8670–8683, 2016 27818585

Vahedi H, Merat S, Rashidioon A, et al: The effect of fluoxetine in patients with pain and con-stipation-predominant irritable bowel syndrome: a double-blind randomized-controlled study. Aliment Pharmacol Ther 22(5):381–385, 2005 16128675

van Beek MH, Oude Voshaar RC, Beek AM, et al: A brief cognitive-behavioral intervention for treating depression and panic disorder in patients with noncardiac chest pain: a 24-week randomized controlled trial. Depress Anxiety 30(7):670–678, 2013 23625592

van der Have M, van der Aalst KS, Kaptein AA, et al: Determinants of health-related quality of life in Crohn's disease: a systematic review and meta-analysis. J Crohns Colitis 8(2):93–106, 2014 23746864

van Soest EM, Dieleman JP, Siersema PD, et al: Tricyclic antidepressants and the risk of reflux esophagitis. Am J Gastroenterol 102(9):1870–1877, 2007 17511756

Vanuytsel T, van Wanrooy S, Vanheel H, et al: Psychological stress and corticotropin-releasing hormone increase intestinal permeability in humans by a mast cell-dependent mechanism. Gut 63(8):1293–1299, 2014 24153250

Vavricka SR, Schoepfer A, Scharl M, et al: Extraintestinal manifestations of inflammatory bowel disease. Inflamm Bowel Dis 21(8):1982–1992, 2015 26154136

Viazis N, Keyoglou A, Kanellopoulos AK, et al: Selective serotonin reuptake inhibitors for the treatment of hypersensitive esophagus: a randomized, double-blind, placebo-controlled study. Am J Gastroenterol 107(11):1662–1667, 2012 21625270

Villa A, Connell CL, Abati S: Diagnosis and management of xerostomia and hyposalivation. Ther Clin Risk Manag 11:45–51, 2014 25653532

Vilstrup H, Amodio P, Bajaj J, et al: Hepatic encephalopathy in chronic liver disease: 2014 prac-tice guideline by the American Association for the Study of Liver Diseases and the Euro-pean Association for the Study of the Liver. Hepatology 60(2):715–735, 2014 25042402

Vinklerová I, Procházka M, Procházka V, Urbánek K: Incidence, severity, and etiology of drug-induced acute pancreatitis. Dig Dis Sci 55(10):2977–2981, 2010 20499176

Viramontes Hörner D, Avery A, Stow R: The effects of probiotics and symbiotics on risk factors for hepatic encephalopathy: a systematic review. J Clin Gastroenterol 51(4):312–323, 2017 28059938

Visser HK, Wigington JL, Keltner NL, Kowalski PC: Biological perspectives: Choking and antipsychotics: is this a significant concern? Perspect Psychiatr Care 50(2):79–82, 2014 24606560

Voican CS, Corruble E, Naveau S, Perlemuter G: Antidepressant-induced liver injury: a review for clinicians. Am J Psychiatry 171(4):404–415, 2014 24362450

Wee TC: Gastrointestinal hemorrhage related to fluoxetine in a patient with stroke. Am J Phys Med Rehabil 96(11):e201–e203, 2017 28141599

Weijenborg PW, de Schepper HS, Smout AJ, Bredenoord AJ: Effects of antidepressants in pa-tients with functional esophageal disorders or gastroesophageal reflux disease: a system-atic review. Clin Gastroenterol Hepatol 13(2):251–259, 2015 24997325

Weijenborg PW, Smout AJ, Bredenoord AJ: Esophageal acid sensitivity and mucosal integrity in patients with functional heartburn. Neurogastroenterol Motil 28(11):1649–1654, 2016 27194216

Weissenborn K: The clinical relevance of minimal hepatic encephalopathy—a critical look. Dig Dis 33(4):555–561, 2015 26159273

Whorwell P, Keefer L, Drossman DA, et al: Centrally mediated disorder of gastrointestinal pain, in Rome IV Functional Gastrointestinal Disorders: Disorders of Gut-Brain Interaction, 4th Edition. Edited by Drossman DA, Chang L, Chey WD, et al. Raleigh, NC, Rome Foundation, 2016, pp 1059–1116

Wijdicks EFM: Hepatic encephalopathy. N Engl J Med 375(17):1660–1670, 2016 27783916

Wirth R, Dziewas R, Beck AM, et al: Oropharyngeal dysphagia in older persons—from pathophysiology to adequate intervention: a review and summary of an international expert meeting. Clin Interv Aging 11:189–208, 2016 26966356

Wolff A, Joshi RK, Ekstrom J, et al: A guide to medications inducing salivary gland dysfunction, xerostomia, and subjective sialorrhea: a systematic review sponsored by the World Workshop on Oral Medicine VI. Drugs R D 17(1):1–28, 2017 27853957

Woodhouse S, Hebbard G, Knowles SR: Psychological controversies in gastroparesis: a systematic review. World J Gastroenterol 23(7):1298–1309, 2017 28275310

Woodman CL, Breen K, Noyes R Jr, et al: The relationship between irritable bowel syndrome and psychiatric illness. A family study. Psychosomatics 39(1):45–54, 1998 9538675

Xie C, Tang Y, Wang Y, et al: Efficacy and safety of antidepressants for the treatment of irritable bowel syndrome: a meta-analysis. PLoS One 10(8):e0127815, 2015 26252008

Yanartas O, Kani HT, Bicakci E, et al: The effects of psychiatric treatment on depression, anxiety, quality of life, and sexual dysfunction in patients with inflammatory bowel disease. Neuropsychiatr Dis Treat 12:673–683, 2016 27069364

Yarlott L, Heald E, Forton D: Hepatitis C virus infection, and neurological and psychiatric disorders—a review. J Adv Res 8(2):139–148, 2017 28149649

Ye Y, Pang Z, Chen W, et al: The epidemiology and risk factors of inflammatory bowel disease. Int J Clin Exp Med 8(12):22529–22542, 2015 26885239

Yin J, Song J, Lei Y, et al: Prokinetic effects of mirtazapine on gastrointestinal transit. Am J Physiol Gastrointest Liver Physiol 306(9):G796–G801, 2014 24627566

Yoon JY, Shin JE, Park SH, et al: Disability due to inflammatory bowel disease is correlated with drug compliance, disease activity, and quality of life. Gut Liver 11(3):370–376, 2017 28208008

You LQ, Liu J, Jia L, et al: Effect of low-dose amitriptyline on globus pharyngeus and its side effects. World J Gastroenterol 19(42):7455–7460, 2013 24259978

Zaccara G, Franciotta D, Perucca E: Idiosyncratic adverse reactions to antiepileptic drugs. Epilepsia 48(7):1223–1244, 2007 17386054

Zakrzewska J, Buchanan JA: Burning mouth syndrome. BMJ Clin Evid pii:1301, 2016 26745781

CHAPTER 20

Renal Disease

Daniel Cukor, Ph.D.

James L. Levenson, M.D.

Deborah Rosenthal-Asher, Ph.D.

Paul L. Kimmel, M.D.

In this chapter, we cover psychiatric issues in chronic kidney disease (CKD) and end-stage renal disease (ESRD), including comorbid psychiatric disorders, social support, sexual dysfunction, treatment adherence, withdrawal from dialysis, renal psychiatric palliative care, psychotherapy and psychopharmacology (including psychiatric adverse effects of renal drugs), and drug interactions. Renal transplantation is also discussed in Chapter 29, "Organ Transplantation," and Chapter 32, "Pediatrics," and hemodialysis for toxic ingestions is covered in Chapter 35, "Medical Toxicology." Electrolyte disorders are discussed in Chapter 21, "Endocrine and Metabolic Disorders."

As the techniques of dialysis and transplantation have advanced, ESRD patients, including those with more severe illnesses and comorbidities, are living somewhat longer. Given that psychiatric disorders are widely prevalent among dialysis and renal transplant populations, mental health professionals can play a vital role in management, including intervention for mental health difficulties and promotion of compliance, as well as in palliative care for dying patients and those who wish to decline or discontinue dialysis.

Nephrology has recognized the need for psychiatric consultation since the initial development of kidney dialysis in the late 1960s and early 1970s. Nearly universal access to treatment in the United States followed passage of the 1972 End-Stage Renal Disease amendment to the Social Security Act, which provided federal subsidy for dialysis. Subsequently, the ESRD population has steadily grown, aged, and become more severely ill (United States Renal Data System 2016). Psychiatry's potential role in the collaborative care of patients with renal disease is increasing.

Each year, approximately 100,000 Americans develop ESRD and more than 650,000 individuals are treated for ESRD (United States Renal Data System 2016). About

430,000 people are receiving maintenance dialysis, and 200,000 have a functioning kidney transplant. The number of patients starting renal replacement therapy in the United States had been growing by 5%–7% each year but is beginning to level off. In addition to the population with ESRD, an estimated 8 million individuals have earlier-stage CKD (United States Renal Data System 2016). The current annual cost of treating CKD is approximately $50 billion, and the Medicare expenditure is about $27 billion for hemodialysis and $4 billion for transplantation (United States Renal Data System 2016).

The major causes of renal failure are diabetes, hypertension, generalized arteriosclerosis, systemic lupus erythematosus, HIV infection, and primary renal diseases such as chronic glomerulonephritis, chronic interstitial nephritis, polycystic kidney disease, and other hereditary and congenital disorders. Diabetes is now found in almost half of ESRD cases. Patients with diabetes are especially likely to have increased morbidity because of its plethora of microvascular and macrovascular complications (Lea and Nicholas 2002).

Renal transplantation is the treatment of choice for many patients. If a transplant is successful, the patient's survival (United States Renal Data System 2016) and quality of life (Franke et al. 2003; Kimmel and Patel 2006) are improved over what they would have been with maintenance dialysis. A major issue in transplantation is the shortage of donor organs. Transplanted kidneys may come from a living donor or through organ donation following death (long-term kidney survival is greater with living donors). More than two-thirds of kidneys transplanted in 2014 were from deceased donors. As of the end of 2014, the kidney transplant waiting list had nearly 90,000 dialysis patients who were candidates, with 83% awaiting their first transplant (United States Renal Data System 2016). Nearly 18,000 kidney transplants were performed in 2014 (United States Renal Data System 2016).

Peritoneal dialysis and hemodialysis are the two forms of dialysis. In peritoneal dialysis, dialysate fluid is introduced into and then removed from the peritoneal space through an indwelling catheter. The peritoneum serves as a semipermeable membrane, and fluid and wastes are removed together with dialysate. Peritoneal dialysis may be performed by a machine in the home at night (continuous cycling peritoneal dialysis [CCPD]) or manually at home four to six times per day (continuous ambulatory peritoneal dialysis [CAPD]). Only 7% of ESRD patients use peritoneal dialysis as the initial mode of renal replacement therapy (United States Renal Data System 2016). Hemodialysis may be conducted at the patient's home but usually takes place at an outpatient dialysis unit for 3- to 4-hour sessions, typically three times per week. Home dialysis requires the participation of another person, who must be available to assist with 12–15 hours of weekly treatment. Although no studies have used random assignment to dialysis modalities, a study using patient surveys reported that those receiving peritoneal dialysis were more likely than those receiving hemodialysis to rate their care as excellent (Rubin et al. 2004).

Psychiatric Disorders in Renal Disease

In a study of 200,000 adult U.S. dialysis patients, almost 9% had been hospitalized with a comorbid psychiatric diagnosis (Kimmel et al. 1998b). Depression and other

mood disorders were the most common diagnoses, followed by delirium and dementia. In a smaller study in an urban hemodialysis population, roughly 70% of the sample had at least one current DSM-IV (American Psychiatric Association 1994) Axis I diagnosis, as determined by the Structured Clinical Interview for DSM-IV Axis I Disorders (SCID-I) (Cukor et al. 2007). Depression and anxiety were the two most prevalent psychiatric disorders, followed by substance abuse and psychosis. A primary diagnosis of depression was more prevalent in ESRD patients than in patients with ischemic heart disease or cerebrovascular disease (Kimmel et al. 1998b).

Depression

Early studies of depression in ESRD reported prevalence rates ranging from 0% to 100%, reflecting widely variable definitions, criteria, and measurement methods (for a review, see Cukor et al. 2006). In the nephrology literature, there is a lack of clarity regarding the term *depression* and whether it refers to the affective symptom or the psychiatric disorder (Cohen 1996). In addition, the evaluation of depression is complicated by the fact that many of the somatic signs and symptoms of ESRD are very similar to signs of depression. For example, many uremic patients have diminished appetite, loss of energy, poor sleep (Losso et al. 2015), and diminished sexual interest (Kimmel 2002; Kimmel et al. 2007; Meyer and Hostetter 2007).

A variety of techniques have been used to improve the diagnostic accuracy of depression in patients with renal disease. Some ESRD research studies have relied exclusively on self-report instruments to determine symptom severity but have adjusted scoring of the measures to account for somatic complaints (Craven et al. 1988; Kimmel et al. 1993; Smith et al. 1985). Other studies (Cukor et al. 2007; Finkelstein and Finkelstein 2000; Hedayati et al. 2006; Watnick et al. 2003) have combined self-report measures with a structured diagnostic interview based on DSM-IV-TR (American Psychiatric Association 2000) criteria or have used multiple measurement points across time (Boulware et al. 2006; Cukor et al. 2008b; Kimmel et al. 2000). Although there has been much less study of depression in patients with CKD before initiation of dialysis, depression rates appear to be elevated in this population as well (Palmer et al. 2013).

Rigorous studies of depression self-report measures in ESRD patients have assessed these measures against structured diagnostic interviews (e.g., SCID-I) to determine optimal cutoff scores for diagnostic accuracy in ESRD. The Beck Depression Inventory (utilizing a cutoff of 14–15), the Patient Health Questionnaire–9 (PHQ-9) (utilizing scores ≥10), and the Center for Epidemiologic Studies Depression Scale (using scores ≥18) have all been used by studies to estimate the prevalence of major depressive disorder (MDD) in ESRD samples. However, despite their utilization of different instruments, studies have reported similar MDD prevalence rates, 20%–27% (Hedayati et al. 2006, 2009; Kimmel 2001; Kimmel et al. 1996, 1998a, 2000; Watnick et al. 2005).

Depression in patients with ESRD is a strong predictor of worse medical outcomes (Fan et al. 2014; Farrokhi et al. 2014). In a study examining the effect of depression on outcomes (time to death or hospitalization) in dialysis patients, Hedayati et al. (2008) found the diagnosis of MDD to be associated with a hazard ratio of 2.07 compared with nondepressed control subjects, after adjustment for other variables. Kimmel et al. (2000) found that tracking multiple measurements of depression produced a more robust association with mortality than did tracking any single measurement in hemo-

dialysis patients. Similarly, Boulware et al. (2006) demonstrated that associations with outcomes existed with multiple measurements of depression that did not exist with baseline data. Cukor et al. (2008b) reassessed SCID-diagnosed depressed and anxious ESRD patients after 16 months and noted a variety of clinical trajectories. A persistent course of depression was associated with significantly lower quality of life and more reported health problems compared with intermittent depression. These data suggest that a single measure of depression at a specific point in time might not be as meaningful as assessment of depression over a longer time span.

Despite the high prevalence of depression in dialysis patients and frequent prescription of antidepressants, there has been little study of the effectiveness of these medications. A 2016 Cochrane review identified only four small clinical trials examining the efficacy of antidepressant in ESRD patients, and rated the evidence as limited and inconclusive (Palmer et al. 2016). A larger trial of sertraline yielded negative findings (Friedli et al. 2017). The utility of antidepressants may be limited by low acceptance rates among hemodialysis patients (Atalay et al. 2010; Friedli et al. 2017; Pena et al. 2017).

In addition to pharmacotherapy, psychotherapy is an appropriate intervention for depressed ESRD patients, with cognitive-behavioral therapy (CBT) receiving the most scientific attention. Both individual (Cukor et al. 2014) and group psychotherapy interventions (Duarte et al. 2009) have been associated with significant improvement of depression in hemodialysis patients in small-scale randomized trials. Despite the significant challenges of studying depression in ESRD populations, including recruitment, screening, outcome measurement, confounding treatment, and overall low acceptance of interventions (Hackett and Jardine 2017), larger-scale rigorous trials investigating interventions for depression are currently under way (Hedayati et al. 2016).

Anxiety and Posttraumatic Stress Symptoms

Anxiety is a complicating comorbid diagnosis for many medical illnesses and often co-occurs with depression in ESRD populations (Cohen et al. 2016; Cukor et al. 2007, 2008a, 2008b). There is relatively little anxiety research specific to ESRD patients, but it appears that an anxiety diagnosis is associated with diminished quality of life (Cukor et al. 2008a, 2013; Sareen et al. 2006). One early study (Nichols and Springford 1984) found that about one-third of hemodialysis patients experienced episodes of moderate anxiety during their first year of dialysis treatment. In a study that assessed psychiatric diagnoses in a sample of 70 predominately African American ESRD patients, about 45% had at least one anxiety disorder. The most common diagnoses identified were phobias and panic disorder (Cukor et al. 2008a). The prevalence of panic disorder was much higher in ESRD patients than in community samples, a finding that may be related to hypervigilance to bodily sensations associated with hemodialysis or fears about the outcome of ESRD treatment.

Posttraumatic stress symptoms related to dialysis experiences, serious medical events, or other traumas are also common among hemodialysis patients (Tagay et al. 2007). Phobias for needles or the sight of blood are common in the general population (see Chapter 10, "Anxiety Disorders"), and such phobias are among the most frequently reported reasons that hemodialysis patients choose self-care treatment in-

stead of in-center dialysis (McLaughlin et al. 2003). There are no published clinical trials of psychopharmacology or psychotherapy for anxiety in patients with ESRD and very few case reports regarding anxiety in this population (Cohen et al. 2016).

Substance Use Disorders

Substance use disorders, such as cocaine or heroin dependence or chronic overuse of nonsteroidal anti-inflammatory drugs (NSAIDs), can lead to CKD (Jaffe and Kimmel 2006; Norris et al. 2001). Substance use may also result in HIV infection, which can secondarily cause renal failure (Kimmel et al. 2003). In a sample of 145 hemodialysis patients, Hegde et al. (2000) found that 28% had difficulty with chronic alcoholism. Those who abused alcohol had poorer nutrition than nonabusers, as demonstrated by serum albumin measurements (Hegde et al. 2000). Another study found cocaine users to be less compliant with dialysis attendance than nonusers (Obialo et al. 2008). There is a high and variable rate of prescription opioid use in dialysis centers (Wyne et al. 2011), which may be of particular concern in the context of the current opioid epidemic. Chronic opioid prescription was found to be associated with greater risk of death, discontinuation of dialysis, and hospitalization in U.S. dialysis patients (Kimmel et al. 2017). Although additional research is needed regarding substance use disorders and dialysis, substance abuse should be taken seriously and addressed with specialist care.

The Disruptive Dialysis Patient

To function well, dialysis units depend on the ability of their staff to provide appropriate patient care. There has been an increase in the number of reported disruptive patients within dialysis units (Hashmi and Moss 2008), with verbal aggression being the most prevalent behavior (Jones et al. 2014). Disruption on the unit may affect the individual, as in the case of noncompliance with treatment. A patient's disruptive behavior may also affect other patients receiving dialysis therapy. A disruptive patient may harm others by coming late to appointments, thus disrupting dialysis scheduling for others, or by threatening the staff (Hashmi and Moss 2008).

The decision to withhold dialysis treatment from a disruptive patient must be carefully considered. Although all patients should be treated equally and with respect, the welfare of a disruptive patient must be balanced against the welfare of health care personnel and other patients. If disruptive behavior affects only the patient him- or herself, the individual should not be refused dialysis treatment. For example, treatment cannot be denied to a patient who is noncompliant with his or her medical regimen but continues to want dialysis. However, in the case of a disruptive patient who continually shows up late to appointments and does not abide by rules of the unit, moving the individual to a different shift or unit might be considered (Hashmi and Moss 2008). Verbal or physical abuse on the unit should not be tolerated, and the welfare of staff and other patients should not be compromised.

Suggested strategies for dealing with disruptive patients include attempting to first create a calm environment, approaching the patient directly about his or her behavior, using reflective listening techniques to help the patient feel understood, attempting to understand the reasons for the patient's responses and behavior, outlining specific goals the patient can pursue in treatment, educating the patient about consequences that may result from his or her behavior (ideally through a behavioral contract), and making a referral to a skilled team member such as a psychologist or social worker (Goldman 2008; Hashmi and Moss 2008; Sukolsky 2004). Two helpful resources addressing dialysis-related disruptive behavior and conflict resolution are the Renal Physicians Association/American Society of Nephrology's "Clinical Practice Guideline on Shared Decision-Making in the Appropriate Initiation of and Withdrawal From Dialysis" (Galla and The Renal Physicians Association and the American Society of Nephrology 2000) and the Decreasing Dialysis Patient–Provider Conflict (DPC) project (for a review, see Goldman 2008).

Cognitive Disorders

The extent to which CKD represents a unique risk factor for dementia (Deckers et al. 2017) and the cognitive impact of hemodialysis are still unclear (Lin et al. 2015); however, cognitive impairment is prevalent in ESRD (Murray et al. 2006). A recent meta-analysis found that hemodialysis patients perform more poorly across cognitive domains compared with the general population, especially on measurements of orientation and attention (O'Lone et al. 2016). Cognitive impairment has been associated with increased mortality in hemodialysis patients (Drew et al. 2015; Griva et al. 2010), with impairment in cognitive abilities potentially impacting decision making and adherence to treatment (Kurella Tamura and Yaffe 2011).

Cognitive impairment in this population may be related to uremia, various medical comorbidities (e.g., electrolyte disturbances, severe malnutrition, impaired metabolism, cerebrovascular disease), or adverse effects of treatment. Uremia is a clinical syndrome resulting from profound loss of renal function and has been associated with cognitive impairment, including difficulty with concentration, memory, and intellectual functioning (Pliskin et al. 1996; Souheaver et al. 1982; Williams et al. 2004). Signs and symptoms of uremia vary considerably, with severity presumably dependent on both the degree of renal failure and the speed with which renal function is lost. Central nervous system symptoms may begin with mild cognitive dysfunction, fatigue, and headache, progressing to hypoactive delirium and, if untreated, coma. Restless legs syndrome, muscle cramps, and sleep disorders are also common in uremic patients (see Chapter 14, "Sleep Disorders"). Other common symptoms include pruritus, anorexia, nausea, and vomiting (Haddy et al. 2008; Meyer and Hostetter 2007; Weisbord et al. 2003). Anemia is also a potential risk factor for impaired cognitive functioning in those with kidney disease (Pereira et al. 2005). A reduction in oxygen due to anemia may result in impaired cognitive function, especially in individuals with neurological or cerebrovascular diseases (Johnson et al. 1990). Depression itself may also be etiologically related to the cognitive deficits (Dong et al. 2016).

The relationship between degree of cognitive impairment and CKD stage is unclear. Kurella et al. (2004) measured cognitive functioning in 80 CKD patients not receiving dialysis and 80 ESRD patients receiving hemodialysis treatment. The authors found a relationship between stage of CKD and degree of cognitive impairment on measures of mental status, executive functioning, and verbal memory. Another study (Elias et al. 2009) also found an association between CKD severity and presence of cognitive impairment. In this study, CKD patients with lower renal function, as well as those with higher serum creatinine levels, showed performance decrements on measures of visuospatial processing, attention, and planning. More recently, Kurella Tamura et al. (2017) examined dialysis initiation and cognitive functioning in 212 patients with advanced CKD. Although there was no change in global cognitive functioning, the study found an association between dialysis initiation and reduced performance on tests of executive functioning. Additionally, patients with advanced CKD who transitioned to dialysis demonstrated poorer executive functioning compared with those who did not initiate dialysis. This study raises the possibility that dialysis treatment itself may negatively affect executive functioning.

Dementia has been identified as a mortality risk factor in ESRD. Hypertension and diabetes, both highly prevalent among ESRD patients, are risk factors for the development of dementia (Saczynski et al. 2008; Semplicini et al. 2006). One large study of hemodialysis patients (Kurella et al. 2006) found a dementia prevalence of 4% in the overall sample. Compared with those without dementia, patients diagnosed with dementia had a higher risk of death (relative risk (RR)=1.48; 95% confidence interval (CI)=1.32–1.66) and were twice as likely (RR=2.01; 95% CI=1.57–2.57) to withdraw from dialysis treatment. Consistent with findings in the general population, older age, black race, lower education, and presence of diabetes or cerebrovascular disease were found to be related to dementia risk in ESRD patients.

Maintaining an optimal level of cognitive function is important for quality of life and is a prerequisite for successful adaptation to dialysis. Further studies are needed to help elucidate the relationships among CKD, dialysis, and cognitive functioning in order to identify and minimize risk factors and develop management and intervention techniques to help decrease the impact cognitive impairment has on this population.

Social Support

ESRD patients can receive social support from family, friends, and individuals on the dialysis unit (e.g., physicians, social workers, nurses, other patients). Increased levels of social support may positively influence outcomes through various mechanisms, including decreased depression, increased patient perception of quality of life, increased access to health care, increased patient adherence to prescribed therapies, and beneficial physiological effects on the immune system (Cohen et al. 2007b). Higher levels of perceived social support are thought to have a positive influence on health outcomes, utilization of health care services, and treatment compliance. Previous research has demonstrated that social support is related to improved health outcomes and lower mortality in ESRD patients (Cohen et al. 2007b; Kimmel et al. 1998a; Untas et al. 2011).

Sexual Dysfunction

The impact of hemodialysis on both male and female sexual functioning is well documented (Levy and Cohen 2001) but often not discussed with patients. One study found that 43% of ESRD patients reported having a decreased interest in sex, and 47% reported trouble getting aroused (Abdel-Kader et al. 2009). Data show that women with ESRD often have decreased sexual desire but do not necessarily identify it as sexual dysfunction (Mor et al. 2014). A meta-analysis found that depression, older age, and diabetes were consistently associated with higher levels of sexual dysfunction (Navaneethan et al. 2010). The relative roles of physical dysfunction, medical illness, medication effects, and psychological function in inducing sexual dysfunction in CKD patients have not been determined. The first line of treatment for erectile dysfunction is typically sildenafil, which appears to be safe in ESRD patients who do not have contraindications to treatment (Palmer 2003), as well as effective (Turk et al. 2010). (See also Chapter 15, "Sexual Dysfunctions.")

Treatment Adherence

Clinical and behavioral indices of adherence in dialysis patients include dialysis attendance, interdialytic weight gain, and medication adherence. Lack of adherence to treatment regimens is believed to be a common cause of inadequate dialysis and poor outcome (Kaveh and Kimmel 2001). Many factors may contribute to nonadherence, including depression, anxiety, cognitive dysfunction, personality traits, the doctor–patient relationship, and financial difficulties. The rate of nonadherence among dialysis patients varies by country as well (Bleyer et al. 1999; Hecking et al. 2004). Common noncompliant behaviors include shortening or missing dialysis sessions and engaging in dietary and medication indiscretions. According to self-reports, 12% of dialysis patients miss one peritoneal dialysis exchange per week, and 5% skip two to three exchanges per week (United States Renal Data System 2016). To maintain optimal health, ESRD patients must adhere to their prescribed treatments. Patients are prescribed regimens for their medications, diet, fluid intake, exercise, medical appointments, and dialysis attendance. Measures of behavioral compliance are clinically meaningful and associated with hard outcomes (Kimmel et al. 1995, 1998a; Leggat 2005). A study that examined medication adherence in ESRD found that 37% of hemodialysis patients reported less-than-perfect adherence to the medication regimen and that increased depressive affect was associated with decreased medication adherence (Cukor et al. 2009). Because adherence was self-reported, the data may be an overestimation of the actual level of adherence, demonstrating the great need for addressing this issue in this population. Similarly, a study looking at 286 patients found depressive symptoms to be associated with missing and shortening dialysis treatment sessions (Weisbord et al. 2014). Another study found that the median daily pill burden of an ESRD cohort was 19. In one-quarter of subjects, it exceeded 25 pills per day. Phosphate binders accounted for about one-half of the daily pill burden, and 62% of the participants were noncompliant with the prescribed phosphate binder therapy (Chiu et al. 2009). A systematic review of studies of adherence to prescribed oral medications in adult chronic hemodialysis patients found that more than half of the included studies reported nonadherence rates of 50% or more, with a mean of 67% (Schmid et al. 2009).

A variety of interventions targeting adherence in ESRD have been studied. Some of these interventions are educational in nature, attempting to increase knowledge of the importance of adherence and the consequences of noncompliance. However, the efficacy of educational interventions that target adherence is questionable. One study found that the hemodialysis patients who demonstrated better knowledge about the importance of monitoring phosphorus levels in their dietary regimens were *less* compliant, as measured by biomarkers and interdialytic weight gain (Durose et al. 2004). Other interventions have included CBT, motivational interviewing, relaxation training, social skills training, self-monitoring, and behavioral reinforcement to increase adherence (Nozaki et al. 2005; Sharp et al. 2005b; Tsay et al. 2005). A small randomized controlled trial of CBT demonstrated an increase in fluid adherence (as measured by interdialytic weight gain) at 10 weeks postbaseline (Sharp et al. 2005a). Another small study (Christensen et al. 2002) compared levels of adherence in hemodialysis patients who participated in a 7-week behavioral self-regulation intervention and matched control hemodialysis patients. The study showed that the intervention patients had higher adherence (as measured by interdialytic weight gain) 8 weeks after completing the intervention compared with the control patients. A more recent similar study did not demonstrate improvement in the behavioral self-regulation group over a placebo support control condition (Howren et al. 2016). A pilot study designed to improve immunosuppressant medication adherence in kidney transplant recipients that utilized a brief intervention based on motivational interviewing and CBT also demonstrated efficacy (Cukor et al. 2017). In a study that was targeting depression (Cukor et al. 2014), patients receiving CBT showed improvements in mood as well as in fluid compliance (as measured by interdialytic weight gain). These studies suggest the potential value of implementing interventions to target adherence, but the studies to date have been small and of short duration and have had bias-prone study designs (Sharp et al. 2005b).

Withdrawal From Dialysis

Withdrawal from dialysis can be viewed as part of the life cycle of the ESRD patient and part of the dying process. In the United States, dialysis withdrawal has been more common among women and older patients and less common among African American and Asian patients, with significant regional variation (Gessert et al. 2013; Kurella Tamura et al. 2010; Munshi et al. 2001). Cognitive impairment has also been associated with the decision to withdraw (Chater et al. 2006). Patients who begin dialysis with high depression scores are more likely to withdraw within the first year of treatment (Lacson et al. 2012).

The topic of dialysis withdrawal is commonly approached in the assessment of patient quality of life versus quantity of life (Hackett and Watnick 2007). Reasons for the decisions of individuals who choose not to initiate or continue dialysis have included concerns about being a burden to family members and mistrust of medical treatment (Ashby et al. 2005). However, withdrawal from dialysis may often be appropriate for a dialysis patient who is failing to thrive or is suffering. Many patients and families choose this option because it allows for a quicker death and the end of suffering (Cohen and Germain 2005; Cohen et al. 2003). The median time to death after stopping dialysis is 7–8 days (O'Connor et al. 2013), and dialysis termination usually does not cause pain or discomfort (Cohen et al. 2000). Withdrawal typically results in lethargy progressing to coma and death. Psychiatrists can assist with determinations of patient capacity and the potential influence of depression or other psychosocial factors. One study that controlled for biomarkers and age found depression to be a unique predictor of withdrawal from dialysis treatment (McDade-Montez et al. 2006). The decision to withdraw from dialysis is complex, and a patient's decision to discontinue does not necessarily constitute suicide. Ideally, the decision should be made when the patient is not in the midst of severe depression, so that the appropriate course is clear (Russ et al. 2007).

Renal Palliative Care

With the goal of providing better end-of-life care for this very ill population, Cohen et al. (2005) have advocated that attention be focused on the following issues:

1. *Early frank discussions concerning prognosis and goals of care*—Ideally, these discussions should include the family and should begin when options for care are discussed. The possibility of not starting dialysis, especially if the burdens of dialysis might outweigh the benefits, should be considered. Patients should also know that they have the option of stopping dialysis if their quality of life diminishes. Written advance directives can help focus the discussion, and do-not-resuscitate orders should be strongly considered when cardiopulmonary resuscitation is likely to be futile (Moss 2000).
2. *Attention to symptoms at all stages of the disease process*—Patients with ESRD have a high burden of symptoms related to dialysis and their comorbid conditions (Cohen and Germain 2005; Weisbord et al. 2008).
3. *Early hospice referrals*—Such referrals can take place in the hospital, home, nursing home, or inpatient hospice unit. All patients who terminate dialysis should be offered referral to hospice.
4. *Maximal palliative care at the end of life*—This care includes aggressive pain control, spiritual and emotional support, and attention to the patient's terminal treatment preferences and goals. Utmost sensitivity is needed in making decisions about withholding or discontinuing care, attending to cultural biases, countertransference, and other complicating factors (Moss 1998, 2000).

Newer models of renal palliative care emphasize integration of dialysis and hospice services (Moss 2017) and specialized training in end-of-life issues for nephrologists (Bristowe et al. 2014). There has also been recent acknowledgment of the systemic barriers in place that prevent adequate renal palliative care from reaching all patients (Grubbs et al. 2014; Tamura and Meier 2013). While the logistics of the incorporation of palliative care vary widely across medical settings, the psychiatrist is often an integral member of the team required to initiate, develop, and then execute a care plan.

Psychopharmacology in Renal Disease

Antidepressants

Among the selective serotonin reuptake inhibitors (SSRIs), citalopram, escitalopram, and sertraline would be expected to have the fewest potential interactions with other medications taken by patients with renal impairment. Paroxetine clearance is reduced in patients with renal insufficiency (Doyle et al. 1989). Some evidence suggests that dosage adjustments may not be needed for citalopram (Spigset et al. 2000) and fluox-etine (Finkelstein and Finkelstein 2000) in patients with renal insufficiency.

While the longest experience has been with the tricyclic antidepressants (TCAs), ESRD patients, especially those with diabetes, are often more sensitive to their side effects. Hydroxylated metabolites of TCAs may be markedly elevated in patients with ESRD and responsible for some TCA side effects. Nortriptyline and desipramine are the preferred TCAs in renal failure because they are less likely to cause anticho-linergic effects or orthostatic hypotension than other TCAs (Gillman 2007).

Limited data are available on the use of newer antidepressants in patients with re-nal failure. The half-life of venlafaxine is prolonged in renal insufficiency; its clearance is reduced by over 50% in patients undergoing dialysis (Troy et al. 1994). Desvenla-faxine undergoes significant renal elimination, so dosage reduction is required in moderate to severe renal impairment. Because antidepressants are typically metabo-lized by the liver and those metabolites are excreted by the kidney, it seems prudent to initially reduce the dose for all antidepressants to minimize the potential accumu-lation of active metabolites (Cohen et al. 2007a). However, ordinary dosages are fre-quently required in ESRD patients and are usually well tolerated (Dev et al. 2014).

A recent, well-designed randomized controlled trial by Hedayati et al. (2017) com-pared the SSRI sertraline against placebo in the pharmacological treatment of de-pressed patients with CKD but not ESRD. Despite having a high rate of medication adherence and no greater than usual amounts of side effects, patients treated with ser-traline had no detectable differences in outcome compared with patients treated with placebo. The reason for this surprising finding may have to do with the role of the pla-cebo effect in behavioral trials (Walther et al. 2017), or it may be related to the overall moderate level of depression in the study sample and the questionable utility of SSRIs for mild to moderate depression (Cukor and Kimmel 2018).

Antipsychotics

Antipsychotics typically do not depend on renal elimination, with the exception of paliperidone, which is largely excreted unchanged in urine and thus requires dosage reduction in patients with renal insufficiency (Vermeir et al. 2008). As with TCAs, ad-verse effects of antipsychotics may be amplified by medical comorbidities such as diabetes, hyperlipidemia, and cerebrovascular disease in ESRD patients.

Anxiolytics and Sedative-Hypnotics

No clinical trials of pharmacotherapy for anxiety in ESRD patients have been pub-lished. The preferred benzodiazepines are those with inactive metabolites (e.g., loraz-epam, oxazepam). Even so, the half-lives of lorazepam and oxazepam may rise signif-icantly in patients with ESRD, and dosage reduction may be required. Other benzo-diazepines with inactive metabolites include clonazepam and temazepam, but less is known about changes in their half-lives in ESRD. SSRIs are typically the first line of treatment for anxiety in ESRD patients, particularly given the high comorbidity of de-pression (Cohen et al. 2016).

Mood Stabilizers

Lithium is almost entirely excreted by the kidneys. It is contraindicated in patients with acute renal failure. Some clinicians consider lithium to be relatively contraindicated in patients with stable renal insufficiency. If used, lithium should be conservatively dosed while monitoring renal function frequently. Despite these cautions and lithium's possible nephrotoxicity (discussed under "Renal Effects of Psychotropics" later in this chapter), there are some bipolar patients who do not respond to or tolerate the alternative mood stabilizers. For these patients, lithium is the only effective drug. Lithium is completely dialyzed and may be given safely as a single oral dose (300–600 mg) following hemodialysis treatment. Lithium levels should not be checked until at least 2–3 hours after dialysis because re-equilibration from tissue stores occurs in the immediate postdialysis period. The dose of gabapentin, pregabalin, lithium, and topiramate should be modified on the basis of creatinine clearance (Levenson and Owen 2017).

Cholinesterase Inhibitors and Memantine

While the data are limited, dosage adjustment of donepezil and rivastigmine is probably unnecessary. Galantamine should be used cautiously in patients with moderate renal insufficiency and is not recommended in patients with severe renal insufficiency. Memantine requires dosage reduction in patients with severe renal insufficiency (Levenson and Owen 2017).

Dopamine Agonists for Restless Legs Syndrome

Dopaminergic therapy (i.e., levodopa or the dopamine receptor agonists pramipexole, ropinirole, and rotigotine) has been recommended as first-line treatment for restless legs syndrome, based on studies in the general population. However, data supporting use of dopamine agonists in individuals with ESRD are very limited, as are data for alternative therapies (e.g., gabapentin, clonazepam, opioids) (Gopaluni et al. 2016).

Renal Effects of Psychotropics

The syndrome of inappropriate antidiuretic hormone secretion (SIADH), resulting in hyponatremia, may be caused by many psychotropic drugs, especially carbamazepine and oxcarbazepine, but also SSRIs, TCAs, and antipsychotics. Hypernatremia due to nephrogenic diabetes insipidus (NDI) may be caused by lithium through inhibition of renal tubular water reabsorption. Most patients receiving lithium have polydipsia and polyuria, reflecting NDI. Adverse effects of lithium-induced NDI vary from mild polyuria to hyperosmolar coma. Amiloride is considered the treatment of choice for lithium-induced NDI, but NDI also has been treated with NSAIDs, thiazides, and sodium restriction (Grünfeld and Rossier 2009).

    The effect of lithium on renal function is controversial, with variable results from recent retrospective and cohort studies (for a review, see Levenson and Owen 2017). Progression to ESRD in patients taking lithium is rare (0.2%–0.7%) and typically requires use for many years (Presne et al. 2003). One meta-analysis concluded that any lithium-induced effect on renal function is quantitatively small and probably clinically insignificant (Paul et al. 2009). A population-based study in Sweden found that renal failure was rare but did occur in patients being treated with lithium (Bendz et al. 2010). However, a larger nationwide Danish study found that maintenance treatment with lithium was associated with an increased rate of CKD, but not an increased rate of ESRD (Kessing et al. 2015). The authors concluded that associations between use of lithium and CKD may be at least partly attributable to bias. Other factors besides lithium use that may contribute to such changes include age, episodes of lithium toxicity, other medications (NSAIDs, substance abuse), and the presence of comorbid disorders (e.g., hypertension, diabetes). Lithium nephrotoxicity is not strongly dose related (Freeman and Freeman 2006). Other psychiatric drugs have not been reported to be associated with kidney injury, except for one recent retrospective study that found moderate (but small absolute) increased risks of acute kidney injury with some, but not all, antipsychotics, with greater risk with atypical than typical antipsychotics (Jiang et al. 2017).

Urological Effects of Psychotropics

Drugs with significant anticholinergic activity, such as TCAs and antipsychotics (both low-potency typical agents and atypical agents), frequently cause urinary retention. Less commonly, urinary retention has been reported to occur with SSRIs, serotonin–norepinephrine reuptake inhibitors, and bupropion. Urinary incontinence and other lower-urinary-tract side effects are very common with clozapine (Jeong et al. 2008). Sexual side effects of psychotropic drugs are reviewed in Chapter 15, "Sexual Dysfunctions."

Psychiatric Adverse Effects of Renal and Urological Agents

Anticholinergic agents commonly used to treat overactive bladder are associated with psychiatric adverse effects, including cognitive impairment, confusion, fatigue and psychosis. Cumulative use of strong anticholinergics, including bladder antimuscarinics, is associated with an increase in incident dementia (Gray et al. 2015). Thiazide diuretics are a common cause of hyponatremia, which when severe can cause lethargy, stupor, confusion, psychosis, irritability, and seizures. The risk may be increased further if the patient is also taking a psychotropic drug that causes hyponatremia, such as an SSRI or carbamazepine. Psychiatric adverse effects of other medications frequently used to treat patients with renal disease are covered elsewhere in this book—corticosteroids for autoimmune nephritis (Chapter 24, "Rheumatology"), antihypertensives (Chapter 17, "Heart Disease"), and immunosuppressants after renal transplantation (Chapter 29, "Organ Transplantation").

Drug–Drug Interactions

A number of pharmacodynamic and pharmacokinetic drug interactions frequently occur between drugs prescribed for renal and urological disorders and psychotropic drugs. Anticholinergic side effects may be increased if anticholinergic psychotropic drugs are given to patients taking urinary antispasmodics. Like other anticholinergics, antispasmodics may block the benefits of cholinesterase inhibitors. As noted in the previous section, the hyponatremic effects of thiazide diuretics may be enhanced in combination with oxcarbazepine and carbamazepine, and to a lesser degree with SSRIs, TCAs, and antipsychotics.

Diuretics variably affect lithium excretion, depending on the type of diuretic and the volume status of the patient. Thiazide diuretics may reduce lithium excretion, resulting in increased lithium levels. Acute administration of loop diuretics (e.g., furosemide, ethacrynic acid, bumetanide) increases lithium excretion, causing a drop in lithium levels, but with chronic use, compensatory changes leave lithium levels somewhat unpredictable but usually not significantly changed. Carbonic anhydrase inhibitors (e.g., acetazolamide) and osmotic diuretics (e.g., mannitol) reduce lithium levels (Levenson and Owen 2017). Potassium-sparing diuretics (e.g., amiloride, triamterene, spironolactone) may increase lithium excretion. Furosemide and amiloride are considered to have the least effects on lithium excretion (Levenson and Owen 2017).

Conclusion

The psychosocial needs of the renal patient are becoming more clearly defined and valued by Centers for Medicare & Medicaid Services guidelines and dialysis care teams. The psychiatric presentation of patients with chronic kidney disease and end-stage renal disease are varied, but depression and anxiety seem to be paramount. More research is needed to identify safe and efficacious treatments in this population and to examine possible confluent mechanisms in patients with comorbid psychiatric difficulty and renal dysfunction. Kidney patients, especially in the advanced stages of the disease, are particularly susceptible to isolation and sexual dysfunction, conditions not often discussed with the medical team. There are multilayered reasons why some kidney patients are nonadherent to treatment recommendations and consider withdrawal from dialysis, and a thorough understanding of the biopsychosocial universe of the patient is often necessary to understand their behavior. The psychiatrist should be an integral member of the treatment team.

References

Abdel-Kader K, Unruh ML, Weisbord SD: Symptom burden, depression, and quality of life in chronic and end-stage kidney disease. Clin J Am Soc Nephrol 4(6):1057–1064, 2009 19423570

American Psychiatric Association: Diagnostic and Statistical Manual of Mental Disorders, 4th Edition, Revised. Washington, DC, American Psychiatric Association, 1994

American Psychiatric Association: Diagnostic and Statistical Manual of Mental Disorders, 4th Edition, Text Revision. Washington, DC, American Psychiatric Association, 2000

Ashby M, op't Hoog C, Kellehear A, et al: Renal dialysis abatement: lessons from a social study. Palliat Med 19(5):389–396, 2005 16111062

Atalay H, Solak Y, Biyik M, et al: Sertraline treatment is associated with an improvement in depression and health-related quality of life in chronic peritoneal dialysis patients. Int Urol Nephrol 42(2):527–536, 2010 19953347

Bendz H, Schön S, Attman PO, et al: Renal failure occurs in chronic lithium treatment but is uncommon. Kidney Int 77(3):219–224, 2010 19940841

Bleyer AJ, Hylander B, Sudo H, et al: An international study of patient compliance with hemodialysis. JAMA 281(13):1211–1213, 1999 10199431

Bristowe K, Shepherd K, Bryan L, et al: The development and piloting of the REnal specific Advanced Communication Training (REACT) programme to improve Advance Care Planning for renal patients. Palliat Med 28(4):360–366, 2014 24201135

Boulware LE, Liu Y, Fink NE, et al: Temporal relation among depression symptoms, cardiovascular disease events, and mortality in end-stage renal disease: contribution of reverse causality. Clin J Am Soc Nephrol 1(3):496–504, 2006 17699251

Chater S, Davison SN, Germain MJ, et al: Withdrawal from dialysis: a palliative care perspective. Clin Nephrol 66(5):364–372, 2006 17140166

Chiu YW, Teitelbaum I, Misra M, et al: Pill burden, adherence, hyperphosphatemia, and quality of life in maintenance dialysis patients. Clin J Am Soc Nephrol 4(6):1089–1096, 2009 19423571

Christensen AJ, Moran PJ, Wiebe JS, et al: Effect of a behavioral self-regulation intervention on patient adherence in hemodialysis. Health Psychol 21(4):393–397, 2002 12090682

Cohen L: Renal disease (Chapter 25: Internal Medicine and Medical Subspecialties), in The American Psychiatric Press Textbook of Consultation-Liaison Psychiatry. Edited by Rundell JR, Wise MG. Washington, DC, American Psychiatric Press, 1996, pp 573–578

Cohen LM, Germain MJ: The psychiatric landscape of withdrawal. Semin Dial 18(2):147–153, 2005 15771660

Cohen LM, Germain M, Poppel DM, et al: Dialysis discontinuation and palliative care. Am J Kidney Dis 36(1):140–144, 2000 10873883

Cohen LM, Germain MJ, Poppel DM: Practical considerations in dialysis withdrawal: "to have that option is a blessing." JAMA 289(16):2113–2119, 2003 12709469

Cohen LM, Levy NB, Tessier EG, et al: Renal disease, in The American Psychiatric Publishing Textbook of Psychosomatic Medicine. Edited by Levenson JL. Washington, DC, American Psychiatric Publishing, 2005, pp 483–493

Cohen SD, Norris L, Acquaviva K, et al: Screening, diagnosis, and treatment of depression in patients with end-stage renal disease. Clin J Am Soc Nephrol 2(6):1332–1342, 2007a 17942763

Cohen SD, Sharma T, Acquaviva K, et al: Social support and chronic kidney disease: an update. Adv Chronic Kidney Dis 14(4):335–344, 2007b 17904500

Cohen SD, Cukor D, Kimmel PL: Anxiety in patients treated with hemodialysis. Clin J Am Soc Nephrol 11(12):2250–2255, 2016 27660303

Craven JL, Rodin GM, Littlefield C: The Beck Depression Inventory as a screening device for major depression in renal dialysis patients. Int J Psychiatry Med 18(4):365–374, 1988 3235282

Cukor D, Kimmel PL: Treatment of depression in CKD patients with an SSRI: why things don't always turn out as you expect. Clin J Am Soc Nephrol April 13, 2018 [Epub ahead of print] 29653958

Cukor D, Peterson RA, Cohen SD, et al: Depression in end-stage renal disease hemodialysis patients. Nat Clin Pract Nephrol 2(12):678–687, 2006 17124525

Cukor D, Coplan J, Brown C, et al: Depression and anxiety in urban hemodialysis patients. Clin J Am Soc Nephrol 2(3):484–490, 2007 17699455

Cukor D, Coplan J, Brown C, et al: Anxiety disorders in adults treated by hemodialysis: a single-center study. Am J Kidney Dis 52(1):128–136, 2008a 18440682

Cukor D, Coplan J, Brown C, et al: Course of depression and anxiety diagnosis in patients treated with hemodialysis: a 16-month follow-up. Clin J Am Soc Nephrol 3(6):1752–1758, 2008b 18684897

Cukor D, Rosenthal DS, Jindal RM, et al: Depression is an important contributor to low medication adherence in hemodialyzed patients and transplant recipients. Kidney Int 75(11):1223–1229, 2009 19242502

Cukor D, Ver Halen N, Fruchter Y: Anxiety and quality of life in ESRD. Semin Dial 26(3):265–268, 2013 23432416

Cukor D, Ver Halen N, Asher DR, et al: Psychosocial intervention improves depression, quality of life, and fluid adherence in hemodialysis. J Am Soc Nephrol 25(1):196–206, 2014 24115478

Cukor D, Ver Halen N, Pencille M, et al: A pilot randomized controlled trial to promote immunosuppressant adherence in adult kidney transplant recipients. Nephron 135(1):6–14, 2017 28049201

Deckers K, Camerino I, van Boxtel MP, et al: Dementia risk in renal dysfunction: a systematic review and meta-analysis of prospective studies. Neurology 88(2):198–208, 2017 27974647

Dev V, Dixon SN, Fleet JL, et al: Higher anti-depressant dose and major adverse outcomes in moderate chronic kidney disease: a retrospective population-based study. BMC Nephrol 15:79, 2014 24884589

Dong J, Pi HC, Xiong ZY, et al: Depression and cognitive impairment in peritoneal dialysis: a multicenter cross-sectional study. Am J Kidney Dis 67(1):111–118, 2016 26255306

Doyle GD, Laher M, Kelly JG, et al: The pharmacokinetics of paroxetine in renal impairment. Acta Psychiatr Scand Suppl 350:89–90, 1989 2530798

Drew DA, Weiner DE, Tighiouart H, et al: Cognitive function and all-cause mortality in maintenance hemodialysis patients. Am J Kidney Dis 65(2):303–311, 2015 25240262

Duarte PS, Miyazaki MC, Blay SL, et al: Cognitive-behavioral group therapy is an effective treatment for major depression in hemodialysis patients. Kidney Int 76(4):414–421, 2009 19455196

Durose CL, Holdsworth M, Watson V, et al: Knowledge of dietary restrictions and the medical consequences of noncompliance by patients on hemodialysis are not predictive of dietary compliance. J Am Diet Assoc 104(1):35–41, 2004 14702581

Elias MF, Elias PK, Seliger SL, et al: Chronic kidney disease, creatinine and cognitive functioning. Nephrol Dial Transplant 24(8):2446–2452, 2009 19297357

Fan L, Sarnak MJ, Tighiouart H, et al: Depression and all-cause mortality in hemodialysis patients. Am J Nephrol 40(1):12–18, 2014 24969267

Farrokhi F, Abedi N, Beyene J, et al: Association between depression and mortality in patients receiving long-term dialysis: a systematic review and meta-analysis. Am J Kidney Dis 63(4):623–635, 2014 24183836

Finkelstein FO, Finkelstein SH: Depression in chronic dialysis patients: assessment and treatment. Nephrol Dial Transplant 15(12):1911–1913, 2000 11096130

Franke GH, Reimer J, Philipp T, et al: Aspects of quality of life through end-stage renal disease. Qual Life Res 12(2):103–115, 2003 12639058

Freeman MP, Freeman SA: Lithium: clinical considerations in internal medicine. Am J Med 119(6):478–481, 2006 16750958

Friedli K, Guirguis A, Almond M, et al: Sertraline versus placebo in patients with major depressive disorder undergoing hemodialysis: a randomized, controlled feasibility trial. Clin J Am Soc Nephrol 12(2):280–286, 2017 28126706

Galla JH; The Renal Physicians Association and the American Society of Nephrology: Clinical practice guideline on shared decision-making in the appropriate initiation of and withdrawal from dialysis. J Am Soc Nephrol 11(7):1340–1342, 2000 10864592

Gessert CE, Haller IV, Johnson BP: Regional variation in care at the end of life: discontinuation of dialysis. BMC Geriatr 13:39, 2013 23635315

Gillman PK: Tricyclic antidepressant pharmacology and therapeutic drug interactions updated. Br J Pharmacol 151(6):737–748, 2007 17471183

Goldman RS: Medical director responsibilities regarding disruptive behavior in the dialysis center—leading effective conflict resolution. Semin Dial 21(3):245–249, 2008 18533968

Gopaluni S, Sherif M, Ahmadouk NA: Interventions for chronic kidney disease-associated restless legs syndrome. Cochrane Database Syst Rev (11):CD010690, 2016 27819409

Gray SL, Anderson ML, Dublin S, et al: Cumulative use of strong anticholinergics and incident dementia: a prospective cohort study. JAMA Intern Med 175(3):401–407, 2015 25621434

Griva K, Stygall J, Hankins M, et al: Cognitive impairment and 7-year mortality in dialysis patients. Am J Kidney Dis 56(4):693–703, 2010 20800327

Grubbs V, Moss AH, Cohen LM, et al; Dialysis Advisory Group of the American Society of Nephrology: A palliative approach to dialysis care: a patient-centered transition to the end of life. J Am Soc Nephrol 9(12):2203–2209, 2014 25104274

Grünfeld JP, Rossier BC: Lithium nephrotoxicity revisited. Nat Rev Nephrol 5(5):270–276, 2009 19384328

Hackett AS, Jardine MJ: We need to talk about depression and dialysis: but what questions should we ask, and does anyone know the answers? Clin J Am Soc Nephrol 12(2):222–224, 2017 28126705

Hackett AS, Watnick SG: Withdrawal from dialysis in end-stage renal disease: medical, social, and psychological issues. Semin Dial 20(1):86–90, 2007 17244129

Haddy FJ, Meyer TW, Hostetter TH: Uremia. N Engl J Med 358(1):95, author reply 95, 2008 18172186

Hashmi A, Moss AH: Treating difficult or disruptive dialysis patients: practical strategies based on ethical principles. Nat Clin Pract Nephrol 4(9):515–520, 2008 18612329

Hecking E, Bragg-Gresham JL, Rayner HC, et al: Haemodialysis prescription, adherence and nutritional indicators in five European countries: results from the Dialysis Outcomes and Practice Patterns Study (DOPPS). Nephrol Dial Transplant 19(1):100–107, 2004 14671045

Hedayati SS, Bosworth HB, Kuchibhatla M, et al: The predictive value of self-report scales compared with physician diagnosis of depression in hemodialysis patients. Kidney Int 69(9):1662–1668, 2006 16598203

Hedayati SS, Bosworth HB, Briley LP, et al: Death or hospitalization of patients on chronic hemodialysis is associated with a physician-based diagnosis of depression. Kidney Int 74(7):930–936, 2008 18580856

Hedayati SS, Minhajuddin AT, Toto RD, et al: Prevalence of major depressive episode in CKD. Am J Kidney Dis 54(3):424–432, 2009 19493599

Hedayati SS, Daniel DM, Cohen S, et al: Rationale and design of a trial of sertraline vs. cognitive behavioral therapy for end-stage renal disease patients with depression (ASCEND). Contemp Clin Trials 47:1–11, 2016 26621218

Hedayati SS, Gregg LP, Carmody T, et al: Effect of sertraline on depressive symptoms in patients with chronic kidney disease without dialysis dependence: the CAST randomized clinical trial. JAMA 318(19):1876–1890, 2017 29101402

Hegde A, Veis JH, Seidman A, et al: High prevalence of alcoholism in dialysis patients. Am J Kidney Dis 35(6):1039–1043, 2000 10845814

Howren MB, Kellerman QD, Hillis SL, et al: Effect of a behavioral self-regulation intervention on patient adherence to fluid-intake restrictions in hemodialysis: a randomized controlled trial. Ann Behav Med 50(2):167–176, 2016 26631085

Jaffe JA, Kimmel PL: Chronic nephropathies of cocaine and heroin abuse: a critical review. Clin J Am Soc Nephrol 1(4):655–667, 2006 17699270

Jeong SH, Kim JH, Ahn YM, et al: A 2-year prospective follow-up study of lower urinary tract symptoms in patients treated with clozapine. J Clin Psychopharmacol 28(6):618–624, 2008 19011429

Jiang Y, McCombs JS, Park SH: A retrospective cohort study of acute kidney injury risk associated with antipsychotics. CNS Drugs 31(4):319–326, 2017 28290080

Johnson WJ, McCarthy JT, Yanagihara T, et al: Effects of recombinant human erythropoietin on cerebral and cutaneous blood flow and on blood coagulability. Kidney Int 38(5):919–924, 1990 2266676

Jones J, Nijman H, Ross J, et al: Aggression on haemodialysis units: a mixed method study. J Ren Care 40(3):180–193, 2014 25042357

Kaveh K, Kimmel PL: Compliance in hemodialysis patients: multidimensional measures in search of a gold standard. Am J Kidney Dis 37(2):244–266, 2001 11157365

Kessing LV, Gerds TA, Feldt-Rasmussen B, et al: Use of lithium and anticonvulsants and the rate of chronic kidney disease: a nationwide population-based study. JAMA Psychiatry 72(12):1182–1191, 2015 26535805

Kimmel PL: Psychosocial factors in dialysis patients. Kidney Int 59(4):1599–1613, 2001 11260433

Kimmel PL: Depression in patients with chronic renal disease: what we know and what we need to know. J Psychosom Res 53(4):951–956, 2002 12377308

Kimmel PL, Patel SS: Quality of life in patients with chronic kidney disease: focus on end-stage renal disease treated with hemodialysis. Semin Nephrol 26(1):68–79, 2006 16412831

Kimmel PL, Weihs K, Peterson RA: Survival in hemodialysis patients: the role of depression. J Am Soc Nephrol 4(1):12–27, 1993 8400064

Kimmel PL, Peterson RA, Weihs KL, et al: Behavioral compliance with dialysis prescription in hemodialysis patients. J Am Soc Nephrol 5(10):1826–1834, 1995 7787151

Kimmel PL, Peterson RA, Weihs KL, et al: Psychologic functioning, quality of life, and behavioral compliance in patients beginning hemodialysis. J Am Soc Nephrol 7(10):2152–2159, 1996 8915975

Kimmel PL, Peterson RA, Weihs KL, et al: Psychosocial factors, behavioral compliance and survival in urban hemodialysis patients. Kidney Int 54(1):245–254, 1998a 9648085

Kimmel PL, Thamer M, Richard CM, et al: Psychiatric illness in patients with end-stage renal disease. Am J Med 105(3):214–221, 1998b 9753024

Kimmel PL, Peterson RA, Weihs KL, et al: Multiple measurements of depression predict mortality in a longitudinal study of chronic hemodialysis outpatients. Kidney Int 57(5):2093–2098, 2000 10792629

Kimmel PL, Barisoni L, Kopp JB: Pathogenesis and treatment of HIV-associated renal diseases: lessons from clinical and animal studies, molecular pathologic correlations, and genetic investigations. Ann Intern Med 139(3):214–226, 2003 12899589

Kimmel PL, Cukor D, Cohen SD, et al: Depression in end-stage renal disease patients: a critical review. Adv Chronic Kidney Dis 14(4):328–334, 2007 17904499

Kimmel PL, Fwu C, Abbot KC, et al: Opioid prescription, morbidity, and mortality of United States dialysis patients. J Am Soc Nephrol 28(12):3658–3670, 2017 28935654

Kurella M, Chertow GM, Luan J, et al: Cognitive impairment in chronic kidney disease. J Am Geriatr Soc 52(11):1863–1869, 2004 15507063

Kurella M, Mapes DL, Port FK, et al: Correlates and outcomes of dementia among dialysis patients: the Dialysis Outcomes and Practice Patterns Study. Nephrol Dial Transplant 21(9):2543–2548, 2006 16751655

Kurella Tamura M, Yaffe K: Dementia and cognitive impairment in ESRD: diagnostic and therapeutic strategies. Kidney Int 79(1):14–22, 2011 20861818

Kurella Tamura M, Goldstein MK, Pérez-Stable EJ: Preferences for dialysis withdrawal and engagement in advance care planning within a diverse sample of dialysis patients. Nephrol Dial Transplant 25(1):237–242, 2010 19734137

Kurella Tamura M, Vittinghoff E, Hsu CY, et al; CRIC Study Investigators: Loss of executive function after dialysis initiation in adults with chronic kidney disease. Kidney Int 91(4):948–953, 2017 28139292

Lacson E Jr, Li NC, Guerra-Dean S, et al: Depressive symptoms associate with high mortality risk and dialysis withdrawal in incident hemodialysis patients. Nephrol Dial Transplant 27(7):2921–2928, 2012 22273670

Lea JP, Nicholas SB: Diabetes mellitus and hypertension: key risk factors for kidney disease. J Natl Med Assoc 94 (8 suppl):7S–15S, 2002 12152917

Leggat JE Jr: Adherence with dialysis: a focus on mortality risk. Semin Dial 18(2):137–141, 2005 15771658

Levenson JL, Owen JA: Renal and urological disorders, in Clinical Manual of Psychopharmacology in the Medically Ill, 2nd Edition. Edited by Levenson JL, Ferrando SJ. Arlington, VA, American Psychiatric Publishing, 2017, pp 195–232

Levy NB, Cohen LM (eds): Central and peripheral nervous systems in uremia, in Textbook of Nephrology, 4th Edition. Edited by Massry SG, Glassock R. Philadelphia, PA, Williams & Wilkins, 2001, pp 1279–1282

Lin YT, Wu PHJ, Kuo MC, et al: Comparison of dementia risk between end stage renal disease patients with hemodialysis and peritoneal dialysis—a population based study. Sci Rep 5:8224, 2015 25703589

Losso RL, Minhoto GR, Riella MC: Sleep disorders in patients with end-stage renal disease undergoing dialysis: comparison between hemodialysis, continuous ambulatory peritoneal dialysis and automated peritoneal dialysis. Int Urol Nephrol 47(2):369–375, 2015 25358390

McDade-Montez EA, Christensen AJ, Cvengros JA, et al: The role of depression symptoms in dialysis withdrawal. Health Psychol 25(2):198–204, 2006 16569111

McLaughlin K, Manns B, Mortis G, et al: Why patients with ESRD do not select self-care dialysis as a treatment option. Am J Kidney Dis 41(2):380–385, 2003 12552500

Meyer TW, Hostetter TH: Uremia. N Engl J Med 357(13):1316–1325, 2007 17898101

Mor MK, Sevick MA, Shields AM, et al: Sexual function, activity, and satisfaction among women receiving maintenance hemodialysis. Clin J Am Soc Nephrol 9(1):128–134, 2014 24357510

Moss AH: "At least we do not feel guilty": Managing conflict with families over dialysis discontinuation. Am J Kidney Dis 31(5):868–883, 1998 9590203

Moss AH: A new clinical practice guideline on initiation and withdrawal of dialysis that makes explicit the role of palliative medicine. J Palliat Med 3(3):253–260, 2000 15859665

Moss AH: Integrating supportive care principles into dialysis decision making: a primer for palliative medicine providers. J Pain Symptom Manage 53(3):656.e1–662.e1, 2017 28065700

Munshi SK, Vijayakumar N, Taub NA, et al: Outcome of renal replacement therapy in the very elderly. Nephrol Dial Transplant 16(1):128–133, 2001 11209006

Murray AM, Tupper DE, Knopman DS, et al: Cognitive impairment in hemodialysis patients is common. Neurology 67(2):216–223, 2006 16864811

Navaneethan SD, Vecchio M, Johnson DW, et al: Prevalence and correlates of self-reported sexual dysfunction in CKD: a meta-analysis of observational studies. Am J Kidney Dis 56(4):670–685, 2010 20801572

Nichols KA, Springford V: The psycho-social stressors associated with survival by dialysis. Behav Res Ther 22(5):563–574, 1984 6508707

Norris KC, Thornhill-Joynes M, Robinson C, et al: Cocaine use, hypertension, and end-stage renal disease. Am J Kidney Dis 38(3):523–528, 2001 11532684

Nozaki C, Oka M, Chaboyer W: The effects of a cognitive behavioural therapy programme for self-care on haemodialysis patients. Int J Nurs Pract 11(5):228–236, 2005 16109047

Obialo CI, Bashir K, Goring S, et al: Dialysis "no-shows" on Saturdays: implications of the weekly hemodialysis schedules on nonadherence and outcomes. J Natl Med Assoc 100(4):412–419, 2008 18481480

O'Connor NR, Dougherty M, Harris PS, et al: Survival after dialysis discontinuation and hospice enrollment for ESRD. Clin J Am Soc Nephrol 8(12):2117–2122, 2013 24202133

O'Lone E, Connors M, Masson P, et al: Cognition in people with end-stage kidney disease treated with hemodialysis: a systematic review and meta-analysis. Am J Kidney Dis 67(6):925–935, 2016 26919914

Palmer BF: Sexual dysfunction in men and women with chronic kidney disease and end-stage kidney disease. Adv Ren Replace Ther 10(1):48–60, 2003 12616463

Palmer S, Vecchio M, Craig JC, et al: Prevalence of depression in chronic kidney disease: systematic review and meta-analysis of observational studies. Kidney Int 84(1):179–191, 2013 23486521

Palmer SC, Natale P, Ruospo M, et al: Antidepressants for treating depression in adults with end-stage kidney disease treated with dialysis. Cochrane Database Syst Rev (5):CD004541, 2016 27210414

Paul R, Minay J, Cardwell C, et al: Meta-analysis of the effects of lithium usage on serum creatinine levels. J Psychopharmacol 24(10):1425–1431, 2009 19395432

Pena J, Mor M, Tohme F, et al: Acceptance of anti-depressant treatment by patients on hemodialysis and their renal providers. Clin J Am Soc Nephrol 12:298–303, 2017 28126707

Pereira AA, Weiner DE, Scott T, et al: Cognitive function in dialysis patients. Am J Kidney Dis 45(3):448–462, 2005 15754267

Pliskin NH, Yurk HM, Ho LT, et al: Neurocognitive function in chronic hemodialysis patients. Kidney Int 49(5):1435–1440, 1996 8731111

Presne C, Fakhouri F, Noël LH, et al: Lithium-induced nephropathy: rate of progression and prognostic factors. Kidney Int 64(2):585–592, 2003 12846754

Rubin HR, Fink NE, Plantinga LC, et al: Patient ratings of dialysis care with peritoneal dialysis vs hemodialysis. JAMA 291(6):697–703, 2004 14871912

Russ AJ, Shim JK, Kaufman SR: The value of "life at any cost": talk about stopping kidney dialysis. Soc Sci Med 64(11):2236–2247, 2007 17418924

Saczynski JS, Jónsdóttir MK, Garcia ME, et al: Cognitive impairment: an increasingly important complication of type 2 diabetes: the age, gene/environment susceptibility—Reykjavik study. Am J Epidemiol 168(10):1132–1139, 2008 18836152

Sareen J, Jacobi F, Cox BJ, et al: Disability and poor quality of life associated with comorbid anxiety disorders and physical conditions. Arch Intern Med 166(19):2109–2116, 2006 17060541

Schmid H, Hartmann B, Schiffl H: Adherence to prescribed oral medication in adult patients undergoing chronic hemodialysis: a critical review of the literature. Eur J Med Res 14(5):185–190, 2009 19541573

Semplicini A, Amodio P, Leonetti G, et al: Diagnostic tools for the study of vascular cognitive dysfunction in hypertension and antihypertensive drug research. Pharmacol Ther 109(1–2):274–283, 2006 16202453

Sharp J, Wild MR, Gumley AI, et al: A cognitive behavioral group approach to enhance adherence to hemodialysis fluid restrictions: a randomized controlled trial. Am J Kidney Dis 45(6):1046–1057, 2005a 15957134

Sharp J, Wild MR, Gumley AI: A systematic review of psychological interventions for the treatment of nonadherence to fluid-intake restrictions in people receiving hemodialysis. Am J Kidney Dis 45(1):15–27, 2005b 15696440

Smith MD, Hong BA, Robson AM: Diagnosis of depression in patients with end-stage renal disease. Comparative analysis. Am J Med 79(2):160–166, 1985 3895906

Souheaver GT, Ryan JJ, DeWolfe AS: Neuropsychological patterns in uremia. J Clin Psychol 38(3):490–496, 1982 7050178

Spigset O, Hägg S, Stegmayr B, et al: Citalopram pharmacokinetics in patients with chronic renal failure and the effect of haemodialysis. Eur J Clin Pharmacol 56(9–10):699–703, 2000 11214779

Sukolsky A: Patients who try our patience. Am J Kidney Dis 44(5):893–901, 2004 15492956

Tagay S, Kribben A, Hohenstein A, et al: Posttraumatic stress disorder in hemodialysis patients. Am J Kidney Dis 50(4):594–601, 2007 17900459

Tamura MK, Meier DE: Five policies to promote palliative care for patients with ESRD. Clin J Am Soc Nephrol 8(10):1783–1790, 2013 2374400

Troy SM, Schultz RW, Parker VD, et al: The effect of renal disease on the disposition of venlafaxine. Clin Pharmacol Ther 56(1):14–21, 1994 8033490

Tsay SL, Lee YC, Lee YC: Effects of an adaptation training programme for patients with end-stage renal disease. J Adv Nurs 50(1):39–46, 2005 15788064

Turk S, Solak Y, Kan S, et al: Effects of sildenafil and vardenafil on erectile dysfunction and health-related quality of life in haemodialysis patients: a prospective randomized crossover study. Nephrol Dial Transplant 25(11):3729–3733, 2010 20466680

United States Renal Data System: USRDS 2015 Annual Report: Atlas of End-Stage Renal Disease in the United States. Bethesda, MD, National Institutes of Health, National Institute of Diabetes and Digestive and Kidney Diseases, 2016

Untas A, Thumma J, Rascle N, et al: The associations of social support and other psychosocial factors with mortality and quality of life in the dialysis outcomes and practice patterns study. Clin J Am Soc Nephrol 6(1):142–152, 2011 20966121

Vermeir M, Naessens I, Remmerie B, et al: Absorption, metabolism, and excretion of paliperidone, a new monoaminergic antagonist, in humans. Drug Metab Dispos 36(4):769–779, 2008 18227146

Walther CP, Shah AA, Winkelmayer WC: Treating depression in patients with advanced CKD: beyond the generalizability frontier. JAMA 318(19):1873–1874, 2017 29101401

Watnick S, Kirwin P, Mahnensmith R, et al: The prevalence and treatment of depression among patients starting dialysis. Am J Kidney Dis 41(1):105–110, 2003 12500227

Watnick S, Wang PL, Demadura T, et al: Validation of 2 depression screening tools in dialysis patients. Am J Kidney Dis 46(5):919–924, 2005 16253733

Weisbord SD, Carmody SS, Bruns FJ, et al: Symptom burden, quality of life, advance care planning and the potential value of palliative care in severely ill haemodialysis patients. Nephrol Dial Transplant 18(7):1345–1352, 2003 12808172

Weisbord SD, Bossola M, Fried LF, et al: Cultural comparison of symptoms in patients on maintenance hemodialysis. Hemodial Int 12(4):434–440, 2008 19090866

Weisbord SD, Mor MK, Sevick MA, et al: Associations of depressive symptoms and pain with dialysis adherence, health resource utilization, and mortality in patients receiving chronic hemodialysis. Clin J Am Soc Nephrol 9(9):1594–1602, 2014 25081360

Williams MA, Sklar AH, Burright RG, et al: Temporal effects of dialysis on cognitive functioning in patients with ESRD. Am J Kidney Dis 43(4):705–711, 2004 15042548

Wyne A, Rai R, Cuerden M, et al: Opioid and benzodiazepine use in end-stage renal disease: a systematic review. Clin J Am Soc Nephrol 6(2):326–333, 2011 21071517

CHAPTER 21

Endocrine and Metabolic Disorders

James L. Levenson, M.D.

Alyson K. Myers, M.D.

The onset, course, and outcomes of endocrine disorders traditionally have been linked to psychological and social factors. A growing body of neuroendocrine research has begun to illuminate important biological mechanisms underlying the interplay of psyche and soma, with important clinical ramifications. In this chapter, we focus primarily on these latter pragmatic issues. Diabetes mellitus is the most common endocrine condition and is growing in epidemic proportions, so it has been given major emphasis. Other topics include disturbances in thyroid, parathyroid, adrenal, growth, prolactin, and gonadal hormones; pheochromocytomas; and metabolic disorders including electrolyte and acid–base disturbances, vitamin deficiencies, osteoporosis, and inherited disorders including the porphyrias.

Diabetes

Type 1 Diabetes

Type 1 diabetes mellitus (T1DM) is a chronic autoimmune disease that affects an estimated 500,000 to 1 million people in the United States. It is most commonly diagnosed in children and young adults (see also Chapter 32, "Pediatrics") but is also diagnosed in middle-aged and older adults (Thomas and Philipson 2015). The exact mechanism of T1DM is unknown; however, it appears that genetic and environmental factors trigger an autoimmune response, which attacks the insulin-producing beta cells of the pancreas.

The Diabetes Control and Complications Trial, a 9-year multicenter intervention study of nearly 1,500 persons with T1DM in the United States and Canada, established that tight glycemic control delays the onset and slows the progression of diabetic complications (Nathan et al. 1993). Therefore, treatment is aimed at lowering and stabilizing blood glucose to near-normal levels through dietary control, exercise, blood glucose monitoring, and insulin therapy. Intensive blood glucose management for T1DM can be achieved by the use of basal–bolus insulin injections or the use of a continuous subcutaneous insulin infusion pump, with the goal of mirroring as closely as possible the physiological patterns of insulin release. In 2014, the U.S. Food and Drug Administration (FDA) approved the use of continuous glucose monitoring (CGM) in lieu of fingerstick testing. CGM has been found to be noninferior to the use of a glucometer when blood sugars are 70–180 mg/dL (Aleppo et al. 2017).

Type 2 Diabetes

In both T1DM and type 2 diabetes mellitus (T2DM), hemoglobin A_{1C} (HbA_{1C}) is used to assess glycemic control, reflecting average blood glucose concentrations over a 2- to 3-month period. The HbA_{1C} can be falsely elevated in coexisting conditions of abnormal red blood cell turnover such as anemia, end-stage renal disease, pregnancy, or a recent blood transfusion (Nathan et al. 2007). For most patients, the target is an HbA_{1C} level less than 7%, but the target may be higher in those who are very old or who have multiple medical comorbidities (American Diabetes Association 2017a).

Approximately 90% of all people with diabetes have T2DM, which is caused by insulin resistance leading to dysglycemia. Insulin resistance leads to progressively increased pancreatic insulin production to achieve normoglycemia. In the early stages, patients can have impaired fasting glucose (IFG) or impaired glucose tolerance (IGT) (Nathan et al. 2007). IFG is diagnosed when the fasting glucose is 100–125 mg/dL and the HbA_{1C} is 5.7%–6.4%, whereas IGT is diagnosed when the postprandial glucose is 140–200 mg/dL 2 hours after a 75-g glucose load (oral glucose tolerance test [OGTT]). Once the fasting glucose is greater than 126 mg/dL and the HbA_{1C} is greater than 6.5%, the diagnosis of diabetes can be made (American Diabetes Association 2017a). After 10–15 years of having T2DM, the pancreas can no longer meet the increased need of insulin production, and exogenous insulin therapy is required. Risk factors for T2DM include IFG/IGT; history of gestational diabetes mellitus (GDM); obesity; black, Hispanic, Native American, or Asian ethnicity; sedentary lifestyle; metabolic syndrome; and chronic use of medications such as corticosteroids or antipsychotics. Onset of T2DM is typically during middle age, but with growing rates of obesity at younger ages, children and adolescents are starting to develop the disease at higher rates.

Stress and Diabetes

The association between stress and diabetes is rooted in biological as well as behavioral causes (Pouwer et al. 2010). Those with high levels of stress tend to have a sedentary lifestyle as well as poor dietary habits. On a biological level, repeated stress leads to overstimulation of the hypothalamic-pituitary-adrenal (HPA) axis. This leads to increases in the cortisol and inflammatory cytokines that play a role in insulin resistance (Golden 2007; Kan et al. 2013). Several studies have shown that glycemic control is poorer in people with diabetes who report more stress (Garay-Sevilla et al. 2000; Lloyd et al. 1999). However, this finding may be limited to certain populations; for example, in the Whitehall II prospective study of workers older than 18 years, obese women with high psychosocial work stress were the only group to show an increased risk of diabetes (Heraclides et al. 2012). This association was not seen in men or in nonobese women. It is still unclear whether stress directly influences metabolic regulation or whether people under stress change their self-care behaviors.

Psychiatric Disorders and Diabetes Management

The Diabetes Control and Complications Trial (DCCT) and U.K. Prospective Diabetes Study (UKPDS) research established that intensive management of T1DM and T2DM improves long-term health outcomes in diabetes (Nathan et al. 1993; U.K. Prospective Diabetes Study [UKPDS] Group 1998a, 1998b). However, the newer approach to diabetes management is to set glycemic targets based on patient goals, psychosocial factors, age, life expectancy, and comorbid conditions (Young-Hyman et al. 2016). For most patients, the goal of glycemic control is an HbA$_{1C}$ level less than 7%, but in persons with severe mental illness, this may not be attainable. Many patients have difficulty sustaining the burden of self-care over time—the stress of coping with a chronic disease is a major risk factor for psychopathology and nonadherence to complex treatment recommendations (Lustman et al. 2000a). There is a growing literature examining the relationship of T1DM and T2DM with psychiatric disorders, especially mood and eating disorders. In both types of diabetes, psychiatric disorders have been linked to treatment nonadherence, worse blood glucose control, and complications. Disease outcomes in diabetes are dependent on patient behaviors, attitudes, and cognitions; thus, optimal treatment is multidisciplinary, including primary care providers, endocrinologists, certified diabetes educators, psychiatrists, and other mental health care professionals.

Depression and Diabetes

The prevalence of depression in both T1DM and T2DM is two to three times higher than that found in the general population (Gendelman et al. 2009; Li et al. 2008). The International Prevalence and Treatment of Diabetes and Depression (INTERPRET-DD) study, currently ongoing in 16 countries, is examining the prevalence of diabetes and depression as well as diagnostic measures, treatment modalities, and clinical outcomes (Lloyd et al. 2015). The consequences of having both diabetes and depression include worse glycemic control (Brieler et al. 2016), more severe diabetic symptoms (Nguyen et al. 2015), and a heightened risk of major diabetic complications (Ciechanowski et al. 2000; de Groot et al. 2001). Complications such as painful neuropathy, sexual dysfunction, and renal disease increase the risk for development of depression (Holt et al. 2014).

However, there have also been studies showing no association between glycemic control and depression. In a population sample, there was no difference in attainment of individual HbA$_{1C}$, blood pressure, or cholesterol goals between diabetic individuals with depression and those without depression; however, those without depression were more likely to reach goals for all three measures (Shah et al. 2015). In a cohort of Black and Latino elderly patients in New York, depression was not associated with worsened glycemic control (Palta et al. 2014).

The association between diabetes and depression is described as bidirectional (Holt et al. 2014), in that individuals with depression have been found to have a 60%

increased risk of developing diabetes (Mezuk et al. 2008), which is due to genetic predisposition as well as poor health behaviors (Park and Reynolds 2015). The converse is also true, in that the stress of diabetes can lead to depression in individuals who have a biological or psychological predisposition to it. In a meta-analysis of 24 studies of depression, hyperglycemia, and diabetes, Lustman et al. (2000a) concluded that hyperglycemia is provoked by depression and also independently contributes to the exacerbation of depression.

Anxiety symptoms are also frequently reported by patients with diabetes and depression but may independently contribute to diminished quality of life (Collins et al. 2009). After accounting for depression, one study found that panic symptoms correlated with elevated HbA_{1C}, higher rates of complications, and lower self-rated functional health (Ludman et al. 2006). In persons with T1DM, isolated anxiety regarding hypoglycemia may also be present, leading to manipulation of insulin dosing in order to maintain blood sugar above 150 mg/dL. Risk factors for fear of hypoglycemia (FOH) include duration of diabetes and history of hypoglycemia and of fluctuating blood sugars (Wild et al. 2007). FOH, as measured by the Hypoglycemia Fear Survey (HFS), is associated with greater symptoms of anxiety and depression (Gonder-Frederick et al. 2011).

Related research has shown that the number of diabetes symptoms reported by patients was more strongly associated with the number of depression symptoms reported than it was with measures of glycemic control and diabetes complications (i.e., HbA_{1C} levels above 8.0% and two or more complications) (Ludman et al. 2004). Depression is associated with increased mortality in diabetes (Black et al. 2003; Katon et al. 2006) as well as an increased risk of self-harm or suicide (Myers and Trivedi 2017).

Diagnosing depression in individuals with diabetes can be complicated, as some symptoms of hyperglycemia overlap with those of depression, including fatigue, poor sleep, and inattention. Standard self-report scales such as the nine-item depression scale of the Patient Health Questionnaire (PHQ-9) or the Beck Depression Inventory–II (BDI-II) can be used for screening (Young-Hyman et al. 2016). In addition, "depressive" symptoms may not fulfill criteria for major depressive disorder; therefore, patients should also be assessed for *diabetes distress* (American Diabetes Association 2017b). The term *diabetes distress* conceptually recognizes that some patients are not depressed, but rather are distressed about their diagnosis of diabetes, and this distress leads to poorer glycemic control and worse health behaviors regarding diet and exercise (Fisher et al. 2012). Providers can use either the Diabetes Distress Scale (DDS) or the Problem Areas in Diabetes (PAID) questionnaire to pinpoint the exact areas of diabetes care that are most distressing to the patient (Young-Hyman et al. 2016).

Evidence is limited by small sample sizes and is somewhat contradictory regarding whether specific treatment of depression can lead to improvements in diabetes treatment adherence and glycemic control. Two small controlled studies reported that nortriptyline and fluoxetine are effective treatments for depression in diabetes. However, nortriptyline improved mood but did not improve glucose regulation, whereas fluoxetine was associated with improvements in mood and a nonsignificant trend for improved HbA_{1C} levels (Lustman et al. 1997, 2000b). Sertraline maintenance also was shown to decrease the risk of recurrence of depression in younger patients with diabetes (Williams et al. 2007). HbA_{1C} was found to improve slightly in relation to symptom improvement and to deteriorate with depression recurrence in those treated with sertraline (Lustman et al. 2006). Paroxetine in individuals with T2DM and mild depression led to statistically but not clinically significant improvement in HbA$_{1C}$ at 3 months of therapy; however, the effect was lost at 6 months (Paile-Hyvärinen et al. 2007). Compared with patients receiving diabetes education only, patients receiving cognitive-behavioral therapy (CBT) to address their depression symptoms showed significant improvements in HbA$_{1C}$ levels (Lustman et al. 1998). A similar study showed improved mood in response to CBT but no change in HbA$_{1C}$ levels either during treatment or 1 year later (Georgiades et al. 2007). In a study of sertraline versus group CBT, remission of depression was more likely for those treated with sertraline; however, despite the improvement in depressive symptoms, only minimal improvements were seen in glycemic control (Petrak et al. 2015). CBT was shown in a small study to improve pain symptoms in individuals with painful diabetic neuropathy, but with minimal change in depressive symptoms (Otis et al. 2013).

It appears that improving glycemic control involves addressing both depression and diabetes during therapy (van der Feltz-Cornelis 2013). As a result, collaborative care studies in which both diabetes and depression are addressed have become more popular. Katon et al. (2010) randomly assigned 214 people with depression and poorly controlled diabetes to care as usual with primary care versus bimonthly to monthly visits with nurses. The nurses were trained by physicians in motivational interviewing and adjusting medications for diabetes, depression, dyslipidemia, and hypertension. Unsurprisingly, the intervention group had better outcomes and satisfaction with care, but at a greater expense (average cost: $1,224 per person). This increased expense was in contrast to a previous study, the Improving Mood—Promoting Access to Collaborative Treatment (IMPACT) trial, which found that treatment of depression in older adults with diabetes contributed to significant clinical benefits without adding to health care costs (Katon et al. 2006). The Diabetes–Depression Care Management Adoption Trial (DCAT) demonstrated an improvement in depression but not glycemic control in participants who received interdisciplinary care by telephone and in person from physician, nurses, and social workers (Wu et al. 2014). Collaborative care interventions have also been delivered by telemedicine. Two studies delivering Web-based interventions targeting depression in adults with T1DM and T2DM reported improvement in both diabetes distress and depressive symptoms, with less-robust improvement in glycemia (Nobis et al. 2015; van Bastelaar et al. 2011).

In summary, the high prevalence of depression and its adverse effects in diabetes, combined with clinically proven treatments, argue for aggressive identification and treatment of depression as early as possible in diabetes. In a meta-analysis of studies delivering interventions with pharmacotherapy and/or psychotherapy, the effect on depression was greater than that on glycemic control (van der Feltz-Cornelis et al. 2010). As a result, there is a need for more research to improve both indices.

Bipolar Disorder, Schizophrenia, and Diabetes

T2DM occurs with significantly increased prevalence in bipolar disorder and schizophrenia. Patients with these disorders have diabetes rates of 10%–15%, which is two to three times higher than rates in the general population (De Hert et al. 2009), and risks are greater in females than in males (Goff et al. 2005). Much of the association appears to be related to obesity—specifically central adiposity—secondary to overstimulation of the HPA axis; poor sleep; a sedentary lifestyle; poor dietary choices;

and the metabolic effects of psychotropic medications (Holt 2015; Calkin et al. 2013). As a result, the American Diabetes Association, American Psychiatric Association, American Association of Clinical Endocrinologists, and North American Association for the Study of Obesity partnered to develop screening guidelines for metabolic syndrome (MetS) in patients taking antipsychotics (American Diabetes Association et al. 2004). These guidelines specify that prior to initiating treatment with a second-generation antipsychotic, all persons should be assessed for family history of diabetes and the components of MetS: weight/body mass index (BMI), blood pressure, fasting glucose, and fasting lipids. Weight should be checked monthly for the first 3 months and then quarterly. Measurements of blood pressure and fasting glucose should be taken again at 12 weeks and then annually. Fasting lipids should be measured again at 12 weeks and then every 5 years. With several of the atypical antipsychotics, the onset of diabetes may occur suddenly, with emergent diabetic ketoacidosis or hyperglycemic hyperosmolar state (Buse 2002; Geller and MacFadden 2003).

Lifestyle or pharmacological interventions aimed at self-management of weight and glycemic targets in patients with schizophrenia and diabetes have shown mixed results. McKibbin et al. (2006) found that adults (>40 years of age) with schizophrenia who received a 24-week lifestyle intervention involving group diabetes education showed improved weight and HbA$_{1C}$ levels compared with control patients who received pamphlets on diabetes; however, those in the intervention had higher baseline levels of HbA$_{1C}$. The STRIDE weight loss and lifestyle intervention study found that 40% of patients with schizophrenia in the treatment arm lost 5% or more of their initial weight; the number of sessions attended correlated with weight loss (Green et al. 2015). A similar result was seen in the ACHIEVE behavioral weight loss intervention study; however, participants completed the intervention at local psychiatric rehabilitation centers as opposed to being responsible for making weekly appointments on their own (Daumit et al. 2013). Other lifestyle interventions studied in this population group involved goals such as 150 minutes of physical activity per week, losing 5%–15% of weight, increasing fiber in the diet, and reducing dietary fat below 30% (Holt 2015).

Medications have also been used to improve glycemic control in individuals with prediabetes. Salsalate has been used in some small studies as a short-term therapy, because its anti-inflammatory properties can decrease the levels of inflammatory markers that contribute to insulin resistance in patients with or without schizophrenia (Goldfine et al. 2008; Keller et al. 2013). In the Diabetes Prevention Program (DPP) study, the insulin sensitizer metformin was found to reduce the onset of diabetes in prediabetic patients by 31% in comparison with placebo; unfortunately, patients with severe mental illness were excluded from this study (Knowler et al. 2002). Acarbose and thiazolidinediones have also been used to reduce the risk of diabetes in prediabetic individuals, although studies have not been conducted in patients with schizophrenia (Holt 2015). Glucagon-like peptide 1 (GLP-1) agonists are another class of drugs being studied for diabetes prevention in patients with schizophrenia treated with olanzapine or clozapine (Larsen et al. 2014). These agents are an attractive option because they induce early satiety.

Antipsychotics as well as mood stabilizers have been implicated in insulin resistance and weight gain through several proposed mechanisms; these include carbohydrate cravings and antagonism of histamine and serotonin$_{2A}$ and serotonin$_{2C}$ receptors (Calkin et al. 2013). In patients with known diabetes, antipsychotics with lower propensities to cause weight gain and glucose intolerance, such as perphenazine, molindone, aripiprazole, and ziprasidone, should be favored (Meyer et al. 2008) (see Chapter 36, "Psychopharmacology," for a full discussion). Unsurprisingly, patients who are adherent to their antipsychotic medications are more likely to adhere to their diabetes medications (Hansen et al. 2012); therefore, good glycemic control warrants a multidisciplinary effort from mental health care professionals, primary care physicians, and diabetologists.

Eating Disorders and Diabetes

Insulin is an anabolic hormone that aids in glycemic control at the expense of weight gain; therefore, a negative side of intensive diabetes management is weight gain (see also Chapter 13, "Eating Disorders"). Disturbed eating behavior (DEB) is common among adolescent girls and young women in the general population, and those with T1DM are more likely than their peers without diabetes to have two or more disturbed eating behaviors (Colton et al. 2004). Olmsted et al. (2008) defined DEB as eating disorder symptomatology not yet at the level of frequency or severity to merit a formal diagnosis; such behaviors include dieting for weight loss, binge eating, calorie purging through self-induced vomiting, laxative or diuretic use, excessive exercise, and insulin restriction (in the case of T1DM). Studies of the natural history of DEB in T1DM indicate that these behaviors persist and increase in severity over time, becoming more common in young adulthood (Colton et al. 2004; Peveler et al. 2005). Evidence suggests that in comparison with women without diabetes, women with T1DM have 2.4 times the risk of developing an eating disorder and 1.9 times the risk of developing subthreshold eating disorders (Jones et al. 2000). Predisposing factors for DEB in adolescents with T1DM, as identified by Peterson et al. (2015), included a preoccupation with food due to the need for teens to count their carbohydrates, weight gain due to the use of insulin, and overeating after episodes of hypoglycemia caused by restrictive behaviors. Other characteristics associated with DEB include valuing others' opinions or needs before one's own (Young-Hyman and Davis 2010), having high levels of diabetes distress, having fears of hypoglycemia, and having poor diabetes self-care behaviors (Goebel-Fabbri et al. 2008). As noted for mood disorders, practitioners should screen patients with T1DM for comorbid eating disorders. In females ages 13–53 years, the Eating Disorders Inventory–3 (Garner 2004) can be used (Young-Hyman et al. 2016).

Women with T1DM may manipulate insulin (e.g., taking reduced insulin doses or omitting necessary doses altogether) as a means of caloric purging. Intentionally induced glucosuria—known as "diabulimia" (Shaban 2013)—is a powerful weight loss behavior and a symptom of eating disorders unique to T1DM. Diabulimia is not intended to describe the subset of people who may omit insulin for reasons other than weight loss (e.g., fear of hypoglycemia) (Weinger and Beverly 2010). Questions such as "Do you ever change your insulin dose or skip insulin doses to influence your weight?" or "How often do you take less insulin than is prescribed?" can be helpful in screening for insulin omission, especially for patients who present with persistently elevated HbA$_{1C}$ levels, repeated episodes of diabetic ketoacidosis, frequent hospitalizations, drastic weight changes, or amenorrhea (Gagnon et al. 2012).

Intermittent insulin omission or dose reduction for weight loss purposes has been found to be a common practice among women with T1DM. As many as 31% of women with T1DM report intentional insulin restriction, with rates of this disturbed eating behavior peaking in late adolescence and early adulthood (40% of women between the ages of 15 and 30 years) (Polonsky et al. 1994). Even subthreshold disturbed eating behaviors can lead to significant medical and psychological consequences in the context of diabetes (Verrotti et al. 1999). In one study, use of insulin restriction was associated with a threefold increased risk of death over the 11-year follow-up period (Goebel-Fabbri et al. 2008).

Binge-eating disorder (BED) with or without inappropriate compensatory behavior is a common problem seen in T2DM. If the binge is accompanied by certain behaviors, then the diagnosis becomes that of bulimia. Behaviors used to compensate for overeating in persons with T1DM include skipping meals, misusing diuretics and/or diet pills, underdosing insulin to induce glucosuria, and self-inducing vomiting (Gagnon et al. 2012). Obesity is a significant risk factor in T2DM, and recurrent binge eating may increase the risk of obesity development (Striegel-Moore et al. 2000). Initial studies of BED and T2DM relied on small, nonrepresentative samples. Kenardy et al. (1994) found that 14% of the patients with newly diagnosed T2DM experienced problems with binge eating, compared with 4% of individuals in the age-, sex-, and weight-matched control group. In a study of Brazilian middle-aged, low-educated individuals with T2DM, there was a 10% prevalence of BED (Papelbaum et al. 2005). Those with both conditions tended to have a family history of mood disorders and a personal history of anxiety disorder. Another study showed higher rates of both depression and anxiety in those with T2DM and BED compared with those with just BED, but the difference was not statistically significant, and HbA_{1C} levels did not differ between the two groups (Crow et al. 2001).

Night-eating symptoms also have been associated with obesity and poor diabetes control. In a survey of adults with T2DM, increased symptoms of night eating were associated with poorer glycemic control and disruptions in eating, sleep, and mood, including a significantly increased likelihood of having HbA_{1C} levels greater than 7% (Hood et al. 2014). In the largest study of its kind to date, more than 5,000 patients with T2DM were evaluated to determine whether binge eating was related to weight loss after a 1-year intervention. Larger weight losses were observed in those patients who never endorsed binge eating or who reported that they were no longer binge eating at 1-year follow-up (Gorin et al. 2008). Thus, recurrent binge eating and night eating symptoms can be expected to make it difficult to control diabetes and weight.

A multidisciplinary team approach, including a diabetologist, nurse educator, nutritionist with eating disorder and diabetes training, and mental health care practitioner, is ideal for the treatment of comorbid eating disorders and diabetes (Kahn et al. 2005; Mitchell et al. 1997). At this time, little research has examined treatment efficacy for eating disorders in the context of diabetes; however, a large research literature on treatment outcomes in bulimia nervosa supports the use of CBT in combination with antidepressant medications as the most effective treatment (Peterson and Mitchell 1999; Walsh and Devlin 1995).

Early in treatment, intensive glycemic management of diabetes is not an appropriate target for a person with diabetes and an eating disorder. Overly intensive diabetes management may actually aggravate obsessional thinking about food and weight in patients with eating disorders. The first goal should focus on medical stabilization. Gradually, the team can build toward increasing doses of insulin, increases in food intake, greater flexibility of meal plans, regularity of eating routine, and more frequent blood glucose monitoring.

Sexual Function and Diabetes

For information on diabetes and sexual function, see Chapter 15, "Sexual Dysfunctions."

Cognitive Functioning and Diabetes

Older persons with diabetes are at increased risk of both cognitive impairment and dementia, and their risk is 50%–100% greater than that in persons without diabetes (Mayeda et al. 2015). Cognitive impairment in diabetes is influenced by glycemic control as well as control of comorbid conditions such as hypertension and dyslipidemia. Most of the studies of cognition have been in T2DM. The American Diabetes Association (2017c) recommends screening persons older than 65 years for mild cognitive impairment with the Mini-Mental State Examination and the Montreal Cognitive Assessment. Managing patients with cognitive dysfunction and diabetes can be difficult, as they may be unable to participate in self-care behaviors such as adhering to a diabetic diet, testing blood sugars, or taking medications. Some of these issues can be mitigated by using alternative methods of nutrition, giving meal insulin after the patient eats, using long-acting medications, or scheduling medication administration/glucose testing for times when the patient is more cooperative (Munshi et al. 2016).

Some risk factors for dementia in diabetic individuals are similar to those in the general population: low level of education, unmarried status, depression, and older age. Some of these risk factors are more common in those with diabetes: chronic severe hyper/hypoglycemia, history of diabetic ulcer or limb amputations, retinopathy, and coronary artery disease (Bruce et al. 2014). The diabetes-specific dementia risk score can be used to predict the 10-year risk of developing dementia in persons with T2DM (Exalto et al. 2013). The most common types of dementia are Alzheimer's and vascular, or a combination of the two (Strachan et al. 2008).

Neurocognitive decline in diabetes is thought to be mediated by chronic hyperglycemia and insulin resistance contributing to the formation of free radicals, inflammation, and advanced glycation end products. These agents then contribute to the formation of neurofibrillary tangles and beta-amyloid deposition, and micro/macrovascular disease, leading to cognitive decline with eventual dementia (Mayeda et al. 2015). Recurrent episodes of hypoglycemia also have been implicated in cognitive decline. In a longitudinal study of elderly persons with T2DM, each visit to the emergency department for hypoglycemia increased the risk of eventual dementia by 2.39% (Whitmer et al. 2009). This study did not track episodes of hypoglycemia that did not require an emergency department visit, so the risk may be even greater. Interestingly enough, the same association is not seen in persons with T1DM, who are at even greater risk of hypoglycemia. In both the DCCT and the Epidemiology of Diabetes Interventions and Complications (EDIC) studies ($N=1,144$), patients randomly assigned to either intense or conventional treatment arms did not have cognitive deficits noted on extensive neuropsychological testing (Diabetes Control and Complications Trial/Epidemiology of Diabetes Interventions and Complications Study Research Group et al. 2007). When the data were reanalyzed after elimination of cohorts with visual impairment, stroke, or severe renal disease, patients in the conventional treatment group showed worsening of psychomotor speed. Another cause of cognitive impairment in diabetes is depression, especially in the elderly (Park and Reynolds 2015). Vitamin B_{12} deficiency should also be considered as a cause of cognitive dysfunction in patients treated with metformin, which decreases B_{12} absorption in the terminal ileum (Biemans et al. 2015). Statins were previously believed to be associated with cognitive dysfunction, but subsequent studies have disproved this association (Ott et al. 2015).

Thyroid Disorders

Hyperthyroidism and hypothyroidism are accompanied by a variety of physiological, psychiatric, and cognitive symptoms. Patients with psychiatric disorders, especially depression, have elevated rates of thyroid disease (Farmer et al. 2008). However, routine screening of psychiatric inpatients for thyroid dysfunction is not warranted, given that cases of dysfunction are not common in the absence of physical signs of hypo- or hyperthyroidism (Garnier et al. 2016).

Hyperthyroidism

Hyperthyroidism is accompanied by a host of physiological symptoms, including nervousness, sweating, fatigue, heat intolerance, weight loss, and muscle weakness. The most common cause of hyperthyroidism is Graves' disease. Less common causes include toxic nodular goiter and thyroid-stimulating hormone (TSH)–secreting pituitary tumors. Graves' disease is an autoimmune disorder that also causes ophthalmopathy and infiltrative dermopathy (pretibial edema). Some evidence shows that stress can precipitate Graves' disease (Vita et al. 2015) and can aggravate treated disease (Fukao et al. 2003). The presentation of hyperthyroidism can vary depending on the age of the patient. In younger patients, hyperthyroidism typically manifests as hyperactivity or anxious dysphoria, whereas in the elderly, it can manifest as apathy or depression (referred to as "apathetic hyperthyroidism"). The best screening test for hyperthyroidism is measurement of serum TSH, but a low TSH level should be followed by a free thyroxine (T_4) test to confirm the diagnosis. Treatment options for hyperthyroidism include antithyroid medications, thyroidectomy, and radioactive iodine.

Patients with hyperthyroidism often present with anxiety, hypomania, depression, and cognitive difficulties. There are many case reports of mania or psychosis in patients with extreme hyperthyroidism (thyrotoxicosis) (Brownlie et al. 2000). Ironically, lithium can precipitate hyperthyroidism. Psychiatric symptoms correlate poorly with thyroid hormone levels (Vogel et al. 2007), and typically resolve with antithyroid therapy or with use of beta-blockers (Trzepacz et al. 1988). Consequently, psychiatric drugs may not be needed and should be reserved for severe mood or psychotic symptoms, or for psychiatric symptoms that persist despite effective antithyroid treatment, as is not uncommon (Cramon et al. 2016). Hyperthyroidism may increase risk for future psychopathology. A Danish study that followed 2,631 patients with hypothyroidism and matched control subjects without the disorder over 6 years found that the patients were more likely than controls to receive psychiatric medications and to be psychiatrically hospitalized by study end (Brandt et al. 2013). A Taiwanese cohort study in 21,574 hyperthyroid patients and matched control subjects found more than twice the risk of bipolar disorder in patients compared with controls (Hu et al. 2013). Even subclinical hyperthyroidism (low TSH, normal T_4) may increase risk for depression (Kvetny et al. 2015).

Hyperthyroid patients have been reported to have a variety of cognitive impairments (e.g., Yuan et al. 2015), although subjective cognitive complaints are not supported by objective evidence (Vogel et al. 2007). A recent meta-analysis of prospective studies concluded that even subclinical hyperthyroidism may be associated with an elevated risk for cognitive decline in the elderly (Rieben et al. 2016), but there is no evidence that antithyroid treatment prevents such decline.

Hypothyroidism

Hypothyroid patients often experience weakness, fatigue, somnolence, cold intolerance, weight gain, constipation, hair loss, hoarseness, stiffness, and muscle aches. The most common cause of hypothyroidism is autoimmune thyroiditis (Hashimoto's thyroiditis). Hypothyroidism is also a side effect of lithium. Radioactive iodine, the most commonly used modality for treating hyperthyroidism (such as in Graves' disease), may cause hypothyroidism, which may go undiagnosed for several years after treatment for hyperthyroidism.

The symptoms of hypothyroidism overlap with retarded depression, and the diagnosis is easy to miss in patients who already have a depression diagnosis. Physical signs of hypothyroidism include weakness, bradycardia, facial puffiness, weight gain, hair loss, hoarseness, and slowed speech. The best screening test for hypothyroidism is measurement of serum TSH concentration, but an elevated TSH level should be followed by a free T_4 determination to confirm the diagnosis. A serum TSH determination will be misleading in patients with secondary hypothyroidism caused by pituitary or hypothalamic disease. In such a patient, a free T_4 measurement is usually diagnostic.

Severe hypothyroidism is relatively rare, although milder hypothyroidism is common. Patients with *overt* hypothyroidism are usually symptomatic and have elevated TSH and low free T_4 concentrations. Patients with *subclinical* hypothyroidism typically have either mild or no symptoms of hypothyroidism, and have an elevated TSH level and a normal free T_4 level. Subclinical hypothyroidism is fairly common, affecting 5%–10% of the population, mainly women, and occurs in 15%–20% of women older than 45 years. Subclinical hypothyroidism is particularly common in elderly women.

Cognitive Function

A variety of cognitive functions may be impaired in overt hypothyroidism, including attention, memory, reaction time, and performance on speeded tests (Miller et al. 2007; Smith et al. 2015). One possible explanation is that cognitive inefficiency in hypothyroidism is a result of secondary depression. However, in some cases, patient perceptions of cognitive difficulty (rather than actual cognitive dysfunction) may be a result of depression or fatigue.

Earlier studies found subtle signs of cognitive dysfunction in patients with subclinical hypothyroidism, but more recent research has generally been less supportive of subclinical hypothyroidism as a cause of cognitive dysfunction (Pasqualetti et al.

2015; Rieben et al. 2016). Whether and when to treat subclinical hypothyroidism remains controversial (Garber et al. 2012).

Depression

Hypothyroidism is a known cause of secondary depression. Concurrent symptoms of depression are extremely common in patients with hypothyroidism (Bathla et al. 2016) but typically do not include reported guilt and lowered self-esteem (Smith et al. 2015). Depressive symptoms are also increased in patients with subclinical hypothyroidism (Blum et al. 2016; Demartini et al. 2010). Whether subclinical hypothyroidism is a risk factor for depression is controversial (de Jongh et al. 2011; Yu et al. 2016).

Triiodothyronine (T_3) has long been used to augment the effects of antidepressants in treatment-resistant depression.

Patients with bipolar disorder with either rapid cycling or mixed episodes have particularly high rates of subclinical hypothyroidism. In one study, almost 40% of rapid-cycling or mixed-episode bipolar patients were found to have subclinical hypothyroidism (Joffe et al. 1988). Although lithium-induced thyroid dysfunction may be the cause in some cases, subclinical hypothyroidism is common in bipolar patients receiving other mood stabilizers (Lambert et al. 2016). Every patient with rapid-cycling bipolar disorder should be evaluated for (subclinical) hypothyroidism and should receive T_4 if TSH levels are elevated. High-dose thyroid supplementation has been advocated in the treatment of bipolar disorder, even if patients are euthyroid, and studies have found that this treatment does not increase the risk of adverse cardiac effects or osteoporosis (Kelly et al. 2016).

Psychosis

Untreated hypothyroidism can result in psychosis, so-called myxedema madness. This condition was fairly common—reported in up to 5% of all hypothyroid patients (Kudrjavcev 1978)—before the widespread use of modern thyroid function tests. It is now rare, although cases continue to be reported. Psychotic symptoms typically remit when TSH and T_4 levels return to normal. Another rare possibility in hypothyroid patients is Hashimoto's encephalopathy, a delirium with psychosis, seizures, and focal neurological signs, which is associated with high serum antithyroid antibody concentrations, responsive to corticosteroids, and thought to be an autoimmune disorder. Most cases of Hashimoto's encephalopathy are euthyroid or mildly hypothyroid (Montagna et al. 2016).

Congenital Hypothyroidism

Congenital hypothyroidism usually occurs as a result of thyroid agenesis or dysgenesis, although inherited defects in thyroid hormone synthesis also may play a role. From a global perspective, iodine deficiency is the most common cause of congenital hypothyroidism. Newborns with untreated hypothyroidism develop the syndrome of cretinism, characterized by mental retardation, short stature, poor motor development, and a characteristic puffiness of the face and hands. Because early treatment is essential to prevent permanent mental retardation, all infants born in the United States are screened for hypothyroidism at birth (American Academy of Pediatrics et al. 2006). Treatment with thyroid hormones before age 3 months can result in normal intellectual development in most infants.

Parathyroid Disorders

Hyperparathyroidism

Hyperparathyroidism can cause bone disease, kidney stones, and hypercalcemia via oversecretion of parathyroid hormone. Symptoms of hypercalcemia include anorexia, thirst, frequent urination, lethargy, fatigue, muscle weakness, joint pain, constipation, and, when severe, depression and eventually coma.

The prevalence of hyperparathyroidism is 0.1%. It is three times more common in women than in men, and its prevalence increases with age. Hyperparathyroidism may occur as a consequence of radiation therapy to the head and neck and is an underrecognized side effect of long-term lithium therapy (Albert et al. 2015). Cessation of lithium often does not correct the hyperparathyroidism, necessitating parathyroidectomy.

With mild hypercalcemia, patients may show personality changes, lack of spontaneity, and lack of initiative. Moderate hypercalcemia (serum calcium concentration = 10–14 mg/dL) may cause dysphoria, anhedonia, apathy, anxiety, irritability, and impairment of concentration and recent memory. In severe hypercalcemia (serum calcium concentration >14 mg/dL), confusion, disorientation, catatonia, agitation, paranoid ideation, delusions, auditory and visual hallucinations, and lethargy progressing to coma may occur. Symptoms of depression, anxiety, and cognitive impairment are very common prior to parathyroidectomy and resolve in most patients following surgery (Kahal et al. 2012; Liu et al. 2016; Weber et al. 2013).

Hypoparathyroidism

Patients with hypoparathyroidism present with hypocalcemia causing increased neuromuscular irritability. Typical symptoms include paresthesias, muscle cramps, carpopedal spasm, and (less commonly) facial grimacing and seizures. Complications include calcification of the basal ganglia and pseudotumor cerebri. Psychiatric symptoms may include anxiety, emotional irritability, and lability. Severe hypocalcemia causes tetany and seizures. Hypoparathyroidism is caused by inadequate parathyroid hormone secretion, most often as a result of parathyroid or thyroid surgery. Hypoparathyroidism is also common in the 22q11.2 deletion syndrome (velocardiofacial syndrome), in which psychosis is common in adults and mood, anxiety, attentional, and behavior disorders are common in children (Radoeva et al. 2017).

Cognitive and neurological deficits, which are common in patients with longstanding hypoparathyroidism, may be irreversible but do not always correlate with the extent of intracranial calcification (Aggarwal et al. 2013).

Osteoporosis

Osteoporosis is a metabolic disturbance of bone resulting in low bone mass, reduced bone strength, and increased risk of fractures. Osteoporosis occurs most commonly in postmenopausal women. The association between depression and osteoporosis is bidirectional; there is evidence that depression is a risk factor for osteoporosis in both women and men (Lee et al. 2015). The causal relationship between depression and osteoporosis is unclear. Some of the association may be the result of antidepressants, especially selective serotonin reuptake inhibitors (SSRIs), which as a class are associated with reduced bone mineral density and increased fracture risk (Bruyère and Reginster 2015). Other risk factors for osteoporosis in depression include hypercortisolism, smoking, alcohol consumption, and physical inactivity. An increased risk of osteoporosis might be expected in patients receiving long-term augmentation of antidepressant therapy with T_3, but whether chronic augmentation of antidepressants with T_3 increases risk of osteoporosis has not been studied. Osteoporosis is common in people with schizophrenia, although the extent to which osteoporosis is due to antipsychotic-induced hyperprolactinemia is unclear (De Hert et al. 2016).

Adrenal Gland Disorders

Cushing's Syndrome

Cushing's syndrome results from abnormally high levels of cortisol and other glucocorticoids. The most common cause is the pharmacological use of corticosteroids, followed by excessive corticotropin secretion (most commonly by a pituitary tumor, referred to as Cushing's disease) and adrenal tumors. Symptoms and signs of Cushing's syndrome include truncal obesity and striae, diabetes, hypertension, hyperglycemia, muscle weakness, osteopenia, skin atrophy and bruising, increased susceptibility to infections, and gonadal dysfunction.

Cushing's syndrome patients commonly experience a range of psychiatric symptoms, including depression, anxiety, hypomania or frank mania, psychosis, and cognitive dysfunction (Pivonello et al. 2015; Starkman 2013), with rates varying widely across studies. Depression is the most prevalent psychiatric disturbance in Cushing's syndrome. A full depressive syndrome has been reported in 50%–80% of cases, accompanied by irritability, insomnia, crying, decreased energy and libido, poor concentration and memory, and suicidal ideation (Pivonello et al. 2015). Although antidepressants are less effective than in regular major depressive disorder, they are helpful until definitive treatment of Cushing's syndrome can be provided. Mood symptoms generally improve with resolution of hypercortisolemia (Pivonello et al. 2015) but may persist in remitted patients (Valassi et al. 2017). There are many case reports of Cushing's syndrome patients presenting with a variety of psychotic symptoms, usually as part of a manic or depressive syndrome (Arnaldi et al. 2003), leading to misdiagnosis of bipolar disorder or a schizophrenia spectrum disorder. Chronic hypercortisolism can impair cognition, with effects on attention, executive performance, and nonverbal memory (Forget et al. 2016) that are not attributable to depression. Cushing's disease causes reduction in hippocampal volume and cerebral atrophy, which may not be entirely reversible after cortisol levels return to normal (Andela et al. 2015). The data are mixed on whether cognitive deficits improve or persist after treatment of Cushing's syndrome (Arnaldi et al. 2003).

The primary treatment for corticotropin-dependent Cushing's syndrome is surgery. However, medical therapies—including inhibitors of steroidogenesis (e.g., etomidate) and glucocorticoid receptor antagonists (e.g., mifepristone)—have a role in reducing psychiatric and other symptoms (Fleseriu et al. 2012).

Adrenal Insufficiency: Addison's Disease and Corticotropin Deficiency

Insufficient production of adrenal corticosteroids can be caused by several mechanisms. Primary adrenal insufficiency, or Addison's disease, results in deficient secretion of mineralocorticoids and glucocorticoids. The major causes of Addison's disease are autoimmune adrenalitis, metastatic cancer, and infection (e.g., tuberculosis, HIV). The most common cause of secondary adrenal insufficiency is suppression of corticotropin (adrenocorticotropic hormone [ACTH]) secretion by chronic glucocorticoid administration. Less common secondary causes include diseases that result in pituitary destruction. In secondary adrenal insufficiency, ACTH levels are low, whereas in Addison's disease, the deficiency in cortisol results in an increase in ACTH. This increase in ACTH can cause hyperpigmentation. The decrease in mineralocorticoid levels results in contraction of the extracellular volume, leading to postural hypotension. Individuals with adrenal insufficiency are prone to hypoglycemia when stressed or fasting. Although electrolytes can be normal in mild Addison's disease, hyponatremia and hyperkalemia are typical. Other manifestations of adrenal insufficiency include anemia, anorexia, nausea, vomiting, diarrhea, abdominal pain, weight loss, and muscle weakness.

Psychiatric symptoms such as apathy, social withdrawal, fatigue, anhedonia, poverty of thought, and negativism are common in patients with Addison's disease. Nonspecific symptoms such as weakness, fatigue, and anorexia often appear before more specific findings, making it difficult to attribute the cause to adrenal insufficiency. Cognitive impairment, especially memory loss, is often present but ephemeral and varying in severity (Tiemensma et al. 2016). During Addisonian crisis, patients may experience delirium, disorientation, confusion, and even psychosis (Anglin et al. 2006). Adrenal insufficiency is particularly likely to be misdiagnosed as primary major depression in patients with chronic medical illness who previously received high doses of corticosteroids, resulting in unrecognized secondary adrenal insufficiency. Another possible psychiatric misdiagnosis is anorexia nervosa.

Although the diagnosis of adrenal insufficiency may be suspected on the basis of a low morning serum cortisol level, definitive diagnosis requires a corticotropin stimulation test. This is typically performed with cosyntropin, a synthetic ACTH analogue. An increase in the serum cortisol concentration to greater than 20 ng/dL following cosyntropin injection excludes the diagnosis of adrenal insufficiency.

The cause of depression in patients with Addison's disease is not clear. Regardless of the etiology of adrenal insufficiency, urgent treatment is indicated. Both glucocorticoid and mineralocorticoid replacement are usually necessary in the treatment of Addison's disease, whereas glucocorticoid replacement alone is sufficient in secondary adrenal insufficiency.

Adrenal insufficiency is also a feature in adrenoleukodystrophy, a rare, X-linked inherited metabolic disease, which also leads to leukoencephalic myeloneuropathy. Adult onset is rare but commonly presents with psychiatric symptoms, including mania, psychosis, and cognitive dysfunction (Rosebush et al. 1999).

Acromegaly

Acromegaly is a disease of excess growth hormone (GH) secretion. Deficiency of GH in children results in short stature, as discussed in Chapter 32, "Pediatrics." The most common cause of acromegaly is a GH-secreting adenoma of the anterior pituitary. Clinical manifestations of acromegaly include headache, cranial nerve palsies, acral enlargement (frontal bossing), increased hand and foot size, prognathism, soft tissue overgrowth (macroglossia), glucose intolerance, and hypertension.

Psychiatric disturbances associated with acromegaly include mood disorders, anxiety, and personality changes, which may persist after treatment (Tiemensma et al. 2010). Psychiatric symptoms and impairment in quality of life have been attributed both to the endocrine disorder itself and to the psychosocial stress of disfigurement (T'Sjoen et al. 2007). However, studies have found that body-image perceptions and quality of life are more reflective of emotional state than of objective measures of the disease (Dimopoulou et al. 2017; Geraedts et al. 2015). Personality changes described in acromegalic patients include loss of initiative and spontaneity, with marked lability in mood (Pantanetti et al. 2002). Cognitive impairments in attention, memory, and executive function are common (Sievers et al. 2012).

Treatment of acromegaly may include surgery, medication, and radiation.

Pheochromocytoma

Pheochromocytomas are rare catecholamine-secreting tumors derived from the adrenal medulla and sympathetic ganglia. The clinical signs and symptoms arise from the release of catecholamines, which leads to increased heart rate, blood pressure, myocardial contractility, and vasoconstriction, resulting in paroxysmal hypertension, headache, palpitations, diaphoresis, anxiety, tremulousness, pallor (rarely flushing), chest and abdominal pain, and often nausea and vomiting (Manger 2009). Because these are nonspecific symptoms, pheochromocytomas may be suspected in patients who actually have anxiety disorders (especially panic disorder), migraine or cluster headaches, stimulant abuse, or alcohol withdrawal. Among patients tested for pheochromocytoma, fewer than 2% are found to have the tumor (Eisenhofer et al. 2008). Many of those with negative tests have unexplained severe symptomatic paroxysmal hypertension, often referred to as "pseudopheochromocytoma," which appears to be triggered by anxiety (Pickering and Clemow 2008). Cases of classic panic attacks in patients with pheochromocytoma have been reported in both adults and children (Manger 2009). There are reports of cases in which antidepressants have "unmasked" silent pheochromocytomas, presumably by inhibiting neuronal intake of circulating catecholamines.

There is still no consensus as to the "best test" for the diagnosis of pheochromocytoma. Some centers rely on 24-hour urine measurement of increased excretion of catecholamines and metanephrines. Plasma metanephrine determinations have an extremely high sensitivity (approaching 99%) and overall specificity (in the 85%–90% range) (Lenders et al. 2002). The finding of elevated urinary catecholamine levels is not specific to pheochromocytoma and can lead to misdiagnosis. Psychological and physiological stressors can elevate levels of urinary catecholamines. Substances that can interfere with testing include drugs (e.g., tricyclic antidepressants, buspirone, L-dopa, antipsychotics, stimulants, decongestants) as well as certain foods.

Multiple cases of factitious pheochromocytoma have been reported and include cases involving vanilla extract ingestion, phenylpropanolamine abuse, injection of catecholamines, and Valsalva maneuvers (Stern and Cremens 1998).

The rare possibility of a pheochromocytoma should be considered in patients with panic attacks, headaches, and labile hypertension, particularly those who do not respond to treatment. It is not necessary to screen for pheochromocytoma in patients who have only psychiatric symptoms; elevated catecholamines are common and likely to be false-positive results. Some psychotropic drugs may cause hypertensive reactions that mimic pheochromocytoma, and in rare cases the drugs may be unmasking an unsuspected pheochromocytoma.

Hyperprolactinemia

Hyperprolactinemia is the most common pituitary hormone hypersecretion syndrome. The differential diagnosis of hyperprolactinemia includes pituitary adenomas, physiological causes (pregnancy and lactation), medication effects, chronic renal failure, primary hypothyroidism, and lesions of the pituitary stalk and the hypothalamus. Clinical signs in women include galactorrhea, menstrual irregularities, infertility, and decreased libido. Men present with diminished libido and rarely with galactorrhea.

Stress induces an increase in prolactin levels. Hyperprolactinemia has been associated with increased depression and anxiety, which resolve with treatment of hyperprolactinemia (Kars et al. 2007). In patients with treatment-resistant depression who have galactorrhea and/or amenorrhea, hyperprolactinemia should be considered as a possible causal factor (Holroyd and Cohen 1990).

Medication-induced hyperprolactinemia has been associated with antipsychotics and, to a lesser extent, antidepressants. Serum prolactin levels in patients taking therapeutic doses of typical antipsychotics are increased six- to tenfold from mean baseline prolactin levels (Arvanitis and Miller 1997). Atypical antipsychotics vary in their effects on prolactin (Ajmal et al. 2014; Peuskens et al. 2014). Most atypicals either cause no increase in prolactin secretion or increase prolactin transiently, but sustained hyperprolactinemia can occur in patients taking risperidone, paliperidone, and amisulpride. Haloperidol raises the serum prolactin concentration by an average of 17 ng/mL, while risperidone may raise it by 45–80 ng/mL, with larger increases in women than in men (David et al. 2000). Aripiprazole may reduce prolactin levels, and several clinical trials have demonstrated that switching from risperidone to aripiprazole, or adding it adjunctively, promptly reduced previously elevated prolactin levels (Chen et al. 2015).

Antidepressants with serotonergic activity, including SSRIs, monoamine oxidase inhibitors, and some tricyclic antidepressants, can cause modest elevations in prolactin (Ajmal et al. 2014) and may further elevate prolactin levels in patients also taking prolactin-elevating antipsychotics.

Patients on long-term regimens of prolactin-elevating antipsychotics are at risk of osteoporosis and should be educated about—and regularly monitored for—signs and symptoms of hyperprolactinemia.

Gonadal Disorders

Premenstrual Disorders and Menopause

For information on premenstrual disorders and disorders of menopause, readers are referred to Chapter 31, "Obstetrics and Gynecology."

Polycystic Ovary Syndrome

Polycystic ovary syndrome (PCOS) is a common disorder, affecting 5%–10% of women of childbearing age. Clinical manifestations include amenorrhea or oligomenorrhea, infrequent or absent ovulation, increased levels of testosterone, infertility, truncal obesity or weight gain, alopecia, hirsutism, acanthosis nigricans, hypertension, and insulin resistance. The cause of the disorder is unknown. The risk of developing PCOS is increased during treatment with valproate and seems to be higher in women with epilepsy than in women with bipolar disorder (Bilo and Meo 2008).

There are adverse psychosocial consequences of PCOS. Elevated rates of clinically significant anxiety and depression in women with PCOS have been documented in numerous studies, including meta-analyses (Barry et al. 2011; Blay et al. 2016; Dokras et al. 2012) and a Taiwanese national cohort study involving more than 5,000 women with PCOS (Hung et al. 2014). Increased risk for a much wider array of psychiatric disorders and suicidality was found in a Swedish national cohort study involving more than 24,000 women with PCOS (Cesta et al. 2016). Possible causal factors—including BMI, insulin resistance (e.g., Greenwood et al. 2015), hormonal differences (e.g., Annagür et al. 2013), hyperlipidemia, hirsutism, acne, infertility, body image, sexual functioning, and relationship satisfaction—have been examined, primarily with respect to depression. Studies to date have been relatively small, and no consistent associations have been found. Although the causal link between psychiatric symptoms and PCOS is not resolved, the frequency of these symptoms points to the importance of screening all PCOS patients for psychiatric syndromes, especially depression.

Testosterone Deficiency

Testosterone deficiency in men can result from diseases affecting the testes, pituitary gland, or hypothalamus. Consequences of testosterone deficiency vary depending on the stage of sexual development. Testosterone production declines naturally with age, so that a relative testosterone deficiency occurs in older men. Hypogonadal disorders of the testes (primary hypogonadism) are most commonly caused by Klinefelter's syndrome, mumps orchitis, trauma, tumor, cancer chemotherapy, or immune testicular failure (see Chapter 26, "Infectious Diseases," for a discussion of hypotestosteronism in HIV infection). Pituitary lesions caused by tumors, hemochromatosis, sarcoidosis, or cranial irradiation can lead to secondary hypogonadism. The classic cause of hypothalamic hypogonadism is Kallmann's syndrome (hypogonadotropic

hypogonadism with hyposmia, sensorineural hearing loss, oral clefts, micropenis, and cryptorchidism). Hypogonadism in childhood is characterized by failure of normal secondary sexual characteristics to develop and diminished muscle mass. In adult men, typical complaints are sexual dysfunction, diminished energy, decreased beard and body hair, muscle loss, and breast enlargement.

Decreasing testosterone levels as men age appear to be associated with changes in mood and cognition, but no clear relation between psychiatric syndromes and testosterone levels has been established. Men with lower testosterone levels are more likely to be depressed (Westley et al. 2015) or to become depressed (Ford et al. 2016), but there are many potential explanations for this finding. The concept of a male climacteric with related mood, anxiety, and cognitive disorders is controversial.

Evidence supports the use of testosterone replacement in hypogonadal men for improvement of body composition and sexual function. Questions remain about the value of testosterone replacement in age-related testosterone decline as well as in the treatment of depressive disorder in hypogonadal men. In some but not all studies, testosterone does seem to improve mood in hypogonadal men. However, results from randomized controlled clinical trials do not support testosterone treatment for major depressive disorder. The risks associated with physiological doses of testosterone appear to be small. The possible increased risk of prostate cancer remains a concern, but the evidence to date does not substantiate it.

Although some studies have found that testosterone deficiency in women is associated with impaired sexual function, low energy, and depression, other studies have found that higher testosterone levels increase the risk of depression (Milman et al. 2015). What level represents deficiency, as well as the indications, risks, and benefits of replacement, is even less well defined in women than it is in men (see Chapter 15, "Sexual Dysfunctions").

Other Metabolic Disorders

Electrolyte and Acid–Base Disturbances

Hyponatremia and Hypernatremia

Hyponatremia's principal manifestations are neuropsychiatric, and their severity is related to both the degree and the rapidity with which the disorder develops. Patients may have lethargy, stupor, confusion, psychosis, irritability, and seizures. Hyponatremia has many different causes, but those of particular psychiatric relevance are the syndrome of inappropriate antidiuretic hormone secretion (SIADH), which can be caused by many psychotropic drugs (especially carbamazepine and oxcarbazepine, but also SSRIs, tricyclic antidepressants, and antipsychotics); and psychogenic polydipsia. Polydipsia leading to hyponatremia in patients with schizophrenia is mediated by a reduced osmotic threshold for the release of vasopressin and by a defect in the osmoregulation of thirst. Acute-onset symptomatic hyponatremia may require emergent treatment with hypertonic (3%) saline. In chronic cases, correction should be gradual to minimize the risk of pontine myelinolysis, relying on fluid restriction and vasopressin receptor antagonists (Siegel 2008).

The signs of hypernatremia are also predominantly neuropsychiatric and include cognitive dysfunction, delirium, seizures, and lethargy progressing to stupor and coma. Similar symptoms are seen with any hyperosmolar state, such as extreme hyperglycemia. Hypernatremia is usually caused by dehydration, with significant total body water deficits. A rare cause is adipsia, the absence of thirst even in the presence of water depletion or sodium excess, usually caused by a hypothalamic lesion (which may result in other psychopathology) (Harrington et al. 2014).

Hypokalemia and Hyperkalemia

Hypokalemia produces muscular weakness and fatigue and, if severe, may cause severe paralysis (hypokalemic periodic paralysis), but central nervous system functions typically are not affected. Nevertheless, patients with symptomatic hypokalemia sometimes receive the misdiagnosis of depression. Hypokalemia is very common in eating disorders (see Chapter 13, "Eating Disorders," for a full discussion of the metabolic complications of eating disorders), chronic alcoholism, and alcohol withdrawal. The adverse effects of hyperkalemia are mainly cardiac, but severe muscle weakness also may occur.

Hypocalcemia and Hypercalcemia; Hypomagnesemia and Hypermagnesemia

Hypocalcemia and hypercalcemia were described earlier in this chapter in the "Parathyroid Disorders" section. Magnesium levels usually rise and fall in concert with calcium levels. Hypomagnesemia can cause anxiety, irritability, tetany, and seizures. Low magnesium levels are very common in alcoholic patients and in refeeding starving patients (including those with anorexia nervosa and catatonia). Cyclosporine causes hypomagnesemia, which can contribute to its neuropsychiatric side effects. Hypermagnesemia is much less common, usually resulting from excessive ingestion of magnesium-containing antacids or cathartics, and causes central nervous system depression.

Hypophosphatemia

Hypophosphatemia causes anxiety, hyperventilation, irritability, weakness, delirium, and, if severe, seizures, coma, and death, in addition to symptoms in many other organ systems. Hypophosphatemia occurs in the same settings as hypomagnesemia.

Acidosis and Alkalosis

Metabolic acidosis results in compensatory hyperventilation. When the acidosis is severe and acute, as in diabetic ketoacidosis, fatigue and delirium are present and may progress to stupor and coma. Acute metabolic acidosis is a complication of a wide variety of overdoses and toxic ingestions. Patients with chronic metabolic acidosis appear depressed, with prominent anorexia and fatigue. Patients with severe metabolic alkalosis present with apathy, confusion, and stupor. Respiratory acidosis results from ventilatory insufficiency, and respiratory alkalosis results from hyperventilation (see Chapter 18, "Lung Disease").

Vitamin Deficiencies

Deficiencies of vitamin B_{12} and folate are discussed in Chapter 23, "Hematology."

Pellagra, originally thought to be a deficiency of niacin, is now recognized to be a complex deficiency of multiple vitamins and amino acids. The classic triad of symptoms is dermatitis, dementia, and diarrhea, but irritability, anxiety, depression, apathy, and psychosis all have been reported (Prakash et al. 2008). Pellagra is now rare in the developed nations, but cases are still reported in anorexia nervosa, inflammatory bowel disease, and alcoholism.

Thiamine deficiency (beriberi) causes cardiac and neuropsychiatric syndromes, including peripheral neuropathy and Wernicke-Korsakoff encephalopathy. Wernicke's consists of vomiting, nystagmus, ophthalmoplegia, fever, ataxia, and confusion that can progress to coma and death. Korsakoff's is a dementia with amnesia, impaired ability to learn, confabulation, and often psychosis. Improvement usually occurs with thiamine replacement but may be slow. Giving intravenous glucose to a thiamine-deficient patient without coadministering thiamine may precipitate acute beriberi. Thiamine deficiency is well known and most frequent in alcoholic patients, but it also occurs in patients undergoing chronic dialysis, patients refeeding after starvation (including patients with anorexia nervosa), and individuals on fad diets.

Pyridoxine (vitamin B_6) deficiency causes peripheral neuropathy and neuropsychiatric disorders, including reports of seizures, migraine, chronic pain, depression, and psychosis. Homocysteine is elevated in B_6 deficiency and may play a role in accelerating vascular disease and dementia. Pyridoxine deficiency is common because many drugs act as its antagonist. Clinical trials of B_6 supplementation in healthy elderly persons and in cognitively impaired subjects to date have not shown improvements in mood or cognition.

Vitamin E deficiency can cause areflexia, ataxia, and decreased vibratory and proprioceptive sensation. Although lower levels of vitamin E have been reported in major depressive disorder, there is no evidence that vitamin E supplementation benefits mood or cognition.

Porphyrias

The porphyrias are a group of rare disorders of heme biosynthesis that can be inherited or acquired. Neuropsychiatric manifestations occur in the two neuroporphyrias (acute intermittent porphyria and plumboporphyria) and two neurocutaneous porphyrias (hereditary coproporphyria and variegate porphyria). Acute intermittent porphyria is the most common. Recurrent acute attacks are typical in all four, with variable manifestations. In acute porphyria, the cardinal signs are abdominal pain, peripheral neuropathy, and psychiatric symptoms, which can be the sole presenting symptoms, including anxiety, depression, psychosis, and delirium. Seizures, autonomic instability, dehydration, electrolyte imbalance, and dermatological changes also may occur. Symptoms may vary considerably among patients and in the same patient over time, and they can mimic symptoms of other psychiatric and medical disorders, making diagnosis a challenge (Kumar 2012). Stress has long been considered a precipitant of acute episodes, but data are lacking. The diagnosis is made by measuring porphyrins and their metabolites in stool and urine during an acute episode. Between episodes, porphyrin levels return to normal. Diagnosis is more likely to be made when the clinician has a high index of suspicion. The diagnosis may be especially difficult because neuropsychiatric symptoms may continue well after the

end of an acute episode. Therapy is primarily supportive and includes identification of precipitants. Although barbiturates clearly can trigger attacks, evidence is inadequate regarding the role of other psychotropic drugs. A comprehensive rating of drugs' risk for porphyrinogenicity is available at the Drug Database for Acute Porphyria (www.drugs-porphyria.org).

Other Genetic Metabolic Disorders

Inborn errors of metabolism usually presenting in neonates or young children may in rare cases first present in adolescence or adulthood as a psychiatric disorder. Such a possibility may be suspected because of family history or because psychiatric symptoms present as part of a more complex clinical picture with systemic, cognitive, or motor signs (Sedel et al. 2007). Such a diagnostic possibility also should be considered when a psychiatric disorder presents atypically with subtle "organic" signs and responds poorly to standard treatments. Some of these disorders present with acute and recurrent attacks of confusion, which may be misdiagnosed as acute psychosis. Examples include urea cycle disorders (e.g., ornithine transcarbamylase deficiency) and homocysteine remethylation defects (e.g., hyperhomocysteinemia). Others may produce chronic psychiatric symptoms (e.g., catatonia, hallucinations), including homocystinuria, Wilson's disease, adrenoleukodystrophy, and some lysosomal disorders (e.g., Gaucher's disease). Mild intellectual disability and late-onset behavioral or personality changes may be a manifestation of homocystinuria, cerebrotendinous xanthomatosis, monoamine oxidase A deficiency, succinic semialdehyde dehydrogenase deficiency, or creatine transporter deficiency. Recognition of such disorders in an adult with only psychiatric symptoms may be very difficult, but earlier recognition and specific intervention can prevent irreversible nervous system (and other organ) injury.

Conclusion

Endocrine and metabolic disorders frequently occur in conjunction with common psychiatric conditions. The causal linkages and mechanisms vary widely. In some situations, the endocrine state manifests in part as a psychiatric condition. In other instances, the psychiatric condition may be a complex biopsychosocial and/or biological response to the endocrine disorder. Psychiatric conditions and their treatment with psychotropic drugs may also increase risk of endocrine disorders.

References

Aggarwal S, Kailash S, Sagar R, et al: Neuropsychological dysfunction in idiopathic hypoparathyroidism and its relationship with intracranial calcification and serum total calcium. Eur J Endocrinol 168(6):895–903, 2013 23482593
Ajmal A, Joffe H, Nachtigall LB: Psychotropic-induced hyperprolactinemia: a clinical review. Psychosomatics 55(1):29–36, 2014 24140188
Albert U, De Cori D, Aguglia A, et al: Effects of maintenance lithium treatment on serum parathyroid hormone and calcium levels: a retrospective longitudinal naturalistic study. Neuropsychiatr Dis Treat 11:1785–1791, 2015 26229473

Aleppo G, Ruedy KJ, Riddlesworth TD, et al; REPLACE-BG Study Group: REPLACE-BG: a randomized trial comparing continuous glucose monitoring with and without routine blood glucose monitoring in adults with well-controlled type 1 diabetes. Diabetes Care 40(4):538–545, 2017 28209654

American Academy of Pediatrics; Section on Endocrinology and Committee on Genetics, American Thyroid Association; Public Health Committee, Lawson Wilkins Pediatric Endocrine Society; et al: Update of newborn screening and therapy for congenital hypothyroidism. Pediatrics 117(6):2290–2303, 2006 16740880

American Diabetes Association: 2. Classification and Diagnosis of Diabetes. Diabetes Care 40 (suppl 1):S11–S24, 2017a 27979889

American Diabetes Association: 4. Lifestyle Management. Diabetes Care 40 (suppl 1):S33–S43, 2017b 27979891

American Diabetes Association: 11. Older Adults. Diabetes Care 40 (suppl 1):S99–S104, 2017c 27979898

American Diabetes Association; American Psychiatric Association; American Association of Clinical Endocrinologists; North American Association for the Study of Obesity: Consensus development conference on antipsychotic drugs and obesity and diabetes. Diabetes Care 27(2):596–601, 2004 14747245

Andela CD, van Haalen FM, Ragnarsson O, et al: Mechanisms in Endocrinology: Cushing's syndrome causes irreversible effects on the human brain: a systematic review of structural and functional magnetic resonance imaging studies. Eur J Endocrinol 173(1):R1–R14, 2015 25650405

Anglin RE, Rosebush PI, Mazurek MF: The neuropsychiatric profile of Addison's disease: revisiting a forgotten phenomenon. J Neuropsychiatry Clin Neurosci 18(4):450–459, 2006 17135373

Annagür BB, Tazegül A, Uguz F, et al: Biological correlates of major depression and generalized anxiety disorder in women with polycystic ovary syndrome. J Psychosom Res 74(3):244–247, 2013 23438716

Arnaldi G, Angeli A, Atkinson AB, et al: Diagnosis and complications of Cushing's syndrome: a consensus statement. J Clin Endocrinol Metab 88(12):5593–5602, 2003 14671138

Arvanitis LA, Miller BG: Multiple fixed doses of "Seroquel" (quetiapine) in patients with acute exacerbation of schizophrenia: a comparison with haloperidol and placebo. The Seroquel Trial 13 Study Group. Biol Psychiatry 42(4):233–246, 1997 9270900

Barry JA, Kuczmierczyk AR, Hardiman PJ: Anxiety and depression in polycystic ovary syndrome: a systematic review and meta-analysis. Hum Reprod 26(9):2442–2451, 2011 21725075

Bathla M, Singh M, Relan P: Prevalence of anxiety and depressive symptoms among patients with hypothyroidism. Indian J Endocrinol Metab 20(4):468–474, 2016 27366712

Biemans E, Hart HE, Rutten GEHM, et al: Cobalamin status and its relation with depression, cognition and neuropathy in patients with type 2 diabetes mellitus using metformin. Acta Diabetol 52(2):383–393, 2015 25315630

Bilo L, Meo R: Polycystic ovary syndrome in women using valproate: a review. Gynecol Endocrinol 24(10):562–570, 2008 19012099

Black SA, Markides KS, Ray LA: Depression predicts increased incidence of adverse health outcomes in older Mexican Americans with type 2 diabetes. Diabetes Care 26(10):2822–2828, 2003 14514586

Blay SL, Aguiar JV, Passos IC: Polycystic ovary syndrome and mental disorders: a systematic review and exploratory meta-analysis. Neuropsychiatr Dis Treat 12:2895–2903, 2016 27877043

Blum MR, Wijsman LW, Virgini VS, et al; PROSPER study group: Subclinical thyroid dysfunction and depressive symptoms among the elderly: a prospective cohort study. Neuroendocrinology 103(3–4):291–299, 2016 26202797

Brandt F, Thvilum M, Almind D, et al: Hyperthyroidism and psychiatric morbidity: evidence from a Danish nationwide register study. Eur J Endocrinol 170(2):341–348, 2013 24282192

Brieler JA, Lustman PJ, Scherrer JF, et al: Antidepressant medication use and glycaemic control in comorbid type 2 diabetes and depression. Fam Pract 33(1):30–36, 2016 26743722

Brownlie BE, Rae AM, Walshe JW, Wells JE: Psychoses associated with thyrotoxicosis—"thyrotoxic psychosis." A report of 18 cases, with statistical analysis of incidence. Eur J Endocrinol 142(5):438–444, 2000 10802519

Bruce DG, Davis WA, Starkstein SE, Davis TM: Mid-life predictors of cognitive impairment and dementia in type 2 diabetes mellitus: the Fremantle Diabetes Study. J Alzheimers Dis 42 (suppl 3):S63–S70, 2014 24840567

Bruyère O, Reginster JY: Osteoporosis in patients taking selective serotonin reuptake inhibitors: a focus on fracture outcome. Endocrine 48(1):65–68, 2015 25091520

Buse JB: Metabolic side effects of antipsychotics: focus on hyperglycemia and diabetes. J Clin Psychiatry 63 (suppl 4):37–41, 2002 11913675

Calkin CV, Gardner DM, Ransom T, Alda M: The relationship between bipolar disorder and type 2 diabetes: more than just co-morbid disorders. Ann Med 45(2):171–181, 2013 22621171

Cesta CE, Månsson M, Palm C, et al: Polycystic ovary syndrome and psychiatric disorders: comorbidity and heritability in a nationwide Swedish cohort. Psychoneuroendocrinology 73:196–203, 2016 27513883

Chen JX, Su YA, Bian QT, et al: Adjunctive aripiprazole in the treatment of risperidone-induced hyperprolactinemia: a randomized, double-blind, placebo-controlled, dose-response study. Psychoneuroendocrinology 58:130–140, 2015 25981348

Ciechanowski PS, Katon WJ, Russo JE: Depression and diabetes: impact of depressive symptoms on adherence, function, and costs. Arch Intern Med 160(21):3278–3285, 2000 11088090

Collins MM, Corcoran P, Perry IJ: Anxiety and depression symptoms in patients with diabetes. Diabet Med 26(2):153–161, 2009 19236618

Colton P, Olmsted M, Daneman D, et al: Disturbed eating behavior and eating disorders in preteen and early teenage girls with type 1 diabetes: a case-controlled study. Diabetes Care 27(7):1654–1659, 2004 15220242

Cramon P, Winther KH, Watt T, et al: Quality-of-life impairments persist six months after treatment of Graves' hyperthyroidism and toxic nodular goiter: a prospective cohort study. Thyroid 26(8):1010–1018, 2016 27370744

Crow S, Kendall D, Praus B, Thuras P: Binge eating and other psychopathology in patients with type II diabetes mellitus. Int J Eat Disord 30(2):222–226, 2001 11449458

Daumit GL, Dickerson FB, Wang N-Y, et al: A behavioral weight-loss intervention in persons with serious mental illness. N Engl J Med 368(17):1594–1602, 2013 23517118

David SR, Taylor CC, Kinon BJ, Breier A: The effects of olanzapine, risperidone, and haloperidol on plasma prolactin levels in patients with schizophrenia. Clin Ther 22(9):1085–1096, 2000 11048906

de Groot M, Anderson R, Freedland KE, et al: Association of depression and diabetes complications: a meta-analysis. Psychosom Med 63(4):619–630, 2001 11485116

De Hert M, Dekker JM, Wood D, et al: Cardiovascular disease and diabetes in people with severe mental illness position statement from the European Psychiatric Association (EPA), supported by the European Association for the Study of Diabetes (EASD) and the European Society of Cardiology (ESC). Eur Psychiatry 24(6):412–424, 2009 19682863

De Hert M, Detraux J, Stubbs B: Relationship between antipsychotic medication, serum prolactin levels and osteoporosis/osteoporotic fractures in patients with schizophrenia: a critical literature review. Expert Opin Drug Saf 15(6):809–823, 2016 26986209

de Jongh RT, Lips P, van Schoor NM, et al: Endogenous subclinical thyroid disorders, physical and cognitive function, depression, and mortality in older individuals. Eur J Endocrinol 165(4):545–554, 2011 21768248

Demartini B, Masu A, Scarone S, et al: Prevalence of depression in patients affected by subclinical hypothyroidism. Panminerva Med 52(4):277–282, 2010 21183887

Diabetes Control and Complications Trial/Epidemiology of Diabetes Interventions and Complications Study Research Group, Jacobson AM, Musen G, et al: Long-term effect of diabetes and its treatment on cognitive function. N Engl J Med 356(18):1842–1852, 2007 [Erratum in: N Engl J Med 361(19):1914, 2009] 17476010

Dimopoulou C, Leistner SM, Ising M, et al: Body image perception in acromegaly is not associated with objective acromegalic changes, but depends on depressive symptoms. Neuroendocrinology 105(2):115–122, 2017 27453978

Dokras A, Clifton S, Futterweit W, Wild R: Increased prevalence of anxiety symptoms in women with polycystic ovary syndrome: systematic review and meta-analysis. Fertil Steril 97(1):225–30.e2, 2012 22127370

Eisenhofer G, Sharabi Y, Pacak K: Unexplained symptomatic paroxysmal hypertension in pseudopheochromocytoma: a stress response disorder? Ann N Y Acad Sci 1148:469–478, 2008 19120143

Exalto LG, Biessels GJ, Karter AJ, et al: Risk score for prediction of 10 year dementia risk in individuals with type 2 diabetes: a cohort study. Lancet Diabetes Endocrinol 1(3):183–190, 2013 24622366

Farmer A, Korszun A, Owen MJ, et al: Medical disorders in people with recurrent depression. Br J Psychiatry 192(5):351–355, 2008 18450658

Fisher L, Hessler DM, Polonsky WH, Mullan J: When is diabetes distress clinically meaningful? Establishing cut points for the Diabetes Distress Scale. Diabetes Care 35(2):259–264, 2012 22228744

Fleseriu M, Biller BM, Findling JW, et al; SEISMIC Study Investigators: Mifepristone, a glucocorticoid receptor antagonist, produces clinical and metabolic benefits in patients with Cushing's syndrome. J Clin Endocrinol Metab 97(6):2039–2049, 2012 22466348

Ford AH, Yeap BB, Flicker L, et al: Prospective longitudinal study of testosterone and incident depression in older men: the Health In Men Study. Psychoneuroendocrinology 64:57–65, 2016 26615472

Forget H, Lacroix A, Bourdeau I, Cohen H: Long-term cognitive effects of glucocorticoid excess in Cushing's syndrome. Psychoneuroendocrinology 65:26–33, 2016 26708069

Fukao A, Takamatsu J, Murakami Y, et al: The relationship of psychological factors to the prognosis of hyperthyroidism in antithyroid drug-treated patients with Graves' disease. Clin Endocrinol (Oxf) 58(5):550–555, 2003 12699435

Gagnon C, Aimé A, Bélanger C, Markowitz JT: Comorbid diabetes and eating disorders in adult patients: assessment and considerations for treatment. Diabetes Educ 38(4):537–542, 2012 22585871

Garay-Sevilla ME, Malacara JM, González-Contreras E, et al: Perceived psychological stress in diabetes mellitus type 2. Rev Invest Clin 52(3):241–245, 2000 10953606

Garber JR, Cobin RH, Gharib H, et al; American Association of Clinical Endocrinologists and American Thyroid Association Taskforce on Hypothyroidism in Adults: Clinical practice guidelines for hypothyroidism in adults: cosponsored by the American Association of Clinical Endocrinologists and the American Thyroid Association. Endocr Pract 18(6):988–1028, 2012 23246686

Garner DM: Eating Disorder Inventory–3: Professional Manual. Odessa, FL, Psychological Assessment Resources, 2004

Garnier KA, Ismail KA, Moylan S, Harvey R: Thyroid function testing in an inpatient mental health unit. Australas Psychiatry 24(3):256–260, 2016 26635375

Geller WK, MacFadden W: Diabetes and atypical neuroleptics. Am J Psychiatry 160(2):388; author reply 389, 2003 12562601

Gendelman N, Snell-Bergeon JK, McFann K, et al: Prevalence and correlates of depression in individuals with and without type 1 diabetes. Diabetes Care 32(4):575–579, 2009 19171719

Georgiades A, Zucker N, Friedman KE, et al: Changes in depressive symptoms and glycemic control in diabetes mellitus. Psychosom Med 69(3):235–241, 2007 17420441

Geraedts VJ, Dimopoulou C, Auer M, et al: Health outcomes in acromegaly: depression and anxiety are promising targets for improving reduced quality of life. Front Endocrinol (Lausanne) 5:229, 2015 25610427

Goebel-Fabbri AE, Fikkan J, Franko DL, et al: Insulin restriction and associated morbidity and mortality in women with type 1 diabetes. Diabetes Care 31(3):415–419, 2008 18070998

Goff DC, Sullivan LM, McEvoy JP, et al: A comparison of ten-year cardiac risk estimates in schizophrenia patients from the CATIE study and matched controls. Schizophr Res 80(1):45–53, 2005 16198088

Golden SH: A review of the evidence for a neuroendocrine link between stress, depression and diabetes mellitus. Curr Diabetes Rev 3(4):252–259, 2007 18220683

Goldfine AB, Silver R, Aldhahi W, et al: Use of salsalate to target inflammation in the treatment of insulin resistance and type 2 diabetes. Clin Transl Sci 1(1):36–43, 2008 19337387

Gonder-Frederick LA, Schmidt KM, Vajda KA, et al: Psychometric properties of the hypoglycemia fear survey–II for adults with type 1 diabetes. Diabetes Care 34(4):801–806, 2011 21346182

Gorin AA, Niemeier HM, Hogan P, et al; Look AHEAD Research Group: Binge eating and weight loss outcomes in overweight and obese individuals with type 2 diabetes: results from the Look AHEAD trial. Arch Gen Psychiatry 65(12):1447–1455, 2008 19047532

Green CA, Yarborough BJH, Leo MC, et al: The STRIDE weight loss and lifestyle intervention for individuals taking antipsychotic medications: a randomized trial. Am J Psychiatry 172(1):71–81, 2015 25219423

Greenwood EA, Pasch LA, Shinkai K, et al: Putative role for insulin resistance in depression risk in polycystic ovary syndrome. Fertil Steril 104(3):707–14.e1, 2015 26054555

Hansen RA, Maciejewski M, Yu-Isenberg K, Farley JF: Adherence to antipsychotics and cardiometabolic medication: association with health care utilization and costs. Psychiatr Serv 63(9):920–928, 2012 22706887

Harrington C, Grossman J, Richman K: Psychogenic adipsia presenting as acute kidney injury: case report and review of disorders of sodium and water metabolism in psychiatric illness. Psychosomatics 55(3):289–295, 2014 24012289

Heraclides AM, Chandola T, Witte DR, Brunner EJ: Work stress, obesity and the risk of type 2 diabetes: gender-specific bidirectional effect in the Whitehall II study. Obesity (Silver Spring) 20(2):428–433, 2012 21593804

Holroyd S, Cohen MJ: Treatment of hyperprolactinemia in major depression. Am J Psychiatry 147(6):810, 1990 2094233

Holt RIG: The prevention of diabetes and cardiovascular disease in people with schizophrenia. Acta Psychiatr Scand 132(2):86–96, 2015 25976975

Holt RIG, de Groot M, Golden SH: Diabetes and depression. Curr Diab Rep 14(6):491, 2014 24743941

Hood MM, Reutrakul S, Crowley SJ: Night eating in patients with type 2 diabetes. Associations with glycemic control, eating patterns, sleep, and mood. Appetite 79:91–96, 2014 24751916

Hu LY, Shen CC, Hu YW, et al: Hyperthyroidism and risk for bipolar disorders: a nationwide population-based study. PLoS One 8(8):e73057, 2013 24023669

Hung JH, Hu LY, Tsai SJ, et al: Risk of psychiatric disorders following polycystic ovary syndrome: a nationwide population-based cohort study. PLoS One 9(5):e97041, 2014 24816764

Joffe RT, Kutcher S, MacDonald C: Thyroid function and bipolar affective disorder. Psychiatry Res 25(2):117–121, 1988 3140257

Jones JM, Lawson ML, Daneman D, et al: Eating disorders in adolescent females with and without type 1 diabetes: cross sectional study. BMJ 320(7249):1563–1566, 2000 10845962

Kahal H, Aye M, Rigby AS, et al: The effect of parathyroidectomy on neuropsychological symptoms and biochemical parameters in patients with asymptomatic primary hyperparathyroidism. Clin Endocrinol (Oxf) 76(2):196–200, 2012 21851373

Kahn CR, Weir GC, King GL, et al: Joslin's Diabetes Mellitus, 14th Edition. New York, Lippincott Williams & Wilkins, 2005

Kan C, Silva N, Golden SH, et al: A systematic review and meta-analysis of the association between depression and insulin resistance. Diabetes Care 36(2):480–489, 2013 23349152

Kars M, van der Klaauw AA, Onstein CS, et al: Quality of life is decreased in female patients treated for microprolactinoma. Eur J Endocrinol 157(2):133–139, 2007 17656590

Katon W, Unützer J, Fan MY, et al: Cost-effectiveness and net benefit of enhanced treatment of depression for older adults with diabetes and depression. Diabetes Care 29(2):265–270, 2006 16443871

Katon WJ, Lin EHB, Von Korff M, et al: Collaborative care for patients with depression and chronic illnesses. N Engl J Med 363(27):2611–2620, 2010 21190455

Keller WR, Fischer BA, McMahon RP, et al: Open-label salsalate for the treatment of pre-diabetes in people with schizophrenia. Schizophr Res 147(2–3):408–409, 2013 23680037

Kelly T, Denmark L, Lieberman DZ: Elevated levels of circulating thyroid hormone do not cause the medical sequelae of hyperthyroidism. Prog Neuropsychopharmacol Biol Psychiatry 71:1–6, 2016 27302764

Kenardy J, Mensch M, Bowen K, Pearson SA: A comparison of eating behaviors in newly diagnosed NIDDM patients and case-matched control subjects. Diabetes Care 17(10):1197–1199, 1994 7821143

Knowler WC, Barrett-Connor E, Fowler SE, et al; Diabetes Prevention Program Research Group: Reduction in the incidence of type 2 diabetes with lifestyle intervention or metformin. N Engl J Med 346(6):393–403, 2002 11832527

Kudrjavcev T: Neurologic complications of thyroid dysfunction. Adv Neurol 19:619–636, 1978 742545

Kumar B: Acute intermittent porphyria presenting solely with psychosis: a case report and discussion. Psychosomatics 53(5):494–498, 2012 22902088

Kvetny J, Ellervik C, Bech P: Is suppressed thyroid-stimulating hormone (TSH) associated with subclinical depression in the Danish General Suburban Population Study? Nord J Psychiatry 69(4):282–286, 2015 25377023

Lambert CG, Mazurie AJ, Lauve NR, et al: Hypothyroidism risk compared among nine common bipolar disorder therapies in a large US cohort. Bipolar Disord 18(3):247–260, 2016 27226264

Larsen JR, Vedtofte L, Holst JJ, et al: Does a GLP-1 receptor agonist change glucose tolerance in patients treated with antipsychotic medications? Design of a randomised, double-blinded, placebo-controlled clinical trial. BMJ Open 4(3):e004227, 2014 24667381

Lee CW, Liao CH, Lin CL, et al: Increased risk of osteoporosis in patients with depression: a population-based retrospective cohort study. Mayo Clin Proc 90(1):63–70, 2015 25572194

Lenders JW, Pacak K, Walther MM, et al: Biochemical diagnosis of pheochromocytoma: which test is best? JAMA 287(11):1427–1434, 2002 11903030

Li C, Ford ES, Strine TW, Mokdad AH: Prevalence of depression among U.S. adults with diabetes: findings from the 2006 Behavioral Risk Factor Surveillance System. Diabetes Care 31(1):105–107, 2008 17934145

Liu JY, Saunders ND, Chen A, et al: Neuropsychological changes in primary hyperparathyroidism after parathyroidectomy. Am Surg 82(9):839–845, 2016 27670574

Lloyd CE, Dyer PH, Lancashire RJ, et al: Association between stress and glycemic control in adults with type 1 (insulin-dependent) diabetes. Diabetes Care 22(8):1278–1283, 1999 10480771

Lloyd CE, Sartorius N, Cimino LC, et al: The INTERPRET-DD study of diabetes and depression: a protocol. Diabet Med 32(7):925–934, 2015 25659409

Ludman EJ, Katon W, Russo J, et al: Depression and diabetes symptom burden. Gen Hosp Psychiatry 26(6):430–436, 2004 15567208

Ludman E, Katon W, Russo J, et al: Panic episodes among patients with diabetes. Gen Hosp Psychiatry 28(6):475–481, 2006 17088162

Lustman PJ, Griffith LS, Clouse RE, et al: Effects of nortriptyline on depression and glycemic control in diabetes: results of a double-blind, placebo-controlled trial. Psychosom Med 59(3):241–250, 1997 9178335

Lustman PJ, Griffith LS, Freedland KE, et al: Cognitive behavior therapy for depression in type 2 diabetes mellitus. A randomized, controlled trial. Ann Intern Med 129(8):613–621, 1998 9786808

Lustman PJ, Anderson RJ, Freedland KE, et al: Depression and poor glycemic control: a meta-analytic review of the literature. Diabetes Care 23(7):934–942, 2000a 10895843

Lustman PJ, Freedland KE, Griffith LS, Clouse RE: Fluoxetine for depression in diabetes: a randomized double-blind placebo-controlled trial. Diabetes Care 23(5):618–623, 2000b 10834419

Lustman PJ, Clouse RE, Nix BD, et al: Sertraline for prevention of depression recurrence in diabetes mellitus: a randomized, double-blind, placebo-controlled trial. Arch Gen Psychiatry 63(5):521–529, 2006 16651509

Manger WM: The protean manifestations of pheochromocytoma. Horm Metab Res 41(9):658–663, 2009 19242899

Mayeda ER, Whitmer RA, Yaffe K: Diabetes and cognition. Clin Geriatr Med 31(1):101–115, 2015 25453304

McKibbin CL, Patterson TL, Norman G, et al: A lifestyle intervention for older schizophrenia patients with diabetes mellitus: a randomized controlled trial. Schizophr Res 86(1–3):36–44, 2006 16842977

Meyer JM, Davis VG, Goff DC, et al: Change in metabolic syndrome parameters with antipsychotic treatment in the CATIE Schizophrenia Trial: prospective data from phase 1. Schizophr Res 101(1–3):273–286, 2008 18258416

Mezuk B, Eaton WW, Albrecht S, Golden SH: Depression and type 2 diabetes over the lifespan: a meta-analysis. Diabetes Care 31(12):2383–2390, 2008 19033418

Miller KJ, Parsons TD, Whybrow PC, et al: Verbal memory retrieval deficits associated with untreated hypothyroidism. J Neuropsychiatry Clin Neurosci 19(2):132–136, 2007 17431058

Milman LW, Sammel MD, Barnhart KT, et al: Higher serum total testosterone levels correlate with increased risk of depressive symptoms in Caucasian women through the entire menopausal transition. Psychoneuroendocrinology 62:107–113, 2015 26280374

Mitchell JE, Pomeroy C, Adson DE: Managing medical complications, in Handbook for Treatment of Eating Disorders. Edited by Garner D, Garfinkel P. New York, Guilford, 1997, pp 383–393

Montagna G, Imperiali M, Agazzi P, et al: Hashimoto's encephalopathy: a rare proteiform disorder. Autoimmun Rev 15(5):466–476, 2016 26849953

Munshi MN, Florez H, Huang ES, et al: Management of diabetes in long-term care and skilled nursing facilities: a position statement of the American Diabetes Association. Diabetes Care 39(2):308–318, 2016 26798150

Myers A, Trivedi MH: Death by insulin: management of self-harm and suicide in diabetes management. Curr Diabetes Rev 13(3):251–262, 2017 27719630

Nathan DM, Genuth S, Lachin J, et al; Diabetes Control and Complications Trial Research Group: The effect of intensive treatment of diabetes on the development and progression of long-term complications in insulin-dependent diabetes mellitus. N Engl J Med 329(14):977–986, 1993 8366922

Nathan DM, Davidson MB, DeFronzo RA, et al; American Diabetes Association: Impaired fasting glucose and impaired glucose tolerance: implications for care. Diabetes Care 30(3):753–759, 2007 17327355

Nguyen AL, Green J, Enguidanos S: The relationship between depressive symptoms, diabetes symptoms, and self-management among an urban, low-income Latino population. J Diabetes Complications 29(8):1003–1008, 2015 26490755

Nobis S, Lehr D, Ebert DD, et al: Efficacy of a web-based intervention with mobile phone support in treating depressive symptoms in adults with type 1 and type 2 diabetes: a randomized controlled trial. Diabetes Care 38(5):776–783, 2015 25710923

Olmsted MP, Colton PA, Daneman D, et al: Prediction of the onset of disturbed eating behavior in adolescent girls with type 1 diabetes. Diabetes Care 31(10):1978–1982, 2008 18628570

Otis JD, Sanderson K, Hardway C, et al: A randomized controlled pilot study of a cognitive-behavioral therapy approach for painful diabetic peripheral neuropathy. J Pain 14(5):475–482, 2013 23452825

Ott BR, Daiello LA, Dahabreh IJ, et al: Do statins impair cognition? A systematic review and meta-analysis of randomized controlled trials. J Gen Intern Med 30(3):348–358, 2015 25575908

Paile-Hyvärinen M, Wahlbeck K, Eriksson JG: Quality of life and metabolic status in mildly depressed patients with type 2 diabetes treated with paroxetine: a double-blind randomised placebo controlled 6-month trial. BMC Fam Pract 8:34, 2007 17570858

Palta P, Golden SH, Teresi JA, et al: Depression is not associated with diabetes control in minority elderly. J Diabetes Complications 28(6):798–804, 2014 25156987

Pantanetti P, Sonino N, Arnaldi G, Boscaro M: Self image and quality of life in acromegaly. Pituitary 5(1):17–19, 2002 12638721

Papelbaum M, Appolinário JC, Moreira Rde O, et al: Prevalence of eating disorders and psychiatric comorbidity in a clinical sample of type 2 diabetes mellitus patients. Rev Bras Psiquiatr 27(2):135–138, 2005 15962139

Park M, Reynolds CF 3rd: Depression among older adults with diabetes mellitus. Clin Geriatr Med 31(1):117–137, ix, 2015 25453305

Pasqualetti G, Pagano G, Rengo G, et al: Subclinical hypothyroidism and cognitive impairment: systematic review and meta-analysis. J Clin Endocrinol Metab 100(11):4240–4248, 2015 26305618

Peterson CB, Mitchell JE: Psychosocial and pharmacological treatment of eating disorders: a review of research findings. J Clin Psychol 55(6):685–697, 1999 10445860

Peterson CM, Fischer S, Young-Hyman D: Topical review: a comprehensive risk model for disordered eating in youth with type 1 diabetes. J Pediatr Psychol 40(4):385–390, 2015 25502449

Petrak F, Herpertz S, Albus C, et al: Cognitive behavioral therapy versus sertraline in patients with depression and poorly controlled diabetes: the Diabetes and Depression (DAD) Study: a randomized controlled multicenter trial. Diabetes Care 38(5):767–775, 2015 25690005

Peuskens J, Pani L, Detraux J, De Hert M: The effects of novel and newly approved antipsychotics on serum prolactin levels: a comprehensive review. CNS Drugs 28(5):421–453, 2014 24677189

Peveler RC, Bryden KS, Neil HA, et al: The relationship of disordered eating habits and attitudes to clinical outcomes in young adult females with type 1 diabetes. Diabetes Care 28(1):84–88, 2005 15616238

Pickering TG, Clemow L: Paroxysmal hypertension: the role of stress and psychological factors. J Clin Hypertens (Greenwich) 10(7):575–581, 2008 18607143

Pivonello R, Simeoli C, De Martino MC, et al: Neuropsychiatric disorders in Cushing's syndrome. Front Neurosci 9:129, 2015 25941467

Polonsky WH, Anderson BJ, Lohrer PA, et al: Insulin omission in women with IDDM. Diabetes Care 17(10):1178–1185, 1994 7821139

Pouwer F, Kupper N, Adriaanse MC: Does emotional stress cause type 2 diabetes mellitus? A review from the European Depression in Diabetes (EDID) Research Consortium. Discov Med 9(45):112–118, 2010 20193636

Prakash R, Gandotra S, Singh LK, et al: Rapid resolution of delusional parasitosis in pellagra with niacin augmentation therapy. Gen Hosp Psychiatry 30(6):581–584, 2008 19061687

Radoeva PD, Fremont W, Antshel KM, Kates WR: Longitudinal study of premorbid adjustment in 22q11.2 deletion (velocardiofacial) syndrome and association with psychosis. Dev Psychopathol 29(1):93–106, 2017 26864886

Rieben C, Segna D, da Costa BR, et al: Subclinical thyroid dysfunction and the risk of cognitive decline: a meta-analysis of prospective cohort studies. J Clin Endocrinol Metab 101(12):4945–4954, 2016 27689250

Rosebush PI, Garside S, Levinson AJ, Mazurek MF: The neuropsychiatry of adult-onset adrenoleukodystrophy. J Neuropsychiatry Clin Neurosci 11(3):315–327, 1999 10440007

Sedel F, Baumann N, Turpin JC, et al: Psychiatric manifestations revealing inborn errors of metabolism in adolescents and adults. J Inherit Metab Dis 30(5):631–641, 2007 17694356

Shaban C: Diabulimia: mental health condition or media hyperbole? Practical Diabetes 30(3):104–105a, 2013

Shah BM, Mezzio DJ, Ho J, Ip EJ: Association of ABC (HbA1c, blood pressure, LDL-cholesterol) goal attainment with depression and health-related quality of life among adults with type 2 diabetes. J Diabetes Complications 29(6):794–800, 2015 25976863

Siegel AJ: Hyponatremia in psychiatric patients: update on evaluation and management. Harv Rev Psychiatry 16(1):13–24, 2008 18306096

Sievers C, Sämann PG, Pfister H, et al: Cognitive function in acromegaly: description and brain volumetric correlates. Pituitary 15(3):350–357, 2012 21735089

Smith CD, Grondin R, LeMaster W, et al: Reversible cognitive, motor, and driving impairments in severe hypothyroidism. Thyroid 25(1):28–36, 2015 25381990

Starkman MN: Neuropsychiatric findings in Cushing syndrome and exogenous glucocorticoid administration. Endocrinol Metab Clin North Am 42(3):477–488, 2013 24011881

Stern TA, Cremens CM: Factitious pheochromocytoma. One patient history and literature review. Psychosomatics 39(3):283–287, 1998 9664776

Strachan MWJ, Reynolds RM, Frier BM, et al: The relationship between type 2 diabetes and dementia. Br Med Bull 88(1):131–146, 2008 19029150

Striegel-Moore RH, Wilfley DE, Pike KM, et al: Recurrent binge eating in black American women. Arch Fam Med 9(1):83–87, 2000 10664648

Thomas CC, Philipson LH: Update on diabetes classification. Med Clin North Am 99(1):1–16, 2015 25456640

Tiemensma J, Biermasz NR, van der Mast RC, et al: Increased psychopathology and maladaptive personality traits, but normal cognitive functioning, in patients after long-term cure of acromegaly. J Clin Endocrinol Metab 95(12):E392–E402, 2010 20843947

Tiemensma J, Andela CD, Biermasz NR, et al: Mild cognitive deficits in patients with primary adrenal insufficiency. Psychoneuroendocrinology 63:170–177, 2016 26454105

Trzepacz PT, McCue M, Klein I, et al: A psychiatric and neuropsychological study of patients with untreated Graves' disease. Gen Hosp Psychiatry 10(1):49–55, 1988 3345907

T'Sjoen G, Bex M, Maiter D, et al: Health-related quality of life in acromegalic subjects: data from AcroBel, the Belgian registry on acromegaly. Eur J Endocrinol 157(4):411–417, 2007 17893254

U.K. Prospective Diabetes Study (UKPDS) Group: Effect of intensive blood-glucose control with metformin on complications in overweight patients with type 2 diabetes (UKPDS 34). Lancet 352(9131):854–865, 1998a 9742977

U.K. Prospective Diabetes Study (UKPDS) Group: Intensive blood-glucose control with sulphonylureas or insulin compared with conventional treatment and risk of complications in patients with type 2 diabetes (UKPDS 33). Lancet 352(9131):837–853, 1998b 9742976

Valassi E, Crespo I, Keevil BG, et al: Affective alterations in patients with Cushing's syndrome in remission are associated with decreased BDNF and cortisone levels. Eur J Endocrinol 176(2):221–231, 2017 27932530

van Bastelaar KM, Pouwer F, Cuijpers P, et al: Web-based depression treatment for type 1 and type 2 diabetic patients: a randomized, controlled trial. Diabetes Care 34(2):320–325, 2011 21216855

van der Feltz-Cornelis CM: Comorbid diabetes and depression: do e-health treatments achieve better diabetes control? Diabetes Management 3(5):379–388, 2013

van der Feltz-Cornelis CM, Nuyen J, Stoop C, et al: Effect of interventions for major depressive disorder and significant depressive symptoms in patients with diabetes mellitus: a systematic review and meta-analysis. Gen Hosp Psychiatry 32(4):380–395, 2010 20633742

Verrotti A, Catino M, De Luca FA, et al: Eating disorders in adolescents with type 1 diabetes mellitus. Acta Diabetol 36(1–2):21–25, 1999 10436248

Vita R, Lapa D, Trimarchi F, Benvenga S: Stress triggers the onset and the recurrences of hyperthyroidism in patients with Graves' disease. Endocrine 48(1):2554–2563, 2015 24853882

Vogel A, Elberling TV, Hørding M, et al: Affective symptoms and cognitive functions in the acute phase of Graves' thyrotoxicosis. Psychoneuroendocrinology 32(1):36–43, 2007 17097812

Walsh BT, Devlin MJ: Pharmacotherapy of bulimia nervosa and binge eating disorder. Addict Behav 20(6):757–764, 1995 8820528

Weber T, Eberle J, Messelhäuser U, et al: Parathyroidectomy, elevated depression scores, and suicidal ideation in patients with primary hyperparathyroidism: results of a prospective multicenter study. JAMA Surg 148(2):109–115, 2013 23560281

Weinger K, Beverly EA: Barriers to achieving glycemic targets: who omits insulin and why? Diabetes Care 33(2):450–452, 2010 20103561

Westley CJ, Amdur RL, Irwig MS: High rates of depression and depressive symptoms among men referred for borderline testosterone levels. J Sex Med 12(8):1753–1760, 2015 26129722

Whitmer RA, Karter AJ, Yaffe K, et al: Hypoglycemic episodes and risk of dementia in older patients with type 2 diabetes mellitus. JAMA 301(15):1565–1572, 2009 19366776

Wild D, von Maltzahn R, Brohan E, et al: A critical review of the literature on fear of hypoglycemia in diabetes: implications for diabetes management and patient education. Patient Educ Couns 68(1):10–15, 2007 17582726

Williams MM, Clouse RE, Nix BD, et al: Efficacy of sertraline in prevention of depression recurrence in older versus younger adults with diabetes. Diabetes Care 30(4):801–806, 2007 17392541

Wu B, Jin H, Vidyanti I, et al: Collaborative depression care among Latino patients in diabetes disease management, Los Angeles, 2011–2013. Prev Chronic Dis 11:E148, 2014 25167093

Young-Hyman DL, Davis CL: Disordered eating behavior in individuals with diabetes: importance of context, evaluation, and classification. Diabetes Care 33(3):683–689, 2010 20190297

Young-Hyman D, de Groot M, Hill-Briggs F, et al: Psychosocial care for people with diabetes: a position statement of the American Diabetes Association. Diabetes Care 39(12):2126–2140, 2016 27879358

Yu J, Tian AJ, Yuan X, Cheng XX: Subclinical hypothyroidism after 131I-treatment of Graves' disease: a risk factor for depression? PLoS One 11(5):e0154846, 2016 27135245

Yuan L, Tian Y, Zhang F, et al: Decision-making in patients with hyperthyroidism: a neuropsychological study. PLoS One 10(6):e0129773, 2015 26090955

CHAPTER 22

Oncology

Kimberley Miller, M.D., FRCPC
Mary Jane Massie, M.D.

Cancer is a major public health problem globally. In 2017, almost 1.7 million new cases of invasive cancer are expected to be diagnosed in the United States, and nearly 600,000 people are expected to die of cancer (American Cancer Society 2017; Siegel et al. 2017). Although one in four deaths is now caused by cancer, death rates have dropped by 25% since 1991, the result of steady reductions in smoking and advances in early detection and treatment, especially in the four most common cancers (prostate, breast, lung, and colorectal). However, as the death rate decreases and the population ages, more people will be living with cancer, with an anticipated doubling from 1.3 million to 2.6 million between the years 2000 and 2050.

In this chapter, we review psychological factors in cancer risk and progression, the most frequently encountered psychiatric disorders in adult cancer patients, psychiatric issues in specific cancers, psychiatric aspects of cancer treatments, psychiatric interventions in cancer patients, and survivor issues (see Chapter 32, "Pediatrics," for additional coverage of cancer in children).

Psychological Factors Affecting Cancer Risk and Progression

Numerous rigorous studies examining the role that major life events, depression, and personality play in cancer onset, progression, and survival have yielded conflicting results in all areas. Studies of psychological factors and cancer outcomes often identify associations rather than clear causality. Distressed individuals may engage in unhealthy lifestyle behaviors (e.g., smoking, heavy alcohol use, sedentary lifestyle, poor dietary choices, delay in health screenings) that must be controlled for in analyses. In addition to multiple confounding factors, methodological differences (including study design and definitions of distress) as well as publication bias are evident limitations, with caution recommended when interpreting results. Various mechanisms linking psychological distress with cancer have been proposed (Batty et al. 2017). Emotional distress could diminish natural killer cell function, which has been implicated in cancer cell control. Symptoms of depression can lead to dysregulation of the hypothalamic-pituitary-adrenal (HPA) axis, increasing cortisol levels and inflammatory responses and impacting cancer defense processes.

Batty et al. (2017) pooled individual participant data from 16 prospective cohort studies initiated between 1994 and 2008. More than 163,000 men and women provided psychological distress scores based on the 12-item General Health Questionnaire (GHQ-12). A pooled analysis of unpublished raw data suggested associations between distress and cancers of the colorectum, prostate, pancreas, and esophagus as well as leukemia. However, in evaluating the effect of psychological distress on cancer outcome, some authors have suggested that associations between patients' self-ratings on distress scales and survival may reflect patients' perceptions of their disease status rather than a causal effect of distress on the cancer process (Groenvold et al. 2007). Studies attempting to control for disease status have yielded both positive (Groenvold et al. 2007) and negative (Coates et al. 2000) results in linking distress with cancer outcome.

Lutgendorf and Sood (2011) found evidence pointing to a relationship between cancer incidence and severe life events, severe distress, or long-term depression, and also concluded that the preponderance of the epidemiological evidence supports a relationship between psychosocial factors and cancer progression. Yet in 1,011 of 8,736 randomly selected Danish patients who subsequently developed cancer, accumulation of stressful life events was associated with an unhealthy lifestyle but not with an increase in cancer incidence (Bergelt et al. 2006). Such variable and contradictory findings are common among studies in this area.

The evidence associating depression with cancer incidence is weaker than that associating depression with cancer progression, although the literature includes contradictory and inconclusive findings for both mechanisms. Mixed results also have been found when examining the possible link between depression and cancer mortality. Both behavioral (e.g., smoking, alcohol use) and biological factors (e.g., cytokines and the HPA axis) are thought to contribute to worse outcomes (Archer et al. 2008). Depression also may affect the course of illness in patients with cancer through its effect on poorer pain control, poorer treatment adherence, and less desire for life-sustaining therapy. Although it remains unclear whether alleviating cancer patients' psychological distress can prolong their survival, it is prudent to intervene to improve quality of life (QoL) and to foster optimal treatment adherence.

In summary, the available evidence on the effects of depression on cancer is quite limited by methodological problems, reflected in the challenges of trying to prove causality in such a complex system. However, we can state that well-designed studies have not confirmed that psychological processes cause cancer.

Psychiatric Disorders in Cancer Patients

A person's ability to manage a cancer diagnosis and treatment commonly changes over the course of the illness and depends on medical, psychological, and social factors: the disease itself (i.e., site, symptoms, clinical course, prognosis, type of treatments required); the prior level of adjustment; the threat that cancer poses to attaining age-appropriate developmental tasks and goals (i.e., adolescence, career, family, retirement); cultural, spiritual, and religious attitudes; the presence of emotionally supportive persons; the potential for physical and psychological rehabilitation; the patient's own personality and coping style; and experience with loss.

Because emotional distress may not always be recognized by oncology professionals, practice guidelines for patient screening have been developed in many countries. North American distress screening guidelines recommend the use of brief tools (e.g., Edmonton Symptom Assessment System Revised [ESASr], Distress Thermometer [DT]) or Patient Health Questionnaire 2 (PHQ-2) screening questions at the initial patient visit and at subsequent intervals as clinically indicated (Andersen et al. 2014; Howell et al. 2015). Patients who score above a specific cutoff (e.g., >4/10) receive a more comprehensive assessment. Proponents of screening recommend that screening be linked to evidence-based and individualized interventions, the effectiveness of which may be monitored by any of the following self-report measures: Patient Health Questionnaire 9-item (PHQ-9) depression screen, Generalized Anxiety Disorder 7-item (GAD-7) scale, Beck Depression Inventory (BDI), Beck Scale for Suicide Ideation (BSI), Center for Epidemiological Studies Depression (CES-D) scale, and Hospital Anxiety and Depression Scale (HADS). Meijer et al. (2013) reviewed reports on the effects of screening for psychological distress followed by pharmacological or psychological interventions to reduce distress on cancer patient outcomes. Because treatment studies demonstrate only modest improvement in distress symptoms and the one study (Maunsell et al. 1996) that assessed effects of screening on psychological outcomes found no improvement, Meijer et al. (2013) concluded that it was premature to recommend routine screening in cancer settings.

Depression

Depressive symptoms in the cancer patient may occur as part of adjustment to different points along the disease trajectory (e.g., diagnosis, initiation and completion of treatment, survivorship, recurrence, palliation) or be caused by the cancer itself (e.g., primary or secondary brain tumors) and its related symptoms (e.g., fatigue or pain) and treatments (e.g., exogenous cytokines, corticosteroids). Individuals with a history of major depressive disorder are at increased risk of a recurrence during their cancer experience. Depressive symptoms may represent a normal reaction, a psychiatric disorder, or a somatic consequence of cancer or its treatment.

People with cancer have a rate of depression that is at least three times higher than that in the general population and similar to rates associated with other serious medical illnesses. Reports of the prevalence of depression in cancer are highly variable, given the lack of standardization of methodology and diagnostic criteria. A meta-analysis of 70 interview-based studies ($N = 10,071$) in oncology or hematology settings revealed a prevalence of depression (defined by Diagnostic and Statistical Manual of Mental Disorders [DSM] or International Classification of Diseases [ICD] criteria) of 16.3%; of DSM-defined major depressive disorder, 14.9%; of DSM-defined minor depressive disorder, 19.2%; of dysthymia (persistent depressive disorder), 2.7%; of adjustment disorder, 19.4%; and of any mood disorder, including anxiety, 38.2%

(Mitchell et al. 2011). Although not recognized in DSM-5 (American Psychiatric Association 2013) as a distinct entity, *demoralization* has recently emerged as a proposed depression spectrum syndrome characterized by symptoms of hopelessness and helplessness caused by a loss of meaning and purpose in life. This syndrome has been found to be clinically significant in 13%–18% of cancer patients (Robinson et al. 2015). Patients who are single, who are isolated or jobless, who have poorly controlled physical symptoms, or who have inadequately treated anxiety and depressive disorders are at increased risk of demoralization.

Many of the somatic symptoms caused by cancer or its treatment overlap with the diagnostic criteria for major depressive disorder; as a result, clinical judgment must be exercised in determining how heavily to weight the somatic versus the psychological symptoms. An inclusive diagnostic approach may be the most sensitive and reliable. Consideration of the pervasiveness and reactivity of mood symptoms may help to distinguish depressive disorders from normative adjustments to cancer and its impacts. Hypoactive delirium may resemble depression in that both conditions can involve a lack of patient engagement, poor motivation to participate in care, and suicidal ideation; however, disturbances in consciousness, attention, cognition, and perception point to delirium. Distinguishing delirium from depression is extremely important, given the differences in causes, risks, and interventions (see Chapter 4, "Delirium," for a more detailed review). Poorly controlled pain, fatigue, or anorexia–cachexia syndrome also may present with a depressive component.

In cancer patients, risk factors for the development of depression include younger age, inadequate social support, insecure attachment style, and advanced disease (Rodin et al. 2007b). The female predominance in major depressive disorder found in the general population is not consistently found in the oncology setting (Pirl 2004; Rodin et al. 2007b; Strong et al. 2007). There are conflicting findings regarding the extent to which tumor location influences emotional distress. Biopsychosocial risk factors most commonly associated with depression in cancer are listed in Table 22–1. Risk factors related to cancer treatment are listed in Table 22–2.

Several barriers to the diagnosis of depression in cancer patients exist. At the physician level, difficulty distinguishing somatic symptoms related to cancer and its treatment from depression, as well as uncertainty about the effectiveness of psychosocial interventions, may contribute to fewer referrals for mental health care services. Lack of access to and poor patient awareness of such services are additional barriers. At the patient level, reluctance to report depressive symptoms may be related to a fear of psychiatric medication side effects, stigma about seeking help, perceived repercussions of expressing "negativity" on the course of the cancer, and social and cultural differences in expression of distress. Recognition and treatment of depression are essential not only for the patient but also for the patient's spouse and family, as marital and family functioning may be negatively affected.

Suicide and Desire for Hastened Death

In the United States, cancer patients have twice the incidence of suicide compared with the general population (Misono et al. 2008). Higher suicide rates are associated with male gender, white race, and older age at diagnosis. The relative risk (RR) of suicide has been found to be very high, at 12.6, within the first week of receiving a cancer

TABLE 22–1. Biopsychosocial risk factors most commonly associated with depression in cancer

Biological	Psychological	Social
Younger age	External locus of control	Low support
Family history of depression	Perceived low support	Poorer social functioning
Personal history of depression	Anxious or avoidant attachment	Recent loss
Cancer-related factors	Poor coping mechanisms (e.g., hopelessness/helplessness traits)	Stressful life events
• Advanced disease	Ambivalence in expressing emotions	History of trauma or abuse
• Low performance status	Low self-esteem	Loneliness
• Physical burden (pain, fatigue, nausea)		Substance use disorders
• Tumor site (?pancreas, head and neck, lung, brain)		
• Inflammatory factors (interleukin-2, interleukin-6, tumor necrosis factor alpha, proinflammatory cytokines)		
• Treatment (see Table 22–2)		

TABLE 22–2.   **Neuropsychiatric side effects of common chemotherapeutic agents**

Hormones

Corticosteroids	Mild to severe insomnia, hyperactivity, anxiety, depression, psychosis with prominent manic features
Tamoxifen	Sleep disorder, irritability

Biologicals

Cytokines	Encephalopathy
Interferon-alpha	Depression, suicidality, mania, psychosis Delirium, akathisia Seizures
Interleukin-2	Dysphoria, delirium, psychosis Seizures

Chemotherapy agents

L-Asparaginase	Somnolence, lethargy, delirium, depression
Chlorambucil	Hallucinations, lethargy, seizures, stupor, coma
Capecitabine	Multifocal leukoencephalopathy Cerebellar ataxia Reversible neuromuscular syndrome: trismus, slurred speech, confusion, ocular abnormalities
Cisplatin	Encephalopathy (rare), sensory neuropathy
Cytarabine	Delirium, seizures Leukoencephalopathy
5-Fluorouracil	Fatigue, rare seizure or confusion, cerebellar syndrome
Gemcitabine	Fatigue
Ifosfamide	Lethargy, seizures, drunkenness, cerebellar signs, delirium, hallucinations
Methotrexate	Intrathecal regimens: possible leukoencephalopathy (acute and delayed forms) High dose: possible transient delirium
Procarbazine	Somnolence, depression, delirium, psychosis, cerebellar disorder
Taxanes	Sensory neuropathy, fatigue, depression
Thalidomide	Fatigue, reversible dementia
Vincristine, vinblastine, vinorelbine	Depression, fatigue, encephalopathy

Multikinase inhibitors

Sorafenib, sunitinib, bevacizumab	Posterior leukoencephalopathy syndrome

diagnosis, dropping to 3.1 during the first year (Fang et al. 2012). The highest risk of suicide has been found in patients who have cancers with poor prognoses (e.g., gastroesophageal, hepatobiliary, lung) or tumors involving the head and neck (Fang et al. 2012; Misono et al. 2008). In large studies of several thousand cancer patients, 6%–8% reported having "thoughts that you would be better off dead or of hurting yourself in some way" (item 9 of the PHQ-9) (Leung et al. 2013; Walker et al. 2008). Among patients who admitted suicidal ideation, only 11%–33% endorsed suicidal intention in the follow-up interview, a finding underscoring the importance of screening for both ideation and intention (Leung et al. 2013; Walker et al. 2011). Clinically significant emotional distress, substantial pain, and older age were associated with these thoughts. Similarly, 9% of patients with advanced cancer reported suicidal thoughts when asked, "In light of your current circumstances, have you ever had thoughts of killing yourself?" (Spencer et al. 2012). Risk factors for suicidal ideation included meeting criteria for panic disorder or posttraumatic stress disorder (PTSD), feeling unsupported, reporting no religious affiliation or spirituality, lacking a sense of self-efficacy, and having more physical symptoms.

An international consensus definition of the wish to hasten death (WTHD)—an overarching term that encompasses suicidal ideation as one type of such a wish—has been developed by 24 experts from Europe, Canada, and the United States: "a reaction to suffering, in the context of a life-threatening condition, from which the patient can see no way out other than to accelerate his or her death. This wish may be expressed spontaneously or after being asked about it, but it must be distinguished from the acceptance of impending death or from a wish to die naturally, although preferably soon" (Balaguer et al. 2016). Desire for hastened death has been positively associated with hopelessness, depression, and higher physical distress and negatively associated with good physical functioning, spiritual well-being, social support, and self-esteem (Chochinov et al. 1998; Rodin et al. 2007a). Individuals closer to death have been found to express the desire for a hastened death more frequently (17%) than do those with a prognosis of greater than 6 months (2%) (Chochinov et al. 1998; Rodin et al. 2007c). Understanding the complex factors contributing to a WTHD in the specific patient can aid in differentiating a depressive illness from a desire to have control over intolerable symptoms, an expression of despair, or even death acceptance (see also Chapter 8, "Suicidality," and Chapter 39, "Palliative Care").

Euthanasia, or physician-assisted suicide (PAS), can be legally practiced in the Netherlands, Belgium, Luxembourg, Columbia, Switzerland, Canada, and five U.S. states (Oregon, Washington, Montana, Vermont, and California). PAS accounts for 0.3%–4.6% of all deaths in these jurisdictions, 70% of which involve patients with cancer (Emanuel et al. 2016). Patients who request PAS are typically older, white, and well educated. Loss of autonomy and dignity and of the ability to enjoy life's activities—not pain—is the primary motivation for seeking PAS.

Anxiety

Anxiety is a normal response to threat, uncertainty, and loss of control. It is common as patients face the existential plight of cancer and the specific threats of deformity, abandonment, pain, and death. The diagnosis and treatment of cancer are stressful and often traumatic. After the initial shock and disbelief of diagnosis, patients typically feel anxious and irritable. They may experience anorexia, insomnia, and difficulty with concentration, with intrusive thoughts about their prognosis. Often this acute anxiety dissipates as a treatment plan is established and prognosis clarified. Anxiety is common at crisis points such as the start of a new treatment or the diagnosis of recurrence or illness progression, but it also occurs before routine follow-up visits without evidence of disease.

Fear of cancer recurrence (FCR) is a common cause of anxiety and is considered to be one of the most prevalent unmet needs among cancer patients. In a systematic review of FCR, 73% of patients reported some degree of FCR, with almost 50% reporting a moderate to high degree of FCR (Simard et al. 2013). FCR may remain stable over time, highlighting the importance of psychosocial care for those with significant levels of distress. Caregivers reported higher levels of FCR than patients (Simard et al. 2013). A systematic review found that the prevalence of anxiety was higher in long-term cancer survivors (≥2 years after diagnosis) and their spouses than in healthy control subjects, unlike depression prevalence, which did not differ for survivors/spouses and healthy control subjects (Mitchell et al. 2013).

Specific phobia, panic disorder with or without agoraphobia, and generalized anxiety disorder are the most commonly reported anxiety disorders in cancer patients, and patients frequently present with anxious symptoms in the context of adjustment disorders. In DSM-based patient-interview studies, 10% were found to have an anxiety disorder (Mitchell et al. 2011). Some forms of anxiety can affect a patient's adherence to treatment. Patients with claustrophobia (i.e., DSM-5 specific phobia, situational) may have difficulty tolerating magnetic resonance imaging scans, radiation therapy, or placement in isolation because of neutropenia. Needle phobia and other health care–related phobias (i.e., DSM-5 specific phobia, blood–injection–injury) (see Chapter 10, "Anxiety Disorders") may delay or prevent patient consent to chemotherapy and/or surgery.

The presence of anxiety disorder in one partner (patient or caregiver) has been associated with a greater likelihood of anxiety disorder in the other. In recent years, improved antiemetic treatments have reduced the number of patients who vomit as a result of chemotherapy, but nausea is still common. Anxiety related to nausea and vomiting from highly emetogenic chemotherapy may develop into a conditioned response, which may persist after cessation of treatment (see also Chapter 19, "Gastrointestinal Disorders"). Evaluation of acute anxiety in cancer patients should include consideration of conditions that mimic anxiety disorders. Antipsychotics, as well as antiemetics such as prochlorperazine and metoclopramide, may cause akathisia. Akathisia's inner feeling of restlessness is frequently misperceived by patients and misdiagnosed by caregivers as anxiety. The abrupt onset of anxiety and dyspnea may signal pulmonary emboli, which are common among cancer patients. Hypoxia related to primary or secondary lung cancer may cause significant anxiety. The experience of severe, intermittent, or uncontrolled pain is associated with acute and chronic anxiety, and the patient's confidence that he or she has the analgesics to control pain alleviates anxiety. Furthermore, anxiety amplifies pain, and the drive behind additional requests for analgesia may be anxiety rather than somatic pain (see also Chapter 10, "Anxiety Disorders," and Chapter 34, "Pain").

Posttraumatic Stress Disorder

Cancer–related PTSD has been reported to occur in 5% of oncology patients, with a lifetime prevalence of 15% in studies using the Structured Clinical Interview for DSM, Fourth Edition (Abbey et al. 2015). Prevalence rates may be affected by the changes to Criterion A in DSM-5: "A life-threatening illness or debilitating medical condition is not necessarily considered a traumatic event. Medical incidents that qualify as traumatic events involve sudden, catastrophic events (e.g., waking during surgery, anaphylactic shock)" (American Psychiatric Association 2013, p. 274). Thus, a diagnosis of cancer, or going through cancer treatment with no adverse events, is not sufficient to qualify for a PTSD diagnosis. Exploration into whether traumatic occurrences were experienced during the course of the cancer is suggested. Additional changes to the DSM-5 criteria include an increase from three to four symptom clusters: re-experiencing, avoidance, dissociative and/or negative emotion, and arousal and reactivity. Risk factors for PTSD in cancer patients include perception of cancer as threatening, a history of trauma, advanced disease, recent completion of treatment, younger age, less social support, and more difficult interactions with medical staff (Abbey et al. 2015; Jim and Jacobsen 2008). Medical sequelae of cancer treatment (e.g., paresthesias because of nerve injury) may act as a trigger for traumatic memories of treatment.

Mania

In cancer patients, corticosteroids are the most common reason for hypomania or mania (psychiatric side effects of corticosteroids are discussed in detail in Chapter 24, "Rheumatology"). Steroids are commonly given as a component of chemotherapy for lymphoma and multiple myeloma as an antiemetic or to prevent hypersensitivity reactions with chemotherapy, to reduce cerebral or spinal edema, or to prevent cerebral edema during cranial radiation therapy. Lower dosages of corticosteroids also may be used in palliative care to improve appetite, energy, and general well-being. Full-blown manic episodes are rare. The psychological symptoms most commonly reported by patients receiving a short-term course of corticosteroids are insomnia and agitation (see also Chapter 9, "Psychosis, Mania, and Catatonia"). The most significant risk factor for the development of neuropsychiatric effects from steroids is higher daily dosage, but a history of neuropsychiatric disorder also conveys risk. Patients exposed to steroids have a greater than fourfold increased rate of becoming manic compared with nonexposed patients (Fardet et al. 2012). Patients with a history of bipolar disorder should be monitored closely if their cancer treatment includes steroids.

Delirium

The prevalence of delirium in cancer patients has been reported as 5%–30%, up to 25%–50% on hospital admission, and as high as 85% in the terminal stages of illness. Advanced age, possible preexisting dementia, and malnutrition are predisposing factors for delirium in cancer, and potential precipitants include intracranial disease, medications (e.g., opioids, benzodiazepines), and systemic disease (e.g., organ failure, infection, and hematological or metabolic abnormalities). There is often more than one etiological factor contributing to delirium. Delirium is associated with greater morbidity and mortality in patients and greater distress in patients, their families, and caregivers.

Early symptoms of delirium are often unrecognized or misdiagnosed by medical or nursing staff because of fluctuation in presentation, presence of a hypoactive subtype of delirium, and lack of mental status examination of the patient. Delirium is frequently misdiagnosed as dementia, depression, anxiety, or other psychiatric disorders. Early recognition of delirium is essential because the etiology may be a treatable complication of cancer or its treatment. In addition to the general causes of delirium (see Chapter 4, "Delirium"), there are particular considerations in cancer patients (Table 22–3). An electroencephalogram to rule out seizures or a lumbar puncture to rule out leptomeningeal disease or meningitis may be indicated. Limbic encephalopathy may present with impaired memory, fluctuating mood, and seizures, as well as a wide variety of psychiatric symptoms including anxiety, depression, psychosis, and personality change. Posterior reversible encephalopathy syndrome may present with headache, confusion, seizures, and visual disturbance and may be caused by variety of treatments, including chemotherapy, targeted therapy, immunosuppressive drugs (e.g., cyclosporine, tacrolimus), and miscellaneous others (e.g., corticosteroids, interferon-alpha) (see also Chapter 30, "Neurology and Neurosurgery").

Interplay of Physical and Psychological Symptoms in Cancer Patients

Pain

Cancer-related pain is highly prevalent (49%–57% of patients with curable cancer and 56%–75% of patients with advanced disease) and can be attributed to the disease or to surgery, radiation, chemotherapy, or endocrine therapy (Hui and Bruera 2014). For patients not experiencing pain, it is often a feared future symptom. Pain may be a sign of cancer progression, which can contribute to significant distress. Unfortunately, despite decades of experience with pain treatment in patients with cancer, pain remains undertreated in many of them. Appropriate treatment in cancer patients and cancer survivors is challenging in the current climate of concerns about opioid abuse potential, diversion of opioids prescribed for cancer pain, and associated deaths. Key risk factors for opioid misuse have been identified: age 45 years or younger, personal history of substance abuse, mental illness, legal problems, and a family history of substance use disorder (Hui and Bruera 2014).

Opioid-based pharmacotherapy remains the first-line strategy for the treatment of moderate or severe chronic pain in patients with active disease. Portenoy and Ahmed (2014) recently summarized the principles of opioid treatment for cancer pain as follows: discussion of selection of drug and route, opioid rotation, management of breakthrough pain, and adverse effects. They also reviewed the topics of nonadherence, drug abuse, addiction, unintentional overdose, and diversion of drugs into the illicit marketplace. Drug-related behavioral problems in the cancer setting are complex, and oncologists, palliative care providers, and pain medicine specialists serve patients best when they consult with appropriate addiction medicine specialists.

Vardy and Agar (2014) have reviewed use of nonopioid drugs (acetaminophen; nonsteroidal anti-inflammatory drugs, corticosteroids; antineuropathic agents including tricyclic antidepressants [TCAs] and anticonvulsants; and bisphosphonates) in the treatment of cancer pain. Forty percent of cancer survivors experience neuropathic pain or painful syndromes that develop and persist after surgery (e.g., mastectomy, thoracotomy, postamputation), chemotherapy, or radiation therapy (Vardy and Agar 2014). TCAs, duloxetine, gabapentin, and pregabalin can be beneficial adjuvants for the treatment of neuropathic pain. Evidence is lacking for the efficacy of cannabinoids in the treatment of cancer pain, although trials are under way.

TABLE 22–3. **Unique causes of delirium in cancer**

Primary and secondary brain tumors (e.g., lung, breast, melanoma)

Leptomeningeal metastases

Nonconvulsive status epilepticus or postictal phase

Paraneoplastic encephalitis (e.g., limbic encephalopathy—most common in small-cell lung cancer)

Posterior reversible encephalopathy syndrome

Cerebral edema after brain irradiation

Opportunistic infections/sepsis (e.g., immunosuppressed patients, especially those with hematological malignancies)

Medication or substance withdrawal (e.g., substance use may be higher in head and neck and esophageal cancer)

Medications (e.g., antibiotics, opioids, anticholinergics, corticosteroids) (see Table 22–2)

Antineoplastic agents (see Table 22–2)

Hypercalcemia (e.g., bone metastases)

Hyperviscosity syndrome (rarely in lymphoma, Waldenström's macroglobulinemia, and multiple myeloma)

Thromboembolic events

Cerebral venous thrombosis (e.g., asparaginase, tamoxifen, thalidomide, erythropoietin)

The contribution of psychological factors to pain and suffering in patients with cancer and their families has been studied over decades. Syrjala et al. (2014) summarized findings relevant to the effects of psychological factors on pain, as well as psychological and behavioral interventions that have been tested to relieve cancer pain. Evidence that depression aggravates pain symptoms, induces fatigue, and disrupts sleep in cancer patients comes predominantly from cross-sectional studies (Syrjala et al. 2014); however, a longitudinal examination of depression and pain in cancer populations found that depression has a stronger impact on pain than pain does on depression (Wang et al. 2012). There is compelling evidence that some psychological and behavioral interventions (e.g., hypnosis, educational strategies providing training in cognitive-behavioral coping skills) are effective in reducing cancer pain (Syrjala et al. 2014).

Pain management is discussed in detail in Chapter 34, "Pain."

Cancer-Related Fatigue

The term *cancer-related fatigue* (CRF) refers to a subjective feeling of tiredness or exhaustion related to cancer or its treatment that is disproportionate to the level of exertion and is not relieved by rest. CRF is one of the most common and distressing symptoms experienced by cancer patients (affecting up to 100% undergoing active treatment and 30%–40% of cancer survivors), lasting in some patients for years after treatment ends (Jones et al. 2016). CRF may arise from the cancer itself; from treatment or treatment effects, such as anemia, cachexia, pain, infections, and deconditioning; or from comorbid psychiatric (e.g., depression, anxiety, sleep disorders) and medical conditions. Proposed mechanisms for the development of CRF include the release of proinflammatory cytokines by cancer and its treatment, resulting in cognitive and behavioral symptoms (Saligan et al. 2015). Patients undergoing radiation often experience a peak in their fatigue near the end of treatment, which gradually improves over subsequent months, whereas those receiving chemotherapy typically experience worsening in fatigue during the first week after a cycle of treatment, which may accumulate with each subsequent cycle, and gradually tapers off during the first year after treatment. In a meta-analysis involving more than 12,000 breast cancer patients, risk factors for severe fatigue included having a more advanced disease stage; being treated with chemotherapy; and being treated with a combination of surgery, radiation, and chemotherapy either with or without hormonal therapy. Having a partner and being treated with surgery or surgery plus radiation reduced the risk of CRF. A relatively large decrease in the prevalence of severe fatigue appeared to occur during the first 6 months after completion of treatment (Abrahams et al. 2016).

In managing CRF, it is important to first rule out any medical (e.g., anemia, nutrition deficiencies) or substance (medication, treatment)–induced causes. Results are mixed and inconclusive for the use of psychostimulants in CRF, with more patients reporting vertigo, anxiety, anorexia, and nausea with these agents compared with placebo (Gong et al. 2014; Minton et al. 2011). Current recommendations include reserving a trial of psychostimulants or low-dose corticosteroids for patients with more advanced disease, those with severe fatigue (Howell et al. 2015; Yennurajalingam and Bruera 2014), and those with symptoms of both fatigue and depression (Conley et al. 2016). A recent meta-analysis comparing interventions for CRF revealed that exercise (aerobic and anaerobic), psychological interventions (cognitive-behavioral, psycho-educational, and eclectic models), and exercise plus psychological interventions improved CRF both during and after treatment, whereas pharmaceutical interventions (methylphenidate, modafinil, paroxetine) did not (Mustian et al. 2017). Howell and colleagues (Howell et al. 2013; Pearson et al. 2018) developed an evidence-based guideline for the management of CRF that recommends education (information about dimensions of fatigue, its etiologies and management, time and energy management, sleep hygiene, coping with emotions); exercise; and nonpharmacological supportive interventions (cognitive-behavioral therapy [CBT]; psychoeducation targeting fatigue, supportive–expressive therapy). A Cochrane review concluded that although we lack a good understanding of how best to encourage people with cancer to follow exercise recommendations (≥150 minutes/week of aerobic activity), interventions using behavior change techniques—such as goal setting, prompting, self-monitoring, and helping patients to think about how they can increase their exercise by incorporating active behaviors into other life settings—may be helpful (Bourke et al. 2013).

Psychiatric Issues in Specific Cancers

Central Nervous System Tumors

Brain tumors are one of the most difficult types of cancer to live with, given the potential impact on neurological, cognitive, and psychological functioning. One's sense of personhood and identity reside in the brain, so to have this organ affected can be devastating. Metastatic brain tumors (originating most commonly from primary breast, lung, melanoma, kidney, and colorectal cancers) are two to three times more common than primary brain tumors, with leptomeningeal spread of tumor indicating end-stage disease. Meningiomas are the most common type of brain tumor, and are usually non-malignant. Glioblastomas represent the most common malignant brain tumor, with median survival rates with treatment of 14 months. Younger patients have slightly higher 5-year survival rates (17%) compared with patients older than 44 years (4%–6%) (American Cancer Society 2017). Common symptoms include slowed cognition, personality and mood changes, and reduced memory and concentration, all exacerbated by the neurotoxic effects of treatment. Acutely, radiation may increase cerebral edema, requiring treatment with steroids, which may bring their own neuropsychiatric side effects. Months to years after radiation, patients may develop progressive and irreversible cognitive impairment due to its late effects. Frontal lobe tumors can potentially cause disinhibition, impulsivity, mood lability, reduced executive functioning, apathy and psychomotor slowing (resembling depression), and poor judgment, while temporal lobe tumors are likely to affect memory and language. Severe behavioral disturbances and mood symptoms may require treatment with antipsychotics, mood stabilizers, or antidepressants. Benzodiazepines should be used sparingly, and at low dosages, due to the risk of worsening disinhibition or agitation.

Genitourinary Malignancies

Prostate Cancer

Prostate cancer is the most common cancer in men in the United States, although incidence rates have dropped significantly, by more than 10% annually from 2010 to 2013. This reduced incidence is attributed to a decrease in prostate-specific antigen (PSA) testing, in response to the U.S. Preventive Services Task Force recommendations against routine screening (Siegel et al. 2017). PSA screening remains controversial because it carries substantial risks, including overdiagnosis and overtreatment (Barry 2009), and may lead to adverse psychological effects (Drummond et al. 2016). A literature review examining psychological distress associated with prostate cancer found that 10%–30% of men reported depression after receiving a diagnosis of prostate cancer (Sharpley et al. 2008). Another literature review in patients with prostate cancer (N=4,494) revealed that prevalences of depression and anxiety were 17% and 27%, respectively, before patients received treatment; decreased to approximately 15% (both outcomes) while patients were undergoing treatment; and then rose again to about 18% (both outcomes) after patients had completed treatment (Watts et al. 2014). Emotional distress may motivate some men with low-risk prostate cancer to choose more aggressive treatment (Orom et al. 2017). However, in a population-based observational cohort study of more than 41,000 men diagnosed with clinically localized prostate cancer, Prasad et al. (2014) found that patients with intermediate-risk or high-risk prostate cancer who had received a diagnosis of depression in the 2 years preceding their prostate cancer diagnosis were less likely than patients without depression to undergo definitive treatment (radiotherapy or prostatectomy), and the depressed patients also experienced worse overall survival. In a study using a large Surveillance, Epidemiology, and End Results (SEER) data set, Dalela et al. (2016) found that men with prostate cancer were at increased risk of suicide and accidental death within the first year of diagnosis when definitive treatment was recommended but not received. Urinary incontinence and erectile dysfunction may contribute to the heightened suicide risk.

Radical prostatectomy or external beam radiation are common treatments for prostate cancer, and both are likely to cause urinary incontinence and impair erectile function. Urinary incontinence and erectile dysfunction (ED) are debilitating, and ED has negative effects on psychological and marital adjustment (Walker et al. 2015). In a study examining the effect of cancer-related symptoms on psychological well-being among 3,348 men who had been treated for prostate cancer, the risk of anxiety and distress was significantly increased in men with higher scores for fatigue and for urinary-related, bowel-related, and androgen-deprivation therapy (ADT)–related symptoms (Sharp et al. 2016).

ADT is the most common form of treatment for metastatic prostate cancer. Although ADT is not considered curative, many men live for years without symptoms of metastatic disease. In a study of more than 78,000 men with stages I–III prostate cancer identified through the SEER–Medicare database from 1992 to 2006, Dinh et al. (2016) found that patients who received ADT (43%) had a higher 3-year cumulative incidence of depression, inpatient psychiatric treatment, and outpatient psychiatric treatment compared with patients who did not receive ADT. The risk of depression increased with the duration of ADT. The authors recommended that clinicians discuss the potential psychiatric effects of ADT with patients before initiating treatment. ADT adversely affects men's self-image, sexual desire, erectile function, ability to become aroused, and ability to achieve orgasm, all of which may hinder a man's sexual function and disrupt sexual relations. Between 73% and 95% of men receiving ADT reported erectile dysfunction, with rates of sexual activity cessation ranging from 80% to 93% (Donovan et al. 2015). Although the negative effects of prostate cancer treatment on sexual function are well documented, in one study only 4% of health care providers reported referring their patients to a sex therapist (Movsas et al. 2016). Realistic information should be provided to patients and their partners about possible challenges in sexual recovery. Early intervention using a couples-based approach is recommended (Walker et al. 2015).

Other Genitourinary Cancers

Testicular cancer affects young men (average age at diagnosis: 33 years), most of whom are cured, even those that present with distant metastases (73%) (American Cancer Society 2017). Sexuality and fertility may be affected by the diagnosis (many men have low sperm counts at diagnosis) or treatment (orchiectomy, chemotherapy, radiation). Infertility most often results from retroperitoneal lymph node dissection (RPLND) leading to retrograde ejaculation. Long-term effects include secondary malignancies, cardiovascular disease, pulmonary toxicity, nephrotoxicity, neurotoxicity, reduced fertility, hypogonadism, and psychosocial problems (Haugnes et al. 2012). QoL of testicular cancer survivors depends on the extent of treatment required, and anxiety is more common than depression (Haugnes et al. 2012). In a study using the SEER database, patients diagnosed with testicular cancer were found to have a 20% increase in risk of suicide compared with the general population (Alanee and Russo 2012).

Bladder cancer affects three to four times more men than women, with an average age at diagnosis of 73 years and an all-stage 5-year survival rate of 77% (American Cancer Society 2017). Smoking is the best-known risk factor. Superficial bladder cancers are treated with transurethral resection of the bladder (TURB), with chemotherapy placed within the bladder during the procedure. More invasive cancers require radical cystectomy, which may result in creation of an external ileal conduit or internal construction of a neobladder. Sexual dysfunction following either operation is common.

Yang et al. (2016), in a cross-sectional study of 489 consecutive patients with newly diagnosed bladder or kidney cancer, found prevalences of depression, anxiety, and PTSD of 77.5%, 69.3%, and 25.2%, respectively, with patients' perceptions of social support significantly associated with all three disorders. In another study, patients with kidney cancer diagnosed within the past 6 months were found to have posttraumatic stress symptoms (PTSS) independent of and comorbid with depressive symptoms. PTSS were correlated with overall cancer symptom burden (Thekdi et al. 2015). Targeted therapies have replaced immunotherapy (e.g., interferon-alpha), reducing the risk of depression as a side effect of treatment, although fatigue remains common with targeted therapies. Because kidney cancer commonly metastasizes to the brain, any change in personality or cognition should prompt an assessment with central nervous system (CNS) imaging.

Breast Cancer

Breast cancer is the most common cancer in women worldwide and the second leading cause (after lung cancer) of cancer-related deaths in women. The number of women diagnosed with breast cancer has fallen as a result of the decline in use of hormone replacement therapy in postmenopausal women, and modest improvements in the death rate are probably attributable to successful treatment of cancers diagnosed at an early stage. Although only 5% of breast cancer occurs in women younger than 40 years, young women carry a disproportionate burden of the psychological morbidity associated with the diagnosis and its treatments (Ribnikar et al. 2015), as they confront difficult decisions and issues such as treatment options; sexual side effects of treatment; concerns about fertility and the safety of future pregnancies; self-image and body image; prophylactic contralateral mastectomy; genetic testing; and the effect of cancer on current or potential relationships, children, or careers. The psychosocial considerations unique to this age group have been reviewed by others (Menen and Hunt 2016; Ronn and Holzer 2015). In a multicenter retrospective cohort study of 333 women with pregnancy after breast cancer treatment, there was no difference in disease-free survival between pregnant and nonpregnant women at 5-year follow-up (Azim et al. 2013). Consensus guidelines recommend that pregnancy not be discouraged after breast cancer treatment (Partridge et al. 2014).

Women are often referred for psychiatric treatment at the time of their breast cancer diagnosis, and psychiatrists can help address unhealthy behaviors that may contribute to a worse prognosis. Women who are obese at the time of breast cancer diagnosis have a poorer prognosis, and those who gain weight during or after treatment of breast cancer are at higher risk of breast cancer–related death (Jiralerspong and Goodwin 2016), although it is unclear whether the prognosis can be improved by weight loss. Those who smoke have a higher risk of cancer recurrence and mortality (Hamer and Warner 2017). Referral to smoking cessation programs, weight loss/nutrition experts, and exercise programs can be useful for cancer patients while awaiting guidance from randomized controlled trials (RCTs) on the benefits of reversing obesity and increasing exercise in patients being treated for cancer.

Treatment and Side Effects

The treatments for breast cancer include surgery, radiation, chemotherapy, antiestrogen therapy, and bisphosphonates. Local control is still critical; the size, location, and aggressiveness of the tumor usually dictate the initial surgery (mastectomy versus limited resection). There is no difference in overall QoL based on type of surgery alone. Increasingly, women who appear to be excellent candidates for limited resection followed by radiation are choosing instead to have unilateral therapeutic mastectomy or therapeutic mastectomy with contralateral prophylactic mastectomy, and some surgeons refer these women for psychiatric consultation. Although data demonstrate that limited resection followed by radiation is equal to or better than mastectomy in terms of survival, many women prefer to consider unilateral or bilateral mastectomy because they know of women who had breast-sparing procedures and then developed contralateral invasive breast cancer. Although a Cochrane review found insufficient evidence that contralateral prophylactic mastectomy improves survival, mastectomy for many confers "peace of mind" and helps women avoid radiation, which some find frightening (Lustumbo et al. 2010). Use of sentinel node mapping reduces but does not eliminate the risk of developing painful, unsightly, and at times disabling lymphedema. Natural tissue or silicone or saline implant breast reconstruction techniques provide satisfactory to excellent results for many women. Compared with women who undergo mastectomy alone, women who elect to have reconstruction after mastectomy are more likely to have early-stage disease, to be younger and partnered, and to be better educated and have a higher income.

Chemotherapy with alkylating agents can cause alopecia, ovarian failure, premature menopause, cognitive changes, and weight gain. Taxanes can cause painful and disabling peripheral neuropathy, arthralgia, or myalgia. Antiestrogen therapy (tamoxifen or aromatase inhibitors), often prescribed for 10 years following breast cancer treatment, may cause insomnia, hot flashes, irritability, and depression in some women. Women taking an aromatase inhibitor have been found to report higher rates of sexual dysfunction (lubrication, dyspareunia, global dissatisfaction with sex life) compared with women taking tamoxifen and women without breast cancer (Baumgart et al. 2013). Hot flashes can cause anxiety and significant impairment of sleep quality, potentially resulting in nonadherence to hormonal therapy—a consequence that highlights the importance of effective management of vasomotor symptoms. Effective pharmacological interventions include antidepressants—selective serotonin reuptake inhibitors (SSRIs; e.g., citalopram 10 g daily, paroxetine 10 mg daily) and serotonin–norepinephrine reuptake inhibitors (SNRIs; e.g., venlafaxine 75 mg daily, desvenlafaxine 100 mg daily)—and anticonvulsants (e.g., gabapentin 900 mg daily, pregabalin 75 mg twice daily) (Leon-Ferre et al. 2017). When choosing a medication, clinicians should consider side-effect profiles and any comorbid psychiatric conditions. Tamoxifen is a prodrug that requires metabolism by cytochrome P450 (CYP) 2D6 to endoxifen, the active form. There is concern that coadministration of antidepressants that inhibit CYP2D6 may block tamoxifen's therapeutic effects, but data are mixed regarding how serious a risk this presents (Leon-Ferre et al. 2017). In a study of more than 4,000 women, Chubak et al. (2016) found that TCAs, SSRIs, and antidepressants as a class were not associated with increased risk of breast cancer recurrence or mortality, although there was some suggestion of an increased recurrence risk associated with concurrent use of paroxetine (a potent CYP2D6 inhibitor) and tamoxifen compared with use of tamoxifen alone. Despite the fact that a large retrospective cohort study of 16,887 breast cancer patients revealed no increased risk of subsequent breast cancer in women using tamoxifen and antidepressants, very few (3%) of these women were taking paroxetine; therefore, it appears prudent to avoid strong CYP2D6 inhibitors (e.g., paroxetine, fluoxetine, high-dosage sertraline, bupropion, duloxetine) in this patient population (Haque et al. 2016). Other options for hot flashes include clonidine (0.1 mg/day), which is less effective, and megestrol acetate, whose safety in this population is unclear. Most studies do not support the use of complementary and/or alternative treatments, apart from acupuncture (Leon-Ferre et al. 2017). Hot flashes are also an issue for men receiving ADT, although much less evidence exists to guide treatment. A systematic review and network meta-analysis of RCTs for hot flashes in breast and prostate cancer patients is currently under way that aims to address this knowledge gap (Hutton et al. 2015).

Psychiatrists in cancer settings can help women with other psychosocial impacts of breast cancer, including psychological discomfort (anxiety, depression, and anger); behavioral changes due to physical discomfort, marital or sexual disruption, and altered activity level; and fears and concerns related to body image, cancer recurrence, or death. Women worry that their emotional adjustment will forever be changed after cancer treatment. A systematic review of 17 studies indicated that depression has a higher prevalence among breast cancer survivors than among women in the general population, and this higher prevalence is still evident more than 5 years after diagnosis (Maass et al. 2015). There was no indication of an increased prevalence of symptoms of anxiety (Maass et al. 2015). Despite the fact that a significant proportion of women with breast cancer have concerns about sexual health (32%–93%) and body image (27%–88%) that affect their sense of self as sexual beings, an overwhelming number report receiving inadequate care in these domains (Male et al. 2016).

Psychological distress and fear of recurrence accompanied by frequent self-examination and demand for excessive testing are common at the conclusion of breast cancer treatment (Custers et al. 2014). Women who experienced more physical symptoms or side effects from treatments have greater posttreatment distress. Many feel vulnerable when they are no longer being seen regularly by their oncologist, and emotional support is often beneficial.

Genetics

The two most significant risk factors for breast cancer are increasing age and family history. Up to 33% of women in their 20s and 22% of women in their 30s have breast cancer that is attributable to genetic mutations. Patients with a BRCA1 or BRCA2 genetic mutation have an elevated lifetime risk of breast cancer (55%–85%) and ovarian cancer (16%–60%). About 5%–10% of all breast and ovarian cancers are caused by genetic mutations. Approximately 10%–15% of patients younger than 35 years have a BRCA mutation. Identifying such a mutation in an individual may impact treatment decisions, raise awareness for family members, initiate discussions about contralateral prophylactic mastectomy and salpingo-oophorectomy, and guide surgical decision making based on assessment of future risk. Prophylactic salpingo-oophorectomy decreases the risk of ovarian cancer by 80%–96% and the risk of BRCA1-associated breast cancers by up to 72%; the procedure is associated with low all-cause, breast cancer–

specific, and ovarian cancer–specific mortality in women who undergo it (Menen and Hunt 2016). Psychiatrists can assist women in thinking through whether and when to have prophylactic mastectomies and salpingo-oophorectomies; whether to bank eggs or embryos; and how to discuss these issues with potential sexual or life partners.

Gastrointestinal and Hepatobiliary Cancers

Colorectal Cancers

Excluding skin cancers, colorectal cancer is the third most common cancer in the United States, and is the third leading cause of cancer-related death in women and the second in men (American Cancer Society 2017). Colorectal cancer has an earlier onset than other gastrointestinal and hepatobiliary cancers and a higher survival rate. Predictors of health-related QoL after colorectal cancer are similar to those after other cancers, but in colorectal cancer, predictors also include the type and extent of surgery and whether a stoma was required. Patients with colostomies may experience embarrassment due to leaks, odor, and flatus, which may lead to concerns about body image and sexual functioning and contribute to social withdrawal. Common symptoms of bowel dysfunction (e.g., diarrhea, constipation, incontinence), rectal bleeding, anorexia, weight loss, and abdominal pain also influence QoL. A conceptual framework to aid in predicting health-related QoL in colorectal cancer survivors has been developed to aid in identifying those at future risk and to help target appropriate behavioral and psychosocial interventions (Bours et al. 2016). Although the evidence is limited in scope and quality, educational interventions, CBT, relaxation training, and supportive–expressive group therapy can improve outcomes in colorectal cancer patients, including length of hospital stay, days to stoma proficiency, hospital anxiety and depression, and QoL (Hoon et al. 2013).

Gastroesophageal Cancers

Cancers of the esophagus and stomach and their treatment have a significant effect on the ability to eat, due to the development of symptoms including dysphagia, gastroesophageal reflux, and early satiety. Gastroesophageal tumors often have a poor prognosis, with high recurrence rates. Surgical complications may include leaks, leading to strictures that require dilatation. As the disease advances, obstruction and bleeding may occur, further increasing distress. Alcohol use disorder is a risk factor for esophageal cancer; therefore, assessment of alcohol intake and risk for postoperative withdrawal is recommended. Suicide rates among patients with gastroesophageal cancers are reported to be the second highest among all cancer patients in the SEER database (Misono et al. 2008), peaking during the first 3 months after diagnosis and remaining elevated for as long as 2 years after diagnosis (Sugawara and Kunieda 2016). Male sex, white race, unmarried status, and distant metastatic disease are associated with an increased risk of suicide, whereas radiotherapy and surgery appear to lower the risk (Sugawara and Kunieda 2016).

Pancreatic Cancer

Pancreatic cancer is one of the leading causes of cancer deaths, and 80% of cases are unresectable at diagnosis, with a 5-year survival rate of 8% (Siegel et al. 2017), contributing to high rates of distress and depression. The symptoms of pancreatic cancer are typically vague and nonspecific and may include abdominal pain, anorexia, weight loss, fatigue, and jaundice. Symptoms of upper gastrointestinal disease occur in 25% of patients 6 months before diagnosis. Anorexia, early satiety, and back pain are features of progressive disease, and diabetes also may develop. Management of pain and discomfort includes palliative chemotherapy and/or radiotherapy, opiates, celiac blocks, stenting procedures, pancreatic enzymes to relieve cramping associated with pancreatic insufficiency, and prevention and treatment of constipation and diarrhea.

Early small studies found that up to 50% of pancreatic cancer patients manifested psychiatric symptoms at least 6 months prior to their cancer diagnosis (Green and Austin 1993; Joffe et al. 1986), suggesting that there may be a direct tumor-induced effect, although this has not been proven. One clinical study reported that depressive thoughts were more common among patients with pancreatic cancer than among those with gastric cancer (Holland et al. 1986), and a retrospective cohort study found that depression preceded pancreatic cancer more often than it preceded other gastrointestinal malignancies (odds ratio [OR]=4.6) (Carney et al. 2003). Larger prospective studies examining distress by cancer site did find pancreatic cancer to be highly distressing, but no more so than other tumor sites with high symptom burden and poor prognosis, such as lung and brain cancer (Carlson et al. 2004; Zabora et al. 2001).

Regardless of whether depression precedes or follows the diagnosis, depressed pancreatic cancer patients require support and treatment, and—in light of the poor prognosis—collaboration with palliative care services.

Lung Cancer

Lung cancer is the second most common cancer in men and women and is the leading cause of cancer death, with more people dying every year from lung cancer than from colon, breast, and prostate cancer combined. Approximately 10%–15% of lung cancer patients have small-cell lung cancer (SCLC), the more aggressive form. Even stage I lung cancers have a relatively poor prognosis, with 5-year survival rates of 45%–49% in non-small-cell lung cancer (NSCLC) and 31% in SCLC; and stage IV lung cancers (both NSCLC and SCLC) have a 5-year survival rate of less than 5% (American Cancer Society 2017). Although lung cancer is the most preventable of all cancers, with 85%–90% of cases linked to cigarette smoking, it is difficult to diagnose early, and more than one-half of cancer cases are diagnosed at an advanced stage. The number of lung cancer patients who have never smoked has been steadily increasing over the past few decades, especially among women. There is potential for lung cancer to be diagnosed at an earlier stage with the use of low-dose computed tomography, which has been shown to reduce lung cancer mortality in long-term smokers.

Five percent to 13% of lung cancer patients develop major depressive disorder, and up to 44% of patients report depressive symptoms, which is higher than rates in patients with other tumor sites (Zabora et al. 2001). In a longitudinal cohort study of patients with lung cancer, having depressive symptoms at baseline was associated with higher mortality rates in patients with early-stage disease (stages I and II) but not in those with late-stage disease (stages III and IV); by contrast, having depressive symptoms at follow-up was associated with higher mortality rates in patients regardless of their disease stage (Sullivan et al. 2016).

Symptoms of lung cancer (e.g., dyspnea) are inherently distressing and anxiety inducing, highlighting the importance of optimal symptom management. SCLC, more than any other tumor, is associated with paraneoplastic syndromes such as Cushing's syndrome, hyponatremia, and autoimmune encephalopathy. Because pulmonary emboli are common during treatment, dyspnea and anxiety should be evaluated carefully. Hypoxia due to preexisting chronic obstructive pulmonary disease and postradiation hypothyroidism may contribute to cognitive dysfunction. Postthoracotomy neuralgic pain is common.

Because many smokers with lung cancer experience feelings of guilt and self-blame, feeling stigmatized as having inflicted the cancer on themselves through choosing to smoke, taking an open and nonjudgmental stance is recommended in exploring this concern. Continued smoking is associated with decreased survival, development of a secondary primary cancer, and increased risk of developing or exacerbating other medical conditions; therefore, providing support and access to smoking-cessation programs is important. Although some health care providers are hesitant to raise the issue of smoking cessation during the stress of initial diagnosis, the literature supports early antismoking intervention with patients and their family members. For a more detailed review of lung cancer, see Chapter 18, "Lung Disease."

Gynecological Cancers

All types of gynecological cancers have the potential to negatively impact sexual functioning and fertility, affecting a woman's sexuality and sense of identity. Removal of ovaries results in immediate surgical menopause, pelvic nerves may be damaged during surgical procedures, and total removal of the clitoris may be required in some resections (see also Chapter 31, "Obstetrics and Gynecology," and Chapter 15, "Sexual Dysfunctions").

Ovarian Cancer

The second most frequent gynecological cancer among women in the United States, ovarian cancer, is the fifth most frequent cause of cancer death in women and has the highest mortality rate of all gynecological cancers (American Cancer Society 2017). Ovarian cancer usually has an insidious onset and progression; 20% of cases are localized at diagnosis. The 5-year survival rate for patients with early-stage disease is high (94%) relative to the rate for all stages (45%). Five percent to 10% of ovarian cancer cases are inherited, most commonly involving the BRCA1 and BRCA2 genetic mutations. BRCA1 confers a 35%–70% risk of developing ovarian cancer; BRCA2 carries a risk of 10%–30%.

Depression and anxiety are both elevated in women with ovarian cancer across the disease trajectory, although depression has been shown to be higher before treatment than after treatment, whereas anxiety shows an increase beginning at treatment completion, consistent with the known high risk of recurrence and related fears about this (Watts et al. 2015). Almost half of women recently diagnosed with gynecological cancers (the bulk of the sample with stage III ovarian cancer) experienced fear of recurrence that persisted for 6 months after diagnosis (Manne et al. 2017). An intervention developed to address this concern—coping and communication-enhancing intervention (CCI)—was found to improve depression, cancer-specific distress, and emotional well-being and to perform significantly better than supportive counseling or usual care. CCI includes education in cognitive-behavioral approaches and coping (problem- and emotion-focused) skills related to fears of recurrence, the details of which can be found elsewhere (Manne et al. 2017).

Cervical Cancer

Precancerous cervical lesions are much more common than invasive cervical cancers, and the death rate from cervical cancer in the United States has been cut by 50% as a result of access to Papanicolaou (PAP) tests. Although the relationship of cervical cancer to human papillomavirus (HPV) infection can lead to stigma and self-blame about the diagnosis, cervical cancer has also become the first cancer to be preventable through use of vaccination. In addition to causing sexual side effects, cervical cancer treatments can also contribute to anorectal symptoms, urinary symptoms, and lymphedema. Radiation may be associated with a worse QoL compared with other treatments (Ye et al. 2014).

Endometrial Cancer

Endometrial cancer is the most common gynecological cancer in the United States, and because patients are often symptomatic in early stages (90% of patients present with postmenopausal bleeding), approximately 75% are diagnosed with stage I or II, which has a 5-year survival rate of 74%–91% (Morice et al. 2016). Women who have higher levels of depression, anxiety, cancer-related distress, and circulating interleukin-6 report more severe pain following surgery for endometrial cancer (Honerlaw et al. 2016). Given that menopausal and lymphedema symptoms are disabling sequelae of surgery for endometrial cancer, ovarian preservation should be considered for premenopausal women (Ferrandina et al. 2014).

Melanoma

Malignant melanomas represent the fifth and sixth most common cancers in men and women, respectively, with rates having increased over the past 30 years. The 5-year relative survival is 92% for all stages due to the fact that most cases are detected at an early stage, with a 5-year relative survival in localized melanomas of 98% (American Cancer Society 2017). Having a history of melanoma is one of the strongest risk factors for a subsequent diagnosis of melanoma; the 10-year risk of developing a second primary melanoma is 13%, and (for those with two melanomas) of developing a third primary is 28%, leaving many survivors with a fear of cancer recurrence (Lyth et al. 2017). Approximately 30% of patients with melanoma report clinically significant levels of distress, with anxiety being more prevalent than depression; risk factors for distress include female sex, younger age, lower education, visibility of affected body site, lack of social support, and negative appraisal of melanoma (Kasparian et al. 2009). Melanoma is the most aggressive and fatal form of skin cancer; it may result in scarring or lymphedema from lymph node sampling, and it can affect mobility if lower extremities are involved.

Structured interventions offering psychoeducational support can reduce distress and enhance active coping strategies (Boesen et al. 2005). A systematic review of psychoeducational interventions showed that educational interventions (consisting of personal instruction in how to perform skin self-examination [SSE] supplemented by written information) led to increased patient satisfaction with clinical care and information provision, as well as increased frequency of SSE lasting up to 4 months, although accuracy and thoroughness of skin examination were rarely reported (McLoone et al. 2013). Participation in psychological interventions (mostly CBT) was associated with reductions in anxiety, health-related distress, and melanoma recurrence rates as well as positive changes in coping, although little detail was provided on the "active ingredients" of the interventions (McLoone et al. 2013).

The development of targeted therapies for melanoma has contributed to improvement in the overall survival of melanoma patients and has reduced the use of interferon (IFN)-alpha, with its attendant burden of psychiatric side effects. For patients who are prescribed IFN-alpha, pretreatment with an SSRI has been shown to significantly reduce the incidence and severity of major depressive disorder during IFN treatment, regardless of treatment duration (12 or 24 weeks) or preexisting psychiatric disorders (Sarkar and Schaefer 2014). Because melanoma commonly metastasizes to the brain, changes in personality or other new neurological symptoms should always prompt the clinician to consider CNS imaging.

Head and Neck Cancers

Head and neck cancers are highly distressing, and together with their treatments often result in facial disfigurement and loss of the ability to speak, eat, taste, or swallow. Affected patients have a suicide rate three times higher than that in the general population (Kam et al. 2015). Specifically, hypopharyngeal cancer is associated with nearly a 12-fold increase in suicide, and laryngeal cancer with a fivefold higher incidence; these anatomic sites are responsible for speaking and/or swallowing, and dependency on tracheostomies or gastrostomy tubes may contribute to suffering, social isolation, and suicidality. With more head and neck cancer patients surviving longer than 5 years, QoL issues become paramount. Distress may be higher in patients whose identity is closely tied to body image or ability to communicate. Treatment is daunting and leads to mucositis, pain, dysphagia, xerostomia, and sticky saliva, all of which make eating difficult and affect social functioning. Hypothyroidism is common following radiation treatment to the neck. Cranial radiation for nasopharyngeal cancer has been associated with the development of radionecrosis, with consequent cognitive dysfunction. Memory, language, motor performance, and executive function may become impaired.

Head and neck cancer patients often have comorbid substance use disorders that place them at high risk for alcohol and nicotine withdrawal when admitted to the hospital. Underlying comorbid psychiatric illness and maladaptive coping styles often accompany substance use. Guilt about the role substance use may have played in the development of their cancer may contribute to distress. Mouth and throat cancers from HPV have increased 56% and 17% in Canadian men and women, respectively, since the mid-1990s and now account for one-third of HPV cancers, tied with cervical cancer (Vogel 2017).

Research has shown that health-related QoL may return to baseline by 1 year posttreatment, but it is not clear whether this improvement is attributable to response shift, posttraumatic growth, or methodological issues. A Cochrane review failed to find good-quality evidence that psychosocial interventions in head and neck cancer can improve QoL, depression, or anxiety (Semple et al. 2013).

Hematological Malignancies

Leukemia, lymphoma, and multiple myeloma account for 9% of all cancers and often require extensive complex treatments, including chemotherapy, radiation, corticosteroids, and/or hematopoietic stem cell transplantation (SCT) (American Cancer Society 2017). Patients with hematological cancers have been found to have unmet psychosocial needs, including fear of recurrence, as well as practical needs (Swash et al. 2014). Acute myelogenous leukemia (AML) accounts for approximately 80% of acute leukemia in adults, with patients often beginning their treatment within a few days of diagnosis. Thus, new patients still in shock from receiving the diagnosis find themselves suddenly also facing life-threatening complications due to the disease and/or arduous treatment protocols. Two-thirds of AML patients receiving induction chemotherapy will go into remission, and with the addition of consolidation chemotherapy, 50% will go into long-term remission (and may be cured). Receiving allogeneic SCT leads to higher success rates but carries higher risk of death as a complication. Acute lymphoblastic leukemia has a 5-year survival rate of less than 50% among adults ages 20–24 years, less than 30% among those ages 50–54 years, and 12% among those older than 65 years (Katz et al. 2015). In one study of newly diagnosed or recently relapsed adults with acute lymphoblastic leukemia, 17.8% had clinically significant depressive symptoms but fewer (8.5%) reported hopelessness (Gheihman et al. 2016). Further study is needed, but this preservation of hope may reflect patients' perceptions of the potential for cure. Rates of moderate to severe depression increase in the early months following hematopoietic SCT.

Two Cochrane reviews found insufficient information to evaluate the effects of yoga or meditation in patients with hematological malignancies (Felbel et al. 2014; Salhofer et al. 2016); however, physical exercise added to standard care can improve QoL in these patients, especially in regard to physical functioning, depression, and fatigue (Bergenthal et al. 2014).

Psychiatric Aspects of Cancer Treatments

Chemotherapy

The news that one will require chemotherapy can be extremely upsetting, and many studies have confirmed that the most feared side effects of chemotherapy are nausea, vomiting, and alopecia, the latter often being a particular concern in women. The fear of alopecia drives some patients to opt for regimens with less favorable outcomes or even to refuse treatment. Effective treatments for nausea and vomiting exist, but there is currently no treatment for preventing hair loss, although early promising results have been found with scalp-cooling or scalp-hypothermia procedures (Nangia et al. 2017; Rugo et al. 2017). Weight loss or weight gain (e.g., due to premedication with corticosteroids) may also occur as an effect of chemotherapy, contributing to challenges with body image.

The neuropsychiatric side effects of common chemotherapeutic agents are listed in Table 22–2. Because most chemotherapeutic agents are metabolized by CYP3A4, careful consideration of drug–drug interactions involving this enzyme is warranted. Both St. John's wort and modafinil induce CYP3A4 and therefore may render chemotherapy less effective, whereas fluoxetine, sertraline, paroxetine, and fluvoxamine may inhibit CYP3A4 and also increase levels of chemotherapy-related toxicity. Chemotherapy commonly contributes to cognitive changes, referred to as "chemo fog" or "chemo brain" (see "Survivor Issues" section later in this chapter).

Tamoxifen, which is used in the prevention of breast cancer recurrence as well as in the metastatic setting, may cause depression. Antidepressants are commonly prescribed to breast cancer patients taking tamoxifen for management of depression and hot flashes. The issue of interactions between tamoxifen and certain antidepressants was discussed earlier in this chapter (see subsection "Treatment and Side Effects" under "Breast Cancer").

Radiation

Radiation treatment requires a patient to remain still on a flat table for 5–10 minutes so that a prescribed dose can be applied to a specific site. Anxiety (especially specific phobia, situational phobia [claustrophobia], or panic attacks), PTSD, or inadequate pain control may limit the patient's ability to undergo treatment. Because fatigue typically peaks during the weeks following radiation treatment, educating patients about this effect may help to prepare and reassure them. Other side effects of radiation depend on which part of the body is being irradiated (e.g., nausea and vomiting with gastrointestinal cancers, vaginal atrophy with gynecological cancers, localized skin burns for breast cancer). Brain irradiation causes more profound fatigue than does treatment of other sites. Concomitant dexamethasone reduces cerebral edema, but late sequelae of brain radiation, including focal radiation necrosis or leukoencephalopathy, may appear. Newer methods to reduce the volume of brain that requires radiation may decrease these risks.

Hematopoietic Stem Cell Transplantation

Hematopoietic SCT broadly includes bone marrow transplantation and SCT from peripheral or umbilical cord blood. With allogeneic SCT, which uses donor stem cells, there is a risk of developing graft-versus-host disease, whereas autologous SCT uses the patient's own cells, thereby eliminating this risk. In a study of 90 inpatients undergoing their first hematopoietic SCT, Fann et al. (2011) found that 50% of patients experienced delirium during the first 30 days after the procedure. Risk factors for delirium included opioid use as well as cognitive, liver, and renal impairment. In one study, although few patients met criteria for significant depression pretransplantation, nearly one-third (31%) met criteria at 6–7 weeks posttransplantation (Artherholt et al. 2014). The risk of psychological distress declines with time since SCT. Sun et al. (2011) evaluated psychological outcomes in 1,065 long-term survivors of hematopoietic SCT compared with their healthy siblings and found that somatic distress, but not psychological distress, differed in the two groups. Risk factors for psychological distress in survivors included low annual household income, impaired health status, and chronic graft-versus-host disease managed with prednisone.

Cancer Surgery

Chapter 28, "Surgery," provides a general discussion of the emotional aspects of surgery, and Chapter 31, "Obstetrics and Gynecology," includes a discussion of gynecological surgery.

Psychosocial Interventions in Cancer

Exploration of how patients understand and make sense of their illness and prognosis, cancer experience, physical symptoms, concurrent stressors, and personal relationships and supports allows development of an individualized psychosocial care plan. Below we discuss the role of psychotherapeutic and pharmacological interventions for the distressed cancer patient, recognizing that the evidence is of variable quality and limited by small sample sizes, high attrition rates (contributing to selection bias), and confounding factors. There is increasing evidence supporting a collaborative care approach that is embedded within oncology settings, allowing dedicated care managers (nurses or social workers) to work closely with psychosocial specialists in providing psychosocial care (e.g., problem-solving therapy [PST]) (Li et al. 2017). Clinical practice guidelines have also been developed to address the unique and multifaceted needs of depressed cancer patients that incorporate a stepped-care approach, including nonpharmacological and pharmacological considerations (Li et al. 2016).

Psychotherapy

Various psychotherapeutic models have been used in alleviating distress in cancer patients, the choice driven by individual and disease-related factors, including type and severity of distress, stage of disease, and current treatment status, functional status, and the patient's reflective capacity. Cancer patients may face issues related to loss of control, uncertainty, and fear of future dependency, suffering, and death. Psychotherapy supports patients in navigating these challenges through individual, couples, family, or group interventions by offering a supportive, validating, and nonjudgmental presence; providing realistic reassurance; and emphasizing prior strengths and coping. Psychoeducation, problem-solving approaches, relaxation strategies, and CBT may be used for individuals recently diagnosed with cancer (Jassim et al. 2015), whereas existential, life narrative, dignity-conserving, or meaning-centered psychotherapies may be more appropriate for patients with more advanced disease (Li et al. 2012).

Evidence for the effectiveness of psychosocial interventions has been mixed and is difficult to interpret due to variability in interventions used, as well as the heterogeneity in disease status and severity of distress. In patients without clinically significant levels of depression, medium to large effect sizes were found in systematic reviews and meta-analyses of psychological interventions (Jacobsen and Jim 2008). A meta-analysis of six studies that delivered psychotherapeutic interventions for depression (e.g., CBT, supportive–expressive psychotherapy, PST) to patients with advanced cancer, including incurable cancer, found improvement in depression scores in non–clinically depressed samples but no improvement in samples with a diagnosis of depression (Akechi et al. 2008). The inherent challenges of conducting an RCT in seriously ill cancer patients include high attrition rates, inability to implement standard randomization designs, and heterogeneity of patient samples, but in a meta-analysis of existing RCTs examining psychological interventions, four studies found a significant improvement in depression scores posttreatment for CBT, social support, PST, brief psycho-oncological support, and short-term psychodynamic psychotherapy (Li et al. 2017), but only up to 12 weeks; these improvements did not persist in longer-term follow-up.

Group therapy and self-help groups facilitate sharing of information and support coping strategies among cancer patients facing similar situations. In a group setting, patients can glean practical tips and see the range of normal reactions to illness, as well as adaptive coping styles and strategies that make adjustment to illness easier. Group therapy helps to decrease the sense of isolation and alienation as the patient and family see that they are not alone adjusting to illness. Groups are often disease specific or targeted to patients at the same stage of illness. Spiegel et al. (1989) developed supportive–expressive group therapy led by trained professionals for women with breast cancer. The goals of supportive–expressive psychotherapy are to help patients with existential concerns and disease-related emotions, to deepen social support and physician–patient relationships, and to provide symptom control.

Manualized individual psychotherapies have been developed for patients with advanced cancer. These manualized interventions include dignity therapy, meaning-centered psychotherapy, and a brief supportive–expressive intervention called CALM (managing cancer and living meaningfully). Compared with patients who received supportive group psychotherapy, those who received meaning-centered group psychotherapy showed significantly greater improvement in spiritual well-being and sense of meaning (Breitbart et al. 2010). Legacy documents created during a 1-hour interview with a terminally ill patient can reduce suffering and depressed mood (Chochinov et al. 2005) (see Chapter 39, "Palliative Care"). A supportive–expressive group therapy intervention was reported to be protective against development of depressive disorders in metastatic breast cancer patients (Kissane et al. 2007).

Earlier studies of the effect of psychosocial interventions suggested that they could prolong survival (Fawzy et al. 1993, 2003; Spiegel et al. 1989). However, replication studies, which have been methodologically more rigorous, have failed to find any survival benefit (Kissane et al. 2007; Spiegel et al. 2007), suggesting that future trials should focus on improving QoL, easing suffering, and optimizing coping (Kissane 2009).

Music therapy may have beneficial effects on anxiety, pain, fatigue, and QoL and, where available, could be included in psychosocial care for cancer patients (Bradt et al. 2016).

Psychopharmacology

Choosing a psychotropic medication for a cancer patient requires consideration of the patient's prior response to treatment, medical comorbidities, potential drug interactions, route of administration, onset of action required with related patient prognostic information, somatic symptom profile (e.g., pain, insomnia, agitation, hot flashes), and adverse-effect profile of the intended psychotropic medication. In cancer patients with thrombocytopenia, intramuscular injections and restraints should be avoided. Patients who are unable to take medications orally because of mucositis or those with gastrointestinal obstruction may require alternative routes of administration (see Chapter 36, "Psychopharmacology").

A recent systematic review and meta-analysis of prescribing practices revealed that antidepressants are increasingly being prescribed for cancer patients (worldwide prevalence, 15.6%; lower in Asia, at 7.4%); this practice was most prevalent for female or breast cancer patients (22.6%) (Sanjida et al. 2016). Although antidepressants are commonly used, the evidence in depressed cancer patients is limited and of low quality, with few trials studying patients with major depressive disorder (Ostuzzi et al. 2015; Rodin et al. 2007a). Therefore, antidepressant therapy considerations in cancer patients are similar to those in other medically ill patients (see Chapter 7, "Depression," and Chapter 36, "Psychopharmacology"). Mirtazapine's antiemetic and appetite-stimulating effects may make it a good choice for anorexic–cachectic depressed cancer patients or those experiencing nausea or vomiting from chemotherapy. Because of their rapid onset of action, psychostimulants are often the preferred choice in terminally ill patients.

Benzodiazepines are frequently given to cancer patients for acute anxiety and/or insomnia and may be prescribed to augment antiemetics during chemotherapy. A detailed discussion of pharmacotherapy for anxiety is provided in Chapter 10, "Anxiety Disorders."

General management of delirium is reviewed in Chapter 4. There are also cancer-specific treatments for delirium—for example, the use of methylene blue or thiamine to treat ifosfamide-induced encephalopathy. In terminally ill patients, a cause for delirium may not be found in up to 50% of patients. One placebo-controlled study of delirium in palliative care patients revealed that those receiving risperidone or haloperidol had worse outcomes than those receiving placebo (Agar et al. 2017). The most common indication for palliative sedation in the terminally ill is delirium, and the medication most commonly used is continuous midazolam. More thorough reviews of delirium in cancer (Breitbart and Alici 2012) and terminal delirium (Chapter 39, "Palliative Care") can be found elsewhere.

Survivor Issues

Advances in cancer treatment over the past 30 years have led to a rapidly growing population of more than 14.5 million long-term survivors in the United States, more than half of whom are age 65 years or older. Although the long-term adjustment of many appears to be largely unimpaired, some cured cancer patients experience delayed medical complications—for example, organ failure, cognitive impairment, infertility, second cancers, fatigue—as well as psychological concerns, such as fear of termination of treatment; fear of cancer recurrence and death; difficulty with reentry into normal life; persistent guilt; difficult adjustment to physical losses, including disabilities that lead to problems with peer acceptance and social integration; diminished self-esteem or self-confidence; changes in work roles or reduced schedules; and fear of job and insurance discrimination (Stanton et al. 2015). Concerns about infertility reappear when treatment concludes. Several elements are necessary to achieve optimal outcomes in cancer survivors: access to state-of-the-art cancer care; active participation or engagement in one's own care (active coping); use of social support or the perception that support is available; and a sense of meaning or purpose in life (Rowland and Massie 2010). Cancer-related PTSD occurs in less than 10% of cancer survivors (French-Rosas et al. 2011).

Survivors' cognitive functioning is also a concern. Some children and adults who have undergone bone marrow transplantation or who have been treated for CNS tumors have residual deficits, including compromised motor and cognitive test performance (Brinkman et al. 2016). Fifteen percent to 61% of adult patients who have received chemotherapy and/or hormonal therapy for solid tumors report cognitive changes (Ahles et al. 2012). These changes in attention, concentration, memory, and executive function are often subtle and have been challenging to study. Possible biological and neural mechanisms contributing to cognitive changes in patients include direct treatment toxicities, systemic pro-inflammatory cytokines, endocrine therapy, and biotherapies. One review of nonpharmacological interventions for cognitive impairment suggested a possible role for cognitive training and compensatory strategy training; however, the quality of the evidence was considered low (Treanor et al. 2016).

References

Abbey G, Thompson SBN, Hickish T, et al: A meta-analysis of prevalence rates and moderating factors for cancer-related post-traumatic stress disorder. Psychooncology 24(4):371–381, 2015 25146298

Abrahams HJG, Gielissen MFM, Schmits IC, et al: Risk factors, prevalence, and course of severe fatigue after breast cancer treatment: a meta-analysis involving 12,327 breast cancer survivors. Ann Oncol 27(6):965–974, 2016 26940687

Agar MR, Lawlor PG, Quinn S, et al: Efficacy of oral risperidone, haloperidol, or placebo for symptoms of delirium among patients in palliative care. A randomized clinical trial. JAMA Intern Med 177(1):34–42, 2017 27918778

Ahles TA, Root JC, Ryan EL: Cancer- and cancer treatment-associated cognitive change: an update on the state of the science. J Clin Oncol 30(30):3675–3686, 2012 23008308

Akechi T, Okuyama T, Onishi J, et al: Psychotherapy for depression among incurable cancer patients. Cochrane Database Syst Rev (2):CD005537, 2008 18425922

Alanee S, Russo P: Suicide in men with testis cancer. Eur J Cancer Care (Engl) 21(6):817–821, 2012 22624649

American Cancer Society: Cancer Facts and Figures 2017 [Internet]. Atlanta, GA, American Cancer Society, 2017. Available at: http://www.cancer.org/research/cancer-facts-statistics.html. Accessed May 30, 2017.

American Psychiatric Association: Diagnostic and Statistical Manual of Mental Disorders, 5th Edition. Arlington, VA, American Psychiatric Association, 2013

Andersen BL, DeRubeis RJ, Berman BS, et al; American Society of Clinical Oncology: Screening, assessment, and care of anxiety and depressive symptoms in adults with cancer: an American Society of Clinical Oncology guideline adaptation. J Clin Oncol 32(15):1605–1619, 2014 24733793

Archer J, Hutchison I, Korszun A: Mood and malignancy: head and neck cancer and depression. J Oral Pathol Med 37(5):255–270, 2008 18312300

Artherholt SB, Hong F, Berry DL, et al: Risk factors for depression in patients undergoing hematopoietic cell transplantation. Biol Blood Marrow Transplant 20(7):946–950, 2014 24650679

Azim HA Jr, Kroman N, Paesmans M, et al: Prognostic impact of pregnancy after breast cancer according to estrogen receptor status: a multicenter retrospective study. J Clin Oncol 31(1):73–79, 2013 23169515

Balaguer A, Monforte-Royo C, Porta-Sales J, et al: An international consensus definition of the wish to hasten death and its related factors. PLoS One 11(1):e0146184, 2016 26726801

Barry MJ: Screening for prostate cancer—the controversy that refuses to die. N Engl J Med 360(13):1351–1354, 2009 19297564

Batty GD, Russ TC, Stamatakis E, et al: Psychological distress in relation to site specific cancer mortality: pooling of unpublished data from 16 prospective cohort studies. BMJ 356:j108, 2017 28122812

Baumgart J, Nilsson K, Evers AS, et al: Sexual dysfunction in women on adjuvant endocrine therapy after breast cancer. Menopause 20(2):162–168, 2013 22990756

Bergelt C, Prescott E, Grønbaek M, et al: Stressful life events and cancer risk. Br J Cancer 95(11):1579–1581, 2006 17106440

Bergenthal N, Will A, Streckmann F, et al: Aerobic physical exercise for adult patients with haematological malignancies. Cochrane Database Syst Rev (11):CD009075, 2014 25386666

Boesen EH, Ross L, Frederiksen K, et al: Psychoeducational intervention for patients with cutaneous malignant melanoma: a replication study. J Clin Oncol 23(6):1270–1277, 2005 15718325

Bourke L, Homer KE, Thaha MA, et al: Interventions for promoting habitual exercise in people living with and beyond cancer. Cochrane Database of Syst Rev (9):CD010192, 2013 24065550

Bours MJL, van der Linden BWA, Winkels RM, et al: Candidate predictors of health-related quality of life of colorectal cancer survivors: a systematic review. Oncologist 21(4):433–452, 2016 26911406

Bradt J, Dileo C, Magill L, et al: Music interventions for improving psychological and physical outcomes in cancer patients. Cochrane Database Syst Rev (8):CD006911, 2016 27524661

Breitbart W, Alici Y: Evidence-based treatment of delirium in patients with cancer. J Clin Oncol 30(11):1206–1214, 2012 22412123

Breitbart W, Rosenfeld B, Gibson C, et al: Meaning-centered group psychotherapy for patients with advanced cancer: a pilot randomized controlled trial. Psychooncology 19(1):21–28, 2010 19274623

Brinkman TM, Krasin MJ, Liu W, et al: Long-term neurocognitive functioning and social attainment in adult survivors of pediatric CNS tumors: results from the St. Jude lifetime cohort study. J Clin Oncol 34(12):1358–1367, 2016 26834063

Carlson LE, Angen M, Cullum J, et al: High levels of untreated distress and fatigue in cancer patients. Br J Cancer 90(12):2297–2304, 2004 15162149

Carney CP, Jones L, Woolson RF, et al: Relationship between depression and pancreatic cancer in the general population. Psychosom Med 65(5):884–888, 2003 14508036

Chochinov HM, Wilson KG, Enns M, et al: Depression, Hopelessness, and suicidal ideation in the terminally ill. Psychosomatics 39(4):366–370, 1998 9691706

Chochinov HM, Hack T, Hassard T, et al: Dignity therapy: a novel psychotherapeutic intervention for patients near the end of life. J Clin Oncol 23(24):5520–5525, 2005 16110012

Chubak J, Bowles EJ, Yu O, et al: Breast cancer recurrence in relation to antidepressant use. Cancer Causes Control 27(1):125–136, 2016 26518198

Coates AS, Hürny C, Peterson HF, et al; International Breast Cancer Study Group: Quality-of-life scores predict outcome in metastatic but not early breast cancer. J Clin Oncol 18(22):3768–3774, 2000 11078489

Conley CC, Kamen CS, Heckler CE, et al: Modafinil moderates the relationship between cancer-related fatigue and depression in 541 patients receiving chemotherapy. J Clin Psychopharmacol 36(1):82–85, 2016 26658264

Custers JA, van den Berg SW, van Laarhoven HW, et al: The Cancer Worry Scale: detecting fear of recurrence in breast cancer survivors. Cancer Nurs 37(1):E44–E50, 2014 23448956

Dalela D, Krishna N, Okwara J, et al: Suicide and accidental deaths among patients with nonmetastatic prostate cancer. BJU Int 118(2):286–297, 2016 26305451

Dinh KT, Reznor G, Muralidhar V, et al: Association of androgen deprivation therapy with depression in localized prostate cancer. J Clin Oncol 34(16):1905–1912, 2016 27069075

Donovan KA, Walker LM, Wassersug RJ, et al: Psychological effects of androgen-deprivation therapy on men with prostate cancer and their partners. Cancer 121(24):4286–4299, 2015 26372364

Drummond FJ, O'Leary E, Gavin A, et al: Mode of prostate cancer detection is associated with the psychological wellbeing of survivors: results from the PiCTure study. Support Care Cancer 24(5):2297–2307, 2016 26594035

Emanuel EJ, Onwuteaka-Philipsen BD, Urwin JW, et al: Attitudes and practices of euthanasia and physician-assisted suicide in the United States, Canada, and Europe. JAMA 316(1):79–90, 2016 27380345

Fang F, Fall K, Mittleman MA, et al: Suicide and cardiovascular death after a cancer diagnosis. N Engl J Med 366(14):1310–1318, 2012 22475594

Fann JR, Hubbard RA, Alfano CM, et al: Pre- and post-transplantation risk factors for delirium onset and severity in patients undergoing hematopoietic stem-cell transplantation. J Clin Oncol 29(7):895–901, 2011 21263081

Fardet L, Petersen I, Nazareth I: Suicidal behavior and severe neuropsychiatric disorders following glucocorticoid therapy in primary care. Am J Psychiatry 169(5):491–497, 2012 22764363

Fawzy FI, Fawzy NW, Hyun CS, et al: Malignant melanoma. Effects of an early structured psychiatric intervention, coping, and affective state on recurrence and survival 6 years later. Arch Gen Psychiatry 50(9):681–689, 1993 8357293

Fawzy FI, Canada AL, Fawzy NW: Malignant melanoma: effects of a brief, structured psychiatric intervention on survival and recurrence at 10-year follow-up. Arch Gen Psychiatry 60(1):100–103, 2003 12511177

Felbel S, Meerpohl JJ, Monsef I, et al: Yoga in addition to standard care for patients with haematological malignancies. Cochrane Database Syst Rev (6):CD010146, 2014 24919720

Ferrandina G, Petrillo M, Mantegna G, et al: Evaluation of quality of life and emotional distress in endometrial cancer patients: a 2-year prospective, longitudinal study. Gynecol Oncol 133(3):518–525, 2014 24637198

French-Rosas LN, Moye J, Naik AD: Improving the recognition and treatment of cancer-related posttraumatic stress disorder. J Psychiatr Pract 17(4):270–276, 2011 21775828

Gheihman G, Zimmermann C, Deckert A, et al: Depression and hopelessness in patients with acute leukemia: the psychological impact of an acute and life-threatening disorder. Psychooncology 25(8):979–989, 2016 26383625

Gong S, Sheng P, Jin H, et al: Effect of methylphenidate in patients with cancer-related fatigue: a systematic review and meta-analysis. PLoS One 9(1):e84391, 2014 24416225

Green AI, Austin CP: Psychopathology of pancreatic cancer. A psychobiologic probe (review). Psychosomatics 34(3):208–221, 1993 8493302

Groenvold M, Petersen MA, Idler E, et al: Psychological distress and fatigue predicted recurrence and survival in primary breast cancer patients. Breast Cancer Res Treat 105(2):209–219, 2007 17203386

Hamer J, Warner E: Lifestyle modifications for patients with breast cancer to improve prognosis and optimize overall health. CMAJ 189(7):E268–E274, 2017 28246240

Haque R, Shi J, Schottinger JE, et al: Tamoxifen and antidepressant drug interaction in a cohort of 16,887 breast cancer survivors. J Natl Cancer Inst 108(3), 2016 26631176

Haugnes HS, Bosl GJ, Boer H, et al: Long-term and late effects of germ cell testicular cancer treatment and implications for follow-up. J Clin Oncol 30(30):3752–3763, 2012 23008318

Holland JC, Korzun AH, Tross S, et al: Comparative psychological disturbance in patients with pancreatic and gastric cancer. Am J Psychiatry 143(8):982–986, 1986 3524279

Honerlaw KR, Rumble ME, Rose SL, et al: Biopsychosocial predictors of pain among women recovering from surgery for endometrial cancer. Gynecol Oncol 140(2):301–306, 2016 26363211

Hoon LS, Chi Sally CW, Hong-Gu H: Effect of psychosocial interventions on outcomes of patients with colorectal cancer: a review of the literature. Eur J Oncol Nurs 17(6):883–891, 2013 23759360

Howell D, Keller-Olaman S, Oliver TK, et al: A pan-Canadian practice guideline and algorithm: screening, assessment, and supportive care of adults with cancer-related fatigue. Curr Oncol 20(3):e233–e246, 2013 23737693

Howell D, Keshavarz H, Esplen MJ, et al: A pan-Canadian practice guideline: screening, assessment, and care of psychosocial distress, depression, and anxiety in adults with cancer. Version 2, Canadian Partnership Against Cancer (Cancer Journey Advisory Group) and the Canadian Association of Psychosocial Oncology, July 2015. Available at: http://www.capo.ca/wp-content/uploads/2015/11/FINAL_Distress_Guideline1.pdf. Accessed May 30, 2017.

Hui D, Bruera E: A personalized approach to assessing and managing pain in patients with cancer. J Clin Oncol 32(16):1640–1646, 2014 24799495

Hutton B, Yazdi F, Bordeleau L, et al: Comparison of physical interventions, behavioral interventions, natural health products, and pharmacologics to manage hot flashes in patients with breast or prostate cancer: protocol for a systematic review incorporating network meta-analyses. Syst Rev 4:114, 2015 26307105

Jacobsen PB, Jim HS: Psychosocial interventions for anxiety and depression in adult cancer patients: achievements and challenges. CA Cancer J Clin 58(4):214–230, 2008 18558664

Jassim GA, Whitford DL, Hickey A, et al: Psychological interventions for women with non-metastatic breast cancer. Cochrane Database Syst Rev (5):CD008729, 2015 26017383

Jim HS, Jacobsen PB: Posttraumatic stress and posttraumatic growth in cancer survivorship: a review. Cancer J 14(6):414–419, 2008 19060607

Jiralerspong S, Goodwin PJ: Obesity and breast cancer prognosis: evidence, challenges and opportunities. J Clin Oncol 34(35):4203–4216, 2016 27903149

Joffe RT, Rubinow DR, Denicoff KD, et al: Depression and carcinoma of the pancreas. Gen Hosp Psychiatry 8(4):241–245, 1986 3744031

Jones JM, Olson K, Catton P, et al: Cancer-related fatigue and associated disability in post-treatment cancer survivors. J Cancer Surviv 10(1):51–61, 2016 25876557

Kam D, Salib A, Gorgy G, et al: Incidence of suicide in patients with head and neck cancer. JAMA Otolaryngol Head Neck Surg 141(12):1075–1081, 2015 26562764

Kasparian NA, McLoone JK, Butow PN: Psychological responses and coping strategies among patients with malignant melanoma: a systematic review of the literature. Arch Dermatol 145:1415–1427, 2009 20026852

Katz AJ, Chia VM, Schoonen WM, et al: Acute lymphoblastic leukemia: an assessment of international incidence, survival, and disease burden. Cancer Causes Control 26(11):1627–1642, 2015 26376890

Kissane D: Beyond the psychotherapy and survival debate: the challenge of social disparity, depression and treatment adherence in psychosocial cancer care. Psychooncology 18(1):1–5, 2009 19097139

Kissane DW, Grabsch B, Clarke DM, et al: Supportive-expressive group therapy for women with metastatic breast cancer: survival and psychosocial outcome from a randomized controlled trial. Psychooncology 16(4):277–286, 2007 17385190

Leon-Ferre RA, Majithia N, Loprinzi CL: Management of hot flashes in women with breast cancer receiving ovarian function suppression. Cancer Treat Rev 52:82–90, 2017 27960127

Leung YW, Li M, Devins G, et al: Routine screening for suicidal intention in patients with cancer. Psychooncology 22(11):2537–2545, 2013 23878040

Li M, Fitzgerald P, Rodin G: Evidence-based treatment of depression in patients with cancer. J Clin Oncol 30(11):1187–1196, 2012 22412144

Li M, Kennedy EB, Byrne N, et al: Management of depression in patients with cancer: a clinical practice guideline. J Oncol Pract 12(8):747–756, 2016 27382000

Li M, Kennedy EB, Byrne N, et al: Systematic review and meta-analysis of collaborative care interventions for depression in patients with cancer. Psychooncology 26(5):573–587, 2017 27643388

Lustumbo L, Carbine NE, Wallace J: Prophylactic mastectomy for prevention of breast cancer. Cochrane Database Syst Rev (11):CD002748, 2010 21069671

Lutgendorf SK, Sood AK: Biobehavioral factors and cancer progression: physiological pathways and mechanisms. Psychosom Med 73(9):724–730, 2011 22021459

Lyth J, Falk M, Maroti M, et al: Prognostic risk factors of first recurrence in patients with primary stages I–II cutaneous malignant melanoma—from the population-based Swedish melanoma register. J Eur Acad Dermatol Venereol 31(9):1468–1474, 2017 28419674

Maass SW, Roorda C, Berendsen AJ, et al: The prevalence of long-term symptoms of depression and anxiety after breast cancer treatment: a systematic review. Maturitas 82(1):100–108, 2015 25998574

Male DA, Fergus KD, Cullen K: Sexual identity after breast cancer: sexuality, body image, and relationship repercussions. Curr Opin Support Palliat Care 10(1):66–74, 2016 26716393

Manne SL, Myers-Virtue S, Kissane D, et al: Group-based trajectory modeling of fear of disease recurrence among women recently diagnosed with gynecological cancers. Psychooncology 26(11):1799–1809, 2017 27421919

Manne SL, Virtue SM, Ozga M, et al: A comparison of two psychological interventions for newly diagnosed gynecological cancer patients. Gynecol Oncol 144(2):354–362, 2017 27887806

Maunsell E, Brisson J, Deschênes L, et al: Randomized trial of a psychologic distress screening program after breast cancer: effects on quality of life. J Clin Oncol 14(10):2747–2755, 1996 8874336

McLoone J, Menzies S, Meiser B, et al: Psycho-educational interventions for melanoma survivors: a systematic review. Psychooncology 22(7):1444–1456, 2013 22933380

Meijer A, Roseman M, Delisle VC, et al: Effects of screening for psychological distress on patient outcomes in cancer: a systematic review. J Psychosom Res 75(1):1–17, 2013 23751231

Menen RS, Hunt KK: Considerations for the treatment of young patients with breast cancer. Breast J 22(6):667–672, 2016 27542172

Minton O, Richardson A, Sharpe M, et al: Psychostimulants for the management of cancer-related fatigue: a systematic review and meta-analysis. J Pain Symptom Manage 41(4):761–767, 2011 21251796

Misono S, Weiss NS, Fann JR, et al: Incidence of suicide in persons with cancer. J Clin Oncol 26(29):4731–4738, 2008 18695257

Mitchell AJ, Chan M, Bhatti H, et al: Prevalence of depression, anxiety, and adjustment disorder in oncological, haematological, and palliative-care settings: a meta-analysis of 94 interview-based studies. Lancet Oncol 12(2):160–174, 2011 21251875

Mitchell AJ, Ferguson DW, Gill J, et al: Depression and anxiety in long-term cancer survivors compared with spouses and healthy controls: a systematic review and meta-analysis. Lancet Oncol 14(8):721–732, 2013 23759376

Morice P, Leary A, Creutzberg C, et al: Endometrial cancer. Lancet 387(10023):1094–1108, 2016 26354523

Movsas TZ, Yechieli R, Movsas B, et al: Partner's perspective on long-term sexual dysfunction after prostate cancer treatment. Am J Clin Oncol 39(3):276–279, 2016 24685887

Mustian KM, Alfano CM, Heckler C, et al: Comparison of pharmaceutical, psychological and exercise treatments for cancer-related fatigue a meta-analysis. JAMA Oncol 3(7):961–968, 2017 28253393

Nangia J, Wang T, Osborne C, et al: Effect of a scalp cooling device on alopecia in women undergoing chemotherapy for breast cancer: the SCALP randomized clinical trial. JAMA 317(6):596–605, 2017 28196254

Orom H, Underwood W 3rd, Biddle C: Emotional distress increases the likelihood of undergoing surgery among men with localized prostate cancer. J Urol 197(2):350–355, 2017 27506694

Ostuzzi G, Matcham F, Dauchy S, et al: Antidepressants for the treatment of depression in people with cancer. Cochrane Database Syst Rev (6):CD011006, 2015 26029972

Partridge AH, Pagani O, Abulkhair O, et al: First international consensus guidelines for breast cancer in young women (BCY1). Breast 23(3):209–220, 2014 24767882

Pearson EJM, Morris ME, DiStefano M, et al: Interventions for cancer-related fatigue: a scoping review. Eur J Cancer Care (Engl) 27(1), 2018 27254272

Pirl WF: Evidence report on the occurrence, assessment, and treatment of depression in cancer patients. J Natl Cancer Inst Monogr 32(32):32–39, 2004 15263039

Portenoy RK, Ahmed E: Principles of opioid use in cancer pain. J Clin Oncol 32(16):1662–1670, 2014 24799466

Prasad SM, Eggener SE, Lipsitz SR, et al: Effect of depression on diagnosis, treatment, and mortality of men with clinically localized prostate cancer. J Clin Oncol 32(23):2471–2478, 2014 25002728

Ribnikar D, Ribeiro JM, Pinto D, et al: Breast cancer under age 40: a different approach. Curr Treat Options Oncol 16(4):16, 2015 25796377

Robinson S, Kissane DW, Brooker J, et al: A systematic review of the demoralization syndrome in individuals with progressive disease and cancer: a decade of research. J Pain Symptom Manage 49(3):595–610, 2015 25131888

Rodin G, Lloyd N, Katz M, et al; Supportive Care Guidelines Group of Cancer Care Ontario Program in Evidence-Based Care: The treatment of depression in cancer patients: a systematic review. Support Care Cancer 15(2):123–136, 2007a 17058100

Rodin G, Walsh A, Zimmermann C, et al: The contribution of attachment security and social support to depressive symptoms in patients with metastatic cancer. Psychooncology 16(12):1080–1091, 2007b 17464942

Rodin G, Zimmermann C, Rydall A, et al: The desire for hastened death in patients with metastatic cancer. J Pain Symptom Manage 33(6):661–675, 2007c 17531909

Ronn R, Holzer H: Breast cancer and fertility: an update. Curr Opin Support Palliat Care 9(3):285–293, 2015 26262832

Rowland JH, Massie MJ: Breast cancer, in Psycho-Oncology, 2nd Edition. Edited by Holland J. New York, Oxford University Press, 2010, pp 177–186

Rugo HS, Klein P, Melin SA, et al: Association between use of scalp cooling device and alopecia after chemotherapy for breast cancer. JAMA 317(6):606–614, 2017 28196257

Salhofer I, Will A, Monsef I, et al: Meditation for adults with haematological malignancies. Cochrane Database Syst Rev (2):CD011157, 2016 26840029

Saligan LN, Olson K, Filler K, et al; Multinational Association of Supportive Care in Cancer Fatigue Study Group–Biomarker Working Group: The biology of cancer-related fatigue: a review of the literature. Support Care Cancer 23(8):2461–2478, 2015 25975676

Sanjida S, Janda M, Kissane D, et al: A systematic review and meta-analysis of prescribing practices of antidepressants in cancer patients. Psychooncology 25(9):1002–1016, 2016 26775715

Sarkar S, Schaefer M: Antidepressant pretreatment for the prevention of interferon alfa-associated depression: a systematic review and meta-analysis. Psychosomatics 55(3):221–234, 2014 24012293

Semple C, Parahoo K, Norman A, et al: Psychosocial interventions for patients with head and neck cancer (review). Cochrane Database Syst Rev (7):CD009441, 2013 23857592

Sharp L, O'Leary E, Kinnear H, et al: Cancer-related symptoms predict psychological wellbeing among prostate cancer survivors: results from the PiCTure study. Psychooncology 25(3):282–291, 2016 26249170

Sharpley CF, Bitsika V, Christie DH: Psychological distress among prostate cancer patients: fact or fiction? Clin Med Oncol 2:563–572, 2008 21892333

Siegel RL, Miller KD, Jemal A: Cancer statistics, 2017. CA Cancer J Clin 67(1):7–30, 2017 28055103

Simard S, Thewes B, Humphris G, et al: Fear of cancer recurrence in adult cancer survivors: a systematic review of quantitative studies. J Cancer Surviv 7(3):300–322, 2013 23475398

Spencer RJ, Ray A, Pirl WF, et al: Clinical correlates of suicidal thoughts in patients with advanced cancer. Am J Geriatr Psychiatry 20(4):327–336, 2012 21989317

Spiegel D, Bloom JR, Kraemer HC, et al: Effect of psychosocial treatment on survival of patients with metastatic breast cancer. Lancet 2(8668):888–891, 1989 2571815

Spiegel D, Butler LD, Giese-Davis J, et al: Effects of supportive-expressive group therapy on survival of patients with metastatic breast cancer: a randomized prospective trial. Cancer 110(5):1130–1138, 2007 17647221

Stanton AL, Rowland JH, Ganz PA: Life after diagnosis and treatment of cancer in adulthood: contributions from psychosocial oncology research. Am Psychol 70(2):159–174, 2015 25730722

Strong V, Waters R, Hibberd C, et al: Emotional distress in cancer patients: the Edinburgh Cancer Centre symptom study. Br J Cancer 96(6):868–874, 2007 17311020

Sugawara A, Kunieda E: Suicide in patients with gastric cancer: a population-based study. Jpn J Clin Oncol 46(9):850–855, 2016 27307574

Sullivan DR, Forsberg CW, Ganzini L, et al: Longitudinal changes in depression symptoms and survival among patients with lung cancer: a national cohort assessment. J Clin Oncol 34(33):3984–3991, 2016 27996350

Sun CL, Francisco L, Baker KS, et al: Adverse psychological outcomes in long-term survivors of hematopoietic cell transplantation: a report from the Bone Marrow Transplant Survivor Study (BMTSS). Blood 118(17):4723–4731, 2011 21821714

Swash B, Hulbert-Williams N, Bramwell R: Unmet psychosocial needs in haematological cancer: a systematic review. Support Care Cancer 22(4):1131–1141, 2014 24464526

Syrjala KL, Jensen MP, Mendoza ME, et al: Psychological and behavioral approaches to cancer pain management. J Clin Oncol 32(16):1703–1711, 2014 24799497

Thekdi SM, Milbury K, Spelman A, et al: Posttraumatic stress and depressive symptoms in renal cell carcinoma: association with quality of life and utility of single-item distress screening. Psychooncology 24(11):1477–1484, 2015 25690556

Treanor CJ, McMenamin UC, O'Neill RF, et al: Non-pharmacological interventions for cognitive impairment due to systemic cancer treatment. Cochrane Database of Syst Rev (8):CD011325, 2016 27529826

Vardy J, Agar M: Nonopioid drugs in the treatment of cancer pain. J Clin Oncol 32(16):1677–1690, 2014 24799483

Vogel L: HPV not just a young woman's problem. CMAJ 189(10):E416–E417, 2017 28385825

Walker J, Waters RA, Murray G, et al: Better off dead: suicidal thoughts in cancer patients. J Clin Oncol 26(29):4725–4730, 2008 18695258

Walker J, Hansen CH, Butcher I, et al: Thoughts of death and suicide reported by cancer patients who endorsed the "suicidal thoughts" item of the PHQ-9 during routine screening for depression. Psychosomatics 52(5):424–427, 2011 21907060

Walker LM, Wassersug RJ, Robinson JW: Psychosocial perspectives on sexual recovery after prostate cancer treatment. Nat Rev Urol 12(3):167–176, 2015 25753250

Wang HL, Kroenke K, Wu J, et al: Predictors of cancer-related pain improvement over time. Psychosom Med 74(6):642–647, 2012 22753637

Watts S, Leydon G, Birch B, et al: Depression and anxiety in prostate cancer: a systematic review and meta-analysis of prevalence rates. BMJ Open 4(3):e003901, 2014 24625637

Watts S, Prescott P, Mason J, et al: Depression and anxiety in ovarian cancer: a systematic review and meta-analysis of prevalence rates. BMJ Open 5(11):e007618, 2015 26621509

Yang YL, Liu L, Li MY, et al: Psychological disorders and psychosocial resources of patients with newly diagnosed bladder and kidney cancer: a cross-sectional study. PLoS One 11(5):e0155607, 2016 27191964

Ye S, Yang J, Cao D, et al: A systematic review of quality of life and sexual function of patients with cervical cancer after treatment. Int J Gynecol Cancer 24(7):1146–1157, 2014 25033255

Yennurajalingam S, Bruera E: Review of clinical trials of pharmacologic interventions for cancer-related fatigue: focus on psychostimulants and steroids. Cancer J 20(5):319–324, 2014 25299141

Zabora J, BrintzenhofeSzoc K, Curbow B, et al: The prevalence of psychological distress by cancer site. Psychooncology 10(1):19–28, 2001 11180574

CHAPTER 23

Hematology

Madeleine Becker, M.D., M.A.

David J. Axelrod, M.D., J.D.

Keira Chism, M.D., M.A.

Robert Bahnsen, M.D.

The consultation psychiatrist is frequently called on to assess patients in medical settings who have primary or secondary hematological disorders. Our review addresses psychiatric issues that are specific to patients who have selected hematological disorders, including iron, B_{12}, or folate deficiency; sickle cell disease; hemophilia; and thalassemia. We discuss the diseases, their unique psychiatric manifestations, and approaches to management. Hematological side effects of psychotropic medications and their drug interactions are also reviewed.

Iron Deficiency Anemia

Iron deficiency anemia (IDA) is the most common nutrient deficiency in the world. The most common etiology of IDA is blood loss. In men and in postmenopausal women, chronic bleeding from the gastrointestinal tract is the most common cause of IDA. Peptic ulcer, hiatal hernia, gastritis, hemorrhoids, vascular anomalies, and neoplasms are the most common causes of gastrointestinal bleeding in adults. Causes of chronic blood loss also include colon cancer, colonic diverticulae, periampullary tumors, leiomyomas, adenomas, and other malignant or benign neoplasms of the intestine (Coban et al. 2003). Intestinal malabsorption of iron is an uncommon cause of iron deficiency except after gastrointestinal surgery and in malabsorption syndromes such as celiac disease (Annibale et al. 2003). In malabsorption syndromes, IDA may take years to develop due to the indolent nature of iron loss.

IDA is highly prevalent in pregnant women as the result of iron loss from diversion of iron to the fetus and from blood loss during delivery. Daily iron demand dramatically increases during pregnancy and continues through to term. Breast-feeding leads to additional iron diversion to the baby. For these reasons, IDA continues or worsens for a significant percentage of women during the postpartum period (Milman 2006).

Clinical Manifestations

Severe IDA is associated with all of the various symptoms of anemia (resulting from both hypoxia and the body's response to hypoxia), including tachycardia, palpitations, pounding in the ears, headache, light-headedness, angina, and retinal hemorrhages and exudates. Less severe anemia presents with fatigue, weakness, headache, irritability, and exercise intolerance. Glossal pain, dry mouth, atrophy of tongue papillae, and alopecia may be more specific to IDA (Trost et al. 2006). Physical findings of chronic IDA include pallor, glossitis (smooth red tongue), stomatitis, and angular cheilitis.

Neuropsychiatric Manifestations

Neuropsychiatric symptoms of IDA include depression, developmental delay, cognitive deficits, restless legs syndrome, and fatigue. One population-based study found an increased risk of mood disorders and autism spectrum disorders in adults with a history of childhood IDA (Chen et al. 2013). IDA may affect processing speed of visual and auditory functions (Hunt et al. 2014). IDA leads to diminished work and exercise performance as well as neurological dysfunction (Cook and Skikne 1989). IDA may also result in cognitive and motor developmental delays in infants and young children (Booth and Aukett 1997). The pathophysiology of these behavioral deficits is not well understood (Lozoff 1988). Even school-age children and adolescents with iron deficiency (with or without anemia) have been shown to have lower standardized math scores compared with children with normal iron status (Halterman et al. 2001).

In adults, IDA impairs cognitive function, limits activity, and causes work paucity (Beard et al. 2005). Mild anemia is independently associated with worse selective attention performance and disease-specific quality-of-life ratings (Lucca et al. 2008). Mildly anemic elderly patients (not limited to those with IDA) score significantly worse than nonanemic control subjects on multiple cognitive, functional, mood, and quality-of-life measures (Lucca et al. 2008).

Patients with IDA may crave both food items and nonfood substances. Pica and particularly pagophagia (craving ice) are specific symptoms that reportedly occur in 50% of patients with IDA (Rector 1989). The mechanism by which IDA produces pica is poorly understood (Federman et al. 1997).

Motor impairment, cognitive dysfunction, and restless legs syndrome probably result from iron deficiency in the central nervous system (CNS) (Krieger and Schroeder 2001). Early studies demonstrated that IDA plays a role in restless legs syndrome and that treatment with iron improves the syndrome (Allen et al. 2013; Krieger and Schroeder 2001). The severity of restless legs syndrome correlates with serum ferritin levels (Sun et al. 1998). Iron deficiency is also a risk factor for neuroleptic malignant syndrome (Rosebush and Mazurek 1991) and may aggravate akathisia and other extrapyramidal movement disorders (Yoshida et al. 2004).

Diagnosis and Treatment

IDA often is discovered incidentally through screening laboratory tests. IDA is a microcytic, hypochromic anemia. Plasma iron concentration and serum ferritin concentration are low, and iron-binding capacity is increased. Ferritin is the single best test. The classic laboratory findings occur consistently only when IDA is far advanced, is unaccompanied by complicating factors (such as infection or cancer), and is untreated (via transfusions or administration of parenteral iron).

Patients should be educated to maintain a diversified diet with adequate iron from foods such as lean meat and seafood, nuts, beans, vegetables, and fortified grain products (National Institutes of Health 2017). Recovery from IDA almost always requires iron supplementation. Therapy should be initiated immediately. Iron can be replaced orally, parenterally, or (rarely) via blood transfusion. Symptom improvement after iron repletion is often realized quickly. Headache, fatigue, paresthesias, and pica rapidly resolve (Rector 1989). The prognosis of IDA is excellent when the cause of iron deficiency is benign.

Vitamin B_{12} and Folate Deficiency

Vitamin B_{12} deficiency and folate deficiency have similar consequences on the nervous system and lead to megaloblastic anemia (Reynolds 2006). Both B_{12} and folate are cofactors for the conversion of homocysteine to methionine. Deficiency of either B_{12} or folate correlates with high homocysteine levels, which have been associated with cardiovascular disease, stroke, dementia, and Alzheimer's disease (Bonetti et al. 2015; Carmel et al. 2003; Ravaglia et al. 2005; Reynolds 2006). Both high homocysteine levels and deficiencies of B_{12} and folate have been associated with depression (Bottiglieri et al. 2000; Petridou et al. 2016).

Vitamin B_{12} Deficiency

Vitamin B_{12} (cobalamin) is found primarily in meat and dairy products. B_{12} is a necessary coenzyme and cofactor in various reactions, including DNA synthesis and the synthesis of methionine from homocysteine. In the duodenum, vitamin B_{12} binds to intrinsic factor. Intrinsic factor is released by parietal cells, which are located in the fundus and body of the stomach. The B_{12} complex is then absorbed in the terminal ileum. There is usually enough B_{12} stored in the liver to supply daily requirements for up to 2–5 years; therefore, it typically takes years to develop B_{12} deficiency (Andrès et al. 2004). In the elderly, the prevalence of B_{12} deficiency, including mild and subclinical cases, may exceed 20% (Andrès et al. 2004; Loikas et al. 2007).

Pernicious anemia is the most common cause of B_{12} deficiency (Toh et al. 1997). Pernicious anemia is an autoimmune disorder resulting in the loss of parietal cells in the stomach and subsequent loss of intrinsic factor production, which is necessary for B_{12} absorption. Pernicious anemia frequently is associated with other autoimmune disorders, including thyroiditis, diabetes mellitus, Addison's disease, Graves' disease, vitiligo, myasthenia gravis, Lambert-Eaton myasthenic syndrome, and hypoparathyroidism (Carmel et al. 2003; Toh et al. 1997).

Dietary B_{12} deficiency is rare but may occur in strict vegans. B_{12} deficiency also can occur in children who are exclusively breast-fed and whose mothers are vegetarians (Chalouhi et al. 2008). In the elderly, deficiency usually is secondary to malabsorption due to gastric atrophy or pernicious anemia (Andrès et al. 2009). Food or oral cobalamin malabsorption may be caused by *Helicobacter pylori* infection, intestinal overgrowth due to antibiotics, chronic use of metformin (Liu et al. 2006) or of antacids, H_2 receptor antagonists, proton pump inhibitors (Valuck and Ruscin 2004), alcoholism, anorexia nervosa, pancreatic failure, and Sjögren's syndrome. Vitamin B_{12} malabsorption also may result from gastrectomy, gastric bypass surgery (Malinowski 2006; Vargas-Ruiz et al. 2008), ileal disease or ileocecal resection, Crohn's disease, and infection with *Diphyllobothrium latum* (tapeworm) or HIV (Andrès et al. 2004). B_{12} deficiency is common in the elderly. It is also quite common in older individuals with mental illness, both those with and those without neurocognitive disorders (Lachner et al. 2014).

Neuropsychiatric Manifestations

Neuropsychiatric manifestations are common in vitamin B_{12} deficiency, especially in the elderly (Andrès et al. 2004). The hematological and neuropsychiatric symptoms of B_{12} deficiency are often disassociated, and neuropsychiatric symptoms may precede hematological signs (Reynolds 2006). Symmetrical peripheral neuropathy can occur, with paresthesias and numbness. Subacute combined degeneration of the spinal cord is less common (Reynolds 2006). Subacute combined degeneration encompasses both posterior column disruption (resulting in loss of vibration and position sense and ataxia with a positive Romberg's sign) and lateral column disruption (causing weakness, spasticity, and extensor plantar responses) (Toh et al. 1997). Rare manifestations of B_{12} deficiency include optic neuritis, optic atrophy, and incontinence. Psychiatric symptoms may include mood changes (including depression), psychosis, cognitive impairment, and obsessive-compulsive disorder (Bauman et al. 2000; Liu et al. 2006; Petridou et al. 2016; Valuck and Ruscin 2004). B_{12} deficiency appears to be a risk factor for dementia (Andrès et al. 2004). In children, vitamin B_{12} deficiency may cause irritability, failure to thrive, apathy, anorexia, abnormal movements, and developmental regression, which generally respond to supplementation. Long-term cognitive and developmental retardation are most dependent on the duration of the deficiency and the severity of symptoms (Chalouhi et al. 2008).

Diagnosis and Treatment

There is no "gold standard," and there are different normal values for cobalamin levels; however, a deficiency is usually defined as a B_{12} level of less than 200 ng/L (Schrier 2016). Elevated serum methylmalonic acid and elevated serum total homocysteine can help establish whether deficiency exists (Carmel et al. 2003). Tests for intrinsic factor antibody and serum gastrin and a Schilling test may be helpful in diagnosing pernicious anemia. Differentiating the causes of B_{12} deficiency yields important clinical information and can guide diagnosis and treatment (Carmel et al. 2003).

In patients with low B_{12} levels, daily injections of 1,000 mcg of hydroxycobalamin or cyanocobalamin are recommended for 1 week, followed by weekly injections of 1 mg for 4 weeks, and then maintenance doses every 1–3 months, depending on the severity of deficiency (Andrès et al. 2009). Oral B_{12} replacement also is effective as treatment (Health Quality Ontario 2013). Remission is typically achieved within weeks, but continued maintenance therapy is recommended to fully replenish body stores and to maintain longer periods of remission. Significant improvement of neuropsychiatric function has been shown after B_{12} administration (Andrès et al. 2009). B_{12} supplementation does not provide any improvement in cognitive function in people who have normal B_{12} levels (Moore et al. 2012).

Folic Acid Deficiency

Folic acid is found in both animal products and leafy green vegetables. Folate is important in mood and cognition, brain growth, and cell differentiation, development, and repair. These mechanisms are likely mediated through nucleotide synthesis and DNA transcription and integrity (Carmel et al. 2003). Adequate folate levels may protect against certain cancers, birth defects (Lucock 2004), and dementia (Wang et al. 2001), presumably by lowering homocysteine (Ravaglia et al. 2005).

Inadequate diet, alcoholism, chronic illness, drugs (e.g., phenytoin, valproic acid, lamotrigine, barbiturates, trimethoprim/sulfamethoxazole, oral contraceptives, and methotrexate), and malabsorption all can cause folate deficiency (Reynolds 2002). Deficiency is more common in the elderly (Reynolds 2006). Low folate levels are more prevalent in psychiatric inpatients than in patients without psychiatric illness, even after controlling for drug and alcohol abuse (Lerner et al. 2006). Folate deficiency has been reported in up to one-third of psychiatric patients and is especially prevalent in those with depression (Bottiglieri et al. 2000). It is unclear how much of folate deficiency can be attributed to the use of psychotropic medications, especially antiepileptic drugs, which are known to decrease folate levels.

Clinical Manifestations

Symptoms of folate deficiency are similar to those of B_{12} deficiency; however, subacute combined degeneration of the spinal cord is specific to B_{12} deficiency, and depression is more common in folate deficiency (Reynolds 2006). The megaloblastic anemia in folate deficiency is identical to that seen in B_{12} deficiency. Folate deficiency is invariably accompanied by a raised plasma homocysteine level), which carries an increased risk of cardiovascular disease, dementia (Ravaglia et al. 2005), and depression (Bottiglieri et al. 2000; Reynolds 2014)

Insufficient folate during conception and early pregnancy may result in neural tube defects. Since 1998, the U.S. Food and Drug Administration has mandated fortification of grains with folate to help lower women's risk of having a pregnancy affected by neural tube defects. This action has led to a reduction in neural tube defects and an improvement of blood folate status and homocysteine levels in adults in the United States (Wolff et al. 2009).

Diagnosis and Treatment

Low red blood cell folate combined with high plasma homocysteine is a good standard for the diagnosis of folate deficiency and is more accurate than measuring serum folate alone. Full treatment response to folate takes many months (Reynolds 2006). Although there are no clear guidelines for the dose or duration of folate supplementation, treatment is generally recommended for at least 6 months; clinical improvement is usually seen within the first few months (Reynolds 2006).

The relationship of vitamin deficiency to depression and dementia is complex and probably bidirectional. Depression has been associated with low baseline levels of both folate and B_{12} (Kim et al. 2008; Petridou et al. 2016). However, supplementation of B_{12} and folate in patients has not been shown to reduce depressive symptoms (de Koning et al. 2016; Okereke et al. 2015; Sharpley et al. 2014). The evidence to date is limited and varied, but provides more support for methylfolate than folic acid as being clinically effective in augmenting antidepressants (Bedson et al. 2014; Papakostas et al. 2012; Sarris et al. 2016). There is increasing interest in the possibility that elevated homocysteine levels are linked to cognitive impairment and dementia. Researchers have debated whether supplementation of either folate or B_{12}, which can lower homocysteine levels, has any effect on cognition or the development of dementia (Clarke et al. 2008). Findings to date have been inconsistent. Multiple studies have shown that folic acid supplementation increases blood folate and decreases homocysteine (Durga et al. 2007; Jacques et al. 1999). Some studies have found that a higher intake of folate, but not of the other B vitamins, is related to a lower risk of Alzheimer's dementia (Luchsinger et al. 2007; Ravaglia et al. 2005) and to better cognitive functioning (Durga et al. 2007). A recent systematic review found that among other risk factors, low folate levels predict conversion from mild cognitive impairment to dementia (Cooper et al. 2015). Several large reviews have demonstrated that supplementation of either folic acid or B_{12} has no significant effect on cognition in individuals with either normal or impaired cognitive functioning (Balk et al. 2007; Health Quality Ontario 2013; van der Zwaluw et al. 2014).

Sickle Cell Disease

Sickle cell disease (SCD) is the most common hemoglobinopathy. The vaso-occlusive crisis is the hallmark of SCD. These recurrent crises, involving acute episodes of severe pain, represent the most common reason that patients seek medical care. Extremes of temperature, infectious illness, dehydration, and physical exertion may precipitate crises, but the majority of crises occur without an identifiable cause. Vaso-occlusion produces acute pain in the short term and end-organ damage in the long term. Vaso-occlusion potentially affects all organ systems but leads to particular damage in bones, kidneys, lungs, eyes, and brain. Many patients suffer from chronic pain as a result of avascular necrosis, leg ulcers, or other poorly understood chronic pain syndromes. The neuropsychiatric manifestations of SCD can be divided into three main categories: 1) depression and anxiety resulting from living with a chronic stigmatizing disease associated with unpredictable, painful crises and high morbidity and mortality; 2) problems related to living with chronic and acute pain (often undertreated), control of which involves long-term use of analgesics, potentially leading to opioid dependency, addiction, and pseudoaddiction; and 3) CNS damage resulting from cerebral vascular accidents, primarily during childhood. These issues are further complicated by difficult psychosocial circumstances.

Depression and Anxiety

As with many chronic diseases, depression and anxiety are common in adult patients with SCD. The prevalence of depression is 21% among individuals with SCD, although as many as 71% have sleep disturbances (Jenerette et al. 2005; Levenson et al. 2008). Rates of depression are higher in children; Jerrell et al. (2011) reported a depression prevalence of 46% in a retrospective cohort study of children and adolescents with SCD. Dysthymic disorder was observed in 90% of a pediatric SCD population (Jerrell et al. 2011). Anxiety disorders occur in about 7% of patients (Levenson et al. 2008). Depression and anxiety predict more daily pain and poorer physical and psychosocial quality of life in adults with SCD and account for more of the variance in all domains of quality of life than does hemoglobin type (Levenson et al. 2008). Studies assessing depression and anxiety in children with SCD have yielded mixed results (Benton et al. 2007). However, children with SCD have a higher prevalence of excessive fatigue, physical complaints, impaired self-esteem, morbid ideation, and feelings of hopelessness (Anie 2005; Yang et al. 1994). These feelings arise in the context of frequent hospitalizations, chronic absences from school, and inability to experience a normal childhood like other children.

The stigma associated with SCD significantly contributes to anxiety and depression (Jenerette et al. 2005). Adults with SCD face physical deformities, the stigma of chronic opioid use and/or mental illness, and biases related to race. The strain of facing these stigmas may have a variety of negative psychological consequences. Physical deformities result from delayed growth and development as a consequence of chronic hemolysis and chronic vaso-occlusion. In comparison with control subjects, pediatric SCD patients weigh less, are shorter, and have delayed puberty (Cepeda et al. 2000). For adolescents, these physical differences may lead to problems with self-esteem, heightened self-consciousness, dissatisfaction with body image, and social isolation (Morgan and Jackson 1986). Participation in athletics is limited due to short stature and fear of initiating a vaso-occlusive crisis. School performance suffers when hospitalizations cause multiple missed school days. Accordingly, adolescents often experience hopelessness and social withdrawal (Hurtig and Park 1989). In the United States, the stigma of SCD is compounded by the disease's predominance in an ethnic minority, African American individuals, that already is vulnerable to racial prejudice and stereotyping (Haywood et al. 2014; Jacob and American Pain Society 2001).

Chronic and Acute Pain and Opioid Use

Individuals with SCD most commonly seek medical care for treatment of their pain. In the Pain in Sickle Cell Epidemiology Study (PiSCES), a prospective cohort study in which adults with SCD completed daily diaries for up to 6 months, participants reported experiencing pain on more than 50% of days, and 29% reported experiencing pain on more than 95% of days. In addition, whereas these patients reported experiencing sickle cell crises on 16% of days, they sought urgent health care for crisis pain on only 3.5% of days (Smith et al. 2008).

Over the past 15 years, opioid treatment has gained mainstream acceptance for the treatment of SCD pain. Opioids help control pain, improve functional capacity, and decrease hospitalizations in patients with SCD (Ballas et al. 2012; Taylor et al. 2010). Chronic opioid use may result in tolerance, physiological dependence as well as substance dependence, and abuse. There is concern among authors that cognitive deficits may occur with opioid use in patients with chronic pain; however, studies have not revealed consistent evidence to support this claim (Chapman et al. 2002).

Substance dependence and addiction behaviors are difficult to define in any chronic pain condition. The few studies that address addiction in SCD report a low prevalence. Despite the lack of evidence in the medical literature for addiction in SCD, medical practitioners often overestimate the prevalence of addiction (Labbé et al. 2005). In surveys of health care practitioners, 63% of nurses believed that addiction was prevalent in SCD (Pack-Mabien et al. 2001), and 53% of emergency department physicians and 23% of hematologists thought that more than 20% of SCD patients were addicted (Shapiro et al. 1997). Some of this misconception results from failure to understand the difference between physiological tolerance and opioid dependence. Even in the face of the opioid abuse epidemic, SCD patients are more at risk of under-treatment than of overtreatment with opioid pain medications (Ballas et al. 2012).

Due to skepticism and fear of introducing iatrogenic addiction, medical practitioners may undertreat pain in patients with SCD (Labbé et al. 2005). As a result of undertreatment, patients may develop a pseudoaddiction, where addiction-like behaviors occur as a result of inadequate pain management (Smith et al. 2011). Some SCD patients may seek out illegal narcotics as a way to manage their painful crises. This behavior can lead to long-term problems with true addiction and illicit substance abuse (Alao et al. 2003). Policy responses to the opioid crisis involve restrictions on duration and quantity of prescribed opioids, risking potentially dangerous withdrawal in opioid-tolerant individuals with SCD.

Ketamine has been used as an adjunctive treatment for acute pain crises among pediatric and adult patients with SCD. Psychiatric side effects, particularly psychosis, may occur, but ketamine alleviates opioid-induced hyperalgesia and may help offset issues with tolerance and perceived or actual abuse (Uprety et al. 2014).

Central Nervous System Damage

Brain injury from SCD complications begins early in life and is associated with neuro-cognitive dysfunction. An estimated 25%–33% of children with SCD have CNS effects from the disease (Schatz and McClellan 2006). Seizures occur in 12%–14% of pediatric patients with SCD and often herald stroke (Adams 1994; Liu et al. 1994). Cerebrovas-cular accidents, often silent, occur in up to 39% of children with SCD (DeBaun and Kirkham 2016). These children demonstrate cognitive deficits ranging from border-line to moderate, reduced language function, and problems with adjustment (Gold et al. 2008). Cognitive deficits in children with SCD can result in intellectual disability and educational problems, as well as problems with attention and concentration, and may lead to dementia later in life (Anie 2005). SCD patients have been found to have lower scores in language skills and auditory discrimination as early as kindergarten; thus, deficits cannot be attributed to school absences (Steen et al. 2002). As individuals with SCD live longer, they also risk acquisition of further intellectual disability by virtue of suffering further cerebrovascular accidents (Strouse et al. 2011).

Hemophilia

Hemophilia is a bleeding disorder caused by a deficiency of one of the coagulation factors essential for blood clotting. Hemophilia A (factor VIII deficiency) and hemophilia B (factor IX deficiency) are the most well-known inherited bleeding disorders.

Hemophilia A and B are X-linked diseases and mainly affect males. Female carriers can experience excessive bleeding, as they may have half the normal amount of clotting factors. Hemophilia A and B are clinically indistinguishable from one another.

Patients with *severe* hemophilia (<1% clotting factor) typically bleed spontaneously into joints, muscles, soft tissues, and body cavities. *Moderate* hemophilia (1%–5% clotting factor) is typically diagnosed by 5 years of age; bleeding episodes occur less frequently in patients with moderate hemophilia. *Mild* hemophilia (>5% clotting factor) is usually diagnosed later in life, following trauma, tooth extraction, or surgery. In patients with mild hemophilia, bleeding episodes typically occur secondary to trauma; spontaneous bleeding is rare (Bolton-Maggs and Pasi 2003; Manco-Johnson 2005).

Since the 1960s, the availability of purified factor VIII has allowed for home-based infusions, improved quality of life, and increased the life expectancy in patients with severe hemophilia. This has reduced the frequency of recurrent bleeds into large joints and muscles, resulting in fewer complications of joint injury and chronic pain.

Compared with the general population, patients with hemophilia have higher rates of depression (Iannone et al. 2012; Witkop et al. 2015), suicidal thinking (Ghanizadeh and Baligh-Jahromi 2009), and anxiety disorders (Bussing and Burket 1993). Chronic pain and other comorbidities are present throughout the life span and negatively affect developmental milestones from childhood through adulthood (Witkop et al. 2015), as well as quality of life in the elderly (von Mackensen et al. 2012). Adults with hemophilia report having to limit daily activities they consider too risky, and they have higher rates of disability and unemployment (Witkop et al. 2015). Many also report difficulty in developing intimate relationships (Witkop et al. 2015).

Physicians who fear inducing drug dependence with opioids are reluctant to prescribe these agents, despite the severe pain associated with joint bleeds. Even adult patients without drug dependence report concern about potential narcotic addiction (Elander and Barry 2003). In actual practice, opioid analgesics may be used safely in most patients with hemophilia. It is important to address patient concerns about becoming opioid dependent in order to provide adequate analgesia (Kunkel et al. 2000).

Individual, group, and family psychotherapy can be useful in addressing mood disorders and interpersonal and functional limitations in people with hemophilia. Caution is needed in prescribing psychotropic agents to individuals with hemophilia. For older patients with impaired liver function from viral hepatitis, dosages of antidepressants, antipsychotics, or opioid analgesics should be reduced. Several psychotropic agents may increase the risk of bleeding, and caution must be exercised when prescribing those agents to hemophiliacs (Casey and Brown 2003; Gerstner et al. 2006).

Thalassemia

Thalassemia, originally termed *thalassa anemia* ("anemia by the sea") due to its link to the Mediterranean region, is an inherited autosomal recessive blood disease (Lorey et al. 1996; Vichinsky et al. 2005). The thalassemias are a heterogeneous group of disorders characterized by various mutations (in either the alpha or the beta globin chain of hemoglobin) that are inherently unstable and precipitate within red blood cells. Clinical manifestations vary, depending on the type and severity of mutations. The complete absence of alpha globin, known as alpha-thalassemia major, is incompatible with life. Other forms of alpha- and beta-thalassemia are either clinically silent or can lead to death in infancy if not properly treated (Cunningham 2008). Significant advances have been made in treatment, and life spans are increasing.

Demographics

Once considered a fatal childhood illness, thalassemia now is considered a chronic adult disease. There has been a decline in Mediterranean-origin patients due to declining immigration from these regions as well as the introduction of genetic counseling programs and prenatal screening. Asian patients now account for at least 50% of the thalassemic population in North America as a result of increased Asian immigration to the United States (Vichinsky et al. 2005).

Clinical Manifestations

Although patients with thalassemia now have improved treatments, better preventive measures, and longer survival, many continue to suffer from various long-term sequelae. Removal of damaged red blood cells results in splenomegaly, which leads to increased trapping of red blood cells and worsening anemia. Increased but ineffective erythropoiesis can cause bony deformities, resulting in severe disfigurement of the pelvis, spine, and skull (Olivieri 1999); facial deformities, including frontal bossing, overgrowth of the maxillae, and a prominent malar eminence (Raiola et al. 2003); and shortening of the limbs. Iron deposition may cause endocrine (hypogonadism, secondary amenorrhea, short stature) and cardiac (arrhythmias, congestive heart failure) complications (Cunningham 2008).

Treatment

In severe forms of thalassemia, patients require repeated red blood cell transfusions to avoid growth retardation, congestive heart failure, severe bony defects, and endocrinopathies (Schrier and Angelucci 2005). Transfusions may be needed more frequently during pregnancy, rapid growth periods, and infection-associated aplastic crises (Borgna-Pignatti 2007; Nassar et al. 2006).

Regular red blood cell transfusions are associated with iron overload and/or hemosiderosis (Schrier and Angelucci 2005), which may result in cirrhosis, diabetes mellitus, hypothyroidism, hypoparathyroidism, growth failure, sexual immaturity, and cardiac dysfunction (Olivieri 1999). To prevent hemosiderosis, patients are treated with iron chelators. Advances in iron chelation therapy have contributed significantly to improved survival in patients with severe forms of thalassemia.

Stem-cell transplantation offers high rates of cure and greater long-term survival for patients with severe forms of thalassemia, and it is recommended that this therapy be offered early and before organ damage occurs. Unfortunately, only a small fraction of patients are able to receive stem-cell therapy as a result of cost and availability factors (Srivastava and Shaji 2017).

Psychosocial Aspects

Patients with severe forms of thalassemia now live longer lives but experience a greater burden from chronic illness. Depression and anxiety are more prevalent in people with thalassemia than in the general population, and quality of life tends to be poorer (Khoury et al. 2012; Yengil et al. 2014). An early-onset chronic illness characterized by frequent hospitalizations, long-term medication use, and a restricted social life, thalassemia can have a profound impact on development and psychological well-being (Ghanizadeh et al. 2006). Common issues that arise in childhood include denial and acting out, body-image concerns, depression, anxiety, and impaired self-esteem (Shakin and Thompson 1991; Vardaki et al. 2004).

Children with thalassemia frequently miss days of school (Di Palma et al. 1998); may have lower mean verbal IQ scores (Sherman et al. 1985); and may demonstrate deficits in multiple cognitive domains, including abstract reasoning, attention and memory, visuospatial skills, and executive functioning (Monastero et al. 2000; Zafeiriou et al. 2006). Individuals with thalassemia are at increased risk of dementia (Chen et al. 2015). Cognitive impairments may accrue with age; individuals with certain forms of thalassemia are susceptible to transient ischemic attacks and silent brain infarctions (Armstrong 2005) as well as iron deposition in the brain due to long-term iron chelation.

Because psychosocial factors likely play a large role in the development of psychological disturbances in patients with thalassemia, most literature supports a multidisciplinary approach to treatment. When medical care is combined with psychosocial support, patients show improved social integration and acceptance. They are more likely to finish school and to go on to higher education (McAnarney 1985). Addressing the psychiatric concerns of patients with thalassemia may improve adherence to medical treatments and thus improve outcomes (Beratis 1989).

It has been recommended that patients receive an annual assessment of their psychological life as part of their routine medical care (Ratip et al. 1995; Tsiantis 1990). Other recommendations include group meetings, support groups for families, patient education, and encouragement of self-management (Masera et al. 1990). It has been found that children with a limited understanding of their disease have poorer psychiatric adjustment (Sherman et al. 1985).

Some, but not all, studies have suggested a link between zinc deficiency (inherent to chronic iron chelation) and depression (Moafi et al. 2008). Cognitive deficits may also lead to depression and anxiety. Monitoring zinc levels and performing routine cognitive testing may be useful in the assessment of patients with thalassemia and mood disorders.

Hematological Side Effects and Drug Interactions of Psychotropic Agents

Antipsychotics and Agranulocytosis

Various psychotropic medications and their potential hematological side effects are listed in Table 23–1; potential interactions with anticoagulants are listed in Table 23–2. Antipsychotic agents with no reported hematological side effects include aripiprazole and ziprasidone. Hematological adverse effects of antipsychotics include agranulocytosis, aplastic anemia, neutropenia, eosinophilia, and thrombocytopenia.

TABLE 23–1.   **Psychotropic medications and hematological side effects**

Psychotropic agent	Hematological side effects
Antipsychotics	
Conventional agents	Agranulocytosis, anemia (aplastic, hemolytic), eosinophilia, leukopenia, thrombocytopenia
Atypical agents	
Clozapine	Agranulocytosis (1%–2%), eosinophilia, leukocytosis, leukopenia, thrombocytopenia
Other atypicals	Anemia, leukopenia, thrombocytopenia
Antidepressants	
Tricyclic antidepressants	Agranulocytosis, eosinophilia, leukopenia, thrombocytopenia
Serotonin–norepinephrine reuptake inhibitors	Impaired platelet aggregation
Monoamine oxidase inhibitors	
Tranylcypromine	Thrombocytopenia
Selective serotonin reuptake inhibitors	Impaired platelet aggregation
Multimodal agents	
Trazodone[a]	Agranulocytosis
Mirtazapine[b]	Agranulocytosis, thrombocytopenia
Benzodiazepines	Agranulocytosis (reported but not proven)
Mood stabilizers	
Carbamazepine	Agranulocytosis, anemia, eosinophilia, leukocytosis, leukopenia, pure red cell aplasia, thrombocytopenia
Gabapentin	Leukopenia, neutropenia
Lamotrigine	Agranulocytosis, anemia, neutropenia, pancytopenia, pure red cell aplasia, thrombocytopenia
Lithium	Leukocytosis, thrombocytosis
Topiramate	Anemia, thrombocytopenia
Valproic acid	Pure red cell aplasia, thrombocytopenia

Note.   Some of the reports are based on single cases, and therefore validity is not certain.
[a]Serotonin$_2$ receptor antagonism with serotonin reuptake blockade.
[b]Alpha$_2$ antagonism plus serotonin$_2$ and serotonin$_3$ antagonism.

Source.   Data from Cimo et al. 1977; Damiani and Christensen 2000; Derbyshire and Martin 2004; Fadul et al. 2002; Lexi-Drugs 2007; Micromedex Healthcare Series 2007; Mosby Drug Consult 2007; Opgen-Rhein and Dettling 2008; Physicians' Desk Reference 2007; Stahl 1998.

Agranulocytosis is rare except with clozapine, but it is the most common and most serious hematological side effect of the antipsychotics (Flanagan and Dunk 2008; Gareri et al. 2008; Rajagopal 2005; Sedky et al. 2005). Low-potency antipsychotics have a higher frequency of agranulocytosis than high-potency ones. Clozapine causes agranulocytosis in 0.8% of patients (Lahdelma and Appelberg 2012). The highest risk of clozapine-induced agranulocytosis is present during the first 6 months of treatment and then decreases significantly. The case fatality rate of clozapine-induced

TABLE 23–2. **Psychotropic medications and their possible interactions with anticoagulants**

Psychotropic agent	Interaction with anticoagulant
Antidepressants	
Tricyclic antidepressants	Increased bleeding with warfarin[a]
Selective serotonin reuptake inhibitors	Increased INR with warfarin (fluvoxamine, fluoxetine, paroxetine)
Mood stabilizers	
Carbamazepine (CBZ)	Reduced INR with warfarin; CBZ increases metabolism of warfarin by inducing hepatic metabolism Warfarin decreases effect of CBZ
Anticonvulsants	
Phenobarbital	Reduces INR by inducing hepatic metabolism

Note. Some of the reports are based on single cases, and therefore validity is not certain.
[a]Although some reports suggest that imipramine may alter the anticoagulant effect of warfarin by an unknown mechanism, a more recent study (Yoo et al. 2009) concluded that there is no allosteric effect or competition between the two drugs. Until additional information is presented, it may be advisable to monitor the international normalized ratio (INR) and clinical response if both drugs are to be administered.

Source. Data from Buckley and Meltzer 1995; Jenkins and Hansen 1995; Physicians' Desk Reference 2007; Rosse et al. 1989.

agranulocytosis is estimated at 4.2%–16%, depending on whether a granulocyte colony stimulating factor (G-CSF) is used (Schulte 2006). A weekly white blood cell (WBC) count is necessary to detect and monitor for clozapine-induced agranulocytosis for the first 6 months of initiation of the drug, then every 2 weeks for the next 6–12 months, and then monthly after 12 months (Clozapine Risk Evaluation and Mitigation Strategy [REMS] Program 2016). A WBC count lower than 2,000/mm^3 or an absolute neutrophil count (ANC) lower than 1,000/mm^3 is an indication for immediate cessation of clozapine. Individuals with benign ethnic neutropenia may initiate clozapine with an ANC as low as 1,000/mm^3 (Clozapine REMS Program 2016). Stopping clozapine usually leads to recovery in WBC counts within 3 weeks (Opgen-Rhein and Dettling 2008). The mortality risk associated with agranulocytosis is significantly increased if infection occurs before the drug is stopped (Gerson and Meltzer 1992; McEvoy et al. 2006). Clozapine causes bone marrow suppression, and G-CSF therapy may help restore normal bone marrow production (Gerson and Meltzer 1992; Lieberman and Alvir 1992; Sedky and Lippmann 2006). Patients with a history of clozapine-induced agranulocytosis should be closely monitored in cases involving reintroduction. However, the level of risk following reintroduction of clozapine is currently unknown.

Antidepressants and Bleeding

Selective serotonin reuptake inhibitors (SSRIs) inhibit platelet function and have been associated with bruising and bleeding, especially if used concomitantly with aspirin or nonsteroidal anti-inflammatory drugs (NSAIDs) (Jiang et al. 2015; Kuo et al. 2014).

SSRIs increase CNS 5-hydroxytryptamine (5-HT; serotonin) and reduce 5-HT in platelets (leading to reduced platelet aggregation). Serotonin–norepinephrine reuptake inhibitors (SNRIs) also pose an increased bleeding risk by virtue of their serotonergic properties. Platelets normally release serotonin at the site of a vascular tear, leading to further platelet aggregation and vasodilatation and permitting the sealing of the tear without thrombosis of the vessel (Mahdanian et al. 2014).

Especially in the elderly, bleeding from the upper gastrointestinal tract may occur at a frequency ranging from 1 in 100 to 1 in 1,000 patient-years of exposure to drugs, such as the SSRIs, that have high affinity to 5-HT (de Abajo et al. 2006). The likelihood of gastrointestinal bleeding with SSRIs is similar to that with low-dose NSAIDs (Weinrieb et al. 2005). Caution is advised in patients at high risk of gastrointestinal bleeding, for whom clinicians may consider prescribing an antidepressant with low serotonin reuptake inhibition. High-risk patients include patients with thrombocytopenia or with platelet disorders (e.g., von Willebrand's disease), patients on multiple antiplatelet agents (e.g., after myocardial infarction), and patients with advanced cirrhosis with coagulopathy. Patients who are at risk for gastrointestinal hemorrhage and who are taking antidepressants with high serotonin reuptake inhibition should generally use smaller doses or avoid aspirin and NSAIDs (Loke et al. 2008; Weinrieb et al. 2005). Whereas some studies have reported no associated risk of increased gastrointestinal bleeding in patients taking both SSRIs and NSAIDs (Schalekamp et al. 2008; Vidal et al. 2008), other studies have reported an increased risk of gastrointestinal bleeding among this group of patients (Loke et al. 2008; Weinrieb et al. 2005). SNRIs, however, do not appear to increase the risk of gastrointestinal bleeding (Cheng et al. 2015).

A cohort study published in 2017 implicated SSRIs as being associated with an increased risk of intracerebral hemorrhage, particularly when used in conjunction with anticoagulants (Renoux et al. 2017). A 2012 meta-analysis concluded that patients exposed to SSRIs have higher rates of intracerebral and intracranial hemorrhage compared with nonexposed control subjects; however, these are extremely rare events (Hackam and Mrkobrada 2012). Pharmacovigilance is prudent when SSRIs are used in patients at high risk for hemorrhagic and vasoconstrictive stroke (Ramasubbu 2004).

As a result of their antiplatelet effects, SSRIs and SNRIs may also increase the risk of perioperative bleeding. A review of 19 studies reporting information on bleeding complications during surgery among patients taking antidepressants (Roose and Rutherford 2016) found inconsistent risks from SSRIs. Based on this finding, clinicians are advised to weigh with patients the risk of bleeding complications versus the risks of discontinuation syndrome and of symptom recurrence before advising discontinuation of SSRIs or SNRIs preoperatively.

Although some reviews have concluded that there is no increased risk from combining SSRIs with warfarin (Kurdyak et al. 2005), there have been case reports of bleeding with concomitant use. Among the SSRIs, fluoxetine is the most commonly reported offending agent (Skop and Brown 1996). The interactions between warfarin and antidepressants can have potentially serious consequences, resulting from either platelet inhibition or inhibition of the cytochrome P450 (CYP) system. Of the antidepressants, fluoxetine, fluvoxamine, and paroxetine appear to have the highest potential for interactions (Duncan et al. 1998; Halperin and Reber 2007), while citalopram and sertraline may be relatively less likely to interact with warfarin (Duncan et al.

1998). In summary, practitioners should proceed cautiously when prescribing SSRIs and SNRIs for patients who have other sources of bleeding risk, including patients who use antiplatelet agents, such as those prescribed in post–myocardial infarction or post–cardiac catheterization patients, and patients with bleeding dyscrasias from liver failure or hematological disease.

Agranulocytosis due to tricyclic antidepressants is a rare, idiosyncratic condition caused by direct bone marrow toxicity, with a lower frequency than is reported for antipsychotics (Oyesanmi et al. 1999). Agranulocytosis has been associated with imipramine (Albertini and Penders 1978), clomipramine (Alderman et al. 1993), and desipramine (Hardin and Conrath 1982).

Lithium

Lithium stimulates leukocytosis with a true proliferative response. In patients on lithium therapy for cluster headaches, Medina and colleagues (Albertini and Penders 1978; Medina et al. 1980) documented increases in the number of platelets and in platelet serotonin and histamine levels. In the past, because of its hematological side effects, lithium therapy was considered for persistent leukopenia and thrombocytopenia following chemotherapy or radiotherapy; however, more effective therapies are now available.

Anticonvulsants and Mood Stabilizers

Carbamazepine should be avoided in individuals with a history of bone marrow depression. Carbamazepine produces a transient reduction in WBC count in approximately 10% of patients during the first 4 months of treatment (Rall and Schleifer 1980). In very rare cases it can cause potentially fatal agranulocytosis and aplastic anemia. Agranulocytosis results from direct toxicity to the bone marrow (Sedky and Lippmann 2006). A baseline complete blood count is always advised before starting a patient on carbamazepine. Carbamazepine should be discontinued if the WBC count drops below 3,500/mm^3. Administration of lithium and carbamazepine concurrently may lower the risk of carbamazepine-induced neutropenia, because lithium stimulates WBC production, predominantly neutrophils (Kramlinger and Post 1990). Carbamazepine induces its own metabolism. Thus, after a person has been taking the drug for a period of time, the amount of carbamazepine in the blood will suddenly decrease. Because carbamazepine induces CYP1A2, 2C, and 3A4, it reduces the anticoagulant effect of warfarin, so both the carbamazepine level and the international normalized ratio will need to be monitored frequently when both drugs are used (Herman et al. 2006; Whiskey and Taylor 2007).

Valproate-induced increases in red blood cell mean corpuscular volume (MCV) and mean corpuscular hemoglobin concentration (MCHC) have been postulated to result from alterations in erythrocyte membrane phospholipids (Ozkara et al. 1993). Potentially fatal hematopoietic complications such as neutropenia, thrombocytopenia, and macrocytic anemia have been associated with valproate (Nasreddine and Beydoun 2008). Lamotrigine also may cause agranulocytosis (de Camargo and Bode 1999; Fadul et al. 2002). All anticonvulsants should be discontinued if the WBC count drops below 3,000/mm^3 (Ramsay 1994).

Acetylcholinesterase Inhibitors

Donepezil is associated with anemia, thrombocythemia, thrombocytopenia, ecchymosis, and eosinophilia. The mechanism for the hematological side effects is unknown. Rivastigmine has been reported to cause anemia, and galantamine can cause epistaxis, purpura, and thrombocytopenia (Mosby Drug Consult 2007).

Conclusion

This chapter has summarized neuropsychiatric effects of the illnesses and treatments associated with some of the major hematological disorders, including iron deficiency anemia, B_{12} and folate deficiency, sickle cell disease, hemophilia, and thalassemia. Mood disorders are common in patients with hematological disorders, either as a direct result of the disorder (as in the vitamin deficiencies) or as a result of the disorder's effect on quality of life (as in some of the more chronic illnesses such as the thalassemias). Neurocognitive deficits may also be significant factors in these disorders, and may be a direct or indirect result of the illness.

It is important that psychiatrists be knowledgeable about the hematological effects of psychotropic medications, especially when working with a medically ill population. Psychiatrists should be aware of the potential for blood dyscrasias in patients taking psychiatric medications. They should also be cognizant of interactions with other medications and their impact on general medical conditions, and this information should be part of the collaborative treatment plan with the patient and other medical providers.

References

Adams RJ: Neurological complications, in Sickle Cell Disease: Basic Principles and Clinical Practice. Edited by Mohandas N, Steinberg MH. New York, Raven, 1994, pp 560–621

Alao AO, Westmoreland N, Jindal S: Drug addiction in sickle cell disease: case report. Int J Psychiatry Med 33(1):97–101, 2003 12906347

Albertini RS, Penders TM: Agranulocytosis associated with tricyclics. J Clin Psychiatry 39(5):483–485, 1978 641026

Alderman CP, Atchison MM, McNeece JI: Concurrent agranulocytosis and hepatitis secondary to clomipramine therapy. Br J Psychiatry 162:688–689, 1993 8149124

Allen RP, Auerbach S, Bahrain H, et al: The prevalence and impact of restless legs syndrome on patients with iron deficiency anemia. Am J Hematol 88(4):261–264, 2013 23494945

Andrès E, Loukili NH, Noel E, et al: Vitamin B12 (cobalamin) deficiency in elderly patients. CMAJ 171(3):251–259, 2004 15289425

Andrès E, Dali-Youcef N, Vogel T, et al: Oral cobalamin (vitamin B(12)) treatment. An update. Int J Lab Hematol 31(1):1–8, 2009 19032377

Anie KA: Psychological complications in sickle cell disease. Br J Haematol 129(6):723–729, 2005 15952997

Anie KA, Green J: Psychological therapies for sickle cell disease and pain. Cochrane Database Syst Rev (5):CD001916, 2015 25966336

Annibale B, Capurso G, Delle Fave G: The stomach and iron deficiency anaemia: a forgotten link. Dig Liver Dis 35(4):288–295, 2003 12801042

Armstrong FD: Thalassemia and learning: neurocognitive functioning in children. Ann N Y Acad Sci 1054:283–289, 2005 16339676

Balk EM, Raman G, Tatsioni A, et al: Vitamin B6, B12, and folic acid supplementation and cognitive function: a systematic review of randomized trials. Arch Intern Med 167(1):21–30, 2007 17210874

Ballas SK, Gupta K, Adams-Graves P: Sickle cell pain: a critical reappraisal. Blood 120(18):3647–3656, 2012 22923496

Bauman WA, Shaw S, Jayatilleke E, et al: Increased intake of calcium reverses vitamin B12 malabsorption induced by metformin. Diabetes Care 23(9):1227–1231, 2000 10977010

Beard JL, Hendricks MK, Perez EM, et al: Maternal iron deficiency anemia affects postpartum emotions and cognition. J Nutr 135(2):267–272, 2005 15671224

Bedson E, Bell D, Carr D, et al: Folate augmentation of treatment—evaluation for depression (FolATED): randomised trial and economic evaluation. Health Technol Assess 18(48):vii–viii, 1–159, 2014 25052890

Benton TD, Ifeagwu JA, Smith-Whitley K: Anxiety and depression in children and adolescents with sickle cell disease. Curr Psychiatry Rep 9(2):114–121, 2007 17389120

Beratis S: Noncompliance with iron chelation therapy in patients with beta thalassaemia. J Psychosom Res 33(6):739–745, 1989 2695624

Bolton-Maggs PH, Pasi KJ: Haemophilias A and B. Lancet 361(9371):1801–1809, 2003 12781551

Bonetti F, Brombo G, Magon S, Zuliani G: Cognitive status according to homocysteine and B-group vitamins in elderly adults. J Am Geriatr Soc 63(6):1158–1163, 2015 26031567

Booth IW, Aukett MA: Iron deficiency anaemia in infancy and early childhood. Arch Dis Child 76(6):549–553, discussion 553–554, 1997 9245860

Borgna-Pignatti C: Modern treatment of thalassaemia intermedia. Br J Haematol 138(3):291–304, 2007 17565568

Bottiglieri T, Laundy M, Crellin R, et al: Homocysteine, folate, methylation, and monoamine metabolism in depression. J Neurol Neurosurg Psychiatry 69(2):228–232, 2000 10896698

Buckley PF, Meltzer HY: Treatment of schizophrenia, in Textbook of Psychopharmacology. Edited by Schatzberg AF, Nemeroff CB. Washington, DC, American Psychiatric Press, 1995, pp 615–639

Bussing R, Burket RC: Anxiety and intrafamilial stress in children with hemophilia after the HIV crisis. J Am Acad Child Adolesc Psychiatry 32(3):562–567, 1993 8496120

Carmel R, Green R, Rosenblatt DS, Watkins D: Update on cobalamin, folate, and homocysteine. Hematology (Am Soc Hematol Educ Program) 62–81, 2003 14633777

Casey RL, Brown RT: Psychological aspects of hematologic diseases. Child Adolesc Psychiatr Clin N Am 12(3):567–584, 2003 12910823

Cepeda ML, Allen FH, Cepeda NJ, Yang YM: Physical growth, sexual maturation, body image and sickle cell disease. J Natl Med Assoc 92(1):10–14, 2000 10800281

Chalouhi C, Faesch S, Anthoine-Milhomme MC, et al: Neurological consequences of vitamin B12 deficiency and its treatment. Pediatr Emerg Care 24(8):538–541, 2008 18708898

Chapman SL, Byas-Smith MG, Reed BA: Effects of intermediate- and long-term use of opioids on cognition in patients with chronic pain. Clin J Pain 18 (4 suppl):S83–S90, 2002 12479258

Chen MH, Su TP, Chen YS, et al: Association between psychiatric disorders and iron deficiency anemia among children and adolescents: a nationwide population-based study. BMC Psychiatry 13:161, 2013 23735056

Chen YG, Lin TY, Chen HJ, et al: Thalassemia and risk of dementia: a nationwide population-based retrospective cohort study. Eur J Intern Med 26(7):554–559, 2015 26051928

Cheng YL, Hu HY, Lin XH, et al: Use of SSRI but not SNRI increased upper and lower gastrointestinal bleeding: a nationwide population-based cohort study in Taiwan. Medicine (Baltimore) 94(46):e2022, 2015 26579809

Cimo PL, Pisciotta AV, Desai RG, et al: Detection of drug-dependent antibodies by the 51Cr platelet lysis test: documentation of immune thrombocytopenia induced by diphenylhydantoin, diazepam, and sulfisoxazole. Am J Hematol 2(1):65–72, 1977 868869

Clarke R, Sherliker P, Hin H, et al: Folate and vitamin B12 status in relation to cognitive impairment and anaemia in the setting of voluntary fortification in the UK. Br J Nutr 100(5):1054–1059, 2008 18341758

Clozapine Risk Evaluation and Mitigation Strategy (REMS) Program (Web site): Important program update as of December 16, 2016. Available at: https://www.clozapinerems.com/CpmgClozapineUI/home.u. Accessed May 28, 2017.

Coban E, Timuragaoglu A, Meriç M: Iron deficiency anemia in the elderly: prevalence and endoscopic evaluation of the gastrointestinal tract in outpatients. Acta Haematol 110(1):25–28, 2003 12975553

Cook JD, Skikne BS: Iron deficiency: definition and diagnosis. J Intern Med 226(5):349–355, 1989 2681511

Cooper C, Sommerlad A, Lyketsos CG, Livingston G: Modifiable predictors of dementia in mild cognitive impairment: a systematic review and meta-analysis. Am J Psychiatry 172(4):323–334, 2015 25698435

Cunningham MJ: Update on thalassemia: clinical care and complications. Pediatr Clin North Am 55(2):447–460, 2008 18381095

Damiani JT, Christensen RC: Lamotrigine-associated neutropenia in a geriatric patient. Am J Geriatr Psychiatry 8(4):346, 2000 11069275

de Abajo FJ, Montero D, Rodriguez LA, Madurga M: Antidepressants and risk of upper gastrointestinal bleeding. Basic Clin Pharmacol Toxicol 98(3):304–310, 2006 16611206

DeBaun MR, Kirkham FJ: Central nervous system complications and management in sickle cell disease. Blood 127(7):829–838, 2016 26758917

de Camargo OA, Bode H: Agranulocytosis associated with lamotrigine. BMJ 318(7192):1179, 1999 10221944

de Koning EJ, van der Zwaluw NL, van Wijngaarden JP, et al: Effects of two-year vitamin B12 and folic acid supplementation on depressive symptoms and quality of life in older adults with elevated homocysteine concentrations: additional results from the B-PROOF study, an RCT. Nutrients 8(11):E748, 2016 27886078

Derbyshire E, Martin D: Neutropenia occurring after starting gabapentin for neuropathic pain. Clin Oncol (R Coll Radiol) 16(8):575–576, 2004 15630852

Di Palma A, Vullo C, Zani B, Facchini A: Psychosocial integration of adolescents and young adults with thalassemia major. Ann N Y Acad Sci 850:355–360, 1998 9668558

Duncan D, Sayal K, McConnell H, Taylor D: Antidepressant interactions with warfarin. Int Clin Psychopharmacol 13(2):87–94, 1998 9669190

Durga J, van Boxtel MP, Schouten EG, et al: Effect of 3-year folic acid supplementation on cognitive function in older adults in the FACIT trial: a randomised, double blind, controlled trial. Lancet 369(9557):208–216, 2007 17240287

Elander J, Barry T: Analgesic use and pain coping among patients with haemophilia. Haemophilia 9(2):202–213, 2003 12614373

Fadul CE, Meyer LP, Jobst BC, et al: Agranulocytosis associated with lamotrigine in a patient with low-grade glioma. Epilepsia 43(2):199–200, 2002 11903469

Federman DG, Kirsner RS, Federman GS: Pica: are you hungry for the facts? Conn Med 61(4):207–209, 1997 9149482

Flanagan RJ, Dunk L: Haematological toxicity of drugs used in psychiatry. Hum Psychopharmacol 23 (suppl 1):27–41, 2008 18098216

Gareri P, De Fazio P, Russo E, et al: The safety of clozapine in the elderly. Expert Opin Drug Saf 7(5):525–538, 2008 18759705

Gerson SL, Meltzer H: Mechanisms of clozapine-induced agranulocytosis. Drug Saf 7 (suppl 1):17–25, 1992 1503673

Gerstner T, Teich M, Bell N, et al: Valproate-associated coagulopathies are frequent and variable in children. Epilepsia 47(7):1136–1143, 2006 16886976

Ghanizadeh A, Baligh-Jahromi P: Depression, anxiety and suicidal behaviour in children and adolescents with haemophilia. Haemophilia 15(2):528–532, 2009 19187190

Ghanizadeh A, Khajavian S, Ashkani H: Prevalence of psychiatric disorders, depression, and suicidal behavior in child and adolescent with thalassemia major. J Pediatr Hematol Oncol 28(12):781–784, 2006 17164645

Gold JI, Johnson CB, Treadwell MJ, et al: Detection and assessment of stroke in patients with sickle cell disease: neuropsychological functioning and magnetic resonance imaging. Pediatr Hematol Oncol 25(5):409–421, 2008 18569843

Hackam DG, Mrkobrada M: Selective serotonin reuptake inhibitors and brain hemorrhage: a meta-analysis. Neurology 79(18):1862–1865, 2012 23077009

Halperin D, Reber G: Influence of antidepressants on hemostasis. Dialogues Clin Neurosci 9(1):47–59, 2007 17506225

Halterman JS, Kaczorowski JM, Aligne CA, et al: Iron deficiency and cognitive achievement among school-aged children and adolescents in the United States. Pediatrics 107(6):1381–1386, 2001 11389261

Hardin TC, Conrath FC: Desipramine-induced agranulocytosis. A case report. Drug Intell Clin Pharm 16(1):62–63, 1982 7053955

Haywood C Jr, Lanzkron S, Bediako S, et al; IMPORT Investigators: Perceived discrimination, patient trust, and adherence to medical recommendations among persons with sickle cell disease. J Gen Intern Med 29(12):1657–1662, 2014 25205621

Health Quality Ontario: Vitamin B12 and cognitive function: an evidence-based analysis. Ont Health Technol Assess Ser 13(23):1–45, 2013 24379897

Herman D, Locatelli I, Grabnar I, et al: The influence of co-treatment with carbamazepine, amiodarone and statins on warfarin metabolism and maintenance dose. Eur J Clin Pharmacol 62(4):291–296, 2006 16552506

Hunt MG, Belfer S, Atuahene B: Pagophagia improves neuropsychological processing speed in iron-deficiency anemia. Med Hypotheses 83(4):473–476, 2014 25169035

Hurtig AL, Park KB: Adjustment and coping in adolescents with sickle cell disease. Ann N Y Acad Sci 565:172–182, 1989 2774423

Iannone M, Pennick L, Tom A, et al: Prevalence of depression in adults with haemophilia. Haemophilia 18(6):868–874, 2012 22642565

Jacob E; American Pain Society: Pain management in sickle cell disease. Pain Manag Nurs 2(4):121–131, 2001 11748547

Jacques PF, Selhub J, Bostom AG, et al: The effect of folic acid fortification on plasma folate and total homocysteine concentrations. N Engl J Med 340(19):1449–1454, 1999 10320382

Jenerette C, Funk M, Murdaugh C: Sickle cell disease: a stigmatizing condition that may lead to depression. Issues Ment Health Nurs 26(10):1081–1101, 2005 16284000

Jenkins SC, Hansen MR: A Pocket Reference for Psychiatrists, 2nd Edition. Washington, DC, American Psychiatric Press, 1995

Jerrell JM, Tripathi A, McIntyre RS: Prevalence and treatment of depression in children and adolescents with sickle cell disease: a retrospective cohort study. Prim Care Companion CNS Disord 13(2):PCC.10m01063, 2011 21977359

Jiang HY, Chen HZ, Hu XJ, et al: Use of selective serotonin reuptake inhibitors and risk of upper gastrointestinal bleeding: a systematic review and meta-analysis. Clin Gastroenterol Hepatol 13(1):42–50.e3, 2015 24993365

Khoury B, Musallam KM, Abi-Habib R, et al: Prevalence of depression and anxiety in adult patients with b-thalassemia major and intermedia. Int J Psychiatry Med 44(4):291–303, 2012 23885513

Kim JM, Stewart R, Kim SW, et al: Predictive value of folate, vitamin B12 and homocysteine levels in late-life depression. Br J Psychiatry 192(4):268–274, 2008 18378986

Kramlinger KG, Post RM: Addition of lithium carbonate to carbamazepine: hematological and thyroid effects. Am J Psychiatry 147(5):615–620, 1990 2109539

Krieger J, Schroeder C: Iron, brain and restless legs syndrome. Sleep Med Rev 5(4):277–286, 2001 12530992

Kunkel EJ, Thompson TL, Abdelgheni MB, et al: Hematologic disorders, in Psychiatric Care of the Medical Patient, 2nd Edition. Edited by Stoudemire A, Fogel BS, Greenberg DB. New York, Oxford University Press, 2000, pp 833–856

Kuo CY, Liao YT, Chen VC: Risk of upper gastrointestinal bleeding when taking SSRIs with NSAIDs or aspirin. Am J Psychiatry 171(5):582, 2014 24788285

Kurdyak PA, Juurlink DN, Kopp A, et al: Antidepressants, warfarin, and the risk of hemor-rhage. J Clin Psychopharmacol 25(6):561–564, 2005 16282838

Labbé E, Herbert D, Haynes J: Physicians' attitude and practices in sickle cell disease pain management. J Palliat Care 21(4):246–251, 2005 16483093

Lachner C, Martin C, John D, et al: Older adult psychiatric inpatients with non-cognitive disorders should be screened for vitamin B12 deficiency. J Nutr Health Aging 18(2):209–212, 2014 24522476

Lahdelma L, Appelberg B: Clozapine-induced agranulocytosis in Finland, 1982–2007: long-term monitoring of patients is still warranted. J Clin Psychiatry 73(6):837–842, 2012 22480452

Lerner V, Kanevsky M, Dwolatzky T, et al: Vitamin B12 and folate serum levels in newly admitted psychiatric patients. Clin Nutr 25(1):60–67, 2006 16216392

Levenson JL, McClish DK, Dahman BA, et al: Depression and anxiety in adults with sickle cell disease: the PiSCES project. Psychosom Med 70(2):192–196, 2008 18158366

Lexi-Drugs [computer program]. Hudson, OH, Lexi-Comp, 2007

Lieberman JA, Alvir JM: A report of clozapine-induced agranulocytosis in the United States. Incidence and risk factors. Drug Saf 7 (suppl 1):1–2, 1992 1503671

Liu JE, Gzesh DJ, Ballas SK: The spectrum of epilepsy in sickle cell anemia. J Neurol Sci 123(1–2):6–10, 1994 8064323

Liu KW, Dai LK, Jean W: Metformin-related vitamin B12 deficiency. Age Ageing 35(2):200–201, 2006 16495296

Loikas S, Koskinen P, Irjala K, et al: Vitamin B12 deficiency in the aged: a population-based study. Age Ageing 36(2):177–183, 2007 17189285

Loke YK, Trivedi AN, Singh S: Meta-analysis: gastrointestinal bleeding due to interaction between selective serotonin uptake inhibitors and non-steroidal anti-inflammatory drugs. Aliment Pharmacol Ther 27(1):31–40, 2008 17919277

Lorey FW, Arnopp J, Cunningham GC: Distribution of hemoglobinopathy variants by ethnicity in a multiethnic state. Genet Epidemiol 13(5):501–512, 1996 8905396

Lozoff B: Behavioral alterations in iron deficiency. Adv Pediatr 35:331–359, 1988 3055862

Lucca U, Tettamanti M, Mosconi P, et al: Association of mild anemia with cognitive, functional, mood and quality of life outcomes in the elderly: the "Health and Anemia" study. PLoS One 3(4):e1920, 2008 18382689

Luchsinger JA, Tang MX, Miller J, et al: Relation of higher folate intake to lower risk of Alzheimer disease in the elderly. Arch Neurol 64(1):86–92, 2007 17210813

Lucock M: Is folic acid the ultimate functional food component for disease prevention? BMJ 328(7433):211–214, 2004 14739191

Mahdanian AA, Rej S, Bacon SL, et al: Serotonergic antidepressants and perioperative bleeding risk: a systematic review. Expert Opin Drug Saf 13(6):695–704, 2014 24717049

Malinowski SS: Nutritional and metabolic complications of bariatric surgery. Am J Med Sci 331(4):219–225, 2006 16617238

Manco-Johnson M: Hemophilia management: optimizing treatment based on patient needs. Curr Opin Pediatr 17(1):3–6, 2005 15659955

Masera G, Monguzzi W, Tornotti G, et al: Psychosocial support in thalassemia major: Monza Center's experience. Haematologica 75 (suppl 5):181–190, 1990 2086377

McAnarney ER: Social maturation. A challenge for handicapped and chronically ill adolescents. J Adolesc Health Care 6(2):90–101, 1985 3156836

McEvoy JP, Lieberman JA, Stroup TS, et al; CATIE Investigators: Effectiveness of clozapine versus olanzapine, quetiapine, and risperidone in patients with chronic schizophrenia who did not respond to prior atypical antipsychotic treatment. Am J Psychiatry 163(4):600–610, 2006 16585434

Medina JL, Fareed J, Diamond S: Lithium carbonate therapy for cluster headache. Changes in number of platelets, and serotonin and histamine levels. Arch Neurol 37(9):559–563, 1980 7417056

Micromedex Healthcare Series [Internet database]. Greenwood Village, CO, Thomson Reuters (Healthcare), 2007

Milman N: Iron and pregnancy—a delicate balance. Ann Hematol 85(9):559–565, 2006 16691399

Moafi A, Mobaraki G, Taheri SS, et al: Zinc in thalassemic patients and its relation with depression. Biol Trace Elem Res 123(1–3):8–13, 2008 18338112

Monastero R, Monastero G, Ciaccio C, et al: Cognitive deficits in beta-thalassemia major. Acta Neurol Scand 102(3):162–168, 2000 10987375

Moore E, Mander A, Ames D, et al: Cognitive impairment and vitamin B12: a review. Int Psychogeriatr 24(4):541–556, 2012 22221769

Morgan SA, Jackson J: Psychological and social concomitants of sickle cell anemia in adolescents. J Pediatr Psychol 11(3):429–440, 1986 3772686

Mosby Drug Consult. St. Louis, MO, Mosby, 2007

Nasreddine W, Beydoun A: Valproate-induced thrombocytopenia: a prospective monotherapy study. Epilepsia 49(3):438–445, 2008 18031547

Nassar AH, Usta IM, Rechdan JB, et al: Pregnancy in patients with beta-thalassemia intermedia: outcome of mothers and newborns. Am J Hematol 81(7):499–502, 2006 16755576

National Institutes of Health: Iron (dietary supplement fact sheet). Available at: https://ods.od.nih.gov/factsheets/Iron-HealthProfessional/. Accessed April 15, 2017.

Okereke OI, Cook NR, Albert CM, et al: Effect of long-term supplementation with folic acid and B vitamins on risk of depression in older women. Br J Psychiatry 206(4):324–331, 2015 25573400

Olivieri NF: The beta-thalassemias. N Engl J Med 341(2):99–109, 1999 10395635

Opgen-Rhein C, Dettling M: Clozapine-induced agranulocytosis and its genetic determinants. Pharmacogenomics 9(8):1101–1111, 2008 18681784

Oyesanmi O, Kunkel EJ, Monti DA, Field HL: Hematologic side effects of psychotropics. Psychosomatics 40(5):414–421, 1999 10479946

Ozkara C, Dreifuss FE, Apperson Hansen C: Changes in red blood cells with valproate therapy. Acta Neurol Scand 88(3):210–212, 1993 8256557

Pack-Mabien A, Labbe E, Herbert D, Haynes J Jr: Nurses' attitudes and practices in sickle cell pain management. Appl Nurs Res 14(4):187–192, 2001 11699021

Papakostas GI, Shelton RC, Zajecka JM, et al: L-methylfolate as adjunctive therapy for SSRI-resistant major depression: results of two randomized, double-blind, parallel-sequential trials. Am J Psychiatry 169(12):1267–1274, 2012 23212058

Petridou ET, Kousoulis AA, Michelakos T, et al: Folate and B12 serum levels in association with depression in the aged: a systematic review and meta-analysis. Aging Ment Health 20(9):965–973, 2016 26055921

Physicians' Desk Reference, 61st Edition. Montvale, NJ, Medical Economics, 2007

Raiola G, Galati MC, De Sanctis V, et al: Growth and puberty in thalassemia major. J Pediatr Endocrinol Metab 16 (suppl 2):259–266, 2003 12729401

Rajagopal S: Clozapine, agranulocytosis, and benign ethnic neutropenia. Postgrad Med J 81(959):545–546, 2005 16143678

Rall TW, Schleifer LS: Drugs effective in the therapy of the epilepsies, in The Pharmacological Basis of Therapeutics, 6th Edition. Edited by Gilman AG, Goldman LG, Gilman A. New York, Macmillan, 1980, pp 448–474

Ramasubbu R: Cerebrovascular effects of selective serotonin reuptake inhibitors: a systematic review. J Clin Psychiatry 65(12):1642–1653, 2004 15641869

Ramsay RE: Clinical efficacy and safety of gabapentin. Neurology 44 (6 suppl 5):S23–S30; discussion S31–S32, 1994 8022537

Ratip S, Skuse D, Porter J, et al: Psychosocial and clinical burden of thalassaemia intermedia and its implications for prenatal diagnosis. Arch Dis Child 72(5):408–412, 1995 7618906

Ravaglia G, Forti P, Maioli F, et al: Homocysteine and folate as risk factors for dementia and Alzheimer disease. Am J Clin Nutr 82(3):636–643, 2005 16155278

Rector WG Jr: Pica: its frequency and significance in patients with iron-deficiency anemia due to chronic gastrointestinal blood loss. J Gen Intern Med 4(6):512–513, 1989 2585159

Renoux C, Vahey S, Dell'Aniello S, Boivin JF: Association of selective serotonin reuptake inhibitors with the risk for spontaneous intracranial hemorrhage. JAMA Neurol 74(2):173–180, 2017 27918771

Reynolds EH: Benefits and risks of folic acid to the nervous system. J Neurol Neurosurg Psychiatry 72(5):567–571, 2002 11971038

Reynolds E: Vitamin B12, folic acid, and the nervous system. Lancet Neurol 5(11):949–960, 2006 17052662

Reynolds EH: The neurology of folic acid deficiency. Handb Clin Neurol 120:927–943, 2014 24365361

Roose SP, Rutherford BR: Selective serotonin reuptake inhibitors and operative bleeding risk: a review of the literature. J Clin Psychopharmacol 36(6):704–709, 2016 27684291

Rosebush PI, Mazurek MF: Serum iron and neuroleptic malignant syndrome. Lancet 338(8760):149–151, 1991 1677067

Rosse RB, Giese AA, Deutsch SI, et al: Hematological measures of potential relevance to psychiatrists, in Concise Guide to Laboratory and Diagnostic Testing in Psychiatry. Washington, DC, American Psychiatric Press, 1989, pp 31–35

Sarris J, Murphy J, Mischoulon D, et al: Adjunctive nutraceuticals for depression: a systematic review and meta-analysis. Am J Psychiatry 173(6):575–587, 2016 27113121

Schalekamp T, Klungel OH, Souverein PC, de Boer A: Increased bleeding risk with concurrent use of selective serotonin reuptake inhibitors and coumarins. Arch Intern Med 168(2):180–185, 2008 18227365

Schatz J, McClellan CB: Sickle cell disease as a neurodevelopmental disorder. Ment Retard Dev Disabil Res Rev 12(3):200–207, 2006 17061284

Schrier SL: Diagnosis and treatment of vitamin B12 and folate deficiency. UpToDate. Literature review current through: April 2017. This topic last updated: September 21, 2016. Available at: https://www.uptodate.com/contents/diagnosis-and-treatment-of-vitamin-b12-and-folate-deficiency. Accessed May 25, 2017.

Schrier SL, Angelucci E: New strategies in the treatment of the thalassemias. Annu Rev Med 56:157–171, 2005 15660507

Schulte P: Risk of clozapine-associated agranulocytosis and mandatory white blood cell monitoring. Ann Pharmacother 40(4):683–688, 2006 16595571

Sedky K, Lippmann S: Psychotropic medications and leukopenia. Curr Drug Targets 7(9):1191–1194, 2006 17017894

Sedky K, Shaughnessy R, Hughes T, Lippmann S: Clozapine-induced agranulocytosis after 11 years of treatment. Am J Psychiatry 162(4):814, 2005 15800170

Shakin EJ, Thompson TL: Psychiatric aspects of hematologic disorders, in Medical-Psychiatric Practice. Edited by Stoudemire A, Fogel BS. Washington, DC, American Psychiatric Press, 1991, pp 193–242

Shakin EJ, Thompson TL: Hematologic disorders, in Psychiatric Care of the Medical Patient. Edited by Stoudemire A, Fogel BS. New York, Oxford University Press, 1993, pp 691–712

Shapiro BS, Benjamin LJ, Payne R, Heidrich G: Sickle cell-related pain: perceptions of medical practitioners. J Pain Symptom Manage 14(3):168–174, 1997 9291703

Sharpley AL, Hockney R, McPeake L, et al: Folic acid supplementation for prevention of mood disorders in young people at familial risk: a randomised, double blind, placebo controlled trial. J Affect Disord 167:306–311, 2014 25010374

Sherman M, Koch D, Giardina P, et al: Thalassemic children's understanding of illness: a study of cognitive and emotional factors. Ann N Y Acad Sci 445:327–336, 1985 3860137

Skop BP, Brown TM: Potential vascular and bleeding complications of treatment with selective serotonin reuptake inhibitors. Psychosomatics 37(1):12–16, 1996 8600488

Smith WR, Penberthy LT, Bovbjerg VE, et al: Daily assessment of pain in adults with sickle cell disease. Ann Intern Med 148(2):94–101, 2008 18195334

Smith WR, Jordan LB, Hassell KL: Frequently asked questions by hospitalists managing pain in adults with sickle cell disease. J Hosp Med 6(5):297–303, 2011 21661104

Srivastava A, Shaji RV: Cure for thalassemia major—from allogeneic hematopoietic stem cell transplantation to gene therapy. Haematologica 102(2):214–223, 2017 27909215

Stahl SM: Basic psychopharmacology of antidepressants, part 1: antidepressants have seven distinct mechanisms of action. J Clin Psychiatry 59 (suppl 4):5–14, 1998 9554316

Steen RG, Hu XJ, Elliott VE, et al: Kindergarten readiness skills in children with sickle cell disease: evidence of early neurocognitive damage? J Child Neurol 17(2):111–116, 2002 11952070

Strouse JJ, Lanzkron S, Urrutia V: The epidemiology, evaluation and treatment of stroke in adults with sickle cell disease. Expert Rev Hematol 4(6):597–606, 2011 22077524

Sun ER, Chen CA, Ho G, et al: Iron and the restless legs syndrome. Sleep 21(4):371–377, 1998 9646381

Taylor LE, Stotts NA, Humphreys J, et al: A review of the literature on the multiple dimensions of chronic pain in adults with sickle cell disease. J Pain Symptom Manage 40(3):416–435, 2010 20656451

Toh BH, van Driel IR, Gleeson PA: Pernicious anemia. N Engl J Med 337(20):1441–1448, 1997 9358143

Trost LB, Bergfeld WF, Calogeras E: The diagnosis and treatment of iron deficiency and its potential relationship to hair loss. J Am Acad Dermatol 54(5):824–844, 2006 16635664

Tsiantis J: Family reactions and relationships in thalassemia. Ann N Y Acad Sci 612:451–461, 1990 2149810

Uprety D, Baber A, Foy M: Ketamine infusion for sickle cell pain crisis refractory to opioids: a case report and review of literature. Ann Hematol 93(5):769–771, 2014 24232306

Valuck RJ, Ruscin JM: A case-control study on adverse effects: H2 blocker or proton pump inhibitor use and risk of vitamin B12 deficiency in older adults. J Clin Epidemiol 57(4):422–428, 2004 15135846

van der Zwaluw NL, Dhonukshe-Rutten RA, van Wijngaarden JP, et al: Results of 2-year vitamin B treatment on cognitive performance: secondary data from an RCT. Neurology 83(23):2158–2166, 2014 25391305

Vardaki MA, Philalithis AE, Vlachonikolis I: Factors associated with the attitudes and expectations of patients suffering from beta-thalassaemia: a cross-sectional study. Scand J Caring Sci 18(2):177–187, 2004 15147481

Vargas-Ruiz AG, Hernández-Rivera G, Herrera MF: Prevalence of iron, folate, and vitamin B12 deficiency anemia after laparoscopic Roux-en-Y gastric bypass. Obes Surg 18(3):288–293, 2008 18214631

Vichinsky EP, MacKlin EA, Waye JS, et al: Changes in the epidemiology of thalassemia in North America: a new minority disease. Pediatrics 116(6):e818–e825, 2005 16291734

Vidal X, Ibáñez L, Vendrell L, et al; Spanish-Italian Collaborative Group for the Epidemiology of Gastrointestinal Bleeding: Risk of upper gastrointestinal bleeding and the degree of serotonin reuptake inhibition by antidepressants: a case-control study. Drug Saf 31(2):159–168, 2008 18217791

von Mackensen S, Gringeri A, Siboni SM, Mannucci PM; Italian Association of Haemophilia Centres (AICE): Health-related quality of life and psychological well-being in elderly patients with haemophilia. Haemophilia 18(3):345–352, 2012 21910788

Wang HX, Wahlin A, Basun H, et al: Vitamin B(12) and folate in relation to the development of Alzheimer's disease. Neurology 56(9):1188–1194, 2001 11342684

Weinrieb RM, Auriacombe M, Lynch KG, Lewis JD: Selective serotonin re-uptake inhibitors and the risk of bleeding. Expert Opin Drug Saf 4(2):337–344, 2005 15794724

Whiskey E, Taylor D: Restarting clozapine after neutropenia: evaluating the possibilities and practicalities. CNS Drugs 21(1):25–35, 2007 17190527

Witkop M, Guelcher C, Forsyth A, et al: Treatment outcomes, quality of life, and impact of hemophilia on young adults (aged 18–30 years) with hemophilia. Am J Hematol 90 (suppl 2):S3–S10, 2015 26619194

Wolff T, Witkop CT, Miller T, Syed SB; U.S. Preventive Services Task Force: Folic acid supplementation for the prevention of neural tube defects: an update of the evidence for the U.S. Preventive Services Task Force. Ann Intern Med 150(9):632–639, 2009 19414843

Yang YM, Cepeda M, Price C, et al: Depression in children and adolescents with sickle-cell disease. Arch Pediatr Adolesc Med 148(5):457–460, 1994 8180634

Yengil E, Acipayam C, Kokacya MH, et al: Anxiety, depression and quality of life in patients with beta thalassemia major and their caregivers. Int J Clin Exp Med 7(8):2165–2172, 2014 25232402

Yoo MJ, Smith QR, Hage DS: Studies of imipramine binding to human serum albumin by high-performance affinity chromatography. J Chromatogr B Analyt Technol Biomed Life Sci 877(11–12):1149–1154, 2009 19328747

Yoshida T, Suzuki G, Nibuya M, et al: Parkinsonism induced by atypical neuroleptics in a patient with severe iron deficiency. Nihon Shinkei Seishin Yakurigaku Zasshi 24(1):29–31, 2004 15027328

Zafeiriou DI, Economou M, Athanasiou-Metaxa M: Neurological complications in beta-thalassemia. Brain Dev 28(8):477–481, 2006 16574362

CHAPTER 24

Rheumatology

James L. Levenson, M.D.
Michael R. Irwin, M.D.

Rheumatological disorders are an overlapping group of autoimmune conditions characterized by chronic inflammation involving connective tissues and organs. The various diseases are differentiated on the basis of the clinical presentation and the patterns of immune disturbance.

In this chapter we describe aspects of the rheumatological disorders relevant to a clinician working in psychosomatic medicine. We devote most of our attention to rheumatoid arthritis (RA) and systemic lupus erythematosus (SLE) because they are the most commonly seen disorders; other disorders, including osteoarthritis, Sjögren's syndrome, systemic sclerosis, temporal arteritis, polymyositis, polyarteritis nodosa, Behçet's syndrome, and granulomatosis with polyangiitis, are also discussed. Psychiatric side effects of medications used in treating rheumatological disorders are addressed as well. Fibromyalgia is covered in Chapter 25, "Chronic Fatigue and Fibromyalgia Syndromes."

Rheumatoid Arthritis

RA affects approximately 0.8% of the population (range=0.3%–2.1%), with women affected approximately three times more frequently than men. RA is a chronic disorder characterized by persistent inflammatory synovitis. Although any synovial joint can be affected, the disease typically involves peripheral small joints in a symmetrical pattern. Inflammation of the synovium can result in destruction of joint cartilage and bony erosions, which can eventually lead to destruction of the joint. Extra-articular manifestations are common, variably including systemic symptoms (e.g., anorexia, weight loss, myalgia); more localized abnormalities such as rheumatoid nodules; or cardiovascular (e.g., vasculitis, pericarditis), respiratory (e.g., pleural effusions, pulmonary fibrosis), or central nervous system (CNS) (e.g., spinal cord compression, peripheral neuropathy) involvement. The typical course of RA is prolonged, characterized by relapses and remissions. As the disease advances, progressive joint destruction results in limitations in joint movements, joint instability and deformities that increase pain, and functional disability.

The main aims of treatment of RA are 1) analgesia, 2) reduction of inflammation, 3) joint protection, 4) maintenance of functional ability, and 5) reduction of systemic manifestations. Pharmacological management of RA involves several classes of drugs:

- Nonsteroidal anti-inflammatory drugs (NSAIDs) control symptoms and signs of local inflammation, although they do not appear to alter the eventual course of the disease.
- Several drugs alter the course of the disease by reducing inflammation (e.g., methotrexate, antimalarials, minocycline, and sulfasalazine); gold and penicillamine are almost never used anymore.
- Corticosteroids can be used to reduce signs of inflammation by systemic administration (oral or parenteral) or by local injection.
- Currently available biological response modifiers include the anti–tumor necrosis factor (TNF)–alpha agents—namely, etanercept, infliximab, adalimumab, and an interleukin-1 (IL-1) receptor antagonist, anakinra.
- Immunosuppressive agents (azathioprine, leflunomide, cyclosporine, and cyclophosphamide) also reduce inflammation in RA, but because of toxicity, their use is limited to patients who do not respond to other agents.

Neuropsychiatric Disorders in Rheumatological Disease

Epidemiology of Neuropsychiatric Disorders in RA

Neuropsychiatric disorders are common in patients with rheumatological diseases, as they are in most chronic illness populations. In a cross-sectional population survey in 17 countries with more than 85,000 participating adults assessed with a structured diagnostic interview, major depressive disorder was about twice as likely to occur in persons with arthritis than in persons without arthritis (odds ratio [OR]=1.9; 95% confidence interval [CI]=1.7–2.1), with similar increased risk for dysthymia (OR=2.4; 95% CI=2.0–2.7) and anxiety disorders (OR=1.9; 95% CI=1.8–2.3) (He et al. 2008). A meta-analysis of 72 studies involving 13,189 RA patients found a prevalence of major depressive disorder of 16.8% (95% CI=10%–24%). Older age was associated with a higher prevalence of depression, and depression predicted poorer RA outcomes (Matcham et al. 2013). Another study of 22,131 RA patients found a depression prevalence of 15.2% (95% CI=14.7%–15.7%); in this study, RA symptom severity and comorbidity were found to be the best predictors of self-reported depression (Wolfe and Michaud 2009). Despite the prevalence and disability of depression, treating rheumatologists underreport depression; for example, the 12-month rate of depression reported by more than 33,000 patients enrolled in the Consortium of Rheumatology Researchers of North America was 11.7%, but a rate of only 1.0% was reported by rheumatologists (Rathbun et al. 2014).

Neuropsychiatric Manifestations in RA: Potential Etiological Factors

Neuropsychiatric manifestations in RA can arise through several processes, including direct CNS involvement, emotional reactions to chronic illness, and possibly secondary effects of the illness (e.g., the CNS effects of inflammatory cytokines).

Involvement of the CNS in RA.　Despite RA's multisystem manifestations, neurological complications are not common. The most common neurological manifestation is peripheral neuropathy. Direct CNS involvement is rare. Atlantoaxial subluxation may occur, resulting in transverse myelitis. Vasculitis in RA can involve cerebral arteries, resulting in cerebral ischemia or infarction, and has been associated with acute and chronic brain syndromes (Bougea et al. 2015). Treatment with corticosteroids usually can alleviate symptoms of vasculitis and cerebral edema, but impairment from the infarction is permanent.

Psychiatric disorders as a reaction to chronic illness.　Major life stressors, especially those involving interpersonal stress and social rejection, are among the strongest proximal risk factors for depression (Slavich and Irwin 2014). The burden of chronic physical symptoms, disability, and personal losses resulting from RA contribute to a increased risk of depression. More than 58% of RA patients experience adversity in three or more domains of socioeconomic or psychosocial functioning (e.g., work, income, required rest time during the day, leisure activity, transport mobility, housing, social dependency) (Albers et al. 1999). Chronic psychosocial and interpersonal stressors not only contribute to depression but also increase cellular and molecular markers of inflammation, which can lead to worsening of RA disease activity and further exacerbation and perpetuation of disease-related stress and depressive symptoms (Margaretten et al. 2009; Slavich and Irwin 2014). Additionally, disease activity and depression can lead to sleep disturbance, causing further impairments in health functioning with reciprocal impacts on disease progression (Nicassio et al. 2012).

Psychiatric symptoms as consequences of RA and associated inflammation. Animal models, cell culture data, and anti-inflammatory cytokine antagonist treatments provide converging evidence that dysregulation of the proinflammatory cytokine network underlies synovial inflammation in patients with RA. Indeed, proinflammatory cytokines show potent additive effects; TNF-alpha strongly induces the production of IL-1 and IL-6, which promote a cascade of processes, such as leukocyte infiltration of synovial tissue, collagenase and prostaglandin E production, and bone resorption. Such immune activation is thought to contribute to the increased prevalence of depression, fatigue, hyperalgesia, and sleep disturbance in RA patients (Slavich and Irwin 2014). Basic research on neural immune signaling has shown that peripheral proinflammatory cytokines exert potent effects on neural processes that lead to a constellation of behavior changes that have been called "sickness behaviors" (defined as a set of behavioral changes—including fatigue, malaise, depression, and hyperalgesia—considered to be an adaptive response to infectious and inflammatory diseases) (Irwin and Cole 2011). In humans, experimental immune activation is found to induce increases in depressed mood, fatigue, and hyperalgesia, especially in women (Moieni et al. 2015). These findings may have particular relevance for RA patients, because the use of medications that block peripheral proinflammatory cyto-kine activity (e.g., TNF antagonists) is associated with a lower prevalence of major de-pressive disorder and anxiety disorders independent of clinical status (Raison and Miller 2013; Uguz et al. 2009). Furthermore, biological treatments that target inflam-mation have been found to reduce disease activity and improve symptoms of fatigue in RA (Genty et al. 2017), consistent with the ability of etanercept to reduce depressive symptoms in patients with psoriasis (Tyring et al. 2006). Finally, in animal studies of sickness behaviors, novel antidepressant drugs that target the inflammatory signal-ing pathways that are activated in RA (e.g., stress-activated/mitogen-activated pro-tein kinases [SAPKs/MAPKs]) may work jointly to reverse behavioral symptoms and reduce inflammation in RA (Malemud and Miller 2008).

Psychiatric and Psychosocial Predictors of Inflammation, RA Symptoms, and Clinical Disease

Depression and Clinical State

Numerous studies have examined the associations of depression with the physical symptoms of RA. Cross-sectional studies show that self-reported depressive symp-toms are associated with the severity of the pain experienced and the degree of func-tional disability (Smedstad et al. 1996; Wolfe and Kong 1999). Prospective data con-firm that daily stressors predict the short-term course of RA disease activity, fatigue, and pain (Evers et al. 2014), and depression severity and inflammation are associated with each other and have independent effects on perceived pain in RA (Kojima et al. 2009). In turn, there is a reciprocal relationship between disease severity and depres-sive symptoms, and in more than 22,000 patients with RA followed for nearly 10 years, self-reported increases in depression were primarily predicted by symptoms of pain and fatigue (Wolfe and Michaud 2009). Despite these findings, several limitations re-quire consideration. Some of the associations observed might be due to the use of de-pression measures such as the Beck Depression Inventory (BDI), in which physical symptoms associated with the RA itself—e.g., disturbed sleep, fatigue, and loss of ap-petite—are rated as indicators of depression. Exclusion of these somatic items leaves smaller but still significant associations between depression and the physical symp-toms of RA (Peck et al. 1989). Among the few longitudinal studies that have examined the reciprocal associations between depression and changes in the severity of RA symptoms, the associations are weaker (Wolfe and Hawley 1993). Finally, the vast majority of the research performed in this area has focused on ambulatory outpa-tients, probably for a combination of ethical and convenience reasons, and the associ-ation between symptoms of RA and psychiatric symptoms may become more pro-nounced in subjects with the most severe disease (Mindham et al. 1981).

Depression may also impair the efficacy of RA treatments. In a systematic review, seven studies were identified that evaluated temporal relationships between depres-sion and RA outcomes comprising disease activity, treatment persistence, and re-sponse to therapy (Rathbun et al. 2013). Not only did depression exacerbate pain and disease activity, but depression was also associated with a decrease in the efficacy of pharmacological and some nonpharmacological (e.g., cognitive-behavioral therapy) RA treatments (Rathbun et al. 2013). For example, in 389 patients enrolled in the

COmbination of Methotrexate and ETanercept in Active Early Rheumatoid Arthritis (COMET) trial over 104 weeks, clinical remission of RA was found to reduce symptoms of depression, and conversely, depression and anxiety symptoms at baseline and over the trial suppressed the efficacy of treatment on patient-reported outcomes (Kekow et al. 2011). More recent evidence supports this conclusion; secondary analysis of clinical trial data of 379 RA patients showed that baseline and persistent symptoms of depression and anxiety were associated with poorer health outcomes over time, as well as reduced treatment response (Matcham et al. 2016). However, studies of the effectiveness of depression treatments in RA patients are limited and have demonstrated only a low to moderate level of evidence, due to risk of bias and availability of only eight trials (six pharmacological, one psychological, one both) to date (Fiest et al. 2017). Finally, it is important to note that depressed RA patients are more likely to report physical symptoms (Murphy et al. 1999), less likely to be reassured by a doctor, and less likely to take medications as directed (Julian et al. 2009), all of which contribute to the health burden and indirect costs of depression (Joyce et al. 2009).

The mechanisms by which depression influences pain and disability are poorly understood. Depression and psychological stress, as well as sleep disturbance, have all been shown to result in increases in cellular and molecular markers of inflammation, including increases in inflammatory signaling pathways such as nuclear factor kappa–B (Irwin 2015; Irwin and Opp 2017; Slavich and Irwin 2014). Furthermore, increases in the cellular production of inflammatory cytokines correlate with self-reported fatigue in RA patients, independent of pain (Davis et al. 2008). Targeting the inflammatory pathways may be an effective strategy to interrupt this feed-forward loop between depressive symptoms and disease severity, as stress-induced activation of inflammatory signaling in RA patients is blocked by treatments that antagonize production of inflammatory cytokines (e.g., TNF-alpha antagonists) (Motivala et al. 2008). Additionally, behavioral interventions that target negative affective and emotion regulation have been found to produce improvements in depression and pain outcomes, which are coupled with a downregulation of cellular production of inflammatory markers (Zautra et al. 2008). Likewise, in another controlled trial of a cognitive-behavioral therapy (CBT) intervention for patients in an early stage of RA, those receiving adjunctive CBT showed improvement in C reactive protein (but not erythrocyte sedimentation rate [ESR]) immediately after therapy, whereas those receiving the control condition did not; however, this effect was lost by 6 months (Sharpe et al. 2001). It remains unclear whether this improvement was a direct effect of the CBT on inflammatory activity or a result of behavior-mediating factors (which seems more likely), such as improved compliance with treatment, in the intensively followed-up group. Indeed, depression in patients with rheumatological disorders is a strong predictor of poor medication and treatment adherence (Julian et al. 2009).

Role of Cognitive Appraisal Mechanisms

How RA patients think about their illness is crucial to understanding the association of depression with pain and disability. Depression is associated with increased worry about illness and conviction of severe disease. Depressed RA patients perceive their illness as being more serious and feel hopeless about a cure compared with nondepressed RA patients (Murphy et al. 1999). Furthermore, depressed patients are more likely to have cognitive distortions relating to the RA (T.W. Smith et al. 1988). These associations remain significant in RA patients even after the extent of disease and pain levels are controlled, indicating that the association between depression and negative appraisals of health status is not simply the result of depressed people having more severe illness.

Other Psychosocial Factors Contributing to Psychiatric Symptoms

Several other psychosocial and behavioral factors that may predispose any RA patient to psychiatric problems have been suggested.

Neuroticism.   Negative affectivity, or *neuroticism,* is associated with increased sensitivity to physical sensations (Larsen 1992), which may contribute to depressed mood. In a prospective study of RA patients, higher scores on neuroticism predicted more chronic distress, regardless of pain intensity (Affleck et al. 1992), and neuroticism predicted anxiety and depressed mood in RA patients after 3 and 5 years, irrespective of other psychosocial and medical factors (Evers et al. 2002).

Social support.   It is recognized that social support is associated with health and good quality of life in the general population. Some studies have found that social support benefits patients with RA. In patients with RA, social support and its actual or perceived availability have been shown to be associated with use of more adaptive coping strategies (Holtzman et al. 2004), greater perception of ability to control the disease (Spitzer et al. 1995), less fatigue (Xu et al. 2017), better quality of life (Pitsilka et al. 2015), and less psychological distress (Zyrianova et al. 2006). Not all social contacts are supportive, however, and critical or punishing comments are associated with increased psychological distress (Griffin et al. 2001).

RA has an adverse effect on the availability of social support, however. Patients with RA have been shown to have reduced social networks and social support (Fyrand et al. 2001). This disruption of social support appears to be greatest in those with disease of the longest duration and with the most severe functional disability, possibly caused by a significant reduction in the availability of important others to patients with RA (Murphy et al. 1988). That may be why longitudinal studies have found that social support's benefits are short term in RA (Demange et al. 2004; Strating et al. 2006). Such subjective social isolation may drive increases in inflammation and contribute to disease activity. Among socially isolated older adults who report high levels of loneliness, the expression of inflammatory response genes increases, which is driven in part by a reduced glucocorticoid receptor sensitivity and a failure of endogenous glucocorticoids to downregulate the inflammatory response (Cole et al. 2007).

Social stresses.   Experiences of social threat and adversity upregulate components of the immune system involved in inflammation, which are thought to contribute to depression, as previously noted (Slavich and Irwin 2014). In 27 independent studies involving more than 3,000 RA patients, stress—defined as minor hassles and life events lasting hours or days—was associated with subsequent increases in disease activity (Straub et al. 2005). In addition, some studies have suggested that social stresses might play an important part in triggering the onset of RA in adults (e.g., Baker and Brewerton 1981).

Sleep disturbance.   Complaints of disturbed sleep are highly prevalent in RA patients. Clinically significant sleep disturbance (as measured by a Pittsburgh Sleep Quality Index [PSQI] score >5) is found in more than 60% of individuals with RA, with evidence of sleep-continuity disturbance, including increases in sleep-onset latency, decreases in sleep efficiency, and increases in wake after sleep onset (WASO), as characterized by polysomnography (Bjurstrom and Irwin 2016). Sleep disturbance is thought to contribute to pain, fatigue, and depressed mood in patients with RA, and several studies have shown that subjective sleep complaints correlate with fatigue, functional disability, greater joint pain, and more depressive symptoms in these patients (Moldofsky 2001). Indeed, sleep difficulties, pain, depressed mood, and fatigue appear to cluster in RA; depression is associated with greater pain, whereas sleep difficulties are associated with fatigue, depression, and pain (Drewes et al. 1998; Nicassio et al. 2002). The relation between sleep disturbance and other symptoms is complex. Sleep disturbance appears to be causally linked to increases in depressed mood and fatigue, as well as heightened pain perception, in RA patients. For example, experimental sleep loss was found to induce exaggerated increases in fatigue, depression, anxiety, and pain in RA patients compared with control subjects (Irwin et al. 2012). Furthermore, sleep loss has been shown to induce increases in disease-specific activity, as indexed by number of painful joints as well as clinician-rated joint counts (Irwin et al. 2012). Among RA patients as compared with pain-free control subjects, sleep disturbance partly mediated mechanisms of CNS pain amplification, as indexed by diminished conditioned pain modulation (Lee et al. 2013).

Both sleep disturbance and depression may be manifestations of an underlying biological disturbance such as an increase in inflammatory activity, which may alter CNS function, as noted previously. For example, sleep loss induces increases in the production of inflammatory markers (Irwin and Opp 2017; Irwin et al. 2016), which then promote pain, fatigue, and affective disturbance. In turn, elevations of proinflammatory cytokines and pain might recursively initiate further difficulties with sleep (Bjurström et al. 2017), leading to a feed-forward vicious circle with progressive deterioration in clinical outcomes. Among RA patients, inflammation is associated with heightened pain sensitivity at joints, whereas poor sleep is associated with diffuse pain sensitivity, suggesting alternative approaches to treating RA pain (Lee et al. 2009).

Given the reciprocal associations between inflammation and sleep disturbance, the ability of cytokine antagonists to improve sleep in RA patients has been examined. In a prospective observational study of RA patients with poor sleep quality, initiation of anti-TNF-alpha therapy led to improvements in sleep efficiency and WASO (Taylor-Gjevre et al. 2011). Other studies have found evidence that anti-TNF-alpha therapy induces acute (within hours) improvement in sleep, as measured by polysomnography (Zamarrón et al. 2004), and that the effects of anti-TNF-alpha therapy on sleep may be more robust in RA patients with high disease activity (Karatas et al. 2017). Likewise, administration of the IL-6 receptor antagonist tocilizumab led to improvements in sleep quality and daytime sleepiness, which were maintained at the 6-month follow-up and were independent of improvements in RA-specific disease activity (Fragiadaki et al. 2012). Such improvements in sleep, along with physical activity, may also mediate improvements in fatigue (Katz et al. 2016).

Osteoarthritis

Osteoarthritis (OA) is the most common joint disease, with the idiopathic form being the most prevalent. Secondary OA arises most frequently as the result of trauma (acute or chronic), although it also may occur in a variety of metabolic and endocrine disorders. The prevalence of OA increases sharply with age: fewer than 2% of women younger than 45 years are affected, compared with 30% of those between 45 and 64 years of age and 68% of those older than 65 years.

A wide variety of mental disorders are associated with an increased risk of OA (Huang et al. 2016). The prevalence of depression is significantly increased in patients with OA (Stubbs et al. 2016), and there is a bidirectional relationship between depression and OA pain, in part mediated by sleep disturbance (Parmelee et al. 2015). Depression in OA patients leads to greater activity limitations, poorer quality of life, and increased health care utilization (Agarwal and Sambamoorthi 2015).

Few intervention studies have examined the efficacy of antidepressants and psychological therapies in OA. Those that have been performed suggest that both antidepressants and CBT are efficacious in the treatment of depression and that improvement of depression is associated with reduced pain and disability from the disease (Lin 2008). There is also a potential role for antidepressants with analgesic effects. Duloxetine (60–120 mg/day) has been shown to be efficacious for knee pain in OA patients in several randomized, placebo-controlled trials (e.g., Micca et al. 2013). CBT for insomnia has also been shown to improve pain in OA in randomized controlled trials (e.g., M.T. Smith et al. 2015).

Systemic Lupus Erythematosus

SLE is an autoimmune disorder of unknown cause characterized by immune dysregulation with tissue damage caused by pathogenic autoantibodies, immune complexes, and T lymphocytes. Approximately 90% of cases are in women, usually of childbearing age. The average incidence is 5.5 cases per 100,000 population, and the prevalence 73 cases per 100,000 population, but rates are much higher in blacks and other ethnic groups compared with whites. The highest reported prevalence rates in the world have been in Alaska and Puerto Rico. Nonwhite patients have more severe disease and higher mortality than whites (Lewis and Jawad 2017). Asian people are also more often affected than white people. At onset, SLE may involve one or multiple organ systems. Common clinical manifestations include cutaneous lesions (e.g., photosensitivity, malar or discoid rash, oral ulcers), constitutional symptoms (e.g., fatigue, weight loss, fevers), arthralgias and frank arthritis, serositis (e.g., pericarditis or pleuritis), renal disease, neuropsychiatric disorders, and hematological disorders (e.g., anemia, leukopenia). Autoantibodies are detectable at presentation in most cases.

The spectrum of treatment options in SLE is similar to that in RA—namely, NSAIDs, antimalarials (e.g., hydroxychloroquine), corticosteroids, and other immunosuppressants (e.g., azathioprine, mycophenolate mofetil, methotrexate, cyclophosphamide). In addition, anticoagulants are used in SLE patients who have antiphospholipid antibodies if the patients have a history of arterial or venous thrombosis.

Neuropsychiatric Manifestations in Systemic Lupus Erythematosus

Neuropsychiatric symptoms of SLE were first reported in 1872 by Kaposi (1872). Depending on the diagnostic methodology used, neuropsychiatric manifestations—ranging from stroke, seizures, headaches, neuropathy, transverse myelitis, and movement disorders to cognitive deficits, depression, mania, anxiety, psychosis, and delirium—have been reported in 22%–95% of SLE patients, although rates were lower (13%–38%) in more systematic observations (Tay and Mak 2016). CNS involvement is a major cause of morbidity in SLE and is second only to renal failure as a cause of death. The pathogenesis of neuropsychiatric syndromes in SLE is complex. (For a more detailed review of psychiatric aspects of SLE, readers are referred to Cohen et al. [2004].)

Pathogenesis of Neuropsychiatric Syndromes in SLE

Psychiatric syndromes in SLE can be caused by 1) direct CNS involvement; 2) infection, other systemic illness, or drug-induced side effects; 3) reaction to chronic illness; or 4) comorbid primary psychiatric illness.

Direct pathophysiological CNS effects. Two major antibody-mediated mechanisms of CNS injury have been proposed: neuronal injury and microvasculopathy (Scolding and Joseph 2002). Autoantibodies may directly damage neurons by either causing cell death or transiently and reversibly impairing neuronal function. Microvascular endothelial injury in the CNS may increase the permeability of the blood–brain barrier, leading to influx of autoantibodies and further CNS damage. Autoimmune antibodies seem to play a much larger role in direct CNS involvement than does immune complex deposition. Antiribosomal P protein antibodies, antineuronal antibodies, anti–N-methyl-D-aspartate (NMDA) receptor antibodies, and other antibodies have been associated with psychosis and severe depression, but not consistently. None of these have proven causal relationships. In contrast, antiphospholipid antibodies (e.g., anticardiolipin) have been demonstrated to cause focal deficits (strokes) and cognitive dysfunction (Coín et al. 2015). Cytokines also appear to be involved in the pathogenesis of neuropsychiatric SLE, although their role remains unclear.

With the possible exception of cognitive dysfunction, all of the major psychiatric manifestations of SLE (i.e., psychosis, depression, mania, anxiety, and delirium) show a degree of reversibility, as does coma. Even the cognitive deficits sometimes respond to corticosteroids (Denburg et al. 1994; Hanly et al. 1997). Because these psychiatric syndromes tend to resolve within 2–3 weeks with corticosteroid treatment (Denburg et al. 1994), they are probably caused by reversible or transient mechanisms rather than irreversible neuronal death. The reversibility of psychiatric dysfunction in SLE stands in contrast to most focal neurological events, which often have no more reversibility than atherosclerotic stroke and are associated with fixed lesions on neuroimaging. Similarly, in some individuals, the progressive nature of the cognitive impairment (Hanly et al. 1997), often with cerebral atrophy, suggests cumulative irreversible CNS damage.

Risk factors for direct CNS involvement in SLE include cutaneous vasculitis and antiphospholipid syndrome and its associated vasculopathy. Patients with mainly articular manifestations or discoid rash have a much lower risk of neuropsychiatric lupus, as do those few who are antinuclear antibody (ANA)–negative and those with drug-induced SLE. Antiphospholipid antibodies may be the single strongest marker of CNS risk because they are associated with stroke, cognitive dysfunction, and epilepsy (Coín et al. 2015).

Psychological effects of coping with SLE.   Coping with SLE is particularly challenging because lupus is a chronic, often debilitating multisystem illness, and its course is unpredictable. Because SLE can involve almost any organ system or include vague systemic symptoms, the diagnosis can be elusive. The inability to make a diagnosis may erode the patient's confidence in the medical system, and when no etiology can be found, the physician may deem the illness psychogenic. Given that SLE can affect many organ systems, patients may worry that the illness pervades their entire body, even when the disease is limited. The diffuse nature of SLE distinguishes it from most other chronic, recurrent diseases, such as asthma or inflammatory bowel disease, which are primarily limited to one organ. SLE patients are often under the care of an entourage of specialists, which may fragment care. One of the most stressful aspects of SLE is its unpredictable course, with sudden exacerbations, remissions, and variable prognoses, resulting in a profound loss of control, as well as a loss of ability to plan for the future.

Psychological reactions to having SLE are common and include grief, depression, anxiety, regression, denial, and invalidism. A feeling of isolation is reinforced by public ignorance about lupus. People with SLE may become socially withdrawn, especially if they are self-conscious about their appearance. Women with a malar rash or discoid lesions may feel branded, as if by the "scarlet letter." The most prevalent fears among SLE patients are worsening disease, disability, and death. In particular, patients fear cognitive impairment, stroke, renal failure, and becoming a burden on their families.

Stress and SLE.   Although stress may cause a lupus flare, it is also likely, if not inevitable, that lupus flares cause stress. Several studies have provided support for stress-induced immune dysregulation in SLE (for a review, see Cohen et al. 2004). A study in Japanese women found that daily psychological stress was associated with almost twice the risk of developing SLE (Takahashi et al. 2014). Daily stress also has been associated with worsening of SLE symptoms (Peralta-Ramírez et al. 2004) and with cognitive dysfunction (Peralta-Ramírez et al. 2006). Stress, insomnia, and less effective coping are intertwined in SLE patients (Palagini et al. 2016).

Whether stress precipitates onset or exacerbation of SLE symptoms has received relatively little study. One controlled study has reported that 20 patients hospitalized for SLE had significantly greater stress prior to the onset of their illness than did the seriously ill hospitalized control subjects (Otto and Mackay 1967). A prospective case–control study found that baseline stress predicted higher SLE disease activity at 4–5 months' follow-up (Jung et al. 2015).

Classification of Neuropsychiatric Disorders in SLE

The literature on neuropsychiatric SLE has been plagued by terminology that has been imprecise and unstandardized. Terms such as *lupus cerebritis* have obfuscated our understanding because they imply a pathogenesis (inflammation) that remains unproven. Furthermore, because there is no gold standard for the diagnosis of neuro-psychiatric SLE, ascertaining which conditions are direct CNS manifestations of SLE and which are a reaction to illness or a co-occurring disorder has been controversial. To rectify these problems, the American College of Rheumatology (ACR) developed a standardized nomenclature and classification defining 19 different neuropsychiat-ric SLE syndromes (12 involving the brain) (American College of Rheumatology Ad Hoc Committee on Neuropsychiatric Lupus Nomenclature 1999). The guidelines de-fined neuropsychiatric lupus as "the neurological syndromes of the central, periph-eral, and autonomic nervous systems, and the psychiatric syndromes observed in pa-tients with SLE in which other causes have been excluded." Psychiatric disorders included psychosis, acute confusional state, cognitive dysfunction, anxiety disorder, and mood disorders.

The ACR criteria significantly broadened the spectrum of syndromes that can be considered neuropsychiatric SLE. A meta-analysis of studies examining the preva-lence of ACR neuropsychiatric SLE syndromes calculated an overall prevalence of 56.3% (95% CI=42.5%–74.7%); neuropsychiatric syndromes with the highest preva-lence were headache, with a prevalence of 28.3%; mood disorders, 20.7%; cognitive dysfunction, 19.7%; seizures, 9.9%; and cerebrovascular disease, 8.0% (Unterman et al. 2011). The ACR criteria have good sensitivity but low specificity, which makes them better suited for identifying all possible cases of neuropsychiatric SLE than for arriving at a specific valid diagnosis. A large international collaborative cohort study in 572 patients who were newly diagnosed with SLE reported that whereas 28% of pa-tients experienced at least one ACR-defined neuropsychiatric event around the time of diagnosis, only a minority of those events were attributable to SLE (Hanly et al. 2007).

A more fundamental problem with the ACR classification system is that it is diffi-cult to apply clinically. To diagnose neuropsychiatric SLE as the cause of the psychi-atric symptoms, one must exclude a primary psychiatric disorder. By contrast, in DSM-5 (American Psychiatric Association 2013), a primary psychiatric disorder can-not be diagnosed unless medical disorders and substance use are ruled out as etiolo-gies. Whereas medical disorders and substance use can be easily excluded, no clinical criteria or laboratory tests are available for excluding all primary psychiatric disor-ders. For example, if a patient with SLE becomes depressed, it is unclear how one would rule out primary depression as the cause.

Prevalence of Neuropsychiatric Disorders in SLE

Estimates of the prevalence of neuropsychiatric disorders in SLE have ranged widely, reflecting differences in terminology, methods, and subjects. A systematic review of 13 studies of psychiatric disorders in SLE found a high frequency of psychiatric co-morbidities, especially mood and anxiety disorders, although there was no consensus regarding the relationship between SLE disease activity and psychiatric disorders. However, patients with active SLE showed a higher risk of developing mood disor-ders than did patients with inactive SLE (Asano et al. 2013). Other studies have found that psychiatric symptoms have no correlation with active disease or with history of psychosis and/or seizures attributable to SLE (Beltrão et al. 2013). Among youth (ages 10–18 years) with SLE, a somewhat lower prevalence of psychiatric diagnoses was found. Diagnoses of depression were present for 19%, anxiety for 7%, acute stress/adjustment for 6%, and other psychiatric disorders for 18%. Interestingly, African Americans were less likely than whites to be diagnosed with depression (OR= 0.56; 95% CI=0.34–0.90) or anxiety (OR=0.49; 95% CI=0.25–0.98), or to be prescribed anxiolytics (OR=0.23; 95% CI=0.11–0.48), findings that might be due to potential racial/ethnic disparities in care (Knight et al. 2016).

Cognitive dysfunction is the most common neuropsychiatric disorder in patients with SLE, with a prevalence estimated at 80% in one systematic review (Meszaros et al. 2012). In a study of 53 pediatric patients with SLE, all (100%) reported symptoms of cognitive dysfunction, with 75% of these patients having psychotic features (Lim et al. 2013). On neuropsychological testing, even patients who have never had overt neuropsychiatric symptoms are often found to have cognitive impairment. Patients with anticardiolipin antibodies have a three- to fourfold increased risk of cognitive impairment, which is often progressive (Hanly et al. 1997). Although cognitive dysfunction often fluctuates and may be reversible (Hanly et al. 1997), presumably when attributable to edema and inflammation, it is irreversible when secondary to multiple infarcts and may culminate in dementia.

Depression is the second most common neuropsychiatric disorder in SLE. Reported prevalences of depression have varied widely, depending on the diagnostic criteria, patient population, and study design. A recent meta-analysis of 59 studies estimated that depression (as assessed with Hospital Anxiety and Depression Scale scores) was present in 30% of patients with SLE (Zhang et al. 2017), similar to the 39% prevalence reported in an earlier systematic review (Meszaros et al. 2012). Depression may be a preexisting primary psychiatric disorder; an iatrogenically induced illness, particularly from corticosteroids; a reaction to having a chronic disease; or, possibly, a direct CNS manifestation of lupus. The question of whether depression is a direct manifestation of CNS SLE or a reaction to the stress and multiple losses associated with having a chronic, debilitating illness remains unresolved (for a discussion of the complexities involved in this question, see Cohen et al. [2004]). Diagnosing depression in SLE is difficult because of the overlap between depressive symptoms and symptoms associated with SLE or its treatment. Hypothyroidism should be ruled out, because it can mimic depression and is more common in SLE patients than in the general population.

Anxiety is quite common in SLE patients, often as a reaction to the illness. In the previously mentioned meta-analysis of 59 studies, the estimated prevalence of anxiety (as assessed in clinical interviews) was 37% (Zhang et al. 2017). The question of whether anxiety is attributable to direct CNS involvement in SLE or is a reaction to chronic illness remains controversial, as with depression.

In patients with SLE, the most common cause of mania is corticosteroid therapy. Psychosis in SLE patients can be a manifestation of direct CNS involvement, and in some but not all studies, it has been linked to antiribosomal P protein antibodies. Distinguishing psychosis caused by CNS lupus from corticosteroid-induced psychosis presents a major diagnostic challenge (see section titled "Corticosteroid-Induced Psychiatric Symptoms" below). Delirium, referred to as "acute confusional state" in the ACR criteria, is common in severe SLE and is a result of CNS lupus, medication, or other medical disorders, as shown in Table 24–1. Personality changes have been reported in SLE patients whose disease has damaged the frontal or temporal lobes, and symptoms are consistent with those resulting from pathology in those brain regions.

TABLE 24–1. Secondary medical and psychiatric causes of neuropsychiatric symptoms in systemic lupus erythematosus and other rheumatological disorders

CNS infections

Systemic infections

Renal failure (e.g., due to lupus nephritis or vasculitis involving the renal artery)

Fluid or electrolyte disturbance

Hypertensive encephalopathy

Hypoxemia

Fever

CNS tumor (e.g., cerebral lymphoma because of immunosuppression)

Medication side effects (see Tables 24–2 and 24–3)

Comorbid medical illness

Psychiatric symptoms in reaction to illness

Comorbid psychiatric illness

Note.   CNS=central nervous system.

Laboratory Detection of CNS Disease Activity in Systemic Lupus Erythematosus

Virtually all patients with SLE have positive ANA titers, but the ANA titer is not specific. In a patient known to have lupus who develops neuropsychiatric symptoms, serum ANA titers need not be obtained, because they do not seem to correlate with CNS lupus activity. Testing for antiphospholipid antibodies (including lupus anticoagulant and anticardiolipin) is important, particularly in patients with focal symptoms, because the results may determine treatment and prognosis (Levine et al. 2002). Patients with antiphospholipid syndrome are treated primarily with anticoagulation rather than corticosteroid or cytotoxic therapy. As noted earlier, antiribosomal P protein antibodies, antineuronal antibodies, and other specific antibodies have been linked to psychosis and/or depression, but their usefulness for diagnosis of SLE is limited by their low positive predictive value (Arnett et al. 1996; Gerli et al. 2002).

Corticosteroid-Induced Psychiatric Symptoms in Systemic Lupus Erythematosus

Corticosteroids have been shown to cause a variety of psychiatric syndromes. In a prospective study of 135 patients treated with corticosteroids for a flare-up of SLE not involving the CNS, 20 new-onset psychiatric episodes occurred, 14 (70%) of which met the strict definition for a corticosteroid-induced psychiatric disorder (including 13 mood episodes [depressive in 2, manic in 9, and mixed in 2] and 1 psychotic episode) (Nishimura et al. 2014). Nevertheless, distinguishing corticosteroid-induced psychiatric reactions from flares of CNS lupus is one of the most challenging aspects of treating SLE. Helpful distinguishing features are summarized in Table 24–2 (Kohen et al. 1993). Given the risk of untreated CNS lupus and the likelihood that corticosteroids will alleviate such flares and only temporarily exacerbate corticosteroid-induced psychiatric reactions, an empirical initiation or increase of corticosteroids is often the most prudent intervention when the etiology is uncertain. (Corticosteroid-induced psychiatric reactions are discussed later in this chapter in the section "Secondary Causes of Neuropsychiatric Symptoms in Rheumatological Disorders.")

Differential Diagnosis of Neuropsychiatric Disorders in Systemic Lupus Erythematosus

Other Medical Disorders

A wide variety of diseases can mimic neuropsychiatric SLE. One group of diseases, associated with a medium to high ANA titer (>1:160), includes Sjögren's syndrome and mixed or undifferentiated connective tissue disease. A second group of diseases, associated with a low ANA titer (<1:160), includes multiple sclerosis and, less commonly, ANA-positive RA, sarcoidosis, and hepatitis C. A third group of diseases, characterized by a negative ANA, also may be mistaken for CNS lupus. This group includes polyarteritis nodosa, microscopic angiitis, Wegener's granulomatosis, chronic fatigue syndrome, fibromyalgia, temporal arteritis, and Behçet's syndrome.

Psychotropic Drug–Induced Lupus

Patients who are receiving antipsychotic drugs, particularly chlorpromazine, may have positive ANA tests and antiphospholipid antibodies; most of these patients do not develop signs of an autoantibody-associated disease. Compared with other (non-psychiatric) drugs known to cause a symptomatic lupus-like syndrome, chlorpromazine and carbamazepine carry low risk, and several other psychotropics (divalproex, other anticonvulsants, and lithium) have very low risk. CNS involvement is usually absent in drug-induced lupus. Laboratory findings may include mild cytopenia and elevated ESR and ANA titers. Antihistone antibodies are positive in up to 95% but are not pathognomonic of drug-induced lupus. After discontinuation of the drug, symptoms and antibody titers decline, usually over a period of weeks; however, the recovery can be relatively slow and may require a year (Vedove et al. 2009).

Somatic Symptom Disorder ("Psychogenic Pseudolupus")

SLE can be misdiagnosed in "somatizing" patients with multisystem complaints and mildly positive ANA tests, which are common in young women.

Factitious SLE

Factitious SLE appears to be rare, but several cases have been reported (Tlacuilo-Parra et al. 2000). Patients have simulated hematuria by pricking a finger surreptitiously to add trace amounts of blood to urine specimens, injected themselves with feces or other contaminants to cause infections, or applied rouge to their cheeks to simulate a malar rash. One patient feigned proteinuria by inserting a packet of protein into her bladder. These patients had no serological evidence of an autoimmune disorder.

Sjögren's Syndrome

Sjögren's syndrome is characterized by lymphocytic infiltration of the exocrine glands. It can occur alone or in association with another autoimmune rheumatic dis-

TABLE 24–2. Differentiation of CNS lupus flares from corticosteroid-induced psychiatric reactions

	Active primary CNS lupus	Corticosteroid-induced psychiatric reaction
Onset	After decrease in corticosteroid dosage or during ongoing low-dose treatment	Generally <2 weeks after increase in corticosteroid dosage (~90% within 6 weeks)
Corticosteroid dosage	Variable	Rare if <40 mg/day, common if >60 mg/day
Psychiatric symptoms	Psychosis, delirium>mood disorders, cognitive impairment (new onset)	Mania, mixed states, or depression (often with psychotic features)>delirium, psychosis
SLE symptoms	Often present; may coincide with onset of psychiatric symptoms	Often present but precede onset of psychiatric symptoms
Laboratory tests	Increases in indices of inflammation	No specific laboratory findings
Response to corticosteroids	Improvement	Exacerbation of symptoms
Response to decreased corticosteroid dosage	Exacerbation	Improvement

Note. CNS=central nervous system; SLE=systemic lupus erythematosus.

ease. The most common symptoms result from drying of the eyes, mouth, and upper respiratory and urogenital tracts, but systemic manifestations can occur in up to one-third of patients. Although Sjögren's syndrome may be difficult to distinguish from CNS SLE (and the two syndromes may overlap), establishing a specific diagnosis is less crucial clinically because the treatment is very similar.

CNS involvement has been reported in 9%–44% of cases of primary Sjögren's syndrome (Bougea et al. 2015). Unlike SLE, CNS involvement is not correlated with titers of autoantibodies (Bougea et al. 2015). The nature of CNS involvement can be focal (e.g., cerebellar ataxia, vertigo, ophthalmoplegia, cranial nerve involvement) or diffuse (e.g., encephalopathy, aseptic meningoencephalitis, dementia, or psychiatric manifestations). Case reports and series most often describe depression, fatigue, diffuse pain, and (rarely) psychosis (Wong et al. 2014). Cognitive symptoms are common but appear to be partly related to depression (Epstein et al. 2014). Patients' depression, worry, and subjective physical complaints—but not objective measures of systemic Sjögren's syndrome activity—are strong predictors of health-related quality of life (Cornec et al. 2017; Kotsis et al. 2014).

Systemic Sclerosis (Scleroderma)

Systemic sclerosis is characterized by thickening of the skin as a result of the accumulation of fibrotic connective tissue and damage to the microvasculature. Multiple body systems can be involved, including the gastrointestinal tract, heart, lungs, and kidneys. CNS involvement in systemic sclerosis is rare, and most neurological complications are peripheral neuropathies.

Psychiatric symptoms are common, with between one-third and two-thirds of patients reporting symptoms of depression (Thombs et al. 2007). Anxiety, fatigue, sleep disruption, pain, pruritus, body image dissatisfaction, and sexual dysfunction are also common (Kwakkenbos et al. 2015). As in many other chronic diseases, impaired psychological functioning is associated with poorer health-related quality of life (Hyphantis et al. 2007).

No known treatment is available to prevent progression of scleroderma (although some medications alleviate symptoms), and the prognosis can be poor because of renal failure and pulmonary hypertension.

Temporal (Giant Cell) Arteritis

Temporal (giant cell) arteritis, a granulomatous arteritis, predominantly affects those older than 60 years. Most of the clinical features arise because of involvement of the carotid artery and its branches. Extradural arteries are most commonly involved, leading to the typical clinical picture of headache, superficial pain, or sensitivity in skin overlying inflamed vessels (e.g., pain on combing hair). Pain overlying the temporal artery with loss of pulsations is characteristic. Pain in the face, mouth, and jaw may occur, the latter worse on eating. Visual problems occur in 25% of untreated patients, and can result in blindness. In 50% of patients, pain and tenderness occur in the proximal limb muscles without affecting joints, which constitutes the diagnosis of polymyalgia rheumatica. Systemic features such as weight loss and malaise can occur. Such patients may be given the misdiagnosis of fibromyalgia, but onset later in life and an elevated ESR point to polymyalgia rheumatica.

Neuropsychiatric manifestations of temporal arteritis arise because of involvement of arteries supplying blood to the CNS. The insults to the CNS in temporal arteritis can be ischemic or hemorrhagic. Clinical presentation depends on the nature and extent of the brain areas affected. Impairments can be focal (e.g., stroke leading to specific motor or sensory deficits) or diffuse, resulting in impairment of consciousness. Visual hallucinations (Charles Bonnet syndrome) are a sign of optic ischemia, and if not quickly treated progress to permanent visual loss. Most psychiatric symptoms in patients with temporal arteritis are a result of corticosteroid therapy. Treatment with high-dose corticosteroids should commence as soon as the diagnosis has been made on clinical grounds, before results of arterial biopsy are available, to prevent disease progression (Buttgereit et al. 2016).

Polymyositis

Polymyositis is a disease of inflammation of muscles. Dermatomyositis is a related condition that includes inflammation of the skin. The disease can occur on its own or as part of other rheumatological diseases. The clinical picture is typically that of symmetrical, proximal muscle weakness. Involvement of the heart (arrhythmias, cardiac failure), gastrointestinal tract (dysphagia, reflux, constipation), and respiratory muscles (breathlessness and respiratory failure) can occur. Vasculitis can occur, rarely affecting the CNS and resulting in neuropsychiatric manifestations, including seizures, cognitive dysfunction, and depression. As with SLE and temporal arteritis, the clinical features of neuropsychiatric involvement secondary to vasculitis depend on the site and extent of the vasculitic lesions. In 20% of patients, an underlying malignancy is present (most commonly, bronchus, breast, stomach, or ovary). Thus, neuropsychiatric manifestations also may occur as the result of secondary spread of malignancy to the CNS.

Polyarteritis Nodosa

Polyarteritis nodosa is a necrotizing arteritis affecting small and medium-sized vessels, often related to hepatitis B virus infection, typically presenting with systemic symptoms (e.g., fatigue, fever, arthralgias) and signs of multisystem involvement (e.g., hypertension, renal insufficiency, neurological dysfunction, abdominal pain). Asymmetric polyneuropathy is common. CNS involvement can include small cerebral infarcts, intracranial aneurysms, and intracranial hemorrhage. There have been case reports of psychosis in polyarteritis nodosa with cerebral vasculitis (e.g., Kohlhaas et al. 2007).

Behçet's Syndrome

Behçet's syndrome is an idiopathic inflammatory disorder occurring primarily in Asia, with the highest incidence in Turkey. In Europe, most cases are in Turkish immigrants. The most common symptoms include oral and genital ulcers, uveitis, and skin lesions. Neuropsychiatric involvement is common, including meningoencephalitis, brain stem syndromes, and vascular thrombosis. Depression is very common, and personality changes and psychosis have been reported (de Oliveira Ribeiro et al. 2014; Talarico et al. 2015). Cognitive dysfunction has been found in patients with Behçet's syndrome without overt neurological involvement (de Oliveira Ribeiro et al. 2014). Acute neuropsychiatric symptoms respond to corticosteroids, but chronic progressive CNS disease does not.

Granulomatosis With Polyangiitis (Wegener's Granulomatosis)

Granulomatosis with polyangiitis is characterized by a granulomatous vasculitis, predominantly affecting the upper and lower respiratory tracts together with glomerulonephritis. Necrotizing vasculitis is its hallmark, involving both small arteries and veins. Any organ in the body can be involved. CNS involvement has included chronic meningitis, hemorrhage, and mass lesions (Huang et al. 2015). Depression has been reported in 22% of patients (Hajj-Ali et al. 2011).

Secondary Causes of Neuropsychiatric Symptoms in Rheumatological Disorders

Infection, Other CNS or Systemic Illness, and Drug-Induced Side Effects

Neuropsychiatric symptoms are often secondary to complications of the rheumatological disorder or its treatment, especially infection. Because some rheumatological disorders or their treatments can be associated with immunosuppression, these disorders predispose individuals to CNS and systemic infections. CNS infections can mimic CNS involvement by the primary disease (e.g., neuropsychiatric lupus). Infections that can cause secondary neuropsychiatric complications include cryptococcal, tubercular, and meningococcal infections and *Listeria* meningitis; herpes encephalitis; neurosyphilis; CNS nocardiosis; toxoplasmosis; brain abscesses; and progressive multifocal leukoencephalopathy (see also Chapter 26, "Infectious Diseases"). Other causes of neuropsychiatric manifestations in rheumatological disorders include uremia, hypertensive encephalopathy, CNS lymphoma, and medication side effects, as well as comorbid medical or psychiatric disorders and psychological reactions to illness (see Tables 24–1 and 24–3).

Corticosteroid-Induced Psychiatric Syndromes

Corticosteroids have psychiatric adverse effects, including mania, depression, mixed states, psychosis, anxiety, insomnia, and delirium. A previous psychiatric reaction to corticosteroids does not necessarily predict recurrent reactions with subsequent ste-

Table 24–3. **Psychiatric side effects of medications used in treating rheumatological disorders**

Medication	Psychiatric side effect(s)
Abatacept	None reported
Adalimumab	None reported
Azathioprine	Delirium
Belimumab	None reported
Corticosteroids	Mood lability, euphoria, irritability, anxiety, insomnia, mania, depression, psychosis, delirium, cognitive disturbance
Cyclophosphamide	Delirium (at high doses) (rare)
Cyclosporine	Anxiety, delirium, visual hallucinations
Etanercept	None reported
Gold	None reported
Hydroxychloroquine	Confusion, psychosis, mania, depression, nightmares, anxiety, aggression, delirium
Immunoglobulin (intravenous)	Delirium, agitation
Infliximab	None reported
Leflunomide	Anxiety
LJP 394[a]	None reported
Methotrexate	Delirium (at high doses) (rare)
Mycophenolate mofetil	Anxiety, depression, sedation (all rare)
NSAIDs (high dose)	Depression, anxiety, paranoia, hallucinations, reduced concentration, hostility, confusion, delirium
Penicillamine	None reported
Rituximab	None reported
Sulfasalazine	Insomnia, depression, hallucinations
Tacrolimus	Anxiety, delirium, insomnia, restlessness
Tocilizumab	None reported
Tofacitinib	None reported

Note. NSAIDs=nonsteroidal anti-inflammatory drugs.
[a]B-cell tolerogen–anti-double-stranded deoxyribonucleic acid (DNA) antibodies.

roids. Mild psychiatric side effects include insomnia, hyperexcitability, mood lability, mild euphoria, irritability, anxiety, agitation, and racing thoughts. Mood disorders, including depression and mania, are the most common psychiatric reaction to corticosteroids. Patients may experience both mania and depression during a single course of corticosteroid therapy. Affective symptoms are often accompanied by psychotic symptoms. The psychiatric symptoms induced by corticosteroids most often resemble those of bipolar disorder, with manic symptoms most often encountered with high-dose, short-term administration and depression most often seen with chronic therapy. Delirium and psychosis (without mood symptoms) are less common. Cognitive dysfunction also has been reported. The most common symptoms in children are agitation and sleep disturbances (Tavassoli et al. 2008).

The incidence of corticosteroid-induced psychiatric symptoms is dose related: 1.3% in patients receiving less than 40 mg/day of prednisone, 4.6% in those receiving 41–80 mg/day, and 18.4% in those receiving greater than 80 mg/day (Boston Collaborative Drug Surveillance Program 1972). For most patients, the onset of psychiatric symptoms is within the first 2 weeks (and in 90%, within the first 6 weeks) of initiating or increasing corticosteroid treatment.

The preferred treatment for corticosteroid-induced psychiatric reactions is tapering of corticosteroids, if possible, resulting in a greater than 90% response rate. However, rapid tapering or discontinuation of corticosteroids also can induce psychiatric reactions by precipitating a flare of the rheumatological disease, iatrogenic adrenal insufficiency, or possibly corticosteroid withdrawal syndrome. Corticosteroid withdrawal syndrome is manifested by headache, fever, myalgias, arthralgias, weakness, anorexia, nausea, weight loss, and orthostatic hypotension, and sometimes depression, anxiety, agitation, or psychosis (Margolin et al. 2007). Symptoms respond to an increase or a resumption of corticosteroid dosage. Adjunctive treatment with antipsychotics, antidepressants, and mood stabilizers can be helpful, depending on the particular psychiatric symptom constellation, but clinical trials are lacking.

Other drugs used in treating rheumatological disorders may cause psychiatric side effects, especially hydroxychloroquine (see Table 24–3).

Conclusion

Rheumatological disorders include an overlapping group of autoimmune conditions characterized by chronic inflammation. Neuropsychiatric disorders, particularly depression, are common in patients with rheumatological diseases, as they are in most chronic illnesses. Depression is both a consequence and a cause of greater physical symptoms and poorer health-related quality of life. Neuropsychiatric manifestations can arise through several pathways, including direct CNS involvement, emotional reactions to chronic illness, secondary effects of inflammation, and side effects of treatment, particularly corticosteroids.

References

Affleck G, Tennen H, Urrows S, et al: Neuroticism and the pain-mood relation in rheumatoid arthritis: insights from a prospective daily study. J Consult Clin Psychol 60(1):119–126, 1992 1556274

Agarwal P, Sambamoorthi U: Healthcare expenditures associated with depression among individuals with osteoarthritis: post-regression linear decomposition approach. J Gen Intern Med 30(12):1803–1811, 2015 25990191

Albers JM, Kuper HH, van Riel PL, et al: Socio-economic consequences of rheumatoid arthritis in the first years of the disease. Rheumatology (Oxford) 38(5):423–430, 1999 10371280

American College of Rheumatology Ad Hoc Committee on Neuropsychiatric Lupus Nomenclature: The American College of Rheumatology nomenclature and case definitions for neuropsychiatric lupus syndromes. Arthritis Rheum 42(4):599–608, 1999 10211873

American Psychiatric Association: Diagnostic and Statistical Manual of Mental Disorders, 5th Edition. Arlington, VA, American Psychiatric Association, 2013

Arnett FC, Reveille JD, Moutsopoulos HM, et al: Ribosomal P autoantibodies in systemic lupus erythematosus. Frequencies in different ethnic groups and clinical and immunogenetic associations. Arthritis Rheum 39(11):1833–1839, 1996 8912505

Asano NM, Coriolano MD, Asano BJ, et al: Psychiatric comorbidities in patients with systemic lupus erythematosus: a systematic review of the last 10 years. Rev Bras Reumatol 53(5):431–437, 2013 24316900

Baker GHB, Brewerton DA: Rheumatoid arthritis: a psychiatric assessment. Br Med J (Clin Res Ed) 282(6281):2014, 1981 6788174

Beltrão SM, Gigante LB, Zimmer DB, et al: Psychiatric symptoms in patients with systemic lupus erythematosus: frequency and association with disease activity using the Adult Psychiatric Morbidity Questionnaire. Rev Bras Reumatol 53(4):328–334, 2013 24217663

Bjurstrom MF, Irwin MR: Polysomnographic characteristics in nonmalignant chronic pain populations: a review of controlled studies. Sleep Med Rev 26:74–86, 2016 26140866

Bjurström MF, Olmstead R, Irwin MR: Reciprocal relationship between sleep macrostructure and evening and morning cellular inflammation in rheumatoid arthritis. Psychosom Med 79(1):24–33, 2017 27428854

Boston Collaborative Drug Surveillance Program: Acute adverse reactions to prednisone in relation to dosage. Clin Pharmacol Ther 13(5):694–698, 1972 5053810

Bougea A, Anagnostou E, Konstantinos G, et al: A systematic review of peripheral and central nervous system involvement of rheumatoid arthritis, systemic lupus erythematosus, primary Sjögren's syndrome, and associated immunological profiles. Int J Chronic Dis 2015:910352, 2015 26688829

Buttgereit F, Dejaco C, Matteson EL, et al: Polymyalgia rheumatica and giant cell arteritis: a systematic review. JAMA 315(22):2442–2458, 2016 27299619

Cohen W, Roberts WN, Levenson JL: Psychiatric aspects of SLE, in Systemic Lupus Erythematosus. Edited by Lahita R. San Diego, CA, Elsevier, 2004, pp 785–825

Coín MA, Vilar-López R, Peralta-Ramírez I, et al: The role of antiphospholipid autoantibodies in the cognitive deficits of patients with systemic lupus erythematosus. Lupus 24(8):875–879, 2015 25697771

Cole SW, Hawkley LC, Arevalo JM, et al: Social regulation of gene expression in human leukocytes. Genome Biol 8(9):R189, 2007 17854483

Cornec D, Devauchelle-Pensec V, Mariette X, et al: Severe health-related quality-of-life impairment in active primary Sjögren's syndrome is driven by patient-reported outcomes: data from a large therapeutic trial. Arthritis Care Res (Hoboken) 69(4):528–535, 2017 27390310

Davis MC, Zautra AJ, Younger J, et al: Chronic stress and regulation of cellular markers of inflammation in rheumatoid arthritis: implications for fatigue. Brain Behav Immun 22(1):24–32, 2008 17706915

de Oliveira Ribeiro NP, de Mello Schier AR, Pessoa TM, et al: Depression as a comorbidity in Behçet's syndrome. CNS Neurol Disord Drug Targets 13(6):1041–1048, 2014 24923340

Demange V, Guillemin F, Baumann M, et al: Are there more than cross-sectional relationships of social support and support networks with functional limitations and psychological distress in early rheumatoid arthritis? The European Research on Incapacitating Diseases and Social Support Longitudinal Study. Arthritis Rheum 51(5):782–791, 2004 15478164

Denburg SD, Carbotte RM, Denburg JA: Corticosteroids and neuropsychological functioning in patients with systemic lupus erythematosus. Arthritis Rheum 37(9):1311–1320, 1994 7945494

Drewes AM, Svendsen L, Taagholt SJ, et al: Sleep in rheumatoid arthritis: a comparison with healthy subjects and studies of sleep/wake interactions. Br J Rheumatol 37(1):71–81, 1998 9487254

Epstein LC, Masse G, Harmatz JS, et al: Characterization of cognitive dysfunction in Sjögren's syndrome patients. Clin Rheumatol 33(4):511–521, 2014 24337727

Evers AW, Kraaimaat FW, Geenen R, et al: Long-term predictors of anxiety and depressed mood in early rheumatoid arthritis: a 3 and 5 year follow-up. J Rheumatol 29(11):2327–2336, 2002 12415588

Evers AW, Verhoeven EW, van Middendorp H, et al: Does stress affect the joints? Daily stressors, stress vulnerability, immune and HPA axis activity, and short-term disease and symptom fluctuations in rheumatoid arthritis. Ann Rheum Dis 73(9):1683–1688, 2014 23838082

Fiest KM, Hitchon CA, Bernstein CN, et al; CIHR Team "Defining the Burden and Managing the Effects of Psychiatric Comorbidity in Chronic Immunoinflammatory Disease": Systematic review and meta-analysis of interventions for depression and anxiety in persons with rheumatoid arthritis. J Clin Rheumatol 23(8):425–434, 2017 28221313

Fragiadaki K, Tektonidou MG, Konsta M, et al: Sleep disturbances and interleukin 6 receptor inhibition in rheumatoid arthritis. J Rheumatol 39(1):60–62, 2012 22133618

Fyrand L, Moum T, Finset A, et al: Social support in female patients with rheumatoid arthritis compared with healthy controls. Psychol Health 6(4):429–439, 2001

Genty M, Combe B, Kostine M, et al: Improvement of fatigue in patients with rheumatoid arthritis treated with biologics: relationship with sleep disorders, depression and clinical efficacy. A prospective, multicentre study. Clin Exp Rheumatol 35(1):85–92, 2017 27749229

Gerli R, Caponi L, Tincani A, et al: Clinical and serological associations of ribosomal P autoantibodies in systemic lupus erythematosus: prospective evaluation in a large cohort of Italian patients. Rheumatology (Oxford) 41(12):1357–1366, 2002 12468814

Griffin KW, Friend R, Kaell AT, et al: Distress and disease status among patients with rheumatoid arthritis: roles of coping styles and perceived responses from support providers. Ann Behav Med 23(2):133–138, 2001 11394555

Hajj-Ali RA, Wilke WS, Calabrese LH, et al: Pilot study to assess the frequency of fibromyalgia, depression, and sleep disorders in patients with granulomatosis with polyangiitis (Wegener's). Arthritis Care Res (Hoboken) 63(6):827–833, 2011 21337530

Hanly JG, Cassell K, Fisk JD: Cognitive function in systemic lupus erythematosus: results of a 5-year prospective study. Arthritis Rheum 40(8):1542–1543, 1997 9259438

Hanly JG, Urowitz MB, Sanchez-Guerrero J, et al; Systemic Lupus International Collaborating Clinics: Neuropsychiatric events at the time of diagnosis of systemic lupus erythematosus: an international inception cohort study. Arthritis Rheum 56(1):265–273, 2007 17195230

He Y, Zhang M, Lin EH, et al: Mental disorders among persons with arthritis: results from the World Mental Health Surveys. Psychol Med 38(11):1639–1650, 2008 18298879

Holtzman S, Newth S, Delongis A: The role of social support in coping with daily pain among patients with rheumatoid arthritis. J Health Psychol 9(5):677–695, 2004 15310421

Huang YH, Ro LS, Lyu RK, et al: Wegener's granulomatosis with nervous system involvement: a hospital-based study. Eur Neurol 73(3–4):197–204, 2015 25791920

Huang SW, Wang WT, Lin LF, et al: Association between psychiatric disorders and osteoarthritis: a nationwide longitudinal population-based study. Medicine (Baltimore) 95(26):e4016, 2016 27368019

Hyphantis TN, Tsifetaki N, Siafaka V, et al: The impact of psychological functioning upon systemic sclerosis patients' quality of life. Semin Arthritis Rheum 37(2):81–92, 2007 17512572

Irwin MR: Why sleep is important for health: a psychoneuroimmunology perspective. Ann Rev Psychol 66:143–172, 2015 25061767

Irwin MR, Cole SW: Reciprocal regulation of the neural and innate immune systems. Nat Rev Immunol 11(9):625–632, 2011 21818124

Irwin MR, Opp MR: Sleep health: reciprocal regulation of sleep and innate immunity. Neuropsychopharmacology 42(1):129–155, 2017 27510422

Irwin MR, Olmstead R, Carrillo C, et al: Sleep loss exacerbates fatigue, depression, and pain in rheumatoid arthritis. Sleep 35(4):537–543, 2012 22467992

Irwin MR, Olmstead R, Carroll JE: Sleep disturbance, sleep duration, and inflammation: a systematic review and meta-analysis of cohort studies and experimental sleep deprivation. Biol Psychiatry 80(1):40–52, 2016 26140821

Joyce AT, Smith P, Khandker R, et al: Hidden cost of rheumatoid arthritis (RA): estimating cost of comorbid cardiovascular disease and depression among patients with RA. J Rheumatol 36(4):743–752, 2009 19228658

Julian LJ, Yelin E, Yazdany J, et al: Depression, medication adherence, and service utilization in systemic lupus erythematosus. Arthritis Rheum 61(2):240–246, 2009 19177526

Jung JY, Nam JY, Kim HA, et al: Elevated salivary alpha-amylase level, association between depression and disease activity, and stress as a predictor of disease flare in systemic lupus erythematosus: a prospective case-control study. Medicine (Baltimore) 94(30):e1184, 2015 26222848

Kaposi M: Neue beitrage zur Kenntnis des lupus erythematosus. Arch Dermatol Syph 4:36–79, 1872

Karatas G, Bal A, Yuceege M, et al: The evaluation of sleep quality and response to anti-tumor necrosis factor α therapy in rheumatoid arthritis patients. Clin Rheumatol 36(1):45–50, 2017 27567629

Katz P, Margaretten M, Trupin L, et al: Role of sleep disturbance, depression, obesity, and physical inactivity in fatigue in rheumatoid arthritis. Arthritis Care Res (Hoboken) 68(1):81–90, 2016 25779719

Kekow J, Moots R, Khandker R, et al: Improvements in patient-reported outcomes, symptoms of depression and anxiety, and their association with clinical remission among patients with moderate-to-severe active early rheumatoid arthritis. Rheumatology (Oxford) 50(2):401–409, 2011 21059675

Knight AM, Xie M, Mandell DS: Disparities in psychiatric diagnosis and treatment for youth with systemic lupus erythematosus: analysis of a national US Medicaid sample. J Rheumatol 43(7):1427–1433, 2016 27134262

Kohen M, Asherson RA, Gharavi AE, et al: Lupus psychosis: differentiation from the steroid-induced state. Clin Exp Rheumatol 11(3):323–326, 1993 8353989

Kohlhaas K, Brechmann T, Vorgerd M: [Hepatitis B associated polyarteritis nodosa with cerebral vasculitis] (in German). Dtsch Med Wochenschr 132(34–35):1748–1752, 2007 17713883

Kojima M, Kojima T, Suzuki S, et al: Depression, inflammation, and pain in patients with rheumatoid arthritis. Arthritis Rheum 61(8):1018–1024, 2009 19644894

Kotsis K, Voulgari PV, Tsifetaki N, et al: Illness perceptions and psychological distress associated with physical health-related quality of life in primary Sjögren's syndrome compared to systemic lupus erythematosus and rheumatoid arthritis. Rheumatol Int 34(12):1671–1681, 2014 24769916

Kwakkenbos L, Delisle VC, Fox RS, et al: Psychosocial Aspects of Scleroderma. Rheum Dis Clin North Am 41(3):519–528, 2015 26210133

Larsen RJ: Neuroticism and selective encoding and recall of symptoms: evidence from a combined concurrent-retrospective study. J Pers Soc Psychol 62(3):480–488, 1992 1560338

Lee YC, Chibnik LB, Lu B, et al: The relationship between disease activity, sleep, psychiatric distress and pain sensitivity in rheumatoid arthritis: a cross-sectional study. Arthritis Res Ther 11(5):R160, 2009 19874580

Lee YC, Lu B, Edwards RR, et al: The role of sleep problems in central pain processing in rheumatoid arthritis. Arthritis Rheum 65(1):59–68, 2013 23124650

Levine JS, Branch DW, Rauch J: The antiphospholipid syndrome. N Engl J Med 346(10):752–763, 2002 11882732

Lewis MJ, Jawad AS: The effect of ethnicity and genetic ancestry on the epidemiology, clinical features and outcome of systemic lupus erythematosus. Rheumatology (Oxford) 56 (suppl 1):i67–i77, 2017 27940583

Lim LS, Lefebvre A, Benseler S, et al: Psychiatric illness of systemic lupus erythematosus in childhood: spectrum of clinically important manifestations. J Rheumatol 40(4):506–512, 2013 23242179

Lin EH: Depression and osteoarthritis. Am J Med 121 (11 suppl 2):S16–S19, 2008 18954588

Malemud CJ, Miller AH: Pro-inflammatory cytokine-induced SAPK/MAPK and JAK/STAT in rheumatoid arthritis and the new anti-depression drugs. Expert Opin Ther Targets 12(2):171–183, 2008 18208366

Margaretten M, Yelin E, Imboden J, et al: Predictors of depression in a multiethnic cohort of patients with rheumatoid arthritis. Arthritis Rheum 61(11):1586–1591, 2009 19877099

Margolin L, Cope DK, Bakst-Sisser R, Greenspan J: The steroid withdrawal syndrome: a review of the implications, etiology, and treatments. J Pain Symptom Manage 33(2):224–228, 2007 17280928

Matcham F, Rayner L, Steer S, et al: The prevalence of depression in rheumatoid arthritis: a systematic review and meta-analysis. Rheumatology (Oxford) 52(12):2136–2148, 2013 24003249

Matcham F, Norton S, Scott DL, et al: Symptoms of depression and anxiety predict treatment response and long-term physical health outcomes in rheumatoid arthritis: secondary analysis of a randomized controlled trial. Rheumatology (Oxford) 55(2):268–278, 2016 26350486

Meszaros ZS, Perl A, Faraone SV: Psychiatric symptoms in systemic lupus erythematosus: a systematic review. J Clin Psychiatry 73(7):993–1001, 2012 22687742

Micca JL, Ruff D, Ahl J, et al: Safety and efficacy of duloxetine treatment in older and younger patients with osteoarthritis knee pain: a post hoc, subgroup analysis of two randomized, placebo-controlled trials. BMC Musculoskelet Disord 14:137, 2013 23590727

Mindham RH, Bagshaw A, James SA, et al: Factors associated with the appearance of psychiatric symptoms in rheumatoid arthritis. J Psychosom Res 25(5):429–435, 1981 7328510

Moieni M, Irwin MR, Jevtic I, et al: Sex differences in depressive and socioemotional responses to an inflammatory challenge: implications for sex differences in depression. Neuropsychopharmacology 40(7):1709–1716, 2015 25598426

Moldofsky H: Sleep and pain. Sleep Med Rev 5(5):385–396, 2001 12531004

Motivala SJ, Khanna D, FitzGerald J, et al: Stress activation of cellular markers of inflammation in rheumatoid arthritis: protective effects of tumor necrosis factor alpha antagonists. Arthritis Rheum 58(2):376–383, 2008 18240230

Murphy H, Dickens C, Creed F, et al: Depression, illness perception and coping in rheumatoid arthritis. J Psychosom Res 46(2):155–164, 1999 10098824

Murphy S, Creed F, Jayson MI: Psychiatric disorder and illness behaviour in rheumatoid arthritis. Br J Rheumatol 27(5):357–363, 1988 3179624

Nicassio PM, Moxham EG, Schuman CE, et al: The contribution of pain, reported sleep quality, and depressive symptoms to fatigue in fibromyalgia. Pain 100(3):271–279, 2002 12467998

Nicassio PM, Ormseth SR, Kay M, et al: The contribution of pain and depression to self-reported sleep disturbance in patients with rheumatoid arthritis. Pain 153(1):107–112, 2012 22051047

Nishimura K, Omori M, Sato E, et al: New-onset psychiatric disorders after corticosteroid therapy in systemic lupus erythematosus: an observational case-series study. J Neurol 261(11):2150–2158, 2014 25142268

Otto R, Mackay IR: Psycho-social and emotional disturbance in systemic lupus erythematosus. Med J Aust 2(11):488–493, 1967 6066095

Palagini L, Mauri M, Faraguna U, et al: Insomnia symptoms, perceived stress and coping strategies in patients with systemic lupus erythematosus. Lupus 25(9):988–996, 2016 26876691

Parmelee PA, Tighe CA, Dautovich ND: Sleep disturbance in osteoarthritis: linkages with pain, disability, and depressive symptoms. Arthritis Care Res (Hoboken) 67(3):358–365, 2015 25283955

Peck JR, Smith TW, Ward JR, et al: Disability and depression in rheumatoid arthritis. A multitrait, multi-method investigation. Arthritis Rheum 32(9):1100–1106, 1989 2528352

Peralta-Ramírez MI, Jimenez-Alonso J, Godoy-Garcia JF, et al: The effects of daily stress and stressful life events on the clinical symptomatology of patients with lupus erythematosus. Psychosom Med 66(5):788–794, 2004 15385708

Peralta-Ramírez MI, Coin-Mejias MA, Jimenez-Alonso J, et al: Stress as a predictor of cognitive functioning in lupus. Lupus 15(12):858–864, 2006 17121991

Pitsilka DA, Kafetsios K, Niakas D: Social support and quality of life in patients with rheumatoid arthritis in Greece. Clin Exp Rheumatol 33(1):27–33, 2015 25437270

Raison CL, Miller AH: Role of inflammation in depression: implications for phenomenology, pathophysiology and treatment. Mod Trends Pharmacopsychiatry 28:33–48, 2013 25224889

Rathbun AM, Reed GW, Harrold LR: The temporal relationship between depression and rheumatoid arthritis disease activity, treatment persistence and response: a systematic review. Rheumatology (Oxford) 52(10):1785–1794, 2013 23236191

Rathbun AM, Harrold LR, Reed GW: A description of patient- and rheumatologist-reported depression symptoms in an American rheumatoid arthritis registry population. Clin Exp Rheumatol 32(4):523–532, 2014 24984165

Scolding NJ, Joseph FG: The neuropathology and pathogenesis of systemic lupus erythematosus. Neuropathol Appl Neurobiol 28(3):173–189, 2002 12060342

Sharpe L, Sensky T, Timberlake N, et al: A blind, randomized, controlled trial of cognitive-behavioural intervention for patients with recent onset rheumatoid arthritis: preventing psychological and physical morbidity. Pain 89(2–3):275–283, 2001 11166484

Slavich GM, Irwin MR: From stress to inflammation and major depressive disorder: a social signal transduction theory of depression. Psychol Bull 140(3):774–815, 2014 24417575

Smedstad LM, Moum T, Guillemin F, et al: Correlates of functional disability in early rheumatoid arthritis: a cross-sectional study of 706 patients in four European countries. Br J Rheumatol 35(8):746–751, 1996 8761186

Smith MT, Finan PH, Buenaver LF, et al: Cognitive-behavioral therapy for insomnia in knee osteoarthritis: a randomized, double-blind, active placebo-controlled clinical trial. Arthritis Rheumatol 67(5):1221–1233, 2015 25623343

Smith TW, Peck JR, Milano RA, et al: Cognitive distortion in rheumatoid arthritis: relation to depression and disability. J Consult Clin Psychol 56(3):412–416, 1988 2969388

Spitzer A, Bar-Tal Y, Golander H: Social support: how does it really work? J Adv Nurs 22(5):850–854, 1995 8568057

Strating MM, Suurmeijer TP, van Schuur WH: Disability, social support, and distress in rheumatoid arthritis: results from a thirteen-year prospective study. Arthritis Rheum 55(5):736–744, 2006 17013871

Straub RH, Dhabhar FS, Bijlsma JW, et al: How psychological stress via hormones and nerve fibers may exacerbate rheumatoid arthritis. Arthritis Rheum 52(1):16–26, 2005 15641084

Stubbs B, Aluko Y, Myint PK, et al: Prevalence of depressive symptoms and anxiety in osteoarthritis: a systematic review and meta-analysis. Age Ageing 45(2):228–235, 2016 26795974

Takahashi H, Washio M, Kiyohara C, et al; Kyushu Sapporo SLE (KYSS) Study Group: Psychological stress in a Japanese population with systemic lupus erythematosus: finding from KYSS study. Mod Rheumatol 24(3):448–452, 2014 24252033

Talarico R, Palagini L, d'Ascanio A, et al: Epidemiology and management of neuropsychiatric disorders in Behçet's syndrome. CNS Drugs 29(3):189–196, 2015 25643894

Tavassoli N, Montastruc-Fournier J, Montastruc JL; French Association of Regional Pharmacovigilance Centres: Psychiatric adverse drug reactions to glucocorticoids in children and adolescents: a much higher risk with elevated doses. Br J Clin Pharmacol 66(4):566–567, 2008 18537961

Tay SH, Mak A: Diagnosing and attributing neuropsychiatric events to systemic lupus erythematosus: time to untie the Gordian knot? Rheumatology (Oxford) 56 (suppl 1):i14–i23, 2016 27744358

Taylor-Gjevre RM, Gjevre JA, Nair BV, et al: Improved sleep efficiency after anti-tumor necrosis factor alpha therapy in rheumatoid arthritis patients. Ther Adv Musculoskelet Dis 3(5):227–233, 2011 22870481

Thombs BD, Taillefer SS, Hudson M, et al: Depression in patients with systemic sclerosis: a systematic review of the evidence. Arthritis Rheum 57(6):1089–1097, 2007 17665491

Tlacuilo-Parra JA, Guevara-Gutierrez E, Garcia-De La Torre I: Factitious disorders mimicking systemic lupus erythematosus. Clin Exp Rheumatol 18(1):89–93, 2000 10728452

Tyring S, Gottlieb A, Papp K, et al: Etanercept and clinical outcomes, fatigue, and depression in psoriasis: double-blind placebo-controlled randomised phase III trial. Lancet 367(9504):29–35, 2006 16399150

Uguz F, Akman C, Kucuksarac S, et al: Anti-tumor necrosis factor-alpha therapy is associated with less frequent mood and anxiety disorders in patients with rheumatoid arthritis. Psychiatry Clin Neurosci 63(1):50–55, 2009 19154212

Unterman A, Nolte JE, Boaz M, et al: Neuropsychiatric syndromes in systemic lupus erythematosus: a meta-analysis. Semin Arthritis Rheum 41(1):1–11, 2011 20965549

Vedove CD, Del Giglio M, Schena D, et al: Drug-induced lupus erythematosus. Arch Dermatol Res 301(1):99–105, 2009 18797892

Wolfe F, Hawley DJ: The relationship between clinical activity and depression in rheumatoid arthritis. J Rheumatol 20(12):2032–2037, 1993 8014930

Wolfe F, Kong SX: Rasch analysis of the Western Ontario MacMaster questionnaire (WOMAC) in 2205 patients with osteoarthritis, rheumatoid arthritis, and fibromyalgia. Ann Rheum Dis 58(9):563–568, 1999 10460190

Wolfe F, Michaud K: Predicting depression in rheumatoid arthritis: the signal importance of pain extent and fatigue, and comorbidity. Arthritis Rheum 61(5):667–673, 2009 19404997

Wong JK, Nortley R, Andrews T, et al: Psychiatric manifestations of primary Sjögren's syndrome: a case report and literature review. BMJ Case Rep May 23:2014, 2014 24859541

Xu N, Zhao S, Xue H, et al: Associations of perceived social support and positive psychological resources with fatigue symptom in patients with rheumatoid arthritis. PLoS One 12(3):e0173293, 2017 28291837

Zamarrón C, Maceiras F, Mera A, et al: Effect of the first infliximab infusion on sleep and alertness in patients with active rheumatoid arthritis. Ann Rheum Dis 63(1):88–90, 2004 14672898

Zautra AJ, Davis MC, Reich JW, et al: Comparison of cognitive behavioral and mindfulness meditation interventions on adaptation to rheumatoid arthritis for patients with and without history of recurrent depression. J Consult Clin Psychol 76(3):408–421, 2008 18540734

Zhang L, Fu T, Yin R, et al: Prevalence of depression and anxiety in systemic lupus erythematosus: a systematic review and meta-analysis. BMC Psychiatry 17(1):70, 2017 28196529

Zyrianova Y, Kelly BD, Gallagher C, et al: Depression and anxiety in rheumatoid arthritis: the role of perceived social support. Ir J Med Sci 175(2):32–36, 2006 16872026

CHAPTER 25

Chronic Fatigue and Fibromyalgia Syndromes

Michael C. Sharpe, M.A., M.D., FRCP, FRCPsych
Patrick G. O'Malley, M.D., M.P.H., FACP

In this chapter, we review two symptom-defined somatic syndromes: chronic fatigue syndrome (CFS) and fibromyalgia syndrome (FMS). The central feature of CFS is the symptom of severe chronic, disabling fatigue, typically exacerbated by exertion and inadequately unexplained by any other medical condition. The central feature of FMS is widespread pain with localized tenderness that is similarly unexplained by any other diagnosis. Although these syndromes have different historical origins, they have much in common (Sullivan et al. 2002). Therefore, in this chapter we consider them together.

CFS, FMS, and other symptom-defined somatic syndromes are conditions whose homes both in medicine (as functional syndromes) and in psychiatry (some will meet criteria for somatic symptom disorders) are rather temporary structures located in unfashionable areas of their respective communities. These so-called functional somatic syndromes (Wessely et al. 1999) are, however, of central concern to psychosomatic medicine. Other functional syndromes covered elsewhere in this volume include noncardiac chest pain (see Chapter 17, "Heart Disease"), hyperventilation syndrome (see Chapter 18, "Lung Disease"), irritable bowel and functional upper gastrointestinal disorders (see Chapter 19, "Gastrointestinal Disorders"), idiopathic pruritus (see Chapter 27, "Dermatology"), migraine (see Chapter 30, "Neurology and Neurosurgery"), chronic pelvic pain and vulvodynia (see Chapter 31, "Obstetrics and Gynecology"), and several other pain syndromes (see Chapter 34, "Pain"). Somatic symptom disorder is also discussed in Chapter 11, "Somatic Symptom Disorder and Illness Anxiety Disorder."

We are grateful to the following for helpful comments on earlier versions of this chapter: Dr. Peter White, Dr. Leslie Arnold, Professor Simon Wessely, Professor Gijs Belijenberg, and Professor Dan Clauw. We also thank Mr. Ben Steward for checking the references.

General Issues

Symptom or Disorder?

Although CFS and FMS are often regarded as discrete conditions, their core symptoms of fatigue and pain are highly prevalent (Croft et al. 1996; Pawlikowska et al. 1994); the case definitions therefore specify clinically significant cutoff points on the severity continua of these symptoms in the general population.

Organic or Psychogenic?

The history of CFS and FMS has been notorious for disputes about whether these disorders are "organic" or "psychogenic" (Asbring and Närvänen 2003). The extreme organic position argues that they will eventually become as firmly based in disease pathology as any other medical condition, whereas the extreme psychogenic view is that they are pseudo-diseases, rooted not in biology but rather in social constructions based on the psychological amplification of somatic sensations (Shorter 1992). Neither of these extreme positions is satisfactorily sustained by the evidence or, indeed, helpful in managing patients. The extreme organic view encourages the doctor to endlessly seek pathology while the patient is left without treatment. The extreme psychological view may encourage the doctor to dismiss the patient's symptoms as "all in the mind." As with most illnesses, an etiologically neutral and integrated perspective that simultaneously recognizes the reality of the symptoms and acknowledges the contribution of biological, psychological, and social factors is the best basis for clinical practice (Engel 1977).

Medical or Psychiatric?

In parallel with the debate about etiology is an argument about whether these conditions are most appropriately regarded as "medical" or as "psychiatric." For a patient with fatigue and pain, the medical diagnosis might include CFS (myalgic encephalomyelitis) or FMS (chronic widespread pain) (see "History" in the following section, "The Syndromes"). However, the very same symptoms may merit a psychiatric diagnosis of anxiety, mood, or somatic symptom disorder. Which diagnosis is correct? We argue that sometimes both medical and psychiatric diagnoses may be needed. For example, the best diagnosis for a patient might be FMS *and* generalized anxiety disorder.

The Syndromes

Chronic Fatigue Syndrome

History

CFS is not a new illness. A similar, if not identical, condition was described as *neurasthenia* over 100 years ago and probably existed long before that (Wessely 1990). The term *chronic fatigue syndrome* was defined in 1988 as a condition characterized by chronic disabling fatigue accompanied by other somatic symptoms (Holmes et al. 1988). The authors of this early definition anticipated that a specific disease cause, possibly infectious, would be found, but such an etiology has still not been established. *Chronic fatigue syndrome* subsumed a multitude of previous terms used to describe patients with similar symptoms, including *chronic Epstein-Barr virus infection* (see Chapter 26, "Infectious Diseases"), *myalgic encephalomyelitis, neurasthenia* (still a specific diagnosis in ICD-10 [World Health Organization 1992]), and *post-viral fatigue syndrome.* The introduction of the term *chronic fatigue syndrome* operationally defined the syndrome and consequently provided a firm basis for replicable scientific research.

Definition

Many operational diagnostic criteria for CFS have been published (Brurberg et al. 2014). The first case definition, by Holmes et al. (1988), was excessively restrictive, making it difficult to fulfill diagnostic criteria, and was therefore not clinically useful. The currently most widely used criteria (shown in Table 25–1) are based on an international consensus case definition published in 1994 (Fukuda et al. 1994) and subsequently further operationalized in 2003 (Reeves et al. 2003). In 2015, the Institute of Medicine proposed a new name—systemic exertion intolerance disease—with an as-yet-untested definition that emphasizes postexertional malaise. All of these definitions have limitations, however, and clinical practice should not be rigidly bound by them.

Clinical Features

The core symptom of CFS is persistent physical and mental fatigue that is exacerbated by exertion. Disrupted and unrefreshing sleep is almost universally described, and widespread pain is common (Prins et al. 2006). Patients often report marked fluctuations in fatigue from week to week and even from day to day. Few patients are so disabled that they cannot attend an outpatient consultation, although some require the aid of wheelchairs and other assistance. A minority of patients remain bedridden and represent an important and neglected group.

Fibromyalgia Syndrome

History

More than 100 years ago, Gowers (1904) coined the term *fibrositis* to describe chronic widespread pain thought to be caused by inflammation of muscles. However, as with CFS, no specific muscle pathology has been confirmed. Other terms, such as *chronic widespread pain* and *myofascial pain syndrome,* have also been used to describe the condition. In 1990, the American College of Rheumatology (ACR) adopted the term *fibromyalgia* and developed criteria for its classification (Wolfe et al. 1990); the criteria were updated in 2010 (Wolfe et al. 2010). The ACR's definition has facilitated replicable research and has been widely adopted.

Definition

The ACR criteria specify widespread pain of at least 3 months' duration. Although the 1990 criteria require tenderness at 11 or more of 18 specific sites on the body, the

---

TABLE 25–1.   **Diagnostic criteria for chronic fatigue syndrome**

Inclusion criteria

1.   Clinically evaluated, medically unexplained fatigue of at least 6 months' duration that is:
  •   Of new onset (not lifelong)
  •   Not the result of ongoing exertion
  •   Not substantially alleviated by rest
  •   Associated with a substantial reduction in previous level of activities
2.   Presence of four or more of the following symptoms:
  •   Subjective memory impairment
  •   Sore throat
  •   Tender lymph nodes
  •   Muscle pain
  •   Joint pain
  •   Headache
  •   Unrefreshing sleep
  •   Postexertional malaise lasting more than 24 hours

Exclusion criteria

Active, unresolved, or suspected medical disease

Psychotic, melancholic, or bipolar depression (but not uncomplicated major depression)

Psychotic disorders

Dementia

Anorexia or bulimia nervosa

Alcohol or other substance misuse

Severe obesity

Source.   Adapted from Fukuda et al. 1994.

2010 update does *not* require the presence of tender points. The two sets of criteria are shown in Table 25–2.

Clinical Features

The core feature of fibromyalgia is chronic widespread pain. Pain occurs typically in all four quadrants of the body and the axial skeleton but also can be regional. Fatigue, sleep disturbance, musculoskeletal tenderness, and subjective cognitive impairment (memory and concentration) are common. As with fatigue in CFS, the report of pain in fibromyalgia is essentially a subjective phenomenon.

Primary or Secondary?

Both CFS and FMS are typically diagnosed when the patient has no evidence of another general medical condition. However, similar symptoms do occur with other medical diagnoses. For example, symptoms of FMS have been reported in patients with systemic lupus erythematosus (Buskila et al. 2003) and rheumatoid arthritis (Wolfe et al. 1984), and symptoms of CFS have been reported in disease-free cancer patients (Servaes et al. 2002) and in patients with multiple sclerosis (Vercoulen et al.

TABLE 25–2.   Comparison of American College of Rheumatology (ACR) 1990 and 2010 criteria for fibromyalgia

ACR criteria for fibromyalgia, 1990	ACR criteria for fibromyalgia, 2010
1. History of widespread pain	**Criteria—the following 3 conditions must be met:**
Definition: Pain is considered widespread when all of the following are present: pain in the right and left sides of the body, pain above and below the waist, axial skeletal pain (cervical spine or anterior chest or thoracic spine or low back). In this definition, shoulder and buttock pain is considered as pain for each involved side. Low back pain is considered lower-segment pain.	1. Widespread pain index (WPI) ≥ 7 and symptom severity (SS) scale score ≥ 5 or WPI 3–6 and SS scale score ≥ 9 2. Symptoms have been present at a similar level for at least 3 months. 3. The patient does not have a disorder that would otherwise explain the pain.
2. Pain in 11 of 18 tender point sites on digital palpation	**Ascertainment**

Definition: Pain, on digital palpation, must be present in at least 11 of 18 specified tender point sites.	1. WPI: In how many areas (of 19 specified sites) has the patient had pain? (Score will be between 0 and 19.)
	2. SS scale score:[a]
	
	For each of the following—a) fatigue, b) waking unrefreshed, and c) cognitive symptoms—indicate the level of severity over the past week using the following scale:
	  0 no problem
	  1 slight or mild problems, generally mild or intermittent
	  2 moderate, considerable problems, often present and/or at a moderate level
	  3 severe: pervasive, continuous, life-disturbing problems
	Considering somatic symptoms in general, indicate whether the patient has:
	  0 no symptoms
	  1 few symptoms
	  2 a moderate number of symptoms
	  3 a great deal of symptoms

[a] The SS scale score is the sum of the severity of the 3 symptoms (fatigue, waking unrefreshed, cognitive symptoms) plus the extent (severity) of somatic symptoms in general. The final score is between 0 and 12.

Source.   Adapted from Wolfe et al. 1990.

Source.   Adapted from Wolfe et al. 2010.

1996a). The terms *primary* (occurring in the absence of another condition) and *secondary* (accompanying a medical condition) have consequently been used.

Same or Different?

Pain and fatigue tend to co-occur in the general population (Creavin et al. 2010). Furthermore, there is an overlap in the symptoms of patients who have been diagnosed with FMS and those diagnosed with CFS. Put simply, CFS is fatigue with pain, and FMS is pain with fatigue. Not only are the symptoms similar, but a patient who has received the diagnosis of one is also likely to meet diagnostic criteria for the other. Whether these conditions will ultimately be found to be distinct entities, overlapping conditions, or just aspects of the same condition currently remains unclear.

Association With Other Symptom-Defined Syndromes

Studies of the comorbidity of CFS and FMS with other symptom-defined syndromes (also known as medically unexplained symptoms or functional somatic syndromes) have found high rates of comorbidity with migraine, irritable bowel syndrome, pelvic pain, temporomandibular joint pain, and other syndromes (Kanaan et al. 2007; Kato et al. 2006; Lacourt et al. 2013). This observation raises the possibility not only that CFS and FMS are similar but also that functional syndromes have more in common than is usually assumed to be the case (Wessely et al. 1999).

Association With Psychiatric Disorders

In clinical practice, many patients who have received a diagnosis of CFS or FMS also meet criteria for a psychiatric diagnosis. In most cases this is a depressive or anxiety disorder (Janssens et al. 2015). Others may meet criteria for somatic symptom disorder as defined in DSM-5 (American Psychiatric Association 2013) or neurasthenia as described in ICD-10 (Sharpe 1996). Some symptoms of CFS or FMS (e.g., fatigue, sleep disturbance, poor concentration) overlap with the symptoms of depression and anxiety, and the observed prevalence of psychiatric disorders in patient populations will therefore depend on whether symptoms are counted toward a diagnosis of a psychiatric disorder or attributed to the diagnosis of CFS or FMS.

Depression

Fatigue is strongly associated with depression. The World Health Organization (WHO) study of more than 5,000 primary care patients in several countries (Sartorius et al. 1993) found that 67% of patients meeting criteria for CFS (defined from survey data) also had a depressive syndrome (Skapinakis et al. 2000). A study of patients with CFS reported that more than 25% had a current DSM major depressive disorder (MDD) diagnosis and 50%–75% had a lifetime diagnosis (Afari and Buchwald 2003).

Chronic pain is also strongly associated with depression in the general population (Ohayon and Schatzberg 2003; see also Chapter 34, "Pain"). In one study of FMS patients in a specialist clinic, 32% had a depressive disorder (22% had MDD) (Epstein et al. 1999). An increased prevalence of lifetime and family history of MDD also has been reported in patients with FMS (Hudson and Pope 1996).

Generalized Anxiety Disorder, Panic Disorder, and Posttraumatic Stress Disorder

Anxiety disorders have been relatively understudied in association with CFS and FMS. One study reported finding generalized anxiety disorder (GAD) in as many as half of clinic patients with CFS or FMS when the hierarchical rules that subsumed GAD under MDD were suspended (Fischler et al. 1997).

Panic disorder is especially common in patients with medically unexplained symptoms. Prevalence rates were 13% in patients with CFS (Manu et al. 1991) and 7% in patients with FMS (Epstein et al. 1999). Panic disorder, which may present with predominantly somatic symptoms (Chen et al. 2009), should be suspected when the reported somatic symptoms are markedly episodic.

The prevalence of posttraumatic stress disorder has also been reported to be higher in patients with CFS (Dansie et al. 2012) and much higher in patients with FMS (Coppens et al. 2017) than in the general population.

Somatic Symptom and Related Disorders

In DSM-5, the diagnosis somatic symptom disorder replaced the DSM-IV (American Psychiatric Association 1994) diagnosis of somatoform disorder. The DSM-5 disorder emphasizes the presence of excessive concern about somatic symptoms rather than the absence of identified physical disease (Dimsdale et al. 2013). Although it could be argued that most patients with FMS or CFS would meet criteria for DSM-IV somatoform disorder, the percentage who would meet criteria for DSM-5 somatic symptom disorder is uncertain but may be considerably smaller (Häuser et al. 2015b).

Summary of Association of CFS/FMS With Psychiatric Disorders

Although depressive and anxiety disorders are prevalent in CFS and FMS, many patients do not meet criteria for these psychiatric disorders (Henningsen et al. 2003). Whether it is appropriate to then make a diagnosis of somatic symptom disorder rather than either CFS or FMS is controversial. DSM-5 states that patients with functional disorders such as irritable bowel syndrome or fibromyalgia should receive a diagnosis of somatic symptom disorder only if they satisfy Criterion B (excessive thoughts, feelings, or behaviors related to the physical symptoms). Symptom syndromes (such as somatic symptom disorder) defined by psychiatry and syndromes (such as CFS and FMS) defined by other medical specialties can be conceptualized either as comorbid conditions or as different perspectives on the same condition. Whichever view one takes, the potential value of making a psychiatric diagnosis lies in its implications for treatment.

Epidemiology

Prevalence of Fatigue and Chronic Fatigue Syndrome

Chronic fatigue is common, but CFS as defined in diagnostic criteria is relatively uncommon. The observed prevalence of Centers for Disease Control and Prevention–

defined CFS is approximately 3% when the diagnosis is based on self-report data and only 0.8% when based on a clinical assessment (Johnston et al. 2013).

Prevalence of Pain and Fibromyalgia Syndrome

Studies of the prevalence of pain and FMS have reported similar findings. Chronic pain is common and has been reported in as much as 10% of the general population (Croft et al. 1993), whereas FMS defined according to the 2010 ACR criteria (see Table 25–2) has an estimated prevalence of only about 2% (Jones et al. 2015).

Associations With Demographic Characteristics

Gender

Both CFS and FMS are more common in women (Jones et al. 2015; Reyes et al. 2003).

Age

The most common age at onset for both CFS and FMS is between 30 and 50 years, although patients who present with FMS are on average 10 years older (Reyes et al. 2003; White et al. 1999). These syndromes are also diagnosed in children.

Socioeconomic Status

Both CFS and FMS are more prevalent in persons of lower socioeconomic status (Jason et al. 1999; White et al. 1999). CFS is 50% more common in semiskilled and unskilled workers than in professionals.

Nationality and Culture

Whereas the symptoms of fatigue and pain are universal, the diagnoses of CFS and FMS are almost entirely restricted to Western nations. It is unclear to what extent this finding reflects differing epidemiology or different diagnostic practice.

Disability and Work

CFS and FMS are both associated with substantial loss of function and work disability (Assefi et al. 2003). Unemployment in patients with CFS and FMS accessing specialist services in the United States is as high as 50% (Bombardier and Buchwald 1996).

Prognosis

The prognosis for patients with CFS or FMS is variable; these illnesses typically have a chronic but fluctuating course. Rehabilitative therapy improves the outcome (see subsection "Nonpharmacological Treatments" later in this chapter).

Prospective studies of CFS and FMS in the general population have reported that in about half of cases, the syndrome is in partial or complete remission by 2–3 years after diagnosis (Granges et al. 1994; Nisenbaum et al. 2003). Poor outcome in CFS and FMS is predicted by longer illness duration, more severe symptoms, older age, depression, and lack of social support (van der Werf et al. 2002), and in CFS by a strong belief in a physical cause (Cairns and Hotopf 2005). Severely disabled patients have a particularly poor prognosis for recovery (Hill et al. 1999; Wolfe 1997). Both CFS and FMS have been associated with a modestly increased risk of suicide but not with an increase in mortality from other causes (Dreyer et al. 2010; Roberts et al. 2016).

Etiology

The etiologies of CFS and FMS remain unknown. Although a wide range of etiological factors have been proposed, none has been unequivocally established. The available evidence suggests that a combination of environmental factors and individual vulnerability initiates a series of biological, psychological, and social processes that lead to the development of CFS or FMS (Table 25–3). Various factors are discussed in the following subsections as predisposing, precipitating, and perpetuating factors. It is worth mentioning that most research in this area is based on small case–control studies with insufficient power to control for confounding, thereby limiting the ability to draw strong causal inferences about any of the findings reported below.

Predisposing Factors

Predisposing factors make an individual vulnerable to developing the illness.

Biological Factors: Genetics

Modest evidence from family and twin studies suggests that genetic factors play a part in predisposing individuals to CFS or to FMS. In a study of 146 female–female twin pairs, one member of which had CFS, the concordance was 55% in monozygotic and 20% in dizygotic twins (Buchwald et al. 2001), suggesting both moderate heritability and the importance of environmental factors. In FMS, a similar familial clustering has been reported (Buskila and Neumann 1997). Claims for the role of specific genes in the etiology of these conditions remain so far unproven.

Psychological and Social Factors

Personality and activity.   Although obsessional or perfectionistic personality type has been proposed as a risk factor for CFS and for chronic pain, there is limited evidence for this. The clinical observation that CFS and FMS patients lead abnormally active lives or have high levels of exercise before becoming ill has some empirical support (Harvey et al. 2008).

History of trauma.   Childhood and adulthood neglect, abuse, and maltreatment have been reported to be more common in groups of individuals with CFS and FMS than in comparison groups (Afari et al. 2014). Both psychological and biological mechanisms for the etiological role of trauma have been suggested.

Socioeconomic status.   Low socioeconomic status and lower levels of education are risk factors for both CFS and FMS (see "Socioeconomic Status" in the "Epidemiology" section earlier in this chapter).

Precipitating Factors

Precipitating factors trigger the illness in vulnerable persons.

TABLE 25–3.   **Possible etiological factors to consider in a formulation of chronic fatigue syndrome or fibromyalgia syndrome**

	Predisposing	Precipitating	Perpetuating
Biological	Genetics	Infection or injury	Deconditioning Sleep abnormalities Neuroendocrine changes Immunological changes
Psychological	Personality and activity History of trauma	Perceived stress	Depression Unhelpful illness beliefs Avoidance of activity
Social	Low socioeconomic status	Life events	Illness-reinforcing information Lack of perceived legitimacy of illness Occupational and financial factors

Biological Factors

Infection.   There is evidence that infection can precipitate CFS, and some, but less, evidence indicates that infection also may trigger FMS (Rea et al. 1999). Specific infections have been found to be associated with subsequent development of CFS in 10%–40% of patients. These infections are Epstein-Barr virus (White et al. 2001), Q fever (Ayres et al. 1998), viral meningitis (Hotopf et al. 1996), viral hepatitis (Berelowitz et al. 1995), and parvovirus (Kerr and Mattey 2008). The etiological mechanism underlying this association remains unclear but may involve stress, immunological factors, and acute reductions in activity (see "Perpetuating Factors" later in this section).

Injury.   The role of physical injury in the etiology of CFS and FMS has been controversial, in part because of the implications for legal liability and compensation. Limited evidence indicates that both conditions may be precipitated by injury, particularly to the neck. If a link exists, it is likely stronger for FMS than for CFS (Al-Allaf et al. 2002).

Psychological and Social Factors

Clinical experience indicates that patients often report that CFS or FMS has an onset during or after a stressful period in their lives. The evidence for life stress or life events as precipitants of FMS and CFS is, however, both limited and retrospective (Anderberg et al. 2000; Theorell et al. 1999). One of the best studies so far published examined 64 patients and a similar number of matched control subjects. An excess of severe life events and difficulties was found in the CFS patients for the year prior to onset. More specifically, a certain type of life event called a *dilemma*—defined as an event in which the person must choose between two equally undesirable responses to circumstances—was reported by one-third of the patients with CFS and none of the control subjects (Hatcher and House 2003).

Perpetuating Factors

Perpetuating factors are those that maintain a condition once it is established. These factors are clinically the most important because they are potential targets for treatment.

Biological Factors

Chronic infection. There has been much interest in the potential role of ongoing infection and associated immunological factors, especially in CFS. It was previously thought that chronic Epstein-Barr virus was a cause of CFS, but that hypothesis has been rejected. There have been numerous reports of evidence of chronic infection with other agents in both CFS and FMS, but none has so far been substantiated.

Immunological abnormalities. Immunological factors, especially cytokines, have been investigated in CFS and FMS, not only because of the possible triggering effect of infection but also because immune-activating agents, such as interferons, are recognized to cause fatigue and myalgia. Systematic reviews, however, have found only suggestive evidence of any consistent immune abnormality in CFS (Blundell et al. 2015; Nijs et al. 2014).

Myopathic or biochemical abnormalities and physiological deconditioning. In patients with CFS or FMS, there are no proven pathological or biochemical abnormalities of muscle or muscle metabolism other than those expected with deconditioning. Deconditioning—the physiological changes that lead to the loss of tolerance of activity after prolonged rest—has been found in many patients with CFS (Nijs et al. 2011) and FMS (Jones et al. 2008). Deconditioning offers one biological explanation for exercise-induced fatigue and muscle pain in patients with CFS and FMS and provides a rationale for treatment with graded activity (see subsection "Nonpharmacological Treatments" later in this chapter).

Sleep abnormalities. Patients with CFS and FMS typically complain of unrefreshing and broken sleep, a symptom that has been confirmed with polysomnography. Abnormalities in sleep may be of etiological importance, especially in FMS. Early work (Moldofsky et al. 1975) identified a specific sleep electroencephalogram abnormality—alpha-wave intrusion into slow-wave sleep (so-called alpha–delta sleep)—as a possible cause of the myalgia. However, attempts to replicate this finding in both CFS and FMS have produced inconsistent results, and the specificity of this sleep anomaly to chronic pain remains unclear (Rains and Penzien 2003).

Neuroendocrine changes. Changes in the level and response of neuroendocrine stress hormones have been found in both CFS and FMS (Tak et al. 2011). Low blood cortisol and poor cortisol response to stress have been reported (Parker et al. 2001). These observations differ from findings in depression (in which blood levels of cortisol are typically elevated) but are similar to findings in other stress and anxiety states. It is not known whether low cortisol is a primary abnormality or a consequence of inactivity or sleep disruption. There is evidence that these low cortisol levels rise in response to successful cognitive-behavioral therapy (CBT) (Roberts et al. 2009) and also that low cortisol at baseline predicts a poorer response to CBT (Roberts et al. 2010).

Postural blood pressure dysregulation. Failure to maintain blood pressure when assuming an erect posture (orthostatic intolerance) and particularly a pattern in which the heart rate increases abnormally (postural orthostatic tachycardia syndrome) have been reported in both CFS (Rowe et al. 1995) and FMS (Bou-Holaigah et al. 1997). These findings have been interpreted as indicating abnormal autonomic nervous system function (Newton et al. 2009). However, postural hypotension commonly occurs in healthy persons after prolonged inactivity (Sandler and Vernikos 1986), and its specificity to CFS and FMS remains unclear (Roerink et al. 2017).

Brain structural changes.   The brains of patients with CFS and FMS are probably structurally normal, although a reduction in gray matter has been reported in both CFS (de Lange et al. 2005) and FMS (Burgmer et al. 2009). Findings have not been consistent between studies, however, and neurological findings in patients with FMS have been nonspecific (Murga et al. 2017). Interestingly, the reduction in gray matter appears to be at least partially reversed by treatment with CBT (de Lange et al. 2008).

Central nervous system functional changes.   Changes in central nervous system function are likely to be key in the etiology of CFS and FMS, and functional brain imaging has great potential to elucidate the biology of the mechanisms of fatigue and pain. However, use of brain imaging in these conditions remains in its infancy and has largely been limited to small poorly controlled studies. There is accumulating evidence of abnormal changes in functional connectivity and increased activation of pain systems in patients with FMS—findings that are consistent with a sensitization model (Cagnie et al. 2014). It is important to note, however, that changes in brain activation or brain reorganization should not be taken to mean that the symptoms are necessarily based in fixed neurological pathology; such changes can potentially be reversed through behavioral rehabilitation and drug therapy (Lazaridou et al. 2017).

Psychological and Social Factors

There is strong evidence that psychological and behavioral factors play a major role in perpetuating both CFS and FMS.

Illness beliefs.   One of the most striking aspects of CFS or FMS relates to the beliefs that many patients hold about the cause of their illness. Three categories of illness beliefs are considered here: 1) cause of symptoms (attributions), 2) significance of symptoms (catastrophizing), and 3) what one can do despite having symptoms (self-efficacy).

Although the causes of CFS and FMS are unknown, patients often strongly attribute their symptoms to a physical disease (Neerinckx et al. 2000). A systematic review of prognostic studies in CFS found that such strong attributions predicted a poorer outcome (Cairns and Hotopf 2005). It may be that such an attribution favors a focusing of attention on symptoms, more passive coping, and greater inactivity (Heijmans 1998) or, alternatively, that such an attribution leads to nonparticipation in potentially effective psychological and behavioral treatment.

Catastrophizing is a tendency to make excessively negative predictions about symptoms, such as "If I do more, my pain or fatigue will keep getting worse and worse." Catastrophizing has been observed in individuals with CFS (Nijs et al. 2008) and FMS (Estévez-López et al. 2016) and is associated with increased symptom vigilance, avoidance of activity, and more severe disability. Furthermore, a reduction in the belief that activity is damaging is associated with recovery during rehabilitative therapy (Chalder et al. 2015), suggesting that catastrophizing may be a critical target for effective rehabilitation.

Low self-efficacy, defined as a patient's lack of belief that he or she will be able to do something, is associated with more severe disability in CFS (Findley et al. 1998) and FMS (Estévez-López et al. 2016). Self-efficacy is therefore another potential target for treatment that aims to improve patient functioning.

Behavioral factors.   The ways in which patients cope with illness will be influenced by their beliefs about it (Silver et al. 2002). A fear-avoidance phenomenon—in which fear of exacerbating symptoms leads to avoidance of activity–has been well described in both CFS and FMS (Nijs et al. 2013). Objective assessment has confirmed that patients with CFS and FMS have reduced overall activity, with a quarter being pervasively inactive. This reduced activity produces deconditioning, and hence inactivity is a target for treatment.

Another potentially important coping behavior is symptom vigilance, defined as the focusing of attention on symptoms (Roelofs et al. 2003). This behavior is associated with catastrophizing beliefs and greater perceived symptom intensity, and therefore offers another target for treatment (Hughes et al. 2017).

Social factors.   Patients' beliefs about their illness, as well as the coping behaviors associated with these beliefs, are influenced by the information they receive from others. A striking social aspect of CFS and FMS is the vocal patient support and advocacy organizations, often supported by social media. These organizations often campaign against rehabilitation and against psychological and psychiatric involvement in patient care, both of which are seen as threats to the "medical status" of their illness (Murphy et al. 2016). Studies have suggested that patients who are members of such advocacy groups have poorer outcomes and poorer response to rehabilitation (Bentall et al. 2002). The beliefs and behavior of a patient's significant other may also influence the severity of disability (Band et al. 2015). Finally, an occupation that is perceived as stressful and financial compensation that is dependent on demonstration of persisting disability may both be barriers to rehabilitation.

Summary of Etiological Evidence

The available evidence suggests that patients are predisposed to develop CFS and FMS by a combination of genetics, previous experience, and possibly lack of social support. Many patients with CFS have a history of preceding infection, and many patients with FMS point to an accident, injury, or trauma as the triggering event. Others can identify no precipitant. Most research has focused on factors associated with established illness, so-called perpetuating factors, because they are more accessible to study and more relevant to treatment of established cases. Many biological factors have been investigated, with interest initially directed at peripheral nerves and muscles and subsequently focused on the functioning of the central nervous system and especially central sensitization to noxious stimuli. Findings have suggested—but have not yet established—a role for immune factors and possibly for ongoing infection. The physiological effects of inactivity may be important. There is good evidence for the importance of psychological and behavioral factors, especially the fear of exacerbating symptoms and the associated avoidance of activity in both CFS and FMS. Social factors are more difficult to study, but sometimes may be of obvious importance in individual cases.

Models of Chronic Fatigue and Fibromyalgia Syndromes

From the findings discussed in the previous section, three potentially complementary explanatory models for CFS and FMS can be discerned. These correspond approximately to biological, psychological, and social perspectives, although in reality elements of all three are probably relevant.

Biological Models

It is well known that the immune system, the central nervous system, and the endocrine system interact and have reciprocal relations with sleep and activity. It is thus possible to construct tentative biological models in which these systems interact to perpetuate the illness (Häuser et al. 2015a; Tomas et al. 2013). Although there appears to be stronger evidence for the role of infection in triggering CFS and for the role of trauma in FMS, it is unclear whether these represent real differences or simply differences in the hypotheses pursued by researchers.

Psychological Models

Whatever the biological aspects of CFS and FMS, psychological models assume that the symptoms and disability are perpetuated, at least in part, by psychological and behavioral factors (Nijs et al. 2013). Biological factors are not excluded from these models but are assumed to be either only partially responsible for the illness or largely reversible. The cognitive-behavioral models for chronic pain and CFS have much in common. Both emphasize the importance of fear of symptoms leading to a focusing on the symptoms, helplessness, and avoidance of activity. These models provide the rationale for behavioral (e.g., graded exercise) and cognitive-behavioral approaches to rehabilitation (see section "Management" later in this chapter).

Social Models

Social models emphasize the role of social factors in shaping CFS and FMS. A fight for the legitimacy of the syndrome as a chronic medical condition is prominent. Patient advocacy has been strongly hostile to psychological and psychiatric involvement, probably because it is seen as undermining legitimacy (Murphy et al. 2016). The social models propose that patient organizations, while providing valuable social support, can also reinforce patients' illness beliefs, medical care preferences, and disability payment seeking in ways that are not conducive to recovery (Shorter 1997).

Diagnostic Evaluation

Effective management of patients with possible CFS or FMS requires that 1) alternative medical and psychiatric diagnoses be considered and 2) all patients receive an adequately comprehensive assessment.

Identification of Medical and Psychiatric Conditions

Medical Differential Diagnosis

The medical differential diagnosis for CFS and FMS is lengthy because so many diseases can present with pain and/or fatigue (Sharpe and Wilks 2002; Yunus 2002; Table 25–4). Both physical and mental status examinations must be performed in every case to assess for alternative medical and psychiatric diagnoses. The duration of symptoms is important, because 75% of patients presenting to primary care with symptoms such as fatigue and pain improve within 2–4 weeks (Kroenke 2003). For persistent symptoms, most of the common medical disorders can be diagnosed from standard history, physical examination, and basic laboratory studies.

Routine investigations. Initial investigation focuses on the clinical signs, symptoms, and time course. When symptom duration exceeds 4–6 weeks, an initial basic screening workup is appropriate. If there are no specific indications for special investigations, the following are adequate as screening tests: thyrotropin, erythrocyte sedimentation rate, or similar measures of inflammation (sensitive for any condition with systemic inflammation), complete blood count, basic chemistries, and withdrawal of potential culprit medications (particularly statins, which typically require 4–6 weeks for symptom resolution after cessation).

Special investigations. Special investigations should be carried out only if clearly indicated by the history or examination. Immunological and virological tests are generally unhelpful. Sleep studies can be useful in excluding sleep apnea, narcolepsy, nocturnal myoclonus, and restless legs syndrome (see Chapter 14, "Sleep Disorders"). If a patient's symptoms are chronic (i.e., lasting more than 3 months) and remain unexplained, the recommended approach is to avoid excessive diagnostic testing, establish regular follow-up, screen for depressive and anxiety disorders, and focus on symptom management.

Medical misdiagnosis. Physicians who are concerned about missing a serious medical diagnosis can be reassured that in most cases, the physician's initial judgment regarding psychiatric or idiopathic etiology is likely to be accurate (Khan et al. 2003). However, there is some evidence that CFS and FMS may be misdiagnosed by primary care physicians (Fitzcharles and Boulos 2003); evaluating psychiatrists should therefore feel able to request a second medical opinion.

Psychiatric Differential Diagnosis

Psychiatric disorders may be missed in patients presenting with symptoms suggestive of CFS or FMS (Torres-Harding et al. 2002), probably because the medical assessment focuses on somatic symptoms. The most important psychiatric diagnoses to consider are depressive and anxiety disorders because of their frequency and their implications for treatment. Panic attacks with agoraphobia may cause intermittent severe fatigue and disability. Somatic symptom and related disorders are common and differ from anxiety disorders in their implications for management. A diagnosis of severe somatic symptom disorder indicates a poor prognosis, and a diagnosis of DSM-IV hypochondriasis warrants special attention to repeated reassurance seeking, which may perpetuate fears of undiagnosed disease (Sharpe and Williams 2001).

TABLE 25–4.   Medical differential diagnosis for patients with chronic fatigue syndrome (CFS) and fibromyalgia syndrome (FMS)

Relative frequency	Diagnoses	Syndrome	Differentiating clinical features	Initial workup
Very common (~1 per 100)	Thyroid disorders	CFS, FMS	Hypothyroidism: cold intolerance, slowed relaxation phase of reflexes, weight gain, elevated cholesterol Hyperthyroidism: heat intolerance, tremor, weight loss	Thyrotropin
	Medications (statins)	CFS, FMS	Symptom resolution with withdrawal of medication	Creatine kinase, aldolase
	Sleep apnea	CFS, FMS	Daytime somnolence, motor vehicle accidents, witnessed nighttime apnea and snoring, hypertension	Sleep study
	Spinal stenosis	FMS	History of osteoarthritis, degenerative disc disease, back pain with radiculopathy, sensory and/or motor deficits, pseudoclaudication	Nerve conduction study, electromyogram, magnetic resonance imaging of spine if neurological deficits
	Anemia	CFS	Pallor	Complete blood cell count
Common (~1 per 1,000)	Chronic infection: HIV, hepatitis C, endocarditis, osteomyelitis, Lyme disease, occult abscess	CFS, FMS	Infection-specific risk factors and signs (e.g., sexual habits, diabetes, fevers, murmur)	Serology, erythrocyte sedimentation rate, liver function tests, serial blood cultures, bone scan, indium scan
	Polymyalgia rheumatica	FMS	Age >60 years	Erythrocyte sedimentation rate
	Cancer	CFS	Pallor, anemia, anorexia, weight loss, cachexia	Complete blood cell count, albumin, age-appropriate cancer screening studies

TABLE 25–4. Medical differential diagnosis for patients with chronic fatigue syndrome (CFS) and fibromyalgia syndrome (FMS) *(continued)*

Relative frequency	Diagnoses	Syndrome	Differentiating clinical features	Initial workup
Common (~1 per 1,000) *(continued)*	Pulmonary condition: asthma, obstructive lung disease, interstitial lung disease	CFS	Shortness of breath, prominent exertional symptoms, smoking history, hypoxia	Chest X ray, pulmonary function tests, oxygenation saturation with exercise
	Rheumatoid arthritis	FMS	Symmetric synovitis, morning stiffness	Rheumatoid factor
	Inflammatory bowel disease (Crohn's)	CFS	Diarrhea, weight loss, fever, anemia	Serial fecal occult blood with endoscopy if positive
	Systemic lupus	FMS	Malar rash, joint pain	Antinuclear antibody, double-stranded DNA
Uncommon (~1 per 2,500–100,000)	Polymyositis, dermatomyositis, myopathy	CFS, FMS	Proximal muscle weakness	Antinuclear antibody, creatine kinase, aldolase
	Myasthenia gravis, multiple sclerosis	CFS	Neurological findings: extinguishing strength with repetitive movements, ptosis, swallowing difficulties, optic neuritis, sensory deficits	Tensilon test, acetylcholine receptor antibodies, magnetic resonance imaging of brain
	Narcolepsy	CFS	Drop attacks, falling asleep during daily activities	Sleep study
	Symptomatic hyperparathyroidism	CFS	Bone pain, nephrolithiasis, pancreatitis, renal insufficiency	Serum calcium and parathyroid hormone

Assessment of the Illness

Other than to make diagnoses, the aims of the assessment are to 1) establish a collaborative relationship with the patient, 2) elicit the patient's own understanding of his or her illness and how he or she copes with it, and 3) identify current family and social factors that may complicate management. It is especially important to inquire fully about the patient's understanding of his or her illness (e.g., "What do you think is wrong with you?" or "What do you think the cause is?"). Patients may be fearful that their symptoms indicate a progressive, not-yet-diagnosed disease or that exertion will cause a long-term worsening of their condition. A formulation that identifies potential predisposing, precipitating, and perpetuating factors (see Table 25–3) is valuable both in providing an individualized explanation to the patient and for targeting interventions.

Management

Diagnosis, Formulation, and Management Plan

Forming a Therapeutic Relationship With the Patient

It is important to understand the patient's expectations of the consultation, which may have been shaped by prior experiences (Asbring and Närvänen 2003). Previous doctors may have given overly biomedical or overly psychological explanations, or even dismissed the patient's complaints completely.

Explaining Psychiatric Involvement

A psychiatrist's involvement in management might be interpreted by patients as indicating that the condition is considered to be "all in the head." Consequently, it is best for the psychiatrist to begin with an assessment of the physical symptoms and only then to introduce a discussion of psychological factors. Explain that treatments commonly associated with psychiatry (particularly antidepressants and CBT) do not necessarily imply that the person has a mental disorder; rather, they can be seen as ways of normalizing brain and bodily functions in conditions that are exacerbated by stress (Sharpe and Carson 2001).

Giving the Diagnosis

Controversy exists about whether giving patients a diagnosis of CFS or FMS is helpful or harmful (Huibers and Wessely 2006). A positive diagnosis may enable patients both to conceptualize their illness and to communicate about it (Sharpe 1998); however, a diagnosis also may pathologize symptoms and increase disability (Hadler 1996). In our clinical experience, a positive diagnosis, if linked to a clear explanation of the potential reversibility of symptoms and a management plan, not only is a positive intervention in itself but also is an essential starting point from which to plan effective management.

Offering an Explanation

Ideally, the explanation offered should be scientifically accurate, acceptable to the patient, and congruent with the management plan. The clinician can explain that although the specific causes of CFS or FMS remain unknown, a combination of vulnerability and environmental stress that have changed the functioning of the brain and endocrine system is most likely. One such explanation is that the illness is probably a disorder of brain *function* rather than *structure* (Stone et al. 2002).

Explaining the Management Plan

The management plan should be explained to the patient as following from the etiological formulation, focusing on illness-perpetuating factors and consisting of elements intended to 1) relieve symptoms such as depression, pain, and sleep disturbance with agents such as antidepressants; 2) assist the patient's efforts at coping by stabilizing activity and retraining the body to function effectively (graded exercise, CBT); and 3) assist the patient in managing the social and financial aspects of his or her illness and, when possible, remaining in or returning to employment (problem solving).

General Measures

Providing Advice on Symptom Management

The clinician should encourage and guide patients in self-management of their illness. The overall aim is to encourage patients to feel that they can do things to manage the condition themselves, to accept the reality of their illness while still planning positively for the future, and to be cautious about seeking potentially harmful and expensive treatments.

Managing Activity and Avoidance

Once a patient's pattern of activity has been stabilized and large fluctuations between excessive rest and unsustainable activity reduced, very gradual increases in activity can be advised. It is critical, however, to distinguish between carefully graded increases carried out in collaboration with the patient and an overambitious exercise regimen.

Managing Occupational and Social Factors

Patients who continue working despite illness may become overstressed by the effort of doing this. Those who have left work because of illness may become inactive and demoralized. These situations require a problem-solving approach to manage work demands, achieve a graded return to work, or plan an alternative career. Ongoing litigation regarding the illness or financial benefits contingent on demonstrating persistent disability may need to be explicitly discussed with the patient.

Pharmacological Treatment

Most pharmacological treatment studies in CFS and FMS have focused on antidepressants, although various other agents have been advocated. None are generally effective (Collatz et al. 2016).

Antidepressants

Antidepressant drug treatment is indicated when patients have depressive and anxiety syndromes. Also, these agents can provide relief from pain and improve sleep, even in the absence of depression. Overall, there is evidence for the short-term efficacy of antidepressants in FMS (Häuser et al. 2009), but less evidence in CFS.

The tricyclic antidepressants (TCAs) are more effective than the selective serotonin reuptake inhibitors (SSRIs) for relieving pain and for inducing sleep. Small dosages (e.g., 25–50 mg/day of amitriptyline) are often adequate for these purposes. SSRIs are generally better tolerated than TCAs. However, in CFS, fluoxetine was found in a large trial to be no more effective than placebo (Vercoulen et al. 1996b), and in FMS, the benefit of SSRIs was reported to be small (Häuser et al. 2009).

Serotonin–norepinephrine reuptake inhibitors (SNRIs) such as venlafaxine, duloxetine, and milnacipran may be of modest benefit in FMS but may be less effective than TCAs in relieving pain (Häuser et al. 2009; Lunn et al. 2014). Other antidepressant agents may have some benefit; for example, some evidence supports the value of mirtazapine in CFS (Stubhaug et al. 2008).

Other Pharmacological Agents

Patients with CFS or FMS frequently take nonsteroidal anti-inflammatory drugs (NSAIDs) to relieve pain. However, no evidence from clinical trials indicates that NSAIDs are effective (Derry et al. 2017).

Opioids are occasionally used for pain relief in patients with CFS and FMS. However, there is little evidence for their efficacy, and adverse effects, including dependence, are major concerns (Chou et al. 2015).

With benzodiazepines, as with opioids, caution is required because of the risk of dependence. Sedative antidepressant drugs are preferable to benzodiazepines for treating insomnia, and benzodiazepines should be reserved for patients with intractable anxiety.

The anticonvulsants gabapentin and pregabalin may be effective in a minority of patients but may cause severe side effects (Cooper et al. 2017; Derry et al. 2016).

Stimulating medications such as bupropion, methylphenidate, dextroamphetamine, modafinil, and amantadine have all been reported to have value for other fatigue states (e.g., in multiple sclerosis) and have been advocated for use in CFS, but the evidence for their efficacy is very limited. Like opioids and benzodiazepines, stimulants pose a risk of dependence and abuse.

Summary of Pharmacological Treatments

Caution is required when prescribing pharmacological therapy for CFS and FMS. The mainstay of drug treatment continues to be the so-called antidepressant drugs, which may be helpful for mood, pain, and sleep (but not fatigue), but which have limited effect on overall outcome. TCAs are preferred for nighttime sedation and pain, but an SSRI or SNRI may be better tolerated. Although patients often receive low dosages of antidepressants, higher dosages may be required to achieve a therapeutic response when these medications are being prescribed to treat depression. In summary, the available evidence suggests that drug therapy currently has a limited role in the management of these conditions, and nonpharmacological therapies are preferred.

Nonpharmacological Treatments

For most patients, a trial of a rehabilitative outpatient program based on initial stabilization followed by appropriately planned increases in activity, either as graded exercise therapy (GET) or as CBT, is indicated.

Graded Exercise Therapy

GET is a structured progressive exercise program administered and carefully moni-tored by an exercise therapist. It also may be given in individual or group form, or even via Skype (Clark et al. 2017). GET follows the basic principles of exercise pre-scription for healthy individuals, adapted to the patient's current capacity. The initial exercise intensity and duration are individualized, sometimes by heart rate monitor-ing. The important principle is to calculate exercise capacity conservatively and tailor the program to the patient's individual exercise tolerance. At each clinic visit, joint planning of the exercise prescription for the following 1–2 weeks is completed. The initial aim is to establish a regular pattern of exercise (usually walking), with exercise 5 days per week. Home exercise sessions should initially last between 5 and 15 min-utes, depending on the patient's ability and exercise tolerance. The duration is in-creased by 1–2 minutes per week up to a maximum of 30 minutes per session. Then the intensity of exercise can be increased gradually. Patients will vary in their exercise tolerance and progress. Overexertion in an attempt to speed recovery can hinder re-covery or cause relapse. GET has been found in systematic reviews to be of benefit in both CFS and FMS (Bidonde et al. 2017; Larun et al. 2017).

Cognitive-Behavioral Therapy

CBT is not a single treatment but rather a family of treatments. In this section, the term refers to a collaborative, psychologically informed type of rehabilitation that aims to achieve both graded increases in activity and changes in unhelpful concerns about symptoms. In the context of CFS and FMS, CBT also may include problem solving for life and occupational dilemmas. CBT can be provided in an individual or a group form or online (Nijhof et al. 2012). The procedure is 1) to elicit each patient's own illness model and ways of coping; 2) to introduce the possibility of alternatives; and 3) to help patients select the beliefs and coping behaviors that they find most helpful by conducting behavioral experiments. A key question for the behavioral experi-ments is "Is it possible for me to make changes in my behavior that will allow me to achieve my goals?" Patients are encouraged to consider the possibility that their con-dition may at least in part be potentially reversible by their own efforts rather than being a fixed disease alterable only by medical intervention, and then to test out this idea. A typical course of therapy takes place over 5 months with 14 sessions (the first lasting 90 minutes, and the rest 50 minutes); the first 4 sessions are weekly and the remainder are biweekly.

In CFS, individually administered CBT has been tested in trials that together have included more than 1,000 patients and has been found to be moderately effective and safe (Marques et al. 2015; Price et al. 2008). CBT is also of moderate benefit for fibro-myalgia (Bernardy et al. 2013).

Patients Who Do Not Respond to Treatment

Most patients with CFS or FMS respond to some degree to rehabilitative therapies, but many will achieve only partial improvement, and some will fail to improve at all. In such cases, the management is the same as for other chronic conditions: maximize functioning and quality of life while minimizing the risk of iatrogenic harm. A bal-ance must be struck between advocating additional treatment and facilitating acceptance of a chronic illness. Many physicians are reluctant to accept chronic disability in patients with CFS or FMS, perhaps because these physicians do not regard them as being true diseases. However, pushing patients beyond their capabilities may only demoralize them and promote invalidism. For such patients, regular supportive long-term follow-up from a single physician is often the best management.

Conclusion

Although sometimes seen as peripheral to both internal medicine and psychiatry, syndromes such as CFS and FMS are common and core to the practice of consultation-liaison psychiatry. The ability of the consultation-liaison psychiatrist to integrate biological, psychological, and social factors is essential to achieve an adequate understanding of these syndromes and to implement effective management.

References

Afari N, Buchwald D: Chronic fatigue syndrome: a review. Am J Psychiatry 160(2):221–236, 2003 12562565

Afari N, Ahumada SM, Wright LJ, et al: Psychological trauma and functional somatic syndromes: a systematic review and meta-analysis. Psychosom Med 76(1):2–11, 2014 24336429

Al-Allaf AW, Dunbar KL, Hallum NS, et al: A case-control study examining the role of physical trauma in the onset of fibromyalgia syndrome. Rheumatology (Oxford) 41(4):450–453, 2002 11961177

American Psychiatric Association: Diagnostic and Statistical Manual of Mental Disorders, 4th Edition. Washington, DC, American Psychiatric Association, 1994

American Psychiatric Association: Diagnostic and Statistical Manual of Mental Disorders, 5th Edition. Arlington, VA, American Psychiatric Association, 2013

Anderberg UM, Marteinsdottir I, Theorell T, et al: The impact of life events in female patients with fibromyalgia and in female healthy controls. Eur Psychiatry 15(5):295–301, 2000 10954873

Asbring P, Närvänen AL: Ideal versus reality: physicians perspectives on patients with chronic fatigue syndrome (CFS) and fibromyalgia. Soc Sci Med 57(4):711–720, 2003 12821018

Assefi NP, Coy TV, Uslan D, et al: Financial, occupational, and personal consequences of disability in patients with chronic fatigue syndrome and fibromyalgia compared to other fatiguing conditions. J Rheumatol 30(4):804–808, 2003 12672203

Ayres JG, Flint N, Smith EG, et al: Post-infection fatigue syndrome following Q fever. QJM 91(2):105–123, 1998 9578893

Band R, Wearden A, Barrowclough C: Patient outcomes in association with significant other responses to chronic fatigue syndrome: a systematic review of the literature. Clin Psychol (New York) 22(1):29–46, 2015 26617440

Bentall RP, Powell P, Nye FJ, et al: Predictors of response to treatment for chronic fatigue syndrome. Br J Psychiatry 181:248–252, 2002 12204931

Berelowitz GJ, Burgess AP, Thanabalasingham T, et al: Post-hepatitis syndrome revisited. J Viral Hepat 2(3):133–138, 1995 7493307

Bernardy K, Klose P, Busch AJ, et al: Cognitive behavioural therapies for fibromyalgia. Cochrane Database Syst Rev (9):CD009796, 2013 24018611

Bidonde J, Busch AJ, Schachter CL, et al: Aerobic exercise training for adults with fibromyalgia. Cochrane Database Syst Rev (6):CD012700, 2017 28636204

Blundell S, Ray KK, Buckland M, et al: Chronic fatigue syndrome and circulating cytokines: a systematic review. Brain Behav Immun 50:186–195, 2015 26148446

Bombardier CH, Buchwald D: Chronic fatigue, chronic fatigue syndrome, and fibromyalgia. Disability and health-care use. Med Care 34(9):924–930, 1996 8792781

Bou-Holaigah I, Calkins H, Flynn JA, et al: Provocation of hypotension and pain during upright tilt table testing in adults with fibromyalgia. Clin Exp Rheumatol 15(3):239–246, 1997 9177917

Brurberg KG, Fønhus MS, Larun L, et al: Case definitions for chronic fatigue syndrome/myalgic encephalomyelitis (CFS/ME): a systematic review. BMJ Open 4(2):e003973, 2014 24508851

Buchwald D, Herrell R, Ashton S, et al: A twin study of chronic fatigue. Psychosom Med 63(6):936–943, 2001 11719632

Burgmer M, Gaubitz M, Konrad C, et al: Decreased gray matter volumes in the cingulo-frontal cortex and the amygdala in patients with fibromyalgia. Psychosom Med 71(5):566–573, 2009 19414621

Buskila D, Neumann L: Fibromyalgia syndrome (FM) and nonarticular tenderness in relatives of patients with FM. J Rheumatol 24(5):941–944, 1997 9150086

Buskila D, Press J, Abu-Shakra M: Fibromyalgia in systemic lupus erythematosus: prevalence and clinical implications. Clin Rev Allergy Immunol 25(1):25–28, 2003 12794258

Cagnie B, Coppieters I, Denecker S, et al: Central sensitization in fibromyalgia? A systematic review on structural and functional brain MRI. Semin Arthritis Rheum 44(1):68–75, 2014 24508406

Cairns R, Hotopf M: A systematic review describing the prognosis of chronic fatigue syndrome. Occup Med (Lond) 55(1):20–31, 2005 15699087

Chalder T, Goldsmith KA, White PD, et al: Rehabilitative therapies for chronic fatigue syndrome: a secondary mediation analysis of the PACE trial. Lancet Psychiatry 2(2):141–152, 2015 26359750

Chen J, Tsuchiya M, Kawakami N, et al: Non-fearful vs. fearful panic attacks: a general population study from the National Comorbidity Survey. J Affect Disord 112(1–3):273–278, 2009 18534684

Chou R, Turner JA, Devine EB, et al: The effectiveness and risks of long-term opioid therapy for chronic pain: a systematic review for a National Institutes of Health Pathways to Prevention Workshop. Ann Intern Med 162(4):276–286, 2015 25581257

Clark LV, Pesola F, Thomas JM, et al: Guided graded exercise self-help plus specialist medical care versus specialist medical care alone for chronic fatigue syndrome (GETSET): a pragmatic randomised controlled trial. Lancet 390(10092):363–373, 2017 28648402

Collatz A, Johnston SC, Staines DR, et al: A systematic review of drug therapies for chronic fatigue syndrome/myalgic encephalomyelitis. Clin Ther 38(6):1263.e9–1271.e9, 2016 27229907

Cooper TE, Derry S, Wiffen PJ, et al: Gabapentin for fibromyalgia pain in adults. Cochrane Database Syst Rev (1):CD012188, 2017 28045473

Coppens E, Van Wambeke P, Morlion B, et al: Prevalence and impact of childhood adversities and post-traumatic stress disorder in women with fibromyalgia and chronic widespread pain. Eur J Pain 21(9):1582–1590, 2017 28543929

Creavin ST, Dunn KM, Mallen CD, et al: Co-occurrence and associations of pain and fatigue in a community sample of Dutch adults. Eur J Pain 14(3):327–334, 2010 19540139

Croft P, Rigby AS, Boswell R, et al: The prevalence of chronic widespread pain in the general population. J Rheumatol 20(4):710–713, 1993 8496870

Croft P, Burt J, Schollum J, et al: More pain, more tender points: is fibromyalgia just one end of a continuous spectrum? Ann Rheum Dis 55(7):482–485, 1996 8774169

Dansie EJ, Heppner P, Furberg H, et al: The comorbidity of self-reported chronic fatigue syndrome, post-traumatic stress disorder, and traumatic symptoms. Psychosomatics 53(3):250–257, 2012 22296866

de Lange FP, Kalkman JS, Bleijenberg G, et al: Gray matter volume reduction in the chronic fatigue syndrome. Neuroimage 26(3):777–781, 2005 15955487

de Lange FP, Koers A, Kalkman JS, et al: Increase in prefrontal cortical volume following cognitive behavioural therapy in patients with chronic fatigue syndrome. Brain 131(Pt 8):2172–2180, 2008 18587150

Derry S, Cording M, Wiffen PJ, et al: Pregabalin for pain in fibromyalgia in adults. Cochrane Database Syst Rev (9):CD011790, 2016 27684492

Derry S, Wiffen PJ, Häuser W, et al: Oral nonsteroidal anti-inflammatory drugs for fibromyalgia in adults. Cochrane Database Syst Rev (3):CD012332, 2017 28349517

Dimsdale JE, Creed F, Escobar J, et al: Somatic symptom disorder: an important change in DSM. J Psychosom Res 75(3):223–228, 2013 23972410

Dreyer L, Kendall S, Danneskiold-Samsøe B, et al: Mortality in a cohort of Danish patients with fibromyalgia: increased frequency of suicide. Arthritis Rheum 62(10):3101–3108, 2010 20583101

Engel GL: The need for a new medical model: a challenge for biomedicine. Science 196(4286):129–136, 1977 847460

Epstein SA, Kay G, Clauw D, et al: Psychiatric disorders in patients with fibromyalgia. A multicenter investigation. Psychosomatics 40(1):57–63, 1999 9989122

Estévez-López F, Álvarez-Gallardo IC, Segura-Jiménez V, et al: The discordance between subjectively and objectively measured physical function in women with fibromyalgia: association with catastrophizing and self-efficacy cognitions. The al-Ándalus project. Disabil Rehabil Dec 15:1–9, 2016 27973914

Findley JC, Kerns R, Weinberg LD, et al: Self-efficacy as a psychological moderator of chronic fatigue syndrome. J Behav Med 21(4):351–362, 1998 9789165

Fischler B, Cluydts R, De Gucht Y, et al: Generalized anxiety disorder in chronic fatigue syndrome. Acta Psychiatr Scand 95(5):405–413, 1997 9197905

Fitzcharles MA, Boulos P: Inaccuracy in the diagnosis of fibromyalgia syndrome: analysis of referrals. Rheumatology (Oxford) 42(2):263–267, 2003 12595620

Fukuda K, Straus SE, Hickie I, et al; International Chronic Fatigue Syndrome Study Group: The chronic fatigue syndrome: a comprehensive approach to its definition and study. Ann Intern Med 121(12):953–959, 1994 7978722

Gowers WR: A lecture on lumbago: its lessons and analogues: delivered at the National Hospital for the Paralysed and Epileptic. BMJ 1(2246):117–121, 1904 20761312

Granges G, Zilko P, Littlejohn GO: Fibromyalgia syndrome: assessment of the severity of the condition 2 years after diagnosis. J Rheumatol 21(3):523–529, 1994 8006897

Hadler NM: If you have to prove you are ill, you can't get well. The object lesson of fibromyalgia. Spine 21(20):2397–2400, 1996 8915080

Harvey SB, Wadsworth M, Wessely S, et al: Etiology of chronic fatigue syndrome: testing popular hypotheses using a national birth cohort study. Psychosom Med 70(4):488–495, 2008 18378866

Hatcher S, House A: Life events, difficulties and dilemmas in the onset of chronic fatigue syndrome: a case-control study. Psychol Med 33(7):1185–1192, 2003 14580073

Häuser W, Bernardy K, Uçeyler N, et al: Treatment of fibromyalgia syndrome with antidepressants: a meta-analysis. JAMA 301(2):198–209, 2009 19141768

Häuser W, Ablin J, Fitzcharles MA, et al: Fibromyalgia. Nat Rev Dis Primers 1:15022, 2015a 27189527

Häuser W, Bialas P, Welsch K, et al: Construct validity and clinical utility of current research criteria of DSM-5 somatic symptom disorder diagnosis in patients with fibromyalgia syndrome. J Psychosom Res 78(6):546–552, 2015b 25864805

Heijmans MJ: Coping and adaptive outcome in chronic fatigue syndrome: importance of illness cognitions. J Psychosom Res 45(1):39–51, 1998 9720854

Henningsen P, Zimmermann T, Sattel H: Medically unexplained physical symptoms, anxiety, and depression: a meta-analytic review. Psychosom Med 65(4):528–533, 2003 12883101

Hill NF, Tiersky LA, Scavalla VR, et al: Natural history of severe chronic fatigue syndrome. Arch Phys Med Rehabil 80(9):1090–1094, 1999 10489014

Holmes GP, Kaplan JE, Gantz NM, et al: Chronic fatigue syndrome: a working case definition. Ann Intern Med 108(3):387–389, 1988 2829679

Hotopf M, Noah N, Wessely S: Chronic fatigue and minor psychiatric morbidity after viral meningitis: a controlled study. J Neurol Neurosurg Psychiatry 60(5):504–509, 1996 8778253

Hudson JI, Pope HG Jr: The relationship between fibromyalgia and major depressive disorder. Rheum Dis Clin North Am 22(2):285–303, 1996 8860800

Hughes AM, Chalder T, Hirsch CR, et al: An attention and interpretation bias for illness-specific information in chronic fatigue syndrome. Psychol Med 47(5):853–865, 2017 27894380

Huibers MJ, Wessely S: The act of diagnosis: pros and cons of labelling chronic fatigue syndrome. Psychol Med 36(7):895–900, 2006 16403245

Institute of Medicine: Beyond Myalgic Encephalomyelitis/Chronic Fatigue Syndrome: Redefining an Illness. Washington, DC, The National Academies Press, 2015

Janssens KA, Zijlema WL, Joustra ML, et al: Mood and anxiety disorders in chronic fatigue syndrome, fibromyalgia, and irritable bowel syndrome: results from the LifeLines cohort study. Psychosom Med 77(4):449–457, 2015 25768845

Jason LA, Richman JA, Rademaker AW, et al: A community-based study of chronic fatigue syndrome. Arch Intern Med 159(18):2129–2137, 1999 10527290

Johnston S, Brenu EW, Staines D, et al: The prevalence of chronic fatigue syndrome/myalgic encephalomyelitis: a meta-analysis. Clin Epidemiol 5:105–110, 2013 23576883

Jones GT, Atzeni F, Beasley M, et al: The prevalence of fibromyalgia in the general population: a comparison of the American College of Rheumatology 1990, 2010, and modified 2010 classification criteria. Arthritis Rheumatol 67(2):568–575, 2015 25323744

Jones J, Rutledge DN, Jones KD, et al: Self-assessed physical function levels of women with fibromyalgia: a national survey. Womens Health Issues 18(5):406–412, 2008 18723374

Kanaan RA, Lepine JP, Wessely SC: The association or otherwise of the functional somatic syndromes. Psychosom Med 69(9):855–859, 2007 18040094

Kato K, Sullivan PF, Evengård B, et al: Chronic widespread pain and its comorbidities: a population-based study. Arch Intern Med 166(15):1649–1654, 2006 16908799

Kerr JR, Mattey DL: Preexisting psychological stress predicts acute and chronic fatigue and arthritis following symptomatic parvovirus B19 infection. Clin Infect Dis 46(9):e83–e87, 2008 18419428

Khan AA, Khan A, Harezlak J, et al: Somatic symptoms in primary care: etiology and outcome. Psychosomatics 44(6):471–478, 2003 14597681

Kroenke K: Patients presenting with somatic complaints: epidemiology, psychiatric comorbidity and management. Int J Methods Psychiatr Res 12(1):34–43, 2003 12830308

Lacourt T, Houtveen J, van Doornen L: "Functional somatic syndromes, one or many?" An answer by cluster analysis. J Psychosom Res 74(1):6–11, 2013 23272982

Larun L, Brurberg KG, Odgaard-Jensen J, Price JR: Exercise therapy for chronic fatigue syndrome. Cochrane Database Syst Rev (4):CD003200, 2017 28444695

Lazaridou A, Kim J, Cahalan CM, et al: Effects of cognitive-behavioral therapy (CBT) on brain connectivity supporting catastrophizing in fibromyalgia. Clin J Pain 33(3):215–221, 2017 27518491

Lunn MP, Hughes RA, Wiffen PJ: Duloxetine for treating painful neuropathy, chronic pain or fibromyalgia. Cochrane Database Syst Rev (1):CD007115, 2014 24385423

Manu P, Matthews DA, Lane TJ: Panic disorder among patients with chronic fatigue. South Med J 84(4):451–456, 1991 2014428

Marques MM, De Gucht V, Gouveia MJ, et al: Differential effects of behavioral interventions with a graded physical activity component in patients suffering from chronic fatigue (syndrome): an updated systematic review and meta-analysis. Clin Psychol Rev 40:123–137, 2015 26112761

Moldofsky H, Scarisbrick P, England R, et al: Musculoskeletal symptoms and non-REM sleep disturbance in patients with "fibrositis syndrome" and healthy subjects. Psychosom Med 37(4):341–351, 1975 169541

Murga I, Guillen V, Lafuente JV: Cerebral magnetic resonance changes associated with fibromyalgia syndrome. Med Clin (Barc) 148(11):511–516, 2017 28450073

Murphy M, Kontos N, Freudenreich O: Electronic support groups: an open line of communication in contested illness. Psychosomatics 57(6):547–555, 2016 27421707

Neerinckx E, Van Houdenhove B, Lysens R, et al: Attributions in chronic fatigue syndrome and fibromyalgia syndrome in tertiary care. J Rheumatol 27(4):1051–1055, 2000 10782836

Newton JL, Sheth A, Shin J, et al: Lower ambulatory blood pressure in chronic fatigue syndrome. Psychosom Med 71(3):361–365, 2009 19297309

Nijhof SL, Bleijenberg G, Uiterwaal CS, et al: Effectiveness of Internet-based cognitive behavioural treatment for adolescents with chronic fatigue syndrome (FITNET): a randomised controlled trial. Lancet 379(9824):1412–1418, 2012 22385683

Nijs J, Van de Putte K, Louckx F, et al: Exercise performance and chronic pain in chronic fatigue syndrome: the role of pain catastrophizing. Pain Med 9(8):1164–1172, 2008 19086101

Nijs J, Aelbrecht S, Meeus M, et al: Tired of being inactive: a systematic literature review of physical activity, physiological exercise capacity and muscle strength in patients with chronic fatigue syndrome. Disabil Rehabil 33(17–18):1493–1500, 2011 21166613

Nijs J, Roussel N, Van Oosterwijck J, et al: Fear of movement and avoidance behaviour toward physical activity in chronic-fatigue syndrome and fibromyalgia: state of the art and implications for clinical practice. Clin Rheumatol 32(8):1121–1129, 2013 23639990

Nijs J, Nees A, Paul L, et al: Altered immune response to exercise in patients with chronic fatigue syndrome/myalgic encephalomyelitis: a systematic literature review. Exerc Immunol Rev 20:94–116, 2014 24974723

Nisenbaum R, Jones JF, Unger ER, et al: A population-based study of the clinical course of chronic fatigue syndrome. Health Qual Life Outcomes 1:49, 2003 14613572

Ohayon MM, Schatzberg AF: Using chronic pain to predict depressive morbidity in the general population. Arch Gen Psychiatry 60(1):39–47, 2003 12511171

Parker AJ, Wessely S, Cleare AJ: The neuroendocrinology of chronic fatigue syndrome and fibromyalgia. Psychol Med 31(8):1331–1345, 2001 11722149

Pawlikowska T, Chalder T, Hirsch SR, et al: Population based study of fatigue and psychological distress. BMJ 308(6931):763–766, 1994 7908238

Price JR, Mitchell E, Tidy E, Hunot V: Cognitive behaviour therapy for chronic fatigue syndrome in adults. Cochrane Database Syst Rev (3):CD001027, 2008 18646067

Prins JB, van der Meer JW, Bleijenberg G: Chronic fatigue syndrome. Lancet 367(9507):346–355, 2006 16443043

Rains JC, Penzien DB: Sleep and chronic pain: challenges to the alpha-EEG sleep pattern as a pain specific sleep anomaly. J Psychosom Res 54(1):77–83, 2003 12505558

Rea T, Russo J, Katon W, et al: A prospective study of tender points and fibromyalgia during and after an acute viral infection. Arch Intern Med 159(8):865–870, 1999 10219933

Reeves WC, Lloyd A, Vernon SD, et al; International Chronic Fatigue Syndrome Study Group: Identification of ambiguities in the 1994 chronic fatigue syndrome research case definition and recommendations for resolution. BMC Health Serv Res 3(1):25, 2003 14702202

Reyes M, Nisenbaum R, Hoaglin DC, et al: Prevalence and incidence of chronic fatigue syndrome in Wichita, Kansas. Arch Intern Med 163(13):1530–1536, 2003 12860574

Roberts AD, Papadopoulos AS, Wessely S, et al: Salivary cortisol output before and after cognitive behavioural therapy for chronic fatigue syndrome. J Affect Disord 115(1–2):280–286, 2009 18937978

Roberts AD, Charler ML, Papadopoulos A, et al: Does hypocortisolism predict a poor response to cognitive behavioural therapy in chronic fatigue syndrome? Psychol Med 40(3):515–522, 2010 19607750

Roberts E, Wessely S, Chalder T, et al: Mortality of people with chronic fatigue syndrome: a retrospective cohort study in England and Wales from the South London and Maudsley NHS Foundation Trust Biomedical Research Centre (SLaM BRC) Clinical Record Interactive Search (CRIS) Register. Lancet 387(10028):1638–1643, 2016 26873808

Roelofs J, Peters ML, McCracken L, et al: The Pain Vigilance and Awareness Questionnaire (PVAQ): further psychometric evaluation in fibromyalgia and other chronic pain syndromes. Pain 101(3):299–306, 2003 12583873

Roerink ME, Lenders JW, Schmits IC, et al: Postural orthostatic tachycardia is not a useful diagnostic marker for chronic fatigue syndrome. J Intern Med 281(2):179–188, 2017 27696568

Rowe PC, Bou-Holaigah I, Kan JS, et al: Is neurally mediated hypotension an unrecognised cause of chronic fatigue? Lancet 345(8950):623–624, 1995 7898182

Russell IJ, Orr MD, Littman B, et al: Elevated cerebrospinal fluid levels of substance P in patients with the fibromyalgia syndrome. Arthritis Rheum 37(11):1593–1601, 1994 7526868

Sandler H, Vernikos J: Inactivity: Physiological Effects. London, Academic Press, 1986

Sartorius N, Üstün TB, Costa e Silva JA, et al: An international study of psychological problems in primary care. Preliminary report from the World Health Organization Collaborative Project on "Psychological Problems in General Health Care." Arch Gen Psychiatry 50(10):819–824, 1993 8215805

Servaes P, Prins J, Verhagen S, et al: Fatigue after breast cancer and in chronic fatigue syndrome: similarities and differences. J Psychosom Res 52(6):453–459, 2002 12069869

Sharpe M: Chronic fatigue syndrome. Psychiatr Clin North Am 19(3):549–573, 1996 8856816

Sharpe M: Doctors' diagnoses and patients' perceptions. Lessons from chronic fatigue syndrome. Gen Hosp Psychiatry 20(6):335–338, 1998 9854644

Sharpe M, Carson A: "Unexplained" somatic symptoms, functional syndromes, and somatization: do we need a paradigm shift? Ann Intern Med 134(9 Pt 2):926–930, 2001 11346330

Sharpe M, Wilks D: Fatigue. BMJ 325(7362):480–483, 2002 12202331

Sharpe M, Williams A: Treating patients with hypochondriasis and somatoform pain disorder, in Psychological Approaches to Pain Management. Edited by Turk DC, Gatchel RJ. New York, Guilford, 2001, pp 515–533

Shorter E: From Paralysis to Fatigue: A History of Psychosomatic Illness in the Modern Era. New York, Free Press, 1992

Shorter E: Somatization and chronic pain in historic perspective. Clin Orthop Relat Res (336):52–60, 1997 9060486

Silver A, Haeney M, Vijayadurai P, et al: The role of fear of physical movement and activity in chronic fatigue syndrome. J Psychosom Res 52(6):485–493, 2002 12069873

Skapinakis P, Lewis G, Meltzer H: Clarifying the relationship between unexplained chronic fatigue and psychiatric morbidity: results from a community survey in Great Britain. Am J Psychiatry 157(9):1492–1498, 2000 10964867

Stone J, Wojcik W, Durrance D, et al: What should we say to patients with symptoms unexplained by disease? The "number needed to offend." BMJ 325(7378):1449–1450, 2002 12493661

Stubhaug B, Lie SA, Ursin H, et al: Cognitive-behavioural therapy v. mirtazapine for chronic fatigue and neurasthenia: randomised placebo-controlled trial. Br J Psychiatry 192(3):217–223, 2008 18310583

Sullivan PF, Smith W, Buchwald D: Latent class analysis of symptoms associated with chronic fatigue syndrome and fibromyalgia. Psychol Med 32(5):881–888, 2002 12171382

Tak LM, Cleare AJ, Ormel J, et al: Meta-analysis and meta-regression of hypothalamic-pituitary-adrenal axis activity in functional somatic disorders. Biol Psychol 87(2):183–194, 2011 21315796

Theorell T, Blomkvist V, Lindh G, et al: Critical life events, infections, and symptoms during the year preceding chronic fatigue syndrome (CFS): an examination of CFS patients and subjects with a nonspecific life crisis. Psychosom Med 61(3):304–310, 1999 10367610

Tomas C, Newton J, Watson S: A review of hypothalamic-pituitary-adrenal axis function in chronic fatigue syndrome. ISRN Neurosci 2013:784520, 2013 24959566

Torres-Harding SR, Jason LA, Cane V, et al: Physicians' diagnoses of psychiatric disorders for people with chronic fatigue syndrome. Int J Psychiatry Med 32(2):109–124, 2002 12269593

van der Werf SP, de Vree B, Alberts M, et al; Netherlands Fatigue Research Group Nijmegen: Natural course and predicting self-reported improvement in patients with chronic fatigue syndrome with a relatively short illness duration. J Psychosom Res 53(3):749–753, 2002 12217448

Vercoulen JH, Hommes OR, Swanink CM, et al: The measurement of fatigue in patients with multiple sclerosis. A multidimensional comparison with patients with chronic fatigue syndrome and healthy subjects. Arch Neurol 53(7):642–649, 1996a 8929171

Vercoulen JH, Swanink CM, Zitman FG, et al: Randomised, double-blind, placebo-controlled study of fluoxetine in chronic fatigue syndrome. Lancet 347(9005):858–861, 1996b 8622391

Wessely S: Old wine in new bottles: neurasthenia and "ME." Psychol Med 20(1):35–53, 1990 2181519

Wessely S, Nimnuan C, Sharpe M: Functional somatic syndromes: one or many? Lancet 354(9182):936–939, 1999 10489969

White KP, Speechley M, Harth M, et al: The London Fibromyalgia Epidemiology Study: the prevalence of fibromyalgia syndrome in London, Ontario. J Rheumatol 26(7):1570–1576, 1999 10405947

White PD, Thomas JM, Kangro HO, et al: Predictions and associations of fatigue syndromes and mood disorders that occur after infectious mononucleosis. Lancet 358(9297):1946–1954, 2001 11747919

Wolfe F: The relation between tender points and fibromyalgia symptom variables: evidence that fibromyalgia is not a discrete disorder in the clinic. Ann Rheum Dis 56(4):268–271, 1997 9166001

Wolfe F, Cathey MA, Kleinheksel SM: Fibrositis (fibromyalgia) in rheumatoid arthritis. J Rheumatol 11(6):814–818, 1984 6596431

Wolfe F, Smythe HA, Yunus MB, et al: The American College of Rheumatology 1990 criteria for the classification of fibromyalgia: report of the Multicenter Criteria Committee. Arthritis Rheum 33(2):160–172, 1990 2306288

Wolfe F, Clauw DJ, Fitzcharles MA, et al: The American College of Rheumatology preliminary diagnostic criteria for fibromyalgia and measurement of symptom severity. Arthritis Care Res (Hoboken) 62(5):600–610, 2010 20461783

World Health Organization: International Statistical Classification of Diseases and Related Health Problems, 10th Revision. Geneva, World Health Organization, 1992

Yunus MB: A comprehensive medical evaluation of patients with fibromyalgia syndrome. Rheum Dis Clin North Am 28(2):201–217, v–vi, 2002 12122914

CHAPTER 26

Infectious Diseases

James L. Levenson, M.D.
Christopher Kogut, M.D.

Psychiatric symptoms are part of the clinical presentation of many systemic and central nervous system (CNS) infectious processes. Rapid cultural and economic changes affecting regional and international mobility, sexuality, and other behaviors have led to the worldwide spread of new epidemics (e.g., HIV, Ebola) and more limited spread of previously geographically isolated diseases (e.g., cysticercosis). Infectious diseases have been considered in the pathogenesis of psychiatric disorders (e.g., viral antibodies in schizophrenia). Associations between specific infections and psychiatric syndromes (e.g., pediatric autoimmune neuropsychiatric disorder associated with streptococcal infection [PANDAS]) provide intriguing models of etiology. Controversy surrounds some attributions of psychopathology to infections (e.g., Lyme disease).

Consulting psychiatrists should carefully consider relevant aspects of patients' histories, including immune status, regions of origin and residence, travel, high-risk sexual behaviors, occupation, and recreational activities. Physicians must consider which infectious diseases are endemic in their area and wherever the patient has traveled or resided. Similar neuropsychiatric symptoms might suggest possible Lyme disease in a hiker in the northeastern United States and neurocysticercosis in an immigrant from Central America.

Many brain diseases or injuries, as well as the effects of aging, render patients more vulnerable to neuropsychiatric effects of even limited infectious diseases. For example, a simple upper respiratory or bladder infection may cause only discomfort in otherwise healthy individuals but may lead to agitation, irritability, and frank delirium in elderly persons, especially those with dementia. The reasons that older age and brain

The authors wish to acknowledge Crystal C. Watkins, M.D., Ph.D.; Niccolo D. Della Penna, M.D.; Andrew A. Angelino, M.D.; and Glenn J. Treisman, M.D., Ph.D., who were authors of the chapter on HIV/AIDS in the previous edition of *The American Psychiatric Publishing Textbook of Psychosomatic Medicine: Psychiatric Care of the Medically Ill.*

disease make patients vulnerable to delirium with minor infections are not understood but may involve changes in immune function and the blood–brain barrier.

Psychological factors may significantly affect the risk for and course of infectious diseases, with HIV as the most studied example. A large Danish cohort study found that among patients hospitalized for infection, 30-day mortality was 52% higher for individuals with a history of severe mental illness than for those without (Ribe et al. 2015). Psychological factors have been shown to influence other infectious diseases as well, from the common cold (Adam et al. 2013) to viral hepatitis infection (Osher et al. 2003). One mechanism for such effects is through poor sleep (Prather et al. 2015).

This chapter offers an overview of bacterial, viral (including prion disease), fungal, and parasitic infections, followed by a review of psychiatric side effects of antimicrobial drugs and their interactions with psychotropic medications. The chapter closes with a discussion of fears of infectious disease and psychiatric aspects of immunization.

Occult Infections

Occult infections, irrespective of location, by definition are concealed, requiring diagnostic detective work. Such infections may occur anywhere in the body (Table 26–1). Psychiatric symptoms may result from even a small focus of chronic infection. The most likely symptoms are subtle cognitive dysfunction or mood change (e.g., irritability) consistent with a mild encephalopathy, but depression, psychosis, and delirium also may occur.

The diagnosis is suggested by secondary signs of infection, specifically fever and increases in white blood cell count, granulocyte count, and sedimentation rate. A careful history and physical examination may identify overlooked clues (e.g., chronic toothache or lymphadenopathy). If repeat history and physical examination are not fruitful, other studies may be needed (e.g., serologies, imaging, cerebrospinal fluid [CSF] examination).

Bacterial Infections

Bacteremia and Sepsis

Bacteremia literally means entry of bacteria into the bloodstream, whereas *sepsis* refers to the systemic inflammatory response to bacteremia. Systemic symptoms of sepsis result from many different mechanisms, including bacterial toxins, release of cytokines, hyperthermia, shock (poor perfusion), acute renal insufficiency, pulmonary failure ("shock lung"), coagulopathy, disruption of the blood–brain barrier, and spread of the organism into the CNS and other organs. An acute change in mental status may be the first sign of impending sepsis and may precede the development of fever. A patient who has an abrupt change in mental status in concert with a shaking chill should be presumed to be at risk for impending sepsis.

Septic encephalopathy is often part of multiorgan failure (Tsuruta and Oda 2016). Standard treatment is initially broad-spectrum antibiotics, followed by agents tailored to the identified organism and its antimicrobial susceptibilities. Symptoms of acute

TABLE 26–1. **Occult infections that may cause psychiatric symptoms**

Sinusitis

Chronic otitis

Abscess (e.g., dental, lung, intra-abdominal, retroperitoneal, perirectal)

Bronchiectasis

Endocarditis

Cholecystitis

Parasitosis

Urinary tract infection

Pelvic inflammatory disease

Osteomyelitis

Subclinical systemic infections (e.g., HIV, tuberculosis)

and posttraumatic stress disorders are very common following septic shock (Wintermann et al. 2015).

Toxic shock syndrome (TSS) typically occurs in otherwise healthy immunocompetent people, caused by either *Streptococcus pyogenes* (most often) or *Staphylococcus aureus*. TSS generally manifests with rapid onset of fever, rash, and hypotension (shock). There may be a prodromal period of 2–3 days of malaise, myalgia, and chills followed by confusion and lethargy. TSS should be suspected in any patient with a recent wound who acutely develops unexplained pain, lethargy, and confusion and may occur even when a surgical wound appears not to be inflamed.

Pediatric Autoimmune Neuropsychiatric Disorder Associated With Streptococcal Infection

Pediatric acute-onset neuropsychiatric syndrome (PANS) refers to a syndrome in children with obsessive-compulsive and tic disorders (Chang et al. 2015; Murphy et al. 2015). Most cases of PANS are suspected to be postinfectious in origin. PANDAS is the term for a subgroup of PANS in which the symptoms appear to have been triggered by an infection with group A beta-hemolytic streptococci (GABHS). PANDAS is defined by early childhood onset of symptoms; an episodic course characterized by abrupt onset of symptoms with frequent relapses and remissions; association with neurological signs, especially tics; and temporal association with GABHS infections (most commonly pharyngitis). The best way to show the association between recent GABHS infection and PANDAS symptoms is to document a rapid rise in antistreptococcal (ASO) titers associated with symptom onset or exacerbation and a decrease in titers associated with symptom resolution or improvement. Children with PANDAS also frequently have other behavioral symptoms, including attention deficits, hyperactivity, separation anxiety, school issues, sleep disturbances, and urinary problems (e.g., Swedo et al. 2015). GABHS may play a role in some cases of Tourette's syndrome as well. A recent large Danish nationwide study with up to 17 years of follow-up found that children with a streptococcal throat infection had elevated risks of mental disorders, particularly obsessive-compulsive disorder (OCD) and tic disorders. However, nonstreptococcal throat infection was also associated with increased risks (although less than streptococcal infections) of OCD and any mental disorder (Orlovska et al. 2017).

In addition to ASO titers, a throat culture should be obtained. Prompt antibiotic treatment may prevent the expected rise in ASO titers, and children with uncomplicated strep infections treated with antibiotics appear to have no increased risk of PANDAS (Perrin et al. 2004). Only two small randomized controlled trials have examined whether antibiotics can prevent exacerbations in children with PANDAS, with mixed results (Garvey et al. 1999; Snider et al. 2005). Immunomodulatory therapies are not recommended as routine treatment of PANDAS. Consensus treatment guidelines for psychiatric and behavioral interventions have recently been published (Thienemann et al. 2017).

PANDAS has been and remains a controversial concept (Chang et al. 2015). Most cases of OCD and tic disorders in children are unrelated to streptococcal infection. Even in children with signs and symptoms meeting PANDAS criteria, most exacerbations of OCD or tic symptoms are not due to GABHS infection (Kurlan et al. 2008). The failure of immune markers to correlate with clinical exacerbations of PANDAS challenges the autoimmune theory of its etiology (Singer et al. 2008). Apart from specialty centers, inadequate diagnostic evaluation has led to unwarranted antibiotic and immunomodulatory treatment in children with OCD or tics (Helm and Blackwood 2015).

Bacterial Endocarditis

Bacterial endocarditis may cause neuropsychiatric symptoms, via focal, systemic, and CNS disease processes. Rheumatic heart disease remains the most common predisposing factor in the developing world, but in affluent countries it has been replaced by senescent valvular disease, prosthetic valves, and intravenous drug use. Malaise and fatigue may occur early, before the infection is evident. CNS symptoms are caused by occlusion of cerebral arteries by septic emboli, mycotic aneurysms, direct infection of meninges, or brain abscess. The most common psychiatric symptoms involve diffuse encephalopathy, which may occur at any stage of infection. Symptom onset may be insidious to acute, paralleling the course of the endocarditis (chronic, subacute, acute).

Diagnosis is based on clinical history and physical examination, particularly looking for new or changing heart murmurs, signs of microembolism (splinter hemorrhages, retinal hemorrhages, microscopic hematuria), and positive blood cultures in a febrile patient. Cardiac echocardiography is a crucial part of evaluation.

Rocky Mountain Spotted Fever

The etiological agent for Rocky Mountain spotted fever (RMSF) is *Rickettsia rickettsii*. RMSF is a tick-borne disease with a seasonal distribution paralleling human contact with ticks, peaking May through September. Its name is misleading because half of U.S. cases are in the South Atlantic region, and rickettsial spotted fevers occur worldwide. RMSF typically (although not invariably) includes fever and a rash characterized by erythematous macules that later progress to maculopapular lesions with central petechiae. Initially appearing as a nonspecific severe febrile illness, the diagnosis is seldom suspected until the rash appears. Only half of RMSF patients report exposure to ticks. *R. rickettsii* causes a diffuse vasculitis in many organs. CNS involvement occurs in 25% of cases and manifests as lethargy, confusion, and occasionally fulminant delirium. Subtle changes such as irritability, personality changes, and apathy may occur before the rash, particularly in children. Abnormalities on brain imaging may include focal lesions, although 80% of RMSF patients with normal scans have symptoms of encephalopathy as well (Bonawitz et al. 1997). Because mortality is high in untreated patients, a provisional clinical diagnosis (e.g., fever, rash in the appropriate season, geographic setting) is sufficient to initiate definitive antimicrobial therapy.

Typhus Fevers

Typhus fevers are caused by two species of Rickettsia. *R. prowazekii* is the cause of mouse-borne and squirrel-borne typhus. *R. typhi* is the cause of flea-borne typhus. Mouse-borne typhus usually occurs in epidemics related to war or famine, when communal hygiene deteriorates. Flea-borne typhus is associated with fleas found on rodents. The annual disease frequency in the United States was 2,000–5,000 cases in the 1940s. It is now fewer than 100, with most cases in Texas. Clinical manifestations, diagnosis, and treatment of typhus are similar to those of RMSF. The psychiatric manifestations are confusion, lethargy, and particularly headache in a febrile illness with rash. Encephalopathy occurs in two-third of patients (Misra et al. 2015). Memory impairment and behavioral alterations can occur and usually are reversible (Carr et al. 2014). The delirium of typhus and typhoid has been classically described as having a peculiar preoccupied nature, with patients picking at the bedclothes and imaginary objects (Verghese 1985). In fact, the word *typhus* in Greek means "cloud" or "mist," a term Hippocrates used to describe clouded mental status in patients with unremitting fevers.

Typhoid Fever

Typhoid fever is an enteric fever caused by salmonellae. The incidence of typhoid fever has steadily declined with improved sanitation, but the illness remains endemic in many parts of the world. Most of the cases in the United States are acquired outside the country.

Abdominal pain, headache, and fever are the classic presentation. However, when typhoid fever is endemic or is not treated promptly, psychiatric symptoms may appear. *Salmonella typhi* enters a bacteremic phase, and the typhoid bacilli can localize in the CNS. The high fever and electrolyte imbalances also may cause encephalopathy, with delirium reported in up to 75% of cases in some parts of the world (Aghanwa and Morakinyo 2001) and very infrequently (2% of cases) in others (Parry et al. 2002). Mental symptoms such as indifference, listlessness, and dullness are common at presentation. Published cases have described persistent psychiatric symptoms, including irritability, personality change, depression, catatonia, and psychosis, but most survivors completely recover following treatment.

Tetanus

Tetanus is uncommon in the United States but remains internationally significant. *Clostridium tetani* produces a potent neurotoxin called *tetanospasmin*, which is the cause of tetanus. The greatest risk factor for tetanus remains lack of up-to-date immunization. Infections generally occur because an open wound comes into contact with soil contaminated with spores from *C. tetani*. After initial inoculation, tetanospasmin is disseminated via blood, lymph, and nerves and produces symptoms by binding to receptors at the neuromuscular junction.

The classic symptom is muscle stiffness, particularly in the muscles of mastication—hence the descriptive term "lockjaw." If the muscle stiffness extends across the entire face, *risus sardonicus* occurs, an expression of continuous grimace. Also, stiffness may progress to the entire body if left untreated.

Tetanospasmin may enter the CNS, causing encephalopathic symptoms. Diagnosis is based on the clinical manifestations and a history of likely exposure. Patients with tetanus have been initially misdiagnosed with an anxiety disorder or a conversion disorder (Treadway and Prange 1967), although more commonly, a conversion disorder is mistakenly thought to be possible tetanus (Barnes and Ware 1993). If the patient had received antipsychotics or antiemetics, one could easily mistake the symptoms as drug-induced acute dystonia.

Brucellosis

Brucellosis is a worldwide zoonosis caused by species of *Brucella,* gram-negative intracellular coccobacilli. Most human cases are acquired from consumption of unpasteurized dairy products from sheep or goats. Brucellosis has become rare in developed countries (about 100 cases per year in the United States) but is likely underdiagnosed because the symptoms are nonspecific. Brucellosis can occur at any age, with insidious or abrupt onset, affecting any organ system, and hence is notorious for mimicking other diseases. Signs of acute brucellosis include fever, diaphoresis, headache, and myalgia. Chronic brucellosis is not always preceded by acute symptoms. Its manifestations include fatigue, depression, subtle cognitive dysfunction, and multiple chronic pains (Eren et al. 2006), so it is not surprising that patients' symptoms may be misdiagnosed as primary psychiatric illness (Sacks and Van Rensburg 1976). CNS involvement has been reported in 5%–50% of cases and may present as meningoencephalitis, psychosis, depression, or cognitive impairment (Shehata et al. 2010; Yetkin et al. 2006). Diagnosis is confirmed by isolation of the organism or serological testing.

Syphilis

Syphilis is a chronic systemic disease caused by the spirochetal bacterium *Treponema pallidum.* Although *T. pallidum* was not identified until 1905, syphilis was described in the medical literature before the sixteenth century. A hundred years ago, syphilis was the leading diagnosis in psychiatric inpatients; the incidence declined as the antibiotic era began. The rates of syphilis have been increasing over the past two decades, in part related to the global pandemic of HIV infection.

The clinical manifestations are varied and mimic those of other diseases. Syphilis was the original "great imitator." In adults, syphilis passes through several stages. If the chancre of *primary syphilis* is untreated, it will disappear, followed 6–24 weeks later by *secondary syphilis.* During this stage, many different organ systems, including the CNS, may become involved. Most symptoms are constitutional (malaise, fatigue, anorexia, and weight loss). Most syphilitic meningitis occurs within the first year of infection. Symptoms of headache, stiff neck, nausea, and vomiting prevail, and focal neurological findings may be present. Often, signs and symptoms of secondary syphilis disappear, and the infection becomes latent.

Tertiary syphilis refers to infection years to decades after initial infection, and neurosyphilis is the predominant form of tertiary syphilis (Gliatto and Caroff 2001).

Neurosyphilis is divided into asymptomatic, meningeal, meningovascular, and parenchymatous forms. Meningeal syphilis may occur early in the course (as previously noted) or late. Meningovascular syphilis typically occurs 4–7 years after infection, with symptoms including changes in memory and personality, dizziness, and other symptoms mimicking atherosclerotic disease (e.g., transient ischemic attack, multi-infarct dementia). Parenchymatous neurosyphilis syndromes are tabes dorsalis and general paresis. Tabes dorsalis occurs 20–25 years after infection and results from demyelination of the posterior columns and dorsal roots. Paresthesias, Argyll Robertson pupils (i.e., pupils that accommodate but do not react to light), impotence, incontinence, and truncal ataxia may develop. General paresis, now the most common form of neurosyphilis (Drago et al. 2016), develops 15–20 years after infection, manifesting as an insidious dementia that can include seizures and personality deterioration. Case reports document initial presentations with psychosis, mania, depression, and catatonia. Diagnosis relies on serological testing. Except in populations where syphilis is common, it is not cost-effective to screen all new psychiatric patients for syphilis (Roberts et al. 1992); screening should focus on patients with unexplained cognitive dysfunction or other neurological symptoms accompanying the psychopathology. Different algorithms have been recommended for HIV-positive and other immunodeficient patients (Wong et al. 2015). The most frequently used tests and their sensitivities are shown in Table 26–2.

Serological testing is based on both nontreponemal and anti-treponemal antibodies. The Venereal Disease Research Laboratory (VDRL) and the rapid plasma reagin (RPR) are the most commonly used tests for detecting nontreponemal (nonspecific) antibodies. The reactivity of these tests depends on the disease stage. In secondary syphilis and early latent syphilis, the nontreponemal tests show reactivity 95%–100% of the time. However, the reactivities in primary syphilis and tertiary syphilis are 76% and 70%, respectively. The fluorescent treponemal antibody absorption (FTA-ABS) test is more sensitive and more specific than the VDRL and RPR. This test is used to confirm the diagnosis when syphilis is suspected and a nontreponemal test was nonreactive, and to confirm a positive nontreponemal test result. The FTA-ABS test is not used as a screening test because its false-positive rate can be as high as 1%. Another treponemal test is the microhemagglutination assay of *T. pallidum* (MHA-TP). This assay is used as a confirmatory test, typically after a positive RPR test result.

False-positive nontreponemal tests—that is, positive VDRL or RPR and negative FTA-ABS and no clinical evidence of disease—are divided into acute (those that revert to normal in less than 6 months) and chronic (those that persist for longer than 6 months). Acute false-positive results occur after some immunizations, during acute infections, and during pregnancy. Chronic false-positive results occur in individuals with autoimmune disease (e.g., lupus), narcotic addiction, or leprosy, as well as in the elderly.

Intravenous penicillin G is the recommended treatment for all forms of neurosyphilis. If a definitive diagnosis cannot be made, it is prudent to treat presumptively. In

TABLE 26–2.   **Sensitivity (%) of diagnostic tests of serum[a] in different stages of syphilis**

Stage of disease	Screening[b]		Confirmatory[c]	
	RPR or VDRL	FTA-ABS	TPI	MHA-TP
Primary	75	85	40	80
Secondary and early latent	95–100	100	98	100
Late latent and tertiary	70	99	95	98

Note.   FTA-ABS=fluorescent treponemal antibody absorption; MHA-TP=microhemagglutination assay of *Treponema pallidum;* RPR=rapid plasma reagin; TPI=*Treponema pallidum* immunofluorescence assay; VDRL=Venereal Disease Research Laboratory.
[a]Sensitivity and specificity cannot be determined on cerebrospinal fluid because no gold standard exists.
[b]Detects nontreponemal antibodies.
[c]Detects treponemal antibodies. Typically, a laboratory performs one of these tests when a screening test result is positive.

many patients with cognitive impairment due to neurosyphilis, the infection appears to have "burned out," and they show no clinical response to penicillin (Moulton and Koychev 2015). There have been no controlled trials of treatment of psychiatric symptoms associated with neurosyphilis. Case reports describe positive responses to antipsychotics and anticonvulsants, and even to electroconvulsive therapy (Pecenak et al. 2015; Sanchez and Zisselman 2007).

Lyme Disease

Lyme disease is caused by the spirochete *Borrelia burgdorferi*, which is transmitted by deer ticks. The risk of contracting Lyme disease from a single tick bite is 3% (Shapiro 2014). Lyme disease occurs worldwide; it is the most common tick-borne disease in the United States, with four times as many cases as reported in Europe. Disease onset is marked by erythema migrans, a characteristic (more than 90% of cases) spreading rash with central clearing. Acute disseminated disease includes fatigue, arthralgia, headache, fever, and stiff neck. If untreated, Lyme disease may disseminate to other organs and produce subacute or chronic disease. Neurological symptoms occur in about 15% of those infected and may include cranial neuropathies (most often, the facial nerve), meningitis, or painful radiculopathy. If still untreated, patients may develop chronic neuroborreliosis, including a mild sensory radiculopathy, cognitive dysfunction, or depression. Typical symptoms of chronic Lyme encephalopathy include difficulty with concentration and memory, fatigue, daytime hypersomnolence, irritability, and depression. Very rarely, Lyme disease has led to chronic encephalomyelitis. Although these chronic syndromes are not distinctive, they are almost always preceded by the classic early symptoms of Lyme disease, such as erythema migrans, arthritis, cranial neuropathy, or radiculopathy (Feder et al. 2007).

Because of the clear relation between Lyme disease psychopathology and another spirochetal disease, syphilis, the possibility that *B. burgdorferi* causes psychiatric syndromes has become a theory of interest and controversy. Many different psychiatric symptoms have been reported to be associated with Lyme disease, including depression, mania, delirium, dementia, psychosis, obsessions or compulsions, panic attacks, catatonia, and personality change (Tager and Fallon 2001). However, association does not allow one to infer causation by Lyme. Patients with Lyme disease who were evaluated 10 and 20 years after treatment showed no significant differences in symptoms or neuropsychological testing compared with control subjects without Lyme disease. Although symptoms such as pain, fatigue, and difficulty with daily activities are common in patients who received treatment for Lyme disease years earlier, the frequencies of such symptoms are similar in control subjects without Lyme disease (Seltzer et al. 2000). Testing patients with nonspecific symptoms for antibodies against *B. burgdorferi* provides no clinically useful information because there is no correlation between symptoms and seropositivity (Markowicz et al. 2015). Studies of cognitive sequelae in children after treated Lyme disease have yielded mixed findings (McAuliffe et al. 2008; Vázquez et al. 2003).

The differential diagnosis of neuroborreliosis in a patient presenting with fatigue, depression, and/or impaired cognition includes fibromyalgia, chronic fatigue syndrome, other infections (e.g., babesiosis or ehrlichiosis), somatic symptom disorder, depression, autoimmune diseases, and multiple sclerosis (Tager and Fallon 2001).

Unfortunately, Lyme disease has been grossly overdiagnosed in individuals with nonspecific cognitive, affective, or other psychiatric symptoms. As noted earlier in this section, numerous reports in the literature attribute a wide variety of psychiatric symptoms to neuroborreliosis on the basis of positive serological testing. As explained later in this section, this is inappropriate. Adverse consequences of overdiagnosis include reinforcement of somatization and creation of invalidism. Overdiagnosis leads to overtreatment. The diagnosis of an infection that can be treated with antibiotics can be very appealing to patients for whom depression or somatic symptom disorder is an unacceptable diagnosis, but this leads to inappropriate diagnostic procedures and inappropriate extended prescription of antibiotics for a putative chronic CNS infection. Chronic antibiotic prescription is not benign and may lead to secondary infections, antibiotic resistance, and drug toxicity (Feder et al. 2007). Even in patients with classic symptomatic Lyme disease confirmed by serological testing, persisting symptoms are usually explained by some illness other than chronic borreliosis if these patients have received adequate antibiotic therapy (Kalish et al. 2001; Seltzer et al. 2000).

Diagnosis is based on the characteristic clinical features. Serological testing (enzyme-linked immunosorbent assay followed by Western blot) (Moore et al. 2016) can support the diagnosis but should never be the primary basis. False-negative and false-positive results are common with serological testing. In a large sample of patients referred to an infectious disease specialist for suspected Lyme disease, 27.5% were found to have a false-positive IgM immunoblot result, and of these patients, 78% had already received inappropriate antibiotic treatment (Seriburi et al. 2012). Even a true-positive test result simply indicates that the patient has had Lyme disease at some point in life, but no conclusion about current disease activity or extent of infection can be drawn on that basis alone. In chronic neuroborreliosis, increased CSF protein and antibodies to the organism occur in more than 50% of patients. Electroencephalograms (EEGs) are typically normal, whereas magnetic resonance imaging (MRI) shows nonspecific white matter lesions in about 25%. Neuropsychological assessment is useful in measuring cognitive dysfunction, but the findings are not specific (Ravdin et al. 1996).

Treatment is straightforward for acute Lyme disease (see Wormser et al. 2006). Neither serological testing nor antibiotic treatment is cost-effective in patients who have a low probability of having the disease (i.e., nonspecific symptoms, low-incidence region) (Nichol et al. 1998). Multiple controlled trials have found no benefit of extended intravenous or oral antibiotics in patients with well-documented, previously treated Lyme disease who had persistent pain, neurocognitive symptoms, dysesthesia, or fatigue (Berende et al. 2016; Kaplan et al. 2003; Klempner et al. 2001; Krupp et al. 2003; Oksi et al. 2007). The consensus of experts is that chronic antibiotic therapy is not indicated for persistent neuropsychiatric symptoms in patients who previously were adequately treated for Lyme (Feder et al. 2007).

Leptospirosis

Leptospirosis is another protean spirochetal disease that occurs globally. The organism is spread through the urine of many species of mammals. Most infections resemble influenza and are relatively benign. The more severe form of leptospirosis is a multiorgan disease affecting liver, kidneys, lung, and brain (e.g., meningoencephalitis, aseptic meningitis). Confusion and delirium are common, and initial presentations with mania and psychosis have also been reported (Semiz et al. 2005).

Bacterial Meningitis

Bacterial meningitis is an acute illness associated with significant morbidity and mortality. Irrespective of the organism, most cases of bacterial meningitis result from hematogenous spread of bacteria from a primary site to the subarachnoid space. Psychiatric symptoms may arise through several mechanisms, including toxic effects of the organism, inflammatory mediators, cerebral edema, and hypoxia.

The classic sign of meningeal inflammation is nuchal rigidity. Headache, nausea, vomiting, confusion, lethargy, and apathy also may occur. Encephalopathy is a harbinger of fulminant meningitis but may initially present as subtle changes in personality, mood, motivation, or mentation. Symptom severity generally correlates with the magnitude of the host's immune response. When the patient cannot mount a full inflammatory response, the classic symptoms may not occur. In infants and in elderly or immunocompromised patients, the only clinical signs may be irritability or minor changes in mentation or personality. Cognitive impairment may persist after recovery from bacterial meningitis, but usually gradually resolves (Lucas et al. 2016).

Once clinically suspected, the diagnosis is usually confirmed by examination of the CSF, which typically shows pleocytosis, low glucose, high protein, and evidence of the offending organism on appropriate staining. Although neuroimaging is routinely performed to rule out other CNS processes, it rarely establishes the diagnosis of bacterial meningitis.

Cat-Scratch Disease

Cat-scratch disease (CSD), which is caused by *Bartonella henselae,* usually manifests as self-limiting lymphadenopathy following a cat scratch or bite. Encephalopathy is one of the common complications, with almost all cases reported in children. Patients with CSD encephalopathy present with combative behavior, lethargy, and seizures;

significant fever may be absent. Diagnosis relies on serology and/or biopsy of skin or lymph node.

Bacterial Brain Abscess

Brain abscesses frequently occur as a complication of bacterial meningitis endocarditis or other bacterial infections, but also occur without an evident source. The classic triad of headache, fever, and focal neurological deficits is present in fewer than half of patients found to have a brain abscess. Seizures are common. Various psychiatric symptoms may occur, depending on the size and location of the abscess(es), how irritating the organism is, and the extent of the inflammatory response.

Mortality rates have markedly declined as a result of improved neuroimaging and antimicrobials, but morbidity remains high. Neuroimaging is very sensitive in demonstrating focal CNS abscesses. Effective treatment includes empirical antibiotics that cross the blood–brain barrier, with primary excision or aspiration of the abscess usually required. After successful treatment of the infection, psychiatric symptoms may persist.

Tuberculosis

Tuberculosis incidence is at an all-time low in the United States but remains a major world health problem, being endemic in many developing countries. Extensively drug-resistant tuberculosis has been reported in more than 80 countries. Where AIDS is prevalent, the epidemiology of tuberculosis has markedly changed. Tuberculosis now represents the most common serious HIV-related complication worldwide. Depression is highly prevalent in patients treated for tuberculosis; in a review of 31 studies from 11 countries (Sweetland et al. 2014), depression was found in almost 50% of subjects. Treating comorbid depression improves tuberculosis outcomes, including adherence to treatment.

In regions where tuberculosis is not endemic, the diagnosis of tuberculous meningitis is often not considered, because the clinical manifestations are frequently nonspecific. Early diagnosis is essential, because delay in treatment is associated with high morbidity and mortality. Tuberculous seeding of the meninges occurs via hematogenous spread following earlier primary or reactivated pulmonary infection.

Early symptoms of tuberculous meningitis are nonspecific and include low-grade fever, generalized malaise, fatigue, and mild headache; symptoms progress to high-grade fever, severe nuchal rigidity, confusion, and delirium. Persons with HIV, the elderly, persons with substance use disorders, and others with impaired immunity are more likely to present without nuchal rigidity and headache. For such patients, there is increased risk of missing the correct diagnosis while attributing the nonspecific symptoms to more common diagnoses such as alcohol withdrawal.

Confirming the diagnosis can be challenging. The organisms are difficult to detect in the CSF. Early on, when symptoms are mild, CSF glucose may be unchanged and CSF protein only marginally elevated. As the disease progresses, CSF glucose declines drastically, and CSF protein becomes markedly elevated, with white blood cell counts typically between 50 and 200 per cubic millimeter (predominantly lymphocytes). Later complications include cerebral vasculitis and cranial nerve involvement. Diffuse meningeal involvement in tuberculosis may be seen on MRI.

Strong suspicion of tuberculous meningitis calls for early treatment, requiring different drug combinations when multidrug-resistant tuberculosis is present.

Whipple's Disease

Whipple's disease is a rare infection caused by the bacterium *Tropheryma whipplei.* Most patients experience arthralgia, diarrhea, and weight loss. Neurological involvement has been reported in 6%–63% of patients, may occur without intestinal involvement (Mohamed et al. 2011), and can mimic almost any neurological syndrome. Psychiatric symptoms (e.g., depression, personality change) are present in about half of patients with neurological involvement. Cognitive deficits are even more common and may extend to dementia. Whipple's disease is treated with antibiotics, but patients with neurological involvement have a poor prognosis (Fenollar et al. 2007).

Viral Infections

Human Immunodeficiency Virus

HIV psychiatry has evolved over time, and dramatically improved treatments have turned what was once a fatal diagnosis into a chronic, manageable illness. Comprehensive textbooks cover HIV psychiatry in depth (Cohen et al. 2017; Joska et al. 2014). In this section we review HIV treatment adherence issues and psychiatric conditions commonly seen in HIV, including neuropsychiatric complications from HIV infection itself and from opportunistic infections in immunocompromised patients. We also consider psychiatric disorders that are often comorbid with HIV.

HIV is a retrovirus; it contains ribonucleic acid (RNA) strands that must be transcribed into deoxyribonucleic acid (DNA) by the enzyme reverse transcriptase, which is not present in uninfected cells. Viral particles contain the enzyme, two viral RNA molecules, and accessory proteins. Viral particles bind to the surface of cells expressing CD4 antigens at the CD4 protein with the help of a second cell surface protein, CCR5. After the virus is internalized, the protein coat dissolves to release the two viral strands and the viral reverse transcriptase enzyme, which then uses the deoxynucleotides present in the cell to make a DNA strand from the viral RNA. The strands are moved to the nucleus, where they are spliced into the DNA by the viral enzyme integrase. If the cell is activated, the DNA template rapidly makes a huge number of viral RNA strands, which then use the cell's own machinery to make and process viral proteins. A viral protease finally cleaves the proteins and allows mature infectious particles to leave the cell. These steps do not occur within normal human cells and are therefore optimal targets for antiviral drugs. Drugs that interfere with cell entry (fusion inhibitors), reverse transcription (nucleoside and nonnucleoside reverse transcriptase inhibitors, also known as NRTIs, or "nucs," and NNRTIs, or "nonnucs," respectively), integrase activity (integrase inhibitors), and viral protease (protease inhibitors) are currently available. Successful treatment with several drugs at once—antiretroviral therapy (ART)—reduces virus production to undetectable levels and should extend life into the normal range for most patients.

About 37 million people worldwide are living with HIV infection, with about 1.2 million in the United States. It is estimated that 1 in 8 individuals are not aware of their infection. About 83% of new infections in the United States are among men who have sex with men, with men of color at greatest risk, followed by women of color, who are most often infected by heterosexual contact. About 6% of new infections are attributed to intravenous drug use. African Americans represent 12% of the U.S. population but account for 45% (17,670) of HIV cases (Centers for Disease Control and Prevention 2016).

Effect of Psychiatric Disorders on HIV Medication Adherence

The single most important factor affecting outcome of HIV treatment is the patient's ability to adhere to a prescribed drug regimen. A study of HIV-infected prisoners reported that under directly observed therapy in a prison setting, 85% of the individuals achieved undetectable viral loads, with prisoners taking approximately 93% of prescribed doses (Kirkland et al. 2002). In contrast, British community studies found that only 42% of treatment-naive patients taking ART attained undetectable viral loads (Lee and Monteiro 2003). ART adherence rates between 54% and 76% have been reported in other general clinic or community samples (Liu et al. 2001; McNabb et al. 2001; Paterson et al. 2000; Wagner and Ghosh-Dastidar 2002), including groups of patients with serious mental illness (Beyer et al. 2007; Wagner et al. 2003).

Psychiatric factors associated with nonadherence include dementia, depression, psychosis, traumatic life experiences, personality traits, and substance use (Mellins et al. 2009). Many studies have shown decreased adherence to ART attributable to depression, and improved outcomes with its treatment (Campos et al. 2010; Koenig et al. 2008; Kumar and Encinosa 2009). Psychotic patients may refuse medications, deny their illness, or be too disorganized to manage adherence. Patients with dementia may forget doses and appointments. Traumatic life experiences, such as childhood sexual abuse (Meade et al. 2009), are associated with poor adherence. Substance use disorders, particularly alcohol abuse (Conen et al. 2009), greatly contribute to poor medication adherence (Malta et al. 2008). Treatment of addictions can improve adherence and outcome (Roux et al. 2008).

Neuropsychiatric and Medical Complications of HIV Infection

Toxoplasmosis. Infection with *Toxoplasma gondii* generally occurs in 30% of patients with fewer than 100 CD4 cells/mm^3 (Kaplan et al. 2009) (see further discussion of toxoplasmosis in the section "Fungal Infections" later in this chapter). In patients with AIDS, toxoplasmosis, affecting between 2% and 4% of the AIDS population, is the most common cause of intracranial masses. Symptoms of CNS infection are fever, reduced alertness, headache, confusion, focal neurological signs (approximately 80% of cases), and partial or generalized seizures (approximately 30% of cases). Head computed tomography (CT) usually shows multiple bilateral, ring-enhancing lesions in the basal ganglia or at the gray–white matter junction. Brain MRI is more sensitive than CT and is the preferred scanning modality for individuals without focal neurological deficits (Kupfer et al. 1990).

Treatment is usually empirical and consists of pyrimethamine and leucovorin. Clinical and radiological improvement is seen in more than 85% of patients by day 7 (Kaplan et al. 2009). Acute treatment (6 weeks) may be followed by continuous prophylaxis to prevent relapse. Current treatment guidelines advise that primary and secondary prophylaxis against CNS toxoplasmosis can be discontinued when CD4+

T cell counts have remained greater than 200 cells/mm^3 for more than 3 months (Panel on Antiretroviral Guidelines for Adults and Adolescents 2016).

Cryptococcal meningitis.   Although meningitis caused by *Cryptococcus neoformans* is rare in immunocompetent persons, it is a devastating illness occurring in approximately 8%–10% of AIDS patients in the United States and in up to 30% of AIDS patients in other parts of the world (Powderly 2000) (see further discussion of Cryptococcus in the section "Fungal Infections" later in this chapter). More recent incidence estimates range from 0.04% to 12% per year among persons with HIV in various regions (Park et al. 2009). Patients generally present with fever and delirium. Meningeal signs are not universally seen. Seizures and focal neurological deficits occur in about 10% of cases, and intracranial pressure is elevated in about 50%.

Treatment of cryptococcal meningitis in HIV requires amphotericin B. Patients who survive must receive prophylaxis against recurrence with oral fluconazole or intermittent intravenous amphotericin B. Secondary prophylaxis may be terminated in patients on ART who have an undetectable viral load, who have CD4 cell counts ≥100 cells/μL, and who have received a minimum of 1 year of azole antifungal maintenance therapy (Panel on Opportunistic Infections in HIV-Infected Adults and Adolescents 2018).

Progressive multifocal leukoencephalopathy.   Progressive multifocal leukoencephalopathy (PML) is a demyelinating disease caused by reactivation of the JC (John Cunningham) virus in immunocompromised patients. Prior to the introduction of HAART (highly active antiretroviral therapy) in 1996, the prevalence of PML in AIDS was between 1% and 10%. AIDS patients account for almost 75% of PML cases in the United States, with significant reductions in the ART era (Engsig et al. 2009). The risk of PML remains significant in AIDS patients with fewer than 100 CD4 cells/mm^3. The clinical syndrome consists of multiple focal neurological deficits, such as mono- or hemiparetic limb weakness, dysarthria, gait disturbances, sensory deficits, and progressive dementia, with eventual coma and death. Occasionally, seizures or loss of vision may occur. The pathology of PML consists of demyelination and death of astrocytes and oligodendroglia. MRI is more useful than CT in diagnosis; multiple areas of attenuated signal are seen on T2 images, primarily in the white matter, although gray matter, brain-stem, cerebellar, and spinal cord lesions are possible. There is no specific treatment for PML other than immune restoration with ART (Panel on Antiretroviral Guidelines for Adults and Adolescents 2016).

Central Nervous System Neoplasms

Lymphoma is the most common neoplasm seen in AIDS patients, affecting between 0.6% and 3%. AIDS is the most common condition associated with primary CNS lymphoma. The patient is generally afebrile; may develop a single lesion with focal neurological signs or small, multifocal lesions; and most commonly presents with mental status change. Seizures occur in about 15% of cases. CNS lymphoma manifests late in the course of HIV infection and has a very poor prognosis.

CNS lymphoma is at times misdiagnosed as toxoplasmosis, HIV dementia, or another encephalopathy. Head CT scan may be normal or show one or multiple hypodense or patchy, nodular enhancing lesions. MRI generally shows enhanced lesions that may be difficult to differentiate from CNS toxoplasmosis. A biopsy is required for confirmation of the diagnosis of CNS lymphoma. Treatment with radiation and chemotherapy is primarily palliative, and the prognosis is generally poor (Robotin et al. 2004).

HIV-Associated Neurocognitive Disorder

HIV-associated neurocognitive disorder (HAND) is the term for the spectrum of cognitive dysfunction due to primary HIV CNS infection, which ranges from asymptomatic changes demonstrable only on neurocognitive testing to HIV-associated dementia (Antinori et al. 2007). In 1986, HIV-associated dementia was reported in up to two-thirds of AIDS patients (Navia et al. 1986), but its frequency has declined dramatically since the advent of more effective treatments for HIV infection. Less severe forms of HAND now predominate, and the most severe form is uncommon (Saylor et al. 2016). Under the current nomenclature, the least severe form, asymptomatic neurocognitive impairment (ANI), affects about 30% of people with HIV and is defined as the presence of deficits greater than one standard deviation from the mean in at least two domains of neuropsychological testing without limitations in daily functioning. Mild neurocognitive disorder (MND), characterized by mild to moderate difficulties in daily functioning, affects 20%–30% of people with HIV. HIV-associated dementia (HAD), defined as marked impairment in testing and functioning, affects 2%–8% of this population (Antinori et al. 2007). HAND is rarely progressive in patients who have undetectable viral loads. Risk factors for HAND include older age, lower CD4 nadir, co-infection with hepatitis C, alcohol and/or substance use, cerebrovascular disease, and psychiatric disorders. Several of these factors are independent risk factors for cognitive impairment as well.

In the pre-ART era, frank encephalitis and neuronal cell loss were frequently found on autopsy in people with HAND, but growing evidence suggests that factors other than neuronal cell death are essential in the disease pathophysiology. Functional disturbances in inflammatory processes are more likely the proximal cause. Activated circulating monocytes likely introduce the virus across the blood–brain barrier, and CNS macrophages, microglia, and astrocytes all become infected. These cells release chemokines and cytokines, which lead to neuronal damage (Williams et al. 2014). There is also evidence for disturbances in glutamate functioning in the CNS, with increased extracellular glutamate leading to excitotoxicity (Vázquez-Santiago et al. 2014).

Clinically, HAND presents with the typical triad of symptoms seen in other subcortical dementias—memory and psychomotor speed impairments, depressive symptoms, and movement disorders. In milder cases, patients may notice slight problems with reading, comprehension, memory, and mathematical skills, but these symptoms are subtle and may be overlooked or discounted as being due to fatigue and illness. Patients may show impairments on timed tests, such as the Trail-Making Test or the grooved pegboard test. Later, patients develop more global dementia, with marked impairments in naming, language, and praxis; mood disturbances; and more profound neurological deficits.

The Modified HIV Dementia Scale has been demonstrated to be the most specific and valid assessment tool, and can be administered serially to document disease progression (Davis et al. 2002). Other recommended screening tools include the Montreal Cognitive Assessment and a computerized assessment, the CogState, which may be more sensitive at earlier stages (Bloch et al. 2016; Brouillette et al. 2015).

To date, no specific treatments for HAND have been demonstrated to be effective, apart from viral suppression with ART. Data have been inconsistent regarding the extent to which antimicrobials with higher penetrance into the CSF might improve outcomes (Saylor et al. 2016). Memantine is not efficacious (Zhao et al. 2010). Psychostimulants have been shown in some studies to improve cognitive performance in patients with HIV (Brown 1995; Hinkin et al. 2001), but others have noted apparent acceleration of HIV-associated dementia following psychostimulant use (Czub et al. 2001; Nath et al. 2001).

Delirium

Delirium is very common among hospitalized patients with advanced disease, including children (Hatherill and Flisher 2009; Sonneville et al. 2011). Hospitalized patients with AIDS were found to have increased mortality if delirium complicated their hospital course (Uldall et al. 2000). The clinical presentation of delirium in HIV-infected patients is the same as in non-HIV-infected patients and is characterized by inattention, disorganized thinking or confusion, and fluctuations in level of consciousness. Emotional changes are common and often unpredictable, and hallucinations and delusions are frequently seen. The differential diagnosis for delirium includes HAND, major depressive disorder, bipolar disorder, panic disorder, and schizophrenia. Delirium usually can be differentiated on the basis of its rapid onset, fluctuating levels of consciousness, and link to medical etiology. The approach to determining cause is similar to that for delirium in general (see Chapter 4, "Delirium"). Particular considerations in HIV-positive patients include hypoxia with *Pneumocystis jirovecii* pneumonia, malnutrition, CNS infections and neoplasms, systemic infections (e.g., mycobacteria, cytomegalovirus, bacterial sepsis), substance intoxication and withdrawal, medication toxicity, and polypharmacy. Variations in hydration or electrolyte status also may profoundly affect patients with HIV who already have cerebral compromise. HIV infection itself also may produce an acute encephalopathy (Vlassova et al. 2009) that can manifest during the early weeks of the initial infection.

Management of delirium in HIV is very similar to that of delirium in general (see Chapter 4, "Delirium") and includes identification and removal of the underlying cause (when possible), nonpharmacological reorientation and environmental interventions, and pharmacotherapy. Low doses of high-potency antipsychotic agents, such as haloperidol, usually are effective. Treatment with antipsychotics requires awareness of the greater susceptibility of patients with HIV to antipsychotic-induced extrapyramidal symptoms (EPS), even with agents having a lower potential for inducing EPS (Kelly et al. 2002).

Depression

Depression is a significant problem among persons with HIV and AIDS. The estimated prevalence of major depressive disorder (MDD) in HIV-infected patients has been reported as 19%–43% (Cysique et al. 2007; Gibbie et al. 2007). Depression has well-documented negative effects on adherence to treatment (Tao et al. 2018), quality of life (Lenz and Demal 2000; Meltzer-Brody and Davidson 2000), and treatment outcomes (Alciati et al. 2007). MDD is a risk factor for HIV infection (McDermott et al. 1994) via intensification of substance abuse, exacerbation of self-destructive behaviors, and promotion of poor sexual partner choice.

HIV increases the risk of developing MDD through a variety of mechanisms, including direct injury to the subcortex, chronic stress, worsening social isolation, and intense demoralization. Patients with AIDS have been recognized as a group at high risk of psychological distress (Himelhoch et al. 2007; Lyketsos et al. 1996). High rates of suicide have been reported among HIV-infected patients (Carrico et al. 2007; Sherr et al. 2008). Factors associated with suicide in HIV patients include depression, hopelessness, alcohol abuse, poor social support, low self-esteem, and history of psychiatric disorder (Carrico et al. 2007; Sherr et al. 2008). Recent diagnosis of HIV or presence of pain also is associated with increased suicidal thoughts (Andraghetti et al. 2001). For further discussion of suicidality in HIV patients, see Chapter 8 ("Suicidality").

The differential diagnosis of depression in HIV includes nonpathological states of grief and mourning (sometimes made quite severe by individual vulnerabilities) and a variety of psychological and physiological disturbances. Patients who report depressive symptoms may have dysthymia, dementia, delirium, demoralization, intoxication, withdrawal, CNS injury or infection, malnutrition, wasting syndromes, medication side effects, or a variety of other conditions. HAND and other HIV-related CNS conditions can produce a flat, apathetic state that is often misdiagnosed as depression.

HIV-infected patients with MDD frequently present to internists and family practitioners with multiple somatic symptoms. Given the burdens of HIV, the medical problems associated with the disease, and the side effects of medications, depression may be very low on the list of considered causes of the patient's symptoms. Even patients reporting depressive symptoms may have their depression overlooked or discounted because of the presence of other problems. Nonspecific somatic symptoms are often the result of depression rather than HIV infection in patients whose infection is early and asymptomatic. Care should be taken in distinguishing between MDD and demoralization (i.e., adjustment disorder) in patients with HIV.

Fatigue has been found to be more associated with depression than with HIV disease progression. Worsening of fatigue and insomnia at 6-month follow-up was highly correlated with worsening depression but not with CD4 cell count, change in CD4 cell count, or disease progression by Centers for Disease Control and Prevention category (Leserman et al. 2008). These findings support the recommendation that somatic symptoms generally suggestive of depression should trigger a full psychiatric evaluation.

Depressive symptoms can be caused by certain HIV-related medical conditions, including CNS infections such as syphilis, toxoplasmosis, and lymphoma. In male HIV-positive patients, some investigators have found significant rates of depressive symptoms, including low mood, poor appetite with loss of weight, decreased libido, and fatigue, to be associated with low testosterone levels (Rabkin et al. 2006). Several drugs used in patients with HIV, including efavirenz, interferon, metoclopramide, sulfonamides, anabolic steroids, and corticosteroids, have been reported to produce depression. These depressive symptoms often respond to discontinuation of the offending drug; when they do not respond to discontinuation or when the drug must be continued, the symptoms should be treated with an appropriate antidepressant. Routine screening for depression in people with HIV can effectively identify cases. Both the Patient Health Questionnaire–9 (PHQ-9) and the Patient Health Questionnaire–2 have been demonstrated to be valid and reliable in screening patients with HIV (Hirshfield et al. 2008; Mao et al. 2009).

Many open-label and double-blind, placebo-controlled clinical trials of antidepressants for depression in patients with HIV have demonstrated that conventional antidepressant therapy is effective. No single antidepressant has been found superior to others. As with all depressed patients, nonadherence is the most common reason for ineffective drug treatment, and adverse effects are the most common reason for treatment nonadherence (Ferrando and Freyberg 2008). The side effects of certain antidepressants can render them advantageous or disadvantageous in particular patients with HIV. For example, selective serotonin reuptake inhibitors (SSRIs) are best avoided in patients with chronic diarrhea. Sedating antidepressants should be avoided in patients with weakness, lethargy, orthostasis, or other risk factors for falls. Tricyclic antidepressants (TCAs) should be avoided with oral candidiasis because of the aggravating effect of dry mouth on thrush. In cases of anorexia or cachexia, antidepressants with appetite-stimulating effects are best selected.

MDD in HIV-positive men with testosterone deficiency has been effectively treated with intramuscular testosterone (Rabkin et al. 2000). Patients should be advised not to take St. John's wort as an alternative to prescribed antidepressants, because it can lower serum levels of protease inhibitors (Di et al. 2008). An important issue is the interaction of antidepressants and ART medications (see Chapter 36, "Psychopharmacology"). Three points deserve emphasis. First, particularly because depression is associated with reductions in adherence to ART, the risks of untreated depression must be weighed against the risks of potential medication interactions. Second, the clinical significance of some drug–drug interactions has not yet been clearly established (i.e., dosage adjustments may not be required), likely because both antidepressants and ART, unlike drugs such as warfarin or digoxin, have wide therapeutic indices. Finally, no evidence indicates that antidepressants cause fluctuations in CD4 cell counts (Kumar and Encinosa 2009; Schroecksnadel et al. 2008).

Although the literature on use of psychotherapy for treatment of depression in HIV-infected patients is extensive, clinical trial data are sparse. Individual and group cognitive-behavioral therapy, interpersonal psychotherapy, and supportive psychotherapy have demonstrated efficacy both alone and in combination with pharmacotherapies (Ferrando and Freyberg 2008). A wide range of intrapsychic or interpersonal issues may be the focus of psychotherapy. Supportive psychotherapy can help patients with depression who interpret their suffering to be a sign of weakness in the face of adversity. These patients may believe that they should pull themselves out of depression and become frustrated when they fail. Education about the disease and the nature of depression, encouragement, and therapeutic optimism all may be helpful. Other issues that arise in psychotherapy include guilt over acquiring HIV, guilt over infecting others, survivor guilt, and anger at the source of disease, at oneself, or at God. The diagnosis of HIV infection may have involved precipitous revelations of hidden sexual or drug abuse behavior, eliciting shame and self-loathing. The stigma of HIV may lead to rejection or abandonment by loved ones, and shunning by wider society, making patients feel like lepers. Despite effective antiretroviral therapies, some patients become hopeless and nihilistic and forgo HIV treatment.

Bipolar Disorder

Patients with bipolar disorder may be more likely to engage in behaviors that place them at risk for HIV infection, including unprotected sex, sex with partners with unknown HIV status, and drug use. Bipolar disorder occurs at higher rates among people with HIV than in the general population (de Sousa Gurgel et al. 2013) and, among HIV-positive patients in treatment, is associated with behaviors that carry a high risk of infection transmission (Meade et al. 2012). The prevalence of mania is higher in patients with AIDS compared with the general population (Atkinson et al. 2009). Some have suggested that mania should be subdivided into primary and secondary types, with patients who have the secondary type showing close temporal proximity to an organic insult, no history of bipolar illness, essentially negative family history, and late age at onset (Nakimuli-Mpungu et al. 2006). Secondary mania would include cases caused by HIV brain disease itself, by antiretroviral drugs, and by other HIV-related conditions or medications. Before the availability of effective ART, patients with low CD4 cell counts often presented with a constellation of symptoms described as "AIDS mania." Irritable mood was often a prominent feature, but elevated mood was observed as well. Sometimes these symptoms were preceded by or presented concurrently with cognitive decline typical of HAND. AIDS mania was usually quite severe in its presentation and malignant in its course (Lyketsos et al. 1993, 1997). It is rarely seen in the ART era.

Treatment of secondary mania has not been extensively studied, but traditional mood stabilizers have been used widely, and practice guidelines recommend lithium, valproic acid, or carbamazepine as standard therapy. In HIV-positive individuals, management of mania with mood stabilizers can be complicated by potential drug interactions. Carbamazepine is contraindicated with several antiretrovirals because of its action as an inducer of metabolism, potentially lowering the levels of antiretrovirals. Protease inhibitors may lower levels of valproic acid and lamotrigine.

Schizophrenia

Patients with severe and chronic mental illnesses, primarily schizophrenia and bipolar disorder, have reported HIV prevalence rates of between 2% and 20% in both inpatient and outpatient samples (De Hert et al. 2009; Senn and Carey 2008). Patients with schizophrenia have significantly less knowledge about HIV infection and transmission than do people without schizophrenia (Kalichman et al. 1995). High comorbidity with substance use puts people with schizophrenia at increased risk of infection (Prince et al. 2012). Treatment of schizophrenia in HIV-infected patients follows the same basic principles as for other patients with schizophrenia—namely, control of symptoms with medications and psychosocial support and rehabilitation. Close collaboration with HIV care providers is strongly suggested so that HIV treatment can be effectively coordinated and adherence enhanced. Patients with schizophrenia are very likely to have difficulties accessing care, affording medication, and adhering to complex ART regimens. Furthermore, protease inhibitors potentially can elevate blood levels of certain antipsychotic medications. This effect is most clearly seen with quetiapine, for which significant adverse events have been reported (Pollack et al. 2009). Drug interactions between antipsychotics and ART are discussed in Chapter 36 ("Psychopharmacology").

Substance Use Disorders

Substance misuse is a primary vector for the spread of HIV infection for individuals who use injection drugs and their sexual partners, as well as those who are disinhibited by intoxication or driven by addiction to unsafe sexual practices. Patients with substance use disorders may not seek health care or may be excluded from or discriminated against in health care settings. Rates of HIV infection among people who inject drugs have fallen over time, with recent data estimating that 1 in 23 women who inject drugs and 1 in 36 men who inject drugs will be diagnosed with HIV in their lifetime (Centers for Disease Control and Prevention 2016). The current epidemic of prescription opioid misuse and abuse has led to rising numbers of injection drug users, placing new populations at increased risk of HIV infection, as illustrated by a recent outbreak in rural Indiana (Conrad et al. 2015). Additionally, methamphetamine has been linked to an upsurge in sexually transmitted HIV among men who have sex with men, particularly in group settings (Semple et al. 2009). Alcohol intoxication also can lead to risky sexual behaviors by way of cognitive impairment and disinhibition (Pearson et al. 2008). Drug use and alcohol use have been shown to reduce medication adherence, the crucial factor in both successful treatment and successful prevention.

Substance use disorders can be successfully treated in individuals at risk of HIV. One of the most extensively studied interventions in risk reduction is opioid substitution therapy, which resulted in sustained reductions in HIV risk and lower incidence of HIV infection in patients on methadone maintenance (Davstad et al. 2009) and reduced injection-related HIV risk in patients on buprenorphine maintenance (Metzger et al. 2015). Methadone or buprenorphine can be linked to directly observed therapy for HIV for patients at high risk of medication nonadherence. Model programs of fully integrated care providing HIV treatment, substance abuse treatment, and psychiatric treatment have been shown to improve outcomes (Himelhoch et al. 2007).

Other Viral Infections

Many viruses are difficult to detect, most viral infections are difficult to treat, and few are cured by treatment. Viruses can produce psychiatric symptoms from primary CNS involvement, from secondary effects of immune activation, or indirectly from systemic effects. Increased titers of antibodies against a number of viruses have been associated with schizophrenia, bipolar disorder, and depression, but causation has not been established. One serious sequela of certain viral infections is acute disseminated encephalomyelitis, which can present with encephalopathy, acute psychosis, seizures, and other CNS dysfunction. Active demyelination is widespread, and the disease may be difficult to distinguish from multiple sclerosis. Residual cognitive dysfunction may occur (Kuni et al. 2012).

Epstein-Barr Virus

Epstein-Barr virus (EBV), one of the herpesviruses, commonly causes infectious mononucleosis ("mono") in children and young adults. The prodromal stage of infectious mononucleosis is characterized by headache, fatigue, and malaise, with progression to fever, sore throat, and lymphadenopathy. Diagnosis is based on the combination of typical clinical symptoms and a positive heterophil antibody test (Monospot). False-negative results may occur in immunosuppressed patients. Most cases completely resolve. Fatigue with EBV commonly persists for a few months, but persistent fatigue can occur with other viral infections as well (Hickie et al. 2006). In the rare, more severe form of infectious mononucleosis, anemia, leukopenia, eosinophilia, thrombocytopenia, pneumonitis, hepatosplenomegaly, uveitis, and an abnormal pattern of serum globulins may be present. EBV can also cause acute encephalitis and other neurological syndromes.

Because EBV may persist for a lifetime in a latent state following acute infection, periodic reactivation may occur. Patients with reactivated EBV infection may report overwhelming fatigue, malaise, depression, low-grade fever, lymphadenopathy, and other nonspecific symptoms—essentially the picture of the chronic fatigue syndrome. However, only a small fraction of chronic fatigue symptoms are attributable to EBV infection. In the past, patients with chronic fatigue and depression (and sometimes their physicians) attributed causation to chronic EBV infection, erroneously confirming this after a positive Monospot test result. It was erroneous because the test result remains positive long after complete resolution of uncomplicated infectious mononucleosis in youth, and most adults have had the infection (see analogous discussion in subsection "Lyme Disease" earlier in this chapter).

Cytomegalovirus

Like EBV, cytomegalovirus (CMV) is a herpesvirus with the ability to develop a lifelong latency in the host, with possible reactivation. Seroprevalence in adults has been reported to be between 40% and 100%. Most CMV infections are subclinical, and they occur across a broader age group than does EBV. In adults, CMV can produce a syndrome identical to infectious mononucleosis, except that heterophil antibody testing is negative, and a sore throat is usually absent. CMV also may cause hepatitis, retinitis, colitis, and pneumonitis. CMV can cause encephalitis in immunocompromised patients (especially in posttransplant patients or those with AIDS), but this outcome is rare in immunocompetent patients. In patients who have recovered from the infection, CMV has been implicated as a cause of depression or dementia. Seropositive transplant recipients are at risk of infection reactivation, and seronegative recipients are at risk of a more serious primary CMV infection if the donor is seropositive. Prophylactic therapy has reduced posttransplant CMV infections but has also delayed their appearance. Without prophylaxis, the symptoms of CMV reactivation usually occur between the first and fourth month after transplantation.

Viral Meningoencephalitis

Most viruses that cause encephalitis cause meningitis as well. Enteroviruses, mumps, and lymphocytic choriomeningitis primarily affect the meninges, with enteroviruses responsible for most identifiable cases. Patients with viral meningitis (often referred to as *aseptic meningitis*) present with headache, fever, nuchal rigidity, malaise, drowsiness, nausea, and photophobia. Typically, the CSF shows pleocytosis, elevated protein, and no evidence of an organism. Treatment for aseptic meningitis is generally supportive.

In viral encephalitis, psychiatric symptoms are very common in the acute phase and are frequent after recovery (Arciniegas and Anderson 2004; Caroff et al. 2001). Occasionally, patients with viral encephalitis may present initially with psychopathology without neurological symptoms. Caroff et al. (2001) reviewed 108 published cases of psychiatric presentation, classified as psychosis (35%), catatonia (33%), psychotic depression (16%), or mania (11%). Such patients are often misdiagnosed and receive inappropriate treatment. Viral encephalitis patients are more vulnerable to adverse effects of antipsychotic medications, including extrapyramidal side effects, catatonia, and neuroleptic malignant syndrome.

For those who survive viral encephalitis, outcomes vary from complete recovery to serious neuropsychiatric sequelae. Psychiatric sequelae, especially mood disorders, are common following recovery from acute viral encephalitis and constitute a major cause of disability. Depression, hypomania, irritability, and disinhibition of anger, aggression, or sexuality are frequently noted months after recovery, and psychosis may occur in rare cases. Depressive symptoms may respond to treatment with antidepressants or stimulants. Hypomania, irritability, and disinhibition have benefited from antipsychotics, mood stabilizers (including lithium), and electroconvulsive therapy (Kogut et al. 2017).

Arboviruses

Arboviruses (short for arthropod-borne viruses) are the most common cause of viral encephalitis worldwide. Of the arboviral diseases, Japanese encephalitis is the most common worldwide and annually causes more than 10,000 deaths in Asia. In the United States, the major types are St. Louis encephalitis, eastern equine encephalomyelitis, western equine encephalomyelitis, California encephalitis, and West Nile virus. Most arboviruses are mosquito-borne. Arboviral encephalitis typically appears in the summer or fall in children (Japanese encephalitis) or young adults (West Nile virus and St. Louis encephalitis), with abrupt onset of fever, headache, nausea, photophobia, and vomiting, and may be fatal. Reduced level of consciousness, flaccid paralysis resembling poliomyelitis, EPS, and seizures are common (Sarkari et al. 2012a, 2012b). Persistent depression and cognitive problems are common after West Nile infection (Nolan et al. 2012; Samaan et al. 2016). Although no specific treatment is available for arboviral encephalitis, rapid diagnosis is important for public health measures, mosquito control, and, where available, vaccines.

Dengue

Dengue, another disease caused by an arbovirus, is transmitted by mosquitoes, endemic in 100 countries, and encountered in temperate developed countries mainly in travelers and new immigrants. The virus causes three syndromes: the relatively more benign dengue fever, which is a painful influenza-like illness, and the serious forms, hemorrhagic dengue and dengue shock syndrome; the latter two are rare in travelers. CNS involvement has been reported in 3%–21% of cases of dengue; in the more serious endemic dengue infections, encephalitis is common, with confusion, delirium, and seizures (Domingues et al. 2008; Sahu et al. 2014). Case reports have described psychosis, mania, and catatonia. Two-thirds of inpatients with acute dengue have clinically significant symptoms of depression and anxiety (Hashmi et al. 2012), and depression is a common persistent symptom after recovery (Tiga et al. 2016).

Herpes Simplex Virus

Herpes encephalitis is the most common cause of sporadic fatal encephalitis worldwide, with more than 90% of cases caused by herpes simplex type 1 virus. Symptoms may include hypomania, personality change, dysphasia, seizures, autonomic dysfunction, ataxia, delirium, psychosis, and focal neurological symptoms (Więdłocha et al. 2015). Herpes simplex virus (HSV) encephalitis differs from arboviral encephalitis by causing more unilateral and focal findings, with a predilection for temporoparietal areas of the brain. HSV encephalitis is more likely than arboviral encephalitis to cause focal seizures, olfactory hallucinations, and personality change. HSV is the most common identified cause of viral encephalitis simulating a primary psychiatric disorder (Arciniegas and Anderson 2004; Caroff et al. 2001). One possible sequela of HSV encephalitis is the Klüver-Bucy syndrome, which includes oral touching compulsions, hypersexuality, amnesia, placidity, agnosia, and hyperphagia. CSF typically shows pleocytosis, red blood cells (because of the hemorrhagic nature of HSV encephalitis), and elevated protein. Glucose is usually normal. Electroencephalography is a sensitive (but not specific) diagnostic test, showing periodic temporal spikes and slow waves as opposed to the more diffuse changes usually seen in other forms of viral encephalitis. MRI may show diffuse inflammation, particularly in the temporoparietal areas. The diagnosis is confirmed by detection of HSV DNA by polymerase chain reaction. Diagnosis based on symptoms and signs alone misses 50% of cases.

Rapid diagnosis is essential because only early treatment improves outcome. HSV encephalitis is treated with intravenous acyclovir, which itself can cause neuropsychiatric adverse effects (see Table 26–3 later in chapter). Although there are no well-defined treatments for the associated cognitive and neuropsychiatric symptoms, case reports describe success with anticonvulsants such as carbamazepine (especially in patients with comorbid seizures), atypical antipsychotics, SSRIs, stimulants, dopamine agonists, clonidine, and cholinesterase inhibitors (Kogut et al. 2017).

Varicella/Herpes Zoster

The varicella/herpes zoster virus causes chickenpox in children and herpes zoster in adults. Most cases of encephalopathy in children with varicella infection were due to Reye's syndrome, although the virus itself can cause encephalitis. Zoster-associated encephalitis in adults typically presents with delirium within days after the appearance of the rash. The most common neurological sequela of herpes zoster is postherpetic neuralgia (see Chapter 34, "Pain"). Depression and anxiety are common in postherpetic neuralgia (Volpi et al. 2008) and may influence the choice of treatment for the neuropathic pain (e.g., tricyclic or serotonin–norepinephrine reuptake inhibitor [SNRI] antidepressant vs. anticonvulsant). Weeks or months after recovery from herpes zoster, encephalitis may appear (mostly in immunosuppressed patients), with headache, altered mental status, psychosis, fever, seizures, and cognitive deficits (Więdłocha et al. 2015).

Measles

Measles can cause postinfectious encephalomyelitis, subacute measles encephalitis, and subacute sclerosing panencephalitis (SSPE). SSPE typically occurs 7–10 years after measles infection, presenting with cognitive dysfunction, behavior change, headache, and myoclonic jerks (Garg 2008). Cases of SSPE presenting with depression, mania, and catatonia have been reported. Most cases have been in children or adolescents, but cases beginning in middle age have also been reported.

Tick-Borne Encephalitis

Tick-borne encephalitis (TBE) is an important human CNS infection that is prevalent throughout Europe and parts of Asia and is caused by a virus (TBEV) that is mainly transmitted by tick bites and rarely by unpasteurized milk (Kaiser 2008). TBE manifests as meningitis or meningoencephalitis. Neurological and psychiatric sequelae, including motor, affective, and cognitive symptoms and personality change, are common in adults (Więdłocha et al. 2015). No specific treatment for TBE is known, but the disease can be prevented by active immunization.

Zika Virus

Zika virus is a mosquito-borne flavivirus that has emerged as a cause of outbreaks of febrile illness with nonspecific symptoms. It is neurotropic and can cause Guillain-Barré syndrome and (rarely) meningoencephalitis (Carteaux et al. 2016; Petersen et al. 2016). Infection during pregnancy may result in microcephaly.

Postencephalitis Syndromes

Following recovery from acute viral encephalitis, psychiatric sequelae are common and constitute a major cause of disability, especially mood disorders. Depression, amnestic disorders, hypomania, irritability, and disinhibition of anger, aggression, or sexuality have been frequently noted months after recovery, and psychosis occurs rarely. Depressive symptoms may respond to treatment with antidepressants or stimulants. Hypomania, irritability, and disinhibition have benefited from mood stabilizers and antipsychotics, and behavior modification also may be helpful for aggressive and sexual behaviors.

The global pandemic encephalitis from 1917 to 1929, known as encephalitis lethargica (von Economo's disease), had an acute encephalitic phase during which lethargy, psychosis, and catatonia were common. This period was followed by a chronic postencephalitic syndrome that included parkinsonism, mania, depression, and apathy in adults, and conduct disorder, emotional lability, and tics in children, with relatively little cognitive impairment (Berger and Vilensky 2014). Similar cases continue to be sporadically reported. Whether encephalitis lethargica was truly related to influenza remains controversial.

Viral Hepatitis

For a discussion of viral hepatitis, see Chapter 19 ("Gastrointestinal Disorders").

Rabies

Rabies is a viral infection of mammals transmitted by bite. In the United States, wild animals (i.e., bats, raccoons) account for most cases of rabies. Worldwide, human mortality from endemic canine rabies is estimated to be about 59,000 deaths annually (Hampson et al. 2015). Transmission to humans is rare in developed countries.

The usual incubation period is 20–60 days but can vary from several days to years. Initial symptoms are nonspecific and include generalized anxiety, fever, agitation, hyperesthesia, and dysesthesia, especially at the site of inoculation. In the United States, rabies has been misdiagnosed as an anxiety disorder (Centers for Disease Control and Prevention 1991) and as alcohol withdrawal (Centers for Disease Control and Prevention 1998). In one case, "mild personality changes" preceded motor symptoms by more than a week (Centers for Disease Control and Prevention 2003). The initial phase is followed by an excitatory phase, in which the classic symptom of hydrophobia may occur. *Hydrophobia* is an aversion to swallowing liquids (not a phobia of water) secondary to the spasmodic contractions of the muscles of swallowing and respiration, resulting in pain and aspiration. The final phase is a general flaccid paralysis that progresses relentlessly to death. Both rabies and the rabies vaccine may cause delirium.

No effective treatment exists once symptoms are evident. After a bite by an infected animal, the rabies vaccine and immunoglobulin should be given as soon as possible.

Prion Diseases

Prions are proteinaceous agents that cause spongiform changes in the brain. Prion diseases are rare and universally fatal, with an incubation period of months to years—hence, the term "slow viruses" (see also Chapter 30, "Neurology and Neurosurgery"). *Kuru* occurs only in Papua, New Guinea. It was spread by the cannibalistic consumption of dead relatives during mourning rituals. Scrapie is a spongiform encephalopathy found in sheep. Although known to have been present in Great Britain for almost three centuries, scrapie has never been shown to cause disease in humans. Bovine spongiform encephalopathy ("mad cow disease") appears to have been transmitted to cattle by the practice of feeding cattle recycled sheep by-products.

Creutzfeldt-Jakob disease occurs sporadically (sCJD) and sometimes familially in humans, with a mean age at onset of 60 years. It also has been transmitted by intracerebral electrodes, grafts of dura mater, corneal transplants, human growth hormone, and gonadotropin, although such iatrogenic transmission is now rare. sCJD is a severe dementia accompanied by psychosis, affective lability, and dramatic myoclonus that rapidly progresses to rigid mutism and death. A retrospective review of 248 cases found psychiatric symptoms in 90% of sCJD patients, mostly present at disease onset (agitation in 64%, hallucinations in 45%, anxiety in 50%, depression in 37%) (Krasnianski et al. 2015).

New-variant CJD (nvCJD) was initially reported mainly in Great Britain but now has been found in many other countries. nvCJD has distinct differences from sCJD. nvCJD patients are considerably younger than sCJD patients, with an average age at onset of about 30 years, and the disease progresses less rapidly. In most cases of nvCJD, psychiatric symptoms appear several months before any neurological symptoms and include depression, irritability, anxiety, and apathy (Heath et al. 2011). nvCJD can be transmitted through the same iatrogenic routes as sCJD, appearing years after initial exposure. Detection of the 14–3–3 protein in CSF supports the diagnosis of sCJD; however, CSF 14-3-3 assays are not as sensitive or specific as was initially thought, and they are insensitive for nvCJD. The EEG is usually abnormal in both forms of CJD, but definitive diagnosis requires brain biopsy.

Fatal familial insomnia is an even rarer prion disease in which progressive insomnia (and sometimes behavior change) (Raggi et al. 2009) appears months before any cognitive, autonomic, or motor symptoms develop. Despite its name, the disease also occurs through sporadic mutation. Patients with this disorder initially may be given misdiagnoses of mood, anxiety, or somatic symptom disorders.

Fungal Infections

The frequency of fungal infection has steadily increased, coincident with the growing population of immunocompromised individuals who are surviving longer. An aging population, more malignancies, AIDS, the use of immunosuppressive and cytotoxic drugs, intravenous catheters, hyperalimentation, illicit drug use, extensive surgery, and the development of burn units also have contributed to the increased frequency of fungal infection. Whether CNS symptoms develop with such infections depends on the size and shape of the fungi. The smallest fungi have access to the cerebral microcirculation and infect the subarachnoid space. Large hyphae obstruct large and intermediate arteries, giving rise to extensive infarcts (e.g., aspergillosis). Fungi with pseudohyphae occlude small blood vessels, producing small infarctions and microabscesses (e.g., *Candida*). Most fungi are opportunistic (as in aspergillosis, mucormycosis, and candidiasis), but some are pathogenic (as in coccidioidomycosis and cryptococcosis) irrespective of the host's defenses. Many systemic fungal infections are treated with amphotericin B, which can cause neuropsychiatric side effects (see Table 26–3 later in chapter).

Aspergillosis

Aspergillus, an opportunistic organism, infects only individuals who are debilitated. CNS involvement usually follows infection of the lungs or gastrointestinal tract. Symptoms of confusion, headache, and lethargy often accompany focal neurological signs.

Cryptococcosis

Cryptococcosis is an infection caused by Cryptococcus species, a pathogen distributed worldwide. Cryptococcus may act as a solo pathogen, but in up to 85% of cases, it is associated with another illness, especially AIDS (see earlier discussion in the "Human Immunodeficiency Virus" section of this chapter). The portal of entry is usually the respiratory tract, from which hematogenous spread occurs (although pulmonary infection may not be evident at the time of presentation).

Cryptococcus is the most common form of fungal meningitis. It is typically insidious in onset and slowly progressive. Headache is present in up to 75% of cases, varying from mild and episodic to progressively incapacitating and constant. Other signs include cerebellar, cranial nerve, and motor deficits; irritability; and lethargy, which may progress to coma. Case reports of cryptococcal meningitis have included presentations with depression, mania, psychosis, and cognitive impairment. Remission and relapse are common in untreated patients. Isolation of the fungi provides a definitive diagnosis. Serological testing of patients with cryptococcal meningitis identifies cryptococcal antigen (in serum, CSF, or both) in about 90% of cases. Treatment is typically a prolonged course of an antifungal agent.

Coccidioidomycosis

Coccidioidomycosis is caused by a soil fungus endemic in warm, dry areas such as the southwestern United States, Mexico, and parts of South America (particularly Argentina and Paraguay). Coccidioides spores are inhaled in infected dust. Initial infection produces a mild febrile illness, often followed by pulmonary symptoms. Dissemination beyond the lung is relatively rare, and the CNS is not the most common extrapulmonary site. When it does occur, CNS infection is typically insidious in onset,

1–3 months after initial infection, presenting with headache associated with confusion, restlessness, hallucinations, lethargy, and transient focal signs.

Histoplasmosis

Histoplasmosis is a respiratory infection that is found throughout the world and is especially common in the central United States. *Histoplasma capsulatum* is inhaled with contaminated dust. Most infections are asymptomatic and involve the lungs or the reticuloendothelial system. The CNS is involved in 5%–10% of patients with progressive disseminated histoplasmosis. Most but not all are immunocompromised. CNS histoplasmosis may cause chronic meningitis, focal brain lesions, stroke due to infected emboli, and diffuse encephalitis (Saccente 2008).

Blastomycosis

Blastomyces dermatitidis is the causal agent of blastomycosis, an uncommon mycotic infection that in rare cases causes CNS infections, mainly in immunocompromised patients. Blastomycosis is co-endemic with histoplasmosis in the central United States. The most common CNS manifestations are stiff neck and headache, eventually progressing to confusion and lethargy.

Mucormycosis

Mucormycosis refers to any infection caused by a member of the family *Mucoraceae,* opportunistic fungi found in common bread and fruit molds. Mucormycosis is notorious for causing an acute fulminant infection in diabetic patients and patients with neutropenia. Mucor directly invades tissue and disseminates by attacking contiguous structures. Any diabetic patient with a purulent, febrile infection of the face or nose should be emergently evaluated for mucormycosis, because it may rapidly erode into the orbit and cerebrum in a matter of hours. Early mild encephalopathy may quickly progress to severe delirium. Aggressive debridement and intravenous antifungal medication are required.

Candidiasis

Candida causes limited local infections (cutaneous, vaginal, oral) in immunocompetent hosts, typically after broad-spectrum antibiotics. Disseminated candidiasis occurs only in immunocompromised patients. Psychiatric symptoms occur from the toxic effects of fungemia or from direct invasion of the CNS. Cerebral lesions generally occur late in the course of disseminated candidiasis. Candida may cause meningitis, micro-abscesses, macro-abscesses, or vasculitis in the CNS. The nonspecific signs include confusion, drowsiness, lethargy, and headache. Sometimes candida can be cultured from blood or CSF, but most cases of CNS candidiasis are not discovered until autopsy. Suggestive neuroimaging findings and isolation of candida from a non-CNS site in an immunocompromised patient should prompt treatment with appropriate antifungal agents.

An alternative medicine belief is that occult systemic candida infection is the cause of a wide array of somatic and psychological symptoms. There is no scientific support for this theory or its advocated treatments.

Parasitic Infections

Neurocysticercosis

One of the world's most common parasitic infections—neurocysticercosis—is an infection of the CNS by the larval form (cysticerci) of *Taenia solium,* also known as "pork tapeworm." For neurocysticercosis to occur, a human must ingest the tapeworm's eggs through contact with infected swine or humans. Once ingested, the eggs hematogenously spread to the CNS and other sites. Cysticercosis is endemic in developing nations. A Venezuelan study found that cysticercosis infection was much more common among psychiatric inpatients—especially those with intellectual disability—than among healthy control subjects (Meza et al. 2005). In the United States, the infection is usually reported in immigrants from Latin America. Neurocysticercosis was reportedly identified in 10% of patients with seizures presenting to an emergency department in Los Angeles, California, and in 6% of those presenting to an emergency department in New Mexico (Ong et al. 2002).

A high percentage of neurocysticercosis infections remain asymptomatic. However, cerebral involvement may produce seizures, stroke, or hydrocephalus, and neurocysticercosis is the leading cause of seizures in adults residing in areas where the disease is endemic. Psychiatric symptoms are frequently reported and include depression and psychosis. Neurocysticercosis is a common cause of dementia in developing nations (Ciampi de Andrade et al. 2010), although the cognitive decline may be reversible (Ramirez-Bermudez et al. 2005).

Through the clinical history, neuroimaging, and serology, a presumptive diagnosis of neurocysticercosis usually can be made. Definitive diagnosis of neurocysticercosis requires a biopsy, but this step is usually impractical. Treatment of neurocysticercosis infection has involved anticonvulsants, steroids, antihelminthics, and shunting for hydrocephalus. However, antihelminthic drugs may actually aggravate neuropsychiatric symptoms in neurocysticercosis, and their use in some forms of the disease is controversial.

Toxoplasmosis

Toxoplasmosis refers to the disease caused by *Toxoplasma gondii,* a parasite ubiquitously affecting all mammals, some birds, and probably some reptiles. It is the most prevalent human infection, with an estimated 30%–50% of the world population infected, and up to 95% in some regions. Latent infection is common, but in immunosuppressed individuals, particularly those with AIDS (also see discussion of toxoplasmosis in the "Human Immunodeficiency Virus" section of this chapter), toxoplasmosis may preferentially infect the CNS, resulting in a wide range of clinical presentations. Mass lesions mimicking tumors or abscesses are most common, but psychosis has been reported as a presenting symptom. Effective antibiotic therapy can produce rapid remission of active infection but must be continued throughout life to prevent recurrence. Maternal or patient toxoplasmosis exposure has been associated with increased risk for schizophrenia and possibly other psychiatric disorders, but no causal relationship has been established (Torrey and Yolken 2017).

Trypanosomiasis

The family of protozoa *Trypanosomatidae* causes two different syndromes: African trypanosomiasis (sleeping sickness) and American trypanosomiasis (Chagas' disease). African trypanosomiasis, which occurs in several sub-Saharan African countries, is caused by a subspecies of *Trypanosoma brucei* and is transmitted to humans and animals by the bite of the tsetse fly. The illness begins with a lesion at the site of the fly bite, followed by headache, fever, malaise, weight loss, and myalgia, and is often misdiagnosed as malaria. Later, the parasite crosses the blood–brain barrier and causes encephalitis with neuropsychiatric, motor, and sensory abnormalities (Blum et al. 2006; Kennedy 2006), with usually fatal outcome. "Sleeping sickness" is a disturbance of the sleep–wake cycle with bouts of fatigue progressing to daytime somnolence and nighttime insomnia. Meningoencephalitis may develop with prominent somnolence—hence the name "sleeping sickness." One report found that psychiatric symptoms such as hallucinations (21.4%) or depression (21.4%) dominated the clinical picture, leading some patients to be psychiatrically hospitalized (Urech et al. 2011). The drug used to treat late-stage disease is very toxic, with an often-fatal encephalopathy the most feared complication of treatment (Blum et al. 2001); for this reason, early detection—permitting less toxic treatment—is important.

American trypanosomiasis, or Chagas' disease, is caused by *Trypanosoma cruzi*, which is carried by insects ("kissing bugs" or "assassin bugs") in Latin America. More than 300,000 persons chronically infected with Chagas' disease now live in the United States. Transmission is so inefficient that years of exposure are required to acquire the infection. Once acquired, infection is typically lifelong but is asymptomatic in most cases (Bern 2015). Following immunosuppression, reactivated disease may present as meningoencephalitis or brain abscesses. In immunocompetent patients, manifestations of CNS Chagas' disease are nonspecific and minor (Wackermann et al. 2008).

On brain imaging, the lesions are indistinguishable from those of toxoplasmosis, and the organism is often not identifiable in blood. Reactivated Chagas' disease should be suspected in immunosuppressed immigrants from endemic areas of Latin America, especially in presumed cases of toxoplasmosis not responsive to chemotherapy.

Malaria

Malaria remains a major cause of morbidity in tropical nations, especially in young children and pregnant women. In other parts of the world, cases occur in immigrants and travelers to malarial areas. *Plasmodium* species are transmitted to humans by the bite of mosquitoes.

Relapsing fever typifies malaria, with temperatures commonly in excess of 41°C (105°F), and delirium is common. *Plasmodium falciparum* causes cerebral malaria, the most catastrophic complication of malaria, with a mortality rate of 15%–20%. Cerebral malaria begins with disorientation, mild stupor, agitation, and psychosis, and rapidly progresses to seizures and coma (Mishra and Newton 2009). Children who survive cerebral malaria are at increased risk of cognitive impairment, developmental delay, and behavioral problems (Idro et al. 2016). Anxiety and depression are common after recovery in adults (Tesfaye et al. 2014). More severe neuropsychiatric signs, including psychosis in patients fully recovered (aparasitemic) from cerebral malaria, are most likely attributable to pharmacotherapy, as antimalarial drugs commonly cause psychiatric side effects (see Table 26–3 later in chapter). Mefloquine in chemo-prophylaxis doses causes severe CNS side effects (e.g., psychosis, seizures) in 0.1% of persons treated, and other adverse psychiatric symptoms (e.g., nightmares, depression, irritability) in 0.02%–0.5%. Vivid dreams occur in 15%–25% (Freedman 2008). Patients who have had cerebral malaria are more vulnerable to mefloquine's psychiatric adverse effects.

Schistosomiasis

Schistosomiasis is an infection caused by blood flukes (trematodes) of the genus *Schistosoma.* Infection by the larval stage usually occurs while the individual is swimming in infected fresh water. The infection affects about 200 million people in 78 countries (*Schistosoma japonicum* in the Far East; *S. mansoni* and *S. haematobium* in Africa). Most infections are asymptomatic. CNS symptoms are uncommon, but once the worms mature and the eggs have been laid, CNS involvement may be observed with any of the clinical forms of schistosomal infection. Eggs in the CNS may induce a granulomatous reaction, but in most cases, eggs in the CNS are clinically silent. Neurological complications of cerebral schistosomiasis include delirium, seizures, dysphasia, visual field impairment, focal motor deficits, and ataxia (Ross et al. 2012). In advanced disease with *S. mansoni* or *S. haematobium*, portal hypertension is a serious complication, with hepatic encephalopathy.

Trichinosis

Trichinosis is a worldwide disease caused by the ingestion of *Trichinella* larvae encysted in the muscles of infected animals. *Trichinella* larvae are most commonly found in pork in the United States and Europe, but 150 species of mammals from all latitudes may acquire the infection. Trichinosis has become rare in most developed nations but still occurs in ethnic populations that habitually consume raw or undercooked pork or wild animals, such as boar, polar bear, or walrus. Typical symptoms of infection include a febrile illness with myalgias and diarrhea, accompanied by marked eosino-philia. CNS involvement occurs in 10%–20% of cases, through a variety of mechanisms, including obstruction, toxicity, inflammation, vasculitis, and allergic reactions, and may result in headache, delirium, insomnia, meningoencephalitis, and seizures. Neuropsychiatric sequelae and chronic fatigue are common after infection (Nemet et al. 2009), and residual cognitive dysfunction may occur (Harms et al. 1993). CT or MRI scans show multiple small hypodense lesions with ringlike enhancement with contrast. A muscle biopsy is usually diagnostic. Treatment in severe cases requires corticosteroids for the inflammation and antihelminthic drugs to kill *Trichinella.*

Amebiasis

Several amoebas cause human disease and are ubiquitous worldwide. CNS infection with amoebas is rare in the United States. Primary amoebic meningoencephalitis is caused by *Naegleria fowleri,* most often infecting healthy young individuals who engage in water sports. Its course is acute and fulminant, with headache, nausea, confusion, and stiff neck followed by coma and death within days. Granulomatous amoebic encephalitis, caused by *Balamuthia mandrillaris* and some species of *Acan-*

thamoeba, usually occurs in debilitated, immunosuppressed (especially in AIDS), or malnourished individuals. The course is more chronic, with personality changes, confusion, and irritability, eventually progressing to seizures and death (Schuster et al. 2009).

Drugs for Infectious Diseases: Adverse Psychiatric Effects and Drug Interactions

That antibiotics can cause delirium and other psychiatric symptoms is not well appreciated. The best-documented psychiatric side effects of drugs for infectious diseases, and of antiretroviral drugs, are listed in Tables 26–3 and 26–4, respectively. Delirium and psychosis have been particularly associated with quinolones (e.g., ciprofloxacin), procaine penicillin, antimalarial and other antiparasitic drugs (especially mefloquine), and the antituberculous drug cycloserine. The most common adverse effect causing discontinuation of interferon has been depression. Metronidazole and tinidazole can cause disulfiram-like reactions after alcohol ingestion. More detailed reviews are available elsewhere (e.g., Kogut et al. 2017).

Table 26–5 shows selected well-established interactions between antimicrobial and psychotropic drugs. Drug interactions between antibiotics and nonpsychiatric drugs also may pose a risk in psychiatric practice. Erythromycin (and similar antibiotics, such as clarithromycin) and ketoconazole (and similar antifungals) may cause QT interval prolongation and ventricular arrhythmias when given to a patient taking other QT-prolonging drugs, including TCAs and many antipsychotics. Linezolid is an irreversible monoamine oxidase A (MAO-A) inhibitor and therefore may cause serotonin syndrome if taken with serotonergic antidepressants, and hypertensive crisis if taken with sympathomimetics. Isoniazid is a weaker MAO inhibitor. Details regarding the effects of antibiotics on psychiatric drugs via cytochrome P450 interactions can be found elsewhere (Kogut et al. 2017).

Fears of Infectious Disease

Infectious diseases historically have been, and remain, frightening, particularly epidemics of previously unrecognized diseases, such as AIDS, severe acute respiratory syndrome (SARS), Ebola virus disease, and Middle Eastern respiratory syndrome (MERS). Both affected patients and health care workers experience fears of the illness and fears of contagion to family and friends, often resulting in posttraumatic stress disorder (Mak et al. 2009). Quarantined patients struggle with loneliness, isolation, and stigmatization. Hysterical and paranoid reactions in the general population have resulted in targeting and shunning not only of those infected but also of stigmatized high-risk groups and exposed health care workers (Gonsalves and Staley 2014). Such reactions are amplified by sensational media coverage. Governmental reactions may range from draconian measures to frank denial. Feared, stigmatized infected individuals may delay seeking care and remain undetected and untreated. Widespread panic may occur in the event of an outbreak, pointing to the need for psychologically informed public health measures (Lau et al. 2007).

TABLE 26–3. Psychiatric side effects of drugs for infectious diseases (excluding antiretroviral drugs)

Drug	Neuropsychiatric adverse effects
Antibacterial	
Cephalosporins	Euphoria, delusions, depersonalization, illusions
Dapsone	Insomnia, agitation, hallucinations, mania, depression
Procaine penicillin[a]	Agitation, depersonalization, fear of imminent death, hallucinations (probably due to procaine)
Quinolones[a]	Psychosis, paranoia, mania, agitation, Tourette-like syndrome
Trimethoprim–sulfamethoxazole	Delirium, psychosis
Gentamicin	Delirium, psychosis
Clarithromycin	Delirium, mania
Antituberculous	
Cycloserine[a]	Agitation, depression, psychosis, anxiety
Isoniazid	Psychosis, mania
Ethionamide	Depression, hallucinations
Antiviral	
Acyclovir, ganciclovir	Psychosis, delirium, depression, anxiety
Amantadine[a]	Psychosis, delirium
Oseltamivir, zanamivir	Psychosis, delirium
Interferon-alfa[a]	Irritability, depression, agitation, paranoia
Interleukin-2	Psychosis, delirium
Antifungal	
Amphotericin	Delirium, psychosis, depression
Antiparasitic	
Antimalarials[a](especially mefloquine)	Confusion, psychosis, mania, depression, anxiety, aggression, delirium
Metronidazole	Depression, delirium
Thiabendazole	Psychosis

Note. See also Brown and Stoudemire 1998.
[a]More significant (more frequent and/or better established) effects.

Source. Adapted from Abouesh et al. 2002; "Drugs That May Cause Psychiatric Symptoms" 2008; Kogut et al. 2017.

Both individual and group reactions to real or imagined threats of infectious diseases may include hysterical and phobic behaviors. Anxiety about acquiring a feared disease may lead to conversion symptoms, hypochondriacal preoccupation, and unnecessary avoidance behaviors. Contamination obsessions and washing compulsions are among the most frequent symptoms in obsessive-compulsive disorder. Delusional fears or beliefs that one is infected also occur in psychotic disorders, including

TABLE 26–4. **Psychiatric side effects of antiretroviral drugs**

Medication	Neuropsychiatric adverse effects
Nucleoside reverse transcriptase inhibitors	
Abacavir	Depression, mania, suicidal ideation, anxiety, psychosis, insomnia, nightmares, fatigue
Didanosine	Nervousness, agitation, mania, insomnia, dizziness, lethargy
Emtricitabine	Depression, abnormal dreams, insomnia, dizziness, confusion, irritability
Interferon-α-2a	Depression, suicidal ideation, anxiety, mania, psychosis, sleep disturbance, fatigue, delirium, cognitive dysfunction
Lamivudine	Depression, insomnia, dizziness, dystonia
Zidovudine	Anxiety, agitation, restlessness, insomnia, mild confusion, mania, psychosis
Nonnucleoside reverse transcriptase inhibitors	
Delavirdine	Anxiety, agitation, amnesia, confusion, dizziness
Efavirenz	Anxiety, insomnia, irritability, depression, suicidal ideation and behavior, psychosis, vivid dreams/nightmares, cognitive dysfunction, dizziness
Nevirapine	Vivid dreams or nightmares, visual hallucinations, delusions, mood changes
Etravirine	Sleep changes, dizziness
Rilpivirine	Abnormal dreams, insomnia, dizziness
Protease inhibitors	
Atazanavir	Depression, insomnia
Fosamprenavir	Depression
Indinavir	Anxiety, agitation, insomnia
Lopinavir and ritonavir	Insomnia
Nelfinavir	Depression, anxiety, insomnia
Ritonavir	Anxiety, agitation, insomnia, confusion, amnesia, emotional lability, euphoria, hallucinations, decreased libido, metallic taste
Saquinavir	Anxiety, agitation, irritability, depression, excessive dreaming, hallucinations, euphoria, confusion, amnesia
Tipranavir	Depression
Integrase inhibitors	
Raltegravir	Depression, suicidal ideation, psychosis, vivid dreams or nightmares, vertigo, dizziness
Elvitegravir	Depression, insomnia, suicidal ideation
Dolutegravir	Insomnia, fatigue
Fusion inhibitors	
Enfuvirtide	Depression, insomnia
Maraviroc	Dizziness, insomnia

Source. Adapted from Abouesh et al. 2002; "Drugs That May Cause Psychiatric Symptoms" 2008; Kogut et al. 2017.

TABLE 26–5.   Selected antimicrobial–psychotropic drug interactions

Antimicrobial	Effect on psychiatric drug
Antimalarials	Increase phenothiazine level
Azoles	Increase alprazolam, midazolam levels
	Increase buspirone level
Clarithromycin, erythromycin	Increase alprazolam, midazolam levels
	Increase carbamazepine level
	Increase buspirone level
	Increase clozapine level
Quinolones	Increase clozapine level
	Increase benzodiazepine level
	Decrease benzodiazepine effect via GABA receptor
Isoniazid	Increases haloperidol level
	Increases carbamazepine level
	With disulfiram, causes ataxia
Linezolid	With serotonergic drugs, causes serotonin syndrome

Note.   GABA=gamma-aminobutyric acid.

schizophrenia, psychotic depression, and delusional disorder, somatic type (e.g., de-lusions of parasitosis; see Chapter 27, "Dermatology"); however, it is important to consider the possibility that a patient with a delusion of infection may actually be in-fected. Unrealistic fears of infection are especially likely with sexually transmitted diseases (particularly HIV disease), serious outbreaks (e.g., meningococcal meningi-tis on campus), and infectious threats given heavy media coverage (e.g., bacterial food contamination, bovine spongiform encephalopathy, anthrax). Of course, how much vigilance and which precautions are optimal may be uncertain even among ex-perts, but the early years of the AIDS epidemic were a clear example of the potential for widespread irrational behaviors among the public, health care professionals, and officials (Gonsalves and Staley 2014).

At times, mass outbreaks of symptoms occur, falsely attributed to a supposed toxic exposure (e.g., bacterial food poisoning, toxic fumes) or infectious disease. There have been hundreds of reports in the literature of such outbreaks of "mass psychogenic" or "mass sociogenic" illness, and they tend to follow trends in societal concerns (e.g., bio-terrorism). They are most likely to occur in groups of young people in close quarters, such as students at schools or military recruits. Social media have amplified the spread of such mass outbreaks of symptoms (Bartholomew et al. 2012). Some aspects of "germ panic" have become socially normative (Tomes 2000)—for example, inappro-priate use of antibiotics such as ciprofloxacin during the anthrax scare, and the wide-spread overuse of antiseptic soaps, mouthwashes, sprays, and cleaning agents.

Psychiatric Aspects of Immunizations

Psychological factors can influence the antibody response to vaccination. Several studies have shown that psychological stress suppresses the secondary (but not primary) antibody response to immunization (Cohen et al. 2001). However, whereas most studies have shown a reduction in antibody response (Pedersen et al. 2009), others have shown enhancement by stress (Edwards et al. 2008).

Mass outbreaks of psychogenic symptoms have been reported numerous times following vaccinations (Huang et al. 2010). Opposition to vaccination dates back to the very first vaccine in the 1800s. In developed countries, fears of vaccine-preventable diseases have waned, and disinformation regarding potential adverse effects of vaccines has been disseminated by the media and on the Web, resulting in widespread vaccine hesitancy and outright refusal to vaccinate children (Jacobson et al. 2015; Peretti-Watel et al. 2013). Lack of vaccination has led to outbreaks of measles and pertussis. Extensive research has conclusively shown that the measles-mumps-rubella vaccination does not cause autism or encephalitis and that thimerosol, a mercury-containing preservative in some vaccines, does not cause neuropsychological deficits (Jain et al. 2015; Maglione et al. 2014).

Conclusion

Many systemic and CNS infections present with psychiatric symptoms, and the psychiatric history should consider patients' immune status, region of origin and residence, travel, high-risk sexual behaviors, occupation, and recreational activities. Associations between specific infections and psychiatric syndromes provide intriguing but controversial attributions of etiology. Psychological factors may significantly affect the risk for and course of infectious diseases. Irrational fears of real or imagined infectious diseases and of immunization are also important clinical concerns deserving psychiatric attention.

References

Abouesh A, Stone C, Hobbs WR: Antimicrobial-induced mania (antiomania): a review of spontaneous reports. J Clin Psychopharmacol 22(1):71–81, 2002 11799346

Adam Y, Meinlschmidt G, Lieb R: Associations between mental disorders and the common cold in adults: a population-based cross-sectional study. J Psychosom Res 74(1):69–73, 2013 23272991

Aghanwa HS, Morakinyo O: Correlates of psychiatric morbidity in typhoid fever in a Nigerian general hospital setting. Gen Hosp Psychiatry 23(3):158–162, 2001 11427249

Alciati A, Gallo L, Monforte AD, et al: Major depression-related immunological changes and combination antiretroviral therapy in HIV-seropositive patients. Hum Psychopharmacol 22(1):33–40, 2007 17191264

Andraghetti R, Foran S, Colebunders R, et al: Euthanasia: from the perspective of HIV infected persons in Europe. HIV Med 2(1):3–10, 2001 11737370

Antinori A, Arendt G, Becker JT, et al: Updated research nosology for HIV-associated neurocognitive disorders. Neurology 69(18):1789–1799, 2007 17914061

Arciniegas DB, Anderson CA: Viral encephalitis: neuropsychiatric and neurobehavioral aspects. Curr Psychiatry Rep 6(5):372–379, 2004 15355760

Atkinson JH, Higgins JA, Vigil O, et al: Psychiatric context of acute/early HIV infection. The NIMH Multisite Acute HIV Infection Study: IV. AIDS Behav 13(6):1061–1067, 2009 19517225

Barnes V, Ware MR: Tetanus, pseudotetanus, or conversion disorder: a diagnostic dilemma? South Med J 86(5):591–592, 1993 8488415

Bartholomew RE, Wessely S, Rubin GJ: Mass psychogenic illness and the social network: is it changing the pattern of outbreaks? J R Soc Med 105(12):509–512, 2012 23288084

Berende A, ter Hofstede HJ, Vos FJ, et al: Randomized trial of longer-term therapy for symptoms attributed to Lyme disease. N Engl J Med 374(13):1209–1220, 2016 27028911

Berger JR, Vilensky JA: Encephalitis lethargica (von Economo's encephalitis). Handb Clin Neurol 123:745–761, 2014 25015515

Bern C: Chagas' disease. N Engl J Med 373(5):456–466, 2015 26222561

Beyer JL, Taylor L, Gersing KR, et al: Prevalence of HIV infection in a general psychiatric outpatient population. Psychosomatics 48(1):31–37, 2007 17209147

Bloch M, Kamminga J, Jayewardene A, et al: A screening strategy for HIV-associated neurocognitive disorders that accurately identifies patients requiring neurological review. Clin Infect Dis 63(5):687–693, 2016 27325690

Blum J, Nkunku S, Burri C: Clinical description of encephalopathic syndromes and risk factors for their occurrence and outcome during melarsoprol treatment of human African trypanosomiasis. Trop Med Int Health 6(5):390–400, 2001 11348533

Blum J, Schmid C, Burri C: Clinical aspects of 2541 patients with second stage human African trypanosomiasis. Acta Trop 97(1):55–64, 2006 16157286

Bonawitz C, Castillo M, Mukherji SK: Comparison of CT and MR features with clinical outcome in patients with Rocky Mountain spotted fever. AJNR Am J Neuroradiol 18(3):459–464, 1997 9090403

Brouillette MJ, Mayo N, Fellows LK, et al: A better screening tool for HIV-associated neurocognitive disorders: is it what clinicians need? AIDS 29(8):895–902, 2015 25291105

Brown GR: The use of methylphenidate for cognitive decline associated with HIV disease. Int J Psychiatry Med 25(1):21–37, 1995 7649716

Brown TM, Stoudemire A: Antibiotics, in Psychiatric Side Effects of Prescription and Over-the-Counter Medications: Recognition and Management. Washington, DC, American Psychiatric Press, 1998, pp 173–208

Campos LN, Guimarães MD, Remien RH: Anxiety and depression symptoms as risk factors for non-adherence to antiretroviral therapy in Brazil. AIDS Behav 14(2):289–299, 2010 18648925

Caroff SN, Mann SC, Glittoo MF, et al: Psychiatric manifestations of acute viral encephalitis. Psychiatr Ann 31(3):193–204, 2001

Carr SB, Bergamo DF, Emmanuel PJ, et al: Murine typhus as a cause of cognitive impairment: case report and a review of the literature. Pediatr Neurol 50(3):265–268, 2014 24321542

Carrico AW, Johnson MO, Morin SF, et al; NIMH Healthy Living Project Team: Correlates of suicidal ideation among HIV-positive persons. AIDS 21(9):1199–1203, 2007 17502730

Carteaux G, Maquart M, Bedet A, et al: Zika virus associated with meningoencephalitis. N Engl J Med 374(16):1595–1596, 2016 26958738

Centers for Disease Control and Prevention: Human rabies—Texas, Arkansas, and Georgia, 1991. MMWR Morb Mortal Wkly Rep 40(44):765–769, 1991 1944123

Centers for Disease Control and Prevention: Human rabies—Texas and New Jersey, 1997. MMWR Morb Mortal Wkly Rep 47(1):1–5, 1998 9450721

Centers for Disease Control and Prevention: First human death associated with raccoon rabies—Virginia, 2003. MMWR Morb Mortal Wkly Rep 52(45):1102–1103, 2003 14614408

Centers for Disease Control and Prevention: Diagnoses of HIV infection in the United States and dependent areas, 2015. HIV Surveillance Report 27, November 2016. Available at: https://www.cdc.gov/hiv/pdf/library/reports/surveillance/cdc-hiv-surveillance-report-2015-vol-27.pdf. Accessed June 9, 2017.

Chang K, Frankovich J, Cooperstock M, et al; PANS Collaborative Consortium: Clinical evaluation of youth with pediatric acute-onset neuropsychiatric syndrome (PANS): recommendations from the 2013 PANS Consensus Conference. J Child Adolesc Psychopharmacol 25(1):3–13, 2015 25325534

Ciampi de Andrade D, Rodrigues CL, Abraham R, et al: Cognitive impairment and dementia in neurocysticercosis: a cross-sectional controlled study. Neurology 74(16):1288–1295, 2010 20404310

Cohen MA, Gorman JM, Letendre SL, et al (eds): Comprehensive Textbook of AIDS Psychiatry, 2nd Edition. New York, Oxford University Press, 2017

Cohen S, Miller GE, Rabin BS: Psychological stress and antibody response to immunization: a critical review of the human literature. Psychosom Med 63(1):7–18, 2001 11211068

Conen A, Fehr J, Glass TR, et al: Self-reported alcohol consumption and its association with adherence and outcome of antiretroviral therapy in the Swiss HIV Cohort Study. Antivir Ther 14(3):349–357, 2009 19474469

Conrad C, Bradley HM, Broz D, et al; Centers for Disease Control and Prevention (CDC): Community outbreak of HIV infection linked to injection drug use of oxymorphone—Indiana, 2015. MMWR Morb Mortal Wkly Rep 64(16):443–444, 2015 25928470

Cysique LA, Deutsch R, Atkinson JH, et al; HNRC Group: Incident major depression does not affect neuropsychological functioning in HIV-infected men. J Int Neuropsychol Soc 13(1):1–11, 2007 17166298

Czub S, Koutsilieri E, Sopper S, et al: Enhancement of central nervous system pathology in early simian immunodeficiency virus infection by dopaminergic drugs. Acta Neuropathol 101:85–91, 2001 11271377

Davis HF, Skolasky R Jr, Selnes OA, et al: Assessing HIV-associated dementia: modified HIV dementia scale versus the grooved pegboard. AIDS Read 12(1):29–31, 38, 2002 11862658

Davstad I, Stenbacka M, Leifman A, et al: An 18-year follow-up of patients admitted to methadone treatment for the first time. J Addict Dis 28(1):39–52, 2009 19197594

De Hert M, Wampers M, Van Eyck D, et al: Prevalence of HIV and hepatitis C infection among patients with schizophrenia. Schizophr Res 108(1–3):307–308, 2009 19091513

de Sousa Gurgel W, da Silva Carneiro AH, Barreto Rebouças D, et al; Affective Disorders Study Group (GETA): Prevalence of bipolar disorder in a HIV-infected outpatient population. AIDS Care 25(12):1499–1503, 2013 23527945

Di YM, Li CG, Xue CC, et al: Clinical drugs that interact with St. John's wort and implication in drug development. Curr Pharm Des 14(17):1723–1742, 2008 18673195

Domingues RB, Kuster GW, Onuki-Castro FL, et al: Involvement of the central nervous system in patients with dengue virus infection. J Neurol Sci 267(1–2):36–40, 2008 17959198

Drago F, Merlo G, Ciccarese G, et al: Changes in neurosyphilis presentation: a survey on 286 patients. J Eur Acad Dermatol Venereol 30(11):1886–1900, 2016 27306850

Drugs That May Cause Psychiatric Symptoms. Med Lett Drugs Ther 50(1301–1302):100–103, 2008 19078866

Edwards KM, Burns VE, Adkins AE, et al: Meningococcal A vaccination response is enhanced by acute stress in men. Psychosom Med 70(2):147–151, 2008 18256346

Engsig FN, Hansen AB, Omland LH, et al: Incidence, clinical presentation, and outcome of progressive multifocal leukoencephalopathy in HIV-infected patients during the highly active antiretroviral therapy era: a nationwide cohort study. J Infect Dis 199(1):77–83, 2009 19007313

Eren S, Bayam G, Ergönül O, et al: Cognitive and emotional changes in neurobrucellosis. J Infect 53(3):184–189, 2006 16647757

Feder HM Jr, Johnson BJ, O'Connell S, et al; Ad Hoc International Lyme Disease Group: A critical appraisal of "chronic Lyme disease." N Engl J Med 357(14):1422–1430, 2007 17914043

Fenollar F, Puéchal X, Raoult D: Whipple's disease. N Engl J Med 356(1):55–66, 2007 17202456

Ferrando SJ, Freyberg Z: Treatment of depression in HIV positive individuals: a critical review. Int Rev Psychiatry 20(1):61–71, 2008 18240063

Freedman DO: Clinical practice. Malaria prevention in short-term travelers. N Engl J Med 359(6):603–612, 2008 18687641

Garg RK: Subacute sclerosing panencephalitis. J Neurol 255(12):1861–1871, 2008 18846316

Garvey MA, Perlmutter SJ, Allen AJ, et al: A pilot study of penicillin prophylaxis for neuropsychiatric exacerbations triggered by streptococcal infections. Biol Psychiatry 45(12):1564–1571, 1999 10376116

Gibbie T, Hay M, Hutchison CW, et al: Depression, social support and adherence to highly active antiretroviral therapy in people living with HIV/AIDS. Sex Health 4(4):227–232, 2007 18082064

Gliatto MF, Caroff SN: Neurosyphilis: a history and clinical review. Psychiatr Ann 31(3):153–161, 2001

Gonsalves G, Staley P: Panic, paranoia, and public health—the AIDS epidemic's lessons for Ebola. N Engl J Med 371(25):2348–2349, 2014 25372947

Hampson K, Coudeville L, Lembo T, et al; Global Alliance for Rabies Control Partners for Rabies Prevention: Estimating the global burden of endemic canine rabies. PLoS Negl Trop Dis 9(4):e0003709, 2015 25881058

Harms G, Binz P, Feldmeier H, et al: Trichinosis: a prospective controlled study of patients ten years after acute infection. Clin Infect Dis 17(4):637–643, 1993 8268344

Hashmi AM, Butt Z, Idrees Z, et al: Anxiety and depression symptoms in patients with dengue fever and their correlation with symptom severity. Int J Psychiatry Med 44(3):199–210, 2012 23586276

Hatherill S, Flisher A: Delirium in children with HIV/AIDS. J Child Neurol 24(7):879–883, 2009 19299649

Heath CA, Cooper SA, Murray K, et al: Diagnosing variant Creutzfeldt-Jakob disease: a retrospective analysis of the first 150 cases in the UK. J Neurol Neurosurg Psychiatry 82(6):646–651, 2011 21172857

Helm CE, Blackwood RA: Pediatric autoimmune neuropsychiatric disorder associated with streptococcal infections (PANDAS): experience at a tertiary referral center. Tremor Other Hyperkinet Mov (NY) 5:270, 2015 26196024

Hickie I, Davenport T, Wakefield D, et al; Dubbo Infection Outcomes Study Group: Post-infective and chronic fatigue syndromes precipitated by viral and non-viral pathogens: prospective cohort study. BMJ 333(7568):575, 2006 16950834

Himelhoch S, McCarthy JF, Ganoczy D, et al: Understanding associations between serious mental illness and HIV among patients in the VA Health System. Psychiatr Serv 58(9):1165–1172, 2007 17766561

Hinkin CH, Castellon SA, Hardy DJ, et al: Methylphenidate improves HIV-1-associated cognitive slowing. J Neuropsychiatry Clin Neurosci 13(2):248–254, 2001 11449032

Hirshfield S, Wolitski RJ, Chiasson MA, et al: Screening for depressive symptoms in an online sample of men who have sex with men. AIDS Care 20(8):904–910, 2008 18720088

Huang WT, Hsu CC, Lee PI, et al: Mass psychogenic illness in nationwide in-school vaccination for pandemic influenza A(H1N1) 2009, Taiwan, November 2009–January 2010. Euro Surveill 15(21):19575, 2010 20519106

Idro R, Kakooza-Mwesige A, Asea B, et al: Cerebral malaria is associated with long-term mental health disorders: a cross sectional survey of a long-term cohort. Malar J 15:184, 2016 27030124

Jacobson RM, St Sauver JL, Finney Rutten LJ: Vaccine hesitancy. Mayo Clin Proc 90(11):1562–1568, 2015 26541249

Jain A, Marshall J, Buikema A, et al: Autism occurrence by MMR vaccine status among US children with older siblings with and without autism. JAMA 313(15):1534–1540, 2015 25898051

Joska JA, Stein DJ, Grant I (eds): HIV/AIDS and Psychiatry. Hoboken, NJ, Wiley-Blackwell, 2014

Kaiser R: Tick-borne encephalitis. Infect Dis Clin North Am 22(3):561–575, x, 2008 18755391

Kalichman SC, Sikkema KJ, Kelly JA, et al: Use of a brief behavioral skills intervention to prevent HIV infection among chronic mentally ill adults. Psychiatr Serv 46(3):275–280, 1995 7796217

Kalish RA, Kaplan RF, Taylor E, et al: Evaluation of study patients with Lyme disease, 10–20-year follow-up. J Infect Dis 183(3):453–460, 2001 11133377

Kaplan JE, Benson C, Holmes KK, et al; Centers for Disease Control and Prevention (CDC); National Institutes of Health; HIV Medicine Association of the Infectious Diseases Society of America: Guidelines for prevention and treatment of opportunistic infections in HIV-infected adults and adolescents: recommendations from CDC, the National Institutes of Health, and the HIV Medicine Association of the Infectious Diseases Society of America. MMWR Recomm Rep 58(RR-4):1–207, quiz CE1–CE4, 2009 19357635

Kaplan RF, Trevino RP, Johnson GM, et al: Cognitive function in post-treatment Lyme disease: do additional antibiotics help? Neurology 60(12):1916–1922, 2003 12821733

Kelly DV, Béïque LC, Bowmer MI: Extrapyramidal symptoms with ritonavir/indinavir plus risperidone. Ann Pharmacother 36(5):827–830, 2002 11978161

Kennedy PG: Human African trypanosomiasis-neurological aspects. J Neurol 253(4):411–416, 2006 16541214

Kirkland LR, Fischl MA, Tashima KT, et al; NZTA4007 Study Team: Response to lamivudine-zidovudine plus abacavir twice daily in antiretroviral-naive, incarcerated patients with HIV infection taking directly observed treatment. Clin Infect Dis 34(4):511–518, 2002 11797179

Klempner MS, Hu LT, Evans J, et al: Two controlled trials of antibiotic treatment in patients with persistent symptoms and a history of Lyme disease. N Engl J Med 345(2):85–92, 2001 11450676

Koenig LJ, Pals SL, Bush T, et al: Randomized controlled trial of an intervention to prevent adherence failure among HIV-infected patients initiating antiretroviral therapy. Health Psychol 27(2):159–169, 2008 18377134

Kogut CP, Ferrando SJ, Levenson JL, et al: Infectious disease, in Clinical Manual of Psychopharmacology in the Medically Ill, 2nd Edition. Edited by Levenson JL, Ferrando SJ. Arlington, VA, American Psychiatric Publishing, 2017, pp 471–514

Krasnianski A, Bohling GT, Harden M, et al: Psychiatric symptoms in patients with sporadic Creutzfeldt-Jakob disease in Germany. J Clin Psychiatry 76(9):1209–1215, 2015 25938948

Krupp LB, Hyman LG, Grimson R, et al: Study and treatment of post Lyme disease (STOP-LD): a randomized double masked clinical trial. Neurology 60(12):1923–1930, 2003 12821734

Kumar V, Encinosa W: Effects of antidepressant treatment on antiretroviral regimen adherence among depressed HIV-infected patients. Psychiatr Q 80(3):131–141, 2009 19387832

Kuni BJ, Banwell BL, Till C: Cognitive and behavioral outcomes in individuals with a history of acute disseminated encephalomyelitis (ADEM). Dev Neuropsychol 37(8):682–696, 2012 23145566

Kupfer MC, Zee CS, Colletti PM, et al: MRI evaluation of AIDS-related encephalopathy: toxoplasmosis vs. lymphoma. Magn Reson Imaging 8(1):51–57, 1990 2325518

Kurlan R, Johnson D, Kaplan EL; Tourette Syndrome Study Group: Streptococcal infection and exacerbations of childhood tics and obsessive-compulsive symptoms: a prospective blinded cohort study. Pediatrics 121(6):1188–1197, 2008 18519489

Lau JT, Kim JH, Tsui H, et al: Perceptions related to human avian influenza and their associations with anticipated psychological and behavioral responses at the onset of outbreak in the Hong Kong Chinese general population. Am J Infect Control 35(1):38–49, 2007 17276790

Lee R, Monteiro EF: Third regional audit of antiretroviral prescribing in HIV patients. Yorkshire Audit Group for HIV Related Diseases. Int J STD AIDS 14(1):58–60, 2003 12590796

Lenz G, Demal U: Quality of life in depression and anxiety disorders: an exploratory follow-up study after intensive inpatient cognitive behaviour therapy. Psychopathology 33(6):297–302, 2000 11060512

Leserman J, Barroso J, Pence BW, et al: Trauma, stressful life events and depression predict HIV-related fatigue. AIDS Care 20(10):1258–1265, 2008 18608079

Liu H, Golin CE, Miller LG, et al: A comparison study of multiple measures of adherence to HIV protease inhibitors. Ann Intern Med 134(10):968–977, 2001 11352698

Lucas MJ, Brouwer MC, van de Beek D: Neurological sequelae of bacterial meningitis. J Infect 73(1):18–27, 2016 27105658

Lyketsos CG, Hanson AL, Fishman M, et al: Manic syndrome early and late in the course of HIV. Am J Psychiatry 150(2):326–327, 1993 8422087

Lyketsos CG, Hoover DR, Guccione M, et al: Changes in depressive symptoms as AIDS develops. The Multicenter AIDS Cohort Study. Am J Psychiatry 153(11):1430–1437, 1996 8890676

Lyketsos CG, Schwartz J, Fishman M, et al: AIDS mania. J Neuropsychiatry Clin Neurosci 9(2):277–279, 1997 9144109

Maglione MA, Das L, Raaen L, et al: Safety of vaccines used for routine immunization of U.S. children: a systematic review. Pediatrics 134(2):325–337, 2014 25086160

Mak IW, Chu CM, Pan PC, et al: Long-term psychiatric morbidities among SARS survivors. Gen Hosp Psychiatry 31(4):318–326, 2009 19555791

Malta M, Strathdee SA, Magnanini MM, et al: Adherence to antiretroviral therapy for human immunodeficiency virus/acquired immune deficiency syndrome among drug users: a systematic review. Addiction 103(8):1242–1257, 2008 18855813

Mao L, Kidd MR, Rogers G, et al: Social factors associated with major depressive disorder in homosexually active, gay men attending general practices in urban Australia. Aust N Z J Public Health 33(1):83–86, 2009 19236365

Markowicz M, Kivaranovic D, Stanek G: Testing patients with non-specific symptoms for antibodies against Borrelia burgdorferi sensu lato does not provide useful clinical information about their aetiology. Clin Microbiol Infect 21(12):1098–1103, 2015 26321669

McAuliffe P, Brassard MR, Fallon B: Memory and executive functions in adolescents with post-treatment Lyme disease. Appl Neuropsychol 15(3):208–219, 2008 18726742

McDermott BE, Sautter FJ, Winstead DK, et al: Diagnosis, health beliefs, and risk of HIV infection in psychiatric patients. Hosp Community Psychiatry 45(6):580–585, 1994 8088793

McNabb J, Ross JW, Abriola K, et al: Adherence to highly active antiretroviral therapy predicts outcome at an inner-city human immunodeficiency virus clinic. Clin Infect Dis 33(5):700–705, 2001 11486292

Meade CS, Hansen NB, Kochman A, et al: Utilization of medical treatments and adherence to antiretroviral therapy among HIV-positive adults with histories of childhood sexual abuse. AIDS Patient Care STDS 23(4):259–266, 2009 19260772

Meade CS, Bevilacqua LA, Key MD: Bipolar disorder is associated with HIV transmission risk behavior among patients in treatment for HIV. AIDS Behav 16(8):2267–2271, 2012 22614744

Mellins CA, Havens JF, McDonnell C, et al: Adherence to antiretroviral medications and medical care in HIV-infected adults diagnosed with mental and substance abuse disorders. AIDS Care 21(2):168–177, 2009 19229685

Meltzer-Brody S, Davidson JR: Completeness of response and quality of life in mood and anxiety disorders. Depress Anxiety 12 (suppl 1):95–101, 2000 11098422

Metzger DS, Donnell D, Celentano DD, et al; HPTN 058 Protocol Team: Expanding substance use treatment options for HIV prevention with buprenorphine-naloxone: HIV Prevention Trials Network 058. J Acquir Immune Defic Syndr 68(5):554–561, 2015 25564105

Meza NW, Rossi NE, Galeazzi TN, et al: Cysticercosis in chronic psychiatric inpatients from a Venezuelan community. Am J Trop Med Hyg 73(3):504–509, 2005 16172472

Mishra SK, Newton CR: Diagnosis and management of the neurological complications of falciparum malaria. Nat Rev Neurol 5(4):189–198, 2009 19347024

Misra UK, Kalita J, Mani VE: Neurological manifestations of scrub typhus. J Neurol Neurosurg Psychiatry 86(7):761–766, 2015 25209416

Mohamed W, Neil E, Kupsky WJ, et al: Isolated intracranial Whipple's disease—report of a rare case and review of the literature. J Neurol Sci 308(1–2):1–8, 2011 21696776

Moore A, Nelson C, Molins C, et al: Current guidelines, common clinical pitfalls, and future directions for laboratory diagnosis of Lyme disease, United States. Emerg Infect Dis 22(7), 2016 27314832

Moulton CD, Koychev I: The effect of penicillin therapy on cognitive outcomes in neurosyphilis: a systematic review of the literature. Gen Hosp Psychiatry 37(1):49–52, 2015 25468254

Murphy TK, Patel PD, McGuire JF, et al: Characterization of the pediatric acute-onset neuropsychiatric syndrome phenotype. J Child Adolesc Psychopharmacol 25(1):14–25, 2015 25314221

Nakimuli-Mpungu E, Musisi S, Mpungu SK, et al: Primary mania versus HIV-related secondary mania in Uganda. Am J Psychiatry 163(8):1349–1354, quiz 1480, 2006 16877646

Nath A, Maragos WF, Avison MJ, et al: Acceleration of HIV dementia with methamphetamine and cocaine. J Neurovirol 7(1):66–71, 2001 11519485

Navia BA, Jordan BD, Price RW: The AIDS dementia complex, I: clinical features. Ann Neurol 19(6):517–524, 1986 3729308

Nemet C, Rogozea L, Dejica R: Results of the follow-up of the former trichinosis patients from Brasov County—Romania. Vet Parasitol 159(3–4):320–323, 2009 19081195

Nichol G, Dennis DT, Steere AC, et al: Test-treatment strategies for patients suspected of having Lyme disease: a cost-effectiveness analysis. Ann Intern Med 128(1):37–48, 1998 9424980

Nolan MS, Hause AM, Murray KO: Findings of long-term depression up to 8 years post infection from West Nile virus. J Clin Psychol 68(7):801–808, 2012 23929558

Oksi J, Nikoskelainen J, Hiekkanen H, et al: Duration of antibiotic treatment in disseminated Lyme borreliosis: a double-blind, randomized, placebo-controlled, multicenter clinical study. Eur J Clin Microbiol Infect Dis 26(8):571–581, 2007 17587070

Ong S, Talan DA, Moran GJ, et al; EMERGEncy ID NET Study Group: Neurocysticercosis in radiographically imaged seizure patients in U.S. emergency departments. Emerg Infect Dis 8(6):608–613, 2002 12023918

Orlovska S, Vestergaard CH, Bech BH, et al: Association of streptococcal throat infection with mental disorders: testing key aspects of the PANDAS hypothesis in a nationwide study. JAMA Psychiatry 74(7):740–746, 2017 28538981

Osher FC, Goldberg RW, McNary SW, et al; Five-Site Health and Risk Study Research Committee: Substance abuse and the transmission of hepatitis C among persons with severe mental illness. Psychiatr Serv 54(6):842–847, 2003 12773598

Panel on Antiretroviral Guidelines for Adults and Adolescents: Guidelines for the use of antiretroviral agents in HIV-1-infected adults and adolescents. Department of Health and Human Services, July 2016. Available at: https://aidsinfo.nih.gov/contentfiles/lvguidelines/AdultandAdolescentGL.pdf. Accessed June 9, 2017.

Panel on Opportunistic Infections in HIV-Infected Adults and Adolescents: Guidelines for the prevention and treatment of opportunistic infections in HIV-infected adults and adolescents: recommendations from the Centers for Disease Control and Prevention, the National Institutes of Health, and the HIV Medicine Association of the Infectious Diseases Society of America. Revised March 7, 2018. Available at https://aidsinfo.nih.gov/contentfiles/lvguidelines/Adult_OI.pdf. Accessed March 30, 2018.

Park BJ, Wannemuehler KA, Marston BJ, et al: Estimation of the current global burden of cryptococcal meningitis among persons living with HIV/AIDS. AIDS 23(4):525–530, 2009 19182676

Parry CM, Hien TT, Dougan G, et al: Typhoid fever. N Engl J Med 347(22):1770–1782, 2002 12456854

Paterson DL, Swindells S, Mohn J, et al: Adherence to protease inhibitor therapy and outcomes in patients with HIV infection. Ann Intern Med 133(1):21–30, 2000 [Erratum in: Ann Intern Med 136(3):253, 2002] 10877736

Pearson FS, Cleland CM, Chaple M, et al: Substance use, mental health problems, and behavior at risk for HIV: evidence from CJDATS. J Psychoactive Drugs 40(4):459–469, 2008 19283950

Pecenak J, Janik P, Vaseckova B, et al: Electroconvulsive therapy treatment in a patient with neurosyphilis and psychotic disorder: case report and literature review. J ECT 31(4):268–270, 2015 25634568

Pedersen AF, Zachariae R, Bovbjerg DH: Psychological stress and antibody response to influenza vaccination: a meta-analysis. Brain Behav Immun 23(4):427–433, 2009 19486657

Peretti-Watel P, Verger P, Raude J, et al: Dramatic change in public attitudes towards vaccination during the 2009 influenza A(H1N1) pandemic in France. Euro Surveill 18(44):20623, 2013 24176658

Perrin EM, Murphy ML, Casey JR, et al: Does group A beta-hemolytic streptococcal infection increase risk for behavioral and neuropsychiatric symptoms in children? Arch Pediatr Adolesc Med 158(9):848–856, 2004 15351749

Petersen LR, Jamieson DJ, Powers AM, et al: Zika virus. N Engl J Med 374(16):1552–1563, 2016 27028561

Pollack TM, McCoy C, Stead W: Clinically significant adverse events from a drug interaction between quetiapine and atazanavir-ritonavir in two patients. Pharmacotherapy 29(11):1386–1391, 2009 19857154

Powderly WG: Cryptococcal meningitis in HIV-infected patients. Curr Infect Dis Rep 2(4):352–357, 2000 11095877

Prather AA, Janicki-Deverts D, Hall MH, et al: Behaviorally assessed sleep and susceptibility to the common cold. Sleep 38(9):1353–1359, 2015 26118561

Prince JD, Walkup J, Akincigil A, et al: Serious mental illness and risk of new HIV/AIDS diagnoses: an analysis of Medicaid beneficiaries in eight states. Psychiatr Serv 63(10):1032–1038, 2012 22855268

Rabkin JG, Wagner GJ, Rabkin R: A double-blind, placebo-controlled trial of testosterone therapy for HIV-positive men with hypogonadal symptoms. Arch Gen Psychiatry 57(2):141–147, discussion 155–156, 2000 10665616

Rabkin JG, McElhiney MC, Rabkin R, et al: Placebo-controlled trial of dehydroepiandrosterone (DHEA) for treatment of nonmajor depression in patients with HIV/AIDS. Am J Psychiatry 163(1):59–66, 2006 16390890

Raggi A, Perani D, Giaccone G, et al: The behavioural features of fatal familial insomnia: a new Italian case with pathological verification. Sleep Med 10(5):581–585, 2009 18824410

Ramirez-Bermudez J, Higuera J, Sosa AL, et al: Is dementia reversible in patients with neurocysticercosis? J Neurol Neurosurg Psychiatry 76(8):1164–1166, 2005 16024900

Ravdin LD, Hilton E, Primeau M, et al: Memory functioning in Lyme borreliosis. J Clin Psychiatry 57(7):282–286, 1996 8666568

Ribe AR, Vestergaard M, Katon W, et al: Thirty-day mortality after infection among persons with severe mental illness: a population-based cohort study in Denmark. Am J Psychiatry 172(8):776–783, 2015 25698437

Roberts MC, Emsley RA, Jordaan GP: Screening for syphilis and neurosyphilis in acute psychiatric admissions. S Afr Med J 82(1):16–18, 1992 1641712

Robotin MC, Law MG, Milliken S, et al: Clinical features and predictors of survival of AIDS-related non-Hodgkin's lymphoma in a population-based case series in Sydney, Australia. HIV Med 5(5):377–384, 2004 15369514

Ross AG, McManus DP, Farrar J, et al: Neuroschistosomiasis. J Neurol 259(1):22–32, 2012 21674195

Roux P, Carrieri MP, Villes V, et al: The impact of methadone or buprenorphine treatment and ongoing injection on highly active antiretroviral therapy (HAART) adherence: evidence from the MANIF2000 cohort study. Addiction 103(11):1828–1836, 2008 18778390

Saccente M: Central nervous system histoplasmosis. Curr Treat Options Neurol 10(3):161–167, 2008 18579019

Sacks N, Van Rensburg AJ: Clinical aspects of chronic brucellosis. S Afr Med J 50(19):725–728, 1976 818722

Sahu R, Verma R, Jain A, et al: Neurologic complications in dengue virus infection: a prospective cohort study. Neurology 83(18):1601–1609, 2014 25253749

Samaan Z, McDermid Vaz S, Bawor M, et al: Neuropsychological impact of West Nile virus infection: an extensive neuropsychiatric assessment of 49 cases in Canada. PLoS One 11(6):e0158364, 2016 27352145

Sanchez FM, Zisselman MH: Treatment of psychiatric symptoms associated with neurosyphilis. Psychosomatics 48(5):440–445, 2007 17878505

Sarkari NB, Thacker AK, Barthwal SP, et al: Japanese encephalitis (JE) part I: clinical profile of 1,282 adult acute cases of four epidemics. J Neurol 259(1):47–57, 2012a 21678123

Sarkari NB, Thacker AK, Barthwal SP, et al: Japanese encephalitis (JE) part II: 14 years' follow-up of survivors. J Neurol 259(1):58–69, 2012b 21681633

Saylor D, Dickens AM, Sacktor N, et al: HIV-associated neurocognitive disorder—pathogenesis and prospects for treatment. Nat Rev Neurol 12(4):234–248, 2016 26965674

Schroecksnadel K, Sarcletti M, Winkler C, et al: Quality of life and immune activation in patients with HIV-infection. Brain Behav Immun 22(6):881–889, 2008 18261883

Schuster FL, Yagi S, Gavali S, et al: Under the radar: balamuthia amebic encephalitis. Clin Infect Dis 48(7):879–887, 2009 19236272

Seltzer EG, Gerber MA, Cartter ML, et al: Long-term outcomes of persons with Lyme disease. JAMA 283(5):609–616, 2000 10665700

Semiz UB, Turhan V, Basoglu C, et al: Leptospirosis presenting with mania and psychosis: four consecutive cases seen in a military hospital in Turkey. Int J Psychiatry Med 35(3):299–305, 2005 16480244

Semple SJ, Zians J, Strathdee SA, et al: Sexual marathons and methamphetamine use among HIV-positive men who have sex with men. Arch Sex Behav 38(4):583–590, 2009 18185990

Senn TE, Carey MP: HIV, STD, and sexual risk reduction for individuals with a severe mental illness: review of the intervention literature. Curr Psychiatry Rev 4(2):87–100, 2008 18584060

Seriburi V, Ndukwe N, Chang Z, et al: High frequency of false positive IgM immunoblots for Borrelia burgdorferi in clinical practice. Clin Microbiol Infect 18(12):1236–1240, 2012 22369185

Shapiro ED: Clinical practice. Lyme disease. N Engl J Med 370(18):1724–1731, 2014 24785207

Shehata GA, Abdel-Baky L, Rashed H, et al: Neuropsychiatric evaluation of patients with brucellosis. J Neurovirol 16(1):48–55, 2010 20151851

Sherr L, Lampe F, Fisher M, et al: Suicidal ideation in UK HIV clinic attenders. AIDS 22(13):1651–1658, 2008 18670226

Singer HS, Gause C, Morris C, et al; Tourette Syndrome Study Group: Serial immune markers do not correlate with clinical exacerbations in pediatric autoimmune neuropsychiatric disorders associated with streptococcal infections. Pediatrics 121(6):1198–1205, 2008 18519490

Snider LA, Lougee L, Slattery M, et al: Antibiotic prophylaxis with azithromycin or penicillin for childhood-onset neuropsychiatric disorders. Biol Psychiatry 57(7):788–792, 2005 15820236

Sonneville R, Ferrand H, Tubach F, et al: Neurological complications of HIV infection in critically ill patients: clinical features and outcomes. J Infect 62(4):301–308, 2011 21329724

Swedo SE, Seidlitz J, Kovacevic M, et al: Clinical presentation of pediatric autoimmune neuropsychiatric disorders associated with streptococcal infections in research and community settings. J Child Adolesc Psychopharmacol 25(1):26–30, 2015 25695941

Sweetland A, Oquendo M, Wickramaratne P, et al: Depression: a silent driver of the global tuberculosis epidemic. World Psychiatry 13(3):325–326, 2014 25273311

Tager FA, Fallon BA: Psychiatric and cognitive features of Lyme disease. Psychiatr Ann 31(3):172–181, 2001

Tao J, Vermund SH, Qian HZ: Association between depression and antiretroviral therapy use among people living with HIV: a meta-analysis. AIDS Behav 22(5):1542–1550, 2018 28439754

Tesfaye M, Hanlon C, Tessema F, et al: Common mental disorder symptoms among patients with malaria attending primary care in Ethiopia: a cross-sectional survey. PLoS One 9(9):e108923, 2014 25268347

Thienemann M, Murphy T, Leckman J, et al: Clinical management of pediatric acute-onset neuropsychiatric syndrome: part I—psychiatric and behavioral interventions. J Child Adolesc Psychopharmacol 27(7):566–573, 2017 28722481

Tiga DC, Undurraga EA, Ramos-Castañeda J, et al: Persistent symptoms of dengue: estimates of the Incremental Disease and Economic Burden in Mexico. Am J Trop Med Hyg 94(5):1085–1089, 2016 26976885

Tomes N: The making of a germ panic, then and now. Am J Public Health 90(2):191–198, 2000 10667179

Torrey EF, Yolken RH: Schizophrenia and infections: the eyes have it. Schizophr Bull 43(2):247–252, 2017 27507268

Treadway CR, Prange AJ Jr: Tetanus mimicking psychophysiologic reaction. Occurrence after dental extraction. JAMA 200(10):891–892, 1967 6071626

Tsuruta R, Oda Y: A clinical perspective of sepsis-associated delirium. J Intensive Care 4:18, 2016 27011789

Uldall KK, Harris VL, Lalonde B: Outcomes associated with delirium in acutely hospitalized acquired immune deficiency syndrome patients. Compr Psychiatry 41(2):88–91, 2000 10741884

Urech K, Neumayr A, Blum J: Sleeping sickness in travelers—do they really sleep? PLoS Negl Trop Dis 5(11):e1358, 2011 22069503

Vázquez M, Sparrow SS, Shapiro ED: Long-term neuropsychologic and health outcomes of children with facial nerve palsy attributable to Lyme disease. Pediatrics 112(2):e93–e97, 2003 12897313

Vázquez-Santiago FJ, Noel RJ Jr, Porter JT, et al: Glutamate metabolism and HIV-associated neurocognitive disorders. J Neurovirol 20(4):315–331, 2014 24867611

Verghese A: The "typhoid state" revisited. Am J Med 79(3):370–372, 1985 3898837

Vlassova N, Angelino AF, Treisman GJ: Update on mental health issues in patients with HIV infection. Curr Infect Dis Rep 11(2):163–169, 2009 19239808

Volpi A, Gatti A, Pica F, et al: Clinical and psychosocial correlates of post-herpetic neuralgia. J Med Virol 80(9):1646–1652, 2008 18649332

Wackermann PV, Fernandes RM, Elias J Jr, et al: Involvement of the central nervous system in the chronic form of Chagas' disease. J Neurol Sci 269(1–2):152–157, 2008 18262567

Wagner GJ, Ghosh-Dastidar B: Electronic monitoring: adherence assessment or intervention? HIV Clin Trials 3(1):45–51, 2002 11819185

Wagner GJ, Kanouse DE, Koegel P, Sullivan G: Adherence to HIV antiretrovirals among persons with serious mental illness. AIDS Patient Care STDS 17(4):179–186, 2003 12737641

Więdłocha M, Marcinowicz P, Stańczykiewicz B: Psychiatric aspects of herpes simplex encephalitis, tick-borne encephalitis and herpes zoster encephalitis among immunocompetent patients. Adv Clin Exp Med 24(2):361–371, 2015 25931371

Williams DW, Veenstra M, Gaskill PJ, et al: Monocytes mediate HIV neuropathogenesis: mechanisms that contribute to HIV associated neurocognitive disorders. Curr HIV Res 12(2):85–96, 2014 24862333

Wintermann GB, Brunkhorst FM, Petrowski K, et al: Stress disorders following prolonged critical illness in survivors of severe sepsis. Crit Care Med 43(6):1213–1222, 2015 25760659

Wong T, Fonseca K, Chernesky MA, et al: Canadian Public Health Laboratory Network laboratory guidelines for the diagnosis of neurosyphilis in Canada. Can J Infect Dis Med Microbiol 26 (suppl A):18A–22A, 2015 25798161

Wormser GP, Dattwyler RJ, Shapiro ED, et al: The clinical assessment, treatment, and prevention of Lyme disease, human granulocytic anaplasmosis, and babesiosis: clinical practice guidelines by the Infectious Diseases Society of America. Clin Infect Dis 43(9):1089–1134, 2006 17029130

Yetkin MA, Bulut C, Erdinc FS, et al: Evaluation of the clinical presentations in neurobrucellosis. Int J Infect Dis 10(6):446–452, 2006 16914346

Zhao Y, Navia BA, Marra CM, et al; Adult Aids Clinical Trial Group (ACTG) 301 Team: Memantine for AIDS dementia complex: open-label report of ACTG 301. HIV Clin Trials 11(1):59–67, 2010 20400412

CHAPTER 27

Dermatology

Madhulika A. Gupta, M.D., M.Sc., FRCPC
James L. Levenson, M.D.

Dermatological disorders are associated with psychiatric and psychosocial comorbidity, as well as psychosocial stress, in 25%–30% of cases (Gupta and Gupta 1996). The skin is the largest organ of the body and functions as a social, psychological, and metabolically active biological interface between the individual and the environment. The skin and its appendages are innervated with a dense network of afferent sensory nerves and efferent autonomic nerves. The afferent sensory nerves convey sensations of touch, pain, itch, temperature, and other physical stimuli. The efferent innervation of the skin is mainly autonomic and sympathetic and plays a role in maintaining cutaneous homeostasis by regulating vasomotor and pilomotor functions and the activity of the apocrine and eccrine sweat glands. This mainly sympathetic efferent innervation makes the skin much more susceptible to react during situations associated with stress (Gupta and Gupta 2014). Autonomic nervous system (ANS) activation and immune dysregulation can lead to exacerbation of immune-mediated dermatological disorders (e.g., psoriasis, atopic dermatitis) and sympathetically mediated symptoms (e.g., pruritus, idiopathic urticaria, hyperhidrosis). Physical stimulation of the skin (e.g., in recurrent body-focused repetitive behaviors or excessive scratching of the skin) can serve as a further means of regulating affect and coping with intense emotional states. The skin plays a central role in thermoregulation and sleep onset, which can be affected by a lack of proper peripheral dissipation of heat (through sweating, vasodilatation) secondary to a dermatological disorder (Gupta and Gupta 2013d).

The skin plays a vital role in attachment, starting in infancy. Freud observed that during early development, the ego was rooted in the body, especially the skin. Bodily sensations and experiences, both internal and from the surface of the body, form the core around which the ego develops. The skin reacts to emotional states such as extreme fear, anxiety, and embarrassment with blanching, increased perspiration, piloerection, flushing, and blushing. Even minimal flaws in the overall appearance of the skin can have a profound effect on body image, especially in adolescents, and can result in body image pathology.

The impact of psychological stress on the skin is mediated by the central nervous system (CNS) as well as by a local cutaneous neuroendocrine system integrated with the CNS regulators of homeostasis (Slominski et al. 2013). The skin (Arck et al. 2006) is both a target and a source of key stress mediators, such as corticotropin-releasing hormone (CRH) and the pro-opiomelanocortin (POMC)–derived peptides, cortisol, catecholamines, prolactin, substance P, and nerve growth factor. An equivalent of the central hypothalamic-pituitary-adrenal (HPA) axis is activated in the skin in response to stress (Slominski et al. 2013). The skin's responses to acute stress include enhanced skin immune function with increased intracutaneous migration of immunocompetent cells, whereas chronic stress may suppress cutaneous immunity, reducing the immune response to vaccines, slowing wound healing, and reactivating latent viral infections such as herpesviruses (Dhabhar 2013). Acute psychological stress, which is associated with increased glucocorticoid levels, adversely affects recovery of skin barrier function after tape stripping and may exacerbate barrier-mediated dermatoses such as psoriasis and atopic dermatitis (Choi et al. 2005).

Classification

Psychodermatological disorders have been generally divided into three major categories (Gupta and Gupta 1996; Medansky and Handler 1981):

1. *Dermatological manifestations of psychiatric disorders* (Table 27–1). This category includes the recurrent body-focused repetitive behaviors (e.g., trichotillomania [hair-pulling disorder], excoriation [skin-picking] disorder, onychophagia).
2. *Functional cutaneous disorders.* This category includes somatoform pruritus, lichen simplex chronicus, prurigo nodularis, and the mucocutaneous dysesthesias and cutaneous sensory disorders (e.g., scalp dysesthesia, burning mouth syndrome, vulvodynia), in which the symptoms sometimes have no apparent diagnosable dermatological basis but are strongly influenced by psychosomatic factors.
3. *Psychological factors in dermatological disorders.* This category includes a wide range of skin conditions and has been further separated into three subcategories:

   a. Disorders that have a primary dermatopathological basis but may be influenced by psychological factors (e.g., psoriasis, hidradenitis suppurativa, atopic dermatitis, urticaria and angioedema, lichen planus, alopecia areata, vitiligo, acne, rosacea, and some cases of viral warts). Most disorders in this group are exacerbated by psychological stress and associated with psychiatric comorbidity.
   b. Disorders and states that represent an accentuated physiological response, such as hyperhidrosis and blushing.
   c. Disorders that result in an emotional reaction secondary to the impact of the skin disorder (e.g., due to cosmetic disfigurement, social stigma, intractable pruritus) on quality of life. This type of secondary emotional reaction can be a factor in many dermatological disorders.

   These three subcategories are not mutually exclusive, and some dermatological disorders may fall into more than one subgroup.

TABLE 27–1.   Dermatological manifestations of psychiatric disorders

Delusions

Delusions of parasitosis

Delusions of being infested by inanimate materials (e.g., fibers, strands) ("Morgellon's disease")

Delusions of bromhidrosis (delusional belief that a foul odor is being emitted)

Delusions of disfigurement

Hallucinations

Tactile or haptic hallucinations

Sensory flashbacks

Distorted perceptions

Amplified or dysesthetic cutaneous sensations (including pain), allodynia

Intractable pruritus

Conversion and dissociation

Unexplained sensory syndromes (e.g., involving cutaneous pain or numbness, other dysesthesias such as burning and pricking sensations)

Unexplained pruritic states

Idiopathic urticaria and angioedema

Self-induced dermatoses (e.g., dermatitis artefacta, trichotillomania, excoriation disorder, onychophagia)

"Psychogenic purpura"

Obsessions and compulsions

Compulsive hand washing

Compulsive rubbing or picking of the skin

Self-excoriation or skin picking

Hair plucking or trichotillomania

Onychophagia and onychotillomania

Anxiety and panic

Unexplained profuse perspiration, night sweats

Flushing reactions

Urticarial reactions

Body image misperceptions related to the skin

Dermatological complaints about imagined or slight "flaws" of the skin

Concern about skin lesions (e.g., wrinkles, scars, acne) out of proportion to their clinical severity

Excessive grooming behaviors (e.g., styling, shaving, plucking)

General Guidelines for Psychiatric Management of the Dermatology Patient

The dermatology patient's psychosocial history and mental state are important to evaluate (Gupta et al. 2005). The role of psychosocial stressors in the onset or exacerbation of the skin disorder, including *daily hassles* associated with having to live with a chronic and disfiguring skin disorder, *major stressful life events* (e.g., divorce, bereavement), and *traumatic life events* that overwhelm the patient's coping abilities (e.g., developmental trauma such as child abuse and neglect, sexual assault, natural disasters), should be specifically assessed (Gupta and Gupta 2013c). The psychiatrist should thoroughly assess the impact of the skin disorder on the patient's quality of life (the extensively used and validated Dermatology Life Quality Index [DLQI; Basra et al. 2008] may be used to assess this parameter), as well as pruritus and sleep disturbance, and should recommend aggressive dermatological treatment of even clinically mild skin disease that is cosmetically disfiguring (especially facial lesions) or socially stigmatizing. Sleep–wake disorders such as insomnia disorder, obstructive sleep apnea (Gupta et al. 2017c), and circadian rhythm sleep–wake disorders can exacerbate pruritus and immune-mediated dermatological disorders such as psoriasis and atopic dermatitis (Gupta and Gupta 2013d) and should be ruled out. Insomnia can also adversely affect cutaneous body image perception (Gupta et al. 2015). Standard psychiatric therapies are indicated to treat psychiatric comorbidity in the dermatology patient. Psychiatric drugs (Kuhn et al. 2017b) are generally used for one of three purposes: 1) management of dermatological manifestations of primary psychiatric disorders, 2) management of psychiatric disorders that are comorbid with primary dermatological disorders, and 3) provision of certain desired pharmacological properties of psychotropic agents (e.g., the antihistaminic effect of doxepin), even in the absence of a comorbid psychiatric disorder. Currently, no orally administered psychotropic agents are approved by the U.S. Food and Drug Administration (FDA) for the treatment of a primary dermatological disorder; 5% topical doxepin cream is FDA approved for short-term (up to 8 days) management of moderate pruritus in adults with conditions such as atopic dermatitis.

The skin is a highly visible and social organ that reacts readily to psychosocial stress, factors that can render a wide range of dermatological disorders vulnerable to the development of chronic psychiatric reactions and *somatic symptom disorder* (Levenson et al. 2017). Feelings of social alienation as a result of a cosmetically disfiguring skin disorder may be associated with suicidal behavior (Gupta and Gupta 2013a). An assessment of *suicide risk* in the dermatology patient is indicated in several situations (Gupta et al. 2017b), including the following:

- Significant psychiatric comorbidity is present (in up to 30% of dermatology patients).
- Psychopathology manifests as dermatological symptoms.
- Major psychosocial stressors (e.g., bereavement, interpersonal violence) are exacerbating a stress-reactive dermatosis.

- There is high disease burden (including chronicity and increased disease severity), especially for chronic intractable pruritus and associated chronic sleep disruption.
- Marked facial lesions or facial scarring is present.
- Dermatological medications that have been associated with suicidal behavior, such as some biologics (e.g., the tumor necrosis factor–alpha [TNF-α] inhibitor adalimumab) and retinoids (e.g., isotretinoin for acne), are being used.

Suicide is the second leading cause of death among the 15- to 29-year age group, among whom certain skin disorders associated with increased suicide risk (e.g., psoriasis, acne, atopic dermatitis) are common. Therefore, co-occurrence of increased suicide risk and a dermatological disorder in this age group does not always imply a causal relationship (Gupta et al. 2017b).

Dermatological Manifestations of Psychiatric Disorders (Psychocutaneous Disorders)

Delusional Infestation

Delusional infestation (DI) (previously *delusional parasitosis*) is classified as a *delusional disorder, somatic type* (American Psychiatric Association 2013), and is characterized by a fixed false belief that one is infested by parasites or other living or inanimate (e.g., fibers, wax, crystals, needles, particles) pathogens that is maintained despite negative clinical and laboratory findings (Foster et al. 2012; Lepping et al. 2015). (DI with inanimate pathogens is also known as *Morgellon's disease.*) DI is rarely encountered by general psychiatrists but is often seen by dermatologists. The mean age at onset is the mid-50s to 60s, with an equal sex distribution among patients younger than 50 years and a female-to-male ratio of about 3:1 among individuals older than 50 years (Foster et al. 2012). Patients with DI typically present the doctor with alleged parasite specimens in a pill bottle, matchbox, adhesive tape, or plastic bag. They tend to treat their skin by scratching and may use disinfectants, repellents, pesticides, and/or antimicrobials. They may consult exterminators or entomologists, repeatedly launder clothing and linens, and discard possessions and even pets (fearing them as the source). Tactile and olfactory hallucinations related to the delusional theme may be present, and patients may report cutaneous sensations of crawling, stinging, and/or biting. Belief of infestation may extend to any body orifice, including the nares, oral cavity, and orbit. Although most cases of DI appear to represent a primary delusional disorder, some can be secondary to other psychiatric disorders—for example, schizophrenia, obsessive-compulsive disorder (OCD), or psychotic depression—or medical disorders (Kimsey 2016)—for example, structural brain disease, delirium, dementia, endocrinopathy (e.g., hypothyroidism), lupus erythematosus, HIV/AIDS, vitamin deficiency (e.g., B_{12} deficiency, pellagra), neuropathies, uremia, hepatic encephalopathy, or other toxic states, especially those resulting from abuse of amphetamines or cocaine and alcoholism. Of course, it is important not to make the diagnosis of DI prematurely, because some patients really do have infestations (e.g., scabies, lice).

Management

Appropriate dermatological/medical evaluation is required to rule out a real infestation, a dermatological disease, and secondary causes of DI. Because patients with DI do not view themselves as having a psychiatric disorder, treatment is best carried out with a psychiatrist providing consultation to a dermatologist. The biggest challenge in the pharmacotherapy of DI is convincing the patient to take a psychiatric drug. DI is often difficult to manage even in a dermatological setting because of limited response to antipsychotics and nonadherence to treatment recommendations (Ahmad and Ramsay 2009a). The clinician should focus on developing a therapeutic relationship (which is likely to enhance adherence to psychopharmacology), empathize with the patient's distress rather than emphasizing the delusional nature of the complaint, and attempt to prevent self-harm (e.g., determine whether the patient is using pesticides) (Lepping et al. 2015).

Both typical and atypical antipsychotics have been effective in DI, and antipsychotics with a strong antihistaminic effect are suggested because they are more likely to help the patient's anxiety and pruritus (Lepping et al. 2015). Evidence based on case series (Lepping et al. 2015) suggests the effectiveness of risperidone (1–2 mg/day), olanzapine (2.5–5 mg/day), amisulpride (200–400 mg/day), or haloperidol (2–5 mg/day). Risperidone and olanzapine have been the most widely used atypical antipsychotics and have led to full or partial remission in 69% and 72% of cases, respectively (Freudenmann and Lepping 2008). There are many reports of the use of pimozide, but no evidence demonstrates the superiority of pimozide over other antipsychotics for DI (Mothi and Sampson 2013). Pimozide is generally started at 1 mg/day and increased by 1 mg every 5–7 days to a maximum of 4 mg/day (Lee 2008). Sudden deaths have been reported with pimozide and are thought to be due to ventricular arrhythmias caused by QTc prolongation. Additive effects on QTc prolongation should be anticipated if pimozide is administered concomitantly with other QTc-prolonging drugs or with cytochrome P450 (CYP) 3A4 inhibitors. Secondary DI is more likely than primary DI to respond to antipsychotics (78% vs. 59%) (Freudenmann and Lepping 2008). Selective serotonin reuptake inhibitors (SSRIs) have sometimes been helpful for patients whose parasite sensations are more obsessional than delusional (Fellner and Majeed 2009).

Obsessive-Compulsive and Related Disorders

In DSM-5 (American Psychiatric Association 2013), the *body-focused repetitive behaviors* (BFRBs)—excoriation (skin-picking) disorder and trichotillomania (hair-pulling disorder)—and *body dysmorphic disorder* (BDD) are grouped in the newly created category of *obsessive-compulsive and related disorders* (OCRDs), which also includes *hoarding disorder* and *obsessive-compulsive disorder*. *Onychophagia (nail-biting)* is a BFRB that is classified as an *unspecified* OCRD (American Psychiatric Association 2013). BFRBs such as trichotillomania, excoriation disorder, and onychophagia often coexist (Gupta and Gupta 2014).

Recurrent Body-Focused Repetitive Behaviors

Excoriation (skin-picking) disorder (SPD) (American Psychiatric Association 2013) (also referred to as *pathological skin picking, neurotic excoriation, psychogenic excoriation, der-*

matillomania, and *acne excoriée*) is characterized by recurrent picking of one's skin, resulting in skin lesions and repeated attempts to decrease or stop the skin picking. The lesions in SPD are usually a few centimeters in diameter, may range in number from a few to several hundred, and are weeping, crusted, or scarred with postinflammatory hypo- or hyperpigmentation. Unlike lesions in dermatitis artefacta (discussed later in this section), the lesions in SPD do not mimic those of other cutaneous disorders but may result in scarring, ulcerations, and infections. Unlike individuals with dermatitis artefacta, patients with SPD typically acknowledge the self-inflicted nature of their lesions (Gupta et al. 1987b). SPD most often begins during adolescence with the onset of dermatological conditions such as acne, and it may present as *acne excoriée.* SPD can occur at any age and may have first onset in a previously active person who loses mobility—for example, because of aging, illness, or accident (Gupta et al. 1986). The most commonly picked regions are the face, arms, and hands, but patients may pick at multiple body regions. The skin picking may be associated with a range of rituals or behaviors involving the skin or scabs, and may initiate the "itch–scratch cycle" and exacerbate a preexisting dermatosis. The BFRBs may be associated with both obsessive-compulsive and dissociative behavioral styles; dissociative features tend to be present in more severe forms of BFRBs (Gupta et al. 2017d). From a treatment perspective, it is important to recognize the dissociative component, because standard approaches to treating obsessive-compulsive behavior with habit-reversal therapy and SSRIs (Kestenbaum 2013) are not sufficient when high levels of dissociation are present.

Trichotillomania (hair-pulling disorder) (TTM) (American Psychiatric Association 2013) is characterized by recurrent pulling out of one's hair, resulting in hair loss and repeated attempts to decrease or stop hair pulling. TTM occurring solely during sleep has been reported (Murphy et al. 2007). TTM should be distinguished from benign hair pulling, which can be associated with thumb sucking and nail biting in children. Hair pulling may occur from any region of the body where hair grows, the most common sites being the scalp, eyebrows, and eyelashes. Hair pulling may be accompanied by various behaviors and rituals involving the hair—for example, *trichorrhizophagia* (i.e., eating the hair root after pulling out the hair), resulting in trichobezoars and gastrointestinal complications (e.g., obstruction, acute pancreatitis). As in the case of SPD, the hair-pulling behavior in some patients involves a more obsessive-compulsive style with focused attention on the hair pulling with preceding tension and relief upon pulling of the hair. Other patients display more dissociative features with automatic behavior in which the hair pulling appears to occur without full awareness. TTM patients tend to have greater dissociative features than patients with SPD (Lochner et al. 2002, 2004). In patients who deny hair pulling, other dermatological causes of alopecia should be ruled out and the denial should not be simply attributed to dissociative amnesia. An affected area in TTM is rarely completely devoid of hair, and hairs of various lengths and irregularly broken hairs are usually partially distributed over the area of alopecia. Dermoscopy of the hair and scalp and histopathological examination may be necessary to confirm the diagnosis.

Management of BFRBs. The BFRBs are often comorbid with other psychiatric disorders (Kuhn et al. 2017a), including BDD, anxiety disorders, major depressive disorder, and posttraumatic stress disorder (PTSD) (Gupta et al. 2017a). Management of

BFRBs requires a complete psychiatric assessment and treatment of comorbid psychopathology where indicated, including treatment of dissociation and conversion symptoms, which tend to be present in the more severe BFRB cases (Gupta et al. 2017d). Psychological models of BFRBs have investigated the role of emotional regulation and have conceptualized the BFRBs as a maladaptive emotional regulation mechanism (Roberts et al. 2013). Cognitive-behavioral/extinction-based treatments, including habit-reversal therapy, and dialectical behavior therapy have significant support for the treatment of BFRBs (Grant and Chamberlain 2016; Schumer et al. 2016; Selles et al. 2016).

Skin-picking disorder.   The patient should be fully investigated for other systemic and local dermatological causes of pruritus (Craig-Müller and Reichenberg 2015). Double-blind trials of fluoxetine and citalopram, and open trials of fluvoxamine, escitalopram, and sertraline, support the use of SSRIs as a potential treatment (Selles et al. 2016). Lamotrigine has been associated with a reduction in SPD severity but was not superior to placebo (Grant et al. 2010). A systematic review (Schumer et al. 2016) concluded that improvement was seen with all interventions for SPD over the course of short-term clinical trials; however, only behavioral treatments demonstrated significant benefits compared with an inactive control condition. A 12-week randomized, placebo-controlled clinical trial (Grant et al. 2016) ($N=66$) of the glutamate modulator N-acetylcysteine (NAC) (dosage range, 1,200–3,000 mg daily) found that NAC was associated with a significant improvement in skin-picking symptoms but not in psychosocial functioning (Grant et al. 2016).

Trichotillomania.   With appropriate treatment, up to 50% of TTM patients can experience symptom reduction, at least in the short term, versus a 14% rate of improvement without treatment (Grant and Chamberlain 2016). A systematic review of seven blinded randomized controlled trials (RCTs) in which the primary outcome measure was mean change in TTM severity revealed that habit-reversal therapy was superior to SSRIs and to clomipramine (Bloch et al. 2007). There are no universally accepted first-line pharmacotherapies for TTM (Grant and Chamberlain 2016). A Cochrane review (Rothbart et al. 2013) that identified eight RCTs of medication versus placebo or other treatment concluded that none of the three SSRI studies involving fluoxetine and sertraline demonstrated a strong treatment effect on any study outcomes (e.g., urge to pull hair, number of hair-pulling episodes). The Cochrane review further identified one study comparing clomipramine with desipramine that demonstrated a treatment effect of clomipramine on two out of three measures of treatment outcome (Swedo et al. 1989); however, a study comparing clomipramine with placebo (Ninan et al. 2000) found no significant difference between the two groups. One placebo-controlled study ($N=25$) of olanzapine (mean±SD dosage 10.8±5.7 mg daily; 85% of olanzapine vs. 17% of placebo were treatment responders; $P=0.001$) (Van Ameringen et al. 2010) and one placebo-controlled study ($N=50$) of NAC (dosage range, 1,200–2,400 mg daily; 56% of NAC vs. 16% of placebo group were treatment responders; $P=0.003$) (Grant et al. 2009) reported statistically significant treatment effects. The Cochrane review concluded that preliminary evidence suggested treatment benefits of clomipramine, olanzapine, and NAC based on three small trials (Rothbart et al. 2013). Some open-label and case studies report the efficacy of anticonvulsant mood stabilizers (Gupta 2013), including valproic acid (Adewuya et al. 2008), topiramate (Lochner et al. 2006), and oxcarbazepine (Leombruni and Gastaldi 2010), as well as lithium (Christenson et al. 1991), in TTM.

Body Dysmorphic Disorder

BDD (American Psychiatric Association 2013), also referred to as "dysmorphophobia" or "dermatologic non-disease" (Cotterill 1981), is characterized by a preoccupation with one or more perceived defects or flaws in physical appearance that are not observable or appear only slight to others. At some time during the course of the disorder, BDD is associated with repetitive behaviors (e.g., mirror checking, excessive grooming, skin picking, reassurance seeking) or mental acts (e.g., comparison of appearance with that of others) in response to the appearance concerns. In about one-third of cases, BDD presents with *absent insight/delusional beliefs.* The preoccupation with appearance can involve one or more body areas, most commonly the skin (e.g., perceived lines, wrinkles, paleness, acne, scars, vascular markings), hair (e.g., thinning of hair, excessive body or facial hair), or nose (e.g., size, shape). BDD has been associated with excessive indoor tanning despite being given a malignant melanoma diagnosis (Petit et al. 2014). In the United States, the prevalence of BDD is 9%–15% among dermatology patients and 7%–8% among cosmetic surgery patients, in comparison with 2.4% among adults in the general population (American Psychiatric Association 2013).

A systematic review of the literature on BDD and suicidal behavior (Angelakis et al. 2016) revealed a statistically significant association between BDD and both suicidal ideation (odds ratio [OR]=2.57; 95% confidence interval [CI]=1.44–3.69) and suicide attempts (OR=3.30; 95% CI=2.18–4.43). The mean age at onset of BDD is 16–17 years, and two-thirds of patients have onset of their symptoms before age 18 years (American Psychiatric Association 2013). The age at onset of BDD has important implications because it overlaps with first onset of cosmetically disfiguring disorders such as acne (which first presents in mid-adolescence) and psoriasis (with one-third of adults reporting onset before age 20 years), both of which are associated with increased suicidality (Cotterill and Cunliffe 1997). The body image concerns and suicidal behavior (Gupta et al. 2017b) in some dermatology patients may not be entirely due to the cosmetic impact of the skin disorder and may be confounded by underlying BDD. According to Crerand et al. (2010), most studies of BDD patients who underwent surgery for cosmetic procedures found that patients either experienced no change in BDD severity or experienced emergence of new BDD-related ideation, and most patients reported dissatisfaction with treatment outcome.

Management of BDD. A Cochrane review (Ipser et al. 2009) of pharmacotherapy, psychotherapy, or their combination for both delusional and nondelusional BDD identified five RCTs, with two RCTs involving fluoxetine or clomipramine and three involving psychotherapy. The 12-week trial of fluoxetine (mean dosage 78 mg/day) versus placebo indicated the medication's overall superiority (56% response with fluoxetine vs. 15% response with placebo), and a 16-week trial of clomipramine (mean dosage 138 mg/day) versus desipramine indicated superiority of clomipramine. There was significant symptom reduction in the two cognitive-behavioral therapy (CBT) trials. The treatment responses in both medication trials were not affected by whether BDD was delusional. Use of pimozide (Phillips 2005) to augment fluoxetine in fluoxetine nonresponders was no more effective than placebo in reducing BDD severity, including delusionality.

Eating Disorders

Patients with *anorexia nervosa* or *bulimia nervosa* can initially present with dermatological symptoms (Gupta et al. 1987a; Strumia 2013) resulting from malnutrition (e.g., lanugo-like body hair, carotenodermia) or abnormal peripheral vascular response (leading to perniosis or *erythema ab igne* [Dessinioti et al. 2016]) or from bingeing and purging (e.g., knuckle calluses or Russell's sign, periorbital petechiae/subconjunctival hemorrhage, gingivitis, perimylolysis, flare-ups of acne), as well as increased cutaneous body image concerns. In a cross-sectional study (Gupta and Gupta 2001a) examining concerns about various aspects of skin appearance among young adult (<30 years) eating disorder patients (*n*=32) and nonclinical control subjects (*n*=34), 81% of the eating disorder patients, versus 56% of the control subjects, reported dissatisfaction with the appearance of their skin (*P*=0.03). The cutaneous attributes of greatest concern among the eating disorder patients were those that are also associated with aging and photodamage (e.g., "darkness" under the eyes, freckles, fine wrinkles, patchy hyperpigmentation), in addition to dryness and roughness of the skin, which are often secondary to the eating disorder. Alternatively, concern about aging of one's appearance has been associated with a drive for thinness and excessive dieting, factors that are important in the pathogenesis of eating disorders (Gupta 1995). Starvation in eating disorders has been associated with pruritus (Gupta et al. 1992b), and rapid refeeding can lead to a flare-up of acne, most likely because of rising androgen levels (Gupta and Gupta 2001b). It has been suggested that anorexia nervosa should be considered in all patients with low body weight and pruritus (Morgan and Lacey 1999). Because patients with eating disorders often tend to minimize or deny their symptoms, the dermatological signs may be the first clinical clue that the patient has an eating disorder.

Dermatitis Artefacta

Dermatitis artefacta (DA) refers to cutaneous lesions that are wholly self-inflicted; however, the patient typically denies responsibility. DA is a complex disorder, and there is ongoing debate about how to best classify it (Gieler et al. 2013). DA is largely impulsive and is generally associated with prominent dissociative symptoms and dissociative amnesia (Gupta et al. 2017d); this may explain why, as noted above, even though DA is entirely self-induced, patients often deny having caused their lesions. DA is a *factitious disorder,* with no underlying motive to provide false information or behave deceptively, and therefore does not represent malingering (Gieler et al. 2013). The lesions in DA vary widely and may present as purpura, blisters, ulcers, erythema, sinuses, edema, or nodules, depending on the means employed to create them; thus, they can mimic a range of cutaneous disorders. The lesions typically occur in regions that are accessible by hand; they may occur at the site of an old scar or surgical wound or appear suddenly in previously normal skin. Self-inflicted lesions are often bizarre, with sharp geometric borders surrounded by normal-looking skin. Full-thickness skin loss or severe scarring from self-inflicted lesions may necessitate extensive plastic surgery or amputation (Gupta et al. 1987b).

Psychiatric Comorbidity

A personality disorder characterized by very immature coping mechanisms is often observed in which the self-induced lesions serve as "an appeal for help." A history of childhood physical, sexual, or psychological abuse or neglect is common in DA (Gieler et al. 2013). In children, many cases may be associated with intellectual disability, and factitious disorder imposed on another should be ruled out (Boyd et al. 2014). Dissociative disorders and PTSD, which are often underrecognized, should also be considered (Gattu et al. 2009; Gupta et al. 2017a). DA may co-occur in mood, anxiety, and psychotic disorders, as well as in malingering (Cohen and Vardy 2006).

Management

Clinicians should always rule out an underlying dermatological disorder, as a patient may self-excoriate a primary dermatological lesion and create secondary artifactual lesions (Ahmad and Ramsay 2009b). Early diagnosis is important, as it may prevent irreversible self-injury, unnecessary surgery, and chronic morbidity (Gupta and Gupta 1996). Patients with DA typically are not able to describe how their lesions evolved, but the lesions heal if an occlusive dressing is used to cover them. Clinicians should maintain a supportive and empathic approach and should avoid direct discussion or confrontation regarding the self-inflicted nature of the lesions. Once a satisfactory therapeutic alliance has been established, a more insight-oriented psychotherapeutic approach may be used (Fabisch 1980). A major psychosocial stressor such as illness, accident, or bereavement may precede DA in about 20%–30% of cases. Recovery may occur through mobilization of social support.

Functional Dermatological Disorders

Mucocutaneous Dysesthesias

The mucocutaneous dysesthesias, also referred to as *cutaneous sensory disorders* (Gupta and Gupta 2013b), are a heterogeneous group of disorders that involve disagreeable skin sensations (e.g., burning, stinging, itching), pain, allodynia, and/or negative sensory symptoms (e.g., numbness, hypoesthesia), with no diagnosable underlying dermatological disorder. One form is *scalp dysesthesia* (Hoss and Segal 1998), in which patients, mostly women, present with complaints of pruritus, pain, trichodynia, and burning and/or stinging sensations of the scalp without objective physical findings. Mucocutaneous dysesthesias are described in region-specific terms, and skin regions that have a greater density of epidermal innervation, such as the scalp (e.g., scalp dysesthesia, "burning scalp"), face (e.g., "burning mouth syndrome," glossodynia, some cases of atypical facial pain), and perineum (e.g., vulvodynia, scrotodynia), tend to be the most susceptible (Oaklander and Siegel 2005). Scalp dysesthesia has been associated with degenerative changes in the cervical spine, especially in the C5–C6 region (Thornsberry and English 2013). The cutaneous dysesthesias represent a complex and often poorly understood interplay among 1) neurobiological factors associated with cutaneous sensation; 2) neuropathic pain and itching; and 3) neurological/psychiatric states such as radiculopathy, stroke, dissociation, depression, and PTSD (Gupta and Gupta 2013b) that can modulate cutaneous sensory perception.

Management

Various psychotherapeutic interventions, including hypnosis and eye movement desensitization and reprocessing (EMDR) (Gupta and Gupta 2002), may be helpful when the cutaneous symptom represents a conversion disorder, a dissociative state, or a sensory flashback in PTSD. The mucocutaneous dysesthesias are usually treated with the same agents used for the treatment of neuropathic pain, such as tricyclic antidepressants (TCAs), serotonin–norepinephrine reuptake inhibitors (SNRIs), or anticonvulsants such as gabapentin (Thornsberry and English 2013), but controlled clinical trials are lacking (see also Chapter 34, "Pain"). Scalp dysesthesia and other idiopathic pruritic conditions may respond to antihistaminic TCAs such as amitriptyline and doxepin (Hoss and Segal 1998). A Cochrane review (McMillan et al. 2016) of studies of intervention versus placebo for burning mouth syndrome identified 23 RCTs but concluded that there was insufficient evidence to support or discourage the use of any specific intervention for this condition.

Pruritus With Psychiatric Factors

Pruritus, or itching, is an unpleasant sensation that elicits a desire to scratch, thereby perpetuating the "itch–scratch cycle." Scratching can lead to problems with skin barrier function, lichenification, and prurigo formation. The International Forum for the Study of Itch (IFSI) has proposed the following classification for *chronic pruritus*, defined as pruritus lasting longer than 6 weeks: group I (pruritus on diseased/inflamed skin), group II (pruritus on nondiseased/noninflamed skin), and group III (pruritus presenting with severe chronic secondary scratch lesions such as prurigo nodularis and lichen simplex chronicus) (Weisshaar et al. 2012). The IFSI classifies the etiology of chronic pruritus as follows: (i) dermatological, (ii) systemic, (iii) neurological, (iv) somatoform, (v) mixed origin, and (vi) "others." Chronic pruritus may occur as a common symptom of primary dermatological disease; in systemic diseases without primary skin lesions, including renal, hepatic, endocrine, infective, hematological, and neurological disorders; and in psychiatric disorders, such as mood disorders, OCD, schizophrenia, dissociative disorders, and eating disorders (Weisshaar et al. 2012). *Somatoform pruritus* is defined as pruritus in which psychological factors play a critical role in the onset, intensity, exacerbation, or persistence of the symptoms (Weisshaar et al. 2012). Patients' perceptions of pruritus, irrespective of its etiology, can be modulated by psychological factors. Persons with mental distress were found to be twice as likely to experience itching as those without (Dalgard et al. 2007).

Management

A complete history and thorough clinical examination (for evaluation of dermatological, systemic, and neuropsychiatric factors and for medication-related causes) are essential in the management of all pruritus patients (Weisshaar et al. 2012). Somatoform pruritus is not a diagnosis of exclusion; the diagnosis can only be made after a thorough psychiatric examination (Weisshaar et al. 2012). Pruritus in which psychological factors play a primary role (somatoform pruritus) rarely disturbs sleep (Weisshaar et al. 2012); however, pruritus due to PTSD is often associated with nocturnal awakenings from traumatic nightmares (Gupta 2006). A range of psychiatric medications may be used to manage symptoms, based on the factors underlying the pruritus

(Shaw et al. 2007). A systematic review of 26 RCTs comparing interventions versus placebo for pruritus (Pongcharoen and Fleischer 2016) found evidence for the efficacy of different classes of drugs depending on the underlying diagnosis, including naltrexone in cholestatic itch and atopic dermatitis, and gabapentin in uremic pruritus. Smaller studies suggested the possible efficacy of sertraline, paroxetine, and oral doxepin (a histamine H_1- and H_2-receptor antagonist), although this evidence requires confirmation in larger studies (Pongcharoen and Fleischer 2016; Stånder et al. 2009). Mirtazapine was reported to be effective for nocturnal pruritus in a case series of three patients with inflammatory skin disorders (Hundley and Yosipovitch 2004). For both generalized and focal idiopathic pruritus, the most commonly prescribed oral medications are antihistamines, which usually provide some short-term relief. Paroxetine has also been reported to be helpful in severe nondermatological pruritus (Zylicz et al. 2003). Anticonvulsants (e.g., gabapentin, pregabalin, carbamazepine, topiramate) have been suggested as possible remedies (Matsuda et al. 2016). It has been observed that treatments for neuropathic and psychogenic itch tend to be similar (Yosipovitch and Samuel 2008). Psychological therapies (Daunton et al. 2016; Evers et al. 2016; Schut et al. 2016), including CBT, relaxation training for arousal reduction, and habit-reversal therapy, may be helpful in interrupting the itch–scratch cycle, and there are reports of the benefits of hypnosis.

Psychogenic Purpura

Psychogenic purpura, also referred to as *autoerythrocyte sensitization syndrome, painful bruising syndrome,* and *Gardner-Diamond syndrome,* is a poorly understood condition that presents as spontaneous, painful ecchymotic bruising. The condition mainly affects adult women, with a few cases affecting men and children. In addition to dermatological symptoms, menorrhagia, epistaxis, and gingival and gastrointestinal bleeding (Ivanov et al. 2009) have been described in two-thirds of patients (Ratnoff 1989). Severe emotional stress, conversion (including religious stigmata) and dissociation symptoms (Gupta et al. 2017d), and other psychological factors (Ivanov et al. 2009; Ratnoff 1980, 1989) have been observed in the majority of cases; however, there is a marked heterogeneity of psychological findings, and the exact role of psychological factors in psychogenic purpura remains unclear. Gardner and Diamond (1955), who described four cases, postulated that patients become sensitized to their own red blood cells. Subcutaneous injection of autologous red blood cells and hemolysate has been shown to reproduce the lesions, suggesting an underlying autoimmune process. Overall, fewer than 200 cases have been described in the literature (Ivanov et al. 2009). Psychogenic purpura should be differentiated from factitious purpura, which is a type of self-induced factitious dermatitis.

Psychiatric Aspects of Selected Dermatological Disorders

Atopic Dermatitis

Atopic dermatitis (AD), which is a form of eczema (Kang et al. 2008), is a chronic relapsing dermatitis associated with intense pruritus. AD is often associated with a personal or family history of atopy, asthma, and/or allergic rhinitis. AD can occur at any age; however, in up to 90% of cases, onset is before the age of 5 years, and there is a 10%–20% estimated prevalence among school-age children in the United States. Pruritus in AD is often worse in the evening and can interfere with nighttime sleep. The rubbing and scratching in response to the pruritus, which typically further exacerbate the AD, can result in excoriations and may produce lichen simplex chronicus and prurigo nodularis.

Stress

The onset or exacerbation of AD often follows stressful life events, such as parental divorce (Suárez et al. 2012). In children, stress as a risk factor interacts with environmental variables such as sweating. AD patients have been shown to exhibit an overactive sympathetic response to histamine-induced itch and scratching compared with non-AD control subjects (Tran et al. 2010). There is attenuated HPA-axis responsiveness, as evidenced by a blunted cortisol response to a stressor in AD (Buske-Kirschbaum et al. 2006). HPA axis hyporesponsiveness in atopy may be associated with the severity of the allergic inflammatory response in AD (Buske-Kirschbaum et al. 2010; Peters 2016).

Psychosocial and Psychiatric Factors

Atopic individuals with emotional problems may develop a vicious cycle between anxiety/depression and dermatological symptoms. Pruritus severity has been directly correlated with the severity of depression in AD (Gupta and Gupta 1999). Suicidal ideation was reported in 2.1% of adult patients with mild to moderate AD in one U.S. sample (Gupta and Gupta 1998). A Japanese study of patients ages 15–49 years reported a suicidal ideation prevalence of 0.21%, 6%, and 19.6%, respectively, for patients with mild, moderate, and severe AD (Kimata 2006). In a population-based study of 72,435 Korean adolescents (Lee and Shin 2017), the overall prevalence of suicidal behaviors was as follows: 16.3% for suicidal ideation, 5.8% suicidal plans, and 4.2% suicide attempt; among the 6.8% of adolescents who had AD, the prevalence of suicidal behaviors was significantly increased, even after controlling for depression, as follows: suicidal ideation, OR=1.26; 95% CI=1.16–1.36; suicide plans, OR=1.28; 95% CI=1.14–1.44; and suicide attempts, OR=1.29; 95% CI=1.13–1.49 (Lee and Shin 2017). AD patients have also been found to have higher state and trait anxiety and greater psychophysiological reactivity that cannot be attributed solely to increased disease activity (Seiffert et al. 2005). AD patients have a greater risk of developing depression and anxiety (Cheng et al. 2015; Simpson et al. 2016). Data from a German population–based administrative database showed a significant association between AD and attention-deficit/hyperactivity disorder (ADHD) in the 6- to 17-year age group (OR=1.54; 95% CI=1.06–2.22) (Schmitt et al. 2009).

   AD has a substantial effect on quality of life in both children and adults (Blome et al. 2016), with pruritus intensity and sleep disruption contributing significantly to the compromised quality of life in AD (Drucker 2017). AD in children can significantly affect their family's quality of life (Blome et al. 2016). Teasing and bullying related to contagion, and use of teasing as an instrument of social exclusion, can lead to significant psychological sequelae in children and adolescents with AD (Senra and Wollenberg 2014). There is an extensive literature documenting disturbed child–family relationships in childhood AD (Howlett 1999). Parents are often reluctant to discipline a child with AD for fear that this could provoke distress and precipitate scratching. Furthermore, parents and sometimes medical professionals may focus more on the care of the skin disorder than on the emotional and developmental needs of the child with AD (Howlett 1999).

Management

Psychotherapy.   A wide variety of psychotherapeutic treatments have been advocated to interrupt the vicious cycle of itching and scratching in AD. There have been several RCTs of psychological and educational interventions (including relaxation training, habit-reversal therapy, cognitive-behavioral techniques, and stress management training) as adjuncts to enhance the effectiveness of topical therapy in children with AD, but the evidence base remains limited regarding their efficacy (Ersser et al. 2014). RCTs have also shown that interventions directed toward the parents of the child with AD can decrease the severity of the skin disease (Ersser et al. 2014). Habit-reversal therapy (Lavda et al. 2012), combined with relaxation training (Daunton et al. 2016) and standard treatments, is beneficial in adults.

Pharmacotherapy.   Pharmacotherapy of AD aims to interrupt the itch–scratch cycle and to optimize nighttime sleep. Topical doxepin (5% cream) is effective in the treatment of pruritus in AD (Drake et al. 1995) and is FDA approved for short-term treatment in adults but not children. Low-dose oral doxepin (e.g., starting at 10 mg at bedtime) is helpful in adults because of its antihistaminic and sedative properties (Kelsay 2006), with dose increases based on response and side effects. There have also been reports suggesting some benefit from bupropion (Modell et al. 2002), mirtazapine (Hundley and Yosipovitch 2004; Mahtani et al. 2005), and trimipramine (Savin et al. 1979). SSRIs (Ständer et al. 2009) have been found to be effective in chronic pruritus due to several conditions, including AD. The strongly antihistaminic antidepressants doxepin, trimipramine, and amitriptyline may also be effective because of their sedative and strong anticholinergic properties, as the eccrine sweat glands in atopic dermatitis have been found to be hypersensitive to acetylcholine. The pruritus in lichen simplex chronicus and prurigo nodularis, which may be encountered in AD, may be alleviated with gabapentin (Gencoglan et al. 2010). A small short-term RCT of nitrazepam did not significantly reduce nocturnal scratching (Ebata et al. 1998), and benzodiazepine withdrawal may further exacerbate pruritus.

Psoriasis

Psoriasis (Van de Kerkhof 2008) is a chronic and recurrent inflammatory disorder characterized by circumscribed erythematous, dry, scaling plaques that are usually covered by silvery white adherent scales. The lesions are typically symmetrical; have a predilection for the scalp, nails, extensor surfaces of the limbs, hands and feet, and sacral and genital regions; and are associated with pruritus. The worldwide prevalence of psoriasis is 2%. Psoriasis can occur at any age; in approximately 75% of patients, onset is before age 40 years. More than one-third of patients have severe disease, and 5%–30% have psoriatic arthritis. Psoriasis is influenced by both genetic and environmental factors, with a concordance rate of about 70% in monozygotic twins. In addition to psychosocial stress, other risk factors and comorbidities in psoriasis include cigarette smoking, alcohol consumption, metabolic syndrome, chronic kidney disease, inflammatory bowel disease, hepatic disease, certain malignancies, and infections (Takeshita et al. 2017). There is an increased prevalence of obstructive sleep apnea (36%–81.8% in psoriasis vs. 2%–4% in the general population) and restless legs syndrome (15.1%–18% in psoriasis vs. 5%–10% in the general population) (Gupta et al. 2016), which likely is related to multiple factors, including comorbidities and possibly a higher underlying sympathetic tone in psoriasis.

Stress

Stress has long been reported to trigger psoriasis (Hunter et al. 2013). Visibility of lesions, presence of lesions in the genital area (Ryan et al. 2015), and severity of scaling and pruritus have the greatest impact on patient quality of life (Gupta et al. 1989) and can lead to psoriasis-related stress, which in turn can exacerbate the psoriasis. A prospective study found that at times of higher daily stress, patients experienced more severe psoriasis and significantly more itching (Verhoeven et al. 2009). Several studies have found a blunted HPA-axis cortisol response to stress and a heightened sympathetic response in psoriasis (Arnetz et al. 1985; Evers et al. 2010; Richards et al. 2005). The blunted cortisol response has been associated with an upregulation of proinflammatory cytokines (Hunter et al. 2013). Not all studies support these findings; one study (Buske-Kirschbaum et al. 2006) found a normal HPA-axis cortisol response to stress but noted an increased sympathetic response similar to that seen in an earlier study (Arnetz et al. 1985). It has been proposed that stress-reactive psoriasis is associated with a hyporesponsive HPA-axis cortisol response and possibly more severe psoriasis (Hunter et al. 2013). A study in 2,490 Vietnam veterans reported an increased risk of psoriasis in those with chronic PTSD (OR=4.7; 95% CI=1.9–11.7) (Boscarino 2004). PTSD has also been associated with a hyporesponsive HPA-axis cortisol response to stress.

Psychosocial and Psychiatric Factors

There is an extensive literature on psychosocial and psychiatric comorbidity in psoriasis (Fortune et al. 2005). A systematic review and meta-analysis of the prevalence of depression in psoriasis concluded that more than 10% of psoriasis patients suffer from clinical depression, and twice as many have depressive symptoms (Dowlatshahi et al. 2014). A multicenter cross-sectional study of dermatology patients in 13 European countries found elevated prevalence rates of depression (13.8%; adjusted odds ratio [AOR]=3.02), anxiety (22.7%; AOR=2.91), and suicidal ideation (17.3%; AOR= 1.94) among psoriasis patients compared with control subjects (Dalgard et al. 2015). The rate of suicidal ideation in psoriasis was higher than the rate in any other dermatological condition, and 67.6% of psoriasis patients attributed their suicidality to their psoriasis. Major depressive disorder has been associated with an increased risk of developing psoriatic arthritis in patients with psoriasis (hazard ratio=1.37; 95% CI= 1.05–1.80) (Lewinson et al. 2017). Depression in psoriasis has been attributed to both the elevated levels of proinflammatory cytokines and the psychosocial impact of psoriasis (Patel et al. 2017). "Biologics" (i.e., biological products such as the TNF-α inhibitor etanercept) that target inflammatory cytokines have been associated with both improvements in the clinical features of psoriasis and reductions in comorbid depression in some cases (Patel et al. 2017). By contrast, pre-marketing data and case studies have reported suicidal behaviors in association with the biologics that are used to treat psoriasis (Gupta et al. 2017b). A diagnosis of psoriasis, which has been independently associated with a higher prevalence of suicidal behaviors, may be a confounding factor in the reports of suicidal behaviors in psoriasis patients using biologics (Gupta et al. 2017b).

Management

Psychotherapy.   Psoriasis patients who experience stigmatization, who have a history of stress as a significant exacerbating factor, or who suffer from psychiatric comorbidities and experience a lower quality of life can benefit from psychological interventions (Janowski and Pietrzak 2008). Psychological distress can undermine the effectiveness of medical therapies. For example, psoriasis patients with high levels of pathological worrying were almost half as likely as low-worrying patients to experience improvement with psoralen plus ultraviolet A (PUVA) photochemotherapy (Fortune et al. 2003). Various interventions have been reported to be effective; such interventions include group therapy, psychoeducation, mindfulness meditation–based stress reduction (Kabat-Zinn et al. 1998), CBT that provides support and targets negative patterns of thinking (Fortune et al. 2005), cognitive-behavioral stress management, relaxation training and symptom control imagery training (Zachariae et al. 1996), hypnosis (Tausk and Whitmore 1999), and EMDR (when psoriasis arises in the context of psychological trauma; Gupta and Gupta 2002). Online CBT sessions have been shown to significantly reduce anxiety and improve quality of life in patients with chronic plaque psoriasis (Bundy et al. 2013). CBT with biofeedback was found to augment the benefits of narrow-band ultraviolet B (UVB) phototherapy in an 8-week intervention in 20 psoriasis patients (Piaserico et al. 2016). Mindfulness-based cognitive therapy has been reported to reduce patient-assessed psoriasis severity and enhance quality of life (Fordham et al. 2015). In a meta-analysis, psychological interventions (i.e., CBT, arousal reduction) for psoriasis were found to be beneficial (medium effect size) (Lavda et al. 2012).

Pharmacotherapy.   The association between psoriasis and comorbidities such as metabolic syndrome (Takeshita et al. 2017) should be taken into consideration when choosing a psychopharmacotherapeutic agent. Treatment of depressive symptoms may reduce pruritus and insomnia in psoriasis (Gupta et al. 1988). In a placebo-controlled trial, the reversible monoamine oxidase inhibitor (MAOI) moclobemide (currently not available in the United States) reduced psoriasis severity and anxiety (Alpsoy et al. 1998). In a small open-label trial, bupropion produced improvement in psoriasis, with return to baseline levels after its discontinuation (Modell et al. 2002), and paroxetine was reported to be effective in two patients with both depression and psoriasis (Luis Blay 2006). The addition of escitalopram 10 mg/day and psychotherapeutic sessions to the existing treatment regimen with TNF-α antagonists in patients with moderate-to-severe psoriasis was associated with a greater improvement in symptoms of depression and anxiety and reductions in pruritus severity (D'Erme et al. 2014). A Swedish population–based cohort study (Thorslund et al. 2013) of 69,830 patients with plaque psoriasis found that psoriasis patients who had been exposed to SSRIs had a significantly decreased risk (OR=0.44; 95% CI=0.28–0.68) of switching to systemic psoriasis treatments. It is noteworthy that shortly after discovery of the antipsychotic properties of chlorpromazine in 1952, oral chlorpromazine (D'Silva and Fisher 1956; Reiss 1956) and perphenazine (Shanon 1958) were reported to be effective in the treatment of psoriasis.

Urticaria and Angioedema

Urticaria (Grattan and Black 2008), or hives, is characterized by transient (usually lasting less than 24 hours) mucosal or skin swellings due to plasma leakage. The superficial swellings are called *wheals;* the deep swellings in the dermis and subcutaneous or submucosal tissue are termed *angioedema* and typically last for 2–3 days. Angioedema can also be a feature of anaphylaxis if the throat is involved. The wheals of urticaria are characteristically pruritic, and the angioedema is often painful. Urticaria's clinical presentation ranges from occasional localized wheals to widespread recurrent whealing and angioedema affecting the skin, mouth, and/or genitalia. Urticaria is found worldwide, with an estimated prevalence of 1%–5%; is more common in women; and can occur at any age (Grattan and Black 2008). All urticarias are acute initially; they are termed chronic when they persist over a period of 6 weeks or longer. The terms *chronic idiopathic urticaria* (most commonly used in North America) and *chronic spontaneous urticaria* (most commonly used outside North America) are used interchangeably. The etiology is not identifiable in about 70% of cases. Psychogenic factors are reported to be important in around 50% of cases (Gupta 2009). Adrenergic urticaria—a rare type of stress-induced physical urticaria (Hogan et al. 2014) that manifests as "halo-hives" or papules surrounded by blanched vasoconstricted skin— is an entity that is largely stress induced; the symptoms can be produced by injection of epinephrine and resolve when treated with propranolol. Cholinergic urticaria can be triggered by strenuous physical activity, high ambient temperatures, and strong emotions (Vadas et al. 2016); clinicians should be aware that the same cholinergic triggers can cause multisystem reactions (e.g., respiratory, cardiovascular), including anaphylaxis (Vadas et al. 2016).

Stress

Severe emotional stress may exacerbate urticarial reactions, regardless of the primary cause. A review of the literature indicated that stressful life events were found to precede the onset of urticaria in 30%–81% of patients (Gupta 2009). In one study of 48 patients (Czubalski and Rudzki 1977), exacerbation from emotional reactions occurred in 77% of patients with cholinergic urticaria and 82% of patients with dermographism, but did not occur in patients with cold urticaria. One possible mediator in the relationship between stress and urticaria is dehydroepiandrosterone sulfate (DHEAS), which plays an important role in modulating an organism's vulnerability to the negative effects of stress (Morgan et al. 2004). Some patients with chronic urticaria have been shown to have lower serum levels of DHEAS during the active period of the disease (Kasperska-Zajac et al. 2008), and low DHEAS levels were associated with greater psychological distress, as exemplified by higher anxiety and depression scores (Brzoza et al. 2008). In a cross-sectional study of 45 chronic urticaria patients and 45 age-matched control subjects, chronic urticaria was associated with increased levels of inflammatory markers (C reactive protein and interleukin-8) and higher scores on measures of stressful life events and daily hassles and lower basal cortisol levels compared with controls (Varghese et al. 2016).

Psychosocial and Psychiatric Factors

Studies in Turkey and Germany have reported that 48%–60% of patients with chronic urticaria have primary psychiatric disorders, with depressive disorders and OCD being the most common (Ozkan et al. 2007; Staubach et al. 2006; Uguz et al. 2008). A study of 27 children with chronic idiopathic urticaria (CIU) and 27 healthy control subjects revealed higher rates of psychiatric diagnoses (most commonly social anxiety disorder, separation anxiety disorder, and specific phobia) in the CIU patients (70% vs. 30% in controls) (Hergüner et al. 2011). A systematic review concluded that psychosocial factors were contributory in 46.09% (95% CI=44.01%–48.08%) of chronic spontaneous urticaria cases (Ben-Shoshan et al. 2013). Pruritus in chronic urticaria has a significant adverse effect on quality of life and has been directly correlated with severity of comorbid depression (Gupta and Gupta 1999). Sixty-two percent of chronic urticaria patients reported that pruritus interfered with their sleep, and itch scores were significantly higher in those who were also depressed (Yosipovitch et al. 2002). Insomnia has been reported to be the most important symptom associated with onset of chronic urticaria and is a mediator of the relationship with stress (Yang et al. 2005). The role of PTSD, which is often chronic, tends to be underrecognized as a contributing factor in chronic urticaria exacerbations (Gupta 2009); a study of 100 chronic urticaria patients and 60 control patients with allergies reported that patients with chronic urticaria were 1.89 times more likely than patients in the control group to have a current diagnosis of PTSD (Chung et al. 2010).

Management

Psychotherapy.   There is an extensive literature on the effect of hypnotic suggestion on urticarial reactions (Shenefelt 2000). For example, hypnotized volunteers were shown to have a significantly reduced flare reaction to the histamine prick test (Shenefelt 2000). In one small pre–post controlled study of hypnosis for CIU, hypnosis in combination with relaxation techniques reduced pruritus severity but not the number of wheals, although at follow-up 5–14 months after therapy, 40% of patients were free of hives and most of the rest reported improvement (Shertzer and Lookingbill 1987). The impact of chronic urticaria on patient quality of life should be assessed (Poon et al. 1999). Individual and group psychotherapy and stress management may be useful adjunctive therapies.

Pharmacotherapy.   In interpreting the chronic urticaria treatment literature, one must first recognize the very high rate of response to placebo (Rudzki et al. 1970). The less-sedating second-generation antihistamines (loratadine, fexofenadine, and cetirizine) are the first-line antihistamines for urticaria, and the first-generation antihistamine diphenhydramine is useful if itching is causing sleep disturbance. A low dose of a sedating antihistaminic antidepressant such as doxepin (Adhya and Karim 2015) is helpful for pruritus in chronic urticaria, especially when pruritus interferes with sleep (Yosipovitch et al. 2002). Two small randomized trials of doxepin demonstrated its efficacy at dosages of 10 mg three times daily (Greene et al. 1985) and 25 mg three times daily (Goldsobel et al. 1986). Doxepin may provide more than symptomatic relief by reducing the urticarial reaction itself (Rao et al. 1988). Combined H_1 plus H_2 antihistamine therapy may be more effective than H_1 antihistamines alone for urticaria, because dermal blood vessels possess both H_1 and H_2 histamine receptors, and the TCAs doxepin, trimipramine, and amitriptyline are potent histamine H_1 and H_2 receptor antagonists. Small studies and case reports have described a beneficial effect from SSRIs, bupropion, mirtazapine, and gabapentin in chronic urticaria (Yasharpour and Randhawa 2011). A case study reported the efficacy of olanzapine, believed to be related to its antihistaminic effect (Girshman et al. 2014). An open-label study (Demitsu et al. 2010) reported the efficacy of reserpine when added to antihistamines, an effect attributed to reserpine blocking the expression of delayed hypersensitivity by depleting tissue mast cell serotonin.

Acne

Acne vulgaris (Zaenglein 2008) is a multifactorial disorder of the pilosebaceous unit characterized by comedones (whiteheads and blackheads), papules, pustules, nodules, cysts, and scars; it affects the face, neck, upper trunk, and upper arms. Acne vulgaris has a peak incidence during adolescence, affects 85% of individuals 12–24 years of age, and continues on into later life in 12% of women and 3% of men. *Acne excoriée* and *acne excoriée des jeunes filles,* which often have significant psychiatric comorbidity, develop when acne comedones and papules are excoriated by patients (often young women), leaving crusted erosions that may scar. These self-excoriation behaviors are classified as skin-picking disorder (American Psychiatric Association 2013), as discussed earlier in this chapter.

Stress

Psychosocial stress can exacerbate acne in more than 60% of cases (Chiu et al. 2003; Harth et al. 2009). A multicenter Italian study (Di Landro et al. 2016) ($N=248$) examining the role of personal and environmental factors in adult ($\geq$25 years) female acne found that having a high level of reported psychological distress was one of the factors associated with acne (OR=2.95; 95% CI=1.57–5.53) in the multivariate model. Alternatively, having to cope with the cosmetic disfigurement associated with acne can be a significant source of stress for some patients, and the relationship between acne and psychological distress can be bidirectional (Wen et al. 2015). The impact of acne on quality of life and acne-related stress often does not correlate directly with the clinical severity of the condition (Gupta and Gupta 2001b).

Psychosocial and Psychiatric Factors

Psychiatric and psychosocial comorbidity is one of the most disabling features of acne and is sometimes the most important factor in deciding whether to institute dermatological therapies. The peak incidence of acne is during middle adolescence, and acne affects 85% of individuals between the ages of 12 and 24 years, an age period when major psychiatric disorders that have been reported to be associated with acne—such as major depressive disorder, eating disorders, and BDD—also have their onset. Social isolation, difficulties in interpersonal relationships, and body image concerns (which may be the consequence of a psychiatric disorder) may be attributed to acne, both by adolescent patients and sometimes by their parents, who may not be ready to acknowledge the possibility that their child has a mental disorder.

The extent of psychiatric morbidity in acne, including the prevalence of suicidal ideation, is not consistently related to the clinical severity of the skin condition. Bullying and teasing related to the cosmetic effects of acne can be a problem for a significant minority of adolescents (Magin et al. 2008), which in turn can lead to anxiety, poor self-esteem, acting out, or aggression. A cross-sectional survey of 9,567 12- to 18-year-olds in New Zealand revealed that self-reported "problem acne" was associated with an increased frequency of depressive symptoms (OR=2.04; 95% CI=1.70–2.45), anxiety (OR=2.3; 95% CI=1.74–3.00), and suicide attempts (OR=1.83; 95% CI=1.51–2.22) (Purvis et al. 2006). Whereas the lifetime rates of suicidal ideation and suicide attempts among 18-year-olds in a New Zealand cohort from the Christchurch Health and Development Study were 22.5% and 5.2%, respectively, these rates among youth ages 12–18 years with "problem acne" were 33.9% and 12.9%, respectively (Purvis et al. 2006). The association of acne with suicide attempts remained after adjustment for depressive symptoms and anxiety (OR=1.50; 95% CI=1.21–1.86) (Purvis et al. 2006). Similar findings were reported in a Norwegian study (Halvorsen et al. 2011) of 3,775 adolescents ages 18–19 years. Relative to adolescents who reported "no/little acne," those who reported "very much" acne reported suicidal ideation about twice as often among the girls (11.9% vs. 25.5%) and three times as often among the boys (6.3% vs. 22.6%), and the association of substantial acne and suicidal ideation remained significant (OR=1.80; 95% CI=1.30–2.50) in a multivariate model that controlled for depressive symptoms and demographics (Halvorsen et al. 2011). The prevalence of suicidal ideation among older acne patients recruited from dermatology clinics has been reported as 5%–7% (Gupta and Gupta 1998; Picardi et al. 2006); in patients who reported suicidal ideation, the extent of psychiatric comorbidity, including suicidal behavior, did not always correlate with the clinical severity of the acne. An analysis of a nationally representative database in the United States reported that in comparison with other dermatological disorders, acne was more likely to be associated with ADHD (OR=2.34; 95% CI=1.06–5.14) (Gupta et al. 2014). Comorbid ADHD could be a factor underlying increased suicidal behavior in some acne patients (Gupta et al. 2014).

Acne and eating disorders often coexist (Strumia 2013), and binge eating can be associated with acne flare-ups, while starvation, which can result in lower androgen levels, may improve acne (Gupta et al. 1992a). Acne is a major concern among patients with BDD, and dermatological treatments are the most frequently sought after and received nonpsychiatric treatments in BDD, the most common being topical acne agents (Crerand et al. 2005). In a study of acne patients ages 16–35 years, 36.7% of patients with clinically "minimal to nonexistent acne" and 32.9% with clinically mild acne met criteria for BDD (Bowe et al. 2007). Patients requiring systemic isotretinoin therapy were twice as likely to have BDD as those who had never used it (Bowe et al. 2007).

Isotretinoin and Psychiatric Side Effects

Isotretinoin, which is generally used to treat severe acne, has been associated with depression, psychosis, suicide, and aggressive behaviors (Physicians' Desk Reference 2016), an association first reported by the FDA in 1998 (Nightingale 1998). The general consensus at present is that the relationship between isotretinoin and psychiatric side effects is unclear, with little supportive evidence available from RCT data (Gorton et al. 2016; Huang and Cheng 2017). In fact, various studies have reported that treatment of acne with isotretinoin is associated with a significant improvement in quality of life and depression (Schrom et al. 2016). The current U.S. prescribing guidelines for isotretinoin (Accutane is one of the trade names) stipulate that "prior to initiation of Accutane therapy, patients and family members should be asked about any history of psychiatric disorder, and at each visit during therapy, patients should be assessed for symptoms of depression, mood disturbance, psychosis, or aggression to determine if further evaluation may be necessary" (Physicians' Desk Reference 2016). Discontinuation of isotretinoin is not necessarily associated with a remission of the psychiatric symptoms. A Swedish retrospective cohort study (Sundström et al. 2010) linking registries of isotretinoin users and causes of deaths concluded that an increased risk of attempted suicide was apparent up to 6 months after the end of treatment with isotretinoin, and recommended close monitoring of patients for suicidal behavior for up to 1 year after the end of treatment. The authors observed, however, that the risk of attempted suicide was already rising before treatment with isotretinoin, so an additional risk due to isotretinoin treatment could not be established (Sundström et al. 2010).

Management

Psychotherapy.   When adolescent acne is untreated, its problems may persist into later life, when acne is no longer normally a problem. BDD patients, who typically express concern about clinically mild acne, tend to resist any psychological explanation for their skin concerns. Some patients pick their skin and self-excoriate their acne to regulate emotions (e.g., in PTSD); underlying trauma issues should be addressed in therapy after the patient is adequately stabilized. Cognitive-behavioral therapies and hypnosis have been used in *acne excoriée* (Shenefelt 2003). Because of the frequent coexistence of eating disorders and acne, it is important to evaluate the potential impact of acne on the patient's body image and eating behavior.

Pharmacotherapy.   Psychotropic medications in acne patients are directed at underlying psychopathology. Some patients taking isotretinoin who develop depression may require standard antidepressants. Case reports attest to the benefits of a wide variety of psychotropic agents for acne, including paroxetine (Moussavian 2001) and olanzapine for *acne excoriée* (Gupta and Gupta 2000), but there are no controlled trials.

Cutaneous Reactions to Psychopharmacological Agents

Adverse cutaneous drug reactions (ACDRs) can be divided into common (usually relatively benign) ACDRs (Table 27–2), rare and life-threatening ACDRs (Table 27–3), and those that are due to precipitation or aggravation of a primary dermatological disorder (Bliss and Warnock 2013; Litt 2013).

Common Adverse Cutaneous Drug Reactions

Common ACDRs include pruritus, exanthematous rashes, urticaria with or without angioedema, fixed drug eruptions, photosensitivity reactions, drug-induced pigmentation, and alopecia/hypertrichosis.

Pruritus is the most common ACDR, encountered with all antipsychotics, antidepressants, and mood stabilizers, and is usually secondary to other ACDRs.

Exanthematous rashes (morbilliform or maculopapular eruptions) can occur with all antipsychotics, antidepressants, and mood stabilizers. The rash usually occurs within the first 3–14 days of starting the drug and may subside without discontinuation of

---

TABLE 27–2. **Most common cutaneous drug reactions to psychotherapeutic agents**

Pruritus and exanthematous rashes

Urticaria with or without angioedema

Fixed drug eruptions

Photosensitivity reactions

Drug-induced pigmentation

Alopecia/hypertrichosis

TABLE 27–3. **Severe and life-threatening cutaneous drug reactions to psychotherapeutic agents**

Erythema multiforme

Stevens-Johnson syndrome

Toxic epidermal necrolysis

Drug hypersensitivity syndrome (also drug eruption with eosinophilia and systemic symptoms [DRESS])

Exfoliative dermatitis

Drug hypersensitivity vasculitis

---

the causative agent. A rash accompanied by painful skin lesions, mucosal lesions, or sore throat may represent the early stages of one of the more severe and life-threatening ACDRs, such as Stevens-Johnson syndrome (SJS).

Urticaria with or without *angioedema* is the second most common ACDR (after pruritus); it occurs within minutes to hours—but sometimes as late as several days—after starting the drug and can lead to laryngeal angioedema and anaphylaxis. Urticaria can occur with all antipsychotics, antidepressants, and anticonvulsants.

Fixed drug eruptions, which theoretically can occur with any drug, characteristically present as sharply demarcated, solitary or occasionally multiple lesions. Eruptions occur within a few to 24 hours after ingestion of the drug and resolve within several weeks of drug discontinuation.

Drug-induced photosensitivity can present either as phototoxicity (i.e., an exaggerated sunburn restricted to sun-exposed skin) or as photoallergy (i.e., a more generalized eruption triggered by sun exposure when a person is on certain drugs). Drug-induced photosensitivity tends to involve only sun-exposed skin, although there may be exceptions. Photosensitivity reactions can be caused by any of the antipsychotics but are much more frequently associated with chlorpromazine (3% incidence). Photosensitivity also occurs with many antidepressants, anticonvulsants, and sedative-hypnotics. Patients should be advised regarding the use of sunscreen and minimization of sun exposure when the medication must be continued. Photosensitivity caused by psychotropic drugs may interfere with PUVA and UVB phototherapy for psoriasis and other pruritic dermatoses.

Drug-induced pigmentation, which may involve the skin and eyes (retina, lens, and cornea), has been reported after long-term (>6 months) high-dose (>500 mg/day) use of low-potency typical antipsychotics, especially chlorpromazine and thioridazine. Pigmentary changes have been associated with some antidepressants, including various TCAs, all SSRIs, venlafaxine (hypopigmentation), and several anticonvulsants (also changes in hair color and texture).

Alopecia has been frequently reported with lithium (>5%) and valproic acid (>5%) and less frequently with the other mood stabilizers. Alopecia has also been associated with most antidepressants and several antipsychotics. Hair loss may occur rapidly or a few months after the drug is started, with recovery generally 2–18 months after drug discontinuation.

Hypertrichosis and *hirsutism* can occur with some antidepressants and benzodiazepines (Lamer et al. 2010; Litt 2013).

Severe and Life-Threatening Adverse Cutaneous Drug Reactions

Severe and life-threatening skin reactions (see Table 27–3) are most often associated with anticonvulsants and include erythema multiforme, SJS, toxic epidermal necrolysis (TEN), drug hypersensitivity syndrome or drug eruption with eosinophilia and systemic symptoms (DRESS), exfoliative dermatitis, and vasculitis (Bliss and Warnock 2013; Litt 2013). Erythema multiforme, SJS, and TEN lie on a continuum of increasing severity. About 16% of SJS/TEN cases have been associated with short-term use of anticonvulsants, with greatest risk for development of TEN within the first 8 weeks of therapy. Use of multiple anticonvulsants and higher dosages increases the risk. Treatment of severe reactions should include immediate discontinuation of the drug and emergency dermatology consultation. Patients typically require fluid and nutritional support as well as infection and pain control, which may involve management in an intensive care unit or burn unit.

Erythema multiforme occurs within days of starting the drug and may present as a polymorphous eruption, with pathognomonic "target lesions" typically involving the extremities and palmoplantar surfaces. The potential for evolution to more serious SJS/TEN should always be considered. Although it has in rare cases been associated with antipsychotics and antidepressants, erythema multiforme is most commonly associated with carbamazepine, valproic acid, lamotrigine, gabapentin, and oxcarbazepine.

Stevens-Johnson syndrome usually occurs within the first few weeks after drug exposure and presents as flu-like symptoms followed by mucocutaneous lesions; it has a mortality rate as high as 5% due to loss of the cutaneous barrier and sepsis. Bullous lesions can involve mucosal surfaces, including the eyes, mouth, and genital tract. SJS is most frequently associated with the same anticonvulsants as erythema multiforme.

Toxic epidermal necrolysis is considered to be an extreme variant of SJS, resulting in epidermal detachment in more than 30% of cases, which occurs within the first 2 months of treatment, with a mortality rate as high as 45% due to sepsis. In 80% of TEN cases, a strong association is made with specific medications (vs. an association with specific medications in 50% of SJS cases), most often anticonvulsants.

Drug hypersensitivity syndrome (DRESS) characteristically occurs 1–8 weeks after starting drug treatment, most commonly presenting as a morbilliform rash, with fever, eosinophilia, lymphadenopathy, and multiple organ involvement. Treatment involves immediate discontinuation of the suspected drug, systemic steroids, and antihistamines. The mortality rate is 10% if symptoms are unrecognized or untreated. The rash can range from a simple exanthem to TEN and is most commonly associated with anticonvulsants, although it has also been associated with bupropion and fluoxetine (Husain et al. 2013).

Exfoliative dermatitis presents as a widespread rash characterized by desquamation, pruritic erythema, fever, and lymphadenopathy within the first few weeks of drug therapy, with a good prognosis if the causative agent is withdrawn immediately. It has been reported with antipsychotics, most TCAs and other antidepressants, mood stabilizers, lithium, sedatives, and hypnotics.

Drug hypersensitivity vasculitis, characterized by inflammation and necrosis of the walls of blood vessels, occurs within a few weeks of starting a drug. Lesions (e.g., palpable purpura) are primarily localized on the lower third of the legs and ankles. The condition has in rare cases occurred with clozapine, maprotiline, trazodone, carbamazepine, lithium, phenobarbital, pentobarbital, diazepam, and chlordiazepoxide.

The risk of developing SJS/TEN with anticonvulsants (most often carbamazepine) is significantly increased in individuals with particular variants of the human leukocyte antigen (HLA) alleles, specifically HLA-B*1502 and HLA-A*3101 (U.S. Food and Drug Administration 2007). The B*1502 allele variant is more common in Asian populations. The FDA has recommended that individuals of Asian (including South Asian Indians) ancestry be screened for the B*1502 variant prior to commencing treatment with carbamazepine (U.S. Food and Drug Administration 2007). This variant also has been associated with SJS/TEN induced by other anticonvulsants, such as oxcarbazepine, lamotrigine, or phenytoin (Hung et al. 2010). The A*3101 variant is found in numerous populations, including Caucasians, and is associated with a number of ACDRs, including SJS/TEN and DRESS. At present, the FDA does not explicitly advocate genotyping for the A*3101 variant prior to commencing carbamazepine; however, some investigators (Amstutz et al. 2014) have recommended screening for the A*3101 allele among all carbamazepine-naive patients.

Drug-Induced Precipitation or Aggravation of a Primary Dermatological Disorder

Psychotropic drugs can precipitate or exacerbate a number of primary dermatological disorders, including acne, psoriasis, seborrheic dermatitis, hyperhidrosis, and porphyria (Litt 2013). Acne has been associated with most antidepressants, lithium, anticonvulsants, and antipsychotics. It is well recognized that lithium can precipitate or exacerbate psoriasis, sometimes within the first few months but usually within the first few years of treatment. The absolute increased risk is quite small (Brauchli et al. 2009). Psoriasis precipitated or exacerbated by lithium is typically resistant to conventional antipsoriatic treatments. When the psoriasis becomes intractable, lithium must be discontinued, and the psoriasis usually remits within a few months. A small RCT showed that inositol supplements had a significant beneficial effect on psoriasis among patients taking lithium (Allan et al. 2004). Although some reports have linked beta-blockers such as propranolol (often used to treat lithium-induced tremors) with psoriasis, other studies have not confirmed this association (Brauchli et al. 2009). Anticonvulsants, atypical antipsychotics, and SSRIs have less commonly been reported to precipitate or aggravate psoriasis.

Seborrheic dermatitis is very common in patients taking long-term phenothiazines and also has been reported with other antipsychotics, lithium, and anticonvulsants.

Hyperhidrosis, often manifesting as night sweats, is common with SSRIs, SNRIs, bupropion, and MAOIs. Sweating is mediated by sympathetic cholinergic innervation of the eccrine sweat glands; however, the more anticholinergic TCAs have also caused hyperhidrosis, and therefore switching to a more anticholinergic antidepressant is not necessarily helpful. Hyperhidrosis has also been reported with antipsychotics and anticonvulsants. Porphyria may be exacerbated by certain drugs (e.g., carbamazepine, valproic acid, many sedative-hypnotics [especially barbiturates]), resulting in acute dermatological, neuropsychiatric, and abdominal pain symptoms. Chlorpromazine, although photosensitizing, is considered to be "safe" and actually was approved by the FDA for use in acute intermittent porphyria.

Interactions Between Dermatology Drugs and Psychopharmacological Agents

Most pharmacokinetic interactions (Litt 2013) between dermatological and psychotropic drugs result from inhibition of CYP2D6 and 3A4 isoenzymes. Selected interactions are listed in Table 27–4.

Conclusion

Psychodermatological disorders are usually classified as dermatological manifestations of a primary psychiatric disorder (also referred to as *psychocutaneous disorders*); as functional cutaneous disorders; or as psychological factors associated with a primary dermatological disorder that is exacerbated by psychosocial stress and that often is comorbid with psychiatric disorders. Psychological trauma, dissociation, and conversion are often factors in the body-focused repetitive behaviors and dermatitis artefacta. Factors that increase psychiatric morbidity (including suicide risk) in dermatological patients include pruritus with sleep difficulties, disease-related stress (largely due to cosmetic disfigurement), associated social stigma resulting in feelings of social exclusion and alienation, and (especially in pediatric patients) appearance-related bullying. The high prevalence of suicidal ideation among dermatology patients is not consistently related to the clinical severity of the skin condition, but may be related to a concurrent psychiatric disorder with onset around the same time as the dermatological disorder. Covert body dysmorphic disorder can also increase suicide risk and treatment resistance. Psychiatrists should thoroughly assess the impact of the skin disorder on the patient's quality of life (including pruritus severity and sleep disturbance) and should recommend aggressive dermatological treatment of even clinically mild skin disease that is cosmetically disfiguring (especially facial lesions) or socially stigmatizing. Standard psychotherapeutic interventions (typically aimed at reducing scratching behaviors and BFRBs, physiological arousal, and dysfunctional illness perceptions), in conjunction with psychopharmacological agents, may be used to treat psychiatric comorbidity. Severe and life-threatening dermatological reactions to psychotropic agents are most frequently associated with the mood-stabilizing anticonvulsants, with the greatest risk of development during the first 2 months of therapy.

TABLE 27–4. Selected dermatological drug–psychotherapeutic drug pharmacokinetic interactions

Medication used in dermatology	Effects on CYP isoenzymes	Effects on psychotropic drug levels
Azole antifungals (oral formulations only) Itraconazole Ketoconazole Macrolide antibiotics Clarithromycin Erythromycin Cyclosporine (both substrate and inhibitor of CYP 3A4)	Inhibition of CYP 3A4	Benzodiazepine serum levels for agents that undergo hepatic oxidative metabolism (e.g., alprazolam, triazolam) may increase. Buspirone levels are increased. Carbamazepine levels are increased. Pimozide levels are increased.
Terbinafine	Inhibition of CYP 2D6	Antidepressant serum levels may increase for CYP 2D6 substrates (e.g., tricyclic antidepressants, paroxetine, venlafaxine, atomoxetine). Antipsychotic serum levels may increase for CYP 2D6 substrates (e.g., phenothiazines, haloperidol, risperidone, olanzapine, clozapine, aripiprazole).

Note.   CYP=cytochrome P450.

References

Adewuya EC, Zinser W, Thomas C: Trichotillomania: a case of response to valproic acid. J Child Adolesc Psychopharmacol 18(5):533–536, 2008 18928419

Adhya Z, Karim Y: Doxepin may be a useful pharmacotherapeutic agent in chronic urticaria. Clin Exp Allergy 45(8):1370, 2015 26040550

Ahmad K, Ramsay B: Delusional parasitosis: lessons learnt. Acta Derm Venereol 89(2):165–168, 2009a 19326002

Ahmad K, Ramsay B: Misdiagnosis of dermatitis artefacta: how did we get it wrong? Clin Exp Dermatol 34(1):113–114, 2009b 19076815

Allan SJ, Kavanagh GM, Herd RM, et al: The effect of inositol supplements on the psoriasis of patients taking lithium: a randomized, placebo-controlled trial. Br J Dermatol 150(5):966–969, 2004 15149510

Alpsoy E, Ozcan E, Cetin L, et al: Is the efficacy of topical corticosteroid therapy for psoriasis vulgaris enhanced by concurrent moclobemide therapy? A double-blind, placebo-controlled study. J Am Acad Dermatol 38(2 Pt 1):197–200, 1998 9486674

American Psychiatric Association: Diagnostic and Statistical Manual of Mental Disorders, 5th Edition. Arlington, VA, American Psychiatric Association, 2013

Amstutz U, Shear NH, Rieder MJ, et al; CPNDS clinical recommendation group: Recommendations for HLA-B*15:02 and HLA-A*31:01 genetic testing to reduce the risk of carbamazepine-induced hypersensitivity reactions. Epilepsia 55(4):496–506, 2014 24597466

Angelakis I, Gooding PA, Panagioti M: Suicidality in body dysmorphic disorder (BDD): a systematic review with meta-analysis. Clin Psychol Rev 49:55–66, 2016 27607741

Arck PC, Slominski A, Theoharides TC, et al: Neuroimmunology of stress: skin takes center stage. J Invest Dermatol 126(8):1697–1704, 2006 16845409

Arnetz BB, Fjellner B, Eneroth P, et al: Stress and psoriasis: psychoendocrine and metabolic reactions in psoriatic patients during standardized stressor exposure. Psychosom Med 47(6):528–541, 1985 4070523

Basra MK, Fenech R, Gatt RM, et al: The Dermatology Life Quality Index 1994–2007: a comprehensive review of validation data and clinical results. Br J Dermatol 159(5):997–1035, 2008 18795920

Ben-Shoshan M, Blinderman I, Raz A: Psychosocial factors and chronic spontaneous urticaria: a systematic review. Allergy 68(2):131–141, 2013 23157275

Bliss SA, Warnock JK: Psychiatric medications: adverse cutaneous drug reactions. Clin Dermatol 31(1):101–109, 2013 23245981

Bloch MH, Landeros-Weisenberger A, Dombrowski P, et al: Systematic review: pharmacological and behavioral treatment for trichotillomania. Biol Psychiatry 62(8):839–846, 2007 17727824

Blome C, Radtke MA, Eissing L, et al: Quality of life in patients with atopic dermatitis: disease burden, measurement, and treatment benefit. Am J Clin Dermatol 17(2):163–169, 2016 26818063

Boscarino JA: Posttraumatic stress disorder and physical illness: results from clinical and epidemiologic studies. Ann N Y Acad Sci 1032:141–153, 2004 15677401

Bowe WP, Leyden JJ, Crerand CE, et al: Body dysmorphic disorder symptoms among patients with acne vulgaris. J Am Acad Dermatol 57(2):222–230, 2007 17498840

Boyd AS, Ritchie C, Likhari S: Munchausen syndrome and Munchausen syndrome by proxy in dermatology. J Am Acad Dermatol 71(2):376–381, 2014 24613506

Brauchli YB, Jick SS, Curtin F, et al: Lithium, antipsychotics, and risk of psoriasis. J Clin Psychopharmacol 29(2):134–140, 2009 19512974

Brzoza Z, Kasperska-Zajac A, Badura-Brzoza K, et al: Decline in dehydroepiandrosterone sulfate observed in chronic urticaria is associated with psychological distress. Psychosom Med 70(6):723–728, 2008 18606731

Bundy C, Pinder B, Bucci S, et al: A novel, web-based, psychological intervention for people with psoriasis: the electronic Targeted Intervention for Psoriasis (eTIPs) study. Br J Dermatol 169(2):329–336, 2013 23551271

Buske-Kirschbaum A, Ebrecht M, Kern S, et al: Endocrine stress responses in TH1-mediated chronic inflammatory skin disease (psoriasis vulgaris)—do they parallel stress-induced endocrine changes in TH2-mediated inflammatory dermatoses (atopic dermatitis)? Psychoneuroendocrinology 31(4):439–446, 2006 16359823

Buske-Kirschbaum A, Ebrecht M, Hellhammer DH: Blunted HPA axis responsiveness to stress in atopic patients is associated with the acuity and severeness of allergic inflammation. Brain Behav Immun 24(8):1347–1353, 2010 20633637

Cheng CM, Hsu JW, Huang KL, et al: Risk of developing major depressive disorder and anxiety disorders among adolescents and adults with atopic dermatitis: a nationwide longitudinal study. J Affect Disord 178:60–65, 2015 25795537

Chiu A, Chon SY, Kimball AB: The response of skin disease to stress: changes in the severity of acne vulgaris as affected by examination stress. Arch Dermatol 139(7):897–900, 2003 12873885

Choi EH, Brown BE, Crumrine D, et al: Mechanisms by which psychologic stress alters cutaneous permeability barrier homeostasis and stratum corneum integrity. J Invest Dermatol 124(3):587–595, 2005 15737200

Christenson GA, Popkin MK, Mackenzie TB, et al: Lithium treatment of chronic hair pulling. J Clin Psychiatry 52(3):116–120, 1991 1900831

Chung MC, Symons C, Gilliam J, et al: The relationship between posttraumatic stress disorder, psychiatric comorbidity, and personality traits among patients with chronic idiopathic urticaria. Compr Psychiatry 51(1):55–63, 2010 19932827

Cohen AD, Vardy DA: Dermatitis artefacta in soldiers. Mil Med 171(6):497–499, 2006 16808128

Cotterill JA: Dermatological non-disease: a common and potentially fatal disturbance of cutaneous body image. Br J Dermatol 104(6):611–619, 1981 7248174

Cotterill JA, Cunliffe WJ: Suicide in dermatological patients. Br J Dermatol 137(2):246–250, 1997 9292074

Craig-Müller SA, Reichenberg JS: The other itch that rashes: a clinical and therapeutic approach to pruritus and skin picking disorders. Curr Allergy Asthma Rep 15(6):31, 2015 26141577

Crerand CE, Phillips KA, Menard W, et al: Nonpsychiatric medical treatment of body dysmorphic disorder. Psychosomatics 46(6):549–555, 2005 16288134

Crerand CE, Menard W, Phillips KA: Surgical and minimally invasive cosmetic procedures among persons with body dysmorphic disorder. Ann Plast Surg 65(1):11–16, 2010 20467296

Czubalski K, Rudzki E: Neuropsychic factors in physical urticaria. Dermatologica 154(1):1–4, 1977 844637

D'Erme AM, Zanieri F, Campolmi E, et al: Therapeutic implications of adding the psychotropic drug escitalopram in the treatment of patients suffering from moderate-severe psoriasis and psychiatric comorbidity: a retrospective study. J Eur Acad Dermatol Venereol 28(2):246–249, 2014 22963277

D'Silva JL, Fisher RA: Chlorpromazine in the management of psoriasis. Ill Med J 110(3):135–136, 1956 13357173

Dalgard F, Lien L, Dalen I: Itch in the community: associations with psychosocial factors among adults. J Eur Acad Dermatol Venereol 21(9):1215–1219, 2007 17894708

Dalgard FJ, Gieler U, Tomas-Aragones L, et al: The psychological burden of skin diseases: a cross-sectional multicenter study among dermatological out-patients in 13 European countries. J Invest Dermatol 135(4):984–991, 2015 25521458

Daunton A, Bridgett C, Goulding JM: Habit reversal for refractory atopic dermatitis: a review. Br J Dermatol 174(3):657–659, 2016 26384717

Demitsu T, Yoneda K, Kakurai M, et al: Clinical efficacy of reserpine as "add-on therapy" to antihistamines in patients with recalcitrant chronic idiopathic urticaria and urticarial vasculitis. J Dermatol 37(9):827–829, 2010 20883370

Dessinioti C, Katsambas A, Tzavela E, et al: Erythema ab igne in three girls with anorexia nervosa. Pediatr Dermatol 33(2):e149–e150, 2016 26822102

Dhabhar FS: Psychological stress and immunoprotection versus immunopathology in the skin. Clin Dermatol 31(1):18–30, 2013 23245970

Di Landro A, Cazzaniga S, Cusano F, et al: Adult female acne and associated risk factors: results of a multicenter case-control study in Italy. J Am Acad Dermatol 75(6):1134.e1–1141.e1, 2016 27542588

Dowlatshahi EA, Wakkee M, Arends LR, et al: The prevalence and odds of depressive symptoms and clinical depression in psoriasis patients: a systematic review and meta-analysis. J Invest Dermatol 134(6):1542–1551, 2014 24284419

Drake LA, Millikan LE; Doxepin Study Group: The antipruritic effect of 5% doxepin cream in patients with eczematous dermatitis. Arch Dermatol 131(12):1403–1408, 1995 7492129

Drucker AM: Atopic dermatitis: burden of illness, quality of life, and associated complications. Allergy Asthma Proc 38(1):3–8, 2017 28052794

Ebata T, Izumi H, Aizawa H, et al: Effects of nitrazepam on nocturnal scratching in adults with atopic dermatitis: a double-blind placebo-controlled crossover study. Br J Dermatol 138(4):631–634, 1998 9640368

Ersser SJ, Cowdell F, Latter S, et al: Psychological and educational interventions for atopic eczema in children. Cochrane Database Syst Rev (1):CD004054, 2014 24399641

Evers AW, Verhoeven EW, Kraaimaat FW, et al: How stress gets under the skin: cortisol and stress reactivity in psoriasis. Br J Dermatol 163(5):986–991, 2010 20716227

Evers AW, Schut C, Gieler U, et al: Itch management: psychotherapeutic approach. Curr Probl Dermatol 50:64–70, 2016 27578073

Fabisch W: Psychiatric aspects of dermatitis artefacta. Br J Dermatol 102(1):29–34, 1980 7378280

Fellner MJ, Majeed MH: Tales of bugs, delusions of parasitosis, and what to do. Clin Dermatol 27(1):135–138, 2009 19095159

Fordham B, Griffiths CE, Bundy C: A pilot study examining mindfulness-based cognitive therapy in psoriasis. Psychol Health Med 20(1):121–127, 2015 24684520

Fortune DG, Richards HL, Kirby B, et al: Psychological distress impairs clearance of psoriasis in patients treated with photochemotherapy. Arch Dermatol 139(6):752–756, 2003 12810506

Fortune DG, Richards HL, Griffiths CE: Psychologic factors in psoriasis: consequences, mechanisms, and interventions. Dermatol Clin 23(4):681–694, 2005 16112445

Foster AA, Hylwa SA, Bury JE, et al: Delusional infestation: clinical presentation in 147 patients seen at Mayo Clinic. J Am Acad Dermatol 67(4):673.e1–673.e10, 2012 22264448

Freudenmann RW, Lepping P: Second-generation antipsychotics in primary and secondary delusional parasitosis: outcome and efficacy. J Clin Psychopharmacol 28(5):500–508, 2008 18794644

Gardner FH, Diamond LK: Autoerythrocyte sensitization: a form of purpura producing painful bruising following autosensitization to red blood cells in certain women. Blood 10(7):675–690, 1955 14389381

Gattu S, Rashid RM, Khachemoune A: Self-induced skin lesions: a review of dermatitis artefacta. Cutis 84(5):247–251, 2009 20099617

Gencoglan G, Inanir I, Gunduz K: Therapeutic hotline: treatment of prurigo nodularis and lichen simplex chronicus with gabapentin. Dermatol Ther (Heidelb) 23(2):194–198, 2010 20415827

Gieler U, Consoli SG, Tomás-Aragones L, et al: Self-inflicted lesions in dermatology: terminology and classification—a position paper from the European Society for Dermatology and Psychiatry (ESDaP). Acta Derm Venereol 93(1):4–12, 2013 23303467

Girshman YJ, Wang Y, Mendelowitz A: Olanzapine for the treatment of psychiatric illness and urticaria: a case report. Psychosomatics 55(6):735–738, 2014 25262038

Goldsobel AB, Rohr AS, Siegel SC, et al: Efficacy of doxepin in the treatment of chronic idiopathic urticaria. J Allergy Clin Immunol 78(5 Pt 1):867–873, 1986 3782654

Gorton HC, Webb RT, Kapur N, et al: Non-psychotropic medication and risk of suicide or attempted suicide: a systematic review. BMJ Open 6(1):e009074, 2016 26769782

Grant JE, Chamberlain SR: Trichotillomania. Am J Psychiatry 173(9):868–874, 2016 27581696

Grant JE, Odlaug BL, Kim SW: N-acetylcysteine, a glutamate modulator, in the treatment of trichotillomania: a double-blind, placebo-controlled study. Arch Gen Psychiatry 66(7):756–763, 2009 19581567

Grant JE, Odlaug BL, Chamberlain SR, et al: A double-blind, placebo-controlled trial of lamotrigine for pathological skin picking: treatment efficacy and neurocognitive predictors of response. J Clin Psychopharmacol 30(4):396–403, 2010 20531220

Grant JE, Chamberlain SR, Redden SA, et al: N-Acetylcysteine in the treatment of excoriation disorder: a randomized clinical trial. JAMA Psychiatry 73(5):490–496, 2016 27007062

Grattan CEH, Black AK: Urticaria and angioedema, in Dermatology, 2nd Edition, Vol 1. Edited by Bolognia JL, Jorizzo JL, Rapini RP. London, Mosby Elsevier, 2008, pp 261–276

Greene SL, Reed CE, Schroeter AL: Double-blind crossover study comparing doxepin with diphenhydramine for the treatment of chronic urticaria. J Am Acad Dermatol 12(4):669–675, 1985 3886724

Gupta MA: Concerns about aging and a drive for thinness: a factor in the biopsychosocial model of eating disorders? Int J Eat Disord 18(4):351–357, 1995 8580921

Gupta MA: Somatization disorders in dermatology. Int Rev Psychiatry 18(1):41–47, 2006 16451879

Gupta MA: Stress and urticaria, in Neuroimmunology of the Skin: Basic Science to Clinical Practice. Edited by Granstein RD, Luger TA. Berlin, Heidelberg, Germany, Springer-Verlag, 2009, pp 209–217

Gupta MA: Emotional regulation, dissociation, and the self-induced dermatoses: clinical features and implications for treatment with mood stabilizers. Clin Dermatol 31(1):110–117, 2013 23245982

Gupta MA, Gupta AK: Psychodermatology: an update. J Am Acad Dermatol 34(6):1030–1046, 1996 8647969

Gupta MA, Gupta AK: Depression and suicidal ideation in dermatology patients with acne, alopecia areata, atopic dermatitis and psoriasis. Br J Dermatol 139(5):846–850, 1998 9892952

Gupta MA, Gupta AK: Depression modulates pruritus perception. A study of pruritus in psoriasis, atopic dermatitis and chronic idiopathic urticaria. Ann N Y Acad Sci 885:394–395, 1999 10816673

Gupta MA, Gupta AK: Olanzapine is effective in the management of some self-induced dermatoses: three case reports. Cutis 66(2):143–146, 2000 10955197

Gupta MA, Gupta AK: Dissatisfaction with skin appearance among patients with eating disorders and non-clinical controls. Br J Dermatol 145(1):110–113, 2001a 11453917

Gupta MA, Gupta AK: The psychological comorbidity in acne. Clin Dermatol 19(3):360–363, 2001b 11479049

Gupta MA, Gupta AK: Use of eye movement desensitization and reprocessing (EMDR) in the treatment of dermatologic disorders. J Cutan Med Surg 6(5):415–421, 2002 12001004

Gupta MA, Gupta AK: Cutaneous body image dissatisfaction and suicidal ideation: mediation by interpersonal sensitivity. J Psychosom Res 75(1):55–59, 2013a 23751239

Gupta MA, Gupta AK: Cutaneous sensory disorder. Semin Cutan Med Surg 32(2):110–118, 2013b 24049969

Gupta MA, Gupta AK: A practical approach to the assessment of psychosocial and psychiatric comorbidity in the dermatology patient. Clin Dermatol 31(1):57–61, 2013c 23245974

Gupta MA, Gupta AK: Sleep-wake disorders and dermatology. Clin Dermatol 31(1):118–126, 2013d 23245983

Gupta MA, Gupta AK: Current concepts in psychodermatology. Curr Psychiatry Rep 16(6):449, 2014 24740235

Gupta MA, Gupta AK, Haberman HF: Neurotic excoriations: a review and some new perspectives. Compr Psychiatry 27(4):381–386, 1986 3731771

Gupta MA, Gupta AK, Haberman HF: Dermatologic signs in anorexia nervosa and bulimia nervosa. Arch Dermatol 123(10):1386–1390, 1987a 3310913

Gupta MA, Gupta AK, Haberman HF: The self-inflicted dermatoses: a critical review. Gen Hosp Psychiatry 9(1):45–52, 1987b 3817460

Gupta MA, Gupta AK, Kirkby S, et al: Pruritus in psoriasis. A prospective study of some psychiatric and dermatologic correlates. Arch Dermatol 124(7):1052–1057, 1988 3389849

Gupta MA, Gupta AK, Kirkby S, et al: A psychocutaneous profile of psoriasis patients who are stress reactors. A study of 127 patients. Gen Hosp Psychiatry 11(3):166–173, 1989 2721939

Gupta MA, Gupta AK, Ellis CN, et al: Bulimia nervosa and acne may be related: a case report. Can J Psychiatry 37(1):58–61, 1992a 1532340

Gupta MA, Gupta AK, Voorhees JJ: Starvation-associated pruritus: a clinical feature of eating disorders. J Am Acad Dermatol 27(1):118–120, 1992b 1619062

Gupta MA, Gupta AK, Ellis CN, et al: Psychiatric evaluation of the dermatology patient. Dermatol Clin 23(4):591–599, 2005 16112434

Gupta MA, Gupta AK, Vujcic B: Increased frequency of attention deficit hyperactivity disorder (ADHD) in acne versus dermatologic controls: analysis of an epidemiologic database from the US. J Dermatolog Treat 25(2):115–118, 2014 23030461

Gupta MA, Gupta AK, Knapp K: Dissatisfaction with cutaneous body image is directly correlated with insomnia severity: a prospective study in a non-clinical sample. J Dermatolog Treat 26(2):193–197, 2015 24511911

Gupta MA, Simpson FC, Gupta AK: Psoriasis and sleep disorders: a systematic review. Sleep Med Rev 29:63–75, 2016 26624228

Gupta MA, Jarosz P, Gupta AK: Posttraumatic stress disorder (PTSD) and the dermatology patient. Clin Dermatol 35(3):260–266, 2017a 28511822

Gupta MA, Pur DR, Vujcic B, et al: Suicidal behaviors in the dermatology patient. Clin Dermatol 35(3):302–311, 2017b 28511829

Gupta MA, Simpson FC, Vujcic B, et al: Obstructive sleep apnea and dermatologic disorders. Clin Dermatol 35(3):319–327, 2017c 28511831

Gupta MA, Vujcic B, Gupta AK: Dissociation and conversion symptoms in dermatology. Clin Dermatol 35(3):267–272, 2017d 28511823

Halvorsen JA, Stern RS, Dalgard F, et al: Suicidal ideation, mental health problems, and social impairment are increased in adolescents with acne: a population-based study. J Invest Dermatol 131(2):363–370, 2011 20844551

Harth W, Gieler U, Kusnir D, et al: Clinical Management in Psychodermatology, 2009 Edition. Berlin, Heidelberg, Germany, Springer-Verlag, 2009

Hergüner S, Kiliç G, Karakoç S, et al: Levels of depression, anxiety and behavioural problems and frequency of psychiatric disorders in children with chronic idiopathic urticaria. Br J Dermatol 164(6):1342–1347, 2011 21083542

Hogan SR, Mandrell J, Eilers D: Adrenergic urticaria: review of the literature and proposed mechanism. J Am Acad Dermatol 70(4):763–766, 2014 24373776

Hoss D, Segal S: Scalp dysesthesia. Arch Dermatol 134(3):327–330, 1998 9521031

Howlett S: Emotional dysfunction, child-family relationships and childhood atopic dermatitis. Br J Dermatol 140(3):381–384, 1999 10233254

Huang YC, Cheng YC: Isotretinoin treatment for acne and risk of depression: a systematic review and meta-analysis. J Am Acad Dermatol 76(6):1068.e9–1076.e9, 2017 28291553

Hundley JL, Yosipovitch G: Mirtazapine for reducing nocturnal itch in patients with chronic pruritus: a pilot study. J Am Acad Dermatol 50(6):889–891, 2004 15153889

Hung SI, Chung WH, Liu ZS, et al: Common risk allele in aromatic antiepileptic-drug induced Stevens-Johnson syndrome and toxic epidermal necrolysis in Han Chinese. Pharmacogenomics 11(3):349–356, 2010 20235791

Hunter HJ, Griffiths CE, Kleyn CE: Does psychosocial stress play a role in the exacerbation of psoriasis? Br J Dermatol 169(5):965–974, 2013 23796214

Husain Z, Reddy BY, Schwartz RA: DRESS syndrome, part I: clinical perspectives. J Am Acad Dermatol 68(5):693.e1–693.e14; quiz 706–708, 2013 23602182

Ipser JC, Sander C, Stein DJ: Pharmacotherapy and psychotherapy for body dysmorphic disorder. Cochrane Database Syst Rev (1):CD005332, 2009 19160252

Ivanov OL, Lvov AN, Michenko AV, et al: Autoerythrocyte sensitization syndrome (Gardner-Diamond syndrome): review of the literature. J Eur Acad Dermatol Venereol 23(5):499–504, 2009 19192020

Janowski K, Pietrzak A: Indications for psychological intervention in patients with psoriasis. Dermatol Ther (Heidelb) 21(5):409–411, 2008 18844719

Kabat-Zinn J, Wheeler E, Light T, et al: Influence of a mindfulness meditation-based stress reduction intervention on rates of skin clearing in patients with moderate to severe psoriasis undergoing phototherapy (UVB) and photochemotherapy (PUVA). Psychosom Med 60(5):625–632, 1998 9773769

Kang KPA, Nedorost ST, Nedorost ST, et al: Atopic dermatitis, in Dermatology, 2nd Edition, Vol 1. Edited by Rapini RP, Jorizzo JL, Bolognia JL. London, Mosby Elsevier, 2008, pp 181–195

Kasperska-Zajac A, Brzoza Z, Rogala B: Lower serum dehydroepiandrosterone sulphate concentration in chronic idiopathic urticaria: a secondary transient phenomenon? Br J Dermatol 159(3):743–744, 2008 18616787

Kelsay K: Management of sleep disturbance associated with atopic dermatitis. J Allergy Clin Immunol 118(1):198–201, 2006 16815155

Kestenbaum T: Obsessive-compulsive disorder in dermatology. Semin Cutan Med Surg 32(2):83–87, 2013 24049965

Kimata H: Prevalence of suicidal ideation in patients with atopic dermatitis. Suicide Life Threat Behav 36(1):120–124, 2006 16676633

Kimsey LS: Delusional infestation and chronic pruritus: a review. Acta Derm Venereol 96(3):298–302, 2016 26337109

Kuhn H, Mennella C, Magid M, et al: Psychocutaneous disease: clinical perspectives. J Am Acad Dermatol 76(5):779–791, 2017a 28411771

Kuhn H, Mennella C, Magid M, et al: Psychocutaneous disease: pharmacotherapy and psychotherapy. J Am Acad Dermatol 76(5):795–808, 2017b 28411772

Lamer V, Lipozenčić J, Turčić P: Adverse cutaneous reactions to psychopharmaceuticals. Acta Dermatovenerol Croat 18(1):56–67, 2010 20361889

Lavda AC, Webb TL, Thompson AR: A meta-analysis of the effectiveness of psychological interventions for adults with skin conditions. Br J Dermatol 167(5):970–979, 2012 22924999

Lee CS: Delusions of parasitosis. Dermatol Ther (Heidelb) 21(1):2–7, 2008 18318879

Lee S, Shin A: Association of atopic dermatitis with depressive symptoms and suicidal behaviors among adolescents in Korea: the 2013 Korean Youth Risk Behavior Survey. BMC Psychiatry 17(1):3, 2017 28049449

Leombruni P, Gastaldi F: Oxcarbazepine for the treatment of trichotillomania. Clin Neuropharmacol 33(2):107–108, 2010 20375658

Lepping P, Huber M, Freudenmann RW: How to approach delusional infestation. BMJ 350:h1328, 2015 25832416

Levenson JL, Sharma AA, Ortega-Loayza AG: Somatic symptom disorder in dermatology. Clin Dermatol 35(3):246–251, 2017 28511820

Lewinson RT, Vallerand IA, Lowerison MW, et al: Depression is associated with an increased risk of psoriatic arthritis among patients with psoriasis: a population-based study. J Invest Dermatol 137(4):828–835, 2017 28237512

Litt JZ: Litt's Drug Eruptions and Reactions Manual: D.E.R.M., 19th Edition. Boca Raton, FL, CRC Press, 2013

Lochner C, Simeon D, Niehaus DJ, et al: Trichotillomania and skin-picking: a phenomenological comparison. Depress Anxiety 15(2):83–86, 2002 11891999

Lochner C, Seedat S, Hemmings SM, et al: Dissociative experiences in obsessive-compulsive disorder and trichotillomania: clinical and genetic findings. Compr Psychiatry 45(5):384–391, 2004 15332202

Lochner C, Seedat S, Niehaus DJ, et al: Topiramate in the treatment of trichotillomania: an open-label pilot study. Int Clin Psychopharmacol 21(5):255–259, 2006 16877895

Luis Blay S: Depression and psoriasis comorbidity. Treatment with paroxetine: two case reports. Ann Clin Psychiatry 18(4):271–272, 2006 17162628

Magin P, Adams J, Heading G, et al: Experiences of appearance-related teasing and bullying in skin diseases and their psychological sequelae: results of a qualitative study. Scand J Caring Sci 22(3):430–436, 2008 18840226

Mahtani R, Parekh N, Mangat I, et al: Alleviating the itch-scratch cycle in atopic dermatitis. Psychosomatics 46(4):373–374, 2005 16000683

Matsuda KM, Sharma D, Schonfeld AR, et al: Gabapentin and pregabalin for the treatment of chronic pruritus. J Am Acad Dermatol 75(3):619.e6–625.e6, 2016 27206757

McMillan R, Forssell H, Buchanan JA, et al: Interventions for treating burning mouth syndrome. Cochrane Database Syst Rev (11):CD002779, 2016 27855478

Medansky RS, Handler RM: Dermatopsychosomatics: classification, physiology, and therapeutic approaches. J Am Acad Dermatol 5(2):125–136, 1981 7021610

Modell JG, Boyce S, Taylor E, et al: Treatment of atopic dermatitis and psoriasis vulgaris with bupropion-SR: a pilot study. Psychosom Med 64(5):835–840, 2002 12271115

Morgan CA3rd, Southwick S, Hazlett G, et al: Relationships among plasma dehydroepiandrosterone sulfate and cortisol levels, symptoms of dissociation, and objective performance in humans exposed to acute stress. Arch Gen Psychiatry 61(8):819–825, 2004 15289280

Morgan JF, Lacey JH: Scratching and fasting: a study of pruritus and anorexia nervosa. Br J Dermatol 140(3):453–456, 1999 10233265

Mothi M, Sampson S: Pimozide for schizophrenia or related psychoses. Cochrane Database Syst Rev (11):CD001949, 2013 24194433

Moussavian H: Improvement of acne in depressed patients treated with paroxetine. J Am Acad Child Adolesc Psychiatry 40(5):505–506, 2001 11349692

Murphy C, Redenius R, O'Neill E, et al: Sleep-isolated trichotillomania: a survey of dermatologists. J Clin Sleep Med 3(7):719–721, 2007 18198806

Nightingale SL: From the Food and Drug Administration. JAMA 279(13):984, 1998 9533484

Ninan PT, Rothbaum BO, Marsteller FA, et al: A placebo-controlled trial of cognitive-behavioral therapy and clomipramine in trichotillomania. J Clin Psychiatry 61(1):47–50, 2000 10695646

Oaklander AL, Siegel SM: Cutaneous innervation: form and function. J Am Acad Dermatol 53(6):1027–1037, 2005 16310064

Ozkan M, Oflaz SB, Kocaman N, et al: Psychiatric morbidity and quality of life in patients with chronic idiopathic urticaria. Ann Allergy Asthma Immunol 99(1):29–33, 2007 17650826

Patel N, Nadkarni A, Cardwell LA, et al: Psoriasis, depression, and inflammatory overlap: a review. Am J Clin Dermatol 18(5):613–620, 2017 28432649

Peters EM: Stressed skin?—a molecular psychosomatic update on stress-causes and effects in dermatologic diseases. J Dtsch Dermatol Ges 14(3):233–252; quiz 253, 2016 26972185

Petit A, Karila L, Chalmin F, et al: Phenomenology and psychopathology of excessive indoor tanning. Int J Dermatol 53(6):664–672, 2014 24601904

Phillips KA: Placebo-controlled study of pimozide augmentation of fluoxetine in body dysmorphic disorder. Am J Psychiatry 162(2):377–379, 2005 15677604

Physicians' Desk Reference, 70th Edition. Montvale, NJ, Thomas Healthcare, 2016

Piaserico S, Marinello E, Dessi A, et al: Efficacy of biofeedback and cognitive-behavioural therapy in psoriatic patients: a single-blind, randomized, and controlled study with added narrow-band ultraviolet B therapy. Acta Derm Venereol 96(217):91–95, 2016 27283367

Picardi A, Mazzotti E, Pasquini P: Prevalence and correlates of suicidal ideation among patients with skin disease. J Am Acad Dermatol 54(3):420–426, 2006 16488292

Pongcharoen P, Fleischer AB Jr: An evidence-based review of systemic treatments for itch. Eur J Pain 20(1):24–31, 2016 26416344

Poon E, Seed PT, Greaves MW, et al: The extent and nature of disability in different urticarial conditions. Br J Dermatol 140(4):667–671, 1999 10233318

Purvis D, Robinson E, Merry S, et al: Acne, anxiety, depression and suicide in teenagers: a cross-sectional survey of New Zealand secondary school students. J Paediatr Child Health 42(12):793–796, 2006 17096715

Rao KS, Menon PK, Hilman BC, et al: Duration of the suppressive effect of tricyclic antidepressants on histamine-induced wheal-and-flare reactions in human skin. J Allergy Clin Immunol 82(5 Pt 1):752–757, 1988 2903876

Ratnoff OD: The psychogenic purpuras: a review of autoerythrocyte sensitization, autosensitization to DNA, "hysterical" and factitial bleeding, and the religious stigmata. Semin Hematol 17(3):192–213, 1980 7006087

Ratnoff OD: Psychogenic purpura (autoerythrocyte sensitization): an unsolved dilemma. Am J Med 87(3N):16N–21N, 1989 2486528

Reiss F: Psoriasis and stress. Dermatologica 113(2):71–78, 1956 13365323

Richards HL, Ray DW, Kirby B, et al: Response of the hypothalamic-pituitary-adrenal axis to psychological stress in patients with psoriasis. Br J Dermatol 153(6):1114–1120, 2005 16307645

Roberts S, O'Connor K, Bélanger C: Emotion regulation and other psychological models for body-focused repetitive behaviors. Clin Psychol Rev 33(6):745–762, 2013 23792470

Rothbart R, Amos T, Siegfried N, et al: Pharmacotherapy for trichotillomania. Cochrane Database Syst Rev (11):CD007662, 2013 24214100

Rudzki E, Borkowski W, Czubalski K: The suggestive effect of placebo on the intensity of chronic urticaria. Acta Allergol 25(1):70–73, 1970 5468243

Ryan C, Sadlier M, De Vol E, et al: Genital psoriasis is associated with significant impairment in quality of life and sexual functioning. J Am Acad Dermatol 72(6):978–983, 2015 25824273

Savin JA, Paterson WD, Adam K, et al: Effects of trimeprazine and trimipramine on nocturnal scratching in patients with atopic eczema. Arch Dermatol 115(3):313–315, 1979 373632

Schmitt J, Romanos M, Schmitt NM, et al: Atopic eczema and attention-deficit/hyperactivity disorder in a population-based sample of children and adolescents. JAMA 301(7):724–726, 2009 19224748

Schrom K, Nagy T, Mostow E: Depression screening using health questionnaires in patients receiving oral isotretinoin for acne vulgaris. J Am Acad Dermatol 75(1):237–239, 2016 27317530

Schumer MC, Bartley CA, Bloch MH: Systematic Review of Pharmacological and Behavioral Treatments for Skin Picking Disorder. J Clin Psychopharmacol 36(2):147–152, 2016 26872117

Schut C, Mollanazar NK, Kupfer J, et al: Psychological interventions in the treatment of chronic itch. Acta Derm Venereol 96(2):157–161, 2016 26073701

Seiffert K, Hilbert E, Schaechinger H, et al: Psychophysiological reactivity under mental stress in atopic dermatitis. Dermatology 210(4):286–293, 2005 15942214

Selles RR, McGuire JF, Small BJ, et al: A systematic review and meta-analysis of psychiatric treatments for excoriation (skin-picking) disorder. Gen Hosp Psychiatry 41:29–37, 2016 27143352

Senra MS, Wollenberg A: Psychodermatological aspects of atopic dermatitis. Br J Dermatol 170 (suppl 1):38–43, 2014 24930567

Shanon J: A dermatologic and psychiatric study of perphenazine (trilafon) in dermatology. AMA Arch Derm 77(1):119–120, 1958 13486946

Shaw RJ, Dayal S, Good J, et al: Psychiatric medications for the treatment of pruritus. Psychosom Med 69(9):970–978, 2007 17991825

Shenefelt PD: Hypnosis in dermatology. Arch Dermatol 136(3):393–399, 2000 10724204

Shenefelt PD: Biofeedback, cognitive-behavioral methods, and hypnosis in dermatology: is it all in your mind? Dermatol Ther (Heidelb) 16(2):114–122, 2003 12919113

Shertzer CL, Lookingbill DP: Effects of relaxation therapy and hypnotizability in chronic urticaria. Arch Dermatol 123(7):913–916, 1987 3300566

Simpson EL, Bieber T, Eckert L, et al: Patient burden of moderate to severe atopic dermatitis (AD): insights from a phase 2b clinical trial of dupilumab in adults. J Am Acad Dermatol 74(3):491–498, 2016 26777100

Slominski AT, Zmijewski MA, Zbytek B, et al: Key role of CRF in the skin stress response system. Endocr Rev 34(6):827–884, 2013 23939821

Ständer S, Böckenholt B, Schürmeyer-Horst F, et al: Treatment of chronic pruritus with the selective serotonin re-uptake inhibitors paroxetine and fluvoxamine: results of an open-labelled, two-arm proof-of-concept study. Acta Derm Venereol 89(1):45–51, 2009 19197541

Staubach P, Eckhardt-Henn A, Dechene M, et al: Quality of life in patients with chronic urticaria is differentially impaired and determined by psychiatric comorbidity. Br J Dermatol 154(2):294–298, 2006 16433799

Strumia R: Eating disorders and the skin. Clin Dermatol 31(1):80–85, 2013 23245978

Suárez AL, Feramisco JD, Koo J, et al: Psychoneuroimmunology of psychological stress and atopic dermatitis: pathophysiologic and therapeutic updates. Acta Derm Venereol 92(1):7–15, 2012 22101513

Sundström A, Alfredsson L, Sjölin-Forsberg G, et al: Association of suicide attempts with acne and treatment with isotretinoin: retrospective Swedish cohort study. BMJ 341:c5812, 2010 21071484

Swedo SE, Leonard HL, Rapoport JL, et al: A double-blind comparison of clomipramine and desipramine in the treatment of trichotillomania (hair pulling). N Engl J Med 321(8):497–501, 1989 2761586

Takeshita J, Grewal S, Langan SM, et al: Psoriasis and comorbid diseases: implications for management. J Am Acad Dermatol 76(3):393–403, 2017 28212760

Tausk F, Whitmore SE: A pilot study of hypnosis in the treatment of patients with psoriasis. Psychother Psychosom 68(4):221–225, 1999 10396014

Thornsberry LA, English JC 3rd: Scalp dysesthesia related to cervical spine disease. JAMA Dermatol 149(2):200–203, 2013 23565509

Thorslund K, Svensson T, Nordlind K, et al: Use of serotonin reuptake inhibitors in patients with psoriasis is associated with a decreased need for systemic psoriasis treatment: a population-based cohort study. J Intern Med 274(3):281–287, 2013 23711088

Tran BW, Papoiu AD, Russoniello CV, et al: Effect of itch, scratching and mental stress on autonomic nervous system function in atopic dermatitis. Acta Derm Venereol 90(4):354–361, 2010 20574599

Uguz F, Engin B, Yilmaz E: Axis I and Axis II diagnoses in patients with chronic idiopathic urticaria. J Psychosom Res 64(2):225–229, 2008 18222137

U.S. Food and Drug Administration: Information for healthcare professionals: dangerous or even fatal skin reactions—carbamazepine (marketed as Carbatrol, Equetro, Tegretol, and generics). December 2007. Available at: https://www.fda.gov/drugs/drugsafety/postmarketdrugsafetyinformationforpatientsandproviders/ucm124718.htm. Accessed June 9, 2017.

Vadas P, Sinilaite A, Chaim M: Cholinergic urticaria with anaphylaxis: an underrecognized clinical entity. J Allergy Clin Immunol Pract 4(2):284–291, 2016 26619922

Van Ameringen M, Mancini C, Patterson B, et al: A randomized, double-blind, placebo-controlled trial of olanzapine in the treatment of trichotillomania. J Clin Psychiatry 71(10):1336–1343, 2010 20441724

Van de Kerkhof PCM: Psoriasis, in Dermatology, 2nd Edition, Vol 1. Edited by Rapini RP, Jorizzo JL, Bolognia JL. London, Mosby Elsevier, 2008, pp 115–135

Varghese R, Rajappa M, Chandrashekar L, et al: Association among stress, hypocortisolism, systemic inflammation, and disease severity in chronic urticaria. Ann Allergy Asthma Immunol 116(4):344.e1–348.e1, 2016 26905640

Verhoeven EW, Kraaimaat FW, de Jong EM, et al: Individual differences in the effect of daily stressors on psoriasis: a prospective study. Br J Dermatol 161(2):295–299, 2009 19438455

Weisshaar E, Szepietowski JC, Darsow U, et al: European guideline on chronic pruritus. Acta Derm Venereol 92(5):563–581, 2012 22790094

Wen L, Jiang G, Zhang X, et al: Relationship between acne and psychological burden evaluated by ASLEC and HADS surveys in high school and college students from central China. Cell Biochem Biophys 71(2):1083–1088, 2015 25331674

Yang HY, Sun CC, Wu YC, et al: Stress, insomnia, and chronic idiopathic urticaria—a case-control study. J Formos Med Assoc 104(4):254–263, 2005 15909063

Yasharpour MR, Randhawa I: Antidepressants in chronic idiopathic urticaria. Allergy Asthma Proc 32(6):419–424, 2011 22221435

Yosipovitch G, Samuel LS: Neuropathic and psychogenic itch. Dermatol Ther (Heidelb) 21(1):32–41, 2008 18318883

Yosipovitch G, Ansari N, Goon A, et al: Clinical characteristics of pruritus in chronic idiopathic urticaria. Br J Dermatol 147(1):32–36, 2002 12100181

Zachariae R, Oster H, Bjerring P, et al: Effects of psychologic intervention on psoriasis: a preliminary report. J Am Acad Dermatol 34(6):1008–1015, 1996 8647966

Zaenglein AL: Acne vulgaris, in Dermatology, 2nd Edition, Vol 1. Edited by Rapini RP, Jorizzo JL, Bolognia JL. London, Mosby Elsevier, 2008, pp 495–508

Zylicz Z, Krajnik M, Sorge AA, et al: Paroxetine in the treatment of severe non-dermatological pruritus: a randomized, controlled trial. J Pain Symptom Manage 26(6):1105–1112, 2003 14654262

Surgery

Sanjeev Sockalingam, M.D.

Raed Hawa, M.D.

Surgery can elicit a range of psychosocial issues, from psychological distress and difficulty coping to new-onset or deteriorating psychiatric illness. A preexisting history of psychiatric illness may be exacerbated by surgery or postoperative stressors or complications. The prevalence of psychiatric illness in surgical patients has been estimated to be as high as 50% (Strain 1982) and may be even higher in specific surgical settings, such as trauma, burn, and intensive care units. The rising numbers of elderly patients further increase the risk of postoperative psychiatric sequelae, including delirium.

Despite these high rates of psychiatric illness, surgeons historically were less likely than other physicians to refer patients to psychiatrists. A large Spanish study of 3,608 consecutive patient referrals to the consultation-liaison (C-L) service of five hospitals showed a lower rate of referral by surgery services (7.3%) compared with internal medicine (17.5%) (Valdés et al. 2000). More recent studies of referrals from surgery to inpatient C-L psychiatry services in North America report higher referral rates of 18%–41% (Kishi et al. 2004; Sockalingam et al. 2016).

Inpatient psychiatric consultations may consist of requests related to fear of surgery or anesthesia, capacity or readiness assessments for surgical interventions, and management of preexisting psychiatric illness. Specific patient populations may be treated in specialized units, such as burn or transplant, that have established liaison services to support patient care perioperatively. As integrated care models are expanded to surgical populations, psychiatrists may be involved in caring for surgical patients in ambulatory settings focusing on long-term rehabilitation and functioning.

This chapter is an update and revision of Powers PS, Santana CA: "Surgery," in *The American Psychiatric Publishing Textbook of Psychosomatic Medicine: Psychiatric Care of the Medically Ill*, Second Edition. Edited by Levenson JL. Arlington, VA, American Psychiatric Publishing, 2011, pp. 691–724.

Types of Surgical Consultation-Liaison Models

Inpatient Surgical Consultation

Inpatient psychiatric consultations for surgical units can either be part of a general C-L service or a specialized integrated liaison model. Examples of specialized liaison services include burn, trauma, and transplant programs. These dedicated services offer an opportunity for integration of psychiatrists within team meetings or rounds and foster interprofessional relationships that can improve team communication. This model can help to reduce the time needed for the psychiatrist to provide consultation, identify appropriate team members for patient care needs, and increase psychiatrists' understanding of team roles.

In contrast, general C-L services provide care to a broad range of surgical patients and teams. Surgeon consultees may spend a significant part of their time in the operating room, which can limit the psychiatric consultant's ability to communicate with them. Therefore, C-L psychiatrists will need to identify mechanisms to enhance communication, which may occur through liaison with the interprofessional team to support implementation of psychiatric recommendations.

Outpatient Consultation–Liaison Services

Within outpatient settings, psychiatrists may fulfill integral roles within specialized services. For example, presurgical psychiatric assessments focusing on transplant or bariatric surgery readiness can make use of specific standardized psychosocial assessment tools to improve prediction of postsurgery outcomes (Maldonado et al. 2015; Thiara et al. 2016). Presurgery psychiatric assessments may be used to identify patients with poorly controlled psychopathology, anticipate and address pre- and postoperative psychosocial challenges, facilitate longitudinal engagement with mental health care providers/services, and help manage risk and liability (Sogg and Friedman 2015). Given these challenges and potential roles, psychiatrists involved in care for these specialized surgical populations must have sufficient knowledge of the unique risks and benefits of the proposed surgery.

With U.S. outpatient surgeries on the rise, patients commonly arrive a few hours before an operation and leave a few hours afterward, a change that has complicated early identification of perisurgical psychiatric issues and follow-up care. The growth of outpatient surgery programs warrants a reconceptualization of how C-L psychiatric services are designed and implemented.

Staff Coping Mechanisms

Given the traumatic context of some surgeries, it is not surprising that surgeons, nurses, and other team members have powerful emotional responses. A qualitative study of surgeons' reactions to surgical complications showed that complications affect almost all surgeons at an emotional level, and that for some, the effects can be long-lasting (Pinto et al. 2013). This emotional distress may extend to the interprofessional team and add to provider burnout. Psychiatrists may be able to assist their colleagues in processing emotional distress related to disturbing surgical scenarios, thereby potentially mitigating team burnout.

Surgeons can also experience distress after an intraoperative death (Taylor et al. 2008) or when palliative surgical care is required. Awareness of such distress is especially important given that nearly two-thirds of surgeons will experience an intraoperative death during the course of their career (Taylor et al. 2013). Effective use of interpersonal and communication skills has been identified as a core competency in surgical practice, and psychiatrists may assist in building surgical residents' communication skills after catastrophic events (Bradley and Brasel 2007; Taylor et al. 2013).

Perioperative Psychiatric Issues

Psychiatric concerns may emerge during the perioperative period, which can be divided into preoperative, intraoperative, and postoperative phases. During the preoperative period, psychiatric consultations often relate to assessment of patient readiness for surgery and identification of psychosocial factors that may affect postsurgery outcomes.

During the perioperative period, psychiatrists are often consulted to assess the capacity of patients who refuse treatment or surgery or whose ability to provide consent is impaired. Moreover, patients who threaten to leave the hospital against medical advice (AMA) can also precipitate a psychiatry referral, with the goal of determining whether the patient has sufficient decisional capacity and whether his or her decision making is affected by psychiatric illness.

Patients may also have specific fears about surgery, anesthesia, needles, or machines, which can result in panic or anxiety attacks and necessitate urgent psychiatric intervention. The emergence of outpatient surgery procedures and use of agents that induce a lighter level of anesthesia have resulted in more patients reporting intraoperative awareness and recollection of perioperative events.

During the postoperative period, the emergence of psychiatric conditions, such as delirium or acute stress disorder (ASD), or an evolving major depressive disorder can limit a patient's ability to participate in rehabilitation and recovery. Psychiatrists can improve outcomes through early identification and modification of specific risk factors and prompt initiation of pharmacotherapy after surgery.

General Preoperative Issues

Capacity and Consent

Informed consent is a mandatory requirement prior to surgery. The frequency of referrals to C-L psychiatrists for capacity assessments has varied from 3% to 29% of total referrals (Appelbaum 2007; Ormont et al. 1997; Sockalingam et al. 2016).

As part of the consent process, patients are provided with information about the surgical procedure, including risks, benefits, and alternatives, to support patients' ability to make an autonomous, informed decision about surgery. C-L psychiatrists may be asked to assess capacity in outpatient presurgery clinics or during inpatient surgical hospitalizations. Specific questions regarding capacity and consent may arise following treatment refusal or when psychiatric illness is suspected to be complicating the decision-making process. The topic of patients who lack capacity is discussed in Chapter 2, "Legal and Ethical Issues."

Preoperative Psychiatric Evaluation

The preoperative period is the ideal time to obtain a psychiatric history. Patients with a history of psychiatric illness may be at risk of illness exacerbation after surgery. Therefore, presurgery assessment of psychiatric symptoms is essential for establishing patients' emotional and behavioral stability and informing psychiatric interventions to mitigate these potential risks. Psychiatrists should anticipate potential absorption issues, NPO (*nil per os*—nothing by mouth) periods, drug–drug interactions, and adverse psychotropic effects prior to surgery. Postoperative treatment plans should be communicated to the surgical team before surgery.

Preoperative psychiatric assessments may be unexpected by surgical patients, who are focused on preparing for their surgical procedure. For this reason, collaborative models in which psychosocial assessment is considered routine are ideal for normalizing psychiatric assessment and emphasizing a team-based approach to care.

Underreferral of surgical patients for psychiatric assessment is a product of underrecognition of psychiatric burden and psychological distress in surgical patients. However, there is increasing attention to psychological distress, specifically anxiety and depression, being paid by surgical and anesthesia teams (Perks et al. 2009). By contrast, some patients are inappropriately or prematurely referred for psychiatric assessment when they express normal emotions, such as crying, which can be uncomfortable for some surgeons. Such referrals may represent a lack of training in or comfort with managing patient emotions, providing an opportunity for psychiatrists to explore and educate.

Psychiatric Disorders in the Perioperative Period

Psychiatric disorders have been linked to impaired quality of life (QoL), worse surgical outcomes, and higher mortality in surgical patients. A study of 183 consecutive patients undergoing general surgery found that patients with active mental illness (mainly posttraumatic stress disorder [PTSD], depression, anxiety, or substance abuse) had higher rates of readmission and emergency room visits than patients with no active mental illness (Lee et al. 2016). Treatment of psychiatric illness can potentially reduce the impact of comorbidity on surgical outcomes.

Depression

Depression has been associated with worse outcomes after a variety of operations. In a prospective study of 309 coronary artery bypass graft (CABG) patients, patients with major depressive disorder had an increased risk of recurrent cardiac events 12 months after surgery (Connerney et al. 2001). Depression has also been associated with worse outcomes after other procedures, including increased mortality after kidney transplant (Novak et al. 2010), increased cardiovascular events following vascular surgery for peripheral artery disease (Cherr et al. 2007), and complicated recovery after colorectal surgery (Balentine et al. 2011).

Approximately 16% of individuals who undergo surgery are taking antidepressants (Scher and Anwar 1999). Preoperative executive dysfunction and depressive symptoms are predictive of postoperative delirium among noncardiac surgical patients (Smith et al. 2009). The decision of whether to continue or discontinue antidepressant medications prior to surgery requires consideration of the length of time the patient will be on NPO status, changes in medication absorption, risk of causing complications postsurgery (e.g., ileus), and risk of depressive relapse. For example, studies have shown that most patients who undergo Roux-en-Y gastric bypass surgery experience significant reductions both in the amount of drug absorbed and in the time window during which absorption occurs for up to 1 year postsurgery (Roerig and Steffen 2015).

In the past, monoamine oxidase inhibitors (MAOIs) were commonly discontinued prior to surgery because of concerns about hemodynamic instability and interactions with anesthesia. However, the use of specific anesthetic techniques has limited these risks. Moreover, a retrospective observational cohort study from eight Dutch hospitals did not find any significant differences among tranylcypromine users, moclobemide (reversible MAOI) users, and a group of non–antidepressant users in terms of adverse hemodynamic intraoperative events such as hypertension, bradycardia, and tachycardia (van Haelst et al. 2012).

Serotonergic antidepressants may also increase the risk of perioperative bleeding and increase the need for blood transfusions, although the data are mixed and based on observational or retrospective studies (Mahdanian et al. 2014). However, a large cohort study of 132,686 patients who underwent CABG did not find an increased risk of bleeding postsurgery in patients exposed to selective serotonin reuptake inhibitors (SSRIs) compared with patients not exposed (Gagne et al. 2015). If bleeding risk is significantly elevated in a specific patient (e.g., if the patient has a coagulopathy) and an antidepressant is needed, it may be advisable to switch to an antidepressant with low serotonergic reuptake.

Schizophrenia

Patients with schizophrenia are less likely than persons in the general population to receive to receive standard care for medical issues that arise in the context of inpatient hospitalization. Retrospective data from the Veterans Health Administration (VHA) showed that patients with serious mental illness, including schizophrenia, were less likely to receive surgery compared with other patients (Copeland et al. 2015). There are many challenges in providing medical care to patients with schizophrenia. Acute psychotic symptoms may interfere with surgical care and frustrate surgical team members. Paranoid delusions may result in refusal of surgery. Thought disorder and impairment in executive functions can hinder treatment adherence and follow-up, evoking countertransference feelings in surgical team members.

Rates of surgical complications (i.e., 30-day postsurgical mortality) are higher in patients with schizophrenia relative to surgical patients without mental disorders and are especially elevated in patients with unstable psychotic illness (Liao et al. 2013). In comparison with healthy control subjects, patients with schizophrenia have been shown to have lower pain sensitivity, which can result in delayed diagnosis and treatment of conditions requiring surgical intervention and can complicate interpretation of postoperative pain (Engels et al. 2014).

Bipolar Disorder

The psychological and physiological stress associated with surgery may result in destabilization of bipolar disorder with relapse of depressive, mixed, or manic symptoms. Mania in the perioperative period can significantly disrupt the surgical team's ability to provide care, increasing the risk of life-threatening complications. Lithium levels may rise or fall perioperatively during periods of NPO status, intravenous saline administration, and other fluid/electrolyte shifts. For patients who are unable to take oral mood stabilizers for extended periods perioperatively, parenteral haloperidol or intravenous valproate may serve as a temporary alternative.

Preoperative Anxiety and Treatment

Preoperative anxiety, or *surgical fear,* refers to an emotional state resulting from anticipation of a threatening event by patients waiting for surgery. The incidence of preoperative anxiety ranges from 11% to 80% in adult patients and also varies among different surgical groups (Maranets and Kain 1999).

Preoperative anxiety may lead to various problems, such as difficulty accessing veins due to peripheral vasoconstriction, autonomic fluctuations (i.e., tachycardia, hypertension, elevated temperature, sweating), delayed jaw relaxation and coughing during induction of anesthesia, and increased anesthetic requirement.

Therefore, steps should be taken to reduce preoperative anxiety. There are both pharmacological and psychotherapeutic options for treating acute procedure anxiety. Sedative premedication is routinely used to reduce preoperative anxiety. Placebo-controlled clinical trials are lacking, and in their absence, selection among treatments for acute procedure anxiety should be guided by clinical experience and the practical circumstances of a patient's procedure.

Several medications have been used to alleviate presurgical anxiety, including diazepam with midazolam (Pekcan et al. 2005), diazepam alone (Levandovski et al. 2008), mirtazapine (Chen et al. 2008), gabapentin (Ménigaux et al. 2005), and clonidine (Caumo et al. 2009). Patients experiencing acute procedure anxiety who regularly use benzodiazepines or alcohol may require a higher-than-usual benzodiazepine dose to offset possible tolerance to these drugs. A substance use disorder is generally not considered a contraindication to one-time use of a benzodiazepine for acute procedure anxiety so long as the patient is not acutely intoxicated with another sedating substance at the time of the procedure and the patient is closely monitored for respiratory depression.

However, sedatives have their own side effects, which can be minimized by the use of nonpharmacological interventions. Information about surgery can reduce anxiety during the preoperative period. A systematic review (Ayyadhah Alanazi 2014) investigated the effectiveness of various preoperative educational interventions in reducing preoperative anxiety. Fourteen interventional trials (12 randomized controlled trials [RCTs] and two pre/post test trials), involving a total of 1,752 participants, were included. Four of these trials used an audiovisual intervention, two used a visual intervention, two used multimedia-supported education, one used a Web site intervention, two used verbal education coupled with informational leaflets, and one used information leaflets only. Of the 14 trials, 8 demonstrated significant reductions in preoperative anxiety from the preoperative education interventions. A Cochrane review (Bradt et al. 2013) of 26 trials and 2,051 participants concluded that music therapy may be beneficial for preoperative anxiety and may provide an alternative to medications.

Preoperative Fears of Anesthesia

Preoperative fears of anesthesia are common. The reasons for these fears have been explored in a number of studies, with no clear consensus, although fear of postoperative pain seems to be a common theme.

A study of preoperative anxiety among patients (N=193) awaiting elective surgery found that patients whose procedures would be performed under general anesthesia were more anxious than patients who would not be going under general anesthesia (Jawaid et al. 2007). The most common factors responsible for preoperative anxiety were concern about family (in 173 [89.6%] patients), fear of complications (in 168 [87%]), anxiety about results of the operation (in 159 [82.4%]), and fear of postoperative pain (in 152 [78.8%]). Only 74 (38.3%) patients were anxious because of possible awareness during surgery.

In a survey of 400 surgical patients during the preoperative anesthesiology visit, 81% reported experiencing preoperative anxiety (Mavridou et al. 2013). The main sources of anxiety were fear of postoperative pain (84%), fear of not waking up after surgery (64.8%), fear of being nauseous or vomiting (60.2%), and fear of drains and needles (59.5%). Women were more likely than men to report being afraid. Another study found that 88% of the presurgical sample (N=400) experienced preoperative fear (Ruhaiyem et al. 2016). The top three sources of patient fears were fear of postoperative pain (77.3%), fear of intraoperative awareness (73.7%), and fear of delayed recovery of consciousness after anesthesia (69.5%). Fewer patients reported fear of drains and needles in the operating room (48%), fear of revealing personal issues under general anesthesia (55.2%), and fear of not waking up after surgery (56.4%). Women (vs. men) and patients older than 40 years (vs. younger patients) were more likely to report fears.

Another prospective cross-sectional study in South India (Bheemanna et al. 2017), a survey of 150 patients scheduled for surgery under regional anesthesia, reported that the most common fears were of pain during surgery and of needles. A study by McCleane and Cooper (1990) of the most common preoperative fears surrounding surgery in patients preoperatively, and after their operation regarding the same fears if they required another operation, showed interesting findings. Postoperative pain (65% before operation, 50% after), not remaining asleep during the procedure (54%, 28%), a long wait for the operation (53%, 41%), sickness and vomiting (48%, 43%), appearing foolish (36%, 28%), not awakening from anesthesia (34%, 21%), and injections (34%, 27%) were the most common concerns. The persistently high percentage of patients who still had the same fears after they had been through surgery warrants concern and suggests the need for better interventions.

Children and Preoperative Anxiety

It is estimated that as many as 6 million children (including 1.5 million infants) undergo anesthesia and surgery annually in the United States, and that as many as 40%–60% experience significant anxiety before surgery. In a comparison of four different interventions for relieving preoperative anxiety in children, Kain et al. (2007) found that the ADVANCE method (a family-centered behavioral approach) was superior to parental presence during induction of anesthesia, oral midazolam, and a control condition (usual care). An evidence-based review (Chundamala et al. 2009) concluded that parental presence does not relieve anxiety in either the child or the parent, and suggested that premedication with midazolam may be helpful. Despite studies concluding that benzodiazepines (especially midazolam) may reduce anxiety, particularly among pediatric dental and oral surgery patients, a Cochrane review (Matharu and Ashley 2007) was unable to reach a definitive conclusion on which was the most effective drug or method of sedation for anxious children.

Many studies suggest that preoperative preparation programs can reduce anxiety and enhance coping in children. McCann and Kain (2001) offered a historical perspective on the evolution of preoperative preparation programs: from provision of an orientation tour and narrative information to development of modeling techniques that allow children to indirectly experience the perioperative course by role rehearsal using dolls or by viewing a video. Although coping preparation was associated with reductions of anxiety in the preoperative holding area, no differences were found among the various preparation programs during anesthesia induction, in the recovery room period, or postoperatively.

Fear of Needles, Blood, or Medical Equipment

Fear of needles is common in children and adults and exists on a continuum, with blood-injection-injury phobia at the severe end of the needle-fear spectrum. The lifetime prevalence of blood-injection-injury phobia is approximately 3%–4.5% (Bienvenu and Eaton 1998). The prevalence rises to 10%–21% when individuals who have a high degree of needle fear, but not a diagnosis of needle-related phobia, are included (Deacon and Abramowitz 2006; Nir et al. 2003). This fear can lead to a host of deleterious consequences, including vaccination noncompliance and avoidance of health care. A systematic review (McMurtry et al. 2015) of 11 RCTs and quasi-RCTs in children, adults, or both with high levels of needle fear found evidence of benefit from exposure-based psychological interventions and applied muscle tension in the reduction of needle fear.

Twin studies have shown a genetic component in unreasonable fears of blood, needles, hospitals, and illness (Neale et al. 1994). A review of treatments for blood-injury-injection phobia concluded that data on effective treatments are limited and that exposure techniques might result in the greatest improvements (Ayala et al. 2009). Some patients are fearful of contracting HIV or hepatitis virus from blood transfusions or contaminated needles; correcting misconceptions and providing accurate information can be helpful in alleviating their concerns.

Blood refusal is common and is usually related to religious beliefs or fear of blood-borne infection. Because Jehovah's Witnesses and others have refused blood transfusions, there has been a rigorous pursuit of alternatives. Many surgeries previously thought to require transfusions are now routinely done without them. A review by Hughes et al. (2008) concluded that increased morbidity and mortality is rarely observed in patients with a hemoglobin concentration greater than 7 g/dL, and the acute hemoglobin threshold for cardiovascular collapse may be as low as 3–6 g/dL. Intravascular volume expanders and acute hypervolemic hemodilution can be acceptable alternatives to blood transfusion.

Intraoperative Issues: Accidental Awareness During Anesthesia

Accidental awareness during anesthesia (AAA) refers to the experience (with or without later recall) of being partially conscious during general anesthesia, which can vary from just being able to hear to experiencing pain while immobilized. This experience can produce acute distress and long-lasting effects (e.g., nightmares, anxiety, depression, PTSD) (Davidson et al. 2011; Kent et al. 2013; Mashour 2010). In children, approximately 50% of AAA experiences are distressing; most last less than 5 minutes; and neuromuscular blockade combined with pain causes the most distress (Sury 2016). Most cases (approximately 70%) occur during anesthesia induction or emergence.

The estimated incidence of AAA with recall, as reported by anesthetists participating in the NAP5 Project (a national U.K. survey of intraoperative awareness during general anesthesia) was 1 in 19,000 general anesthetics. However, because of the voluntary nature of the reporting, this rate should be interpreted with caution (Pandit et al. 2014). According to the NAP5 Project, factors increasing the risk of AAA included female sex, younger adult age, obesity, anesthetist inexperience (junior trainees), previous AAA, emergencies, out-of-hours operating, type of surgery (cardiac, obstetric), and use of neuromuscular blocking agents. Acute and longer-term distress occurred across the full range of experiences but were particularly likely when the patient experienced paralysis (with or without pain).

Risk factors for intraoperative awareness, according to findings from epidemiological studies, have been classified by Nunes et al. (2012) into three main groups: 1) *patient-related* (females are more susceptible, as are children, the elderly, patients with a history of substance use, patients with an American Society of Anesthesiologists [ASA] classification of III ["patient with severe systemic disease"] or IV ["patient with severe systemic disease that is a constant threat to life"], and patients with difficult-to-intubate airways); 2) *procedure-related* (obstetric, cardiac, and trauma surgeries convey a higher incidence); and 3) *anesthetic technique–related.* Even though it is not possible to prevent all cases of intraoperative awareness (and it may be even more difficult as outpatient surgery becomes more common), preoperative preparation of the patient for the unlikely possibility of AAA may be helpful.

General Postoperative Issues

Substance Use Disorders

Substance use disorders are particularly common in surgical patients. Substance (especially alcohol) use is often a cause of trauma; individuals injured while under the influence of alcohol account for nearly half of all occupied trauma beds (Gentilello et al. 1995; Spies et al. 1996). Therefore, trauma patients should undergo screening during admission to reduce the potential for postoperative complications, to monitor and treat any withdrawal syndromes, and to refer individuals for substance use treatment postoperatively. Surgical patients with chronic alcoholism have a two to four

times greater rate of morbidity and mortality resulting from infections, cardiopulmonary insufficiency, and bleeding disorders (Spies and Rommelspacher 1999). A meta-
analysis of 55 studies examining the association between preoperative alcohol consumption and postoperative complications found that preexisting alcohol use con-
ferred an increased relative risk (RR) of general morbidity (RR=1.56), general infections (RR=1.73), wound complications (RR=1.23), pulmonary complications (RR=
1.80), prolonged hospital stays (RR=1.24), and admissions to intensive care units
(ICUs) (RR=2.68) (Eliasen et al. 2013). The associations between alcohol use and mortality and morbidity were strongest for thoracic surgery and head and neck surgery,
respectively. A longitudinal study of 27,399 patients discharged from trauma centers
between 1983 and 1995 found that patients with a blood alcohol concentration (BAC)
greater than zero at admission were nearly twice as likely to die from a subsequent
injury compared with patients with an admission BAC of zero (Dischinger et al.
2001). Mechanisms that may potentially explain these associations include alcohol-
induced reductions in immune function, leading to infections (Spies et al. 2004);
heightened endocrine stress response to surgery, worsening medical conditions (Tønnesen et al. 1992); and impaired coagulation from alcoholic liver disease, increasing
the risk of bleeding and impairing wound healing (Tønnesen and Kehlet 1999). Methods for screening medical–surgical patients for alcohol misuse and treatment of substance use disorders are discussed in Chapter 16, "Substance-Related Disorders."

Chronic alcohol use can also complicate perioperative anesthesia through alcohol's
effect of enhancing or reducing sensitivity to anesthetics, related to the amount of alcohol consumed, the affinity of alcohol versus other drugs for microsomal enzymes, and
the degree of liver injury and impairment (Lieber 1995). Furthermore, surgical procedures carry higher morbidity and mortality risks in patients with alcohol use disorder
complications such as cirrhosis, seizures, pancreatitis, or cardiomyopathy.

A history of opioid misuse, including receipt of agonist therapy with methadone
or buprenorphine, in surgical patients can pose additional challenges. Patients with
opioid-related disorders who are given "normal" doses of opioids often report insufficient pain relief and, as a result, are considered to be "drug seeking" when in reality
they are being undertreated. For a discussion of pain management in patients with
opioid-related disorders, see Chapter 16 and Chapter 34, "Pain").

Postoperative Delirium

Delirium is common after surgery, with higher rates in specific patient populations
and types of surgery. In a recent review of 34 studies involving a total of 7,738 patients, 21.5% of patients developed incident postoperative delirium, and the mortality
rate after surgery was 21% and 8.7% for delirious and nondelirious patients, respectively (Hamilton et al. 2017). However, when the review authors controlled for pre-
specified confounders, postoperative delirium was no longer associated with increased mortality after surgery. Studies in high-risk populations, such as hip surgery
patients, have reported a postoperative delirium incidence of 24% (Yang et al. 2017).
It is clear that delirium is highly prevalent in surgical populations, and the broader
delirium literature has documented increased morbidity and mortality from delirium
(see Chapter 4, "Delirium").

Because of advances in surgical interventions, such as laparoscopic and endovascular surgery, older patients and patients with more complex illnesses are now being considered for surgery, which can impact postoperative delirium risk.

Risk Factors and Preoperative Screening Strategies

Risk factors for postoperative delirium include patient variables and surgical variables. Presurgical patient risk factors include dementia, advanced age, cognitive impairment, sensory impairment, and depression (Greene et al. 2009; Inouye et al. 2015; Kazmierski et al. 2008). Four key patient characteristics at the time of hospital admission—visual impairment, severe medical illness, cognitive impairment, and dehydration—have been associated with delirium in medical and surgical patients. In a cohort of elderly patients scheduled for hip surgery, high-risk patients, defined as having three or four of these delirium risk factors, had a delirium incidence of 37.1%, compared with an incidence of 3.8% in patients without these risk factors (Kalisvaart et al. 2006). Surgical factors, such as surgeon expertise, surgical team functioning, type of anesthetic used, and type of surgery, may also influence the risk of delirium. Methods for screening and diagnosing delirium are reviewed in Chapter 4.

C-L psychiatrists are at times involved in the care of children postoperatively because of the frequent emergence of delirium. The risk of delirium is multifactorial; influencing factors include invasiveness of the procedure (Joo et al. 2014), severity of pain, and choice of anesthesia and premedication (Costi et al. 2014).

Prevention and Treatment of Postoperative Delirium

Several agents have been studied in the prevention of delirium, with most studies being conducted in surgical populations (see Chapter 4 for a full discussion). Early RCTs in surgical patients suggested that low-dose haloperidol could prevent postoperative delirium (Kaneko et al. 1999) or reduce its severity and duration (Kalisvaart et al. 2005). An RCT in cardiac surgery patients found that 1 mg risperidone given preoperatively reduced the incidence of postoperative delirium significantly (11.1% in the risperidone group vs. 31.7% in the placebo group) (Prakanrattana and Prapaitrakool 2007). Two more recent meta-analyses concluded that there is no clear evidence that administration of antipsychotic medications, cholinesterase inhibitors, or melatonin prior to surgery significantly reduces the incidence of delirium postoperatively (Neufeld et al. 2016; Tremblay and Gold 2016). However, a Cochrane review of 39 studies, including 32 studies from non-ICU surgical populations, suggested that atypical antipsychotics may have some effect in reducing the incidence of delirium (Siddiqi et al. 2016). This review included a single RCT of orthopedic patients who received a 5-mg dose of olanzapine before and after undergoing elective knee- or hip-replacement surgery (Larsen et al. 2010). In this trial, prophylactic olanzapine treatment reduced the incidence of delirium but also resulted in longer and more severe delirium for those patients who developed delirium.

Nonpharmacological approaches may also be helpful in preventing postoperative delirium. Multicomponent interventions consisting of individualized care, education, early mobilization, reorientation, and attention to sensory deprivation are known to reduce the incidence of delirium after surgery (Siddiqi et al. 2016). Moreover, the risk of postoperative delirium can be further reduced by use of team-based approaches to delirium care, consisting of collaboration between geriatric nurses and consultants (Gurlit and Möllmann 2008; Marcantonio et al. 2001).

In ICUs, dexmedetomidine may be a suitable alternative to antipsychotic medications to reduce the incidence and/or duration of postoperative delirium, especially for patients considered to be at high risk. In a study of patients undergoing elective cardiac surgery, patients randomly assigned to receive dexmedetomidine after surgery had a 3% incidence of delirium, which was significantly lower than the delirium incidence with midazolam (50%) or propofol (50%) (Maldonado et al. 2009). A meta-analysis of 16 RCTs ($N=1,994$ patients) comparing dexmedetomidine with other sedative agents (i.e., lorazepam, midazolam, or propofol) in ICU patients found significant reductions in ICU length of stay, mechanical ventilation duration, and delirium incidence in patients receiving dexmedetomidine (Constantin et al. 2016).

Posttraumatic Stress Disorder in the Postoperative Period

PTSD is highly prevalent in physical trauma patients (Klein et al. 2003) and is also a prevalent condition after cardiac surgery and neurosurgery (Powell et al. 2002; Schelling et al. 2003). Among patients receiving follow-up medical and surgical care after experiencing physical trauma, approximately 25% develop PTSD (Alarcon et al. 2012; Warren et al. 2014). Children who experience traumatic disfiguring injuries seem to be at particular risk, with up to 82% showing some symptoms of PTSD 1 month after the event (Rusch et al. 2002). Furthermore, QoL is significantly impaired in patients who develop PTSD after trauma or surgery compared with those who do not develop PTSD (Zatzick et al. 2002).

Several studies have tried to identify factors that predict the emergence of PTSD. As expected, better prior emotional adjustment and social support are relatively protective. Neither severity of the physical injury nor severity of the illness requiring surgery is clearly correlated with emergence of PTSD. The evidence for alcohol use as a predictive factor for PTSD after surgery is mixed. A systematic review of 44 studies examining predictors of PTSD after motor vehicle accidents identified the following risk factors: rumination about the trauma, perceived threat to life, lower social support, higher ASD symptom severity, persistent physical health issues, previous emotional problems, history of an anxiety disorder, and involvement of litigation/compensation (Heron-Delaney et al. 2013). Perhaps the best predictor of PTSD at 1 year is the presence of ASD symptoms during the acute ICU hospitalization (Davydow et al. 2013). Although most studies show that symptoms decrease over time, approximately 15% of patients are still experiencing PTSD symptoms 1 year after their ICU admission.

Additional risk factors for PTSD that have been explored include type of surgery and presence of hypothalamic-pituitary-adrenal (HPA) axis abnormalities. In a study examining pretreatment predictors of psychiatric morbidity (including depression, anxiety, and PTSD) in 216 patients with an abdominal aortic aneurysm or aortoiliac occlusive disease who were treated in surgical clinics, open surgeries (versus conservative medication management or endovascular repair) and elevated baseline cortisol levels were each associated with an increased risk of new-onset psychiatric symptoms posttreatment (King et al. 2015). Research investigating the role of corticosteroids in preventing PTSD in surgical populations (e.g., cardiac surgery patients) has shown potential benefit for these agent in reducing stress and PTSD symptoms;

however, the evidence is of moderate quality and warrants further study (Amos et al. 2014; Schelling et al. 2004).

Diagnosing ASD and PTSD can be difficult in surgical trauma or postoperative patients in the context of delirium and/or substance withdrawal. For the diagnosis of PTSD, the duration criterion is often not met in hospitalized individuals because of relatively short hospital stays. Following hospital discharge, PTSD symptoms may manifest in more subtle ways, such as avoidance of the hospital and outpatient visits, intense fears about future illness, preoccupation with somatic symptoms, preoccupation with memories of delusional experiences in the ICU, confusion about events in the ICU, social isolation related to fear of "germs," and reactivity to noises reminiscent of the ICU (e.g., beeping noises) (Jackson et al. 2016). Given the persistence of PTSD symptoms beyond the initial months after discharge from the hospital, early PTSD screening and intervention may have the potential to mitigate chronic PTSD after injury.

Few studies of PTSD treatment have specifically targeted surgical patients, but general principles appear applicable. Guidelines support the use of pharmacotherapy, specifically the use of SSRIs, as adjuncts to psychological interventions for PTSD (Bernardy and Friedman 2015). Cognitive-behavioral therapy (CBT) has been shown to be more effective than a wait-list control condition or supportive psychotherapy for PTSD among motor vehicle accident survivors (Blanchard et al. 2003). In children, there is general agreement (although not much evidence) that psychotherapy should be the primary treatment for trauma-related PTSD and that SSRIs should be adjunctive (Putnam and Hulsmann 2002). Patient diaries may also help reduce the incidence of PTSD after ICU admission, preventing psychological distress in both patients and family members (Garrouste-Orgeas et al. 2012; Jones et al. 2010).

Postoperative Pain

National survey data suggest that approximately 86% of patients experience pain after surgery and that 74% are still experiencing pain at the time of hospital discharge (Gan et al. 2014). Although it is imperative that patients receive timely and effective pain management after surgery to mitigate the long-term negative impacts of pain on recovery, QoL, and functioning, it is also important to avoid chronic opioid prescription. The American Pain Society outlined a multimodal approach to postoperative pain management in its 2016 guidelines (Chou et al. 2016). For further approaches to management of acute and chronic pain, see Chapter 34.

General Determinants of Functional Outcome

A critical component of surgical care is postsurgery functional outcomes, specifically the ability to perform activities of daily living and to function in one's presurgery role. In addition, many surgeries are proposed with the goal of eventual recovery and improved QoL. The actual severity and extent of the underlying trauma does not necessarily predict postsurgical quality of life. For example, the percentage of total body surface area burned does not correlate with the likelihood of subsequent PTSD. Postoperative functioning as measured by QoL is best predicted by presurgery QoL and psychological well-being across a range of surgery types (McKenzie et al. 2010; Wimmelmann et al. 2014). Therefore, presurgical assessment of mental health, social supports, and coping skills can assist in anticipating postsurgery recovery and functional outcomes.

Several factors over the course of surgery may influence functional outcomes, including the condition requiring surgical intervention and the nature of the surgery. Treatment factors that may help improve outcomes include preparation of the patient and family for surgery, screening for and management of preoperative fears, a respectful attitude on the part of surgeons and operating room personnel during surgery, appropriate treatment of pain, and management of various psychiatric problems following surgery, including delirium and PTSD.

Specific Topics in Surgery

Burn Trauma

According to the American Burn Association (2016), an estimated 486,000 people receive medical treatment for burns each year in the United States. In 2014, there were approximately 3,300 burn-related deaths, with 2,745 of these from residential fires. In 2015, there were 40,000 hospitalizations for burn injuries, which included 30,000 hospital admissions to 128 specialized burn centers (which are typically staffed by physicians, nurses, physical and occupational therapists, pain specialists, mental health professionals, social workers, and chaplains).

Psychiatric Disorders in Burn Patients

Psychiatric disorders are highly prevalent in burn patients, with substance use disorders and mood disorders among the most common. A study using American Burn Association–National Burn Registry (ABA-NBR) data reported that 12.3% of patients admitted to burn centers had psychiatric disorders (Thombs et al. 2007). Of these, alcohol abuse accounted for 5.8%, drug abuse for 3.3%, dementia for 0.3%, and other psychiatric disorders for 2.9%. The percentage of psychiatric disorders in this sample was substantially lower than that in other reports and likely represents an underestimate because of methodological limitations. A study of burn victims 1–4 years postinjury using a structured psychiatric interview found a prevalence rate of 39% for any psychiatric disorder, and noted that 57% of all postburn-onset psychiatric disorders appeared within the first year (Ter Smitten et al. 2011). In this study, postburn prevalence rates of mood disorders, anxiety disorders, and substance use disorders were 11%, 19%, and 10%, respectively.

Assessment of psychosocial outcomes in burned children is confounded by the fact that many children who are burned have preexisting psychiatric disorders and psychosocial problems that influence long-term outcomes. A study from the United Kingdom by James-Ellison et al. (2009) found that one-third of children younger than 3 years who sustained burns had been referred to social services by their sixth birthday, and 9.7% had been abused or neglected, compared with 1.4% of control subjects.

Psychiatric comorbidity has been associated with worse postburn outcomes. Thombs et al. (2007), after controlling for demographic and burn injury characteristics, found that preexisting alcohol abuse was a significant predictor of mortality in the burn unit, and that preexisting dementia, psychiatric diagnosis, alcohol abuse, and drug abuse were all significantly associated with an increased length of hospital stay. Many smaller studies from single burn centers have found that many patients have preexisting maladaptive coping mechanisms or dysfunctional families, and these factors are known to predispose to poorer functional outcomes.

In addition, scarring from burns may also contribute to poorer functioning, QoL, and self-esteem. The prevalence of postburn hypertrophic scarring ranges from 32% to 72% across studies (Lawrence et al. 2012). In general, severity of burn scarring is weakly correlated with body image, depression, and social comfort; however, these correlations are stronger for subjective burn severity ratings (e.g., patient-perceived severity) than for objective burn severity measures (e.g., total body surface area [TBSA] burned) (Lawrence et al. 2012). Psychosocial interventions addressing emotional distress related to burn scars—specifically, social skills training and application of a spray-on skin camouflage product—have not been shown to be more effective than control interventions (Blakeney et al. 2005; Martin et al. 2008). Based on evidence from other medical populations with body image disturbances, CBT may be beneficial, although its efficacy in patients with burn scars requires further study.

Several factors may contribute to patient recovery and rehabilitation after severe burns. Another group from England and Australia (Falder et al. 2009) identified seven core domains of outcome for adult burn survivors, four of which are particularly relevant to psychiatrists: 1) sensory and pain, 2) psychological function (PTSD and depression), 3) community participation (social integration), and 4) perceived QoL. In their extensive review, Falder et al. (2009) evaluated questionnaires and instruments that have been used to diagnose common psychiatric complications following burn injuries. Clinicians may consider using either clinician-administered instruments (e.g. Clinician-Administered PTSD Scale, Structured Clinical Interview for DSM) or self-report measures (e.g., Impact of Events Scale, Davidson Trauma Scale). The assessment of depression in the acute phase of burn treatment should focus on differentiating symptoms of depression from symptoms of delirium and physiological symptoms related to the burn injuries (Falder et al. 2009). In summary, a comprehensive and longitudinal assessment of common psychiatric complications is needed for early identification and management of these conditions to support patient recovery and rehabilitation postburn.

Burns and Substance Use Disorders

McKibben et al. (2009) reviewed rates of alcohol and substance use disorders in different samples of patients admitted to burn units. Alcohol misuse rates at admission varied from 32% to 41%, and drug misuse from 6% to 24%, with differences likely due to differences in nationality and methodology. One study (Jones et al. 1991) found that 27% of admitted patients had been intoxicated at the time of the burn, and 90% of these were then identified as having an alcohol abuse diagnosis, compared with 11% of the nonintoxicated burn patients. In a study of 67 consecutive burn patients who were assessed a mean of 4.6 years after burn injury, 25% reported at-risk drinking at follow-up (Sveen and Öster 2015).

Alcohol use has been found to be associated with several adverse outcomes related to burn injury. Alcohol use is related to increases in percentage of TBSA burned, mortality, hospital lengths of stay, and medical costs in burn injury patients (Jones et al. 1991; Powers et al. 1994). In a case–control study in which 14 burn patients with an admission BAC greater than 30 mg/dL were matched with 14 burn patients with an undetectable BAC according to age, sex, and percentage TBSA burned, patients with elevated BACs had longer durations of mechanical ventilation, longer lengths of stay in the ICU, and higher hospital charges compared with patients with undetectable BACs (Silver et al. 2008). Furthermore, studies suggest that alcohol intoxication before burn injury suppresses intestinal immune defense, impairs gut barrier functions, and increases bacterial growth, all of which may contribute to postburn injury infections (Choudhry and Chaudry 2008).

Even though burn patients have a high rate of preexisting drug abuse, they should receive sufficient doses of opioids for analgesia.

Self-Inflicted Burn Injuries

Self-immolation, the act of intentionally lighting oneself on fire or immersing oneself in flames, varies from nation to nation. Self-immolation as a method of suicide is less common in the United States and Europe, with rates ranging from 1% to 6% of all suicides in comparison with rates as high as 11% in developing countries (Peck 2012). The characteristics of individuals who self-immolate vary based on culture (for a review, see Peck 2012), with fewer gender differences in high-income countries. In low-income countries, individuals who self-immolate are more likely to be young women without a psychiatric disorder who are experiencing marital discord and/or family conflict (Ahmadi and Ytterstad 2007; Ahmadi et al. 2008, 2010). Political protest is a rare but dramatic motivation for self-immolation in low-income countries.

In the United States, most patients with self-inflicted severe burns have a preexisting psychiatric disorder, usually a psychotic disorder (Mulholland et al. 2008). In a retrospective review of all patients admitted to a Scottish regional burn unit over an 11-year period, 53 self-immolation patients were compared with 49 accidentally burned patients. The self-immolation patients were more likely to be unemployed, to live alone, and to have a previous psychiatric diagnosis. They also had more severe burns and longer hospital stays and were more likely to undergo surgery (Conlin et al. 2016).

Patients with self-inflicted burns often elicit intense reactions in staff members, including those in the psychiatric team. It is helpful to remember that most patients (at least in the United States) with self-inflicted burns have a chronic mental illness, and that appropriate psychiatric care may not have been available to or effective for these patients.

PTSD in Burn Patients

The reported prevalence of PTSD among burn patients varies across studies, with rates of 3.3%–35.1% in patients during burn hospitalization and rates up to 25% in patients 2 years after the burn injury (Giannoni-Pastor et al. 2016). Zatzick et al. (2007) found that more than 20% of trauma survivors had symptoms of PTSD 12 months after acute inpatient care. In a large prospective multisite cohort study of major burn injury survivors, psychological stress was common and tended to persist (Fauerbach et al. 2007). The diagnoses of ASD and PTSD in burn patients may be missed because of the confounding effects of delirium and mild traumatic brain injury, and as a result of patients being discharged from the hospital before the duration criterion of 1 month has been met. Nonetheless, many patients do develop the full syndrome of PTSD, and many more have subthreshold PTSD symptoms, predominantly in the reexperiencing symptom cluster (Low et al. 2006). Psychological trauma from extreme pain related to debridement and dressing changes can also elicit posttraumatic distress symptoms.

Several attempts have been made to identify factors predictive of PTSD development among burn patients. In a recent review, the strongest risk factors for development of PTSD after burn injury were perception of a life threat associated with the burn, acute intrusion symptoms, and greater pain severity (Giannoni-Pastor et al. 2016). Additional risk factors for PTSD after a burn injury were being of low socioeconomic status, being unmarried, having a history of mental illness, and experiencing symptoms of psychiatric illness (e.g., substance use disorders, anxiety, depression) during the recovery phase (Giannoni-Pastor et al. 2016). Furthermore, Gaylord et al. (2009) found that there was no difference in risk of PTSD between military personnel and civilians who suffered burn injuries; in this study, factors that predicted PTSD were percentage TBSA burned and Injury Severity Score (Baker et al. 1974).

Acute stress symptoms postburn are a risk factor for developing PTSD. A large prospective cohort study of survivors of major burn injuries found that a very high percentage of these patients (34%) experienced acute stress reactions—consisting of feelings of "alienation" and anxiety—while in the hospital, and that for a large proportion of patients, these symptoms persisted for at least 2 years postburn (Fauerbach et al. 2007). In another prospective study of 178 patients hospitalized for a burn injury (McKibben et al. 2008), the prevalence of in-hospital ASD was 23.6%, and 35.1%, 33.3%, 28.6%, and 25.4% of the patients had symptoms that met PTSD criteria at 1, 6, 12, and 24 months, respectively.

Although not well studied, treatment of PTSD in burn patients is likely to be similar to treatment of PTSD in other patients. Overall, the evidence for benefit from pharmacotherapy and psychotherapy in PTSD related to burns is very limited. In a small RCT involving children with burn injuries, sertraline was found to be safe and showed some benefit in parent-reported, but not child-reported, PTSD and depressive symptoms (Stoddard et al. 2011). Interventions that increase patients' sense of control and alleviate pain, especially during the acute phase of treatment in the burn center, may be helpful in reducing the incidence and severity of distress symptoms. However, superficial psychological interventions can increase emotional distress, as demonstrated in an RCT of a single session of psychological debriefing to prevent ASD in adult burn patients (Bisson et al. 1997).

Burn Pain Management

There are several procedures, including dressing changes and wound debridement, that can result in substantial pain in addition to the injury itself. Pain is often undertreated in burn units, and poorly controlled pain can precipitate or exacerbate delirium, anxiety, and depression. The bidirectional relationship between depression and pain can result in long-term functional and psychological impairment and poorer QoL (Ullrich et al. 2009).

Potent opioids form the basis of pharmacological pain control in patients with extensive burns. However, nonsteroidal anti-inflammatory agents and acetaminophen are still of value when combined with opioids, as the analgesia they provide lessens the dosage requirements for opioids. Because burn pain has well-defined components (i.e., background, procedural, breakthrough, and postoperative pain), pharmacological choices for analgesia should target each pain pattern individually. Analgesic regimens should be continuously evaluated and reassessed to avoid under- or over-medication. If there are sleep and anxiety concerns, then benzodiazepines may provide benefit. Nonpharmacological strategies, including music, relaxation therapy, hypnosis, and virtual reality techniques, may contribute to the alleviation of pain, but they should be adjunctive to the appropriate, flexible use of opioids (Wiechman Askay et al. 2009). Hypnosis has long been used in burn units for pain in adults and children, but the evidence is all anecdotal (Patterson et al. 1996). A meta-analysis of 17 studies examining music treatment in burn patients showed benefit in reducing pain and anxiety (Li et al. 2017).

Guidance for the management of psychiatric disorders in the context of burn care is limited; however, there is increasing recognition of the importance of involving patients' families in their burn care. Sacco et al. (2009) proposed "family-inclusive care" to engage families in the planning and treatment process as part of burn recovery.

Prostatectomy

Accepted therapies for prostate cancer include watchful waiting, radical prostatectomy, radiotherapy, hormonal therapy, orchiectomy, and antineoplastic drug therapy. The ProtecT trial, which followed 1,643 patients with the diagnosis of localized prostate cancer for a median of 10 years, showed that prostatectomy and radiotherapy were associated with lower rates of disease progression than active monitoring (Hamdy et al. 2016).

Physicians may underestimate the degree of emotional distress associated with reduced libido, feelings of unattractiveness, impotence, and incontinence. Although most impotence is treatment-related, for some men, psychogenic factors may be partly responsible, and psychiatric intervention may be important (van Heeringen et al. 1988). Etiology of erectile dysfunction after prostate cancer therapy is probably multifactorial. Veno-occlusive/cavernosal pathology predominates among men undergoing radical prostatectomy. Although most patients report problems in sexual/urinary function, global QoL does not appear to be compromised after prostatectomy (Zelefsky and Eid 1998). Some men may occasionally lose a little urine when lifting objects or coughing (i.e., stress incontinence). Other men are left with very little control over urine flow. Social isolation and embarrassment are understandable consequences and should be attended to. A prospective study of 329 prostate cancer patients in Germany who underwent radical prostatectomy found that approximately 8%–20% of patients experienced psychological distress postsurgery that warranted mental health support (Köhler et al. 2014). Both psychological distress before prostatectomy and urinary symptoms were found to be predictors of distress after surgery. (See Chapter 15, "Sexual Dysfunctions" and Chapter 22, "Oncology," for additional information.)

Ostomies

Many patients with colorectal cancer and inflammatory bowel disease receive intestinal stomas as part of their treatment; however, patients with stomas face many problems, both physical and psychosocial. Ostomy-related issues, including sexual problems, depressive symptoms, gas and/or constipation, dissatisfaction with appearance, clothing adaptations, travel difficulties, fatigue, and worry about noises from the ostomy, were summarized in a recent review by Vonk-Klaassen et al. (2016).

Approximately one-quarter of stoma patients experience clinically significant psychological symptoms postoperatively. Past psychiatric history, dissatisfaction with preoperative preparation for surgery, postoperative physical symptomatology, and the presence of negative stoma-related thoughts/beliefs have all been shown to be significantly associated with psychological morbidity after surgery. These findings suggest that health care professionals should ask all patients about these factors before and after surgery. Questionnaires can be used to screen for difficulties, and/or staff can be trained to detect psychological morbidity and to strengthen links with liaison mental health services (White and Hunt 1997).

Studies examining the impact of ostomies on QoL have yielded inconsistent results. A study in more than 4,700 Crohn's disease patients compared those who had an ostomy for a minimum of 6 months and those without an ostomy. Patients with an ostomy were more likely to be in remission, but there were no differences in overall health-related QoL, anxiety, depression, sleep disturbances, sexual interest and satisfaction, and social satisfaction (Abdalla et al. 2016). In contrast, a survey of rectal cancer survivors 1–10 years after diagnosis (Mols et al. 2014) found that patients with an ostomy had poorer QoL, worse illness perceptions, and higher health care consumption compared with those without an ostomy. Patients with stomas may also experience sexuality and intimacy concerns that merit special attention (Reese et al. 2014). Successful adjustment to ostomies depends on receipt of education on self-care, provision of psychosocial support to help accept changes in body image, and presence of a social support network (Piwonka and Merino 1999).

Bariatric Surgery

Obesity affects more than one-third of adults in the United States and is associated with multiple medical conditions, including coronary artery disease, type 2 diabetes, hyperlipidemia, hypertension, and sleep apnea (Ogden et al. 2013). Morbidity and mortality related to obesity are also a significant concern in mental health populations, with obesity prevalence rates as high as 60% among patients with severe mental illness (Allison et al. 2009).

Bariatric surgery is now recognized as a durable treatment for severe obesity; an RCT in obese patients with type 2 diabetes demonstrated greater sustained weight loss and resolution of metabolic comorbidities with bariatric surgery than with intensive medical therapy (Schauer et al. 2017). The current weight criterion for bariatric (or obesity) surgery is a body mass index (BMI) greater than 40 or a BMI greater than 35 with severe obesity-related comorbidities (e.g., type 2 diabetes mellitus, obstructive sleep apnea) (Mechanick et al. 2013).

There are three main bariatric surgery procedures currently offered in North America: laparoscopic adjustable gastric banding, sleeve gastrectomy, and laparoscopic Roux-en-Y gastric bypass (LRYGB) (Figures 28–1 through 28–3). LRYBG involves creation of a small gastric pouch with a small outlet; the malabsorptive element involves bypass of the distal stomach, the entire duodenum, and about 20–40 cm of the proximal jejunum. Bariatric surgery promotes weight loss through two primary mecha-

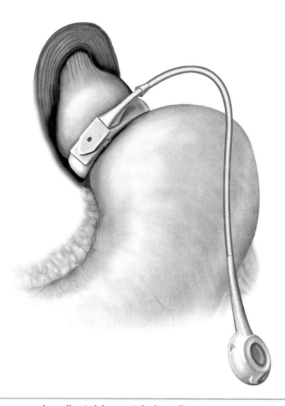

FIGURE 28–1.   Laparoscopic adjustable gastric banding.

Source.   Illustration reprinted, with permission, from Jones DB, Schneider BE, Olbers T: *Atlas of Metabolic and Weight Loss Surgery.* Woodbury, CT, Ciné-Med, 2010. Copyright of the book and illustrations are retained by Ciné-Med.

nisms—namely, restriction and malabsorption. LRYGB uses both restriction and malabsorption and has been shown to result in greater sustained weight loss and more durable resolution of metabolic comorbidities compared with the other two common bariatric surgical procedures. Data from the 2011 American College of Surgeons Bariatric Surgery Centre Network (Hutter et al. 2011) demonstrated that laparoscopic adjustable gastric banding and, to a certain degree, sleeve gastrectomy were less effective than LRYGB (Table 28–1). Data from two 5-year randomized controlled trials comparing weight and obesity-related comorbidity outcomes for sleeve gastrectomy and LRYGB showed comparable diabetes outcomes and only slightly better weight loss outcomes with LRYGB (absolute excess BMI loss −7.2%; absolute excess weight loss −8.2%) (Peterli et al. 2018; Salminen et al. 2018).

A fourth procedure, the biliopancreatic bypass with duodenal switch, removes a large portion of the stomach (to restrict meal sizes), reroutes food away from much of the small intestine (to prevent absorption), and reroutes bile (which impairs digestion). There are no clear indications for this procedure, but it is usually considered only for morbidly obese patients, given its superior weight-loss results but higher complication rates compared with LRYGB (SAGES Guidelines Committee 2008).

Long-term data on patients who have undergone bariatric surgery document the full range of outcomes. In the Swedish Obese Subjects Study (Sjöström 2008), a prospective controlled study of 1,845 bariatric surgical patients compared with 1,660 con-

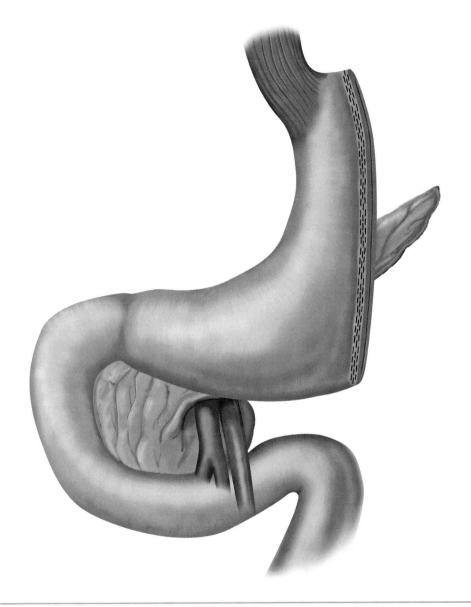

FIGURE 28–2. Sleeve gastrectomy.

Source. Illustration reprinted, with permission, from Jones DB, Schneider BE, Olbers T: *Atlas of Metabolic and Weight Loss Surgery.* Woodbury, CT, Ciné-Med, 2010. Copyright of the book and illustrations are retained by Ciné-Med.

trol patients, weight loss at 2 years was 23.4% in the surgical patients versus a weight gain of 0.1% in the control patients. Among participants still in the study at 15-year follow-up (676 bariatric surgery patients and 556 control patients), weight loss percentages for gastric bypass, vertical banded gastroplasty, and banding were 27%, 18%, and 13%, respectively, in the surgical patients versus an average weight change of ±3% in the control patients (Sjöström 2013).

A meta-analysis of six studies reporting long-term health-related QoL outcomes in patients after bariatric surgery showed significant improvement in physical and men-

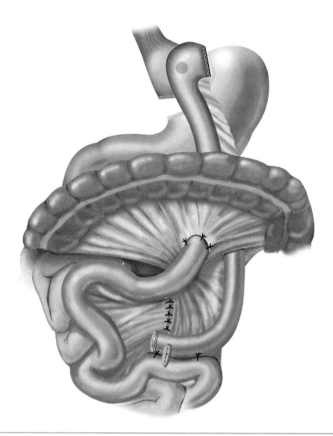

FIGURE 28–3.   Laparoscopic Roux-en-Y gastric bypass.

Source.   Illustration reprinted, with permission, from Jones DB, Schneider BE, Olbers T: *Atlas of Metabolic and Weight Loss Surgery.* Woodbury, CT, Ciné-Med, 2010. Copyright of the book and illustrations are retained by Ciné-Med.

tal health domains 5 or more years after surgery in comparison with individuals in the general population living with obesity or subjects in a surgery wait-list control condition (Driscoll et al. 2016). The degree of improvement in mental health domains was not as large as the degree of improvement in physical health domains. Despite the interest in identifying psychosocial predictors of bariatric surgery outcomes, it is clear that presurgery psychiatric illness is not a reliable predictor of weight loss and QoL (Dawes et al. 2016). Poor eating adaptation and depression may predict lower long-term weight loss after surgery (Sheets et al. 2015). However, several studies have demonstrated that weight-loss outcomes after bariatric surgery for patients with severe mental illness, specifically bipolar disorder, are comparable to outcomes for patients with other psychiatric disorders (Ahmed et al. 2013; Thomson et al. 2016).

Eating Disorders and Bariatric Surgery

Presurgical eating disorders are common in bariatric surgery candidates. In a review of 25 studies (Dawes et al. 2016), the lifetime prevalence of binge-eating disorder in patients seeking bariatric surgery was 17%, which is higher than the lifetime prevalence in the general population. In addition, night-eating syndrome (an eating disorder characterized by a delayed circadian pattern of food intake and manifesting as

TABLE 28–1. Improvements in body mass index (BMI) and obesity-related comorbidities as assessed at 1 year: comparison of three bariatric surgery procedures

Variable	LRYGB	Lap-sleeve gastrectomy	LAGB
Change in BMI (kg/m^2)	–15.34	–11.87	–7.05
Percentage of patients showing resolution or improvement of comorbid condition			
Diabetes	83%	55%	44%
Hyperlipidemia	66%	35%	33%
Hypertension	79%	68%	44%
Obstructive sleep apnea	66%	62%	38%
GERD	70%	50%	64%

Note. GERD=gastroesophageal reflux disorder; LAGB=laparoscopic adjustable gastric banding; LRYGB=laparoscopic Roux-en-Y gastric bypass.

Source. Data from Hutter et al. 2011.

episodes of uncontrolled overeating without the use of compensatory behaviors) is observed in approximately 9% of patients presenting for bariatric surgery (Allison et al. 2006) and is also associated with loss of control over eating (Royal et al. 2015). Other common eating problems after bariatric surgery include grazing behavior (eating small quantities of food continuously over a long period of time), compulsive eating, and emotional eating.

Very little is known about the prevalence of bulimia nervosa and anorexia nervosa among bariatric patients prior to surgery, perhaps because candidates may deny or minimize their disordered eating out fear of surgical ineligibility. There have been reports of development of bulimia nervosa postoperatively, but the actual rates are unknown (Mechanick et al. 2013). Also, anorexia nervosa–like presentations are seen in certain patients, with significant weight loss accompanied by fear of weight regain, dietary restriction, and disturbance in body image (Marino et al. 2012).

Clinically, it is important to mention that certain behaviors or concerns commonly reported after gastric bypass surgery—such as vomiting in response to early adjustment to decreased intake capacity or the sensation that food is "stuck" in the pouch—should not be confused with disordered eating.

Psychiatric Care in Bariatric Surgery

Psychiatrists are often asked to conduct pre–bariatric surgery readiness assessments, and recommendations regarding psychiatrists' role in this process have been summarized in an American Psychiatric Association resource document (Sockalingam et al. 2017). Psychiatric assessment for bariatric surgery should include a thorough weight history (including psychosocial factors influencing weight gain), eating psychopathology, psychosocial history (including social support and developmental history), and health-related behaviors, such as substance use (Sogg et al. 2016). Several standardized pre–bariatric surgery assessment tools have been developed, including the Toronto Bariatric Interprofessional Psychosocial Assessment Suitability Scale

(BIPASS; Thiara et al. 2016) and the Cleveland Clinic Behavioral Rating System for weight loss surgery (Heinberg et al. 2010). These tools can be useful resources for interprofessional bariatric surgery teams to support standardized preoperative assessment and to identify areas for presurgery stabilization.

Following LRYGB surgery, patients are at risk of impaired alcohol metabolism, requiring more time to become sober after ingesting alcohol. In a case–crossover study comparing pre- and postsurgical alcohol metabolism (assessed by measuring breath alcohol content [BrAC] every 5 minutes after drinking 5 oz of red wine) in 19 LRYGB patients, significantly higher BrAC levels were found 6 months after surgery compared with presurgery levels (Woodard et al. 2011). Patients who underwent LRYGB surgery, compared with those who underwent other types of bariatric surgery, were shown to have a higher risk of problematic alcohol use long-term, with approximately 9.6% of patients developing new-onset alcohol use disorder 2 years after bariatric surgery (King et al. 2012). Risk factors for developing alcohol use disorder after bariatric surgery include younger age, male sex, presurgery alcohol use, history of an alcohol use disorder within the past 12 months, presurgery nicotine use, and postsurgery recreational drug use. Literature is limited on opioid use disorders after bariatric surgery; however, one study found that among patients who were chronic opioid users before surgery, 77% continued chronic opioid use, in greater amounts, in the year following surgery (Raebel et al. 2013). Therefore, patients should receive presurgery education on potential substance use risk, especially regarding the changes in alcohol metabolism after bariatric surgery. Close postsurgery screening and monitoring for substance use disorders is recommended in high-risk patients undergoing LRYGB.

Given that nearly 40% of bariatric surgery candidates are taking psychotropic medications, psychiatrists may be consulted for advice on psychiatric medication adjustments in the context of malabsorptive bariatric procedures, mainly the gastric bypass. A limited number of studies are available to inform postsurgery dosage adjustment recommendations. Patients undergoing bariatric surgery who are treated with lithium for mood stabilization should be educated on potential shifts in their medication levels and should be managed using lithium protocols to prevent toxicity (Bingham et al. 2016). Postoperative psychiatric assessment and integrated treatment approaches are needed to mitigate potential postoperative psychosocial complications and to support patients with health benefits resulting from surgery.

Limb Amputation

Nearly 2 million individuals live with limb loss in the United States, with approximately 40% of limb loss secondary to vascular disease with comorbid diabetes mellitus (Ziegler-Graham et al. 2008). Data on the prevalence of psychiatric disorders after limb amputation are limited. Psychological distress, specifically anxiety and depression, may be acutely elevated after limb amputation. Research suggests that these symptoms may improve in the months after rehabilitation; however, additional elevations in anxiety and depression may emerge 2–3 years later (Singh et al. 2009).

Body Integrity Identity Disorder

Rarely, patients may request that a healthy limb be amputated, usually in the context of body integrity identity disorder (BIID). BIID is an extreme form of body image disturbance in which patients experience a sense of alienation and "overcompleteness" in regard to a specific limb (First 2005). Individuals with BIID do not suffer from delusions or psychosis and have insight into the bizarre nature of their wish. As a result, patients with BIID often seek surgical consultation for amputation or in extreme cases resort to self-amputation when they have not found a surgeon to perform the procedure. There are several case reports and one case series (First 2005) describing a group of 52 self-identified patients desiring an amputation, 9 of whom did have amputations (either from their own efforts or after enlisting a surgeon), and 6 of whom reported feeling better afterward. C-L psychiatrists are asked to evaluate patients presenting with this specific problem. A multidisciplinary approach to understanding and managing BIID patients is recommended (Bou Khalil and Richa 2012).

Phantom Limb Pain

The term *phantom limb* refers to the experience of feeling as if an amputated part is still present. Phantom limb pain was first described by Ambrose Paré (1649). Many amputees experience phantom limb sensations, which range from pleasant warmth to discomfort such as pain, paresthesias, and itching. Chronic phantom limb pain occurs in up to 85% of amputees and is a cause of significant disability and impaired QoL (see Brodie et al. 2007 for summary).

Many previous studies of phantom limb pain were complicated by a failure to distinguish between stump pain and various types of phantom limb phenomena (Richardson et al. 2006). *Stump pain* is defined as pain located in the residual portion of the stump, whereas *phantom limb pain* stems from painful sensations in the part of the limb that no longer exists. Risk factors for phantom limb pain include female sex, upper-extremity amputation, presence of preamputation pain, and experience of residual pain in the remaining limb. Time after amputation is also a factor, with peaks in prevalence occurring within the first month postamputation and after the first year postamputation (Subedi and Grossberg 2011).

The etiology of phantom limb pain is complex and not well understood. While there are several hypotheses, phantom limb pain is categorized as *neuropathic* rather than *nociceptive.* Neuropathic treatment approaches have given rise to novel strategies such as "mirror therapy" (Brodie et al. 2007; Chan et al. 2007; Darnall 2009) and the "rubber hand illusion" technique (Ehrsson et al. 2008), as well as a range of pharmacological options. A systematic review of psychopharmacological treatments for phantom limb pain suggests that morphine, ketamine, and gabapentin offer short-term benefit; however, the long-term effectiveness of pharmacological treatments remains unclear (Alviar et al. 2016) (see also Chapter 34).

Ophthalmological Surgery

Cataract Surgery

Cataract is the leading cause of blindness in the world, and cataract surgery is the most common procedure performed by ophthalmologists. Depression is common among patients who have cataracts. A recent systematic review and meta-analysis demonstrated that the prevalence of depression was 23% for cataract patients (Zheng et al. 2017).

Satisfaction with surgery appears to be closely related to expectations prior to surgery, which should be carefully explored during the consent process (Pager 2004). Studies have documented the influence of comorbid psychiatric disorders on postoperative recovery time and satisfaction. Patients' own reports of visual function, dry eye, and health anxiety were found to be stronger predictors of postoperative satisfaction than were objective measures of visual acuity and dry eye (Szakáts et al. 2017). Comorbid PTSD in veterans undergoing cataract surgery was associated with higher pain scores, more intraoperative analgesia, and longer operative times (Rapoport et al. 2017).

A prospective study of 50 patients who underwent cataract surgery with intraocular lens (IOL) implantation studied the factors contributing to preoperative, intraoperative, and postoperative anxiety (Chaudhury et al. 1995). A good doctor–patient relationship, confidence in the surgeon, and knowledge of successful surgery in an acquaintance were the major anxiety-relieving factors. The main anxiety-provoking factors were concerns about the success of the surgery and about remaining immobile and covered with surgical drapes during surgery. Detailed technical knowledge about the surgery was anxiety provoking, and the majority of the patients did not desire it.

The benefits of cataract surgery extend beyond vision and include lower risks of falls (Harwood et al. 2005), fewer motor vehicle accidents (Owsley et al. 2002), and even reductions in mental health visits for depression and/or anxiety (Meuleners et al. 2013).

Stigma and Eye Abnormalities

Several studies have confirmed that eye abnormalities can significantly influence QoL and affect interpersonal perceptions. Preoperative and postoperative photographs of patients with bilateral blepharoptosis and/or dermatochalasis were rated by 210 study subjects on the basis of 11 different personal characteristics, such as intelligence, friendliness, attractiveness, and happiness. The preoperative photographs were rated more negatively than the postoperative photographs on all 11 characteristics for both male and female patients by the study subjects. These psychosocial attitudes may lead to stigma toward affected patients, and surgical correction likely provides benefits beyond improved visual function (Bullock et al. 2001). A study in Chinese children ages 6–17 years found that those with strabismus had a significantly higher prevalence of self-reported alcohol use, depression, and anxiety compared with those without strabismus (Lin et al. 2014).

In a study in which patients with childhood-onset strabismus were evaluated prior to corrective surgery at ages 15–25 years (Menon et al. 2002), more than 75% of the patients reported experiencing social problems because of their continuous squint, being ridiculed at school and work, and having fewer employment opportunities. After the corrective surgery, more than 90% reported improved self-confidence and self-esteem. Similar positive effects were reported by the parents of children with strabismus in another study (Archer et al. 2005), with significant improvements observed in social, emotional, and functional measures of children's health status following strabismus surgery. Another study in 128 patients with childhood-onset strabismus found that strabismus surgery that restored ocular alignment had significant positive effects on patients' reported self-esteem, self-confidence, and perceived intelligence scores (Nelson et al. 2008).

Eye Removal

Self-removal of the eye (*autoenucleation*) is a rare form of self-mutilation that in various psychological theories has been attributed to religious or sexual ideation, symbolism, guilt, and displacement. Autoenucleation has been associated with a variety of psychiatric disorders, including schizophrenia, drug-induced psychosis, depression, obsessive-compulsive disorder, and intellectual disability. Other organic illnesses implicated include neurosyphilis, Lesch-Nyhan syndrome, and structural brain lesions (Patton 2004). A review of 50 cases found a high (39%) incidence of bilateral autoenucleation (Dilly and Imes 2001).

Cosmetic Surgery

The popularity of both surgical and nonsurgical cosmetic procedures is growing. In 2016, the American Society for Aesthetic Plastic Surgery (ASAPS) reported that Americans spent more than $15 billion on combined 1,979,595 surgical and 11,674,754 nonsurgical aesthetic procedures, accounting for an 11% increase over the past year alone (American Society for Aesthetic Plastic Surgery 2016). Surgical procedures accounted for 56% and nonsurgical procedures for 44% of the total. The most common surgical cosmetic procedures were liposuction, breast augmentation, abdominoplasty, blepharoplasty, and breast lift. ASAPS data reflect emerging trends in relatively new surgical procedures, including fat transfer to the breast (up 41.4% since 2015), fat transfer to the face (up 16.7% since 2015), and labiaplasty (up 23.2% since 2015). Women had 91% of the cosmetic procedures.

Research suggests that many patients who seek consultation for a cosmetic procedure meet criteria for a psychiatric disorder such as body dysmorphic disorder, narcissistic personality disorder, or histrionic personality disorder (Ishigooka et al. 1998). Those who undergo a cosmetic procedure and remain dissatisfied despite a clinically satisfactory outcome may pursue additional aesthetic procedures and are at risk of experiencing or exacerbating further psychiatric symptoms. Several studies (Litner et al. 2008; Sabino Neto et al. 2008; Stuerz et al. 2008) have proposed that improvements in body image and self-esteem as a result of cosmetic surgery can lead to improvement in QoL for these patients.

Preoperative Assessment

Limited systematic data are available to help clinicians predict who will do poorly psychologically following a cosmetic procedure. However, studies do provide some guidance for cosmetic specialists (Grossbart and Sarwer 1999; Sarwer and Didie 2002).

Patients should be asked about their specific appearance concerns in detail, including for how long they have had the concern and what precipitated the request for surgery. Past cosmetic interventions should be explored, as the literature suggests that previous surgery with which the patient was dissatisfied is a risk factor for poor outcome. Any history of lawsuits, threats, or violence toward previous cosmetic surgeons should obviously raise significant concern.

Because the literature suggests that unrealistic expectations regarding the outcome of a procedure may also predict a poor response, surgeons should assess patients' expectations regarding both the proposed procedure and the desired outcome. A distinction can usefully be made between expectations regarding the self (e.g., to improve body image) and expectations regarding external parameters (e.g., enhancement of one's social network, establishing a relationship, getting a job).

Most patient dissatisfaction with aesthetic surgery is based on failures of communication and patient selection criteria (Ward 1998). A careful psychosocial history is an essential part of patient selection and provides a way to establish rapport and ensure that the right operation is performed on the right patient. Blackburn and Blackburn (2008) have devised a method for assessing whether a proposed surgery is likely to be successful and satisfactory to the patient. The acronym *SAGA,* which stands for *S*ensitization (the patient's sensitivity to the deformity arising from internal or external sources), *A*esthetic self-assessment (the patient's own private evaluation of the feature about which he or she has a complaint), peer *G*roup comparison (how a patient compares the feature with the same feature in other people), and *A*voidance behavior (strategies used by the patient to camouflage or avoid exposure of the feature of complaint), can be used for that purpose. Wade's Patient Satisfaction Questionnaire (PSQ), a widely used self-administered satisfaction survey for general patient populations, has been modified to make the domains more relevant to plastic surgery, with satisfaction issues categorized into one of five domains: provider-related issues, aesthetic outcomes, functional outcomes, psychological outcomes, and an "all other issues" category (Clapham et al. 2010). Wildgoose et al. (2013) has systematically reviewed available psychological screening measures for use in cosmetic surgery patients.

Body Dysmorphic Disorder

Body dysmorphic disorder (BDD) is one of the most common psychiatric diagnoses in patients seeking cosmetic and dermatological surgery (see also Chapter 27, "Dermatology"). In a systematic review of 33 studies examining the prevalence of BDD in plastic surgery and dermatology patients, BDD was found in 15% (range, 2.21%–56.67%) of plastic surgery patients (mean age, 35 years; 74% women) and 13% (range, 4.52%–35.16%) of dermatology patients (mean age, 28 years; 76% women) (Ribeiro 2017).

Most individuals with BDD continue to be dissatisfied with their appearance following cosmetic treatment. In a sample of 200 patients with BDD who received cosmetic surgery, the most common outcome was no change in the severity of BDD symptoms (Phillips et al. 2001). Another 5-year follow-up study showed that cosmetic surgery had no significant effects on BDD diagnosis, disability, or psychiatric comorbidity (Tignol et al. 2007). In a sample of individuals with BDD who received surgical and minimally invasive procedures for their appearance concerns, 25% showed a longer-term improvement in their preoccupation with the treated body part, but only 2.3% of surgical and minimally invasive procedures led to longer-term improvement in overall BDD symptoms (Crerand et al. 2010).

One area of concern is the risk of suicidality and violent behavior in some individuals with BDD who seek cosmetic treatments. Rates of suicidality—including suicidal ideation and suicide attempts—in individuals with BDD are quite high. In some cases, individuals with BDD can become depressed following cosmetic treatments, because they are upset about the lack of improvement in their symptoms or what they perceive to be a procedure that made their appearance look worse. Although there is little research on the association between cosmetic treatments and suicide risk, studies of women who have sought breast augmentation have shown suicide rates that were two to three times higher than rates in the general population (Lipworth et al. 2007). Higher rates of suicidality in this population may be related to BDD psychopathology, although a direct link has not been made. In addition, there is an increased risk of violence toward physicians providing cosmetic treatments. In one study, 2% of cosmetic surgeons indicated that they had been physically threatened by a patient with BDD (Sarwer 2002).

Because of the legal and personal-safety issues associated with treating persons with BDD, coupled with the evidence that cosmetic treatments rarely improve BDD symptoms, there is growing consensus that BDD should be considered a contraindication to cosmetic treatments. It is important for surgeons to recognize patients with BDD who are seeking surgery and to be able to communicate with empathy that their distress is a result of a body image problem consisting of being overly concerned about and affected by how they think they look. Unfortunately, many patients with BDD decline psychiatric assessment or follow-up.

Conclusion

A variety of psychiatric issues can emerge over the course of patients' surgical care. In this chapter, we have highlighted potential psychiatric problems across a range of surgical populations, from preoperative assessment to postoperative care. Preoperative issues related to readiness for surgery, capacity and consent, and modifiable risk factors, including treatment of preexisting psychiatric conditions, should be addressed to support surgical recovery, improve outcomes, and prevent future mental health problems. Intraoperative awareness can result in significant distress, which may be mitigated through effective presurgery preparation. Acute postoperative issues, such as poorly controlled delirium, acute pain, or acute stress reactions, may predispose individuals to long-term psychiatric complications. Although surgical care may be episodic and focused on acute management, psychiatrists should advocate and support long-term monitoring and timely management of psychopathology, ideally through integrated care models. As summarized in this chapter, there is a growing interest in research focused on the psychiatric care of patients undergoing surgery. As standards and guidelines emerge, psychiatrists should continue to advocate for integration of psychiatric care into surgical programs, especially for high-risk patients, in order to improve clinical outcomes and QoL.

References

Abdalla MI, Sandler RS, Kappelman MD, et al: The impact of ostomy on quality of life and functional status of Crohn's disease patients. Inflamm Bowel Dis 22(11):2658–2664, 2016 27661669

Ahmadi A, Ytterstad B: Prevention of self-immolation by community-based intervention. Burns 33(8):1032–1040, 2007 17544221

Ahmadi A, Mohammadi R, Stavrinos D, et al: Self-immolation in Iran. J Burn Care Res 29(3):451–460, 2008 18388564

Ahmadi A, Mohammadi R, Schwebel DC, et al: Psychiatric disorders (Axis I and Axis II) and self-immolation: a case-control study from Iran. J Forensic Sci 55(2):447–450, 2010 20070465

Ahmed AT, Warton EM, Schaefer CA, et al: The effect of bariatric surgery on psychiatric course among patients with bipolar disorder. Bipolar Disord 15(7):753–763, 2013 23909994

Alarcon LH, Germain A, Clontz AS, et al: Predictors of acute posttraumatic stress disorder symptoms following civilian trauma: highest incidence and severity of symptoms after assault. J Trauma Acute Care Surg 72(3):629–635, discussion 635–637, 2012 22491546

Allison DB, Newcomer JW, Dunn AL, et al: Obesity among those with mental disorders: a National Institute of Mental Health meeting report. Am J Prev Med 36(4):341–350, 2009 19285199

Allison KC, Wadden TA, Sarwer DB, et al: Night eating syndrome and binge eating disorder among persons seeking bariatric surgery: prevalence and related features. Obesity (Silver Spring) 14 (suppl 2):77S–82S, 2006 16648598

Alviar MJ, Hale T, Dungca M: Pharmacologic interventions for treating phantom limb pain. Cochrane Database Syst Rev (10):CD006380, 2016 27737513

American Burn Association: Burn Incidence Fact Sheet: Burn Incidence and Treatment in the US: 2016. Chicago, IL, American Burn Association, 2016. Available at: http://ameriburn.org/who-we-are/media/burn-incidence-fact-sheet/. Accessed December 22, 2017.

American Society for Aesthetic Plastic Surgery: 2016 Cosmetic Surgery National Data Bank Statistics. 2016. Available at: https://www.surgery.org/sites/default/files/ASAPS-Stats2016.pdf. Accessed December 5, 2017.

Amos T, Stein DJ, Ipser JC: Pharmacological interventions for preventing post-traumatic stress disorder (PTSD). Cochrane Database Syst Rev (7):CD006239, 2014 25001071

Appelbaum PS: Clinical practice. Assessment of patients' competence to consent to treatment. N Engl J Med 357(18):1834–1840, 2007 17978292

Archer SM, Musch DC, Wren PA, et al: Social and emotional impact of strabismus surgery on quality of life in children. J AAPOS 9(2):148–151, 2005 15838442

Ayala ES, Meuret AE, Ritz T: Treatments for blood-injury-injection phobia: a critical review of current evidence. J Psychiatr Res 43(15):1235–1242, 2009 19464700

Ayyadhah Alanazi A: Reducing anxiety in preoperative patients: a systematic review. Br J Nurs 23(7):387–393, 2014 24732993

Baker SP, O'Neill B, Haddon W Jr, Long WB: The injury severity score: a method for describing patients with multiple injuries and evaluating emergency care. J Trauma 14(3):187–196, 1974 4814394

Balentine CJ, Hermosillo-Rodriguez J, Robinson CN, et al: Depression is associated with prolonged and complicated recovery following colorectal surgery. J Gastrointest Surg 15(10):1712–1717, 2011 21786060

Bernardy NC, Friedman MJ: Psychopharmacological strategies in the management of posttraumatic stress disorder (PTSD): what have we learned? Curr Psychiatry Rep 17(4):564, 2015 25749751

Bheemanna NK, Channaiah SRD, Gowda PKV, et al: Fears and perceptions associated with regional anesthesia: a study from a tertiary care hospital in South India. Anesth Essays Res 11(2):483–488, 2017 28663646

Bienvenu OJ, Eaton WW: The epidemiology of blood-injection-injury phobia. Psychol Med 28(5):1129–1136, 1998 9794020

Bingham KS, Thoma J, Hawa R, Sockalingam S: Perioperative lithium use in a bariatric surgery: a case series and literature review. Psychosomatics 57(6):638–644, 2016 27726858

Bisson JI, Jenkins PL, Alexander J, Bannister C: Randomised controlled trial of psychological debriefing for victims of acute burn trauma. Br J Psychiatry 171:78–81, 1997 9328501

Blackburn VF, Blackburn AV: Taking a history in aesthetic surgery: SAGA—the surgeon's tool for patient selection. J Plast Reconstr Aesthet Surg 61(7):723–729, 2008 18374638

Blakeney P, Thomas C, Holzer C 3rd, et al: Efficacy of a short-term, intensive social skills training program for burned adolescents. J Burn Care Rehabil 26(6):546–555, 2005 16278574

Blanchard EB, Hickling EJ, Devineni T, et al: A controlled evaluation of cognitive behavioural therapy for posttraumatic stress in motor vehicle accident survivors. Behav Res Ther 41(1):79–96, 2003 12488121

Bou Khalil R, Richa S: Apotemnophilia or body integrity identity disorder: a case report review. Int J Low Extrem Wounds 11(4):313–319, 2012 23089967

Bradley CT, Brasel KJ: Core competencies in palliative care for surgeons: interpersonal and communication skills. Am J Hosp Palliat Care 24(6):499–507, 2007 18182636

Bradt J, Dileo C, Shim M: Music interventions for preoperative anxiety. Cochrane Database Syst Rev (6):CD006908, 2013 23740695

Brodie EE, Whyte A, Niven CA: Analgesia through the looking-glass? A randomized controlled trial investigating the effect of viewing a "virtual" limb upon phantom limb pain, sensation and movement. Eur J Pain 11(4):428–436, 2007 16857400

Bullock JD, Warwar RE, Bienenfeld DG, et al: Psychosocial implications of blepharoptosis and dermatochalasis. Trans Am Ophthalmol Soc 99:65–71, discussion 71–72, 2001 11797321

Caumo W, Levandovski R, Hidalgo MP: Preoperative anxiolytic effect of melatonin and clonidine on postoperative pain and morphine consumption in patients undergoing abdominal hysterectomy: a double-blind, randomized, placebo-controlled study. J Pain 10(1):100–108, 2009 19010741

Chan BL, Witt R, Charrow AP, et al: Mirror therapy for phantom limb pain. N Engl J Med 357(21):2206–2207, 2007 18032777

Chaudhury S, Chakraborty PK, Gurunadh VS, Ratha P: Psychological reactions to cataract surgery with intraocular lens implantation. Indian J Psychiatry 37(4):165–168, 1995 21743743

Chen CC, Lin CS, Ko YP, et al: Premedication with mirtazapine reduces preoperative anxiety and postoperative nausea and vomiting. Anesth Analg 106(1):109–113, 2008 18165563

Cherr GS, Wang J, Zimmerman PM, Dosluoglu HH: Depression is associated with worse patency and recurrent leg symptoms after lower extremity revascularization. J Vasc Surg 45(4):744–750, 2007 17303367

Chou R, Gordon DB, de Leon-Casasola OA, et al: Management of postoperative pain: a clinical practice guideline from the American Pain Society, the American Society of Regional Anesthesia and Pain Medicine, and the American Society of Anesthesiologists' Committee on Regional Anesthesia, Executive Committee, and Administrative Council. J Pain 17(2):131–157, 2016 26827847

Choudhry MA, Chaudry IH: Alcohol, burn injury, and the intestine. J Emerg Trauma Shock 1(2):81–87, 2008 19561986

Chundamala J, Wright JG, Kemp SM: An evidence-based review of parental presence during anesthesia induction and parent/child anxiety. Can J Anaesth 56(1):57–70, 2009 19247779

Clapham PJ, Pushman AG, Chung KC: A systematic review of applying patient satisfaction outcomes in plastic surgery. Plast Reconstr Surg 125(6):1826–1833, 2010 20517109

Conlin S, Littlechild J, Aditya H, Bahia H: Surgical and psychiatric profile of patients who self-harm by burning in a regional burn unit over an 11-year period. Scott Med J 61(1):17–25, 2016 27334530

Connerney I, Shapiro PA, McLaughlin JS, et al: Relation between depression after coronary artery bypass surgery and 12-month outcome: a prospective study. Lancet 358(9295):1766–1771, 2001 11734233

Constantin JM, Momon A, Mantz J, et al: Efficacy and safety of sedation with dexmedetomidine in critical care patients: a meta-analysis of randomized controlled trials. Anaesth Crit Care Pain Med 35(1):7–15, 2016 26700947

Copeland LA, Zeber JE, Sako EY, et al: Serious mental illnesses associated with receipt of surgery in retrospective analysis of patients in the Veterans Health Administration. BMC Surg 15:74, 2015 26084521

Costi D, Cyna AM, Ahmed S, et al: Effects of sevoflurane versus other general anaesthesia on emergence agitation in children. Cochrane Database Syst Rev (9):CD007084, 2014 25212274

Crerand CE, Menard W, Phillips KA: Surgical and minimally invasive cosmetic procedures among persons with body dysmorphic disorder. Ann Plast Surg 65(1):11–16, 2010 20467296

Darnall BD: Self-delivered home-based mirror therapy for lower limb phantom pain. Am J Phys Med Rehabil 88(1):78–81, 2009 19096290

Davidson AJ, Smith KR, Blussé van Oud-Alblas HJ, et al: Awareness in children: a secondary analysis of five cohort studies. Anaesthesia 66(6):446–454, 2011 21501128

Davydow DS, Zatzick D, Hough CL, Katon WJ: A longitudinal investigation of posttraumatic stress and depressive symptoms over the course of the year following medical-surgical intensive care unit admission. Gen Hosp Psychiatry 35(3):226–232, 2013 23369507

Dawes AJ, Maggard-Gibbons M, Maher AR, et al: Mental health conditions among patients seeking and undergoing bariatric surgery: a meta-analysis. JAMA 315(2):150–163, 2016 26757464

Deacon B, Abramowitz J: Fear of needles and vasovagal reactions among phlebotomy patients. J Anxiety Disord 20(7):946–960, 2006 16460906

Dilly JS, Imes RK: Autoenucleation of a blind eye. J Neuroophthalmol 21(1):30–31, 2001 11315978

Dischinger PC, Mitchell KA, Kufera JA, et al: A longitudinal study of former trauma center patients: the association between toxicology status and subsequent injury mortality. J Trauma 51(5):877–884, discussion 884–886, 2001 11706334

Driscoll S, Gregory DM, Fardy JM, Twells LK: Long-term health-related quality of life in bariatric surgery patients: a systematic review and meta-analysis. Obesity (Silver Spring) 24(1):60–70, 2016 26638116

Ehrsson HH, Rosén B, Stockselius A, et al: Upper limb amputees can be induced to experience a rubber hand as their own. Brain 131(Pt 12):3443–3452, 2008 19074189

Eliasen M, Grønkjær M, Skov-Ettrup LS, et al: Preoperative alcohol consumption and postoperative complications: a systematic review and meta-analysis. Ann Surg 258(6):930–942, 2013 23732268

Engels G, Francke AL, van Meijel B, et al: Clinical pain in schizophrenia: a systematic review. J Pain 15(5):457–467, 2014 24365324

Falder S, Browne A, Edgar D, et al: Core outcomes for adult burn survivors: a clinical overview. Burns 35(5):618–641, 2009 19111399

Fauerbach JA, McKibben J, Bienvenu OJ, et al: Psychological distress after major burn injury. Psychosom Med 69(5):473–482, 2007 17585064

First MB: Desire for amputation of a limb: paraphilia, psychosis, or a new type of identity disorder. Psychol Med 35(6):919–928, 2005 15997612

Gagne JJ, Polinski JM, Rassen JA, et al: Selective serotonin reuptake inhibitor use and perioperative bleeding and mortality in patients undergoing coronary artery bypass grafting: a cohort study. Drug Saf 38(11):1075–1082, 2015 26188765

Gan TJ, Habib AS, Miller TE, et al: Incidence, patient satisfaction, and perceptions of post-surgical pain: results from a US national survey. Curr Med Res Opin 30(1):149–160, 2014 24237004

Garrouste-Orgeas M, Coquet I, Périer A, et al: Impact of an intensive care unit diary on psychological distress in patients and relatives. Crit Care Med 40(7):2033–2040, 2012 22584757

Gaylord KM, Holcomb JB, Zolezzi ME: A comparison of posttraumatic stress disorder between combat casualties and civilians treated at a military burn center. J Trauma 66 (4 suppl):S191–S195, 2009 19359965

Gentilello LM, Donovan DM, Dunn CW, Rivara FP: Alcohol interventions in trauma centers. Current practice and future directions. JAMA 274(13):1043–1048, 1995 7563455

Giannoni-Pastor A, Eiroa-Orosa FJ, Fidel Kinori SG, et al: Prevalence and predictors of posttraumatic stress symptomatology among burn survivors: a systematic review and meta-analysis. J Burn Care Res 37(1):e79–e89, 2016 25970798

Greene NH, Attix DK, Weldon BC, et al: Measures of executive function and depression identify patients at risk for postoperative delirium. Anesthesiology 110(4):788–795, 2009 19326494

Grossbart TA, Sarwer DB: Cosmetic surgery: surgical tools—psychosocial goals. Semin Cutan Med Surg 18(2):101–111, 1999 10385278

Gurlit S, Möllmann M: How to prevent perioperative delirium in the elderly? Z Gerontol Geriatr 41(6):447–452, 2008 19190867

Hamdy FC, Donovan JL, Lane JA, et al; ProtecT Study Group: 10-year outcomes after monitoring, surgery, or radiotherapy for localized prostate cancer. N Engl J Med 375(15):1415–1424, 2016 27626136

Hamilton GM, Wheeler K, Di Michele J, et al: A systematic review and meta-analysis examining the impact of incident postoperative delirium on mortality. Anesthesiology 127(1):78–88, 2017 28459734

Harwood RH, Foss AJ, Osborn F, et al: Falls and health status in elderly women following first eye cataract surgery: a randomised controlled trial. Br J Ophthalmol 89(1):53–59, 2005 15615747

Heinberg LJ, Ashton K, Windover A: Moving beyond dichotomous psychological evaluation: the Cleveland Clinic Behavioral Rating System for weight loss surgery. Surg Obes Relat Dis 6(2):185–190, 2010 20096644

Heron-Delaney M, Kenardy J, Charlton E, Matsuoka Y: A systematic review of predictors of posttraumatic stress disorder (PTSD) for adult road traffic crash survivors. Injury 44(11):1413–1422, 2013 23916902

Hughes DB, Ullery BW, Barie PS: The contemporary approach to the care of Jehovah's witnesses. J Trauma 65(1):237–247, 2008 18580506

Hutter MM, Schirmer BD, Jones DB, et al: First report from the American College of Surgeons Bariatric Surgery Center Network: laparoscopic sleeve gastrectomy has morbidity and effectiveness positioned between the band and the bypass. Ann Surg 254(3):410–420, discussion 420–422, 2011 21865942

Inouye SK, Robinson T, Blaum C, et al; American Geriatrics Society Expert Panel on Postoperative Delirium in Older Adults: Postoperative delirium in older adults: best practice statement from the American Geriatrics Society. J Am Coll Surg 220(2):136–48.e1, 2015 25535170

Ishigooka J, Iwao M, Suzuki M, et al: Demographic features of patients seeking cosmetic surgery. Psychiatry Clin Neurosci 52(3):283–287, 1998 9681579

Jackson JC, Jutte JE, Hunter CH, et al: Posttraumatic stress disorder (PTSD) after critical illness: a conceptual review of distinct clinical issues and their implications. Rehabil Psychol 61(2):132–140, 2016 27196856

James-Ellison M, Barnes P, Maddocks A, et al: Social health outcomes following thermal injuries: a retrospective matched cohort study. Arch Dis Child 94(9):663–667, 2009 19531525

Jawaid M, Mushtaq A, Mukhtar S, Khan Z: Preoperative anxiety before elective surgery. Neurosciences (Riyadh) 12(2):145–148, 2007 21857597

Jones C, Bäckman C, Capuzzo M, et al; RACHEL Group: Intensive care diaries reduce new onset post traumatic stress disorder following critical illness: a randomised, controlled trial. Crit Care 14(5):R168, 2010 20843344

Jones JD, Barber B, Engrav L, Heimbach D: Alcohol use and burn injury. J Burn Care Rehabil 12(2):148–152, 1991 2050723

Joo J, Lee S, Lee Y: Emergence delirium is related to the invasiveness of strabismus surgery in preschool-age children. J Int Med Res 42(6):1311–1322, 2014 25298011

Kain ZN, Caldwell-Andrews AA, Mayes LC, et al: Family-centered preparation for surgery improves perioperative outcomes in children: a randomized controlled trial. Anesthesiology 106(1):65–74, 2007 17197846

Kalisvaart KJ, de Jonghe JF, Bogaards MJ, et al: Haloperidol prophylaxis for elderly hip-surgery patients at risk for delirium: a randomized placebo-controlled study. J Am Geriatr Soc 53(10):1658–1666, 2005 16181163

Kalisvaart KJ, Vreeswijk R, de Jonghe JF, et al: Risk factors and prediction of postoperative delirium in elderly hip-surgery patients: implementation and validation of a medical risk factor model. J Am Geriatr Soc 54(5):817–822, 2006 16696749

Kaneko T, Cai J, Ishikura T, et al: Prophylactic consecutive administration of haloperidol can reduce the occurrence of postoperative delirium in gastrointestinal surgery. Yonago Acta Med 42(3):179–184, 1999

Kazmierski J, Kowman M, Banach M, et al: Clinical utility and use of DSM-IV and ICD-10 criteria and the Memorial Delirium Assessment Scale in establishing a diagnosis of delirium after cardiac surgery. Psychosomatics 49(1):73–76, 2008 18212180

Kent CD, Mashour GA, Metzger NA, et al: Psychological impact of unexpected explicit recall of events occurring during surgery performed under sedation, regional anaesthesia, and general anaesthesia: data from the Anesthesia Awareness Registry. Br J Anaesth 110(3):381–387, 2013 23161356

King AP, Abelson JL, Gholami B, et al: Presurgical psychological and neuroendocrine predictors of psychiatric morbidity after major vascular surgery: a prospective longitudinal study. Psychosom Med 77(9):993–1005, 2015 26461854

King WC, Chen JY, Mitchell JE, et al: Prevalence of alcohol use disorders before and after bariatric surgery. JAMA 307(23):2516–2525, 2012 22710289

Kishi Y, Meller WH, Kathol RG, Swigart SE: Factors affecting the relationship between the timing of psychiatric consultation and general hospital length of stay. Psychosomatics 45(6):470–476, 2004 15546823

Klein E, Koren D, Arnon I, Lavie P: Sleep complaints are not corroborated by objective sleep measures in post-traumatic stress disorder: a 1-year prospective study in survivors of motor vehicle crashes. J Sleep Res 12(1):35–41, 2003 12603785

Köhler N, Friedrich M, Gansera L, et al: Psychological distress and adjustment to disease in patients before and after radical prostatectomy. Results of a prospective multi-centre study. Eur J Cancer Care (Engl) 23(6):795–802, 2014 24661440

Kunkel EJS, Bakker JR, Myers RE, et al: Biopsychosocial aspects of prostate cancer. Psychosomatics 41(2):85–94, 2000 10749945

Larsen KA, Kelly SE, Stern TA, et al: Administration of olanzapine to prevent postoperative delirium in elderly joint-replacement patients: a randomized, controlled trial. Psychosomatics 51(5):409–418, 2010 20833940

Lawrence JW, Mason ST, Schomer K, Klein MB: Epidemiology and impact of scarring after burn injury: a systematic review of the literature. J Burn Care Res 33(1):136–146, 2012 22138807

Lee DS, Marsh L, Garcia-Altieri MA, et al: Active mental illnesses adversely affect surgical outcomes. Am Surg 82(12):1238–1243, 2016 28234191

Levandovski R, Ferreira MB, Hidalgo MP, et al: Impact of preoperative anxiolytic on surgical site infection in patients undergoing abdominal hysterectomy. Am J Infect Control 36(10):718–726, 2008 18834731

Li J, Zhou L, Wang Y: The effects of music intervention on burn patients during treatment procedures: a systematic review and meta-analysis of randomized controlled trials. BMC Complement Altern Med 17(1):158, 2017 28302117

Liao CC, Shen WW, Chang CC, et al: Surgical adverse outcomes in patients with schizophrenia: a population-based study. Ann Surg 257(3):433–438, 2013 23241870

Lieber CS: Medical disorders of alcoholism. N Engl J Med 333(16):1058–1065, 1995 7675050

Lin S, Congdon N, Yam JC, et al: Alcohol use and positive screening results for depression and anxiety are highly prevalent among Chinese children with strabismus. Am J Ophthalmol 157(4):894–900.e1, 2014 24445033

Lipworth L, Nyren O, Ye W, et al: Excess mortality from suicide and other external causes of death among women with cosmetic breast implants. Ann Plast Surg 59(2):119–123, discussion 124–125, 2007 17667401

Litner JA, Rotenberg BW, Dennis M, Adamson PA: Impact of cosmetic facial surgery on satisfaction with appearance and quality of life. Arch Facial Plast Surg 10(2):79–83, 2008 18347233

Low AJ, Dyster-Aas J, Kildal M, et al: The presence of nightmares as a screening tool for symptoms of posttraumatic stress disorder in burn survivors. J Burn Care Res 27(5):727–733, 2006 16998407

Mahdanian AA, Rej S, Bacon SL, et al: Serotonergic antidepressants and perioperative bleeding risk: a systematic review. Expert Opin Drug Saf 13(6):695–704, 2014 24717049

Maldonado JR, Wysong A, van der Starre PJ, et al: Dexmedetomidine and the reduction of postoperative delirium after cardiac surgery. Psychosomatics 50(3):206–217, 2009 19567759

Maldonado JR, Sher Y, Lolak S, et al: The Stanford Integrated Psychosocial Assessment for Transplantation: a prospective study of medical and psychosocial outcomes. Psychosom Med 77(9):1018–1030, 2015 26517474

Maranets I, Kain ZN: Preoperative anxiety and intraoperative anesthetic requirements. Anesth Analg 89(6):1346–1351, 1999 10589606

Marcantonio ER, Flacker JM, Wright RJ, Resnick NM: Reducing delirium after hip fracture: a randomized trial. J Am Geriatr Soc 49(5):516–522, 2001 11380742

Marino JM, Ertelt TW, Lancaster K, et al: The emergence of eating pathology after bariatric surgery: a rare outcome with important clinical implications. Int J Eat Disord 45(2):179–184, 2012 21495051

Martin G, Swannell S, Mill J, et al: Spray on skin improves psychosocial functioning in pediatric burns patients: a randomized controlled trial. Burns 34(4):498–504, 2008 18082960

Mashour GA: Posttraumatic stress disorder after intraoperative awareness and high-risk surgery. Anesth Analg 110(3):668–670, 2010 20185646

Matharu LL, Ashley PF: What is the evidence for paediatric dental sedation? J Dent 35(1):2–20, 2007 17010493

Mavridou P, Dimitriou V, Manataki A, et al: Patient's anxiety and fear of anesthesia: effect of gender, age, education, and previous experience of anesthesia. A survey of 400 patients. J Anesth 27(1):104–108, 2013 22864564

McCann ME, Kain ZN: The management of preoperative anxiety in children: an update. Anesth Analg 93(1):98–105, 2001 11429348

McCleane GJ, Cooper R: The nature of pre-operative anxiety. Anaesthesia 45(2):153–155, 1990 2321720

McKenzie LH, Simpson J, Stewart M: A systematic review of pre-operative predictors of post-operative depression and anxiety in individuals who have undergone coronary artery bypass graft surgery. Psychol Health Med 15(1):74–93, 2010 20391226

McKibben JB, Bresnick MG, Wiechman Askay SA, Fauerbach JA: Acute stress disorder and posttraumatic stress disorder: a prospective study of prevalence, course, and predictors in a sample with major burn injuries. J Burn Care Res 29(1):22–35, 2008 18182894

McKibben JB, Ekselius L, Girasek DC, et al: Epidemiology of burn injuries, II: psychiatric and behavioural perspectives. Int Rev Psychiatry 21(6):512–521, 2009 19919204

McMurtry CM, Noel M, Taddio A, et al; HELPinKids&Adults Team: Interventions for individuals with high levels of needle fear: systematic review of randomized controlled trials and quasi-randomized controlled trials. Clin J Pain 31 (10 suppl):S109–S123, 2015 26352916

Mechanick JI, Youdim A, Jones DB, et al: Clinical practice guidelines for the perioperative nutritional, metabolic, and nonsurgical support of the bariatric surgery patient—2013 update: cosponsored by American Association of Clinical Endocrinologists, the Obesity Society, and American Society for Metabolic & Bariatric Surgery. Surg Obes Relat Dis 9(2):159–191, 2013 23537696

Ménigaux C, Adam F, Guignard B, et al: Preoperative gabapentin decreases anxiety and improves early functional recovery from knee surgery. Anesth Analg 100(5):1394–1399, 2005 15845693

Menon V, Saha J, Tandon R, et al: Study of the psychosocial aspects of strabismus. J Pediatr Ophthalmol Strabismus 39(4):203–208, 2002 12148552

Meuleners LB, Hendrie D, Fraser ML, et al: The impact of first eye cataract surgery on mental health contacts for depression and/or anxiety: a population-based study using linked data. Acta Ophthalmol 91(6):e445–e449, 2013 23586972

Mols F, Lemmens V, Bosscha K, et al: Living with the physical and mental consequences of an ostomy: a study among 1–10-year rectal cancer survivors from the population-based PROFILES registry. Psychooncology 23(9):998–1004, 2014 24664891

Mulholland R, Green L, Longstaff C, et al: Deliberate self-harm by burning: a retrospective case controlled study. J Burn Care Res 29(4):644–649, 2008 18535468

Neale MC, Walters EE, Eaves LJ, et al: Genetics of blood-injury fears and phobias: a population-based twin study. Am J Med Genet 54(4):326–334, 1994 7726205

Nelson BA, Gunton KB, Lasker JN, et al: The psychosocial aspects of strabismus in teenagers and adults and the impact of surgical correction. J AAPOS 12(1):72–76.e1, 2008 18314071

Neufeld KJ, Yue J, Robinson TN, et al: Antipsychotics for prevention and treatment of delirium in hospitalized adults: a systematic review and meta-analysis. J Am Geriatr Soc 64(4):705–714, 2016 27004732

Nir Y, Paz A, Sabo E, Potasman I: Fear of injections in young adults: prevalence and associations. Am J Trop Med Hyg 68(3):341–344, 2003 12685642

Novak M, Molnar MZ, Szeifert L, et al: Depressive symptoms and mortality in patients after kidney transplantation: a prospective prevalent cohort study. Psychosom Med 72(6):527–534, 2010 20410250

Nunes RR, Porto VC, Miranda VT, et al: Risk factor for intraoperative awareness. Rev Bras Anestesiol 62(3):365–374, 2012 22656682

Ogden CL, Carroll MD, Kit BK, Flegal KM: Prevalence of obesity among adults: United States, 2011–2012. NCHS Data Brief (131):1–8, 2013 24152742

Ormont MA, Weisman HW, Heller SS, et al: The timing of psychiatric consultation requests: utilization, liaison, and diagnostic considerations. Psychosomatics 38(1):38–44, 1997 8997115

Owsley C, McGwin G Jr, Sloane M, et al: Impact of cataract surgery on motor vehicle crash involvement by older adults. JAMA 288(7):841–849, 2002 12186601

Pager CK: Assessment of visual satisfaction and function after cataract surgery. J Cataract Refract Surg 30(12):2510–2516, 2004 15617917

Pandit JJ, Andrade J, Bogod DG, et al; Royal College of Anaesthetists; Association of Anaesthetists of Great Britain and Ireland: 5th National Audit Project (NAP5) on accidental awareness during general anaesthesia: summary of main findings and risk factors. Br J Anaesth 113(4):549–559, 2014 25204697

Paré A: The Works of That Famous Chirurgion, Ambrose Parey. Translated from the Latin and compared with the French by T. Johnson. London, Cotes, 1649

Patterson DR, Goldberg ML, Ehde DM: Hypnosis in the treatment of patients with severe burns. Am J Clin Hypn 38(3):200–212, discussion 213, 1996 8712163

Patton N: Self-inflicted eye injuries: a review. Eye (Lond) 18(9):867–872, 2004 15002007

Peck MD: Epidemiology of burns throughout the world, part II: intentional burns in adults. Burns 38(5):630–637, 2012 22325849

Pekcan M, Celebioglu B, Demir B, et al: The effect of premedication on preoperative anxiety. Middle East J Anaesthesiol 18(2):421–433, 2005 16438017

Perks A, Chakravarti S, Manninen P: Preoperative anxiety in neurosurgical patients. J Neurosurg Anesthesiol 21(2):127–130, 2009 19295391

Peterli R, Wölnerhanssen BK, Peters T, et al: Effect of laparoscopic sleeve gastrectomy vs laparoscopic Roux-en-Y gastric bypass on weight loss in patients with morbid obesity: the SM-BOSS randomized clinical trial. JAMA 319(3):255–265, 2018 29340679

Phillips KA, Grant J, Siniscalchi J, Albertini RS: Surgical and nonpsychiatric medical treatment of patients with body dysmorphic disorder. Psychosomatics 42(6):504–510, 2001 11815686

Pinto A, Faiz O, Bicknell C, Vincent C: Surgical complications and their implications for surgeons' well-being. Br J Surg 100(13):1748–1755, 2013 24227360

Piwonka MA, Merino JM: A multidimensional modeling of predictors influencing the adjustment to a colostomy. J Wound Ostomy Continence Nurs 26(6):298–305, 1999 10865614

Powell J, Kitchen N, Heslin J, Greenwood R: Psychosocial outcomes at three and nine months after good neurological recovery from aneurysmal subarachnoid haemorrhage: predictors and prognosis. J Neurol Neurosurg Psychiatry 72(6):772–781, 2002 12023423

Powers PS: Practice guideline for psychiatric disorders. Paper presented at the 15th Regional Burn Meeting, Lexington, KY, December 2002

Powers PS, Stevens B, Arias F, et al: Alcohol disorders among patients with burns: crisis and opportunity. J Burn Care Rehabil 15(4):386–391, 1994 7929524

Prakanrattana U, Prapaitrakool S: Efficacy of risperidone for prevention of postoperative delirium in cardiac surgery. Anaesth Intensive Care 35(5):714–719, 2007 17933157

Putnam FW, Hulsmann JE: Pharmacotherapy for survivors of childhood trauma. Semin Clin Neuropsychiatry 7(2):129–136, 2002 11953937

Raebel MA, Newcomer SR, Reifler LM, et al: Chronic use of opioid medications before and after bariatric surgery. JAMA 310(13):1369–1376, 2013 24084922

Rapoport Y, Wayman LL, Chomsky AS: The effect of post-traumatic-stress-disorder on intra-operative analgesia in a veteran population during cataract procedures carried out using retrobulbar or topical anesthesia: a retrospective study. BMC Ophthalmol 17(1):85, 2017 28592279

Reese JB, Finan PH, Haythornthwaite JA, et al: Gastrointestinal ostomies and sexual outcomes: a comparison of colorectal cancer patients by ostomy status. Support Care Cancer 22(2):461–468, 2014 24091721

Ribeiro RVE: Prevalence of body dysmorphic disorder in plastic surgery and dermatology patients: a systematic review with meta-analysis. Aesthetic Plast Surg 41(4):964–970, 2017 28411353

Richardson C, Glenn S, Nurmikko T, Horgan M: Incidence of phantom phenomena including phantom limb pain 6 months after major lower limb amputation in patients with peripheral vascular disease. Clin J Pain 22(4):353–358, 2006 16691088

Roerig JL, Steffen K: Psychopharmacology and bariatric surgery. Eur Eat Disord Rev 23(6):463–469, 2015 26338011

Royal S, Wnuk S, Warwick K, et al: Night eating and loss of control over eating in bariatric surgery candidates. J Clin Psychol Med Settings 22(1):14–19, 2015 25450651

Ruhaiyem ME, Alshehri AA, Saade M, et al: Fear of going under general anesthesia: a cross-sectional study. Saudi J Anaesth 10(3):317–321, 2016 27375388

Rusch MD, Gould LJ, Dzwierzynski WW, Larson DL: Psychological impact of traumatic injuries: what the surgeon can do. Plast Reconstr Surg 109(1):18–24, 2002 11786786

Sabino Neto M, Demattê MF, Freire M, et al: Self-esteem and functional capacity outcomes following reduction mammaplasty. Aesthet Surg J 28(4):417–420, 2008 19083555

Sacco TL, Stapleton MF, Ingersoll GL: Support groups facilitated by families of former patients: creating family-inclusive critical care units. Crit Care Nurse 29(3):36–45, 2009 19487779

SAGES Guidelines Committee: SAGES guideline for clinical application of laparoscopic bariatric surgery. Surg Endosc 22(10):2281–2300, 2008 18791862

Salminen P, Helmiö M, Ovaska J, et al: Effect of laparoscopic sleeve gastrectomy vs laparoscopic Roux-en-Y Gastric bypass on weight loss at 5 years among patients with morbid obesity: the SLEEVEPASS randomized clinical trial. JAMA 319(3):241–254, 2018 29340676

Sarwer DB: Awareness and identification of body dysmorphic disorder by aesthetic surgeons: results of a survey of American Society for Aesthetic Plastic Surgery Members. Aesthet Surg J 22(6):531–535, 2002 19332010

Sarwer DB, Didie ER: Body image in cosmetic surgical and dermatological practice, in Disorders of Body Image. Edited by Castle DJ, Phillips KA. Hampshire, UK, Wrightson Biomedical, 2002, pp 37–53

Schauer PR, Bhatt DL, Kirwan JP, et al; STAMPEDE Investigators: Bariatric surgery versus intensive medical therapy for diabetes—5-year outcomes. N Engl J Med 376(7):641–651, 2017 28199805

Schelling G, Richter M, Roozendaal B, et al: Exposure to high stress in the intensive care unit may have negative effects on health-related quality-of-life outcomes after cardiac surgery. Crit Care Med 31(7):1971–1980, 2003 12847391

Schelling G, Kilger E, Roozendaal B, et al: Stress doses of hydrocortisone, traumatic memories, and symptoms of posttraumatic stress disorder in patients after cardiac surgery: a randomized study. Biol Psychiatry 55(6):627–633, 2004 15013832

Scher CS, Anwar M: The self-reporting of psychiatric medications in patients scheduled for elective surgery. J Clin Anesth 11(8):619–621, 1999 10680101

Sheets CS, Peat CM, Berg KC, et al: Post-operative psychosocial predictors of outcome in bariatric surgery. Obes Surg 25(2):330–345, 2015 25381119

Siddiqi N, Harrison JK, Clegg A, et al: Interventions for preventing delirium in hospitalised non-ICU patients. Cochrane Database Syst Rev (3):CD005563, 2016 26967259

Silver GM, Albright JM, Schermer CR, et al: Adverse clinical outcomes associated with elevated blood alcohol levels at the time of burn injury. J Burn Care Res 29(5):784–789, 2008 18695611

Singh R, Ripley D, Pentland B, et al: Depression and anxiety symptoms after lower limb amputation: the rise and fall. Clin Rehabil 23(3):281–286, 2009 19218302

Sjöström L: Bariatric surgery and reduction in morbidity and mortality: experiences from the SOS study. Int J Obes 32 (suppl 7):S93–S97, 2008 19136998

Sjöström L: Review of the key results from the Swedish Obese Subjects (SOS) trial—a prospective controlled intervention study of bariatric surgery. J Intern Med 273(3):219–234, 2013 23163728

Smith PJ, Attix DK, Weldon BC, et al: Executive function and depression as independent risk factors for postoperative delirium. Anesthesiology 110(4):781–787, 2009 19326492

Sockalingam S, Alzahrani A, Meaney C, et al: Time to consultation-liaison psychiatry service referral as a predictor of length of stay. Psychosomatics 57(3):264–272, 2016 27005725

Sockalingam S, Micula-Gondek W, Lundblad W, et al; Council on Psychosomatic Medicine: Bariatric surgery and psychiatric care. Am J Psychiatry 174(1):81–82, 2017 28041006

Sogg S, Friedman KE: Getting off the right foot: the many roles of the psychosocial evaluation in the bariatric surgery practice. Eur Eat Disord Rev 23(6):451–456, 2015 26294256

Sogg S, Lauretti J, West-Smith L: Recommendations for the presurgical psychosocial evaluation of bariatric surgery patients. Surg Obes Relat Dis 12(4):731–749, 2016 27179400

Spies CD, Rommelspacher H: Alcohol withdrawal in the surgical patient: prevention and treatment. Anesth Analg 88(4):946–954, 1999 10195555

Spies CD, Neuner B, Neumann T, et al: Intercurrent complications in chronic alcoholic men admitted to the intensive care unit following trauma. Intensive Care Med 22(4):286–293, 1996 8708164

Spies CD, von Dossow V, Eggers V, et al: Altered cell-mediated immunity and increased postoperative infection rate in long-term alcoholic patients. Anesthesiology 100(5):1088–1100, 2004 15114205

Stoddard FJ Jr, Luthra R, Sorrentino EA, et al: A randomized controlled trial of sertraline to prevent posttraumatic stress disorder in burned children. J Child Adolesc Psychopharmacol 21(5):469–477, 2011 22040192

Strain JJ: Needs for psychiatry in the general hospital. Hosp Community Psychiatry 33(12):996–1001, 1982 7152502

Stuerz K, Piza H, Niermann K, Kinzl JF: Psychosocial impact of abdominoplasty. Obes Surg 18(1):34–38, 2008 18080729

Subedi B, Grossberg GT: Phantom limb pain: mechanisms and treatment approaches. Pain Res Treat 2011:864605, 2011 22110933

Sury MR: Accidental awareness during anesthesia in children. Paediatr Anaesth 26(5):468–474, 2016 27059416

Sveen J, Öster C: Alcohol consumption after severe burn: a prospective study. Psychosomatics 56(4):390–396, 2015 25553819

Szakáts I, Sebestyén M, Tóth É, Purebl G: Dry eye symptoms, patient-reported visual functioning, and health anxiety influencing patient satisfaction after cataract surgery. Curr Eye Res 42(6):832–836, 2017 28129000

Taylor D, Hassan MA, Luterman A, Rodning CB: Unexpected intraoperative patient death: the imperatives of family- and surgeon-centered care. Arch Surg 143(1):87–92, 2008 18209158

Taylor D, Luterman A, Richards WO, et al: Application of the core competencies after unexpected patient death: consolation of the grieved. J Surg Educ 70(1):37–47, 2013 23337669

Ter Smitten MH, de Graaf R, Van Loey NE: Prevalence and co-morbidity of psychiatric disorders 1–4 years after burn. Burns 37(5):753–761, 2011 21334824

Thiara G, Yanofsky R, Abdul-Kader S, et al: Toronto Bariatric Interprofessional Psychosocial Assessment Suitability Scale: evaluating a new clinical assessment tool for bariatric surgery candidates. Psychosomatics 57(2):165–173, 2016 26895728

Thombs BD, Singh VA, Halonen J, et al: The effects of preexisting medical comorbidities on mortality and length of hospital stay in acute burn injury: evidence from a national sample of 31,338 adult patients. Ann Surg 245(4):629–634, 2007 17414613

Thomson L, Sheehan KA, Meaney C, et al: Prospective study of psychiatric illness as a predictor of weight loss and health related quality of life one year after bariatric surgery. J Psychosom Res 86:7–12, 2016 27302540

Tignol J, Biraben-Gotzamanis L, Martin-Guehl C, et al: Body dysmorphic disorder and cosmetic surgery: evolution of 24 subjects with a minimal defect in appearance 5 years after their request for cosmetic surgery. Eur Psychiatry 22(8):520–524, 2007 17900876

Tønnesen H, Kehlet H: Preoperative alcoholism and postoperative morbidity. Br J Surg 86(7):869–874, 1999 10417555

Tønnesen H, Petersen KR, Højgaard L, et al: Postoperative morbidity among symptom-free alcohol misusers. Lancet 340(8815):334–337, 1992 1353805

Tremblay P, Gold S: Prevention of post-operative delirium in the elderly using pharmacological agents. Can Geriatr J 19(3):113–126, 2016 27729950

Ullrich PM, Askay SW, Patterson DR: Pain, depression, and physical functioning following burn injury. Rehabil Psychol 54(2):211–216, 2009 19469612

Valdés M, de Pablo J, Campos R, et al: El proyecto multinacional europeo y multicéntrico español de mejora de calidad asistencial en psiquiatría de enlace en el hospital general: el perfil clínico en España (in Spanish) [Multinational European project and multicenter Spanish study of quality improvement of assistance on consultation-liaison psychiatry in general hospital: clinical profile in Spain]. Med Clin (Barc) 115(18):690–694, 2000 11141428

van Haelst IM, van Klei WA, Doodeman HJ, et al; MAOI Study Group: Antidepressive treatment with monoamine oxidase inhibitors and the occurrence of intraoperative hemodynamic events: a retrospective observational cohort study. J Clin Psychiatry 73(8):1103–1109, 2012 22938842

van Heeringen C, De Schryver A, Verbeek E: Sexual function disorders after local radiotherapy for carcinoma of the prostate. Radiother Oncol 13(1):47–52, 1988 3141980

Vonk-Klaassen SM, de Vocht HM, den Ouden MEM, et al: Ostomy-related problems and their impact on quality of life of colorectal cancer ostomates: a systematic review. Qual Life Res 25(1):125–133, 2016 26123983

Ward CM: Consenting and consulting for cosmetic surgery. Br J Plast Surg 51(7):547–550, 1998 9924410

Warren AM, Foreman ML, Bennett MM, et al: Posttraumatic stress disorder following traumatic injury at 6 months: associations with alcohol use and depression. J Trauma Acute Care Surg 76(2):517–522, 2014 24458060

White CA, Hunt JC: Psychological factors in postoperative adjustment to stoma surgery. Ann R Coll Surg Engl 79(1):3–7, 1997 9038488

Wiechman Askay S, Patterson DR, Sharar SR, et al: Pain management in patients with burn injuries. Int Rev Psychiatry 21(6):522–530, 2009 19919205

Wildgoose P, Scott A, Pusic AL, et al: Psychological screening measures for cosmetic plastic surgery patients: a systematic review. Aesthet Surg J 33(1):152–159, 2013 23277623

Wimmelmann CL, Dela F, Mortensen EL: Psychological predictors of mental health and health-related quality of life after bariatric surgery: a review of the recent research. Obes Res Clin Pract 8(4):e314–e324, 2014 25091352

Woodard GA, Downey J, Hernandez-Boussard T, Morton JM: Impaired alcohol metabolism after gastric bypass surgery: a case-crossover trial. J Am Coll Surg 212(2):209–214, 2011 21183366

Yang Y, Zhao X, Dong T, et al: Risk factors for postoperative delirium following hip fracture repair in elderly patients: a systematic review and meta-analysis. Aging Clin Exp Res 29(2):115–126, 2017 26873816

Zatzick DF, Jurkovich GJ, Gentilello L, et al: Posttraumatic stress, problem drinking, and functional outcomes after injury. Arch Surg 137(2):200–205, 2002 11822960

Zatzick DF, Rivara FP, Nathens AB, et al: A nationwide US study of post-traumatic stress after hospitalization for physical injury. Psychol Med 37(10):1469–1480, 2007 17559704

Zelefsky MJ, Eid JF: Elucidating the etiology of erectile dysfunction after definitive therapy for prostatic cancer. Int J Radiat Oncol Biol Phys 40(1):129–133, 1998 9422568

Zheng Y, Wu X, Lin X, Lin H: The prevalence of depression and depressive symptoms among eye disease patients: a systematic review and meta-analysis. Sci Rep 7:46453, 2017 28401923

Ziegler-Graham K, MacKenzie EJ, Ephraim PL, et al: Estimating the prevalence of limb loss in the United States: 2005 to 2050. Arch Phys Med Rehabil 89(3):422–429, 2008 18295618

CHAPTER 29

Organ Transplantation

Andrea F. DiMartini, M.D.
Akhil Shenoy, M.D.
Mary Amanda Dew, Ph.D.

Solid organ transplantation began in 1954, with a successful kidney transplant in a patient whose identical twin was the donor. For most patients, however, an identical-twin donor was not an option, and more than a decade passed before immunosuppressive medications were available to conquer the immunological barrier. In 1967, the first successful liver transplant was performed, followed a year later by the first successful heart transplant. Even though surgical challenges of solid organ transplantation had been overcome, it was not until the early 1980s, with the advent of improved immunosuppression, that organ transplantation changed from an experimental procedure to a standard of care for many types of end-stage organ disease.

In that decade, the National Organ Transplant Act established the framework for a U.S. national system of organ transplantation, and the United Network for Organ Sharing (UNOS) began to administer the nation's only Organ Procurement and Transplantation Network. In addition to facilitating organ matching and allocation, UNOS collects data about every transplant performed in the United States and maintains information on every organ type (e.g., wait-list counts, survival rates) in an extensive database available online (https://optn.transplant.hrsa.gov).

Although immunological barriers still exist, the greatest obstacle to receiving a transplant is the shortage of donated organs. The number of wait-listed individuals has increased far beyond the availability of donated organs. Currently, nearly 130,000 persons are active on the U.S. waiting list. Patients awaiting kidney transplant (the most common transplant performed) account for 80% of wait-listed patients. By contrast, slightly less than 15,000 patients are waiting for a liver, 4,000 for a heart, and nearly 1,500 for a lung. The numbers of patients receiving transplants in 2016 for each solid organ type (Organ Procurement and Transplantation Network 2017a) were as follows: 147 for intestine, 215 for isolated pancreas, 2,327 for lung, 3,191 for heart,

859

7,841 for liver, and 19,060 for kidney. In Europe, Eurotransplant, an international collaborative of eight European countries, reported 14,533 wait-listed candidates in 2016 but only 6,129 transplants performed in that year, with kidney candidates representing 72% of the wait list and over 50% of transplants (https://eurotransplant.org/cms/index.php?page=home).

For some transplant types (e.g., kidney, liver), living organ donation has become an option to address the organ shortage (see subsection "Living Donor Transplantation" later in this chapter). Although the percentage of living donors who have died due to donation is less than 1%, the numbers of living kidney donors have somewhat declined in recent years. Initiatives to increase the number of kidney donors have met with limited success. Following several highly publicized U.S. liver donor deaths beginning in 2002, the numbers of living liver donors decreased by about 50%. It appears that liver donation rates are beginning to rebound somewhat. In the absence of an identified living donor, transplant candidates may wait years for an organ. The median wait-listed time depends on the organ type and the recipient's blood type and severity of illness and, for some organs, body size. Kidney candidates have the longest wait times, with a median wait of 4.2 years, whereas the median wait for lung candidates is only 4 months (Organ Procurement and Transplantation Network 2017a). While on the waiting list, 4%–10% of organ candidates become medically unsuitable and are removed from the list, and 10%–15% die (Organ Procurement and Transplantation Network 2017a).

Following transplantation, living-donor kidney and liver recipients experience the highest long-term survival rates (78% and 73%, respectively, are still alive at 10 years posttransplantation) (Figure 29–1) (US DHHS Health Resources and Services Administration 2012). Recipients of deceased-donor kidneys, livers, and hearts have somewhat lower 10-year survival rates (63%, 61%, and 58%, respectively), and intestine and lung recipients have the poorest 10-year survival rates (47% and 30%, respectively) (Organ Procurement and Transplantation Network 2017a). Advances in technology, immunosuppression, and medical care will most likely provide better survival rates for future recipients. However, overall graft survival rates are significantly lower than patient survival rates (e.g., graft survival rates after 10 years are 49% for kidneys and 45% for livers), which means that many transplant recipients may have to face a second transplant 5–10 years after their first (Organ Procurement and Transplantation Network 2017a). In addition, among other risk factors, chronic exposure to nephrotoxic immunosuppressive medication contributes to a 7%–21% 5-year risk of chronic renal failure after transplantation of a nonrenal organ (Ojo et al. 2003), requiring some patients to pursue an additional kidney transplant.

These stark facts highlight the enormous stresses facing transplant candidates, recipients, and their caregivers. These issues have also created an environment in which hospitals must evaluate, treat, and select patients for organ transplantation. The scarcity of donated organs has driven efforts to select candidates believed to have the best chance for optimal posttransplant outcomes.

Pretransplant psychosocial evaluations are commonly requested to assist in candidate and living donor selection, and psychiatric consultation is often needed for clinical input during the pre- and posttransplant phases. A wide body of knowledge on the clinical care of transplant candidates and recipients has been accumulated, and longitudinal research is increasingly available to answer questions about long-term

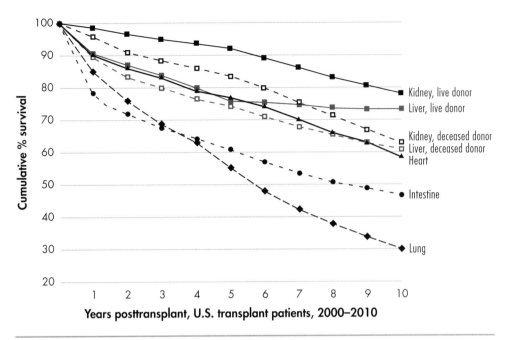

FIGURE 29–1. Survival rates of transplant recipients, by organ type.

Source. U.S. Department of Health and Human Services, Health Resources and Services Administration, Scientific Registry of Transplant Recipients: Organ Procurement and Transplantation Network (OPTN) and Scientific Registry of Transplant Recipients (SRTR) 2011 Annual Data Report. Rockville, MD, U.S. Department of Health and Human Services, Health Resources and Services Administration, Healthcare Systems Bureau, Division of Transplantation, 2012. Available at: https://srtr.transplant.hrsa.gov/annual_reports/2011/Default.aspx. Accessed September 26, 2017.

outcomes and the impact of psychiatric factors—whether assessed pretransplant or in the early years posttransplantation—on outcomes. Research has focused primarily on kidney, heart, and liver transplantation.

In this chapter, we outline the essential information for psychiatric consultants and other mental health clinicians involved in the care of transplant patients—pretransplant assessment and candidate selection, emotional and psychological aspects of the transplant process, therapeutic issues, patients with complex or controversial features, psychopharmacological treatment, and neuropsychiatric side effects of immunosuppressive medications. Specific transplantation issues are also discussed in Chapter 17, "Heart Disease"; Chapter 18, "Lung Disease"; Chapter 19, "Gastrointestinal Disorders"; Chapter 20, "Renal Disease"; and Chapter 32, "Pediatrics."

Pretransplantation Issues

Psychosocial/Psychiatric Assessment

Pretransplant psychosocial assessment has been a traditional role of consultation–liaison psychiatrists. These assessments are frequently used to assist in the determination of a candidate's eligibility for transplantation and to identify psychiatric and/or psychosocial problems and needs that must be addressed to prepare the candidate and family for transplantation. These evaluations are also critical for identifying psychiatric, behavioral, and psychosocial risk factors that may portend poor transplant outcomes (Crone and Wise 1999; Dew et al. 2000, 2015).

Transplant programs often refer for pretransplant psychosocial evaluation those candidates with a known history of psychiatric problems, substance use disorders (including tobacco), and other poor health conditions and behaviors (e.g., obesity, treatment noncompliance). The process and conduct of the psychosocial evaluation varies by program and available staff. Social workers often provide an initial screening, and candidates identified as having psychiatric issues are referred to the mental health team for further evaluation. Some centers employ screening batteries of patient-rated measures to identify candidates with elevated levels of psychological distress, who then undergo a full psychiatric evaluation. Screening instruments can provide baseline cognitive, affective, and psychosocial information on candidates; use of these instruments may help maximize staff resources and minimize costs. For example, using this strategy, Jowsey et al. (2002) identified 20%–44% of potential liver transplant candidates who endorsed symptoms on a range of screening measures, which prompted a higher level of evaluation.

Transplant programs vary considerably in their psychosocial assessment criteria and procedures (see Levenson and Olbrisch 2000 for a review of methodological and philosophical issues). In general, however, psychosocial evaluations have 10 objectives (although a given assessment may not include all 10), as enumerated in Table 29–1 (see Levenson and Olbrisch 2000).

Because information on all of these domains may not be obtainable during a single clinical interview, a follow-up interview and reassessment may be necessary to clarify relevant issues, solidify a working relationship with the patient and family, and resolve problems. Collateral information may be required from the medical record and other medical and psychiatric providers. A multidisciplinary approach is often used, with input from psychiatrists, psychologists, psychiatric nurse clinical specialists, addiction specialists, social workers, transplant physicians, and transplant coordinators, to construct a comprehensive picture of the patient and develop a coordinated treatment plan. As in any psychiatric evaluation, verbal feedback provided to the patient and family will serve to reiterate the expectations of the transplant team and the requirements of the patient for transplant listing. Some centers also use written "contracts" to formalize these recommendations (Cupples and Steslowe 2001; DiMartini et al. 2011; Masson et al. 2014). In difficult cases, these contracts document expectations, thereby minimizing misinterpretation. These contracts are particularly useful with candidates who have substance use disorders, because they specify the transplant program's requirements for addiction treatment, monitoring of adherence (e.g., documented random negative blood alcohol levels), and length of abstinence (see subsection "Alcohol" under "Substance Use Disorders" later in this chapter). Potential candidates may be requested to engage in treatment and return for reevaluation to determine if transplant treatment goals have been met.

Psychosocial Instruments and Measures

Instruments that have been used to evaluate transplant candidates and monitor their posttransplant recovery include transplant-specific instruments (e.g., Psychosocial

TABLE 29–1. **Goals of psychosocial screening**

1. Assess coping skills; intervene with patients who appear to be unable to cope effectively.

2. Diagnose comorbid psychiatric conditions; provide for pre- and posttransplant monitoring and treatment.

3. Determine the candidate's capacity to understand the transplant process and to provide informed consent.

4. Evaluate the candidate's ability to collaborate with the transplant team and to adhere to treatment.

5. Assess substance use/abuse history, recovery, and ability to maintain long-term abstinence.

6. Identify health behaviors that may influence posttransplant morbidity and mortality (e.g., tobacco use, poor eating or exercise habits) and evaluate the candidate's ability to modify these behaviors over the long term.

7. Help the transplant team to understand the patient better as a person.

8. Evaluate the level of social support available to the candidate for pre- and posttransplant phases (including stable family/others committed to assisting the candidate, adequate insurance and financial resources, and logistical support).

9. Determine the psychosocial needs of the patient and family and plan for services during the waiting, recovery, and rehabilitation phases of the transplant process.

10. Establish baseline measures of mental functioning in order to be able to monitor postoperative changes.

Source. Adapted from Levenson J, Olbrisch ME: "Psychosocial Screening and Selection of Candidates for Organ Transplantation," in *The Transplant Patient.* Cambridge, UK, Cambridge University Press, 2000, p. 23. Used with permission.

Assessment of Candidates for Transplantation [PACT; Olbrisch et al. 1989], Transplant Evaluation Rating Scale [TERS; Twillman et al. 1993], Stanford Integrated Psychosocial Assessment for Transplant [SIPAT; Maldonado et al. 2008]); disease-specific instruments (e.g., Miller Health Attitude Scale for cardiac disease [Miller et al. 1982], Chronic Respiratory Disease Questionnaire [Guyatt et al. 1987]); and disorder-specific instruments (e.g., High-Risk Alcohol Relapse Scale for alcoholism [Yates et al. 1993]). These instruments have been used in conjunction with general instruments for rating behavior, coping, cognitive and affective states, and quality of life (QOL) (Corbett et al. 2013). Psychosocial instruments can be used to identify individuals who require further assessment (as described in the previous subsection) or to pursue evaluation of patients already identified as requiring additional screening. The evaluator's purpose for using such instruments will determine the type and specificity of the instruments chosen (e.g., the use of neuropsychiatric tests to aid in the identification of cognitive impairment). Some instruments are more applicable to transplant populations than others. For example, although many instruments and measures are available for assessing alcoholism, they all are focused on general issues of detection and treatment of addiction rather than on issues important in evaluating appropriateness for transplantation. Formal cognitive testing may be appropriate to delineate cognitive deficits, taking into consideration the potential contribution of deficits that may be transient and related to the current degree of illness (e.g., delirium; see subsection "Cognitive Disorders and Delirium" later in this chapter). (For a systematic review of the utility of psychological measures in predicting liver transplant outcomes, see Fineberg et al. 2016.)

Because psychosocial selection criteria differ significantly by program and organ type, development and use of structured evaluation instruments may help to direct and standardize the transplant selection protocols used nationally. The Structured Interview for Renal Transplantation (SIRT; Mori et al. 2000) is a structured yet flexible interview tool designed to guide the clinician efficiently through a comprehensive interview of pertinent information for potential renal transplant candidates. Use of the SIRT requires sound clinical judgment. The instrument can also be used for training clinicians and for research (Mori et al. 2000). This instrument is not scored, and there are no ratings for transplant candidacy. Three other instruments commonly used to assess candidates for transplantation are the PACT, the TERS, and the SIPAT. Different from structured interviews with specific items or questions, these instruments can serve as heuristic tools to aid clinicians in considering and integrating the data gathered from their interviews in the candidacy determination.

Unique Role of the Psychiatric Consultant

Unlike in most clinical interviews, the psychiatrist performing the pre-transplant assessment while identifying the needs of the transplant candidate will also be proposing what psychiatric issues, if any, are conditional for listing. These requirements may be specific to transplantation, and the psychiatric consultant must be candid with the patient about the consultant's role of providing the transplant team with psychiatric recommendations regarding the patient's candidacy. Careful delineation of specific transplant-related expectations, explanation of the importance of these requirements to the success of transplantation, and exploration of the implications of these criteria for the individual candidate serve to establish a meaningful dialogue with the patient from which the therapeutic alliance necessary for future intervention can develop.

For the clinician, this role can be uncomfortable or even anxiety provoking. This is especially true if the clinician is not recommending the candidate for transplantation. Fortunately, many programs do not reject patients outright for psychosocial reasons; rather, they offer such patients the opportunity to work to bring their problematic areas into alignment with the recommendations (i.e., through addiction counseling, behavioral changes, psychiatric treatment, identification of appropriate social supports) and to then undergo reevaluation for candidacy. In these cases, the psychiatric consultant can often function as an advocate for the patient and assist in referral for appropriate treatment if indicated. Rather than being a "gatekeeper," the mental health clinician has the role of optimizing the preparation of the patient. A team makes a determination regarding whether a patient with complex psychosocial issues can be successfully transplanted at their program. Nevertheless, some patients will be unable to comply with the specified transplant requirements or will not survive to complete their efforts to meet candidacy requirements.

Philosophical, moral, ethical, legal, and therapeutic dilemmas are inherent in the role of transplant psychiatrist, as conflicting team opinions present themselves with potential transplant candidates. Team discussions and consultation with other colleagues are the rule in complicated cases. In these instances, team discussions not only aid in resolving candidacy quandaries but also can help alleviate team members' anxiety and discomfort over declining a patient for transplantation. Group or team debriefing may also be desirable, and occasionally consultation with the ethics committee (or consult service), risk management, and/or the legal department of the hospital is needed (e.g., when a candidate is challenging candidacy requirements or the team's candidacy decision). Thorough documentation is essential in order to delineate the issues involved, the expectations of the team for transplantation candidacy, and the efforts to work with the patient.

Psychological and Psychiatric Issues in Organ Transplantation

Psychiatric Symptoms and Disorders in Transplant Patients

Similar to other medically ill populations, transplant candidates and recipients experience a significant amount of psychological distress and are at heightened risk of developing psychiatric disorders. Following transplantation, 20% of kidney, 30% of liver, and up to 60% of heart recipients develop mood and anxiety disorders within the first year (Corbett et al. 2013). Reported prevalence rates for anxiety disorders after transplantation have ranged from 3% to 33% (Dew 2003; Dew et al. 2000), but there are too few studies to identify rates for specific anxiety disorders. Clinicians should consider and screen for posttraumatic stress disorder (PTSD) related to the transplant experience; studies estimate that 3%–15% of transplant recipients develop PTSD or posttraumatic stress symptoms, with associated poorer QOL (Baranyi et al. 2013; Corbett et al. 2013; Jin et al. 2012). In a prospective study that followed 178 lung recipients and 126 heart recipients for the first 2 years after transplantation, the cumulative prevalence rates for psychiatric disorders were 58% and 47%, respectively, for any disorder, including 25% and 30%, respectively, for major depressive disorder; 18% and 8%, respectively, for panic disorder; and 15% and 14%, respectively, for PTSD (Dew et al. 2012). Whereas new onset of panic disorder or PTSD was limited to the first year posttransplantation, new onset of major depressive disorder occurred over the entire 2-year period. Lung recipients were at significantly heightened risk for panic disorder. Other factors that increased the cumulative risk for psychiatric disorders included a pretransplant psychiatric history, female gender, longer wait for transplant, early posttransplant health problems, and psychosocial characteristics (e.g., poorer caregiver support, use of avoidant coping). Studies have found that a pattern of high depression rates in candidates awaiting transplant (across all organ types), with improvements in the short term after transplantation, was associated with better QOL (Akman et al. 2004; Fusar-Poli et al. 2007; Miller et al. 2013). However, dramatic increases in depressive symptoms can accompany early graft loss (Akman et al. 2004) or can develop with long-term (>3 years) decline in functional status (Dew and DiMartini 2011; Fusar-Poli et al. 2005, 2007). In lung transplant recipients, contributors to depression included male gender, comorbid personality disorders, poor coping strategies, life stressors, physical complications, corticosteroid use in the short term after transplantation, and lack of psychosocial support (Fusar-Poli et al. 2007).

Studies show that clinically significant depression or depressive symptoms, whether assessed prior to (Smith et al. 2014) or following transplant (Farmer et al. 2013; Smith et al. 2014), can be associated with negative clinical outcomes following transplant. In one of the few prospective studies to focus on this topic, Rosenberger et al. (2016) used a structured DSM-IV-TR (American Psychiatric Association 2000) interview to identify anxiety and depression in a cohort of lung transplant recipients; they found that posttransplant depression predicted not only poorer patient and graft survival but also the development of chronic rejection (bronchiolitis obliterans syndrome). Anxiety, however, was not associated with poorer outcomes. A meta-analysis of studies examining whether depression or anxiety affected risk for posttransplant morbidity and mortality found that depression, either pre- or posttransplant, predicted poorer survival (Dew et al. 2015). Morbidity was less often studied than mortality but also appeared to be negatively affected by depression, especially death-censored graft loss. In the meta-analysis, few studies examined the effects of anxiety; although anxiety was modestly associated with increased mortality, the association did not reach significance (Dew et al. 2015). A study of heart transplant recipients found that pretransplant major depressive disorder was a significant independent predictor of posttransplant malignancies (Favaro et al. 2011). It is unclear whether treatment of psychiatric disorders will affect patient outcomes, although one study suggested that adequate psychotropic treatment of depression may improve patient outcomes (Rogal et al. 2013). Regardless of whether treatment improves medical outcomes, the role of the psychiatrist in evaluating, diagnosing, and treating psychiatric disorders both pre- and posttransplantation remains critical.

Adaptation to Transplantation

Transplant candidates typically experience a series of adaptive challenges as they proceed through evaluation, waiting, perioperative management, postoperative recuperation, and long-term adaptation to life with a transplant (Dew and DiMartini 2011; Olbrisch et al. 2002; Rosenberger et al. 2012) (Figure 29–2). With chronic illness, there can be progressive debility and gradual loss of vitality and of physical and social functioning. Patients may progressively lose their ability to work, participate in social/family activities, and drive, and may even require assistance with activities of daily living. With these losses of functioning will come the loss of important roles in the family (e.g., breadwinner, parent, spouse, caregiver). Adapting to these changes can elicit anxiety, depression, anger, avoidance, and denial and requires the working through of grief (Olbrisch et al. 2002). Patients may express their distress or ambivalence by missing appointments or procedures or by failing to complete requirements for transplant listing. Patients who are wait-listed may develop contraindications to transplantation (e.g., infection, serious stroke, progressive organ dysfunction), and both patients and families should be made aware that a candidate's eligibility can change over time for many reasons (Stevenson 2002). During this phase, psychiatrists may provide counseling to patients and families to help them navigate these transitions and prepare for either transplantation or death.

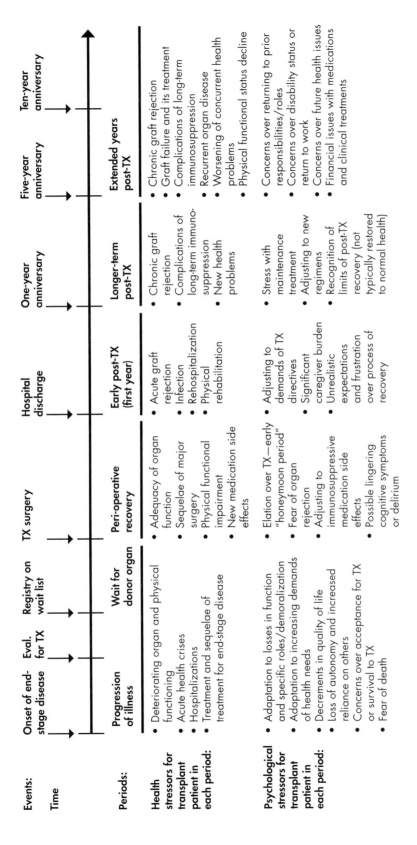

FIGURE 29–2. Organ transplantation timeline: discrete time periods with attendant issues for transplant patients.

Note. Eval.=evaluation; TX=treatment, specifically transplantation.

Source. Adapted from Dew MA, DiMartini AF, Kormos RL: "Organ Transplantation, Stress of," in *Encyclopedia of Stress,* 2nd Edition, Vol 3. Edited by Fink G. Oxford, UK, Academic Press/Elsevier, 2007b, pp. 35–44.

The summons for transplantation can evoke a mixture of elation and great fear. Patients can develop anticipatory anxiety while waiting for the call from the transplant team. Patients may experience panic when they are called for transplantation, and some—due to anxiety, fear, ambivalence, or not feeling ready—may even decline the offer of an organ.

Much of illness behavior depends on the coping strategies and personality style of the individual. In our experience, the adaptive styles of adult transplant recipients often depend on whether patients' pretransplant illness experience was chronic or acute, as delineated in the following broadly generalized profiles.

Patients who have dealt with chronic illness for years may adapt psychologically to the sick role and can develop coping strategies that perpetuate a dependency on being ill (Olbrisch et al. 2002). For these patients, transplantation may psychologically represent a transition from one state of illness to another, and such patients can have difficulty adjusting to or transitioning into a "state of health." They often complain that the transplant team is expecting too fast a recovery from them, and they may describe feeling pressured to get better. Some patients may develop unexplained chronic pain or other somatic complaints or may begin to evince nonadherence to transplant team directives.

For patients with good premorbid functioning who become acutely ill, with only a short period of pretransplant infirmity, the transplant can be an unwelcome event. These patients can experience a heightened sense of vulnerability, and they may deny the seriousness of their medical situation (Olbrisch et al. 2002). They often wish to return to normal functioning as quickly as possible posttransplantation, and they may recover more rapidly than the transplant team expects; however, they may suffer later as a result of pushing themselves too much (e.g., returning to work before they are physically ready). They may resent being transplant recipients, with the inherent restrictions and regimens, and may act out their anger or denial in episodes of nonadherence (Olbrisch et al. 2002).

Treatment Modalities With a Focus on Transplant-Specific Issues

Patients with psychological or psychiatric issues can benefit from traditional psychotherapies (reviewed in this section) and pharmacotherapy (reviewed later in chapter). Many programs employ educational groups to prepare patients for transplant and recovery. Patients identified as having psychosocial problems during these sessions or during the psychosocial evaluation are commonly referred to local providers for assistance. Psychotherapeutic treatments will likely focus on transplant-specific issues, and because local transplant expertise may not be available, consultation psychiatrists may need to educate therapists on how to address these issues. For example, in a prospective study of kidney transplant recipients, three recurring psychological themes were expressed by patients: 1) fear of organ rejection, 2) feelings of paradoxical loss after surgery despite successful transplantation, and 3) psychological adaptation to the new kidney (Baines et al. 2002). The study demonstrated that individual psychotherapy was effective in resolving transplant-related emotional problems, with significant reductions in depressive symptoms after therapy. Other transplant-specific themes, such as perceiving a loss of control over outcomes and/or attributing outcomes to chance, can be associated with depressed affect (Cukor et al. 2008) and may offer a focus for intervention.

In addition to traditional therapies, various innovative strategies have been employed to deal with specific transplantation issues and also to address logistical issues (e.g., distance from program, transportation, physical debility, lack of local expertise) and staffing resources. Two studies of wait-listed candidates successfully demonstrated the use of telephone therapy to overcome logistical barriers and deal with transplant-specific themes (e.g., uncertainty management, QOL, caregiver support) (Bailey et al. 2017; Rodrigue et al. 2011). Peer mentoring has become increasingly popular and is available at some transplant programs and through online resources (e.g., http://www.americantransplantfoundation.org/programs/mentorship-program-2/). Mentorship by a transplant recipient can augment patient care by providing information and support from a peer perspective (Wright et al. 2001). At the University of Toronto mentoring program, the four topics most commonly discussed between mentors and mentees were postoperative complications, medications, wait on the transplant list, and the surgery itself (L. Wright et al. 2001). To increase patient satisfaction with a mentor program, Wright et al. (2001) recommend early introduction of a mentor and matching of mentors with mentees according to demographics and clinical course. One innovative three-pronged intervention was designed to improve kidney recipients' QOL using 1) proactive, patient-initiated care to prevent transplant-related morbidities (education on self-assessment, Web-based and learning library materials); 2) employment/vocational counseling with a rehabilitation counselor; and 3) enhancement of social support (trained peer-mentors, support group, social worker counseling on support network) (Chang et al. 2004). Not only was the intervention cost-effective, but the patients in the intervention had significantly better QOL and had more quality-adjusted treatment-free days.

Group psychotherapy for organ transplant patients and family members has also been successfully used. Abbey and Farrow (1998) described a program in which group psychotherapy was organized along three dimensions: course of illness (pre- vs. posttransplantation), homogeneous versus heterogeneous group membership (e.g., separate groups for patients and caregivers vs. integrated groups, organ-specific groups vs. cross-organ groups), and group focus (issue-specific vs. unstructured). Group therapy participants reported decreases in negative affect, increases in positive affect and happiness, less illness intrusiveness, and improved QOL. Transplant coordinators also reported that patients in group therapy required less contact, both in clinic and by telephone for social support.

Internet resources for transplant patient information and support are increasing, but few studies have examined the impact of Internet-delivered transplant interventions for mental health issues. Dew et al. (2004) designed and evaluated an Internet-based psychosocial intervention for heart transplant recipients and their families. This multifaceted intervention included stress and medical regimen management workshops, monitored discussion groups, access to electronic communication with the transplant team, and information on transplant-related health issues. Compared with recipients without access to the Web site, intervention patients and their caregivers reported significant reductions in symptoms of mental distress, and patients also experienced improvements in QOL and medication adherence (Dew et al. 2004). A recent review of studies examining mobile health interventions for organ transplant patients identified several apps designed to improve pretransplant knowledge and QOL, as well as educational apps targeting posttransplant medication regimen adherence, but the studies were limited to measuring feasibility and identifying themes for future interventional studies (Fleming et al. 2017). Most mobile apps target adherence to transplant directives (see "Posttransplant Regimen Adherence" subsection below).

Patients With Complex or Controversial Psychosocial and Psychiatric Issues

The stringency of selection criteria for transplantation appears to depend on the type of organ transplant being considered, and transplant programs often have strongly ingrained beliefs about the suitability of candidates with certain types of mental illness. Cardiac transplant programs are more likely than liver transplant programs to consider psychosocial issues as contraindications, and liver transplant programs in turn are more stringent than kidney transplant programs (Butt et al. 2014b). These differences may be attributable to the relative availability of specific types of organs (Yates et al. 1993); alternatively, the extent of experience with specific organ transplants may allow programs to feel more comfortable with less stringent criteria (e.g., kidney transplantation, with more than three decades of experience and more than 400,000 kidney transplants performed in the United States) (Organ Procurement and Transplantation Network 2017a). In addition, for kidney transplantation, cost-effectiveness research has clearly demonstrated the long-term cost savings of kidney transplantation relative to dialysis; with such unequivocal evidence, insurance payers have a strong financial incentive to refer patients early for preemptive transplantation, before the high costs of dialysis begin to accumulate (Eggers 1992). In such a setting, psychosocial factors may have less impact on transplantation candidacy. Other issues influencing the selection process include moral and ethical beliefs, societal views, personal beliefs, and even financial constraints. One study of kidney candidates found that those with a history of mental disorders or nonadherence were less likely to even complete the transplant workup within 2 years of referral (Mucsi et al. 2017).

Although each additional indicator of poor prognosis present during the perioperative period may increase the risk of nonadherence posttransplantation (Fine et al. 2009; Nevins et al. 2017; see "Posttransplant Regimen Adherence" below), it should be emphasized that candidates with any one of these features are not categorically poor recipients and, conversely, that patients without any of these features do not categorically make the best candidates. However, clinical assumptions that patients with certain personality disorders, substance use disorders, poor coping skills, poor adherence, and poor social supports will have worse posttransplant outcomes are increasingly supported by research. Nevertheless, case reports have demonstrated that even some patients who might seem inappropriate for transplant—for example, patients with active psychosis (DiMartini and Twillman 1994; Shapiro 2005), severe personality disorders (Carlson et al. 2000), or intellectual disability (Samelson-Jones et al. 2012)—can successfully undergo transplantation and maintain adequate adherence to medication regimens after the procedure. Patients with such conditions should be carefully assessed before transplantation, with optimization of their condition followed by ongoing psychiatric monitoring and treatment after transplantation. These cases demonstrate that with expert management, good social support, and a longitudinal relationship with the transplant team, even complicated patients, such as those with severe psychiatric disorders, can have positive long-term outcomes. An analysis of 822 solid organ transplants in the U.S. Veterans Administration system found that 17% of transplant recipients suffered from a serious mental illness (including schizophrenia and other psychotic disorders, bipolar disorder, major depressive disorder, and severe PTSD), and another 30% carried other psychiatric diagnoses (Evans et al. 2015). The investigators found no differences among those with serious mental illnesses, other mental illness, and no mental health diagnosis in attendance at follow-up appointments, frequency of filling immunosuppressant prescriptions, or 3-year mortality. On the other hand, if optimal management is not provided in complex cases, patient and graft survival can be adversely affected (Abbott et al. 2003).

Posttransplant Regimen Adherence

Lifelong immunosuppression is a prerequisite for maintaining graft function, and nonadherence to immunosuppressive medication regimens is often associated with late acute rejection episodes, chronic rejection, graft loss, and death. It might be assumed that transplant patients, in general, constitute a highly motivated group and that their adherence levels would be high. Unfortunately, in common with other patients living with chronic disease, organ recipients often experience difficulty in maintaining high levels of adherence to the multiple components of their regimens (DeVito Dabbs et al. 2016; Dew et al. 2007a). In a meta-analysis involving nearly 150 studies of all organ types, average annual nonadherence rates ranged from 1–4 cases per 100 patients for substance use (including tobacco, alcohol, and illicit drugs) to 19–25 cases per 100 patients for a variety of other areas of noncompliance (immunosuppressant medication, diet, exercise, and other transplant health care requirements) (Dew et al. 2007a). Medication nonadherence was especially high, and clinicians can expect to see 23 nonadherent patients for every 100 individuals seen during a given year of follow-up. Immunosuppressant nonadherence was highest in kidney recipients (36 cases per 100 patients annually, vs. 7–15 cases per 100 patients for recipients of other organs).

Nonadherence to immunosuppressive medications impairs both life quality and life span; it is a major risk factor for graft-rejection episodes and may be responsible for up to 36% of graft loss after the initial recovery period (Fine et al. 2009; Laederach-Hofmann and Bunzel 2000). Nonadherence leads to waste, as it reduces the potential benefits of therapy and adds to the costs of treating avoidable consequent morbidity. Graft loss from nonadherence is also tragic, given the large numbers of patients on the waiting lists. Global assessment of posttransplant regimen adherence is difficult, and patients can manifest varying degrees of adherence to medical recommendations. Moreover, the medical recommendations pertain to a multifaceted regimen of care. For transplant recipients, adherence to immunosuppressants is typically the chief area of focus. Even occasional missing of a dose can have deleterious consequences, with some studies suggesting that less than 95% adherence is sufficient to produce poorer outcomes (Fine et al. 2009; Nevins et al. 2017). Studies using electronic monitoring of pill taking through special medicine containers have demonstrated that medication nonadherence can begin shortly after transplant and increases over time (Fine et al. 2009; Nevins et al. 2017).

Given the extent and critical nature of nonadherence, research has focused on efforts to predict and prevent it. Factors associated with posttransplantation nonadherence include younger age (i.e., adolescence or young adulthood), pretransplant nonadherence, depression and anxiety, substance misuse, poor coping, poorer perceived self-efficacy, poorer perceived health, poor support, poor health literacy, lower socioeconomic status, greater regimen complexity, and differences in health care systems (Calia et al. 2015; Dew et al. 2007a; Fine et al. 2009; Nevins et al. 2017). One study revealed that when risk factors accumulate, adherence problems are likely to rise dramatically (Dew et al. 1996). However, clinical observation of individual patients reveals that there can be many reasons for nonadherence, and an attempt to identify, understand, and correct the reasons is required. Patients may require ongoing or remedial education about the need for lifelong adherence to immunosuppressants. Often, the symptoms of chronic rejection are silent, and recipients may not recognize that they are developing complications because they do not initially feel any adverse effects from discontinuing their medications. Discomfort with medication side effects should be elicited and alleviated if possible. Problems with insurance prescription coverage or other financial issues should be assessed. Additionally, symptoms of depression and anxiety should be identified and treated. Methods to identify nonadherence, measures of medication taking, and tools to explore barriers to adherence have been reviewed by Lam and Fresco (2015). Although self-report can overestimate adherence, it is the most commonly used technique and can provide critical information (Nevins et al. 2017) (Table 29–2).

Adherence in Pediatric Populations

Adherence in pediatric transplant recipients can be additionally complicated by developmental stage, attempts at autonomy/individuation, parental control/support, and parental stress. In a meta-analysis, Dew et al. (2009) found (across all organ types) that nonadherence to clinic appointments and tests was the most common type of nonadherence in pediatric patients, at 12.9 cases per 100 patients annually. The rate of nonadherence to immunosuppressants was 6 cases per 100 patients annually. Older age of the child, worse family functioning (e.g., greater parental distress, lower family cohesion), and poorer psychological status of the child (e.g., poorer behavioral functioning, greater distress) were significantly but only modestly correlated with poorer adherence.

Nonadherent adolescents report poorer health perceptions, lower self-esteem, and more limitations in social and school activities (Fredericks et al. 2008). Better knowledge of medication regimens, using a pillbox to organize medications, and parental involvement in medication administration all contribute to improved adherence among adolescent renal transplant candidates (Zelikovsky et al. 2008).

In an attempt to develop a clinically useful measure of adherence in adolescents and children, Stuber et al. (2008) calculated the standard deviation of tacrolimus blood levels over a 1-year period and found that rather than a one-time "snapshot" or a single abnormal blood level, a threshold-value standard deviation of 2.5 in the tacrolimus level over the year predicted rejection episodes. The reader is also referred to Chapter 32, "Pediatrics," for additional information on adherence in adolescents.

TABLE 29–2.   **Recommendations to clinicians for assessing adherence in transplant recipients**

Inquire about patients' adherence routinely, both early posttransplant and in ensuing years. Consider asking:

How often did you miss a dose of your immunosuppressive medication in the past 4 weeks?

Did you miss more than 1 consecutive dose of your immunosuppressive medication in the past 4 weeks?

Recognize that posttransplant adherence involves multiple activities:

Taking medication

Attending clinic appointments

Self-monitoring of symptoms and vital signs

Completing required tests

Adhering to lifestyle requirements (e.g., diet, exercise)

Avoiding alcohol, illicit drugs, and tobacco

Collect evidence from multiple sources: the patient, spouse/significant other/family, transplant coordinator, laboratory data, and pharmacy records.

Inquire about correlates of nonadherence (e.g., psychological distress/psychiatric disorders, patient/family supports, insurance/financial issues).

Consider psychological, characterological, and other behavioral factors and coping strategies that are possibly playing a role in nonadherence.

Keep in mind that solutions may require multifaceted interventions to address not only nonadherence but also these other contributory factors.

Source.   Adapted from Dew et al. 2009 and Nevins et al. 2017.

Interventions to Improve Medication Adherence

A systematic review of the literature on interventions intended to improve medication adherence in transplant patients found that a combination of cognitive, educational, counseling, and psychological interventions at the patient, health care provider, setting, and system levels was more likely than any single intervention to be effective in the long term (De Bleser et al. 2009). This finding is consistent with the intent underlying the multimodal collaborative approach to chronic disease management. Other studies emphasize the need for patient involvement in the selection of strategies to improve adherence, the importance of patient education, and the value of allowing patients with support to make their own decisions about their care (Chisholm-Burns et al. 2013; Dobbels et al. 2017; Joost et al. 2014; Popoola et al. 2014). Patients may benefit from motivational interviewing or problem-solving therapies to address barriers to adherence. Technology-based strategies for monitoring and supporting adherence are gaining popularity. These strategies include a variety of mobile phone apps, electronic pill monitoring with feedback, and automated text messaging, all of which are well accepted by transplant patients and have been demonstrated to improve adherence (DeVito Dabbs et al. 2009; Dobbels et al. 2017; McGillicuddy et al. 2013; Reese et al. 2017). However, because adherence tends to deteriorate over time

(De Geest et al. 2014), interventions without booster sessions or a maintenance plan are not likely to be effective over the long term.

Substance Use and Disorders

Alcohol

Compared with other solid-organ transplant candidates, liver transplant (LT) candidates more often require psychiatric consultation for substance abuse assessment, due to the prevalence of alcoholic liver disease (ALD) and viral hepatitis transmitted through contaminated needles. An estimated 50% of LT recipients have a pre-LT history of alcohol and/or drug abuse/dependence (DiMartini et al. 2002). ALD is the leading indication for liver transplant in Europe. Although it remains the second most common indication for liver transplant in the United States, it could become the leading indication in the next decade, because of more effective treatment for hepatitis C. Moreover, there are high rates of alcohol use disorder in patients who undergo transplantation for viral hepatitis. The outcomes for patients who undergo liver transplantation for ALD are better than those for patients who undergo transplantation for hepatitis C and are similar to those for transplant patients with all other conditions (Lucey 2014).

In the optimal situation, the psychiatrist is an integral member of the transplant team and can identify problems and integrate the addiction treatment plan into the patient's pre- and posttransplant care. In a prospective study of alcohol consumption follow-up after liver transplantation in which patients were consecutively evaluated by their hepatologist and an addiction specialist, the addiction specialist was able to uncover problematic alcohol use in 41% of posttransplant patients irrespective of the reason for their transplant; in contrast, the identification rate was 22% by the hepatologist (Donnadieu-Rigole et al. 2017). Psychiatric consultation provides a thorough evaluation of the candidate's substance history, the stability of his or her recovery, the candidate's understanding of his or her substance use (especially in the context of his or her health and need for transplantation, lifelong abstinence, and further or ongoing addiction treatment), and the presence of other psychiatric disorders. Family and social support for patients' continued abstinence both pre- and posttransplantation must also be evaluated. The identification of alcohol use disorder in the context of transplantation is complex. Psychological barriers that are common in this disorder, such as shame, guilt, and denial, are heightened in patients seeking transplantation (DiMartini and Dew 2012). The Alcohol Use Disorders Identification Test—Consumption (AUDIT-C; Bush et al. 1998) is a screening tool used at some centers, but collateral information and random toxicological screening are essential for identification of pre- and posttransplant alcohol use. Hepatic encephalopathy and other conditions affecting cognition, such as alcoholic brain damage, can also interfere with the assessment. These transplant candidates often do not perceive a need for help with their addiction because they are focused on the end-organ damage and its management. Motivational enhancement therapy can aid in overcoming resistance to treatment (Weinrieb et al. 2011). Although there is no evidence that an "alcohol contract" confirming the transplant candidate's commitment to abstinence affects alcohol consumption after liver transplant (Masson et al. 2014), not surprisingly those who receive addiction treatment before and after transplant may have the lowest relapse rates (Rodrigue et al.

2013). In one LT center, the introduction of an embedded alcohol addiction unit was associated with a decrease in posttransplant relapse rates (16.4% after vs. 35.1% before introduction of the unit) and an improvement in the 5-year mortality rate in patients who underwent LT for alcoholic cirrhosis (Addolorato et al. 2013).

Relapse rates of 15%–25% have been reported in wait-listed LT candidates, with most relapses identified by biological testing (DiMartini and Dew 2012; Webzell et al. 2011). Blood alcohol level is the most widely used and available test, but due to the fast elimination of ethanol, this test can only detect very recent use. Methanol may provide a longer window of detection and retain specificity, whereas carbohydrate-deficient transferrin can be falsely elevated in liver disease. Ethyl glucuronide, tested in hair, may be useful in LT candidates (Sterneck et al. 2014); this test can detect alcohol use for up to a week and is highly specific. Ultimately, a combination of patient interviews, independent caregiver reports, and biochemical monitoring may be the optimal strategy for identification of alcohol and other substance use in transplant candidates.

A meta-analysis of 50 studies of LT recipients identified an average annual rate of 5.6% for any alcohol use after transplant and 2.5% for heavy use (Dew et al. 2008). Although these rates may appear relatively low, they are cumulative over time, such that by 5 years after transplant, 28% of recipients with ALD will have relapsed to at least some alcohol use, and 12.5% will have engaged in heavy use. Studies from single centers have reported rates of relapse to harmful drinking that can impact outcomes of around 20%–25% (Cuadrado et al. 2005; DiMartini et al. 2010; Dumortier et al. 2015). In one study, one-third of liver recipients who relapsed to heavy alcohol use developed cirrhosis in less than 5 years (Dumortier et al. 2015). In a retrospective study, excessive drinking was associated with increased graft damage and worsened long-term survival (Rice et al. 2013). In another study, by 10 years posttransplant, relapsers drinking more than 30 grams of ethanol a day had significantly poorer survival compared with nonrelapsers (45.1% vs. 85.5%) (Cuadrado et al. 2005). Thus, whereas mild to moderate drinking may not affect outcomes, heavy drinking has demonstrated negative effects. Additionally, in light of the organ shortage, any return to drinking may adversely affect public perceptions of the suitability of allocating organs to patients at high risk for relapse (Neuberger et al. 1998), and transplant teams' morale can be negatively impacted by related poor outcomes (Lee et al. 2017).

Predictors of posttransplant alcohol use have been difficult to identify. This may be due to the heterogeneity of the ALD transplant population and the potential for selection bias (whereby the most stable candidates are chosen), making this population different from the general population of individuals with alcohol abuse/dependence (DiMartini et al. 2002). In addition to the presence of alcohol use disorder, risk factors for relapse include shorter duration of pretransplant sobriety, family history of alcoholism, a diagnosis of alcohol dependence, and low social support (Dew et al. 2008; DiMartini et al. 2010; Rustad et al. 2015). With regard to duration of sobriety, the commonly used 6-month cut point does not appear to be definitive. In general, the longer the duration of sobriety, the lower the risk, with no clear threshold. In some cases, good outcomes are possible with shorter lengths of sobriety. For example, in patients with severe alcoholic hepatitis at high risk for mortality without transplantation, liver transplantation in highly selected cases has resulted in survival and relapse rates comparable to rates of patients in sustained remission (Im et al. 2016; Mathurin et al. 2011).

After transplantation, maintaining an open, nonjudgmental dialogue with transplant recipients may be the most effective way to identify alcohol and/or other substance use, and most recipients are open to discussing their substance use habits with the transplant team (DiMartini et al. 2001; Weinrieb et al. 2000). A review of liver enzymes and biopsy results and a candid discussion of the damage caused by alcohol and other substances provide an opportunity to explore the patient's denial of the consequences of their use. Even in the most difficult cases, patients wish to maintain their health and are willing to listen to advice and recommendations on addiction treatment. In our experience, transplant team personnel are able to establish powerful emotional bonds with recipients. Many patients who have resumed substance use were relieved to learn that the transplant team would not abandon them. On the other hand, it is important not to condone or dismiss small amounts of alcohol or other substance use. What may seem supportive can be distorted by the patient with an addiction and become a tacit permission to use more regularly.

Medications that may reduce cravings and potentially diminish relapse risk for alcohol (e.g., acamprosate, ondansetron, naltrexone) or for opioids (e.g., naltrexone) have not been studied in transplant patients. One study that attempted to use naltrexone in actively alcohol-relapsing LT recipients found that patients were reluctant to use naltrexone because of its potential, albeit small, risk of hepatotoxicity (Weinrieb et al. 2001). Naltrexone can be a direct hepatotoxin at dosages higher than recommended (>300 mg/day) and is not recommended for patients with active hepatitis or liver failure. Baclofen was found in a randomized controlled trial to be safe and efficacious in patients with end-stage liver disease (Addolorato et al. 2007). In nontransplant populations, selective serotonin reuptake inhibitors (SSRIs) and tricyclic antidepressants (TCAs) can stabilize mood and improve abstinence rates in depressed relapsing alcoholic individuals (Cornelius et al. 2003). Anecdotally, acamprosate has been safely used in a number of LT recipients, with some success in decreasing cravings and alcohol use. Because acamprosate is renally excreted, the dosage must be adjusted in renal insufficiency.

Tobacco

Smoking by organ transplant patients has a major impact on outcomes. Despite the availability of effective counseling and pharmacotherapies for smoking cessation, rates of return to smoking after transplant remain high, at 10%–40% (Corbett et al. 2012; Duerinckx et al. 2016). Two meta-analyses of posttransplantation adherence reported annual tobacco use rates of 3.4% among patients in the general transplant population and 10% among transplant recipients with substance use histories (Dew et al. 2007a, 2008). Tobacco use coupled with immunosuppressive therapy, which also increases cancer risk (Nabel 1999), results in higher rates of oropharyngeal and lung cancers, as well as of other malignancies. Tobacco suppresses immunity and can aggravate many disease states, resulting in higher rates of infections, vascular thrombosis, and atherosclerosis. Atherosclerosis is especially problematic for transplant recipients already at risk for hypertension, hyperlipidemia, and hyperglycemia induced by immunosuppressive medication. A meta-analysis across all organ types found that posttransplant smokers had higher rates of newly developed cardiovascular disease and nonskin malignancies, shorter survival times, and higher odds of mortality (Duerinckx et al. 2016).

Studies of heart transplant recipients have reported that 27%–50% of smokers resume smoking after transplantation (Botha et al. 2008; Corbett et al. 2012). Compared with nonsmokers, smokers had higher rates of vasculopathy, malignancies, and renal dysfunction, and significantly worse survival (Arora et al. 2009; Corbett et al. 2012; Duerinckx et al. 2016). Graft coronary artery disease and malignancy attributable to tobacco use have been found to be frequent causes of death following cardiac transplant (Botha et al. 2008). A study of heart transplant recipients found that elevated posttransplant anxiety was associated with a higher risk of resuming smoking (Dew et al. 1996).

A cross-sectional retrospective study of renal transplant recipients identified cigarette smoking as a factor in the progression of kidney disease (Zitt et al. 2007). Compared with nonsmokers, smokers had significant increases in the risk of cardiovascular events, renal fibrosis, graft rejection and graft failure, diabetes, and malignancies (Corbett et al. 2012; Zitt et al. 2007), and showed a fourfold increase in the risk of arteriopathy (Zitt et al. 2007). Previous smoking was also found to be a risk factor for graft failure after kidney transplant (Van Laecke et al. 2017). A study of LT recipients found that smoking cessation 2 years prior to transplantation reduced the incidence of vascular complications by 58% (Pungpapong et al. 2002).

Although historically most cardiothoracic transplant teams have required tobacco and even nicotine discontinuation prior to transplant, only slightly more than 20% of abdominal transplant programs now consider current smoking to be an absolute contraindication to transplant (Butt et al. 2014a). However, given that tobacco use is a modifiable risk factor that has demonstrated significant and negative effects on both patient and graft outcomes and survival, psychiatric consultants should make tobacco use a routine part of their assessments and should provide smoking cessation assistance when necessary. Given the beneficial effects on outcomes, cessation of all tobacco use prior to transplantation is strongly recommended, with close posttransplant monitoring because of the high risk that patients will resume use posttransplantation. Similar to findings regarding pretransplant alcohol use, the shorter the period of pretransplant tobacco abstinence, the higher the risk of relapse posttransplant (Corbett et al. 2012; Duerinckx et al. 2016; Ruttens et al. 2014). Self-reported tobacco use underrepresents actual use, and measurement of urinary cotinine, a metabolite of nicotine, can aid in identification (Corbett et al. 2012; Duerinckx et al. 2016). Treatments for smoking cessation include varenicline, bupropion, nicotine replacement (patches, gum, lozenges, and aerosolized formulations), and behavioral therapies (Hurt et al. 1997; Jorenby et al. 1999). Nicotine replacement strategies have been safely used in patients with advanced liver and lung disease, but severe renal disease may affect nicotine clearance. Nicotine replacement is relatively contraindicated in patients with serious heart disease due to the potential for worsening angina, increasing heart rate, and possibly exacerbating arrhythmias. When nicotine replacement therapy has been combined with bupropion, cases of severe hypertension have been reported, so careful monitoring of blood pressure is indicated. Bupropion should be used cautiously in transplant recipients, who are already at increased risk for seizures from immunosuppressive medications, specifically during the early posttransplant period, when immunosuppressive levels are higher. Because varenicline is eliminated by renal clearance, dosage reductions are necessary for patients with renal insufficiency or on dialysis. Varenicline's side effects of nausea and vomiting may be problematic in transplant patients.

Other Substances

Compared with LT candidates with alcohol dependence, LT candidates with polysubstance dependence are more likely to have multiple prior addiction treatments; more likely to be diagnosed with personality disorders, especially those in Cluster B (antisocial, narcissistic, histrionic, borderline); and less likely to have stable housing, a consistent work history, or reliable social support (Fireman 2000). Despite evidence that this specific population could be at higher risk for relapse, there are few outcome studies addressing posttransplant nonalcohol substance use. Most studies have investigated the rates of relapse only in ALD recipients who also had a nonalcohol substance use disorder. One of the few studies to investigate all patients with a pre-LT addiction history found not only that patients with a pre-LT history of polysubstance use disorders had a higher relapse rate compared with those with alcohol dependence alone (38% vs. 20%) but also that the majority of polysubstance users demonstrated ongoing post-LT substance use (Fireman 2000). In a meta-analysis of eight studies including liver, kidney, and heart recipients, the annual rate of relapse to illicit drug use was 3.7% (Dew et al. 2008). Interestingly, this rate was significantly lower in liver recipients versus other organ recipients (1.9% vs. 6.1%).

Transplant program acceptance of opioid-dependent patients receiving methadone maintenance treatment (MMT) is a controversial issue. Several studies have examined candidate selection processes and posttransplant outcomes for this population. A survey of LT programs (Koch and Banys 2001) found that of the 56% of programs that reported accepting patients for evaluation who were taking methadone, a surprising 32% required patients to discontinue their methadone use prior to transplantation. Of even more concern was the overall lack of experience that programs had with such patients (i.e., only 10% of the programs had treated more than five MMT patients). Although there are no studies of pretransplant methadone cessation in LT patients, abundant evidence suggests that tapering methadone in stable methadone-maintained patients results in relapse to illicit opiate use in up to 82% of these individuals (Ball and Ross 1991). In our opinion, an attempt to taper a recovering opiate addict from methadone should not be made at a time when the patient is struggling with the stresses and pain associated with end-stage liver disease. Until data to the contrary emerge, requiring methadone tapering in stable opiate-dependent patients as a prerequisite for transplant candidacy could be considered unethical. Tapering heightens the risk for relapse, and those who relapse would be denied transplantation.

In regard to posttransplant outcomes of MMT patients, Koch and Banys (2001) found that among approximately 180 transplant patients on MMT, fewer than 10% relapsed to illicit opiate use. In general, regardless of patients' illicit drug use, the transplant programs did not consider that immunosuppressive medication nonadherence (with rates <23%) necessarily affected outcomes, and the transplant coordinators' impressions were that only 7 of the 180 patients had poor outcomes (Koch and Banys 2001). In two small series of MMT LT recipients (N=5 for each), overall long-term patient and graft survival in these recipients were found to be comparable to those in other LT recipients at the transplant centers, with none of the MMT patients evidencing posttransplant nonadherence or relapse to illicit drug use (Hails and Kanchana 2000; Kanchana et al. 2002). Liu et al. (2003), in a study of the largest single cohort

(*N*=36) of MMT LT recipients to date, concluded that patient and graft survival were comparable to national averages (this study did not use a control group, however). Although four patients (11%) reported isolated episodes of heroin use posttransplantation, relapses were not considered to have resulted in poorer outcomes.

An important clinical consideration is pain management for patients on MMT. These patients may require higher-than-average doses of narcotic analgesics postoperatively. In one specific example, patients on MMT in whom methadone was also used as the posthospitalization pain medication required an average methadone dose increase of 60% posttransplantation, presumably to adjust for chronic downregulation of μ opioid pain receptors from chronic methadone exposure (Weinrieb et al. 2004) and improvement in metabolism after transplantation. Many clinicians consider methadone to be a useful choice for pain management rather than introducing another narcotic that may inadvertently precipitate a relapse.

Listing patients with active marijuana use has also led to controversy, partly because few data exist about the effects of marijuana in transplant recipients. In a large survey of heart transplant providers from 26 countries, two-thirds supported listing patients who use legal medical marijuana, but just under one-third supported listing patients who use legal recreational marijuana (Neyer et al. 2016). In 2015, California passed the Medical Cannabis Organ Transplant Act, which prohibits discrimination against medical cannabis patients in the organ transplant process unless a doctor has determined that medical cannabis use is clinically harmful in transplant. Several other states have followed this example. In the Neyer et al. (2016) survey, there was considerable heterogeneity in providers' individual opinions about denying transplant to medical marijuana users despite being from regions that prohibit such practice. Smoked cannabis, however, may expose immunocompromised patients to infectious agents, as suggested by a number of case reports of fungal lung infections in cannabis smoking transplant recipients (Coffman 2008; Marks et al. 1996). New evidence suggests that inhaled/vaporized marijuana may be the source of these infections (Thompson et al. 2017). A recent study of medicinal dispensaries cultured multiple fungi (including *Aspergillus* and *Cryptococcus*) and bacteria (including *Klebsiella, Enterobacter, Pseudomonas,* and *Bacillus*) from their cannabis samples (Thompson et al. 2017), confirming that viable infectious organisms can be recovered from cannabis. Because medicinal dispensaries do not have quality/purity oversight (Wilkinson and D'Souza 2014), their marijuana can raise risks for immunocompromised patients.

Personality Disorders

Personality disorders are characterized by persisting and inflexible maladaptive patterns of subjective experience and behavior that may create emotional distress and interfere with an individual's interpersonal relationships and social functioning. The requirements of successful transplantation can be too difficult for such individuals, as the process requires a series of adaptations to changes in physical and social functioning and significant ability to work constructively with both caregivers and the transplant team. By identifying personality disorders, the psychiatrist can potentially predict patterns of behavior, recommend treatment, develop a behavioral plan with the team to work constructively with the patient, and render an opinion as to the candidate's ability to proceed with transplantation. Patients with personality disorders can require excessive amounts of time from the transplant team, which raises the issue of resource allocation as a potential selection criterion (Carlson et al. 2000). Not all personality disorders should be viewed similarly, however, because the behavioral and coping styles of different disorders can present varying degrees of concordance with the needs of transplantation. For example, the need for structure and orderliness of a candidate with obsessive-compulsive personality disorder would be more adaptive to the demands of transplantation than the coping style of a patient with borderline personality disorder.

The incidence of personality disorders in transplant populations is similar to that in the general population, ranging from 10% to 26% (Chacko et al. 1996; Dobbels et al. 2000), although in some cohorts, estimates have been as high as 33% (in a cohort of heart and lung transplant recipients) (Stilley et al. 2005) or even 57% (predominantly in those with a history of substance abuse) (Stilley et al. 1997). Case reports of patients with severe character pathology demonstrate the extent of adherence problems that can arise from these disorders, resulting in significant morbidity and mortality (Surman and Purtilo 1992; Weitzner et al. 1999). The disturbances in interpersonal relationships that can occur with personality disorders also can decrease the likelihood that patients will have stable and reliable social supports during the pre- and posttransplant phases (Yates et al. 1998). Of the personality disorders, borderline personality disorder is considered to represent the highest risk for posttransplant nonadherence (Laederach-Hofmann and Bunzel 2000). Among internal medicine outpatients, those with borderline personality symptoms had poorer adherence across a range of health care behaviors than those without (Sansone et al. 2015).

Sociopathy has not consistently been associated with substance relapse in the addiction literature (Vaillant 1997). However, in a study of 91 patients transplanted for ALD and followed for up to 3 years, 50% of the 18 patients who were identified as exhibiting antisocial behavior returned to either alcohol ($n=6$) or prescription narcotic addiction ($n=3$) posttransplantation, a rate that was significantly higher than the 19.8% return to alcohol use by the total group (Coffman et al. 1997). In a prospective study of 125 heart transplant recipients, personality disorders were associated with posttransplant adherence problems and a higher incidence of graft rejection (Shapiro et al. 1995).

Using the Type D (for "distressed") personality construct (based on two broad and stable personality traits—negative affectivity and social inhibition), Denollet et al. (2007) found significantly higher rates of mortality and early allograft rejection in heart recipients with Type D personality than for those with non–Type D personality. Although Pedersen et al. (2006) found that those with Type D personality were also more likely to have worse physical and mental health–related QOL (3 and 6 times greater risk, respectively), the connection between this personality and posttransplant outcomes has not been further studied.

Patients with personality disorders do best with ongoing pre- and posttransplant psychotherapy, specifically cognitive and behavioral interventions to promote adherence to the care regimen and to establish a working alliance with transplant team members (Dobbels et al. 2000). These patients should be given clear and consistent instructions on rules and requirements of transplantation, reinforced by regular outpatient appointments. A limited number of transplant center personnel should maintain contact with each patient, and staff members should communicate regularly among themselves and with the outpatient psychiatric team (Carlson et al. 2000) to coordinate care and to reduce opportunities for cognitive distortions and splitting by the patient. A formal written contract can document the expectations of the transplant team and serve as a therapeutic treatment plan whereby the patient and team agree to work together toward common goals for the transplant recipient's health (Dobbels et al. 2000).

Psychotic Disorders

Although chronic and active psychosis is thought by many to be incompatible with successful transplantation, case reports (Goracci et al. 2008; Krahn et al. 1998; Shapiro 2005) and a case series of 10 transplant recipients (Zimbrean and Emre 2015) demonstrate that carefully selected patients with psychosis can successfully undergo transplantation and with expert management survive after the procedure. Two sources—a survey of transplant psychiatrists at 12 national and international transplant programs (which identified only 35 cases of pretransplant psychotic disorders in transplant recipients) (Coffman and Crone 2002) and a historical cohort study of transplant recipients in the U.S. Renal Data System (which showed a 1.5% prevalence of psychosis requiring hospitalization among renal transplant recipients) (Abbott et al. 2003)—suggest that such patients are highly underrepresented among transplant recipients. The survey confirmed previously expressed stipulations that patients with psychotic disorders should be carefully screened before acceptance. Candidates should have demonstrated good adherence to both medical and psychiatric follow-up requirements; possess adequate social supports, especially in-residence support; and be capable of establishing a working relationship with the transplant team.

The survey by Coffman and Crone (2002) found that risk factors for problems with adherence after transplantation included antisocial or borderline personality disorder features, a history of assault, living alone, positive psychotic symptoms, and a family history of schizophrenia. Posttransplant nonadherence to nonpsychiatric medications was found in 20% of patients (7 of 35), and noncompliance with laboratory tests was found in 17% (6 of 35); however, these numbers are similar to percentages of medication and laboratory testing nonadherence in general transplant populations. Overall, nonadherence was responsible for rejection episodes in 5 patients (14%) and reduced graft function or loss in 4 patients (12%). Thirty-seven percent of patients experienced psychotic or manic episodes posttransplantation (not necessarily associated with immunosuppression), 20% attempted suicide (with two completed suicides), 20% experienced severe depression or catatonia, 5.7% committed assaults, 5.7% were arrested for disorderly conduct, and 8.6% required psychiatric commitment.

A recent review found no evidence of poorer posttransplant adherence in patients with psychotic disorders than in patients without (Price et al. 2014). A review of the Irish National Renal Transplant Programme database identified fewer than 1% of kidney recipients with bipolar disorder or schizophrenia, with no significant differences between these recipients and the general renal transplant group in length of transplant hospitalization, frequency of acute rejection episodes, graft function, or patient or graft survival (Butler et al. 2017). However, a historical cohort study of 39,628 renal transplant recipients in the U.S. Renal Data System showed substantially higher rates of death, graft loss, and nonadherence-related graft loss among patients hospitalized for psychosis, a finding that may have been at least partially mediated by undertreatment by medical providers or patient nonadherence (Abbott et al. 2003).

Concerns have been raised in regard to the potential of immunosuppressive medications to produce or exacerbate psychotic symptoms in patients with a prior psychiatric history. Antipsychotics are usually adequate to manage these symptoms if they emerge. Because transplant teams often overlook the early postoperative reinstitution of antipsychotics, it is essential that the psychiatrist devote careful attention to this issue. If quick reintegration of patients into their pretransplant outpatient psychiatric treatment regimen is not possible because of infirmity, interim in-home psychiatric follow-up care may be needed.

Special Issues in Transplantation

Intestinal Transplantation

Isolated small-bowel transplantation and multivisceral transplantation including the bowel are still relatively uncommon procedures, with total parenteral nutrition (TPN) remaining the primary therapeutic option for short-gut syndrome (Ceulemans et al. 2016). Candidates for intestinal transplantation typically have experienced complications such as repeated episodes of sepsis or dehydration, early liver disease, or loss of central venous access (Fishbein 2009). For parenteral-nutrition-dependent patients without complications who seek to improve their QOL, the decision to transplant is controversial, and the limited data suggesting improvements in QOL are from studies with less-than-optimal methodological rigor (Ceulemans et al. 2016). A review by the Intestinal Transplant Registry, representing 82 international intestinal transplant programs covering 2,887 transplants prior to 2013, reported survival rates of 76%, 56%, and 43% at 1, 5, and 10 years, respectively (Grant et al. 2015). Perhaps because of small numbers and poor long-term survival of patients, few studies have investigated outcomes beyond the immediate postoperative course and survival. Earlier studies examining psychiatric characteristics in the patient population showed patients to be a complex group, often with character pathology and drug and/or alcohol dependence histories and with iatrogenic dependence on high-dose narcotics (DiMartini et al. 1996). Some of these features could be ascribed to the difficulties of living with a chronic debilitating illness prior to transplantation, the severity and extent of the transplant surgery, and the prolonged posttransplantation hospitalizations marked by frequent setbacks.

Patients and their caregivers should be prepared for long and frequent hospitalizations, especially during the first years following transplantation (DiMartini et al. 1996), although substantial reductions in length of the initial hospitalization and need for readmission have occurred in recent years (Grant et al. 2015; Langnas 2004). A literature review of QOL in adults who had undergone intestinal transplant found that patients experienced improvement in QOL compared with pretransplant, as well as further improvement with longer posttransplant follow-up. Compared with TPN patients, patients who underwent transplant had fewer gastrointestinal symptoms and better energy, social functioning, and travel ability (Ceulemans et al. 2016; Pironi et al. 2012). For candidates or recipients who lack adequate gut absorption, the use of psychotropics without parenteral formulations is challenging, and other nonenteral routes of administration may need to be considered (Thompson and DiMartini 1999; see also "Alternative Routes of Administration" in Chapter 36, "Psychopharmacology"). Weaning patients from high-dose narcotics following successful transplantation may be difficult (DiMartini et al. 1996).

Cognitive Disorders and Delirium

Throughout the pre- to posttransplant phases, patients frequently experience cognitive dysfunction ranging from subclinical or mild symptoms to frank delirium. Impairment in cognitive function often results from physiological consequences of end-stage organ disease but may also be secondary to other comorbid disease processes (e.g., cerebrovascular disease from diabetes or hypertension), damage from prior alcohol or drug exposures, or previous structural damage to the brain (e.g., head trauma). (See Chapter 4, "Delirium," for a general review of the evaluation and treatment of delirium.) The reversibility or progression of deficits may in part depend on age, the homeostatic reserve of the brain, prior central nervous system (CNS) insults, and the ability to withstand future transplant-related stressors (e.g., prolonged anesthesia, use of cardiac bypass, hemodynamic fluctuations, posttransplant immunosuppressive medications). Identification of cognitive impairment is critical to evaluating the candidate's capacity to comprehend, make decisions, and follow medical directives. Caregivers also are impacted by the patient's cognitive deficits, because they may be responsible for providing oversight, direct patient care, or assistance with activities of daily living. Although the restoration of normal organ function and physiology after transplantation may be expected to correct reversible cognitive impairments, such deficits may take months to years to resolve and may not resolve completely (Kramer et al. 1996; Sotil et al. 2009).

In heart failure, low cardiac output and CNS hypoperfusion can contribute to cognitive impairment. Even in the absence of acute cerebrovascular events, impaired cerebrovascular reactivity and ischemia may result. CNS microemboli are common in pre–heart transplant patients, especially in those on ventricular assist devices (VADs). In renal disease, accumulation of uremic toxins—in addition to hormonal elevations, electrolyte imbalances, malnutrition, and decreased γ-aminobutyric acid (GABA) and glycine activity—contributes to encephalopathy. Removal of uremic toxins via hemodialysis, correction of electrolyte imbalances and anemia, and treatment of malnutrition can improve cognition. For patients with end-stage lung disease, hypoxia and hypercapnia may cause mild to severe cognitive deficits, particularly in executive functions, attention, and memory (Parekh et al. 2005). Oxygen therapy may improve cognitive function for some lung candidates, and these patients can benefit from lung transplantation, but the extent to which these deficits are reversible is unclear (Parekh et al. 2005). Hepatic encephalopathy and adverse events related to VADs are two specific areas considered in detail below.

Hepatic Encephalopathy

Hepatic encephalopathy (HE), a neuropsychiatric syndrome commonly encountered in LT candidates, manifests a constellation of signs and symptoms, including alterations of consciousness (including stupor or coma), cognitive impairment, confusion/

disorientation, affective/emotional dysregulation, psychosis, behavioral disturbances, bioregulatory disturbances, and physical signs such as asterixis. (HE is also addressed in Chapter 19, "Gastrointestinal Disorders.") Identification of HE is important, because it directly affects patient quality and quantity of life; fulminant HE is associated with intracranial hypertension, cerebral edema, and death pretransplant (Ferenci et al. 2002). Even subclinical HE is clinically important, because it can impair patient safety (Schomerus et al. 1981) and is associated with persistent cognitive deficits post-LT (Tarter et al. 1990). By definition, subclinical HE is not identifiable on a typical clinical examination; detection may require additional neuropsychological tests of psychomotor speed, praxis, concentration, and attention. The Trail Making Test and the Digit Symbol and Block Design subtests from the Wechsler Adult Intelligence Scale—Revised are commonly used to identify subclinical HE, but neurocognitive testing is often not employed in gastrointestinal clinics due to lack of time and expertise. One study validated a smartphone application for delivering the Stroop cognitive screening test to detect minimal HE (Bajaj et al. 2013). A self-scoring algorithm and mobile device app potentially allow prospective monitoring even from home (Bajaj et al. 2013).

Because of their facility with cognitive examinations and testing, psychiatric consultants are often the clinicians who recognize and monitor HE symptoms and make recommendations regarding initiation of or improvement in treatment. Patients who undergo shunting procedures to relieve portal hypertension are at increased risk of ammonia buildup with subsequent HE (in one study, 45% of patients had at least one episode of HE following a shunting procedure [Riggio et al. 2008]), and they and their caregivers should be educated on monitoring for HE. Treatment should strive to normalize ammonia levels, despite the fact that blood ammonia levels are not well correlated with symptoms of HE (Riordan and Williams 1997). Treatment strategies include administration of lactulose (an osmotic laxative to flush out ammonia) and nonabsorbable antibiotics (to reduce levels of intestinal bacteria that convert protein to ammonia). Medications that potentially contribute to symptoms of encephalopathy—anticholinergic drugs, tranquilizers, and sedatives—should be avoided.

Ventricular Assist Devices in Heart Transplantation

Progress in the development of mechanical circulatory support (MCS) devices, including VADs and total artificial hearts, has dramatically improved both the physical and the psychological health of potential cardiac transplant candidates, and MCS devices are increasingly used as bridges to transplant or as permanent therapy in patients who do not meet criteria for transplant. (See also Chapter 17, "Heart Disease.") These devices can reduce cognitive impairment from low cardiac output but also can cause adverse neurological and psychiatric events. The newer nonpulsatile continuous-flow MCS devices provide improved survival and reduced morbidity compared with the older pulsatile devices and are half as likely to lead to neuropsychiatric sequelae (Kirklin et al. 2013). A small prospective study that followed patients with heart failure before and after VAD implantation found no psychopathology (e.g., anxiety or depression), and patients' memory actually improved, while other cognitive domains remained stable (Mapelli et al. 2014). MCS patients often experience improvements in QOL within months postimplantation, and these improvements are sustained (Grady and Dew 2012; Park et al. 2012).

Patients on MCS devices can undergo physical and physiological rehabilitation, develop exercise tolerance, and rebuild muscle mass, thus stabilizing their cardiac condition (Eshelman et al. 2009; Grady and Dew 2012). The lack of mobility restriction means that patients often can return to work and engage in activities such as dancing and driving (Catanese et al. 1996). With the urgency for transplantation diminished, the transplant team can wait for an optimal donor organ.

However, there continue to be risks and drawbacks with either temporary or permanent MCS therapy. The logistics of arranging outpatient care require a well-trained medical team whose members are available at all times, resulting in significant patient, caregiver, and medical system burden. Patient and caregiver responsibilities for MCS require the ability to perform daily inspections and as-needed maintenance, monitor for complications, and respond to alarms (for comprehensive reviews, see Caro et al. 2016 and Eshelman et al. 2009). Although patients using MCS devices have improved cerebral perfusion, they are at high risk of microembolic events. These events may be clinically silent (Thoennissen et al. 2005), but their cumulative effects on cognitive function may be significant over time, and periodic cognitive testing may be helpful in monitoring changes (Komoda et al. 2005). The risk of such events appears to be lower with the newer-generation MCS devices, but given that implantation periods have lengthened, routine care of MCS recipients requires consideration of cognitive status and identification of any developing deficits (see also Chapter 17, "Heart Disease").

In posttransplantation comparisons with heart recipients who did not receive a VAD (either biventricular or left ventricular assist device), patients who were bridged to transplantation with a VAD showed similar improvements in physical functioning and emotional well-being, significantly lower rates of anxiety, but poorer cognitive status (Dew et al. 2001). The cognitive impairments observed in these VAD recipients were believed to be attributable to neurological events (e.g., microemboli, strokes) that occurred during the period of VAD support, and these events occurred at a higher rate among VAD recipients relative to non-VAD patients during the waiting period before transplantation. Although mild, these impairments appeared to persist during the first year following transplantation and were associated with a reduced likelihood of returning to employment.

Living Donor Transplantation

Despite the physical risks, discomfort and pain, expense and inconvenience, and potential psychological consequences of donating an organ, significant numbers of people volunteer to become living donors. Given the organ shortage and the improved survival rates of recipients of living organ donations, transplant programs are increasingly considering living donation. Living kidney donations are the most common type of living organ donation in the United States, accounting for more than one-third of all kidney transplants each year (around 5,600 donations per year). It is also possible to donate a portion of the liver and (in rare instances) a lobe of a lung or a portion of the pancreas or intestine (Organ Procurement and Transplantation Network 2017a).

Donation of an organ—putting one's life at risk to help another—is an incredibly generous and altruistic gift. Yet the evaluation of such donors is a complex process requiring assessment of the circumstances and motives of the donor, the dynamics of the relationship between donor and recipient, the severity of the recipient's illness, and family and societal forces. Current practice guidelines require a psychosocial evaluation for each potential donor to thoroughly examine these and other issues (Table 29–3) (Dew et al. 2007b, 2007c; Olbrisch et al. 2001; Surman 2002). In all U.S. centers, living-donor medical evaluation protocols include a predonation psychosocial assessment (performed by a psychiatrist, a psychologist, or a master's-level or licensed clinical social worker) documenting the elements listed in Table 29–3 (Organ Procurement and Transplantation Network 2017b). The Live Donor Assessment Tool was developed to cover all of the potential areas of assessment and is being tested prospectively for validity (Iacoviello et al. 2017). Also, the recently developed Donor Cognition Instrument has been found to be reliable in assessing cognitions surrounding living organ donation (e.g., donor benefits, idealistic incentives, gratitude, worries about donation), which may facilitate psychosocial donor evaluation by mental health care professionals (Wirken et al. 2017). Donor assessments are designed to screen out potential donors with significant psychiatric morbidity (including substance abuse or dependence) and those unwilling or unable to give informed consent (due to the presence of coercion, likely financial gain, and/or impaired cognitive capacity). This screening process, combined with rigorous medical evaluation, ensures that living donors are very healthy before donation. Additionally, donors must be fully willing, independently motivated, and completely informed about the surgery. For all donors, and for liver donors in particular, long-term sequelae that may affect the donor's future health, functioning, and even ability to obtain health insurance (due to the presence of a preexisting condition) are not fully known. Donor decision-making aids, standardized computerized education, and other educational interventions can lead to better-informed donors (Freeman et al. 2013) and living donor recipients (Waterman et al. 2014).

Living liver donation is a much more surgically complex and invasive procedure than kidney donation and is therefore potentially more dangerous. Although mortality rates have been less than 1% for both kidney and liver donors (both adult-to-adult and adult-to-child) (Abecassis et al. 2012; Dew et al. 2017), nearly 40% of liver donors have complications within the first year, and serious complications occur in 3%–16% of donors (Abecassis et al. 2012; Dew et al. 2017). In the United States, transplant programs are required to have an independent living-donor advocate (i.e., someone who is not a member of the transplant team responsible for the recipient's care and who is independent of the decision to transplant the potential recipient) to serve as a safeguard for patient autonomy, readiness to donate, and informed consent (Abecassis et al. 2000; Conti et al. 2002) to avoid conflicts of interest. The qualifications of these advocates must include knowledge of living organ donation, transplantation, medical ethics, informed consent, and the potential impact of family or other external pressures on the potential living donor's donation decision (Organ Procurement and Transplantation Network 2017b).

Kidney donors should expect to miss 4–6 weeks of work and liver donors 8–12 weeks of work, especially if their jobs involve heavy lifting. Laparoscopic donor nephrectomy can result in overall quicker recovery times, as well as more favorable cosmetic results. For all donor types, the issue of donor financial hardship is becoming an increasingly prominent concern. Although recipients' insurance covers the evaluation and immediate postoperative medical care, donors frequently report out-of-

TABLE 29–3. Components of living donor evaluation

Psychosocial areas of assessment	Specific requirements for U.S. living donation from Organ Procurement and Transplantation Network policy 14[a]
Donor's knowledge about the surgery	The determination that the living donor understands the short- and long-term medical and psychosocial risks for both the living donor and the recipient associated with living donation Identification of factors that warrant educational intervention prior to final donation decision
Motivation Ambivalence Evidence of coercion/inducement	An assessment of whether the decision to donate is free of inducement, coercion, and other undue pressure by exploring the reasons for donating and the nature of the relationship, if any, to the transplant candidate
Attitudes of significant others toward the donation	
Availability of support Financial resources Work- and/or school-related issues (if applicable)	A review of the donor's occupation, employment status, health insurance status, living arrangements, and social support The determination that the donor understands the potential financial implications of living donation
Psychiatric disorders Personality disorders Coping resources/styles Pain syndromes Prior psychological trauma/abuse Substance use/abuse	An evaluation of the donor's psychological health, including any mental health issues that might complicate the donor's recovery and that could be identified as risk factors for a poor psychosocial outcome Identification of factors that warrant therapeutic intervention prior to final donation decision An assessment for the presence of behaviors that may increase risk of disease transmission, as defined by the U.S. Public Health Service (Seem et al. 2013) A review of the living donor's history of smoking and of alcohol and drug use, including past or present substance use disorders
Ability to provide informed consent	An assessment of the living donor's ability to make an informed decision and ability to cope with the major surgery and related stress; this includes evaluating whether the donor has a realistic plan for donation and recovery, with social, emotional, and financial support available as recommended

[a]Adapted from Organ Procurement and Transplantation Network 2017b.

pocket costs, and some may have difficulties in obtaining or retaining health and life insurance (Boyarsky et al. 2014; Dew et al. 2007c; DiMartini et al. 2017). In a multisite study of liver donors ($N=271$), 44% reported that the out-of-pockets costs were burdensome, and 5% had difficulty getting or keeping health insurance (DiMartini et al. 2017). Kidney donors reported financial stresses from lost work and wages for both themselves and their family caregivers; costs incurred for household services they could not perform by themselves while recovering; and direct costs incurred for dependent care, transportation, and housing, with 30% reporting a loss exceeding $2,500 U.S. dollars (Rodrigue et al. 2015, 2016).

Living donors almost uniformly report that they do not regret having donated, that they would donate again if that were possible, and that they feel a deep sense of gratification at being able to help another person (Dew et al. 2014b). Moreover, generic health-related QOL assessments show that—at least in the early years postdonation—donors' well-being, on average, meets or exceeds that reported in the general population (Dew et al. 2014b, 2017).

In a large multicenter study ("Adult-to-Adult Living Donor Liver Transplantation Cohort Study [A2ALL]" 2003) that prospectively followed hundreds of liver donors for up to 10 years after donation, 30% of donors reported improved family/spousal relationships, and more than 50% reported an improved relationship with the recipient (DiMartini et al. 2017). Some donors reported experiencing personal psychological growth as a result of the donation experience (Dew et al. 2016). The study also identified low rates (generally <5%) of major depressive, alcohol abuse, and anxiety syndromes in the first 2 years following donation (Butt et al. 2017). However, while 90% of donors surveyed 3–10 years (average 6 years) after donation felt positive about donation and would make the same decision again to donate, nearly 50% reported concerns about donation-related health issues, and 15% reported current donation-related health problems (Dew et al. 2016). A similar large multicenter study—the Renal and Lung Donors Evaluation Study—found that the majority of kidney donors reported being satisfied with their lives postdonation (Messersmith et al. 2014) and that depression rates in donors were comparable to rates in the general population (Jowsey et al. 2014). Predictors of depressive symptoms included nonwhite race, younger age at donation, longer duration of recovery after donation, greater financial burden, and feeling morally obligated to donate (Jowsey et al. 2014). A predonation intervention targeting donor risk factors for poorer psychosocial outcomes showed that donors in the intervention experienced lower rates of physical and psychological symptoms following donation (Dew et al. 2013). However, an alarming finding from a large multicenter study was that three liver donors had attempted suicide, with one completed suicide, following donation (Trotter et al. 2007). Trotter et al. (2007) estimated the suicide rate in liver donors at 2 cases per 1,000 donors, although the contribution of the donation to these events is unclear.

Altruistic (or *nondirected*) donors—individuals who donate an organ to an unknown recipient—pose one of the most complex challenges to transplant evaluation. In these cases, the psychosocial evaluation has particular importance in determining the suitability of the donor, and some believe that the medical standards for such donors should be higher (Ross 2002). These donors account for 1%–2% of all living organ donations (Organ Procurement and Transplantation Network 2017a). Altruistic donors are commonly viewed with some skepticism and are evaluated with greater caution than are related donors (Kazley et al. 2016). A detailed evaluation is critical, both to understand the motives of the donor and the psychological meaning of the donation to the donor and to identify any financial or other types of compensation expected for the donation. (See Dew et al. [2007b] and Dew et al. [2014a] for issues and guidelines relevant to the psychosocial evaluation and informed consent of unrelated donors.) One study of nondirected donors reported 360 inquiries over a 6-year period, of which 60 were declined on preliminary telephone interview (22% declined for psychosocial reasons); of the 51 serious candidates who came for partial or full evaluations, 8 (16%) were declined for psychosocial reasons (Jacobs et al. 2004). A postdonation study of directed and nondirected kidney donors found no differences in depression, anxiety, stress, self-esteem, physical outcomes, regret, or well-being between the groups, but nondirected donors were more engaged in other altruistic behaviors ($P<0.001$) (Maple et al. 2014).

Posttransplant Organ Function and Pharmacological Considerations

Although many transplant-specific psychological stresses can be appropriately managed with psychotherapeutic techniques, pharmacotherapy is an essential component in the psychiatric care of transplant patients. Given the high prevalence of psychiatric disorders in transplant candidates and recipients and the potential for untreated psychiatric disorders to influence outcomes, including adherence, pharmacological treatment is often required. Unfortunately, psychotropic medications are often not provided because of concerns about their potential risks and patients' medical fragility. End-stage organ disease alters most aspects of drug pharmacokinetics, including absorption, bioavailability, metabolism, and clearance. For a full review of the pharmacokinetics of psychotropic drugs in general, and of pharmacokinetic changes in hepatic, renal, bowel, heart, and lung disease in particular, see Chapter 36, "Psychopharmacology"; see also Robinson and Levenson (2001) and Trzepacz et al. (2000). Here we discuss important aspects of pharmacokinetics in the newly transplanted patient during the recovery period (see Fireman et al. 2017 for further pharmacological considerations in transplant patients).

Although organ function may deteriorate slowly over the time before transplantation, following transplantation, for the majority of recipients, the newly transplanted organ functions immediately, so that normal physiological parameters are quickly restored and pharmacokinetic abnormalities resolve. Within the first month following transplantation for patients who have stable liver or kidney function, the clearance and steady-state volume of distribution of drugs can be similar to those in healthy volunteers (Hebert et al. 2003). Many transplant recipients can be treated with normal therapeutic drug dosing once they have recovered from immediate postoperative complications (e.g., delirium, sedation, ileus). With the resumption of normal organ function after transplantation, any psychotropic medications prescribed at lower dosages prior to transplant to accommodate diminished metabolism or elimination may need to be adjusted to higher levels.

For some transplant recipients, however, the transplanted organ does not assume normal autonomous physiological function immediately, or the organ may slowly regain normal function over time. Studies of posttransplantation pharmacokinetics have been mostly conducted in liver and kidney recipients due to the relevance of these organs to drug pharmacokinetics. Additionally, these studies have focused exclusively on immunosuppressive medications because of the need to achieve and maintain stable immunosuppressive medication levels to prevent organ rejection, the ability to monitor serum levels, and the narrow therapeutic range of these drugs. Nevertheless, data from these studies provide general guidelines on medication prescribing for specific types of posttransplant organ dysfunction.

Delayed Graft Function and Rejection

The most common allograft complication affecting pharmacokinetics in the immediate posttransplantation period is delayed graft function (DGF). DGF occurs in 10%–25% of liver and kidney recipients, although rates can reach 50% of cases if marginal organs are used (Angelico 2005; Shoskes and Cecka 1998; U.S. Renal Data System 2008). Liver recipients with DGF may require one-half of the typical immunosuppressive medication dose (Hebert et al. 2003; Lück et al. 2004). For kidney transplant recipients, DGF is deemed to have occurred if the recipient requires dialysis within the first week after transplant. For kidney recipients, DGF alters pharmacokinetics by mechanisms that increase the free fraction of parent drugs and renally excreted metabolites (Shaw et al. 1998). Severe or acute impairment in renal function after transplant can result in immunosuppressive levels 3–6 times higher than those in nonimpaired recipients for renally excreted drugs and their metabolites (Bullingham et al. 1998; Shaw et al. 1998). Acute cellular rejection occurs in 20%–70% of LT recipients, typically within the first 3 weeks posttransplant, resulting in transient graft dysfunction. Sixty-five percent to 80% of cases are effectively treated with high-dose steroids, and most episodes do not lead to clinically significant alterations in liver histology or architecture (Lake 2003). Chronic graft rejection, which occurs in 5%–10% of liver recipients, tends to respond poorly to treatment. Loss of liver synthetic function may not occur until very late in the course of chronic rejection (Lake 2003).

Among kidney recipients, 25%–60% will experience acute rejection, most often within the first 6 months after transplantation. Treatment of an identified rejection episode typically restores prerejection functioning; however, subclinical rejection that remains undetected can lead to gradually worsening renal function over time, with eventual graft loss (Rush et al. 1998).

If the episode of graft rejection is acute and resolves quickly, no specific changes in psychotropic dosages would be required (this is true across all organ types). Chronic rejection tends to evolve over time, with gradual deterioration in organ function and eventual loss of metabolic/elimination capacity. For all organ types, chronic graft rejection is potentially reversible in the early stages but not once chronic dysfunction has set in and progressive graft failure occurs. In these cases, pharmacokinetics may be similar to those in the pretransplant state.

General Issues

In addition to DGF or acute rejection, some recipients will experience transient physiological abnormalities in the weeks following transplant that could also affect pharmacokinetics (e.g., liver congestion and/or renal hypoperfusion in heart recipients, fluid overload in renal recipients, resolving hepatorenal syndrome in liver recipients). The mechanisms causing these derangements are complex and can include perioperative hemodynamic and fluid instability; graft-related factors such as graft harvesting; ischemic or reperfusion injury; or use of marginal organs. Thus, in addition to the status of the transplanted organ, evaluation of the recipients' total physiological status is important in drug consideration and dosing.

Finally, in transplants of all organ types, calcineurin-inhibiting immunosuppressants are nephrotoxic with chronic use. Although there may be cumulative causes for renal failure in organ recipients, chronic use of immunosuppressants leads to renal failure in 7%–21% of recipients by 5 years posttransplant (Ojo et al. 2003). Thus, the state of the patient's renal function should always be considered in decisions about medication usage, particularly in long-term transplant recipients and especially if the medication chosen requires renal clearance.

Neuropsychiatric Side Effects of Immunosuppressive Agents

Advances in the understanding of immunology and the development of newer strategies for immunosuppression may significantly reduce the need for—if not obviate completely—long-term maintenance immunosuppression. In the future, transplant recipients of all organ types may require immunosuppressant dosages only one or two times a week, or not at all (Starzl 2002). This achievement would remove the final obstacle to long-term successful outcomes for transplant recipients, given that the majority of long-term morbidity and mortality is due to chronic immunosuppression (e.g., infections, renal failure, cancer). Additionally, reduced requirements for immunosuppressants would facilitate medication adherence and would relieve some of the financial burden of long-term immunosuppression. However, for now, transplant recipients will continue to require immunosuppressive therapy and to be subject to these drugs' potential neurotoxic and neuropsychiatric side effects. Psychiatrists should be familiar with the signs, symptoms, differential diagnosis, neuroimaging findings, and management of immunosuppressive neurotoxicity and secondary psychiatric disorders in solid organ recipients (Strouse et al. 1998) (see DiMartini et al. 2010 for further discussion of neuropsychiatric side effects of immunosuppressants).

Calcineurin-Inhibiting Immunosuppressive Medications

Cyclosporine

Cyclosporine is used as a primary immunosuppressive agent. Side effects are usually mild and include tremor, restlessness, and headache (Wijdicks et al. 1999). About 12% of patients on cyclosporine experience more serious neurotoxicity, characterized by acute confusional states, psychosis, seizures, speech apraxia, cortical blindness, and coma (de Groen et al. 1987; Wijdicks et al. 1995, 1996; Wilson et al. 1988).

Serious neurological side effects are associated with intravenous administration and higher dosages (Wijdicks et al. 1999). Cyclosporine trough levels correlate poorly with cyclosporine neurotoxicity, although in most studies, symptoms resolved when cyclosporine was discontinued and subsequently reinstated at a lower dosage (Wijdicks et al. 1999). Anticonvulsants can successfully treat cyclosporine-induced seizures but are not required long-term (Wijdicks et al. 1996), and seizures may cease with dosage reduction or discontinuation of cyclosporine. A few patients with serious clinical neurotoxic side effects have been found to have diffuse white matter abnormalities, predominantly in the occipitoparietal region, on computed tomography (CT) scans (de Groen et al. 1987; Gijtenbeek et al. 1999; Wijdicks et al. 1995) (see discussion of posterior reversible [leuko]encephalopathy syndrome [PRES] in the next subsection). In one case, symptoms of cyclosporine-induced cortical blindness resolved with drug discontinuation, although pathological evidence of CNS demyelination persisted for months after the episode (Wilson et al. 1988).

Tacrolimus

Tacrolimus is used as primary immunosuppressive therapy, as rescue therapy for patients who fail to respond to cyclosporine, and as treatment for graft-versus-host disease. In response to evidence that higher frequency of dosing was associated with poorer medication adherence (Weng et al. 2005), extended-release formulations were developed. Although tacrolimus is more potent and possibly less toxic than cyclosporine, the neuropsychiatric side effects of the two drugs appear to be similar (DiMartini et al. 1991; Freise et al. 1991). With tacrolimus, as with cyclosporine, neuropsychiatric side effects are more common with intravenous administration and diminish with oral administration and dosage reduction. Common symptoms include tremulousness, headache, restlessness, insomnia, vivid dreams, hyperesthesias, anxiety, and agitation (Fung et al. 1991). Cognitive impairment, coma, seizures, dysarthria, and delirium occur less often (8.4%) and are associated with higher plasma levels (DiMartini et al. 1997; Fung et al. 1991). Tacrolimus can produce symptoms of akathisia (Bernstein and Daviss 1992).

Tacrolimus is believed to cross the blood–brain barrier in humans. More serious neurotoxic side effects (e.g., focal neurological abnormalities, speech disturbances, hemiplegia, cortical blindness) may occur from higher CNS levels in patients who have a disrupted blood–brain barrier (Eidelman et al. 1991). In a study of 294 consecutive transplant recipients taking tacrolimus, those with preexisting CNS damage (e.g., from stroke, multiple sclerosis) were at higher risk of neurotoxic side effects (Eidelman et al. 1991). Both cyclosporine and tacrolimus are associated with posterior reversible (leuko)encephalopathy syndrome (PRES), an uncommon neurotoxic syndrome involving demyelination (particularly in the parieto-occipital region and centrum semiovale) (Ahn et al. 2003; Bartynski and Boardman 2007; Small et al. 1996). PRES typically occurs early postoperatively, often within the first months (Cruz et al. 2012), but can also occur years later. The presentation is variable and can include mental status changes, focal neurological symptoms, or generalized seizures without a clear metabolic etiology. Thus, moderate to serious symptoms of neurotoxicity warrant investigation with brain imaging. Characteristic neuroradiological abnormalities (low attenuation of white matter on CT scan or hyperintense lesions on T2-weighted magnetic resonance imaging [MRI]) are most commonly seen in the cortical and subcortical white matter, typically involving the posterior lobes (parietal and/or occipital), although cases have been reported involving the anterior brain, cerebellum, and brain stem (Bartynski and Boardman 2007). MRI may be better than CT for identifying the radiographic changes that characterize PRES (DiMartini et al. 2008). Like other serious neurotoxic side effects, PRES is not associated with the absolute serum level of tacrolimus but does resolve on discontinuation of the drug (Small et al. 1996). Multifocal sensorimotor polyneuropathy can occur with long-term immunosuppressive medication use and may require either dosage reduction (if possible) or medication treatment for painful peripheral neuropathy.

Other Agents for Adjunctive Immunosuppression or Treatment of Graft Rejection

Corticosteroids

Although chronic corticosteroid use has become less essential in immunosuppression for most patients posttransplantation, high dosages of corticosteroids are still employed in the early postoperative phase and also as "pulsed" dosages to treat acute rejection. Behavioral and psychiatric side effects of corticosteroids are common, but conclusions regarding the incidence or characteristics of these effects—or the specific dosages required to cause such effects—are not well established. These side effects are reviewed elsewhere in this volume, particularly in Chapter 7, "Depression"; Chapter 9, "Psychosis, Mania, and Catatonia"; Chapter 21, "Endocrine and Metabolic Disorders"; and Chapter 24, "Rheumatology."

Sirolimus and Everolimus

The side effects of sirolimus and its analog everolimus do not include neurotoxicity (Watson et al. 1999). However, a systematic evaluation of sirolimus neurotoxicity has yet to be conducted.

Azathioprine

Azathioprine is primarily used as an adjunctive immunosuppressant and is less widely used today. Specific neuropsychiatric side effects have not been reported. Several reports of depressive symptoms in patients receiving azathioprine have been confounded by the concurrent use of other medications (specifically cyclosporine and prednisone) that may have contributed to the mood disturbance.

Mycophenolate Mofetil

Few neuropsychiatric symptoms have been reported with mycophenolate mofetil. Adverse reported CNS events (with incidence ranging from >3% to <20%) included anxiety, depression, delirium, seizures, agitation, hypertonia, paresthesias, neuropathy, psychosis, and somnolence (Roche Pharmaceuticals 2003); however, because the patients in whom these symptoms occurred were receiving mycophenolate mofetil in combination with cyclosporine and corticosteroids, the precise contribution of mycophenolate mofetil to the symptoms is difficult to interpret.

Monoclonal Antibodies

Monoclonal antibodies to T cells are used for induction immunosuppression or adjunctive therapy when a transplant recipient is experiencing an episode of rejection. Neuropsychiatric side effects, including headache, weakness, dizziness, tremor, and anxiety, are generally mild for these agents, with the exception of muromonab-CD3

(OKT3), which often causes more severe headache, tremor, agitation, and depression. OKT3 may also cause cerebral edema and encephalopathy, with confusion, disorientation, hallucinations, and seizures (Alloway et al. 1998). Rituximab has been associated with progressive multifocal leukoencephalopathy (Kranick et al. 2007). Basiliximab has been associated with insomnia, tremor, and headaches in more than 10% of patients.

Drug Interactions Between Psychotropic and Immunosuppressive Medications

Most of the immunosuppressants (e.g., tacrolimus, cyclosporine, sirolimus, everolimus, mycophenolate mofetil and corticosteroids) are metabolized by cytochrome P450 3A4 (CYP3A4); thus, psychotropics that strongly interact with CYP3A4 should be used cautiously or avoided in patients taking these immunosuppressants. Most immunosuppressants have significant toxicities and narrow therapeutic indices. Inhibitors and inducers of CYP3A4 may cause clinically significant drug-level changes, resulting in either toxicity or inadequate immunosuppression. Specific CYP3A4 inhibitors capable of interacting adversely with immunosuppressants, in decreasing order of inhibition, are as follows: fluvoxamine, nefazodone > fluoxetine > sertraline, TCAs, paroxetine > venlafaxine. Nefazodone has been implicated in several case reports (Campo et al. 1998; Helms-Smith et al. 1996; Wright et al. 1999) as causing toxic calcineurin inhibitor immunosuppressant levels, leading to acute renal insufficiency and delirium, and in two cases as causing elevated liver enzymes (Garton 2002). In a case report of a patient on stable dosages of nefazodone and sirolimus with therapeutic sirolimus levels, blood levels of sirolimus became undetectable when the nefazodone was stopped (Michalski et al. 2011). In a study in which fluoxetine or TCAs were used to treat depressed transplant recipients, no differences in cyclosporine blood level–dosage ratios and dose–response relationships were found between those treated and those not treated with antidepressants (Strouse et al. 1996). This finding suggests that antidepressants with less CYP3A4 inhibition may not have clinically meaningful drug interactions with immunosuppressants. Potent inducers of CYP3A4 (e.g., modafinil, St. John's wort, carbamazepine) may lower the levels of immunosuppressive medications and thereby increase the risk of graft rejection (Fireman et al. 2017).

Several side effects relevant to immunosuppressant–psychotropic combinations deserve mention. Gastrointestinal symptoms (e.g., nausea, vomiting, diarrhea) are common adverse effects of immunosuppressants, occurring in more than 60% of patients, and additional requirements for supplemental magnesium may aggravate these symptoms (Pescovitz and Navarro 2001); therefore, use of psychotropic medications with similar gastrointestinal adverse effects (e.g., SSRIs, venlafaxine) should be avoided. Immunosuppressants have significant metabolic side effects (e.g., weight gain, glucose intolerance, hyperlipidemia), suggesting the need to avoid psychotropics that cause these same metabolic effects. Tacrolimus and other immunosuppressants are associated with QT prolongation (Ikitimur et al. 2015) and should be used carefully in combination with QT-prolonging psychotropics.

References

Abbey S, Farrow S: Group therapy and organ transplantation. Int J Group Psychother 48(2):163–185, 1998 9563237

Abbott KC, Agodoa LY, O'Malley PG: Hospitalized psychoses after renal transplantation in the United States: incidence, risk factors, and prognosis. J Am Soc Nephrol 14(6):1628–1635, 2003 12761265

Abecassis M, Adams M, Adams P, et al; Live Organ Donor Consensus Group: Consensus statement on the live organ donor. JAMA 284(22):2919–2926, 2000 11187711

Abecassis MM, Fisher RA, Olthoff KM, et al: Complications of living donor hepatic lobectomy—a comprehensive report. Am J Transplant 12:1208–1217, 2012 22335782

Addolorato G, Leggio L, Ferrulli A, et al: Effectiveness and safety of baclofen for maintenance of alcohol abstinence in alcohol-dependent patients with liver cirrhosis: randomised, double-blind controlled study. Lancet 370(9603):1915–1922, 2007 18068515

Addolorato G, Mirijello A, Leggio L, et al; Gemelli OLT Group: Liver transplantation in alcoholic patients: impact of an alcohol addiction unit within a liver transplant center. Alcohol Clin Exp Res 37(9):1601–1608, 2013 23578009

Adult-to-adult living donor liver transplantation cohort study (A2ALL). Hepatology 38(4):792, 2003 14512864

Ahn KJ, Lee JW, Hahn ST, et al: Diffusion-weighted MRI and ADC mapping in FK506 neurotoxicity. Br J Radiol 76(912):916–919, 2003 14711782

Akman B, Ozdemir FN, Sezer S, et al: Depression levels before and after renal transplantation. Transplant Proc 36(1):111–113, 2004 15013316

Alloway RR, Holt C, Somerville KT: Solid organ transplant, in Pharmacotherapy Self-Assessment Program, 3rd Edition. Kansas City, MO, American College of Clinical Pharmacy, 1998, pp 219–272

American Psychiatric Association: Diagnostic and Statistical Manual of Mental Disorders, 4th Edition, Text Revision. Washington, DC, American Psychiatric Association, 2000

Angelico M: Donor liver steatosis and graft selection for liver transplantation: a short review. Eur Rev Med Pharmacol Sci 9(5):295–297, 2005 16231593

Arora S, Aukrust P, Andreassen A, et al: The prognostic importance of modifiable risk factors after heart transplantation. Am Heart J 158(3):431–436, 2009 19699867

Bailey DE Jr, Hendrix CC, Steinhauser KE, et al: Randomized trial of an uncertainty self-management telephone intervention for patients awaiting liver transplant. Patient Educ Couns 100(3):509–517, 2017 28277289

Baines LS, Joseph JT, Jindal RM: Emotional issues after kidney transplantation: a prospective psychotherapeutic study. Clin Transplant 16(6):455–460, 2002 12437627

Bajaj JS, Thacker LR, Heuman DM, et al: The Stroop smartphone application is a short and valid method to screen for minimal hepatic encephalopathy. Hepatology 58(3):1122–1132, 2013 23389962

Ball J, Ross A: The Effectiveness of Methadone Maintenance Treatment. New York, Springer-Verlag, 1991

Baranyi A, Krauseneck T, Rothenhäusler HB: Posttraumatic stress symptoms after solid-organ transplantation: preoperative risk factors and the impact on health-related quality of life and life satisfaction. Health Qual Life Outcomes 11:111, 2013 23822659

Bartynski WS, Boardman JF: Distinct imaging patterns and lesion distribution in posterior reversible encephalopathy syndrome. AJNR Am J Neuroradiol 28(7):1320–1327, 2007 17698535

Bernstein L, Daviss SR: Organic anxiety disorder with symptoms of akathisia in a patient treated with the immunosuppressant FK506. Gen Hosp Psychiatry 14(3):210–211, 1992 1376291

Botha P, Peaston R, White K, et al: Smoking after cardiac transplantation. Am J Transplant 8(4):866–871, 2008 18324978

Boyarsky BJ, Massie AB, Alejo JL, et al: Experiences obtaining insurance after live kidney donation. Am J Transplant 14(9):2168–2172, 2014 25041695

Bullingham RES, Nicholls AJ, Kamm BR: Clinical pharmacokinetics of mycophenolate mofetil. Clin Pharmacokinet 34(6):429–455, 1998 9646007

Bush K, Kivlahan DR, McDonell MB, et al: The AUDIT alcohol consumption questions (AUDIT-C): an effective brief screening test for problem drinking. Ambulatory Care Quality Improvement Project (ACQUIP). Alcohol Use Disorders Identification Test. Arch Intern Med 158(16):1789–1795, 1998 9738608

Butler MI, McCartan D, Cooney A, et al: Outcomes of renal transplantation in patients with bipolar affective disorder and schizophrenia: a national retrospective cohort study. Psychosomatics 58(1):69–76, 2017 27887740

Butt Z, Levenson J, Olbrisch ME: Policies on tobacco and marijuana smoking among U.S. cardiac, kidney, and liver transplant programs. Presentation at the annual meeting of the Society of Behavioral Medicine, April 26, 2014a

Butt Z, Levenson J, Olbrisch ME: Psychosocial screening practices and criteria for kidney transplantation: a survey of U.S. transplant centers. Presentation at the annual meeting of the Society of Behavioral Medicine, April 26, 2014b

Butt Z, Dew MA, Liu Q, et al: Psychological outcomes of living liver donors from a multicenter prospective study: results from the Adult-to-Adult Living Donor Liver Transplantation Cohort Study2 (A2ALL-2). Am J Transplant 17(5):1267–1277, 2017 27865040

Calia R, Lai C, Aceto P, et al: Emotional self-efficacy and alexithymia may affect compliance, renal function and quality of life in kidney transplant recipients: results from a preliminary cross-sectional study. Physiol Behav 142:152–154, 2015 25680476

Campo JV, Smith C, Perel JM: Tacrolimus toxic reaction associated with the use of nefazodone: paroxetine as an alternative agent. Arch Gen Psychiatry 55(11):1050–1052, 1998 9819077

Carlson J, Potter L, Pennington S, et al: Liver transplantation in a patient at psychosocial risk. Prog Transplant 10(4):209–214, 2000 11232551

Caro MA, Rosenthal JL, Kendall K, et al: What the psychiatrist needs to know about ventricular assist devices: a comprehensive review. Psychosomatics 57(3):229–237, 2016 27005723

Catanese KA, Goldstein DJ, Williams DL, et al: Outpatient left ventricular assist device support: a destination rather than a bridge. Ann Thorac Surg 62(3):646–652, discussion 653, 1996 8783988

Ceulemans LJ, Lomme C, Pirenne J, et al: Systematic literature review on self-reported quality of life in adult intestinal transplantation. Transplant Rev (Orlando) 30(2):109–118, 2016 27066940

Chacko RC, Harper RG, Gotto J, et al: Psychiatric interview and psychometric predictors of cardiac transplant survival. Am J Psychiatry 153(12):1607–1612, 1996 8942458

Chang CF, Winsett RP, Gaber AO, et al: Cost-effectiveness of post-transplantation quality of life intervention among kidney recipients. Clin Transplant 18(4):407–414, 2004 15233818

Chisholm-Burns MA, Spivey CA, Graff Zivin J, et al: Improving outcomes of renal transplant recipients with behavioral adherence contracts: a randomized controlled trial. Am J Transplant 13(9):2364–2373, 2013 23819827

Coffman KL: The debate about marijuana usage in transplant candidates: recent medical evidence on marijuana health effects. Curr Opin Organ Transplant 13(2):189–195, 2008 18685302

Coffman KL, Crone C: Rational guidelines for transplantation in patients with psychotic disorders. Curr Opin Organ Transplant 7(4):385–388, 2002

Coffman KL, Hoffman A, Sher L, et al: Treatment of the postoperative alcoholic liver transplant recipient with other addictions. Liver Transpl Surg 3(3):322–327, 1997 9346758

Conti DJ, Delmonico FL, Dubler N, et al: New York State Committee on Quality Improvement in Living Liver Donation: a Report to New York State Transplant Council and New York State Department of Health. December 2002. Available at: https://www.health.ny.gov/professionals/patients/donation/organ/liver/. Accessed September 26, 2007.

Corbett C, Armstrong MJ, Neuberger J: Tobacco smoking and solid organ transplantation. Transplantation 94(10):979–987, 2012 23169222

Corbett C, Armstrong MJ, Parker R, et al: Mental health disorders and solid-organ transplant recipients. Transplantation 96(7):593–600, 2013 23743726

Cornelius JR, Bukstein O, Salloum I, et al: Alcohol and psychiatric comorbidity. Recent Dev Alcohol 16:361–374, 2003 12638646

Crone CC, Wise TN: Psychiatric aspects of transplantation, I: evaluation and selection of candidates. Crit Care Nurse 19(1):79–87, 1999 10401293

Cruz RJ Jr, DiMartini A, Akhavanheidari M, et al: Posterior reversible encephalopathy syndrome in liver transplant patients: clinical presentation, risk factors and initial management. Am J Transplant 12(8):2228–2236, 2012 22494636

Cuadrado A, Fábrega E, Casafont F, et al: Alcohol recidivism impairs long-term patient survival after orthotopic liver transplantation for alcoholic liver disease. Liver Transpl 11(4):420–426, 2005 15776421

Cukor D, Newville H, Jindal R: Depression and immunosuppressive medication adherence in kidney transplant patients. Gen Hosp Psychiatry 30(4):386–387, 2008 18585547

Cupples SA, Steslow B: Use of behavioral contingency contracting with heart transplant candidates. Prog Transplant 11(2):137–144, 2001 11871049

De Bleser L, Matteson M, Dobbels F, et al: Interventions to improve medication-adherence after transplantation: a systematic review. Transpl Int 22(8):780–797, 2009 19386076

De Geest S, Burkhalter H, Bogert L, et al; Psychosocial Interest Group; Swiss Transplant Cohort Study: Describing the evolution of medication nonadherence from pretransplant until 3 years post-transplant and determining pretransplant medication nonadherence as risk factor for post-transplant nonadherence to immunosuppressives: the Swiss Transplant Cohort Study. Transpl Int 27(7):657–666, 2014 24628915

de Groen PC, Aksamit AJ, Rakela J, et al: Central nervous system toxicity after liver transplantation. The role of cyclosporine and cholesterol. N Engl J Med 317(14):861–866, 1987 3306386

Denollet J, Holmes RVF, Vrints CJ, et al: Unfavorable outcome of heart transplantation in recipients with type D personality. J Heart Lung Transplant 26(2):152–158, 2007 17258149

DeVito Dabbs A, Dew MA, Myers B, et al: Evaluation of a hand-held, computer-based intervention to promote early self-care behaviors after lung transplant. Clin Transplant 23(4):537–545, 2009 19473201

DeVito Dabbs A, Song MK, Myers BA, et al: A randomized controlled trial of a mobile health intervention to promote self-management after lung transplantation. Am J Transplant 16(7):2172–2180, 2016 26729617

Dew MA: Anxiety and depression following transplantation. Presented at the Contemporary Forums Conference on Advances in Transplantation, Chicago, IL, September 2003

Dew MA, DiMartini AF: Transplantation, in Oxford Handbook of Health Psychology. Edited by Friedman HS. New York, Oxford University Press, 2011, pp 522–559

Dew MA, Roth LH, Thompson ME, et al: Medical compliance and its predictors in the first year after heart transplantation. J Heart Lung Transplant 15(6):631–645, 1996 8794030

Dew MA, Switzer GE, DiMartini AF, et al: Psychosocial assessments and outcomes in organ transplantation. Prog Transplant 10(4):239–259, quiz 260–261, 2000 11232552

Dew MA, Kormos RL, Winowich S, et al: Quality of life outcomes after heart transplantation in individuals bridged to transplant with ventricular assist devices. J Heart Lung Transplant 20(11):1199–1212, 2001 11704480

Dew MA, Goycoolea JM, Harris RC, et al: An Internet-based intervention to improve psychosocial outcomes in heart transplant recipients and family caregivers: development and evaluation. J Heart Lung Transplant 23(6):745–758, 2004 15366436

Dew MA, DiMartini AF, De Vito Dabbs A, et al: Rates and risk factors for nonadherence to the medical regimen after adult solid organ transplantation. Transplantation 83(7):858–873, 2007a 17460556

Dew MA, Jacobs CL, Jowsey SG, et al; United Network for Organ Sharing (UNOS); American Society of Transplant Surgeons; American Society of Transplantation: Guidelines for the psychosocial evaluation of living unrelated kidney donors in the United States. Am J Transplant 7(5):1047–1054, 2007b 17359510

Dew MA, Switzer GE, DiMartini AF, et al: Psychosocial aspects of living organ donation, in Living Donor Organ Transplantation. Edited by Tan HP, Marcos A, Shapiro R. New York, Taylor & Francis, 2007c, pp 7–26

Dew MA, DiMartini AF, Steel J, et al: Meta-analysis of risk for relapse to substance use after transplantation of the liver or other solid organs. Liver Transpl 14(2):159–172, 2008 18236389

Dew MA, Dabbs AD, Myaskovsky L, et al: Meta-analysis of medical regimen adherence outcomes in pediatric solid organ transplantation. Transplantation 88(5):736–746, 2009 19741474

Dew MA, DiMartini AF, DeVito Dabbs AJ, et al: Onset and risk factors for anxiety and depression during the first 2 years after lung transplantation. Gen Hosp Psychiatry 34(2):127–138, 2012 22245165

Dew MA, DiMartini AF, DeVito Dabbs AJ, et al: Preventive intervention for living donor psychosocial outcomes: feasibility and efficacy in a randomized controlled trial. Am J Transplant 13(10):2672–2684, 2013 23924065

Dew MA, Boneysteele G, DiMartini A: Unrelated donors, in Living Donor Advocacy: An Evolving Role Within Transplantation. Edited by Steel JL. New York, Springer, 2014a, pp 149–167

Dew MA, Myaskovsky L, Steel JL, et al: Managing the psychosocial and financial consequences of living donation. Curr Transplant Rep 1(1):24–34, 2014b 24592353

Dew MA, Rosenberger EM, Myaskovsky L, et al: Depression and anxiety as risk factors for morbidity and mortality after organ transplantation: a systematic review and meta-analysis. Transplantation 100(5):988–1003, 2015 26492128

Dew MA, DiMartini AF, Ladner DP, et al: Psychosocial outcomes 3 to 10 years after donation in the Adult to Adult Living Donor Liver Transplantation Cohort Study. Transplantation 100(6):1257–1269, 2016 27152918

Dew MA, Butt Z, Humar A, et al: Long-term medical and psychosocial outcomes in living liver donors. Am J Transplant 17(4):880–892, 2017 27862972

DiMartini AF, Dew MA: Monitoring alcohol use on the liver transplant wait list: therapeutic and practical issues. Liver Transpl 18(11):1267–1269, 2012 22887916

DiMartini A, Twillman R: Organ transplantation in paranoid schizophrenia. Psychosomatics 35(2):159–161, 1994 8171175

DiMartini A, Pajer K, Trzepacz P, et al: Psychiatric morbidity in liver transplant patients. Transplant Proc 23(6):3179–3180, 1991 1721399

DiMartini A, Fitzgerald MG, Magill J, et al: Psychiatric evaluations of small intestine transplantation patients. Gen Hosp Psychiatry 18 (6 suppl):25S–29S, 1996 8937920

DiMartini A, Trzepacz PT, Pajer KA, et al: Neuropsychiatric side effects of FK506 vs. cyclosporine A. First-week postoperative findings. Psychosomatics 38(6):565–569, 1997 9427854

DiMartini A, Day N, Dew MA, et al: Alcohol use following liver transplantation: a comparison of follow-up methods. Psychosomatics 42(1):55–62, 2001 11161122

DiMartini A, Weinrieb R, Fireman M: Liver transplantation in patients with alcohol and other substance use disorders. Psychiatr Clin North Am 25(1):195–209, 2002 11912940

DiMartini A, Fontes P, Dew MA, et al: Age, model for end-stage liver disease score, and organ functioning predict posttransplant tacrolimus neurotoxicity. Liver Transpl 14:815–822, 2008 18508372

DiMartini A, Dew MA, Day N, et al: Trajectories of alcohol consumption following liver transplantation. Am J Transplant 10(10):2305–2312, 2010 20726963

DiMartini A, Crone C, Dew MA: Alcohol and substance use in liver transplant patients. Clin Liver Dis 15(4):727–751, 2011 22032526

DiMartini A, Dew MA, Liu Q, et al: Social and financial outcomes of living liver donation: a prospective investigation within the Adult-to-Adult Living Liver Cohort Study-2 (A2ALL-2). Am J Transplant 17(4):1081–1096, 2017 27647626

Dobbels F, Put C, Vanhaecke J: Personality disorders: a challenge for transplantation. Prog Transplant 10(4):226–232, 2000 11216178

Dobbels F, De Bleser L, Berben L, et al: Efficacy of a medication adherence enhancing intervention in transplantation: the MAESTRO-Tx trial. J Heart Lung Transplant 36(5):499–508, 2017 28162931

Donnadieu-Rigole H, Olive L, Nalpas B, et al: Follow up of alcohol consumption after liver transplantation: interest of an addiction team? Alcohol Clin Exp Res 41(1):165–170, 2017 27936489

Duerinckx N, Burkhalter H, Engberg SJ, et al; B-SERIOUS consortium: Correlates and outcomes of post-transplant smoking in solid organ transplant recipients: a systematic literature review and meta-analysis. Transplantation 100(11):2252–2263, 2016 27479162

Dumortier J, Dharancy S, Cannesson A, et al: Recurrent alcoholic cirrhosis in severe alcoholic relapse after liver transplantation: a frequent and serious complication. Am J Gastroenterol 110(8):1160–1166, quiz 1167, 2015 26169514

Eggers P: Comparison of treatment costs between dialysis and transplantation. Semin Nephrol 12(3):284–289, 1992 1615249

Eidelman BH, Abu-Elmagd K, Wilson J, et al: Neurologic complications of FK 506. Transplant Proc 23(6):3175–3178, 1991 1721398

Eshelman AK, Mason S, Nemeh H, et al: LVAD destination therapy: applying what we know about psychiatric evaluation and management from cardiac failure and transplant. Heart Fail Rev 14(1):21–28, 2009 18214674

Evans LD, Stock EM, Zeber JE, et al: Post-transplantation outcomes in veterans with serious mental illness transplantation. Transplantation 99(8):e57–e65, 2015 25706275

Farmer SA, Grady KL, Wang E, et al: Demographic, psychosocial, and behavioral factors associated with survival after heart transplantation. Ann Thorac Surg 95(3):876–883, 2013 23374446

Favaro A, Gerosa G, Caforio AL, et al: Posttraumatic stress disorder and depression in heart transplantation recipients: the relationship with outcome and adherence to medical treatment. Gen Hosp Psychiatry 33(1):1–7, 2011 21353121

Ferenci P, Lockwood A, Mullen K, et al: Hepatic encephalopathy—definition, nomenclature, diagnosis, and quantification: final report of the working party at the 11th World Congresses of Gastroenterology, Vienna, 1998. Hepatology 35(3):716–721, 2002 11870389

Fine RN, Becker Y, De Geest S, et al: Nonadherence consensus conference summary report. Am J Transplant 9(1):35–41, 2009 19133930

Fineberg SK, West A, Na PJ, et al: Utility of pretransplant psychological measures to predict posttransplant outcomes in liver transplant patients: a systematic review. Gen Hosp Psychiatry 40:4–11, 2016 26947255

Fireman M: Outcome of liver transplantation in patients with alcohol and polysubstance dependence. Presented at Research Society on Alcoholism: Symposium on Liver Transplantation for the Alcohol Dependent Patient, Denver, CO, June 2000

Fireman M, DiMartini A, Crone C: Organ transplantation, in Psychopharmacology of the Medically Ill, 2nd Edition. Edited by Ferrando SJ, Levenson JL. Arlington, VA, American Psychiatric Publishing, 2017, pp 597–632

Fishbein TM: Intestinal transplantation. N Engl J Med 361(10):998–1008, 2009 19726774

Fleming JN, Taber DJ, McElligott J, et al: Mobile health in solid organ transplant: the time is now. Am J Transplant 17(9):2263–2276, 2017 28188681

Fredericks EM, Magee JC, Opipari-Arrigan L, et al: Adherence and health-related quality of life in adolescent liver transplant recipients. Pediatr Transplant 12(3):289–299, 2008 18282211

Freeman J, Emond J, Gillespie BW, et al; A2ALL Study Group: Computerized assessment of competence-related abilities in living liver donors: the Adult-to-Adult Living Donor Liver Transplantation Cohort Study. Clin Transplant 27(4):633–645, 2013 23859354

Freise CE, Rowley H, Lake J, et al: Similar clinical presentation of neurotoxicity following FK 506 and cyclosporine in a liver transplant recipient. Transplant Proc 23(6):3173–3174, 1991 1721397

Fung JJ, Alessiani M, Abu-Elmagd K, et al: Adverse effects associated with the use of FK 506. Transplant Proc 23(6):3105–3108, 1991 1721372

Fusar-Poli P, Martinelli V, Klersy C, et al: Depression and quality of life in patients living 10 to 18 years beyond heart transplantation. J Heart Lung Transplant 24(12):2269–2278, 2005 16364881

Fusar-Poli P, Lazzaretti M, Ceruti M, et al: Depression after lung transplantation: causes and treatment. Lung 185(2):55–65, 2007 17393235

Garton T: Nefazodone and CYP450 3A4 interactions with cyclosporine and tacrolimus1. Transplantation 74(5):745, 2002 12352898

Gijtenbeek JM, van den Bent MJ, Vecht CJ: Cyclosporine neurotoxicity: a review. J Neurol 246(5):339–346, 1999 10399863

Goracci A, Fagiolini A, Calossi S, et al: Quetiapine in post-transplant acute mania/bipolar disorder NOS. Int J Neuropsychopharmacol 11(5):723–724, 2008 18346295

Grady KL, Dew MA: Psychosocial issues in mechanical circulatory support, in Mechanical Circulatory Support: A Companion to Braunwald's Heart Disease. Edited by Kormos RL, Miller LW. Philadelphia, PA, Elsevier, 2012, pp 194–205

Grant D, Abu-Elmagd K, Mazariegos G, et al; Intestinal Transplant Association: Intestinal Transplant Registry report: global activity and trends. Am J Transplant 15(1):210–219, 2015 25438622

Guyatt GH, Berman LB, Townsend M, et al: A measure of quality of life for clinical trials in chronic lung disease. Thorax 42(10):773–778, 1987 3321537

Hails KC, Kanchana T: Outcome of liver transplants for patients on methadone. Poster presented at the 153rd annual meeting of the American Psychiatric Association, Chicago, IL, May 13–18, 2000

Hebert MF, Wacher VJ, Roberts JP, et al: Pharmacokinetics of cyclosporine pre- and post-liver transplantation. J Clin Pharmacol 43(1):38–42, 2003 12520626

Helms-Smith KM, Curtis SL, Hatton RC: Apparent interaction between nefazodone and cyclosporine (letter). Ann Intern Med 125(5):424, 1996 8702104

Hurt RD, Sachs DP, Glover ED, et al: A comparison of sustained-release bupropion and placebo for smoking cessation. N Engl J Med 337(17):1195–1202, 1997 9337378

Iacoviello BM, Shenoy A, Hunt J, et al: A prospective study of the reliability and validity of the Live Donor Assessment Tool. Psychosomatics 58(5):519–526, 2017 28526401

Ikitimur B, Cosansu K, Karadag B, et al: Long-term impact of different immunosuppressive drugs on QT and PR intervals in renal transplant patients. Ann Noninvasive Electrocardiol 20(5):426–432, 2015 25367596

Im GY, Kim-Schluger L, Shenoy A, et al: Early liver transplantation for severe alcoholic hepatitis in the United States—a single-center experience. Am J Transplant 16(3):841–849, 2016 26710309

Jacobs CL, Roman D, Garvey C, et al: Twenty-two nondirected kidney donors: an update on a single center's experience. Am J Transplant 4(7):1110–1116, 2004 15196069

Jin SG, Yan LN, Xiang B, et al: Posttraumatic stress disorder after liver transplantation. Hepatobiliary Pancreat Dis Int 11(1):28–33, 2012 22251467

Joost R, Dörje F, Schwitulla J, et al: Intensified pharmaceutical care is improving immunosuppressive medication adherence in kidney transplant recipients during the first post-transplant year: a quasi-experimental study. Nephrol Dial Transplant 29(8):1597–1607, 2014 24914089

Jorenby DE, Leischow SJ, Nides MA, et al: A controlled trial of sustained-release bupropion, a nicotine patch, or both for smoking cessation. N Engl J Med 340(9):685–691, 1999 10053177

Jowsey SG, Taylor M, Trenerry MR: Special topics in transplantation: psychometric screening of transplant candidates. Oral presentation presented at the annual meeting of the Academy of Psychosomatic Medicine, Tucson, AZ, November 2002

Jowsey SG, Jacobs C, Gross CR, et al; RELIVE Study Group: Emotional well-being of living kidney donors: findings from the RELIVE Study. Am J Transplant 14(11):2535–2544, 2014 25293374

Kanchana TP, Kaul V, Manzarbeitia C, et al: Liver transplantation for patients on methadone maintenance. Liver Transpl 8(9):778–782, 2002 12200777

Kazley AS, Amarnath R, Palanisamy A, et al: Anonymous altruistic living kidney donation in the US: reality and practice. International Journal of Transplant Research and Medicine 2(2):021, 2016

Kirklin JK, Naftel DC, Kormos RL, et al: Fifth INTERMACS annual report: risk factor analysis from more than 6000 mechanical circulatory support patients. J Heart Lung Transplant 32(2):141–156, 2013 23352390

Koch M, Banys P: Liver transplantation and opioid dependence. JAMA 285(8):1056–1058, 2001 11209177

Komoda T, Drews T, Sakuraba S, et al: Executive cognitive dysfunction without stroke after long-term mechanical circulatory support. ASAIO J 51(6):764–768, 2005 16340365

Krahn LE, Santoscoy G, Van Loon JA: A schizophrenic patient's attempt to resume dialysis following renal transplantation. Psychosomatics 39(5):470–473, 1998 9775708

Kramer L, Madl C, Stockenhuber F, et al: Beneficial effect of renal transplantation on cognitive brain function. Kidney Int 49(3):833–838, 1996 8648927

Kranick SM, Mowry EM, Rosenfeld MR: Progressive multifocal leukoencephalopathy after rituximab in a case of non-Hodgkin lymphoma. Neurology 69(7):704–706, 2007 17698796

Laederach-Hofmann K, Bunzel B: Noncompliance in organ transplant recipients: a literature review. Gen Hosp Psychiatry 22(6):412–424, 2000 11072057

Lake JR: Liver transplantation, in Current Diagnosis and Treatment in Gastroenterology, 2nd Edition. Edited by Friedman SL, McQuaid KR, Grendell JH. New York, McGraw-Hill, 2003, pp 813–834

Lam WY, Fresco P: Medication adherence measures: an overview. Biomed Res Int 2015:217047, 2015 26539470

Langnas AN: Advances in small-intestine transplantation. Transplantation 77 (9 suppl):S75–S78, 2004 15201690

Lee BP, Chen P-H, Haugen C, et al: Three-year results of a pilot program in early liver transplantation for severe alcoholic hepatitis. Ann Surg 265(1):20–29, 2017 27280501

Levenson J, Olbrisch ME: Psychosocial screening and selection of candidates for organ transplantation, in The Transplant Patient. Edited by Trzepacz PT, DiMartini AF. Cambridge, UK, Cambridge University Press, 2000, pp 21–41

Liu LU, Schiano TD, Lau N, et al: Survival and risk of recidivism in methadone-dependent patients undergoing liver transplantation. Am J Transplant 3(10):1273–1277, 2003 14510701

Lucey MR: Liver transplantation for alcoholic liver disease. Nat Rev Gastroenterol Hepatol 11(5):300–307, 2014 24393837

Lück R, Böger J, Kuse E, et al: Achieving adequate cyclosporine exposure in liver transplant recipients: a novel strategy for monitoring and dosing using intravenous therapy. Liver Transpl 10(5):686–691, 2004 15108262

Maldonado J, Plante R, David E: The Stanford Integrated Psychosocial Assessment for Transplantation (SIPAT). Oral presentation presented at the annual meeting of the Academy of Psychosomatic Medicine, Miami, FL, November 22, 2008

Mapelli D, Cavazzana A, Cavalli C, et al: Clinical psychological and neuropsychological issues with left ventricular assist devices (LVADs). Ann Cardiothorac Surg 3(5):480–489, 2014 25452908

Maple H, Chilcot J, Burnapp L, et al: Motivations, outcomes, and characteristics of unspecified (nondirected altruistic) kidney donors in the United Kingdom. Transplantation 98(11):1182–1189, 2014 25099701

Marks WH, Florence L, Lieberman J, et al: Successfully treated invasive pulmonary aspergillosis associated with smoking marijuana in a renal transplant recipient. Transplantation 61(12):1771–1774, 1996 8685958

Masson S, Marrow B, Kendrick S, et al: An "alcohol contract" has no significant effect on return to drinking after liver transplantation for alcoholic liver disease. Transpl Int 27(5):475–481, 2014 24533687

Mathurin P, Moreno C, Samuel D, et al: Early liver transplantation for severe alcoholic hepatitis. N Engl J Med 365(19):1790–1800, 2011 22070476

McGillicuddy JW, Gregoski MJ, Weiland AK, et al: Mobile health medication adherence and blood pressure control in renal transplant recipients: a proof-of-concept randomized controlled trial. JMIR Res Protoc 2(2):e32, 2013 24004517

Messersmith EE, Gross CR, Beil CA, et al; RELIVE Study Group: Satisfaction with life among living kidney donors: a RELIVE study of long-term donor outcomes. Transplantation 98(12):1294–1399, 2014 25136843

Michalski LS, Bhuva D, Pakrasi A, et al: Sirolimus and nefazodone interaction in a renal transplant patient. Eur J Psychiatry 25(3):119–121, 2011

Miller LR, Paulson D, Eshelman A, et al: Mental health affects the quality of life and recovery after liver transplantation. Liver Transpl 19(11):1272–1278, 2013 23959592

Miller P, Wikoff R, McMahon M, et al: Development of a health attitude scale. Nurs Res 31(3):132–136, 1982 6918917

Mori DL, Gallagher P, Milne J: The Structured Interview for Renal Transplantation—SIRT. Psychosomatics 41(5):393–406, 2000 11015625

Mucsi I, Bansal A, Jeannette M, et al: Mental health and behavioral barriers in access to kidney transplantation: a Canadian cohort study. Transplantation 101(6):1182–1190, 2017 27467541

Nabel GJ: A transformed view of cyclosporine. Nature 397(6719):471–472, 1999 10028962

Neuberger J, Adams D, MacMaster P, et al: Assessing priorities for allocation of donor liver grafts: survey of public and clinicians. BMJ 317(7152):172–175, 1998 9665895

Nevins TE, Nickerson PW, Dew MA: Understanding medication nonadherence after kidney transplantation. J Am Soc Nephrol 28(8):2290–2301, 2017 28630231

Neyer J, Uberoi A, Hamilton M, et al: Marijuana and listing for heart transplant: a survey of transplant providers. Circ Heart Fail 9(7):e002851, 2016 27413036

Ojo AO, Held PJ, Port FK, et al: Chronic renal failure after transplantation of a nonrenal organ. N Engl J Med 349(10):931–940, 2003 12954741

Olbrisch ME, Levenson JL, Hamer R: The PACT: a rating scale for the study of clinical decision making in psychosocial screening of organ transplant candidates. Clinical Transplantation 3(3):164–169, 1989

Olbrisch ME, Benedict SM, Haller DL, et al: Psychosocial assessment of living organ donors: clinical and ethical considerations. Prog Transplant 11(1):40–49, 2001 11357556

Olbrisch ME, Benedict SM, Ashe K, et al: Psychological assessment and care of organ transplant patients. J Consult Clin Psychol 70(3):771–783, 2002 12090382

Organ Procurement and Transplantation Network: Data. 2017a. Available at: https://optn.transplant.hrsa.gov/data/. Accessed September 26, 2017.

Organ Procurement and Transplantation Network: Policies. 2017b. Available at: https://optn.transplant.hrsa.gov/governance/policies/. Accessed September 26, 2017.

Parekh PI, Blumenthal JA, Babyak MA, et al; INSPIRE Investigators: Gas exchange and exercise capacity affect neurocognitive performance in patients with lung disease. Psychosom Med 67(3):425–432, 2005 15911906

Park SJ, Milano CA, Tatooles AJ, et al; HeartMate II Clinical Investigators: Outcomes in advanced heart failure patients with left ventricular assist devices for destination therapy. Circ Heart Fail 5(2):241–248, 2012 22282104

Pedersen SS, Holkamp PG, Caliskan K, et al: Type D personality is associated with impaired health-related quality of life 7 years following heart transplantation. J Psychosom Res 61(6):791–795, 2006 17141667

Pescovitz MD, Navarro MT: Immunosuppressive therapy and post-transplantation diarrhea. Clin Transplant 15 (suppl 4):23–28, 2001 11778784

Pironi L, Baxter JP, Lauro A, et al: Assessment of quality of life on home parenteral nutrition and after intestinal transplantation using treatment-specific questionnaires. Am J Transplant 12 (suppl 4):S60–S66, 2012 22958831

Popoola J, Greene H, Kyegombe M, et al: Patient involvement in selection of immunosuppressive regimen following transplantation. Patient Prefer Adherence 8:1705–1712, 2014 25525347

Price A, Whitwell S, Henderson M: Impact of psychotic disorder on transplant eligibility and outcomes. Curr Opin Organ Transplant 19(2):196–200, 2014 24553499

Pungpapong S, Manzarbeitia C, Ortiz J, et al: Cigarette smoking is associated with an increased incidence of vascular complications after liver transplantation. Liver Transpl 8(7):582–587, 2002 12089709

Reese PP, Bloom RD, Trofe-Clark J, et al: Automated reminders and physician notification to promote immunosuppression adherence among kidney transplant recipients: a randomized trial. Am J Kidney Dis 69(3):400–409, 2017 27940063

Rice JP, Eickhoff J, Agni R, et al: Abusive drinking after liver transplantation is associated with allograft loss and advanced allograft fibrosis. Liver Transpl 19(12):1377–1386, 2013 24115392

Riggio O, Angeloni S, Salvatori FM, et al: Incidence, natural history, and risk factors of hepatic encephalopathy after transjugular intrahepatic portosystemic shunt with polytetrafluoroethylene-covered stent grafts. Am J Gastroenterol 103(11):2738–2746, 2008 18775022

Riordan SM, Williams R: Treatment of hepatic encephalopathy. N Engl J Med 337(7):473–479, 1997 9250851

Robinson MJ, Levenson JL: Psychopharmacology in transplant patients, in Biopsychosocial Perspectives on Transplantation. Edited by Rodrigue JR. New York, Kluwer Academic/Plenum, 2001, pp 151–172

Roche Pharmaceuticals: CellCept (Mycophenolate Mofetil) Product Information. Nutley, NJ, Roche Laboratories, 2003

Rodrigue JR, Mandelbrot DA, Pavlakis M: A psychological intervention to improve quality of life and reduce psychological distress in adults awaiting kidney transplantation. Nephrol Dial Transplant 26(2):709–715, 2011 20603243

Rodrigue JR, Hanto DW, Curry MP: The Alcohol Relapse Risk Assessment: a scoring system to predict the risk of relapse to any alcohol use after liver transplant. Prog Transplant 23(4):310–318, 2013 24311394

Rodrigue JR, Schold JD, Morrissey P, et al; KDOC Study Group: Predonation direct and indirect costs incurred by adults who donated a kidney: findings from the KDOC study. Am J Transplant 15(9):2387–2393, 2015 25943721

Rodrigue JR, Schold JD, Morrissey P, et al; KDOC Study Group: Direct and indirect costs following living kidney donation: findings from the KDOC study. Am J Transplant 16(3):869–876, 2016 26845630

Rogal SS, Dew MA, Fontes P, DiMartini AF: Early treatment of depressive symptoms and long-term survival after liver transplantation. Am J Transplant 13(4):928–935, 2013 23425326

Rosenberger EM, Dew MA, DiMartini AF, et al: Psychosocial issues facing lung transplant candidates, recipients and family caregivers. Thorac Surg Clin 22(4):517–529, 2012 23084615

Rosenberger EM, DiMartini AF, DeVito Dabbs AJ, et al: Psychiatric predictors of long-term transplant-related outcomes in lung transplant recipients. Transplantation 100(1):239–247, 2016 26177087

Ross LF: All donations should not be treated equally: a response to Jeffrey Kahn's commentary. J Law Med Ethics 30(3):448–451, 2002 12497705

Rush D, Nickerson P, Gough J, et al: Beneficial effects of treatment of early subclinical rejection: a randomized study. J Am Soc Nephrol 9(11):2129–2134, 1998 9808101

Rustad JK, Stern TA, Prabhakar M, Musselman D: Risk factors for alcohol relapse following orthotopic liver transplantation: a systematic review. Psychosomatics 56(1):21–35, 2015 25619671

Ruttens D, Verleden SE, Goeminne PC, et al: Smoking resumption after lung transplantation: standardised screening and importance for long-term outcome. Eur Respir J 43(1):300–303, 2014 23988766

Samelson-Jones E, Mancini DM, Shapiro PA: Cardiac transplantation in adult patients with mental retardation: do outcomes support consensus guidelines? Psychosomatics 53(2):133–138, 2012 22424161

Sansone RA, Bohinc RJ, Wiederman MW: Borderline personality symptomatology and compliance with general health care among internal medicine outpatients. Int J Psychiatry Clin Pract 19(2):132–136, 2015 25410155

Schomerus H, Hamster W, Blunck H, et al: Latent portasystemic encephalopathy, I: nature of cerebral functional defects and their effect on fitness to drive. Dig Dis Sci 26(7):622–630, 1981 7249898

Seem DL, Lee I, Umscheid CA, Kuehnert MJ; United States Public Health Service: PHS guideline for reducing human immunodeficiency virus, hepatitis B virus, and hepatitis C virus transmission through organ transplantation. Public Health Rep 128(4):247–343, 2013 23814319

Shapiro PA: Heart transplantation in a schizophrenia patient. Am J Psychiatry 162(11):2194–2195, 2005 16263872

Shapiro PA, Williams DL, Foray AT, et al: Psychosocial evaluation and prediction of compliance problems and morbidity after heart transplantation. Transplantation 60(12):1462–1466, 1995 8545875

Shaw LM, Mick R, Nowak I, et al: Pharmacokinetics of mycophenolic acid in renal transplant patients with delayed graft function. J Clin Pharmacol 38(3):268–275, 1998 9549665

Shoskes DA, Cecka JM: Deleterious effects of delayed graft function in cadaveric renal transplant recipients independent of acute rejection. Transplantation 66(12):1697–1701, 1998 9884262

Small SL, Fukui MB, Bramblett GT, et al: Immunosuppression-induced leukoencephalopathy from tacrolimus (FK506). Ann Neurol 40(4):575–580, 1996 8871576

Smith PJ, Blumenthal JA, Carney RM, et al: Neurobehavioral functioning and survival following lung transplantation. Chest 145(3):604–611, 2014 24233282

Sotil EU, Gottstein J, Ayala E, et al: Impact of preoperative overt hepatic encephalopathy on neurocognitive function after liver transplantation. Liver Transpl 15(2):184–192, 2009 19177446

Starzl TE: The saga of liver replacement, with particular reference to the reciprocal influence of liver and kidney transplantation (1955–1967). J Am Coll Surg 195(5):587–610, 2002 12437245

Sterneck M, Yegles M, Rothkirch von G, et al: Determination of ethyl glucuronide in hair improves evaluation of long-term alcohol abstention in liver transplant candidates. Liver Int 34(3):469–476, 2014 23829409

Stevenson LW: Indications for listing and de-listing patients for cardiac transplantation (Chapter 233 [Cardiac Transplantation], reviews and editorials), in Harrison's Online. 2002. Available at: http://harrisons.accessmedicine.com. Accessed September 26, 2017.

Stilley CS, Miller DJ, Tarter RE: Measuring psychological distress in candidates for liver transplantation: a pilot study. J Clin Psychol 53(5):459–464, 1997 9257224

Stilley CS, Dew MA, Pilkonis P, et al: Personality characteristics among cardiothoracic transplant recipients. Gen Hosp Psychiatry 27(2):113–118, 2005 15763122

Strouse TB, Fairbanks LA, Skotzko CE, et al: Fluoxetine and cyclosporine in organ transplantation. Failure to detect significant drug interactions or adverse clinical events in depressed organ recipients. Psychosomatics 37(1):23–30, 1996 8600490

Strouse TB, el-Saden SM, Glaser NE, et al: Immunosuppressant neurotoxicity in liver transplant recipients. Clinical challenges for the consultation-liaison psychiatrist. Psychosomatics 39(2):124–133, 1998 9584538

Stuber ML, Shemesh E, Seacord D, et al: Evaluating non-adherence to immunosuppressant medications in pediatric liver transplant recipients. Pediatr Transplant 12(3):284–288, 2008 18331387

Surman OS: The ethics of partial-liver donation (comment). N Engl J Med 346(14):1038, 2002 11932469

Surman OS, Purtilo R: Reevaluation of organ transplantation criteria. Allocation of scarce resources to borderline candidates. Psychosomatics 33(2):202–212, 1992 1557485

Tarter RE, Switala JA, Arria A, et al: Subclinical hepatic encephalopathy. Comparison before and after orthotopic liver transplantation. Transplantation 50(4):632–637, 1990 2219286

Thoennissen NH, Schneider M, Allroggen A, et al: High level of cerebral microembolization in patients supported with the DeBakey left ventricular assist device. J Thorac Cardiovasc Surg 130(4):1159–1166, 2005 16214534

Thompson D, DiMartini A: Nonenteral routes of administration for psychiatric medications. A literature review. Psychosomatics 40:185–192, 1999 10341530

Thompson GR3rd, Tuscano JM, Dennis M, et al: A microbiome assessment of medical marijuana. Clin Microbiol Infect 23(4):269–270, 2017 27956269

Trotter JF, Hill-Callahan MM, Gillespie BW, et al; A2ALL Study Group: Severe psychiatric problems in right hepatic lobe donors for living donor liver transplantation. Transplantation 83(11):1506–1508, 2007 17565325

Trzepacz PT, DiMartini AF, Gupta B: Psychopharmacologic issues in transplantation, in The Transplant Patient. Edited by Trzepacz P, DiMartini A. Cambridge, UK, Cambridge University Press, 2000, pp 187–213

Twillman RK, Manetto C, Wellisch DK, et al: The Transplant Evaluation Rating Scale. A revision of the psychosocial levels system for evaluating organ transplant candidates. Psychosomatics 34(2):144–153, 1993 8456157

U.S. Department of Health and Human Services, Health Resources and Services Administration, Healthcare Systems Bureau, Division of Transplantation: Organ Procurement and Transplantation Network (OPTN) and Scientific Registry of Transplant Recipients (SRTR) 2011 Annual Data Report. Rockville, MD, U.S. Department of Health and Human Services, Health Resources and Services Administration, Healthcare Systems Bureau, Division of Transplantation, 2012. Available at: https://srtr.transplant.hrsa.gov/annual_reports/2011/Default.aspx. Accessed September 26, 2017.

U.S. Renal Data System: USRDS 2008 annual data report: atlas of chronic kidney disease and end-stage renal disease in the United States. Bethesda, MD, National Institutes of Health, National Institute of Diabetes and Digestive and Kidney Diseases, 2008. Available at: https://www.usrds.org/atlas08.aspx. Accessed September 26, 2017.

Vaillant GE: The natural history of alcoholism and its relationship to liver transplantation. Liver Transpl Surg 3(3):304–310, 1997 9346756

Van Laecke S, Nagler EV, Peeters P, et al: Former smoking and early and long-term graft outcome in renal transplant recipients: a retrospective cohort study. Transpl Int 30(2):187–195, 2017 27896857

Waterman AD, Robbins ML, Paiva AL, et al: Your Path to Transplant: a randomized controlled trial of a tailored computer education intervention to increase living donor kidney transplant. BMC Nephrol 15:166, 2014 25315644

Watson CJ, Friend PJ, Jamieson NV, et al: Sirolimus: a potent new immunosuppressant for liver transplantation. Transplantation 67(4):505–509, 1999 10071017

Webzell I, Ball D, Bell J, et al: Substance use by liver transplant candidates: an anonymous urinalysis study. Liver Transpl 17(10):1200–1204, 2011 21744466

Weinrieb RM, Van Horn DH, McLellan AT, et al: Interpreting the significance of drinking by alcohol-dependent liver transplant patients: fostering candor is the key to recovery. Liver Transpl 6(6):769–776, 2000 11084066

Weinrieb RM, Van Horn DH, McLellan AT, et al: Alcoholism treatment after liver transplantation: lessons learned from a clinical trial that failed. Psychosomatics 42(2):110–116, 2001 11239123

Weinrieb RM, Barnett R, Lynch KG, et al: A matched comparison study of medical and psychiatric complications and anesthesia and analgesia requirements in methadone-maintained liver transplant recipients. Liver Transpl 10(1):97–106, 2004 14755785

Weinrieb RM, Van Horn DH, Lynch KG, Lucey MR: A randomized, controlled study of treatment for alcohol dependence in patients awaiting liver transplantation. Liver Transpl 17(5):539–547, 2011 21506242

Weitzner MA, Lehninger F, Sullivan D, et al: Borderline personality disorder and bone marrow transplantation: ethical considerations and review. Psychooncology 8(1):46–54, 1999 10202782

Weng FL, Israni AK, Joffe MM, et al: Race and electronically measured adherence to immuno-suppressive medications after deceased donor renal transplantation. J Am Soc Nephrol 16(6):1839–1848, 2005 15800121

Wijdicks EF, Wiesner RH, Krom RA: Neurotoxicity in liver transplant recipients with cyclosporine immunosuppression. Neurology 45(11):1962–1964, 1995 7501141

Wijdicks EF, Plevak DJ, Wiesner RH, et al: Causes and outcome of seizures in liver transplant recipients. Neurology 47(6):1523–1525, 1996 8960738

Wijdicks EF, Dahlke LJ, Wiesner RH: Oral cyclosporine decreases severity of neurotoxicity in liver transplant recipients. Neurology 52(8):1708–1710, 1999 10331708

Wilkinson ST, D'Souza DC: Problems with the medicalization of marijuana. JAMA 311(23):2377–2378, 2014 24845238

Wilson SE, de Groen PC, Aksamit AJ, et al: Cyclosporin A-induced reversible cortical blindness. J Clin Neuroophthalmol 8(4):215–220, 1988 2977135

Wirken L, van Middendorp H, Hooghof CW, et al: Pre-donation cognitions of potential living organ donors: the development of the Donation Cognition Instrument in potential kidney donors. Nephrol Dial Transplant 32(3):573–580, 2017 28160472

Wright DH, Lake KD, Bruhn PS, Emery RW Jr: Nefazodone and cyclosporine drug-drug interaction. J Heart Lung Transplant 18(9):913–915, 1999 10528754

Wright L, Pennington JJ, Abbey S, et al: Evaluation of a mentorship program for heart transplant patients. J Heart Lung Transplant 20(9):1030–1033, 2001 11557200

Yates WR, Booth BM, Reed DA, et al: Descriptive and predictive validity of a high-risk alcoholism relapse model. J Stud Alcohol 54(6):645–651, 1993 8271799

Yates WR, LaBrecque DR, Pfab D: Personality disorder as a contraindication for liver transplantation in alcoholic cirrhosis. Psychosomatics 39(6):501–511, 1998 9819950

Zelikovsky N, Schast AP, Palmer J, et al: Perceived barriers to adherence among adolescent renal transplant candidates. Pediatr Transplant 12(3):300–308, 2008 18194352

Zimbrean P, Emre S: Patients with psychotic disorders in solid-organ transplant. Prog Transplant 25(4):289–296, 2015 26645920

Zitt N, Kollerits B, Neyer U, et al: Cigarette smoking and chronic allograft nephropathy. Nephrol Dial Transplant 22(10):3034–3039, 2007 17517794

CHAPTER 30

Neurology and Neurosurgery

Alan J. Carson, M.Phil., M.D., FRCPsych, FRCP

Adam Zeman, M.A., D.M., FRCP

Jon Stone, Ph.D., FRCP

The divide between neurology and psychiatry is viewed by some as a historical artifact (Baker et al. 2002). New developments in neuroscience are bringing an understanding of the mechanisms of interactions among biological, psychological, and social aspects of illness, making this one of the most intellectually fascinating areas of work for a psychiatrist. Psychiatrists working in a clinical neurosciences center are likely to be required to address four main categories of clinical problems:

1. Cognitive impairment—either as a primary presentation or as a secondary complication of a known condition such as multiple sclerosis
2. Neurological disease accompanied by emotional and behavioral disturbance in excess of the clinical norm
3. Neurological symptoms that do not correspond to any recognized pattern of neurological disease
4. Post-neurosurgery complications—usually involving behavioral, cognitive, or emotional disturbance

In this chapter, we concentrate on commonly encountered neurological conditions. The principles of assessment applicable to these disorders are also relevant to other, rarer neurological conditions. Psychopharmacological and psychological treatments are not discussed in detail here because they are covered in other chapters. Although we refer to drug therapies, we wish to remind the reader that for many neuropsychiatric conditions, behavioral management and environmental manipulation are of equal importance.

Neuropsychiatric topics covered elsewhere in this book include the mental status examination (Chapter 1, "Psychiatric Assessment and Consultation"), delirium (Chapter 4, "Delirium"), dementia (Chapter 5, "Dementia"), traumatic brain and spinal cord injuries (Chapter 33, "Physical Medicine and Rehabilitation"), pain syndromes (Chapter 34, "Pain"), and psychopharmacological interventions in neurological disease (Chapter 36, "Psychopharmacology").

Stroke

Stroke is defined as "a clinical syndrome which is characterized by an acute loss of focal cerebral function with symptoms lasting more than 24 hours or leading to death, and which is thought to be due to either spontaneous hemorrhage into the brain substance (hemorrhagic stroke) or inadequate cerebral blood supply to a part of the brain (ischemic stroke) as a result of low blood flow, thrombosis or embolism associated with diseases of the blood vessels (arteries or veins), heart or blood" (Warlow et al. 2008, p. 35). Infarctions account for 85% of stroke cases and, as a result of a lower immediate fatality rate than hemorrhage, are a much greater source of enduring disability, with a 1-year survival rate of approximately 75%, compared with 33% survival after a hemorrhagic stroke. Strokes are the third most common cause of death in the Western world. The Oxfordshire Community Stroke Project (OCSP) reported a population incidence of 2 per 1,000 for first-ever stroke (Bamford et al. 1988). Age is the major risk factor, although one-quarter of persons affected are younger than 65 years. Stroke occurs more commonly in men.

Clinical Features

Stroke and its associated syndromes are normally categorized according to the OCSP classification (Table 30–1).

Cognitive Impairment and Delirium

Delirium affects 30%–40% of patients during the first week after a stroke, especially after a hemorrhagic stroke (Gustafson et al. 1993; Langhorne et al. 2000; Rahkonen et al. 2000). If not specifically inquired about, it will often be missed. It is important to distinguish delirium from focal cognitive deficits affecting declarative memory. Some clinicians recommend the use of structured scales such as the Confusion Assessment Method or the Delirium Rating Scale (McManus et al. 2009a). Predictors of delirium include preexisting dementia, older age, impaired vision, impaired swallowing, and inability to raise both arms (McManus et al. 2009b; Sheng et al. 2006). The presence of delirium after stroke is associated with poorer prognosis, longer duration of hospitalization, increased mortality, increased risk of dementia, and institutionalization (Shi et al. 2012).

Dementia following stroke is common; dementia is found to be present in up to one-third of patients at 3 months poststroke (Mijajlović et al. 2017), and its risk is independent of prior cognitive function (Reitz et al. 2008). The incidence rises significantly if focal impairments are also considered. *Vascular dementia* is an imprecise term referring to a heterogeneous group of dementing disorders caused by impairment of

TABLE 30–1. **Oxfordshire Community Stroke Project classification of stroke syndromes**

Total anterior circulation syndrome (TACS)	1) Motor
	    Hemiplegia and/ or facial weakness or severe hemiparesis ± hemisensory deficit
	2) Higher cerebral
	    Dysphasia (dominant hemisphere)
	    Visuospatial deficit or neglect (nondominant hemisphere)
	3) Visual field
	    Homonymous hemianopsia

Partial anterior circulation syndrome (PACS)	Two of the above *[1) 2) 3)]*

Lacunar syndrome (LACS)	Pure motor stroke
	    Unilateral weakness must involve at least two out of three areas of the face, whole arm, and leg
	Pure sensory stroke
	    Ataxic hemiparesis
	    Sensorimotor stroke
	    No visual field defect; no impairment in higher cerebral function

Posterior circulation syndrome (POCS)	Any of the following:
	    Ipsilateral cranial nerve (III–XII) palsy with contralateral motor and/or sensory deficit
	    Bilateral motor and/or sensory deficit
	    Disorder of conjugate eye movement
	    Cerebellar dysfunction
	    Isolated hemianopia or cortical blindness

Source. Content adapted from Warlow et al. 2008.

the brain's blood supply. These disorders fall into three principal categories: subcortical ischemic dementia, multi-infarct dementia, and dementia due to focal "strategic" infarction. Most authorities agree that poststroke dementia combines features of vascular insult with the more typical neurodegenerative features (Mijajlović et al. 2017). Although the Montreal Cognitive Assessment (MoCa) is the generally recommended screening tool, it has relatively poor sensitivity. We consider that the extra time spent to use Addenbooke's Cognitive Examination (Hsieh et al. 2013)—20 minutes as opposed to 10—is time well spent for such an important clinical consideration (Mijajlović et al. 2017). Treatment trials to date have not been encouraging, and a range of strategies—including secondary prevention with antihypertensives and statins, lifestyle modifications (e.g., exercise), treatment with cognitive enhancers, and cognitive rehabilitation—have failed to show convincing benefits (Mijajlović et al. 2017). The next wave of interventions, targeting pathophysiological mechanisms such as tau processes or inflammatory mediators, may have more to offer. In the meantime, primary prevention of stroke holds the most promise (Mijajlović et al. 2017).

The common occurrence of relatively subtle cognitive decline, falling short of frank dementia, in the context of cerebrovascular disease has given rise to the broader concept of "vascular cognitive impairment." Subcortical ischemic dementia and multi-infarct dementia are described in more detail in Chapter 5. The term *strategic infarction* refers to the occurrence of unexpectedly severe cognitive impairment following limited infarction, often in the absence of classic signs such as hemiplegia. Sites at which infarctions can have such an effect include the thalamus, especially the medial thalamus; the inferior genu of the internal capsule; the basal ganglia; the left angular gyrus (causing Gerstmann's syndrome of agraphia, acalculia, left–right disorientation, and finger agnosia); the basal forebrain; and the territory of the posterior cerebral arteries.

Behavioral Changes

The diverse behavioral changes following stroke are not unique to this condition and can therefore serve as a helpful model for understanding the clinical consequences of focal cerebral lesions of other causes (Bogousslavsky and Cummings 2000).

Aphasia

Global aphasia leads to the abolition of all linguistic faculties, and the mental state examination must rely on inferences from the patient's behavior and nonverbal communication. Aphasia is often accompanied by intense emotional frustration (Carota et al. 2000). Wernicke's aphasia is characterized by a lack of insight, with the patient unable to comprehend that he or she cannot communicate (Lazar et al. 2000).

Anosognosia

Anosognosia refers to partial or complete unawareness of a deficit. This phenomenon occurs more frequently with right-sided lesions, particularly those in the region of the middle cerebral artery (Breier et al. 1995; Jehkonen et al. 2006). It may coexist with depression (Starkstein et al. 1990), a finding that both implicates separate neural systems for different aspects of emotions (Damasio 1994) and suggests that depression after stroke cannot be explained solely as a psychological reaction to disability (Ramasubbu 1994). Anosognosia for hemiplegia is perhaps the most often described form of the condition; however, anosognosia can occur with reference to any function, and it is commonly associated with visual and language dysfunction. Patients with anosognosia have no spontaneous complaints and may, for instance, claim normal movements in the paralyzed limb. Patients may attempt to walk normally despite the hemiplegia, yet paradoxically accept a wheelchair, all while continuing to maintain that their functioning is intact. In extreme cases, ownership of the limb is denied—or, exceptionally, "extra" phantom limb sensations ("somatoparaphrenia") can occur. There is no established effective treatment for somatoparaphrenia, although in research settings the use of mirrors to create the illusion of normal movement in the affected hand seems to transiently restore a sense of limb ownership (Fotopoulou et al. 2011).

Affective Dysprosody

Affective dysprosody involves impairment in the production and comprehension of language components used to communicate inner emotional states in speech. These components include stresses, pauses, cadence, accent, melody, and intonation. Affective dysprosody is not associated with an actual deficit in the ability to *experience* emotions. It is particularly associated with right-hemispheric lesions. A depressed patient with dysprosody will appear depressed and say that he or she is depressed, but the patient will not "sound" depressed. This is in contrast to a patient with anosognosia, who will both appear and sound depressed but may deny that he or she is depressed.

Apathy

Apathy is common after stroke, affecting up to 25% of patients, and appears to be distinct from depression (van Dalen et al. 2013). Patients with apathy show little spontaneous action or speech; their responses may be delayed, short, slow, or absent (Fisher 1995). Apathy is often associated with hypophonia, perseveration, grasp reflex, compulsive motor manipulations, cognitive impairment, and older age; it is also associated with poor functional outcomes (Hama et al. 2007). Disruption to fronto-subcortical circuits is the most commonly implicated mechanism in poststroke apathy.

Depression

Although depression following stroke is commonly defined according to DSM-5 (American Psychiatric Association 2013) or ICD-10 criteria (Starkstein and Robinson 1989), imposition of these categorical diagnoses on patients who have suffered a stroke is problematic because it is often unclear which symptoms are attributable to the stroke and which are attributable to depression (Gainotti et al. 1997, 1999). Which definition or diagnostic method is adopted has a substantive effect on reported prevalence rates of depressive illness after stroke. Most studies suggest that poststroke depression is a common problem, affecting about one-quarter of stroke patients, although some high-quality studies have reported significantly lower prevalence rates (Ferro et al. 2016). We take a pragmatic approach, treating depression if the patient has symptoms suggestive of low mood or anhedonia accompanied by some somatic symptoms (e.g., insomnia, anorexia) as well as signs of lack of engagement with the environment (e.g., poor participation in physiotherapy).

Most epidemiological studies have suggested an association between depression and increased disability and mortality. However, the direction of causality is unclear and is most probably circular. Some, but not all, pharmacological treatment studies have suggested that effective treatment of the depression leads to a reduction in overall disability. The role of selective serotonin reuptake inhibitors (SSRIs) in improving outcome after stroke independent of depression is a subject of ongoing studies (Ferro et al. 2016).

There has been much speculation over the etiological mechanisms of depression after stroke, and emphasis has been placed on the site of the stroke lesion. One hypothesis put forward is that left frontal lesions are associated with an increased rate of depressive illness (Starkstein and Robinson 1989); however, a meta-analysis concluded that the available scientific literature did not support the left frontal hypothesis (Carson et al. 2000a). More consensus has developed around subcortical small-vessel disease, large infarct volumes, and silent infarcts as risk factors for poststroke depression (Ferro et al. 2016). Serotonin transporter gene and brain-derived neurotrophic factor gene polymorphisms appear to carry significant risk.

There is clear evidence—based on a Cochrane review of 56 randomized controlled trials (RCTs) and 4,059 patients (Mead et al. 2012)—that SSRIs are effective in treating depression after stroke (Ferro et al. 2016). In addition, adoption of a care management approach appears to confer significant advantages in the delivery of treatment (Williams et al. 2007). Psychological treatment—in particular, cognitive-behavioral therapy (CBT)—offers a potential solution for patients in whom pharmacotherapy is ineffective or contraindicated, but thus far, trials have shown disappointing outcomes (Ferro et al. 2016). Furthermore, it is likely that only a minority of patients with poststroke depression are suitable for such treatment (Lincoln et al. 1997). Our own experience is that only a limited number of patients can actually cope with the rigor of CBT therapy after a stroke, but in those who can, the treatment shows promise, so the poor tolerability of CBT is possibly responsible for poor trial results. A number of studies have examined the effectiveness of early interventions intended to prevent development of depression after stroke. One Cochrane review found antidepressant drugs to be ineffective for poststroke depression (Hackett et al. 2008), although there have been dissenting voices (Chen et al. 2007), and there may be modest benefits to be gained from problem-solving therapy (Hackett et al. 2008). However, a randomized controlled trial that compared the antidepressant drug escitalopram and problem-solving therapy found the former to be more efficacious (Robinson et al. 2008); the trial itself and the relative effectiveness of treatments remain a controversial issue (Leo and Lacasse 2009; Robinson and Arndt 2009; Robinson and Penningworth 2009), and further studies are clearly required.

Anxiety and Posttraumatic Stress Disorders

Anxiety disorders are common after stroke and probably share the same risk factors as depression (Aström 1996). Estimates of prevalence have varied markedly, depending on whether the investigators subsumed anxiety symptoms within the construct of major depressive disorder. The reported prevalence of poststroke anxiety is around 20% (Ferro et al. 2016); however, there has been little effort to date to break down anxiety symptoms into separate disorders, despite the fact that different anxiety disorders (e.g., phobia and generalized anxiety disorder) require very different therapeutic approaches. Burvill et al. (1995) reported a prevalence of 5%–10% for phobic states in poststroke patients, with an excess found in women. Female gender, a history of anxiety or depression, alcohol misuse, and social isolation all seem to increase the risk of poststroke anxiety disorders. Our own experience is that fear of falls is particularly important as a risk factor for poststroke anxiety.

Stroke is a sudden and unpredictable life-threatening stressor and, not surprisingly, a highly aversive experience (McEwen 1996). Poststroke anxiety states may include posttraumatic stress symptoms, with compulsive and intrusive revisiting of the event, as well as health worries, with checking and reassurance-seeking about the risk of recurrence (Lindesay 1991). These worries can be associated with agoraphobia and with a tendency to misinterpret somatic anxiety symptoms, especially headache and dizziness, as evidence of recurrence. Around 10% of stroke patients report posttraumatic stress symptoms (Ferro et al. 2016).

Emotional Lability

Emotionalism, or emotional lability—uncontrollable episodes of laughing or crying that occur with little or no warning—is common in acute stroke but can also have a delayed onset (Berthier et al. 1996; Cummings et al. 2006). There is no consistent approach to diagnosis; as a result, estimates of prevalence vary considerably. However, higher-quality studies suggest a prevalence of between 8% and 30% in the first 6 months after stroke, and a reduction in frequency thereafter (Hackett et al. 2014).

Some authors have suggested that the neurological basis of emotional lability is in serotonergic systems and that there is a specific response to SSRIs (Andersen et al. 1994; Choi-Kwon et al. 2006), while others point to disruption in fronto-subcortical circuits (Hackett et al. 2014). In truth, the basis for emotionalism is poorly understood, and there is little consistency in findings. SSRIs remain the first-line therapy (Hackett et al. 2014), despite some advocating use of dextromethorphan–quinidine on the basis of small trials suggesting its efficacy in treating pseudobulbar affect in multiple sclerosis and amyotrophic lateral sclerosis (Pioro et al. 2010).

Catastrophic Reactions

Catastrophic reactions manifest as disruptive emotional behavior, typically self-directed anger or frustration, precipitated when a patient finds a task unsolvable (Goldstein 1939). This symptom is often associated with aphasia, and it has been suggested that damage to language areas is a critical part of the etiology (Carota et al. 2001). Many patients who show early catastrophic reactions go on to develop depression (Starkstein et al. 1993).

Psychosis

Psychosis—and, in particular, mania—has been observed following acute stroke. Its true incidence is unknown, although a rate of 1% has been reported (Starkstein et al. 1987). Psychotic symptoms have generally been associated with right-sided lesions (Cummings and Mendez 1984; Lampl et al. 2005), although we would suggest caution in accepting such claims. Old age and preexisting degenerative disease seem to increase the risk (Starkstein 1998) (see Chapter 9, "Psychosis, Mania, and Catatonia," for further details and treatment considerations). Reduplicative paramnesias can occur: one memorable patient believed that he was being treated on a cruise liner; on looking out of the window and seeing hospital porters delivering goods, he surmised that the ship must be in "dry dock." Such paramnesias are usually short-lived, although a small number of chronic cases have been reported (Vighetto et al. 1980).

Obsessive-Compulsive Disorder

Obsessive-compulsive disorder has been reported after cerebral infarctions, particularly those affecting the basal ganglia (Maraganore et al. 1991; Nighoghossian et al. 2006; Rodrigo Escalona et al. 1997).

Hyposexuality

Hyposexuality is a common complaint after stroke in both men and women (see also Chapter 15, "Sexual Dysfunctions"). The symptoms generally are nonspecific, although health worries concerning body image and fear of recurrence may also be relevant. A relationship between reduced libido and emotionalism has also been proposed, suggesting a common serotonergic dysfunction (Kim and Choi-Kwon 2000). Boller et al. (2015) offer a detailed review of this topic.

Executive Function Impairment

Executive function, including decision making, judgment, and social cognition, is regulated by complex systems that are relatively resistant to damage after stroke

(Carota et al. 2002; Zinn et al. 2007). Although executive function is commonly impaired as part of a general dementia, isolated dysexecutive syndromes are rare.

Inhibition Dyscontrol

Deficits in inhibition control occur with impulsive behavior. The most striking examples of inhibition dyscontrol are grasp reflexes in patients with frontal lesions, but utilization behavior (a tendency to use objects present in the environment automatically), hyperphasia, and hypergraphia have all been described. Such behavior tends to improve during the first few months after stroke (Carota et al. 2002).

Loss of Empathy

Loss of empathy has been reported after bilateral orbitofrontal lesions (Stone et al. 1998). It has been suggested that this difficulty in understanding and adapting to the needs of others may underlie many of the personality changes associated with frontal lesions. These changes include lack of tact, inappropriate familiarity, loss of initiative and spontaneity, childish behavior, sexual disinhibition, and poverty of emotional expression (Carota et al. 2002).

Parkinson's Disease

Parkinson's disease (PD) is a degenerative condition traditionally characterized by motor features of tremor, rigidity, and bradykinesia. The nonmotor features are numerous and include cognitive and psychiatric symptoms.

Incidence

Two incidence studies of PD, one from Minnesota (Bower et al. 1999) and one from Finland (Kuopio et al. 1999), estimated the incidence as 10.8 cases per 100,000 person-years and 17.2 cases per 100,000 population, respectively. Both studies found a slight excess in men and confirmed that incidence increases with age, leveling off after age 80 years. Recent meta-analyses have reported similar findings (Hirsch et al. 2016). The Finnish study also suggested that PD was more common in rural areas.

Etiology

The cause of PD remains unknown. Genetic forms of the disease have been described, but the implicated genes are not identified in most patients. Similarly, environmental causes have been suggested, but no single exposure has been consistently replicated, with the exception of cases associated with MPTP (1-methyl-4-phenyl-1,2,3,6-tetrahydropyridine) (Tanner and Aston 2000). Cigarette smoking is associated with decreased risk (Gorell et al. 1999).

Clinical Features

The core feature of PD is the triad of tremor, rigidity, and bradykinesia (Sethi 2002). Bradykinesia—usually of insidious onset and easily misdiagnosed as depression or boredom—is the most common initial sign and ultimately is the most disabling symptom. Resting tremor is the most characteristic feature of PD, affecting more than

70% of patients. In the early stages of the disease, the tremor is described as "pill-rolling." The rigidity manifests as fixed abnormalities of posture and resistance to passive movement throughout the range of motion, often with a "cogwheel" effect. Postural instability is a common additional feature, giving rise to an increasing liability to falls as the disorder progresses. Abnormal involuntary movements are a result both of the disease process and of dopaminergic therapy. As the disease progresses, patients can fluctuate between phases of good motor control accompanied by excess involuntary movements ("on" periods) and phases of immobility and incapacity ("off" periods). Freezing of gait is particularly distressing to patients, but it is one of the most poorly understood features of PD. Because such freezing may occur in response to visual cues (especially freezing during "off" periods), it can be misdiagnosed as willful behavior.

Nonmotor manifestations are common in PD and include autonomic (in particular, orthostatic hypotension and bladder and gastrointestinal dysfunction), sensory (pain), sleep, cognitive, olfactory, and other psychiatric symptoms.

Anosmia, rapid eye movement (REM) sleep behavior disorder, and chronic constipation commonly precede the onset of motor symptoms by around 15 years.

Cognitive Features (Including Psychotic Symptoms)

Dementia with Lewy bodies (DLB), PD, and PD with dementia share common features, motor symptoms, and responses to treatment. The boundaries between these disorders are not distinct. Hallucinations and delusions occur in 57%–76% of DLB cases, in 29%–54% of cases of PD with dementia, and in 7%–14% of cases of PD without dementia (Aarsland et al. 2001). Hallucinations usually are visual, are characterized by intact insight, and are phenomenologically similar to those of Charles Bonnet syndrome (Diederich et al. 2000). Typically, hallucinations are nonthreatening, are worse at night, and involve children or animals (Papapetropoulos et al. 2008). Delusions are much less common, but when present, they are often paranoid in type and mainly involve persecution and jealousy.

Evidence suggests that the most likely etiology of psychosis in PD is a combination of cortical PD pathology and age-related loss of central cholinergic function (Ffytche 2004; Wolters and Berendse 2001). Cognitive impairment and sleep disruption are predictive of the development of psychosis (Arnulf et al. 2000). Imaging in PD patients without dementia suggests that psychosis is associated with decreased gray matter volume in right inferior frontal regions, in left temporal regions, and in the thalamus (Shin et al. 2012). Clinically, one should seek to distinguish PD psychosis from delirium of acute onset with disorientation, impaired attention, perceptive and cognitive disturbance, and alterations in the sleep–wake cycle. True dopaminomimetic psychosis is a subacute, gradually progressive psychotic state unaccompanied by a primary deficit of attention. Delirium may be induced by drugs used in the treatment of PD, such as selegiline and anticholinergic medication.

The evidence surrounding dopamine and dopamine agonists as an etiological factor in PD psychosis is more controversial. There are conflicting results from studies. On balance, the evidence appears to suggest that whereas dopamine agonists may increase the risk of hallucinations in the early stages of PD, cognitive impairment and deterioration of cholinergic pathways become more important contributors to psychosis as the disease progresses (Morgante et al. 2012). Active treatment of dopaminomimetic psychosis is recommended only if symptoms begin to interfere with daily functioning. Dosage reduction of dopaminomimetic drugs is seldom effective, and antipsychotic drugs are often required (Wolters and Berendse 2001). The atypical antipsychotic drug clozapine is the only antipsychotic that has been demonstrated in RCTs to reduce psychosis without worsening motor symptoms (Cummings 1999; Rabinstein and Shulman 2000). Quetiapine is ineffective (Shotbolt et al. 2010), and high-potency typical antipsychotics and risperidone should be avoided (see Chapter 9). Secondary analyses of data from PD dementia trials suggest that cholinesterase inhibitors may have a role in the treatment of PD psychosis (Emre et al. 2004), as well as a good safety profile and an action that targets visual hallucinations that result from loss of central cholinergic function. There has been recent interest in and promising results for the use of pimavanserin, a selective serotonin 2A (5-HT$_{2A}$) inverse agonist (Cummings et al. 2014), to treat PD psychosis. Pimavanserin produced substantial reductions in symptoms and showed a good side-effect profile in motor and nonmotor domains, but its cost may limit widespread use (Kianirad and Simuni 2017).

Emotional Symptoms

Depressive symptoms are common in PD, with a prevalence of around 40%–50%, and major depressive disorder has a prevalence of around 23% (Marsh 2013). Timing of onset shows a bimodal distribution, with peaks during early and late stages of the disease. Several large-scale studies have demonstrated that depression is one of the major determinants of quality of life in PD and, in particular, predicts early worsening of motor function and early commencement of levodopa therapy (Marsh 2013). Depression is now regarded as an integral part of PD rather than a comorbidity (Berg et al. 2014). It is likely that both the neurodegenerative process of PD and the psychological problems of managing the illness contribute to depressive symptoms in PD. A prevailing model for the development of depression proposes that degeneration of mesocortical and mesolimbic dopaminergic neurons causes orbitofrontal dysfunction, which disrupts serotonergic neurons in the dorsal raphe and leads to dysfunction of depression-related orbitofrontal–basal ganglia–thalamic circuits.

The diagnosis of depression in PD is difficult, because many depressive symptoms overlap with the core features of PD—motor retardation, attention deficit, sleep disturbance, hypophonia, impotence, weight loss, fatigue, preoccupation with health, and reduced facial expression. Therefore, anhedonia and sustained sadness are important diagnostic features, particularly if they are out of proportion to the severity of motor symptoms (Brooks and Doder 2001).

Mood changes can accompany the late-stage fluctuations in response to levodopa (known as "on–off" phenomena), and some patients have symptoms that fulfill criteria for major depressive disorder during the "off" phase but not during the "on" phase. There is currently insufficient evidence to offer definitive recommendations for treatment of depression in PD. A 2013 meta-analysis (Rocha et al. 2013) found only six studies of usable quality. The meta-analysis suggested that antidepressants were probably superior to placebo but could not recommend any particular class. SSRIs are the most popular, although some have questioned whether their mechanism of action is suitable in PD patients (De Deurwaerdère and Ding 2016). In addition, case reports have described exacerbation of motor symptoms with fluoxetine, citalopram, or paroxetine (Ceravolo et al. 2000; Chouinard and Sultan 1992; Leo 1996; Steur 1993; Tesei et al. 2000); however, a more recent RCT did not find evidence of worsened motor function (Richard et al. 2012). Our own clinical experience suggests that SSRIs can exert this effect in a minority of cases, but we would suggest vigilance rather than avoidance. In small-scale trials, tricyclic antidepressants (TCAs) have led to better motor outcomes than have SSRIs; however, TCAs with marked anticholinergic activity (e.g., amitriptyline) should be used with caution because of their potential to produce adverse effects on cognition and autonomic function, particularly constipation (Olanow et al. 2001). Drugs such as mirtazapine may offer a compromise (Pact and Giduz 1999), but there is a disappointing lack of data to offer guidance. Indeed, a recent systematic review found more guidelines on management than well-conducted trials addressing the topic (Goodarzi et al. 2016).

There has been some support for the use of CBT, with a well-conducted study showing promising results (Dobkin et al. 2011) and a much weaker study suggesting that it may be deliverable by telephone (Veazey et al. 2009).

Case report data suggest that both electroconvulsive therapy (ECT) (Borisovskaya et al. 2016) and transcranial magnetic stimulation (TMS) can be used to treat depression in PD, although TMS is associated with short-lived adverse effects and seizures (Fregni et al. 2004; George et al. 1996; Olanow et al. 2001). The use of ECT in PD is reviewed in Chapter 38, "Electroconvulsive Therapy and Other Brain Stimulation Therapies."

Anxiety phenomena are common in PD; they tend to occur later in the disease process than depression and are more closely associated with severity of motor symptoms (Witjas et al. 2002). In particular, marked anticipatory anxiety related to freezing of gait is common. Treatment with antidepressant drugs (Olanow et al. 2001) and CBT, particularly if delivered in conjunction with an active physiotherapy program, can be helpful. Occasionally, benzodiazepines may be required.

Medication-Related Impulse-Control Disorders

There has been increased recognition of complex behavioral problems associated with dopamine receptor stimulation in PD (Weintraub et al. 2006). These behavioral problems include pathological gambling, hypersexuality, punding (i.e., intense fascination with repetitive handling, examining, sorting, and arranging of objects), compulsive shopping, and compulsive medication use. These behaviors, which are sometimes described as impulse-control disorders (Voon et al. 2007), appear to affect up to 14% of patients with PD (Grall-Bronnec et al. 2017). Many patients are secretive about these impulsive behaviors and will not volunteer the symptoms unless specifically asked.

The etiology of these impulsive behaviors is believed to be linked to dopamine agonist use, although there is not a clear dose-related effect. It has been postulated that neuronal sensitization (particularly in mesolimbic dopaminergic tracts) to intermittent administration of dopamine agonists leads to an increased behavioral response to similar levels of psychostimulation (Evans et al. 2006; Pessiglione et al. 2006). This sensitization process can be modified by a genetic predisposition to risk taking (there is a general association between PD and low risk-taking traits) as well as by environmental factors. It is believed that younger age at onset, right-sided onset, and executive cognitive impairments can all facilitate this process.

Management of medication-related impulsivity involves transitioning patients from dopamine agonists to levodopa and, if possible, reducing the total levodopa dosage. Small trials have suggested some benefits from SSRIs and antiandrogens in hypersexuality. In one case series, subthalamic deep brain stimulation (DBS) showed very encouraging results (Ardouin et al. 2006), but a meta-analysis cautioned that a history of impulse-control disorders was a risk factor for postoperative suicide (Voon et al. 2007). Okun and Weintraub (2013) concluded that impulse-control disorders were not a primary indication for DBS, although the matter remains controversial (Kasemsuk et al. 2017).

Two syndromes related to impulse-control disorders in PD are the dopamine dysregulation syndrome (DDS) and the dopamine agonist withdrawal syndrome (DAWS). DDS refers to a compulsive pattern of levodopa misuse in PD patients, usually in more advanced states of the disease. Patients with DDS often present with excessive demands, and cravings, for increases in dopamine in conjunction with behavioral abnormalities, abnormal requests for assistance from carers/nursing staff, and unusually severe "off" periods that appear conflated with panic and often a phobic fear of their occurrence. Drug-induced psychosis can occur, with predominantly paranoid delusions similar to those associated with cocaine (Cilia et al. 2013). DDS is associated with more severe "off" periods earlier in the disease and is believed to be linked to particularly severe deterioration in nigrostriatal motor pathways. Treatment is very difficult and often unsuccessful. A high degree of vigilance and prevention is key.

DAWS involves psychiatric symptoms such as panic, irritability, anxiety, insomnia, pain, fatigue, and drug cravings accompanied by autonomic signs of orthostatic hypotension, dizziness, nausea, and diaphoresis. It is similar to other psychostimulant withdrawal syndromes. It appears to be closely associated with impulse-control disorders (Pondal et al. 2012). Like DDS, DAWS is very difficult to treat once established, and prevention is key. As Edwards (2013) aptly described, all clinicians need to be very aware of the "perils of flicking the dopamine 'switch.'"

Clinicians must avoid abrupt discontinuation of levodopa and dopamine agonists, because it can trigger the rare but potentially fatal complication of parkinsonism hyperpyrexia syndrome (Newman et al. 2009).

Sleep Disorders

Sleep disturbance is a very common symptom in PD. REM sleep behavior disorder (RBD), in which the sufferer acts out his or her dreams, may precede the onset of motor symptoms in PD by many years (Postuma et al. 2006). Indeed, RBD is now regarded as a potential disease marker for early-phase neuroprotective trials (Postuma et al. 2015), because around half of patients reporting primary RBD will develop PD over a 15-year period, with others developing other disorders related to Lewy body pathology and only 10% having isolated RBD. Looked at in the other direction, around a quarter of PD patients have suffered from RBD (Zhang et al. 2017). Daytime somnolence may also be a problem. There is increasing recognition that sudden somnolence can occur in PD, especially in relation to dopaminergic medication. Patients should therefore be warned about this possibility.

Multiple Sclerosis

Multiple sclerosis (MS) is a demyelinating disorder of the central nervous system (CNS) that causes some degree of cognitive impairment in almost half of cases and that can manifest with subcortical dementia. It can also be accompanied by affective disorders. The presence of high signal abnormalities on T2-weighted magnetic resonance imaging (MRI) and of oligoclonal bands of immunoglobulin in the cerebrospinal fluid (CSF) helps to confirm the diagnosis.

Onset of MS can occur at any age, but the median age at onset is 24 years, with a tendency for relapsing–remitting disease to present earlier than primary progressive MS. MS is more common in women. Epidemiological studies suggest that an exogenous or environmental factor, possibly viral infection, plays a part, although its nature remains unclear. The prevalence of the disorder rises with increasing distance from the equator, a finding that has given rise to theories that vitamin D deficiency may be a factor. Genetic factors appear to influence susceptibility. A family history in a first-degree relative increases the risk some 30- to 50-fold; the risk for siblings is usually estimated to be 3%–5%, with that for children slightly lower (Franklin and Nelson 2003).

Neurological syndromes that commonly occur at or close to the onset of MS include optic neuritis (unilateral visual impairment, usually painful), evolving sensory loss, and upper motor neuron or cerebellar disorders of the limbs and gait. These deficits typically develop and remit over the course of weeks and result from conduction block in regions of CNS inflammation. Transient worsening of function, lasting for minutes, can occur in partially demyelinated axons as a result of physiological changes (e.g., increase in body temperature). Positive symptoms, including Lhermitte's phenomenon (electric shock–like sensations on flexing the neck) and trigeminal neuralgia, can also occur. Over time, the remissions and relapses of MS tend to give way to a progressive worsening of disability. A minority of patients present with a primary progressive form of the disease, with gradual worsening from onset without remissions (McDonald et al. 2001).

MS is characterized by multifocal areas of inflammatory demyelinating white matter lesions with glial scar formation and (as now recognized) axonal loss (Trapp et al. 1998). However, growing evidence of extensive gray matter and subpial pathology in the disorder has led to a theoretical shift toward regarding MS as an inflammatory neurodegenerative condition (Stadelmann et al. 2008). This shift to a neurodegenerative profile is particularly relevant to the neuropsychiatric clinical features of MS.

Cognitive Impairment

Cognitive impairment affects at least half of all patients with MS (Beatty et al. 1989; Heaton et al. 1985; Rao 1986; Rao et al. 1991). Impairment, when present, is generally a "subcortical dementia," with impaired attention and speed of processing as the hallmark signs. Executive function deficits are common. Deficits in working, semantic, and episodic memory are reported, but procedural and implicit memory functions are generally preserved. Cortical syndromes such as aphasia, apraxia, and agnosia are relatively rare. Neuropsychological tests such as the Paced Auditory Serial Addition Test (PASAT) appear most sensitive to changes in cognitive function (Hoffmann et al.

2007). At the bedside, tests such as verbal fluency are of most value. In general, speed of test completion is usually more impaired than accuracy (Henry and Beatty 2006). MRI studies show that cognitive impairment in MS correlates with general atrophy, but attempts to link specific cognitive deficits with particular gray or white matter lesions have led to conflicting results (Rovaris et al. 2006), and attempts to gain clarity have not been notable successful in the past decade (Sbardella et al. 2013), although it is increasingly clear that cerebellar lesions are involved (D'Ambrosio et al. 2016; Weier et al. 2014). However, this type of region-of-interest approach is at odds with brain function, a circumstance that likely explains the limitations in findings. More recent studies examining degradations of functional networks offer a more promising strategy (Meijer et al. 2017). Not surprisingly, cognitive outcomes are worse in the more progressive forms of MS (Planche et al. 2016), but beyond this type of staging, attempts at early detection of individuals at risk of poorer cognitive outcomes have been disappointing (Uher et al. 2017). It remains unclear whether disease-modifying agents can help prevent cognitive decline, and trials of therapeutics for existing cognitive impairment have been disappointing (Niccolai et al. 2017). In contrast, there is slightly more robust evidence showing the utility of treating comorbid depression when present (Feinstein 2006).

Psychosis

Well-conducted population studies have challenged the perceived orthodoxy that MS is not associated with an increased risk of psychosis. Patten et al. (2005b) reported that the population baseline rate of psychosis (1%) was increased in MS to 2%–3%, with the highest prevalence (4%) in the 15- to 24-year-old population. Interestingly, however, MS is associated with a decreased incidence of schizophrenia (Johansson et al. 2014), and MS psychoses typically involve much less elaborate delusional schema than are seen in schizophrenia. Bipolar states and mania occur at far higher than predicted rates, with one systematic study suggesting an odds ratio for an association as high as 44 (Carta et al. 2014). We suspect that this is an overestimate, but the contribution of corticosteroids and antidepressants in a significant number of bipolar II disorder cases does seem likely and warrants appropriate caution.

Mood Disorders

Mood disorders are common in MS, with more than half of MS patients reporting depressive symptoms. A recent systematic review found a pooled prevalence rate of depression of 30.5% (Boeschoten et al. 2017). Depression may be a direct physiologically mediated consequence of the disease, a psychological reaction to the illness, a complication of pharmacotherapy, or coincidental. Mania and emotional lability are also frequently reported (Joffe et al. 1987; Sadovnick et al. 1996) (see also Chapter 7, "Depression," and Chapter 9). It is important to distinguish depression from the fatigue and pain that are commonly associated with MS (see subsections "Fatigue" and "Pain" below).

There have been an increasing number of studies trying to understand the underlying mechanism of the risk for depression in MS. It is clear that risk is multifactorial, with a range of social contributors—including low socioeconomic status, limited social support, and loss of recreational activities—seen as important (Ghaffar and Feinstein 2007). Psychologically, poor coping mechanisms, hopelessness, and uncertainty over prognosis all increase the risk of depression and are associated with suicidal ideation (Haussleiter et al. 2009; Lynch et al. 2001). Biologically, around half of depressed MS patients have a failure of cortisol suppression in response to dexamethasone (Chwastiak and Ehde 2007). Structurally, there is an association between increased lesion load and risk of depression, and more recent connectome analyses have suggested abnormalities in white matter connectivity between the frontal lobes and the limbic system (Murphy et al. 2017).

RCTs of antidepressants in MS suggest moderate efficacy (Murphy et al. 2017), similar to antidepressants' efficacy in depression associated with neurological illness in general (Price et al. 2011). It has been suggested that SSRIs may be particularly useful, because they reduce axonal degradation via induction of glycogenolysis in astrocytes, thereby potentially increasing the energy source to neurons and reducing the development of new lesions (Mostert et al. 2008; Murphy et al. 2017; Sijens et al. 2008).

A number of small trials have suggested efficacy for CBT (Hind et al. 2014), but our clinical experience with this treatment modality has been disappointing.

Interferon-beta therapy was reported to cause depression (and fatigue) in 40% of MS patients in an open-label trial (Neilley et al. 1996). However, depression is highly prevalent in untreated MS, and more recent systematic studies have found no increase in depression following interferon-beta therapy (Schippling et al. 2016). This discrepancy may lie in the fact that interferon-beta may cause symptoms, particularly early in therapy, that are mislabeled as depression (Patten et al. 2005a).

Anxiety Disorders

There has been far less focus on anxiety in MS in comparison with depression or psychosis. The rates of anxiety disorder in MS seem similar to the rates in other neurological conditions (Chwastiak and Ehde 2007). A recent systematic review found a pooled prevalence rate of anxiety of 22.1% (Boeschoten et al. 2017). Not surprisingly, new diagnoses and relapses are particular risks (Korostil and Feinstein 2007). Following the development of self-injectable disease-modifying agents, a substantial proportion of patients developed a specific phobia to injecting themselves. This seems to respond well to CBT along a specific phobia model (Mohr et al. 2002).

Substance Misuse

Misuse of substances, particularly alcohol, is relatively common in MS, with rates of 13%–19% (Choy et al. 1995; Ó Donnchadha et al. 2013). Cannabis use is common among patients with more severe MS (Chong et al. 2006). Indeed, Δ-9-tetrahydrocannabinol/cannabidiol oromucosal spray has been approved in Europe as an add-on therapy for spasticity in MS patients.

Fatigue

Fatigue is the most common single symptom in MS, affecting up to 80% of individuals with the disease. It is generally a disabling and aversive experience and affects motivation as well as physical strength. It is important to differentiate fatigue from depression, sleepiness, adverse medication side effects, or pure physical exhaustion secondary to gait abnormalities. The pathophysiology of fatigue is poorly understood and almost certainly multifactorial. Comorbidity in MS fatigue is common and includes depression and anxiety, as well as functional disorders such as irritable bowel syndrome and migraine (Fiest et al. 2016). Daytime sleepiness secondary to comorbid sleep disorders (e.g., sleep apnea), which often go unrecognized and untreated in MS as in other populations, may be erroneously attributed to fatigue related to MS (Popp et al. 2017). A number of agents have been advocated for the treatment of MS fatigue, including amantadine, aminopyridines, psychostimulants, modafinil, and bupropion. A recent meta-analysis concluded that only amantadine had relatively sufficient evidence of effectiveness (Yang et al. 2017); however, our experience with the drug has not been encouraging. Another recent meta-analysis concluded that CBT provides moderately positive short-term benefits (van den Akker et al. 2016); our own experience has been that the benefits of CBT are modest and that multidisciplinary rehabilitation with emphasis on maximizing function has been more productive.

Pain

Pain, both acute and chronic, is a common and disabling complication of MS. One study found that one-quarter of MS patients in a large community-based sample had severe chronic pain (Ehde et al. 2003). Mechanisms may include dysesthesia, altered cognitive function, and other MS complications such as spasticity. Of the acute pain syndromes, trigeminal neuralgia is the most common and usually responds to carbamazepine (Thompson 1998). Widespread chronic pain is more frequent than acute pain and is harder to manage. Small RCTs have shown some benefit from lamotrigine (Breuer et al. 2007), levetiracetam (Rossi et al. 2009), and cannabinoids (Rog et al. 2005) for central pain syndromes in MS. Dysesthetic limb pain is particularly troublesome; treatment is usually with amitriptyline or gabapentin (Samkoff et al. 1997). Pain in the lumbar area, by contrast, tends to respond better to physiotherapy than to analgesia (Thompson 1998; see also Chapter 34).

Amnestic Syndromes

The amnestic (or amnesic) syndrome is an abnormal mental state in which learning and memory are affected out of proportion to other cognitive functions in an otherwise alert and responsive individual. The most common cause of amnestic states is Wernicke-Korsakoff syndrome, which results from nutritional depletion, particularly thiamine deficiency. Other causes of amnestic syndromes include carbon monoxide poisoning, herpes simplex encephalitis and other CNS infections, limbic encephalitis, hypoxic and other acquired brain injuries, stroke, deep midline cerebral tumors, and surgical resections, particularly for epilepsy. In the majority of cases, the pathology lies in midline or medial temporal structures, but there are also case reports of amnestic disorder following frontal lobe lesions.

Wernicke-Korsakoff Syndrome

Wernicke-Korsakoff syndrome results from thiamine depletion, and any cause of such depletion—including hyperemesis gravidarum and gastric bypass surgery—can lead to the syndrome. However, the overwhelming majority of cases are associated with chronic alcohol abuse, which results in both decreased intake and decreased absorption of thiamine.

The syndrome presents acutely with Wernicke's encephalopathy, which is characterized by confusion, ataxia, nystagmus, and ophthalmoplegia. Peripheral neuropathy can also be present. Parenteral administration of high-dose B vitamins is required as *emergency* treatment if the chronic state of Korsakoff's syndrome is to be avoided. The majority of cases of Korsakoff's syndrome occur following Wernicke's encephalopathy.

On clinical examination, patients with Korsakoff's syndrome may perform well on standard tasks of attention and working memory (e.g., serial sevens and reverse digit span) (Kopelman 1985) but may struggle on more complex tasks involving shifting and dividing attention. A severe memory impairment involving both anterograde and retrograde deficits is present (Kopelman et al. 1999). Defective encoding of new information is the core component of this memory disorder (Meudell and Mayes 1982). In addition to a dense anterograde amnesia affecting declarative functions, there is inconsistent, poorly organized retrieval of retrograde memories, with a temporal gradient (i.e., more impairment for relatively recent than for more remote memories). A limited degree of new learning may be possible, particularly if the patient is given a strategy to follow. Confabulation commonly occurs, particularly early in the disorder. Procedural memory remains relatively intact (Schacter 1987).

Other cognitive impairments and behavioral changes may accompany the amnesia. Executive functions are commonly mildly affected, but this impairment may be secondary to chronic alcoholism rather than representing a specific deficit. Disorientation and apathy, often with lack of curiosity about the past, are common, yet such disengaged patients frequently demonstrate labile irritability.

The pathological process in Wernicke-Korsakoff syndrome involves neuronal loss, microhemorrhages, and gliosis in the paraventricular and periaqueductal gray matter (Victor et al. 1971). The mammillary bodies, mammillothalamic tract, and anterior thalamus are the main structures affected (Mair et al. 1979; Mayes et al. 1988). There is often a degree of generalized cortical atrophy that is more marked in the frontal lobes (Jacobson and Lishman 1990). The atrophy may, however, be nonspecific and secondary to alcohol abuse. MRI reveals specific atrophy in diencephalic structures (Colchester et al. 2001; Sullivan and Pfefferbaum 2009).

With vitamin replacement and abstinence from alcohol, the prognosis for Wernicke-Korsakoff syndrome is fair: one-quarter of patients will recover, half will improve but retain some persistent impairment, and one-quarter will show no change (Victor et al. 1971). High-dose B vitamins should be given to all patients acutely and should probably be continued, but it is unclear how long this therapy should be maintained.

Transient Amnestic Syndromes

Transient amnesia can occur in several contexts. Transient global amnesia (TGA) is a distinctive benign disorder affecting middle-aged or elderly persons, who become amnestic for recent events and unable to form new memories for a period of around 4 hours (Arena and Rabinstein 2015; Hodges and Ward 1989). Repetitive questioning by patients of their companions is a characteristic feature. Episodes can be provoked by physical or emotional stress and are usually isolated; the medium-term recurrence rate is 3% per year (Arena and Rabinstein 2015; Hodges 1991). There is good evidence that TGA results from reversible medial temporal lobe dysfunction, but the etiological mechanism is uncertain (Stillhard et al. 1990). Although temporal lobe epilepsy occasionally mimics TGA ("transient epileptic amnesia"), TGA episodes typically are briefer (lasting less than an hour) and recurrent (several per year) and tend to occur on waking (Butler et al. 2007; Zeman and Butler 2010; Zeman et al. 1998). Other causes of transient amnesia include transient cerebral ischemia (usually accompanied by other neurological symptoms and signs), migraine, drug ingestion, head injury, and dissociative disorders.

Dementias Accompanied by Neurological Signs

Dementia refers to a deterioration of intellectual faculties, such as memory, concentration, and judgment, sometimes accompanied by emotional disturbance and personality changes. Approaches to management of dementing conditions (including Alzheimer's disease, vascular dementia, Lewy body dementia, frontotemporal dementia (FTD), Huntington's disease, Parkinson's disease, and normal-pressure hydrocephalus) are described in detail in Chapter 5. In this section, we concentrate on neurocognitive disorders that are particularly likely to manifest with other neurological symptoms, often a movement disorder. Other causes of dementia are also discussed elsewhere in this volume.

Huntington's Disease

Huntington's disease (HD), also known as Huntington's chorea, was first described in Long Island in 1872 by George Huntington. This dominantly inherited disorder causes a combination of progressive motor, cognitive, psychiatric, and behavioral dysfunction.

Epidemiology

HD has a prevalence of 5–7 cases per 100,000 population in the United States, with wide regional variations (Chua and Chiu 1994). The sexes are affected equally. Onset can be at any age but most commonly is in young or middle adulthood (Adams et al. 1988; Farrer and Conneally 1985). The disorder exhibits the phenomenon of *anticipation*, in which the age at onset tends to decrease over the generations, especially with paternal transmission (Brinkman et al. 1997).

Clinical Features

Chorea—involuntary fidgety movements of the face and limbs—is the characteristic motor disorder in HD. As the disease progresses, other extrapyramidal features can develop, including rigidity, dystonia, and bradykinesia, as well as dysphagia, dysarthria, and pyramidal signs (Harper 1991). Childhood-onset HD tends to be dominated by rigidity and myoclonus (i.e., the "Westphal variant" of HD). Epilepsy can occur. Cognitive dysfunction goes hand in hand with the motor disorder. The dementia of HD is predominantly "subcortical," with impairment of attention, executive function, processing speed, and memory (Zakzanis 1998). Psychiatric symptoms and behavioral changes are the norm (Mendez 1994; Zappacosta et al. 1996), with depression, apathy, and aggressiveness present in most cases (Burns et al. 1990; Levy et al. 1998), and psychosis, obsessional behavior, and suicidal behavior in a significant minority of cases (Almqvist et al. 1999; Cummings and Cunningham 1992; Folstein et al. 1979). Obsessive behavior appears to be a trait marker in persons who are gene carriers. Depression and irritability frequently precede the development of motor and cognitive symptoms. Psychosis, by contrast, rarely precedes the development of motor symptoms. Apathy tends to correlate positively with disease progression (Paulsen et al. 2005; van Duijn et al. 2007). Progression to a state of immobility and dementia typically occurs over a period of 15–20 years (Feigin et al. 1995). Cognitive and behavioral changes may predate the clear-cut emergence of symptomatic HD (Kirkwood et al. 1999).

The onset of the condition in individuals known to be gene positive can be predicted by taking into account the CAG (cytosine–adenine–guanine) repeat length, presence of subtle motor abnormalities, deterioration in Stroop Color and Word Test scores, and reductions in size of the putamen (Paulsen et al. 2014). Reductions in caudate volume and in whole-brain volume are associated with clinical progression (Tabrizi et al. 2011). Neuropsychiatric changes consistent with frontostriatal loss correlate with functional declines (Tabrizi et al. 2013).

Pathology and Etiology

The key pathological processes in HD occur in the striatum, caudate, and putamen. The loss of small neurons in the striatum is accompanied by neuronal loss in the cerebral cortex, cerebral atrophy, ventricular dilatation, and, eventually, neuronal depletion throughout the basal ganglia (de la Monte et al. 1988; Vonsattel and DiFiglia 1998).

The underlying genetic abnormality in HD is expansion of a "base triplet repeat"—CAG—in the *IT15* gene on chromosome 4, which codes for the huntingtin protein.

Investigation and Differential Diagnosis

A number of disorders can cause the combination of chorea and cognitive change seen in HD, including other inherited disorders such as neuroacanthocytosis and dentatorubral-pallidoluysian atrophy (DRPLA) and acquired disorders such as systemic lupus erythematosus. However, the diagnosis of HD can now be made with confidence via DNA analysis. Counseling by a clinical geneticist is mandatory before presymptomatic testing and should be considered in other circumstances as well (Nance 2017).

Management

Chorea may require treatment, although patients often are not as concerned about the symptom as their caregivers are. A range of agents have been suggested, with tetrabenazine having the most supportive evidence of benefit (de Tommaso et al. 2011). However, given the cognitive and/or extrapyramidal side effects of antipsychotics, dopamine depleters like tetrabenazine, and benzodiazepines, it is often best to avoid use of these agents (Rosenblatt et al. 1999). Other psychiatric symptoms should be treated along standard lines (Leroi and Michalon 1998).

Wilson's Disease (Hepatolenticular Degeneration)

First described by Samuel Wilson in 1912, Wilson's disease is a very rare autosomal-recessive, progressive degenerative brain disease caused by a disorder of copper metabolism, which produces personality change, cognitive decline, extrapyramidal signs, and cirrhosis of the liver.

Clinical Features

The onset of Wilson's disease is most commonly in childhood or adolescence but can be as late as the fifth decade. Patients may present to psychiatrists with personality change, behavioral disturbance, depression, irritability, or dementia, or to neurologists with a variety of extrapyramidal signs, including tremor, dysarthria and drooling, rigidity, bradykinesia, and dystonia. Although commonly featured in psychiatry textbooks, schizophreniform psychosis is in fact rare (Shanmugiah et al. 2008). Careful examination reveals these features, and also, in virtually all symptomatic cases, the presence of *Kayser-Fleischer rings*—rings of greenish-brown copper pigment at the edge of the cornea, often requiring slit lamp examination by an ophthalmologist for detection. The liver failure and the neuropsychiatric syndrome can occur together or independently.

Pathology and Etiology

The causative genetic mutation leads to excessive copper deposition in the brain, cornea, liver, and kidneys and increased copper excretion in urine. The caudate and putamen are the brain regions most severely affected, but other parts of the basal ganglia and the cerebral cortex are also involved.

Investigation and Differential Diagnosis

Ninety-five percent of patients with Wilson's disease have low serum levels of the copper-binding protein ceruloplasmin. Normal ceruloplasmin levels and an absence of Kayser-Fleischer rings render the diagnosis very unlikely in cases with neuropsychiatric features (Ferenci et al. 1998). Uncertain cases may require measurement of urinary copper excretion and liver biopsy for measurement of copper content (Pfeil and Lynn 1999). The differential diagnosis varies with the type of presentation.

Management

Several copper-chelating agents (e.g., penicillamine, tetraethylenetetramine, zinc acetate) are available to treat patients with Wilson's disease, but the risk of significant side effects mandates care by a specialist (Pfeil and Lynn 1999).

Leukodystrophies

Leukodystrophies—recessively inherited or X-linked disorders of myelination—can be accompanied by neuropsychiatric syndromes, including psychosis and mania, usually with associated neurological features. Metachromatic leukodystrophy, caused by a deficiency of the enzyme arylsulfatase A (Hyde et al. 1992), and adrenoleukodystrophy, an X-linked disorder associated with abnormalities of very-long-chain fatty acids (James et al. 1984), are the most commonly encountered leukodystrophies.

Progressive Supranuclear Palsy

Progressive supranuclear palsy (PSP) is characterized by supranuclear gaze palsy (an inability to direct eye movements voluntarily, especially vertical eye movements, in the presence of normal reflex eye movements); truncal rigidity, akinesia, postural instability, and early falls; bulbar features, with dysarthria and dysphagia; subcortical dementia; and alterations in mood (including pathological crying and laughing), personality, and behavior (de Bruin and Lees 1992). Neuropsychiatric symptoms frequently precede the more obvious parkinsonism, and the nonspecific behavioral changes and apathy can be difficult to diagnose (Bruns and Josephs 2013).

Corticobasal Degeneration

Corticobasal degeneration typically manifests as a combination of limb apraxia (usually asymmetric at onset), alien limb phenomena, limb myoclonus, parkinsonism, and cognitive decline (Rinne et al. 1994). The neuropsychiatric features tend to be those characteristic of "frontal" disorders. Interestingly, unlike in other parkinsonian syndromes, visual hallucinations appear to be rare (Bruns and Josephs 2013; Geda et al. 2007). MRI usually reveals frontoparietal atrophy.

Transmissible Spongiform Encephalopathies (Prion Dementias)

The transmissible spongiform encephalopathies are a group of rare dementias caused by an accumulation of abnormal prion protein within the brain. Sporadic Creutzfeldt-Jakob disease (CJD) is the most common human-transmissible spongiform encephalopathy; variant CJD usually occurs in younger individuals. Three other varieties of human transmissible spongiform encephalopathy have been described: 1) *kuru,* a cerebellar syndrome with progression to dementia caused by cannibalism in Papua New Guinea; 2) *Gerstmann-Sträussler-Scheinker syndrome,* an autosomal dominant prion dementia characterized by cerebellar dysfunction and a protracted clinical course; and 3) *fatal familial insomnia,* a very rare autosomal dominant prion disorder with severe insomnia and dysautonomia. Prion diseases are discussed in Chapter 26, "Infectious Diseases."

Other Dementias Due to Infectious Diseases

Dementia is a common manifestation of tertiary (untreated) syphilis. Both acute and chronic infections with a variety of organisms may result in dementia and other neurological symptoms. Whipple's disease is rare but is important as a cause of neuropsychiatric symptoms, because it is a treatable multisystem infection. Subacute sclerosing panencephalitis is a rare complication of childhood measles. Progressive multifocal leukoencephalopathy is caused by reactivation of JC virus (John Cunningham virus; also known as papovavirus) in the CNS in immunocompromised patients. These conditions and their complications are all discussed in Chapter 26.

Autoimmune Encephalitis

Limbic encephalitis (LE) is an autoimmune-mediated inflammation centered on the limbic system. Patients with LE can present with a range of neuropsychiatric signs, including focal seizures, memory impairment, confusion, and alterations in mood, personality, and behavior (Schott 2006). LE may occur as a paraneoplastic phenomenon or (more often) as a primary autoimmune disease. The diagnosis is supported by MRI, which sometimes shows increased signal in the medial temporal lobes. The CSF often contains oligoclonal bands of immunoglobulin.

Paraneoplastic LE is most commonly caused by small-cell lung cancer, but breast, ovarian, renal, and testicular carcinoma and lymphoma can also be responsible. The tumor may be quite small and sometimes is initially undetectable by imaging. A range of antineuronal antibodies in serum or CSF may be found, most commonly "anti-Hu." Forty percent of paraneoplastic LE cases are antibody-negative (Darnell and Posner 2003).

Primary autoimmune LE normally presents subacutely, often over a couple of weeks but occasionally over a period as long as 3 months, with mood changes and sometimes psychosis evolving into confusion with seizures. Progressive impairment of working memory is thought to be a hallmark symptom. CSF shows a lymphocytic pleocytosis (usually <100 white blood cells per mm^3) in the majority of patients, and may also show an elevated immunoglobulin G (IgG) index or oligoclonal bands. MRI often reveals increased signal on T2-weighted fluid-attenuated inversion recovery (FLAIR) imaging in one or both medial temporal lobes. Focal CNS findings on examination are common (Graus et al. 2016).

Anti–NMDA (N-methyl-D-aspartate) receptor encephalitis is particularly common, occurring in association with an occult ovarian teratoma in young women in about one-third of cases. It has a rapid onset, with psychiatric and cognitive disturbance, pressured speech or verbal reduction/mutism, movement disorder or dyskinesias or rigidity/abnormal posture, decreased level of consciousness, autonomic dysfunction, or central hypoventilation. Because of the initial psychiatric prodrome, patients may first present to psychiatrists, but the encephalopathic features quickly become apparent. The electroencephalogram (EEG) may show abnormalities such as focal or diffuse slow or disorganized activity; epilepsy; or extreme "delta brush" (Graus et al. 2016).

Diagnosis and Treatment of Autoimmune Encephalitis

Diagnosis of autoimmune encephalitis is usually confirmed by testing of serum or CSF for presence of antibodies, but there are often delays of several weeks before test results are available, and treatment with steroids or intravenous immunoglobulin (IVIG) is normally started empirically in probable cases. Positive antibodies are not always found in autoimmune encephalitis, and the diagnosis can be made on the basis of typical clinical features, MRI or CSF findings, and reasonable exclusion of alternative causes—in particular, well-defined encephalitic syndromes such as typical limbic encephalitis, Bickerstaff's brainstem encephalitis, and acute disseminated encephalomyelitis (Graus et al. 2016).

Autoimmune encephalitis is often associated with a remote tumor that requires targeted investigation. Common antibodies and associated tumors are shown in Table 30–2. Just over half of patients do well with first-line treatments (i.e., steroids, plasmapheresis, or IVIG), showing improvement within 4 weeks. The rest may require more prolonged immunosuppression with rituximab or cyclophosphamide. Eighty percent will have a good long-term outcome (Titulaer et al. 2013). In patients with poorer outcomes, deficits in episodic memory, executive function, and processing speed are noted at long-term follow-up (McKeon et al. 2017). A particular problem for psychi-

TABLE 30–2. **Antibodies associated with autoimmune encephalitis**

Antibody	Syndrome	Associated malignancy
Hu (ANNA-1)	Limbic encephalitis	Small-cell lung carcinoma
Ma2	Limbic encephalitis	Testicular seminoma
GAD	Limbic encephalitis	Thymoma, small-cell lung carcinoma
NMDA receptor	Anti–NMDA receptor encephalitis	Ovarian teratoma
AMPA receptor	Limbic encephalitis	Thymoma, small-cell lung carcinoma
$GABA_B$ receptor	Limbic encephalitis	Small-cell lung carcinoma
$GABA_A$ receptor	Encephalitis	Thymoma
mGluR5	Encephalitis	Hodgkin's lymphoma
Dopamine$_2$ receptor	Basal ganglia encephalitis	—
LGI1	Limbic encephalitis	Thymoma
CASPR2	Morvan's syndrome or limbic encephalitis	Thymoma
DPPX	Encephalitis	Lymphoma
MOG	Acute disseminated encephalomyelitis	—
Aquaporin 4	Encephalitis	—
GQ1b	Bickerstaff's brainstem encephalitis	—

Note. AMPA=α-amino-3-hydroxy-5-methyl-4-isoxazolepropionic acid; ANNA-1=type I anti-neuronal nuclear antibody; CASPR2=contactin associated protein 2; DPPX=dipeptidyl-peptidase-like protein–6; GABA=γ-aminobutyric acid; GAD=glutamic acid decarboxylase; LGI1=leucine-rich glioma inactivated 1; mGluR5=metabotropic glutamate receptor 5; MOG=myelin oligodendrocyte glycoprotein; NMDA= N-methyl-D-aspartate.

Source. Graus et al. 2016.

atrists is dealing with acute behavioral disturbance and prolonged psychotic symptoms. Primary management should be treatment of the underlying condition, but when adjunctive intervention is required, close nursing support and antipsychotics are usually the mainstays. No trial evidence is available to guide antipsychotic use, but we follow standard dosage regimens for new-onset psychosis, keeping a close eye on potential adverse effects, particularly neuroleptic malignant syndrome. Patients with autoimmune encephalitis can deteriorate very suddenly, and the need for close observation and a safe nursing environment cannot be overemphasized.

The presence of psychotic symptoms prior to the onset of more characteristic encephalitic features has led investigators to question whether an exclusively psychiatric presentation of the condition is possible. Antibodies associated with autoimmune encephalitis—in particular, antibodies against the NMDA receptor—were found in 9% of newly presenting psychotic patients in general psychiatric settings (Lennox et al. 2017). The clinical phenotype of antibody-positive patients was indistinguishable from other psychoses. It remains unknown whether the presence of the antibodies is pathogenic (Lennox et al. 2017; Zandi et al. 2011).

Steroid-Responsive Encephalopathy With Autoimmune Thyroiditis (Hashimoto's Encephalopathy)

Hashimoto's encephalopathy is a severe encephalopathic illness, manifesting in the presence of high serum antithyroid antibody concentrations, that responds dramatically to steroids. Seizures, psychosis, confusion, stroke-like episodes, and elevated levels of CSF protein, often with normal MRI findings, are the common features. There is controversy regarding whether the thyroid antibodies are causal or epiphenomenal (Laurent et al. 2016).

Amyotrophic Lateral Sclerosis (Motor Neurone Disease)

Amyotrophic lateral sclerosis (ALS) (known as *motor neurone disease* in Europe) is a neurodegenerative disorder, usually of unknown etiology, in which the affected person typically presents in the seventh decade with progressive weakness either of limbs (limb onset) or of speech and swallowing (bulbar onset). In 5%–10% of cases, there is a genetic basis. The diagnosis is made on the basis of progressive mixed upper and lower motor neuron signs in three limbs or in two limbs with bulbar symptoms (Brooks et al. 2000). Although the effects of ALS were traditionally thought to be confined to the motor system, it is now clear that at least some patients with the disease will experience specific neuropsychiatric complications.

In approximately 5% of sporadic ALS cases and 15% of familial ALS cases, the patient develops FTD, which manifests either as a typical frontal syndrome (with impaired executive function, apathy, and breakdown of social behavior) or as a more specific focal dementia (especially primary progressive aphasia and semantic dementia). A large proportion of patients with ALS are found to have subtle executive function deficits on testing in the absence of symptoms (Abrahams et al. 2005). Emotional lability is also common in ALS, affecting up to 20% of patients (Palmieri et al. 2009).

The 2011 discovery of hexanucleotide repeat expansions in the *C9orf72* gene was a landmark moment in understanding the relationship between ALS and FTD. Repeat expansions in *C9orf72* were quickly established as the most common cause in both FTD and ALS. The repeat expansion not only is found in familial cases of both conditions but also occurs sporadically. The neurodegenerative mechanisms associated with the gene are not understood (Rohrer et al. 2015). The penetrance of the mutation is also poorly understood, and while genetic counseling is advised in all cases of ALS and FTD with a family history, it is difficult to know how to characterize genetic risk in patients in whom the repeat expansions have occurred sporadically (Rohrer et al. 2015).

The *C9orf72* mutation is of particular interest to psychiatrists because of the phenotype of behavioral-variant FTD (the most common FTD presentation), which includes apathy, disinhibition, loss of empathy, socially inappropriate behavior, and abnormal eating patterns. Also of particular interest is the mutation's strong association with psychosis; hallucinations or delusions were present in 25%–50% of patients with repeat expansions in *C9orf72*, compared with around 10% of those without expansions. The symptoms of psychosis can predate other manifestations of FTD or ALS and can lead to a misdiagnosis of schizophrenia, bipolar disorder, or depressive pseudodementia. FTD due to the *C9orf72* mutation can also involve impairments in episodic memory, making it difficult to distinguish from Alzheimer's disease. Among carriers of the *C9orf72* mutation, general psychiatric morbidity can be present for many years before any signs of atrophy are detectable on neuroimaging (Rohrer et al. 2015).

CNS Tumors, Hydrocephalus, and Subdural Hematoma

CNS tumors, hydrocephalus, and subdural hematoma are discussed in the section "Neurosurgical Issues" later in this chapter.

Epilepsy

Epileptic seizures are transient cerebral dysfunctions resulting from an excessive and abnormal electrical discharge of neurons. The clinical manifestations are numerous. As a result, psychiatrists commonly deal with epilepsy, both when considering whether epilepsy is the primary cause of paroxysmal psychiatric symptoms and when treating its significant psychiatric complications.

Epidemiology

Problems with case definition and ascertainment complicate epidemiological estimates of epilepsy. However, incidence rates of 40–70 cases per 100,000 population in developed countries and 100–190 cases per 100,000 population in developing countries are generally accepted. The prevalence of active epilepsy is around 7 cases per 1,000 population in developed countries (Abramovici and Bagić 2016). The higher incidence of epilepsy in developing nations is thought to be related to increased rates of birth trauma and head injury and lack of health services to manage them, as well as poor sanitation leading to high rates of CNS infection (e.g., cysticercosis; see Chapter 26). Most studies show a bimodal distribution for incidence by age, with increased rates in persons younger than 10 years and older than 60 years. Epilepsy is more common in men than in women.

A specific etiological mechanism is identified in fewer than one-third of epilepsy cases; potential mechanisms include perinatal disorders, cerebral palsy, head trauma, CNS infection, cerebrovascular disease, brain tumors, Alzheimer's disease, and substance misuse. In addition, many so-called idiopathic seizures are likely to have a genetic basis.

Estimates of seizure recurrence after a first event are widely varied and depend on the population being studied. However, if seizures are going to recur, they usually do so within 6 months of the first event; the prognosis improves as the seizure-free period lengthens. In patients with established epilepsy, the prognosis is extremely variable. In some benign childhood epilepsies, anticonvulsants are unnecessary and remission is the rule. In the majority of patients with epilepsy, remission occurs with treatment, and it may be possible to withdraw treatment in the long term. In some epilepsy syndromes, such as juvenile myoclonic epilepsy, treatment is effective but must be continued indefinitely. In around one-third of patients with epilepsy, anticonvulsants fail to provide adequate control of seizures. This is particularly likely in patients with aggressive pediatric epilepsy syndromes (e.g., infantile spasms, Lennox-Gastaut syndrome) or in patients whose epilepsy has a defined structural or congenital cause.

Clinical Features

Epilepsy's clinical features reflect the diversity of its causes. The key clinical distinction is between seizures with a focal cerebral origin and those with a generalized origin. The former are more likely to be associated with a detectable and potentially remediable cerebral lesion, whereas the latter are more likely to start in childhood or adolescence and to be familial. Despite the wide variety of possible seizure manifestations, an individual patient's seizures are usually stereotyped. Their clinical features result from a recurrent pattern of cortical hyperactivity during the ictal event followed by hypoactivity in the same area postictally. Documentation of the clinical features of the seizure is the key to diagnosis. Because firsthand observation is seldom possible unless seizures are very frequent, the history of the episode, including an eyewitness account (or a home/mobile phone video), is of paramount importance.

Tonic-Clonic Seizures

Tonic-clonic seizures are the most dramatic manifestation of epilepsy and are characterized by motor activity and sudden loss of consciousness. In a typical seizure, a patient has no warning (with the possible exception of a couple of myoclonic jerks) of its onset. The seizure begins with sudden loss of consciousness and a tonic phase of sustained muscle contractions lasting 10–20 seconds. This is followed by a clonic phase of repetitive muscle contractions lasting approximately 30 seconds. A number of autonomic changes, including blood pressure and pulse rate increases, apnea, mydriasis, incontinence, piloerection, cyanosis, and perspiration, may also occur. In the postictal period, the patient is drowsy and confused, and abnormal neurological signs are often elicited.

Partial Seizures

Partial seizures are categorized according to whether they are *simple* (without impairment in consciousness) or *complex* (with impairment of consciousness). This classification may be difficult to apply in practice, however.

Simple partial seizures.   The clinical features of simple partial seizures depend on the brain region activated. Although the initial area is relatively localized, it is common for the abnormal activity to spread to adjacent areas, producing a progression of seizure pattern. If the activity originates in the motor cortex, there will be jerking movements in the contralateral body part.

Seizures originating in the *parietal lobe* can cause tingling or numbness in a bodily region or more complex sensory experiences. Seizures in the inferior regions of the parietal lobe can cause severe vertigo and disorientation in space. Dominant-hemisphere parietal lobe seizures can cause language disturbance.

Seizures of the *occipital lobe* are associated with visual symptoms, which are usually elementary (e.g., simple flashing lights). However, if the seizure occurs at the border with the temporal lobe, more complex experiences can occur, including micropsia and macropsia, as well as visual hallucinations.

Seizures affecting the *temporal lobe* can be the most difficult to diagnose, but this lobe is also the most common site of onset. Symptoms may include auditory hallucinations (ranging from simple sounds to complex language) and olfactory hallucinations (usually involving unpleasant odors). Seizures in the Sylvian fissure or operculum will cause gustatory sensations; ictal epigastric sensations such as nausea or emptiness generally have a temporal lobe origin. The well-known emotional and psychic phenomena of temporal lobe seizures can be present in simple seizures but are much more common in complex partial seizures.

Complex partial seizures.   In a complex partial seizure, the patient frequently experiences an aura at the onset of the seizure. An aura is a simple partial seizure lasting seconds to minutes. It should be distinguished from a *prodrome,* which is not an ictal event and which can last for hours or even days before a seizure. Prodromes usually consist of a sense of nervousness or irritability. The content of the aura will depend on the location of the abnormal discharge within the brain; thus, it may contain motor, sensory, visceral, or psychic elements. Auras may include hallucinations; intense fear, depression, panic, or depersonalization, as well as cognitive symptoms such as aphasia. Distortions of memory can include dreamy states, flashbacks, and distortions of familiarity with events (déjà vu or jamais vu). Rage is rare; when it does occur, it is characterized by lack of provocation and abrupt abatement. This phase is followed by impairment of consciousness and a seizure (usually lasting 60–90 seconds) that may generalize. Automatisms may occur and can involve an extension of the patient's actions prior to seizure onset. Common facial automatisms include chewing or swallowing, lip smacking, and grimacing; automatisms in the extremities include fumbling with objects, walking, or trying to stand up. Postictal confusion is usually significant and typically lasts 10 minutes or longer.

Complex partial seizures of frontal lobe origin tend to begin and end abruptly, with minimal postictal confusion. They often occur in clusters. The attacks are usually bizarre, with motor automatisms such as bicycling or with sexual automatisms and vocalizations.

Absence Seizures

Absence seizures are well-defined clinical and EEG events. The essential feature is an abrupt, brief episode of decreased awareness that occurs without any warning, aura, or postictal symptoms. At the onset there is a disruption of activity.

A *simple* absence seizure involves only an alteration in consciousness; the patient remains mobile, breathing is unaffected, and there is no color change and no loss of postural tone. The ending is abrupt, and the patient resumes previous activity immediately, often unaware that a seizure has occurred. An attack usually lasts around 15 seconds. A *complex* absence seizure involves additional symptoms, such as alterations in postural tone, clonic jerks, minor automatisms, and autonomic symptoms.

Violent Behavior

Epilepsy, in particular epilepsy involving the temporal lobe, may cause emotional symptoms and very occasionally can result in undirected violent behavior. However, in the majority of cases of epilepsy-related violence, the behavior occurs in response to being restrained during a seizure. One should be very cautious in attributing other violence to a seizure. Indeed, a systematic review concluded that overall, patients with epilepsy have a reduced risk for violence compared with control subjects without epilepsy (Fazel et al. 2009). This issue is discussed in greater detail in Chapter 6, "Aggression and Violence," which includes criteria for determining whether a violent act resulted from an epileptic seizure.

Differential Diagnosis

Differentiating epilepsy from psychogenic nonepileptic seizures (dissociative seizures) and syncope can be difficult. Other paroxysmal disorders should also be considered; these include transient ischemic attacks, hypoglycemia, migraine, transient global amnesia, cataplexy, paroxysmal movement disorders, and paroxysmal symptoms in MS. Diagnosis of attacks that occur during sleep can pose particular problems, as informant reports are less useful.

Dissociative Seizures (Psychogenic Nonepileptic Seizures)

Dissociative seizures—also called "pseudoseizures," "nonepileptic attack disorder," and "psychogenic seizures"—constitute the most common alternative diagnosis, accounting for about 30% of patients presenting to clinics with suspected epilepsy (Reuber and Elger 2003), and having a reported community prevalence of 33 cases per 100,000 population (Benbadis and Allen Hauser 2000). The terminology is confusing, and it is unclear whether the term *dissociative seizures* describes a specific diagnosis or is a collective term for a number of psychiatric diagnoses or symptoms that may cause seizure-like spells, including conversion, panic attacks, hyperventilation syndrome (see Chapter 18, "Lung Disease"), posttraumatic stress disorder, and catatonia. We personally favor the view that dissociative seizures are often a variant of panic disorder with prominent dissociation (Goldstein and Mellers 2006). Although patients with dissociative seizures are more likely than those with epilepsy to have concurrent psychiatric disorders (Diprose et al. 2016), they are also paradoxically more likely to have an external health locus of control and to deny that psychological factors might contribute to their illness (Stone et al. 2004). Some patients have both epilepsy and nonepileptic attacks, but probably only around 10% of individuals with dissociative seizures fall into this category (Benbadis et al. 2001; Reuber et al. 2002). Many of these patients are learning disabled and at increased risk of both epilepsy and psychiatric disorders.

The diagnosis of dissociative seizures can often be made on the basis of a careful history and examination. At the core of this syndrome is a distinct seizure semiology (with tremulous movements, often of varying frequency) that differs from the evolving jerky movements of epilepsy. Breathing is maintained. Some patients fall down and lie still without movement for prolonged periods. Clinical clues include a preexisting somatoform disorder; atypical varieties of seizure, especially the occurrence of frequent and prolonged seizures in the face of normal intellectual function and normal interictal EEG; a preponderance of seizures in public places, especially in clinics and hospitals; and behavior during an apparent generalized seizure that suggests preservation of awareness (e.g., resistance to attempted eye opening). Compared with patients who have epilepsy, those with recent-onset dissociative seizures are more likely to believe that psychological factors are less important than somatic ones and have a greater tendency to deny nonhealth life stresses (Stone et al. 2004). Eye closure during the spell has been considered to be a reliable indicator that the spell is not epileptic (Chung et al. 2006), although this belief has been challenged (Syed et al. 2008). A history of childhood sexual abuse is common but not universal among those with the diagnosis (Binzer et al. 2004). When doubt remains after careful clinical assessment and standard investigations, the gold standard for diagnosis is observation of attacks via video telemetry. A normal EEG during or immediately following an apparent generalized seizure also strongly suggests a dissociative seizure. However, surface EEG may be normal during focal seizures.

The diagnosis of dissociative seizures is regarded as distinct from deliberate falsification of attacks (i.e., malingering or factitious disorder). The majority of patients will be cooperative with investigation and diagnosis, even when they know in advance that the purpose is to confirm dissociative seizures and rule out epilepsy (McGonigal et al. 2002).

Treatment begins with a clear diagnosis, including explanation of the nature of the attacks and reassurance about their benign albeit disabling nature. Treatment should include taking the patient seriously, giving the problem a diagnostic label, explaining the rationale for the diagnosis, discussing to some degree how the symptoms arise, emphasizing expectation of recovery, and making a referral for other treatment where appropriate (Stone et al. 2016). Comorbid emotional disorders should be treated with standard pharmacological and psychological approaches. The attacks themselves may benefit from a range of psychotherapies, with CBT having the best evidence, but case series suggest that psychodynamic and group therapies may also have a role (Goldstein and Mellers 2016). There is some weak evidence that SSRIs may have a direct treatment effect on the attacks (LaFrance et al. 2014).

Syncope

Syncope, usually due to temporary interruption of the blood supply to the brain, is often accompanied by myoclonic jerks that are frequently regarded as epileptic by lay and medical onlookers (Lempert et al. 1994). The occurrence of more complex movements, eye deviation, eyelid flicker, or vocalizations can confuse the diagnosis further, as can aura symptoms, which are recalled by the majority of subjects and which include epigastric, vertiginous, visual, and somatosensory experiences (Benke et al. 1997).

Sleep Disorders

Sleep disorders—including sleepwalking, night terrors, and confusional arousals, all of which occur during slow-wave sleep; REM sleep behavior disorder; and a variety of other parasomnias, including bruxism, rhythmic movement disorder, and periodic limb movements—must all be distinguished from epilepsy (see Chapter 14, "Sleep Disorders").

Investigation of Seizures

Epilepsy is above all a clinical diagnosis, and the use and interpretation of tests should reflect this. Routine blood tests should include a complete blood count and routine chemistries, including serum calcium and magnesium. An electrocardiogram should always be performed. An EEG is helpful in confirming the diagnosis and in clarifying the type of epilepsy (i.e., generalized versus focal, a distinction particularly relevant for children and adolescents). However, the EEG is insensitive; a single interictal EEG will detect clearly epileptiform abnormalities in only about 30% of patients with epilepsy. Therefore, a normal EEG does not exclude epilepsy, just as minor nonspecific abnormalities do not confirm it. Serial recordings, including sleep-deprived recordings, increase the diagnostic yield to around 80% (Chabolla and Cascino 1997).

EEG can be supplemented with video recording to allow examination of the correlation between the clinical symptoms and the EEG abnormalities (video telemetry). Twenty-four-hour ambulatory monitoring is sometimes helpful.

Some form of neuroimaging should be performed in all patients with epilepsy, unless EEG has clearly demonstrated a syndrome of primary generalized epilepsy in a young patient. Computed tomography (CT) is adequate to exclude tumors and major structural abnormalities; however, CT may miss subtle pathologies. MRI is undoubtedly the imaging modality of choice, capable of detecting pathological abnormalities in up to 90% of patients with intractable epilepsy, including mesial temporal sclerosis (Spencer 1994). It can, however, be difficult to access in some countries.

Prolactin will rise after a generalized seizure but not, as a rule, after a nonepileptic attack. However, interpretation of the test requires knowledge of the basal prolactin and concurrent drug treatment (e.g., antipsychotics). Partial seizures and syncope can also elevate prolactin (Oribe et al. 1996; Pohlmann-Eden et al. 1997).

Additional cardiac investigations that may be helpful in selected cases include 24-hour ambulatory electrocardiography to identify cardiac dysrhythmias, echocardiography to identify structural cardiac abnormalities, and tilt-table testing to help confirm orthostatic syncope.

Psychiatric Complications

Record-linkage studies (Bredkjaer et al. 1998; Jalava and Sillanpää 1996) have reported a higher prevalence of psychotic symptoms, particularly schizophreniform and paranoid psychoses, in men, but not women, with epilepsy. Studies have also shown that patients (both men and woman) with epilepsy had a fourfold increased risk of psychiatric disorders compared with individuals in the general population, but not compared with patients with other medical diagnoses (Jalava and Sillanpää 1996).

Psychosis

Psychotic symptoms may be categorized as either transient postictal psychosis or chronic interictal psychosis. A meta-analysis found an overall prevalence of psychosis of 5.6% in epilepsy and of 7% in temporal lobe epilepsy. The prevalences of interictal psychosis and postictal psychosis were 5.2% and 2%, respectively (Clancy et al. 2014). In general, psychotic episodes do not begin immediately after a seizure, but instead occur after a lucid interval of 2–72 hours. Psychosis in epilepsy is discussed in Chapter 9.

Psychosis is also a potential side effect of anticonvulsants; it is most frequently associated with levetiracetam and topiramate but also occurs with phenytoin, valproate, lamotrigine, zonisamide, pregabalin, and vigabatrin (Mula et al. 2003). This effect occurs more commonly in patients with a history of psychiatric illness.

Cognitive Disorders

Cognitive disorders are commonly associated with epilepsy (Hermann and Seidenberg 2007). Mild generalized cognitive deficits, especially in memory, can be detected within months of seizure onset, and in children, academic records suggest that these deficits may predate seizure onset (Oostrom et al. 2003). Quantitative volumetric MRI studies suggest associations of cognitive deficits with temporal lobe abnormalities (Bonilha et al. 2004). The impairment can be progressive, although this is not inevitable, and patients can be reassured that the impairment will not lead to dementia. Poor seizure control and cumulative effects of medication appear to be risk factors for deterioration. The direct impairments can be compounded by the indirect effects of epilepsy on scholastic achievement.

Depressive and Anxiety Disorders

It is well established that epilepsy is a significant risk factor for depressive illness. A meta-analysis examining depression in people with epilepsy reported an overall prevalence of current or past-year depression of 23.1%, which was 2.77 times the rate in people without epilepsy (Fiest et al. 2013). Depression arising from learned helplessness may occur in patients with epilepsy as a consequence of repeatedly experiencing unpredictable and unavoidable seizures (Weigartz et al. 1999). The stress of having to live with a stigmatized chronic illness may also be relevant. Finally, anticonvulsants can themselves be a cause of depression. The relationship between depression and epilepsy is bidirectional (i.e., each is a risk factor for the other). Depression is an independent risk factor for unprovoked seizures (Hesdorffer et al. 2000). The contribution of depression to risk appears to be particularly marked for partial seizures. However, data from three population-based studies have also shown that depression is associated with a four- to sevenfold increased risk for developing epilepsy (Kanner 2006). This bidirectional relationship does not imply causality but rather suggests common pathogenic mechanisms shared by both conditions (Kanner 2006). Depressive symptoms not only affect onset of epilepsy but also are associated with poorer response to treatment and poorer quality of life.

Depressive disorders can be typical of their DSM mood disorder description (Jones et al. 2005), can be characterized by their relationship to the ictal event, or can present as "interictal dysphoric disorder" (Kanner et al. 2000). The last-mentioned concept was introduced originally by Kraepelin and then Bleuler, describing a pleomorphic pattern of symptoms consisting of prominent irritability intermixed with euphoria, anxiety, anergia, insomnia, and pain. Interictal dysphoric disorder is said to have a chronic relapsing–remitting course but to respond well to antidepressants. However, it is a controversial diagnosis whose validity has been questioned (Amiri and Hansen 2015).

There has been increasing interest in screening for depression in epilepsy patients. A recent systematic review of 16 screening instruments singled out the Neurological Disorders Depression Inventory for Epilepsy as the most extensively validated screening tool; this instrument is free, easy to administer, and validated in multiple languages (Gill et al. 2017). The importance of depression as a predictor of pharmacoresistance in epilepsy was highlighted in a study describing the development of a predictive model using MRI scans, genomic information, and the A-B Neuropsychological Assessment Schedule (ABNAS) (Hitiris et al. 2007). The role of depression in exacerbating seizure risk is important, because many psychiatrists worry that antidepressant use will worsen epilepsy, when in fact it is the persistence of untreated depression that carries the greater threat.

Similarly, anxiety in epilepsy may have a complex etiology (Goldstein and Harden 2000). Anticipatory anxiety about having a seizure without warning can lead to agoraphobic-like behavior. A recent meta-analysis reported a pooled prevalence of anxiety disorders in epilepsy patients of 20.2%. That patients' physicians frequently miss the diagnosis is suggested by the finding that the prevalence based on unstructured clinician assessment was 8.1%, compared with a prevalence of 27.3% based on a structured clinical interview (Scott et al. 2017).

Treatment of depressive and anxiety disorders in epilepsy patients is generally the same as that of anxiety and depression in the medically ill (see Chapter 7 and Chapter 10, "Anxiety Disorders"). Certain psychiatric drugs can lower the seizure threshold, thereby increasing the risk of seizures (see Chapter 36 for a review). However, this risk is often exaggerated, and in general, undertreatment has caused far more problems than overtreatment. In particular, the risk of seizures with bupropion has been overstated in many sources; a systematic review concluded that the risk was lower than that associated with TCAs (Ruffmann et al. 2006).

A 2008 U.S. Food and Drug Administration investigation of antiepileptic drugs and suicide (U.S. Department of Health and Human Services et al. 2008) concluded that all classes of antiepileptic drugs (AEDs) were associated with an increased risk of suicide; suicidal behaviors were found in 0.43% of patients taking AEDs, compared with 0.24% of placebo control subjects. However, to date there is no consensus across studies regarding which anticonvulsants carry the most risk, and the mechanism of this relationship is poorly understood. The elevated rates of psychiatric comorbidity in epilepsy likely account for at least some of the increased risk (Grimaldi-Bensouda et al. 2017). The benefits of AEDs in patients with epilepsy far outweigh the risks. The complexity of this issue highlights the need for good neuropsychiatric care in all patients with epilepsy.

Approximately 20%–30% of patients do not achieve seizure control with AED therapy. In carefully selected cases, surgery can be dramatically effective. Most studies investigating outcomes of consecutive patients undergoing surgery report seizure freedom for at least 1 year in 50%–85% (Spencer and Huh 2008). Criteria for selection generally include presence of a focal lesion on neuroimaging, evidence from video telemetry that the lesion is the source of the habitual seizures, and neuropsychological evidence that resection of the lesion should not cause major cognitive deficits. Psychological factors are also often relevant in the decision to perform surgery (see section "Neurosurgical Issues" later in this chapter).

Vagal nerve stimulation has been shown to reduce seizure frequency in some patients with refractory epilepsy (Privitera et al. 2002), but it probably is no more effective than the addition of the newer anticonvulsants to established therapy.

Tic Disorders

Tics are habitual spasmodic muscular movements or contractions, usually of the face or extremities, that are associated with a variety of disorders.

Gilles de la Tourette's syndrome (GTS) is characterized by a combination of multiple waxing and waning motor and vocal tics. These vary from simple twitches and grunts to complex stereotypies. Premonitory sensory sensations in the body parts that "need to tic" are a common feature and complicate the picture, because their temporary suppressibility lends them a voluntary component. Other features are echolalia and coprolalia, particularly in severe cases. GTS is strongly associated with obsessive-compulsive disorder (OCD), but many claim that the GTS-associated disorder is qualitatively different from pure OCD, with a greater focus on symmetry, aggressive thoughts, forced touching, and fear of harming oneself in OCD-GTS versus a more frequent focus on hygiene and cleanliness in pure OCD. Depressive symptoms in GTS are common (Cavanna et al. 2009). The prevalence of GTS is about 5 cases per 10,000 population, with a male:female ratio of 4:1. A debate exists as to whether OCD in itself constitutes a specific psychopathological entity comorbid with GTS or whether diverse pathological disorders—including attention-deficit/hyperactivity disorder (ADHD), eating disorders, anxiety disorders, and substance misuse— should also be considered to be part of the phenotype. Genetic studies suggest a strong hereditary component in the disorder. The neurobiology of GTS remains elusive, with evidence supporting dysfunctions in dopaminergic basal ganglia circuitry receiving the most attention. Structural-imaging findings in GTS are usually normal; functional imaging data are contradictory. Early-childhood abrupt onset of OCD accompanied by tics may represent the syndrome designated *pediatric autoimmune neuropsychiatric disorders associated with streptococcal infection* (PANDAS), which is discussed in Chapter 26.

Management of GTS is multidisciplinary, with a clear need to address the educational, social, and family consequences of the disorder. Dopamine antagonists remain the mainstay of pharmacological management. Haloperidol has been the most widely used antipsychotic, but many authors advocate use of atypical antipsychotics on the basis of fewer extrapyramidal side effects (Budman 2014). Clonidine is used widely in the United States, but in the United Kingdom its use is generally restricted to patients with comorbid ADHD symptoms (Leckman et al. 1991). DBS has been used in severe GTS, although it carries the usual risks of functional neurosurgery and as yet has not been proven in a sham controlled trial (Servello et al. 2016). Behavioral treatments, including habit reversal, have also shown promise (Wilhelm et al. 2003). In establishing treatment priorities, psychiatrists should bear in mind that the associated OCD and ADHD symptoms probably cause more functional and educational disability than do the tics themselves. For many patients, tics are only a problem because of the attitudes of others.

Dystonias

The dystonias are a group of disorders characterized by involuntary twisting and repetitive movements and abnormal postures. The traditional clinical categorization is based on age at onset, distribution of symptoms, and site. Early-onset dystonia often starts in one limb, tends to generalize, and frequently has a genetic origin. By contrast, adult-onset dystonias usually spare the lower limbs, frequently involve the cervical or cranial muscles, and tend to remain focal. They appear sporadic in most cases. Dystonias tend to improve with relaxation, hypnosis, and sleep. With the exception of cervical dystonia, pain is uncommon. Erroneous attribution of dystonia to a psychogenic cause was common because of the fluctuating nature of the symptoms, their often dramatic appearance, the ability of patients to use "tricks" to suppress them, and their association with task-specific symptoms (e.g., writer's cramp). Dystonic movements may, however, be seen as the presentation of a conversion disorder. Psychogenic dystonia typically presents as a fixed posture, usually a clenched fist or inverted plantar-flexed foot, and onset is often associated with physical trauma (Schrag et al. 2004). It is important to remember the role of exposure to medications (e.g., antipsychotics, antiemetics) in the development of both acute and tardive dystonias (Sweet et al. 1995).

Generalized dystonia is associated with an expanding range of largely autosomal dominant genetic mutations (Geyer and Bressman 2006). The most common of these is *primary torsion dystonia*, which is caused by a mutation in the *DYT1* gene. The dystonia usually begins in childhood in one limb and subsequently generalizes to other body parts.

Focal dystonia is the most prevalent form. It starts in adulthood and usually remains localized (e.g., as in isolated torticollis [focal cervical dystonia], writer's cramp, blepharospasm, and musician's dystonia). The majority of cases are sporadic, although some family pedigree studies have shown an increased risk of focal dystonias in other family members.

Dopa-responsive dystonia is characterized by childhood onset, diurnal fluctuation of symptoms, and a dramatic response to levodopa therapy. It may be confused with spastic paraparesis, leading to diagnostic delay. It generally has autosomal dominant inheritance associated with a mutation in the *DYT5* gene.

Medical treatment of dystonia involves botulinum injections, oral drugs, and potentially neurosurgery; detailed reviews have been published on treatment issues in adults (Termsarasab et al. 2016) and in children (Luc and Querubin 2017). Comorbid psychiatric disorders—particularly OCD, panic disorder, and depression—are commonly associated with dystonias and should be actively treated in their own right.

Headache

Acute Headache

Headache of abrupt onset that is very severe and prolonged can be due to *subarachnoid hemorrhage,* usually from a ruptured aneurysm, or to migraine, meningitis, or another cranial infection (e.g., otitis media, sinusitis). The diagnosis of subarachnoid hemorrhage is suggested by the rapidity of onset ("thunderclap" headache, at its worst within the first minute or so) and associated loss of consciousness, photophobia, vomiting, and neck stiffness. A headache with these features requires immediate neurological referral for assessment. Psychiatrists are predominantly involved in the management of the associated brain injury following subarachnoid hemorrhage. (For a further discussion of these management principles, see the section "Stroke" earlier in this chapter; see also Chapter 33.)

Migraine can mimic subarachnoid hemorrhage. The diagnosis is usually suggested by a history of more typical intermittent headaches with evolving prodromal visual (or other focal neurological) disturbance and a hemicranial throbbing headache, worse on exercise, with photophobia and nausea or vomiting. *Meningitis* is suggested by a severe headache, usually worsening over hours, with photophobia, nausea, and neck stiffness in association with fever and other features of infection. There are many other causes of acute headache, such as spontaneous intracranial hypotension and venous sinus thrombosis.

Chronic Headache

Headache is an almost universal experience (see also Chapter 34). The exhaustive International Headache Society classification of headaches is available free online (Headache Classification Committee of the International Headache Society 2018). *Migraine with aura* (previously classical migraine) has the features described above. In *migraine without aura* (previously common migraine), there is throbbing hemicranial pain in the absence of focal neurological symptoms such as visual disturbance. *Tension-type headache* is familiar to most of us as a global headache, usually of mild to moderate severity, sometimes with a "band like" or pressing quality. It often worsens as the day goes on or following stress and has few associated symptoms. *Chronic tension-type headache*, defined as more than 15 headache days a month, is one type of chronic daily headache (CDH). Most patients with CDH have underlying migraine that is often made worse by *analgesic overuse headache.* Prolonged exposure to any analgesic (not just opioids) can lead to analgesic overuse headache, and withdrawal of these agents often leads to improvement, although this must be done with careful explanation to the patient (Weatherall 2007). It is important in CDH, therefore, to assess how much of the problem is migraine versus tension-type headache versus analgesic overuse headache.

A large literature has shown a close, probably bidirectional, association between CDH and psychiatric comorbidity, especially depression and anxiety (Hamelsky and Lipton 2006). The presence of psychiatric comorbidity is associated with poorer outcomes. Treatment of comorbid mood disorders with antidepressants and CBT can be helpful (Kroenke and Swindle 2000).

Patients with chronic migraine headaches have been described as having a "typical" personality characterized by conscientiousness, perfectionism, ambitiousness, rigidity, tenseness, and resentfulness; however, controlled studies have not consistently supported this profile (Davis et al. 2013). Specific personality traits in migraine appear more likely to be a consequence rather than a cause of suffering from recurrent headaches (Pompili et al. 2009). It has been difficult to disentangle personality traits from manifestations of comorbid depression and anxiety (which are highly prevalent in this patient population).

Cervicogenic headache is strictly defined by the International Headache Society as headache arising from clearly defined pathology such as tumors, fractures, infections, and rheumatoid arthritis. *Temporal arteritis* is a disorder of older people that causes scalp pain and tenderness, jaw claudication, malaise, and an elevated erythrocyte sedimentation rate (see Chapter 24, "Rheumatology"). *Raised intracranial pressure* typically causes a headache that is worse on lying down and relieved by standing; disturbs sleep; and is present in the mornings. The pressure eventually causes nausea and vomiting. The raised pressure can result from space-occupying lesions, hydrocephalus, or idiopathic intracranial hypertension. *Low CSF volume headache* is an increasingly well-recognized syndrome with features inverse to those of the headache of raised intracranial pressure: the headache comes on after getting up and is relieved by lying down. This type of headache is often iatrogenic (e.g., following lumbar puncture), but it can also occur as a result of spontaneous CSF leaks.

Certain "headaches" are felt mainly in the face. *Cluster headache,* a rare type of headache that is more common in young men, gives rise to severe retro-orbital pain occurring in bursts lasting an hour or so that recur over a period of days to weeks (the "cluster"). The headache often wakes the sufferer in the middle of the night and usually makes him or her extremely restless (in contrast to migraine, which sends sufferers to their beds). *Trigeminal neuralgia* causes stabs of lancinating pain in one of the three divisions of the trigeminal nerve. *Atypical facial pain* is a diagnosis of exclusion, the facial equivalent of chronic daily headache.

Conversion (Functional Neurological Symptom) Disorder in Neurology

Conversion (functional neurological symptom) disorder describes patients with motor and/or sensory symptoms or blackouts that suggest a neurological or other general medical condition who display symptoms and signs that are inconsistent or incongruent with pathophysiology. Patients prefer the term *functional disorder* (Stone et al. 2002), and the name *functional neurological disorder* has been universally adopted by the emerging patient charities (which enjoy notably positive relationships with both neurologists and psychiatrists who are interested in the field). In DSM-5, the requirement that psychological factors be judged to be associated with the symptoms was eliminated from the diagnostic criteria for conversion disorder, given that the theoretical basis of the requirement remains unconfirmed and that a proportion of patients do not appear to experience such stressors. Furthermore, because psychological factors are common in all neurological presentations, the requirement is nonspecific and likely to be diagnostically unreliable. Common conversion symptoms include paralysis, weakness, seizures, anesthesia, aphonia, blindness, amnesia, and stupor. (The epidemiology and clinical features of nonepileptic attacks were discussed earlier in this chapter in the section "Epilepsy.")

Epidemiology

Neurological symptoms in the absence of neurological disease or disproportionate to disease are observed in approximately one-third of patients seen in neurology clinics (Carson and Lehn 2016; Carson et al. 2000b). The incidence of functional weakness and paralysis is estimated to be at least 5 cases per 100,000 population (Binzer and Kullgren 1998), and patients with these symptoms account for around 3% of new referrals to neurology outpatient clinics, a rate similar to that of new referrals of patients with MS. The belief that conversion disorder is predominantly found in populations living in rural settings and characterized by low educational levels and low socioeconomic status is not consistent with the evidence (Carson and Lehn 2016). Approximately 10% of patients with functional motor symptoms make a complete recovery, and about half improve over long-term follow-up (Gelauff et al. 2013). Predictors of poor outcome include early expectation of nonrecovery, nonattribution of symptoms to psychological factors, and receipt of health-related benefits at the time of the initial consultation (Sharpe et al. 2010). A two-nation surveillance study of conversion symptoms among children ages 7–15 years reported a 1-year incidence of 1.30 cases per 100,000 population (Ani et al. 2013), but transient conversion symptoms are well recognized in children.

Clinical Features

Diagnosis requires taking a careful history, first concentrating on the somatic symptoms, and then exploring psychological and social factors. A detailed description of the approach to assessment is provided by Carson et al. (2016a). In considering the diagnosis, particular attention should be paid to the presence of multiple somatic symptoms and of depression or anxiety (particularly panic), as well as a history of functional symptoms. However, patient experience should be the key focus—patients with functional disorders tend to have similar patterns of symptom onset and development and to use similar language to describe their experiences. Childhood abuse and neglect, personality factors, recent stressful life events, secondary gain (financial or otherwise), and strong beliefs about the causation may all be relevant to management, but these factors occur in all kinds of disease, and their presence does not allow one to infer a diagnosis of conversion disorder (Stone et al. 2005a). The presence of *la belle indifférence* was classically considered to be highly suggestive of the disorder; however, this attitude is seen in only a minority of patients with conversion, and with equal frequency in patients with organic neurological disorders (Stone et al. 2006).

Patients with conversion weakness will often describe symptoms suggestive of depersonalization or derealization at the time of onset. Symptom onset is most commonly associated with a physical trauma (often minor) (Pareés et al. 2014), a panic attack, or an unexpected physiological event (e.g., postmicturitional syncope, sleep paralysis) (Stone et al. 2009).

The neurological examination has a crucial role in the diagnosis of conversion disorder. Because of the difficulties in relying on features in the history, the diagnosis requires the presence of positive physical signs of internal inconsistency or marked incongruity with recognized neurological disorders. Helpful indicators include Hoover's sign (Ziv et al. 1998), collapsing ("giveaway") weakness, and co-contraction (Knutsson and Mårtensson 1985); however, none of these signs should be interpreted in isolation, because there may be false positives. A conversion tremor typically demonstrates variable frequency and marked attenuation with distraction and entrainment (in which the frequency entrains to a contralateral limb voluntarily, making a 3- to 4-Hz movement). *Fixed dystonia* is a term used to describe the sustained posture of a limb, usually a clenched hand or an inverted, plantar-flexed foot (Hallett et al. 2005; Schrag et al. 2004). There are many tests of visual conversion symptoms (Beatty 1999), and the finding of a tubular visual field deficit at the bedside or a spiral on perimetry testing is suggestive. All of these signs can be demonstrated to patients in a collaborative, rather than confrontational, manner (Stone et al. 2005a). The full range of presentations has been reviewed in detail by Hallett et al. (2016).

Pathology and Etiology

The etiology of conversion disorder is gradually being elucidated. Over the past decade, studies have increasingly focused on mechanisms of symptom production rather than background risk factors of aversive experience. Central to this change in focus is an improved understanding of the role of conscious effort in motor processing. What we think of as our conscious experience of controlling movement almost certainly relates to the feedback stage rather than the feedforward initial activation. Converging evidence suggests that initiation of movement begins at a preconscious level, an idea that opens up the possibility that this early preconscious initiation of movement may be disrupted in conversion disorder, allowing an explanation of why a disorder of voluntary movement may be perceived as involuntary. The disruption of preconscious processes in conversion disorder is believed to be facilitated by rigidly held cognitive models and expectations, coupled with alterations in attention. These phenomena can be understood in Bayesian predictive brain coding terms as excessively strong "top down" expectations (or "priors") overriding "bottom up" sensory feedback and distorting the sense of "agency." These ideas have been outlined in detail in a seminal paper by Edwards et al. (2012). This increasing interest in mechanism does not mean that previously considered risk factors of traumatic childhood and adult experiences are no longer relevant. On the contrary, functional imaging studies are beginning to disclose how aversive memories might contribute to creation of conversion symptoms; for example, functional MRI studies have demonstrated that enhanced amygdalar activity in response to a perceived threat exerts an unusually strong influence on premotor planning areas (Aybek et al. 2014).

Investigation and Differential Diagnosis

Further imaging or neurophysiological testing may be required, depending on the symptoms present, but ultimately the diagnosis of conversion disorder should be made on the basis of clear positive features of neurological signs that are inconsistent or incongruent with neurological disease and not on the basis of negative (normal) imaging findings. However, functional disorders and neurological disease are not mutually exclusive, and some degree of "workup" may be required to rule out important comorbidities—thus, we would normally image all patients with clear functional gait disorders. Diagnostic error has been a cause for concern among psychiatrists, based in part on an often-quoted study published more than 50 years ago, and subsequently discredited, that cautioned that many patients diagnosed with conversion disorder subsequently received a diagnosis of a neurological or medical condition. By contrast, a systematic review of 27 studies found that the error rate since 1970 has been on average 4% (Stone et al. 2005b). This is better than the diagnostic error rates for most neurological and psychiatric conditions (Carson et al. 2003; Stone et al. 2005b, 2009). Presentations that can result in misdiagnosis are discussed in detail by Stone et al. (2013). Although clinicians tend to worry about missing "organic" disease and therefore are often very conservative in making a diagnosis of conversion disorder, the Scottish Neurological Symptoms Study indicated that the reverse was a more significant problem (Stone et al. 2009). In our experience, this reluctance to diagnose conversion disorder leads to iatrogenic complications of unneeded treatment and invalidism. Interestingly, several medical negligence suits are now being brought for delays in making a correct diagnosis of functional disorder.

Management

The foundation of treatment for conversion disorder is an explicit acceptance of the reality of the symptoms and a nonstigmatizing, positive explanation of the diagnosis that emphasizes the potential reversibility of the problem. Explanation about how the diagnosis has been made and why it indicates the absence of neurological disease is likely to be more successful than simple reassurance alone (Stone et al. 2005a, 2016).

Dismissing the symptoms as "nothing wrong" risks antagonizing or humiliating the patient and is rarely a good basis for collaborative management. Only after the patient and the physician are reasonably satisfied that the diagnosis is correct can further treatment continue. In our own experience, conceptualizing the symptoms as functional symptoms—a problem with the functioning of the nervous system, as opposed to a structural disorder—works both theoretically and practically with patients (Sharpe and Carson 2001). This approach—which Carson et al. (2016b) have outlined in detail—involves a collaborative and open encounter in which the physician provides a clear diagnosis in terms of what is wrong (e.g., "You have functional neurological symptoms"), shows patients their clinical signs and demonstrates reversibility, explains underlying mechanisms in terms of attention and processing, and (if appropriate) concludes with a discussion of the role played by risk factors such as aversive experiences. We think this approach preferable to the current common practice of inverting the typical transcript of the consultation by stating what is *not* wrong and then adding vague comments about what the problem might be. We regard a clear explanation in positive terms, as the foundation stone of treatment, and for some patients, that is all that may be required. In regard to symptom-focused treatment, there is evidence for the efficacy of CBT (Goldstein and Mellers 2016), including an abbreviated form (Sharpe et al. 2011), as well as for inpatient rehabilitation and physiotherapy (Williams et al. 2016).

The development of specific physiotherapies is of particular interest because treatment is based on an understanding of etiological mechanisms (Nielsen et al. 2015, 2016). Interpersonal therapies and hypnosis also show some promise. There is no evidence to support pharmacological treatment of conversion disorder per se, although there are good reasons to consider that pharmacological strategies might be similar to those used in somatic symptom–related disorders in general, and our clinical experience is that a TCA can be a useful adjunct to treatment, particularly for pain. Comorbid mood disorders should be treated in the usual way. There has been a revival of interest in the use of therapeutic sedation—that is, sedation targeted toward demonstrating reversibility of symptoms rather than uncovering repressed emotions (Stone et al. 2014).

Neurosurgical Issues

Many of the psychiatric issues arising in neurosurgical settings are described in other chapters in this book. Of particular relevance are Chapters 4, 28 ("Surgery"), and Chapter 33 (which discusses brain injury). High dosages of corticosteroids are used by neurosurgeons to reduce elevated intracranial pressure; the psychiatric adverse effects of corticosteroids are reviewed in Chapter 24. Mood disorders are common after neurosurgery, and their assessment should be guided by the principles discussed in earlier sections of this chapter, particularly the section on stroke.

Central Nervous System Tumors

Psychiatric aspects of cancer are reviewed in Chapter 22, "Oncology." Psychiatrists generally become involved in neuro-oncology cases after tumor diagnosis when clinical issues—such as adjustment difficulties, mood disorders, or cognitive impairment—are present. Patients with primary and metastatic CNS tumors typically present with headache, focal neurological signs, or seizures, but these tumors can also cause cognitive impairment, and occasionally their presentation mimics a dementing illness (Lishman 1997). Some brain tumors present with predominantly psychiatric symptoms, including depression, panic attacks, psychosis, disordered eating, and personality changes. CT scanning should reveal tumor presence, although diffusely infiltrating tumors are sometimes missed in the early stages.

Hydrocephalus

Hydrocephalus is caused by dilatation of the ventricles within the brain resulting from elevation of CSF pressure. Hydrocephalus is termed *communicating* when the blockage to CSF flow is outside the ventricular system, and *noncommunicating* when the blockage is within the ventricles. In "compensated" hydrocephalus, the clinical signs and CSF dynamics stabilize at an elevated level of CSF pressure. *Normal-pressure hydrocephalus* (NPH) describes ventricular enlargement in the presence of normal CSF pressure, possibly as the result of persistent elevation or intermittent surges of high pressure.

Clinical Features

Hydrocephalus can cause a wide range of symptoms and signs. These include enlargement of the head (if the condition is present in infancy), depression, headache, progressive visual failure, gait disturbance (often "gait apraxia"), incontinence, subcortical cognitive impairment progressing to dementia, and acute elevations of intracranial pressure ("hydrocephalic attacks") causing sudden death. NPH in older individuals is associated with the classic triad of gait apraxia, incontinence, and cognitive decline. However, this triad is not specific to NPH and may occur in vascular dementia or other neurodegenerative diseases. Depression commonly occurs in NPH (Israelsson et al. 2016).

Diagnosis

In younger persons, the radiological signs of hydrocephalus are usually clear-cut on CT scanning. This may also be the case in some elderly patients, but in other older patients apparent hydrocephalus is often due to ex vacuo atrophy of the subcortical white matter. The presence of easily visible cortical sulci should alert the clinician to this possibility. When enlargement of the ventricles raises the suspicion of communicating hydrocephalus in an older person, determination of whether imaging findings are clinically meaningful requires specialized studies—usually either serial lumbar punctures with observation of the clinical effects or neurosurgical studies of CSF pressure. However, there is no one test that can confirm a diagnosis of NPH or predict the response to shunting, which means that appropriate investigations for NPH are controversial (Shprecher et al. 2008). Ultimately, only the insertion of a shunt can reliably determine whether a patient will benefit from shunting.

Management

Shunting to treat hydrocephalus—surgery to divert CSF to the venous system or peritoneum—can be beneficial in the long term (Pujari et al. 2008), potentially yielding significant improvement in cognition (Peterson et al. 2016). However, the procedure leads to complications—including subdural hematoma and shunt infection—in nearly half of patients (Hebb and Cusimano 2001) and therefore should not be undertaken lightly.

Subdural Hematoma

Subdural hematoma is caused by accumulations of blood and blood products in the space between the fibrous dura mater and the more delicate arachnoid membrane that encloses the brain. Acute subdural hematomas accumulate rapidly following head injury; chronic hematomas can often (although not always) be traced back to a head injury.

Clinical Features

Acute subdural hematomas are, by definition, diagnosed close to the time of trauma, as a result of symptoms present at the time—headache, depressed level of consciousness, focal neurological signs—or seen on CT scan. Chronic subdural hematomas give rise to more gradually evolving symptoms and signs. Although they also can cause headache, depressed consciousness, and focal signs, chronic subdural hematomas sometimes result in predominantly cognitive features, including confusion and dementia, which may be reversed with surgery (Ishikawa et al. 2002). Marked variability of the mental state, and sometimes also of the neurological features, is often a clue to the diagnosis. Seizures can occur. Both acute and chronic subdural hematomas are especially common in alcoholic individuals, who frequently do not recall having experienced head trauma.

Pathology

The variability of the clinical features is explained by the tendency of the size of a chronic subdural hematoma to wax and wane as a result of alternating phases of bleeding and of breakdown of the contents of the hematoma. Subdural hematomas exert their effects both by local compression and irritation of adjacent cortical tissue and by global "brain shift" (with the risk of brain herniation and secondary brain stem compression).

Investigation and Differential Diagnosis

Subdural hematomas can generally be diagnosed via CT scanning. They are occasionally "isodense" with brain and therefore easily missed, especially if bilateral. It is important to recognize that a small subdural hematoma can be an incidental finding; for example, cerebral atrophy occurring in the course of a dementing illness predisposes to subdural hematoma as vulnerable bridging veins are stretched between the dura and the arachnoid. In these circumstances, treatment of the subdural hematoma is unlikely to be helpful.

Management

Small subdural hematomas often resorb spontaneously. If a subdural hematoma is considered to be relevant to a patient's problems and drainage is required, several surgical approaches are available.

Subarachnoid Hemorrhage

Severe, prolonged headache of abrupt onset can be due to a subarachnoid hemorrhage, usually arising from a ruptured berry aneurysm. A diagnosis of subarachnoid hemorrhage is suggested by the rapidity of onset ("thunderclap" headache, at its worst within the first minute or so) and associated loss of consciousness, photophobia, vomiting, and neck stiffness (Al-Shahi et al. 2006). Psychiatrists are rarely involved in the diagnosis of subarachnoid hemorrhage but are frequently asked to evaluate patients in the postacute phase, as for stroke. In the first 21 days after a subarachnoid hemorrhage, one-third of patients may develop a fluctuating clinical course due to cerebral vasospasm (Wintermark et al. 2006). Symptoms and signs vary according to the territory affected, but variable akinetic mutism is particularly common in patients with vasospasm after an anterior cerebral artery aneursymal hemorrhage.

Fitness for Surgery

Psychiatrists may be requested to assess patients' fitness for neurosurgery. Such requests occur most commonly for patients with epilepsy or Parkinson's disease. A general assessment of capacity (see Chapter 2, "Legal and Ethical Issues") and consideration of specific issues relevant to the operation in question are required, necessitating special attention when the operation is considered investigational.

Epilepsy Surgery

A psychiatric opinion should be sought prior to surgery if there are significant associated behavioral or social problems. Such problems include anticipated noncompliance with medication, severe personality disturbance, psychosis, severe mood disorder, unrealistic expectations of surgery, and an absence of social support. The presence of intellectual disability is not an absolute contraindication to surgery but can complicate postsurgical care. The most commonly performed procedures are temporal lobectomy and amygdalohippocampectomy. Other procedures include extratemporal cortical resections, hemispherectomy, and white matter transactions, including corpus callosotomy (Engel 1993). Around two-thirds of patients will become seizure free after surgery. Mortality is exceptionally rare, and the rate of neurological complications has lowered significantly over the last 2 years, with hemiparesis now being exceptionally rare (Spencer and Huh 2008). Reported rates of complications after temporal lobectomies (including partial hemianopsia, aphasia, and cranial nerve palsies) are 0.4%–4% (Spencer and Huh 2008). Cognitive changes—in particular, decline in verbal memory—are reported in around one-third of patients (Spencer and Huh 2008). The risk of new onset of a mood disorder after surgery is most closely related to presurgical mental state and whether the patient is seizure free (Spencer and Huh 2008). De novo development of psychosis is recognized, but the risk factors for its development are not (Spencer and Huh 2008). It is noteworthy that poor psychological outcomes occasionally accompany good postoperative seizure control, and some patients need considerable psychological help in adjusting to life without seizures.

Parkinson's Disease Surgery

Subthalamic DBS is an effective neurosurgical treatment for motor symptoms in advanced Parkinson's disease. However, neuropsychiatric symptoms—including executive function impairments, reduced verbal fluency, delirium, depression, mania, apathy, psychosis, and impulse-control problems—have been reported to occur during optimization of stimulation parameters. Most of these symptoms are short-lived (Abulseoud et al. 2016). Compared with younger patients (mean age of 52.9 years), older patients (mean age of 63.2 years) were found to be at higher risk of experiencing psychotic symptoms post-DBS (Cozac et al. 2016). Impulsivity symptoms (e.g., pathological gambling, sexual disinhibition) after DBS for Parkinson's disease are similar to those associated with dopamine agonists. (See section "Medication-Related Impulse-Control Disorders" earlier in this chapter.)

Conclusion

The practice of psychiatry in a neurological or neurosurgical setting is both challenging and rewarding. In this chapter we have outlined general principles of assessment and management in relation to the more commonly encountered conditions. These same principles apply to the more rarely encountered problems. Working closely with colleagues who share an interest in disorders of the brain can be very rewarding, and new developments in neuroscience are providing a greater understanding of the mechanisms by which biological, psychological, and social factors interact to cause both neurological and psychiatric illness. Consequently, the interface between these specialties is rapidly becoming one of the most intellectually fascinating areas of work for the specialist in psychosomatic medicine.

References

Aarsland D, Ballard C, Larsen JP, et al: A comparative study of psychiatric symptoms in dementia with Lewy bodies and Parkinson's disease with and without dementia. Int J Geriatr Psychiatry 16(5):528–536, 2001 11376470

Abrahams S, Goldstein LH, Leigh PN: Cognitive change in amyotrophic lateral sclerosis: a prospective study. Neurology 64:1222–1226, 2005 15824350

Abramovici S, Bagić A: Epidemiology of epilepsy. Handb Clin Neurol 138:159–171, 2016 27637958

Abulseoud OA, Kasasbeh A, Min HK, et al: Stimulation-induced transient nonmotor psychiatric symptoms following subthalamic deep brain stimulation in patients with Parkinson's disease: association with clinical outcomes and neuroanatomical correlates. Stereotact Funct Neurosurg 94(2):93–101, 2016 27093641

Adams P, Falek A, Arnold J: Huntington disease in Georgia: age at onset. Am J Hum Genet 43(5):695–704, 1988 2973230

Almqvist EW, Bloch M, Brinkman R, et al: A worldwide assessment of the frequency of suicide, suicide attempts, or psychiatric hospitalization after predictive testing for Huntington disease. Am J Hum Genet 64(5):1293–1304, 1999 10205260

Al-Shahi R, White PM, Davenport RJ, et al: Subarachnoid haemorrhage. BMJ 333(7561):235–240, 2006 16873858

American Psychiatric Association: Diagnostic and Statistical Manual of Mental Disorders, 5th Edition. Arlington, VA, American Psychiatric Association, 2013

Amiri M, Hansen CP: The interictal dysphoric disorder in patients with epilepsy: a doubtful disorder lacking diagnostic tools. Seizure 24:70–76, 2015 25246233

Andersen G, Vestergaard K, Lauritzen L: Effective treatment of poststroke depression with the selective serotonin reuptake inhibitor citalopram. Stroke 25(6):1099–1104, 1994 8202964

Ani C, Reading R, Lynn R, et al: Incidence and 12-month outcome of non-transient childhood conversion disorder in the U.K. and Ireland. Br J Psychiatry 202:413–418, 2013 23620449

Ardouin C, Voon V, Worbe Y, et al: Pathological gambling in Parkinson's disease improves on chronic subthalamic nucleus stimulation. Mov Disord 21(11):1941–1946, 2006 16972268

Arena JE, Rabinstein AA: Transient global amnesia. Mayo Clin Proc 90(2):264–272, 2015 25659242

Arnulf I, Bonnet AM, Damier P, et al: Hallucinations, REM sleep, and Parkinson's disease: a medical hypothesis. Neurology 55(2):281–288, 2000 10908906

Aström M: Generalized anxiety disorder in stroke patients. A 3-year longitudinal study. Stroke 27(2):270–275, 1996 8571422

Aybek S, Nicholson TR, Zelaya F, et al: Neural correlates of recall of life events in conversion disorder. JAMA Psychiatry 71(1):52–60, 2014 24258270

Baker MG, Kale R, Menken M: The wall between neurology and psychiatry. BMJ 324(7352):1468–1469, 2002 12077018

Bamford J, Sandercock P, Dennis M, et al: A prospective study of acute cerebrovascular disease in the community: the Oxfordshire Community Stroke Project 1981–86, I: methodology, demography and incident cases of first-ever stroke. J Neurol Neurosurg Psychiatry 51(11):1373–1380, 1988 3266234

Beatty S: Non-organic visual loss. Postgrad Med J 75(882):201–207, 1999 10715758

Beatty WW, Goodkin DE, Beatty PA, et al: Frontal lobe dysfunction and memory impairment in patients with chronic progressive multiple sclerosis. Brain Cogn 11(1):73–86, 1989 2789818

Benbadis SR, Allen Hauser W: An estimate of the prevalence of psychogenic non-epileptic seizures. Seizure 9(4):280–281, 2000 10880289

Benbadis SR, Agrawal V, Tatum WO 4th: How many patients with psychogenic nonepileptic seizures also have epilepsy? Neurology 57(5):915–917, 2001 11552032

Benke T, Hochleitner M, Bauer G: Aura phenomena during syncope. Eur Neurol 37(1):28–32, 1997 9018029

Berg D, Postuma RB, Bloem B, et al: Time to redefine PD? Introductory statement of the MDS Task Force on the definition of Parkinson's disease. Mov Disord 29(4):454–462, 2014 24619848

Berthier ML, Kulisevsky J, Gironell A, et al: Poststroke bipolar affective disorder: clinical subtypes, concurrent movement disorders, and anatomical correlates. J Neuropsychiatry Clin Neurosci 8(2):160–167, 1996 9081551

Binzer M, Kullgren G: Motor conversion disorder. A prospective 2- to 5-year follow-up study. Psychosomatics 39(6):519–527, 1998 9819952

Binzer M, Stone J, Sharpe M: Recent onset pseudoseizures—clues to aetiology. Seizure 13(3):146–155, 2004 15010051

Boeschoten RE, Braamse AMJ, Beekman ATF, et al: Prevalence of depression and anxiety in multiple sclerosis: a systematic review and meta-analysis. J Neurol Sci 372:331–341, 2017 28017241

Bogousslavsky J, Cummings JL: Behavior and Mood Disorders in Focal Brain Lesions. New York, Cambridge University Press, 2000

Boller F, Agrawal K, Romano A: Sexual function after strokes. Handb Clin Neurol 130:289–295, 2015 26003250

Bonilha L, Rorden C, Castellano G, et al: Voxel-based morphometry reveals gray matter network atrophy in refractory medial temporal lobe epilepsy. Arch Neurol 61(9):1379–1384, 2004 15364683

Borisovskaya A, Bryson WC, Buchholz J, et al: Electroconvulsive therapy for depression in Parkinson's disease: systematic review of evidence and recommendations. Neurodegener Dis Manag 6(2):161–176, 2016 27033556

Bower JH, Maraganore DM, McDonnell SK, et al: Incidence and distribution of parkinsonism in Olmsted County, Minnesota, 1976–1990. Neurology 52(6):1214–1220, 1999 10214746

Bredkjaer SR, Mortensen PB, Parnas J: Epilepsy and non-organic non-affective psychosis. National epidemiologic study. Br J Psychiatry 172:235–238, 1998 9614472

Breier JI, Adair JC, Gold M, et al: Dissociation of anosognosia for hemiplegia and aphasia during left-hemisphere anesthesia. Neurology 45(1):65–67, 1995 7824138

Breuer B, Pappagallo M, Knotkova H, et al: A randomized, double-blind, placebo-controlled, two-period, crossover, pilot trial of lamotrigine in patients with central pain due to multiple sclerosis. Clin Ther 29(9):2022–2030, 2007 18035201

Brinkman RR, Mezei MM, Theilmann J, et al: The likelihood of being affected with Huntington disease by a particular age, for a specific CAG size. Am J Hum Genet 60(5):1202–1210, 1997 9150168

Brooks BR, Miller RG, Swash M, et al; World Federation of Neurology Research Group on Motor Neuron Diseases: El Escorial revisited: revised criteria for the diagnosis of amyotrophic lateral sclerosis. Amyotroph Lateral Scler Other Motor Neuron Disord 1(5):293–299, 2000 11464847

Brooks DJ, Doder M: Depression in Parkinson's disease. Curr Opin Neurol 14(4):465–470, 2001 11470962

Bruns MB, Josephs KA: Neuropsychiatry of corticobasal degeneration and progressive supranuclear palsy. Int Rev Psychiatry 25(2):197–209, 2013 23611349

Budman CL: The role of atypical antipsychotics for treatment of Tourette's syndrome: an overview. Drugs 74(11):1177–1193, 2014 25034359

Burns A, Folstein S, Brandt J, et al: Clinical assessment of irritability, aggression, and apathy in Huntington and Alzheimer disease. J Nerv Ment Dis 178(1):20–26, 1990 2136908

Burvill PW, Johnson GA, Jamrozik KD, et al: Anxiety disorders after stroke: results from the Perth Community Stroke Study. Br J Psychiatry 166(3):328–332, 1995 7788124

Butler CR, Graham KS, Hodges JR, et al: The syndrome of transient epileptic amnesia. Ann Neurol 61(6):587–598, 2007 17444534

Carota A, Nicola A, Aybek S, et al: Aphasia-related emotional behaviors in acute stroke. Neurology 54:A244, 2000

Carota A, Rossetti AO, Karapanayiotides T, et al: Catastrophic reaction in acute stroke: a reflex behavior in aphasic patients. Neurology 57(10):1902–1905, 2001 11723287

Carota A, Staub F, Bogousslavsky J: Emotions, behaviours and mood changes in stroke. Curr Opin Neurol 15(1):57–69, 2002 11796952

Carson AJ, Lehn A: Epidemiology, in Functional Neurologic Disorders. Edited by Hallett M, Stone J, Carson A (Handbook of Neurology, Vol 139, 3rd Series, Aminoff MJ, Boller F, Swaab DJ, series eds). New York, Elsevier, 2016, pp 47–60

Carson AJ, MacHale S, Allen K, et al: Depression after stroke and lesion location: a systematic review. Lancet 356(9224):122–126, 2000a 10963248

Carson AJ, Ringbauer B, Stone J, et al: Do medically unexplained symptoms matter? A prospective cohort study of 300 new referrals to neurology outpatient clinics. J Neurol Neurosurg Psychiatry 68:207–210, 2000b 10644789

Carson AJ, Best S, Postma K, et al: The outcome of neurology outpatients with medically unexplained symptoms: a prospective cohort study. J Neurol Neurosurg Psychiatry 74(7):897–900, 2003 12810775

Carson AJ, Hallett M, Stone J: Assessment of patients with functional neurologic disorders, in Functional Neurologic Disorders. Edited by Hallett M, Stone J, Carson A (Handbook of Neurology, Vol 139, 3rd Series, Aminoff MJ, Boller F, Swaab DJ, series eds). New York, Elsevier, 2016a, pp 169–188

Carson AJ, Lehn A, Ludwig L, et al: Explaining functional disorders in the neurology clinic: a photo story. Practical Neurology 16(1):56–61, 2016b 26769761

Carta MG, Moro MF, Lorefice L, et al: The risk of bipolar disorders in multiple sclerosis. J Affect Disord 155:255–260, 2014 24295600

Cavanna AE, Servo S, Monaco F, et al: The behavioral spectrum of Gilles de la Tourette syndrome. J Neuropsychiatry Clin Neurosci 21(1):13–23, 2009 19359447

Ceravolo R, Nuti A, Piccinni A, et al: Paroxetine in Parkinson's disease: effects on motor and depressive symptoms. Neurology 55(8):1216–1218, 2000 11071504

Chabolla DR, Cascino GD: Interpretation of extracranial EEG, in The Treatment of Epilepsy: Principles and Practice, 2nd Edition. Edited by Wylie E. Baltimore, MD, Williams & Wilkins, 1997, pp 264–279

Chen Y, Patel NC, Guo JJ, et al: Antidepressant prophylaxis for poststroke depression: a meta-analysis. Int Clin Psychopharmacol 22(3):159–166, 2007 17414742

Choi-Kwon S, Han SW, Kwon SU, et al: Fluoxetine treatment in poststroke depression, emotional incontinence, and anger proneness: a double-blind, placebo-controlled study. Stroke 37(1):156–161, 2006 16306470

Chong MS, Wolff K, Wise K, et al: Cannabis use in patients with multiple sclerosis. Mult Scler 12(5):646–651, 2006 17086912

Chouinard G, Sultan S: A case of Parkinson's disease exacerbated by fluoxetine. Hum Psychopharmacol 7(1):63–66, 1992

Choy W, Gerstein DR, Ghadialy R, et al: National Household Survey on Drug Abuse: Main Findings, 1992. Rockville, MD, Substance Abuse and Mental Health Services Administration, 1995

Chua P, Chiu E: Huntington's disease, in Dementia. Edited by Burns A, Levy R. London, Chapman & Hall, 1994, pp 827–844

Chung SS, Gerber P, Kirlin KA: Ictal eye closure is a reliable indicator for psychogenic nonepileptic seizures. Neurology 66(11):1730–1731, 2006 16769949

Chwastiak LA, Ehde DM: Psychiatric issues in multiple sclerosis. Psychiatr Clin North Am 30(4):803–817, 2007 17938046

Cilia R, Siri C, Canesi M, et al: Dopamine dysregulation syndrome in Parkinson's disease: from clinical and neuropsychological characterisation to management and long-term outcome. J Neurol Neurosurg Psychiatry 85(3):311–318, 2013 23591553

Clancy MJ, Clarke MC, Connor DJ, et al: The prevalence of psychosis in epilepsy: a systematic review and meta-analysis. BMC Psychiatry 14:75, 2014 24625201

Colchester A, Kingsley D, Lasserson D, et al: Structural MRI volumetric analysis in patients with organic amnesia, 1: methods and comparative findings across diagnostic groups. J Neurol Neurosurg Psychiatry 71(1):13–22, 2001 11413256

Cozac VV, Ehrensperger MM, Gschwandtner U, et al: Older candidates for subthalamic deep brain stimulation in Parkinson's disease have a higher incidence of psychiatric serious adverse events. Front Aging Neurosci 8:132, 2016 27375478

Cummings JL: Managing psychosis in patients with Parkinson's disease. N Engl J Med 340(10):801–803, 1999 10072418

Cummings JL, Cunningham K: Obsessive-compulsive disorder in Huntington's disease. Biol Psychiatry 31(3):263–270, 1992 1532132

Cummings JL, Mendez MF: Secondary mania with focal cerebrovascular lesions. Am J Psychiatry 141(9):1084–1087, 1984 6465386

Cummings JL, Arciniegas DB, Brooks BR, et al: Defining and diagnosing involuntary emotional expression disorder. CNS Spectr 11(S6):1–7, 2006 16816786

Cummings J, Isaacson S, Mills R, et al: Pimavanserin for patients with Parkinson's disease psychosis: a randomised, placebo-controlled phase 3 trial. Lancet 383(9916):533–540, 2014 24183563

Damasio AR: Emotion, Reason, and the Human Brain. New York, GP Putnam & Sons, 1994

D'Ambrosio A, Pagani E, Riccitelli G, et al: Cerebellar contribution to motor and cognitive impairment in multiple sclerosis patients: an MRI sub-regional structural analysis. Mult Scler 23(9):1194–1203, 2016 27760859

Darnell RB, Posner JB: Paraneoplastic syndromes involving the nervous system. N Engl J Med 349(16):1543–1554, 2003 14561798

Davis RE, Smitherman TA, Baskin SM: Personality traits, personality disorders, and migraine: a review. Neurol Sci 34 (suppl 1):S7–S10, 2013 23695036

de Bruin VMS, Lees AJ: The clinical features of 67 patients with clinically definite Steele-Richardson-Olszewski syndrome. Behav Neurol 5(4):229–232, 1992 24487808

De Deurwaerdère P, Ding Y: Antiparkinsonian treatment for depression in Parkinson's disease: are selective serotonin reuptake inhibitors recommended? Translational Neuroscience and Clinics 2(2):138–149, 2016 de la Monte SM, Vonsattel JP, Richardson EP Jr: Morphometric demonstration of atrophic changes in the cerebral cortex, white matter, and neostriatum in Huntington's disease. J Neuropathol Exp Neurol 47(5):516–525, 1988 2971785

de Tommaso M, Serpino C, Sciruicchio V: Management of Huntington's disease: role of tetrabenazine. Ther Clin Risk Manag 7:123–129, 2011 21479143

Diederich NJ, Pieri V, Goetz CG: [Visual hallucinations in Parkinson and Charles Bonnet Syndrome patients. A phenomenological and pathogenetic comparison] [in German]. Fortschr Neurol Psychiatr 68(3):129–136, 2000 10758844

Diprose W, Sundram F, Menkes DB: Psychiatric comorbidity in psychogenic nonepileptic seizures compared with epilepsy. Epilepsy Behav 56:123–130, 2016 26874243

Dobkin RD, Menza M, Allen LA, et al: Cognitive-behavioral therapy for depression in Parkinson's disease: a randomized, controlled trial. Am J Psychiatry 168(10):1066–1074, 2011 21676990

Edwards MJ: Dopamine agonist withdrawal syndrome (DAWS): perils of flicking the dopamine "switch." J Neurol Neurosurg Psychiatry 84(2):120, 2013 22993451

Edwards MJ, Rick A, Adams HB, et al: A Bayesian account of "hysteria." Brain 135(Pt 11):3495–3512, 2012 22641838

Ehde DM, Gibbons LE, Chwastiak L, et al: Chronic pain in a large community sample of persons with multiple sclerosis. Mult Scler 9(6):605–611, 2003 14664474

Emre M, Aarsland D, Albanese A, et al: Rivastigmine for dementia associated with Parkinson's disease. N Engl J Med 351(24):2509–2518, 2004 15590953

Engel J Jr: Clinical neurophysiology, neuroimaging, and the surgical treatment of epilepsy. Curr Opin Neurol Neurosurg 6(2):240–249, 1993 8481567

Evans AH, Pavese N, Lawrence AD, et al: Compulsive drug use linked to sensitized ventral striatal dopamine transmission. Ann Neurol 59(5):852–858, 2006 16557571

Farrer LA, Conneally PM: A genetic model for age at onset in Huntington disease. Am J Hum Genet 37(2):350–357, 1985 3157315

Fazel S, Philipson J, Gardiner L, et al: Neurological disorders and violence: a systematic review and meta-analysis with a focus on epilepsy and traumatic brain injury. J Neurol 256(10):1591–1602, 2009 19353216

Feigin A, Kieburtz K, Bordwell K, et al: Functional decline in Huntington's disease. Mov Disord 10(2):211–214, 1995 7753064

Feinstein A: Mood disorders in multiple sclerosis and the effects on cognition. J Neurol Sci 245(1–2):63–66, 2006 16643952

Ferenci P, Puéchal X, Raoult D: Wilson's disease. Clin Liver Dis 2(1):31–49, v–vi, 1998 15560044

Ferro JM, Caeiro L, Figueira ML: Neuropsychiatric sequelae of stroke. Nat Rev Neurol 12(5):269–280, 2016 27063107

Ffytche D: Visual hallucination and illusion disorders: a clinical guide. Adv Clin Neurosci Rehabil 4(2):16–18, 2004

Fiest KM, Dykeman J, Patten SB, et al: Depression in epilepsy: a systematic review and meta-analysis. Neurology 80(6):590–599, 2013 23175727

Fiest KM, Fisk JD, Patten SB, et al; CIHR Team in the Epidemiology and Impact of Comorbidity on Multiple Sclerosis (ECoMS): Fatigue and Comorbidities in Multiple Sclerosis. Int J MS Care 18(2):96–104, 2016 27134583

Fisher CM: Abulia, in Stroke Syndromes. Edited by Bogousslavsky J, Caplan L. Cambridge, UK, Cambridge University Press, 1995, pp 182–187

Folstein SE, Folstein MF, McHugh PR: Psychiatric syndromes in Huntington's disease, in Advances in Neurology, Vol 23: Huntington's Disease. Edited by Wexler TN, Barbeau NS, Chase A. New York, Raven, 1979, pp 281–289

Fotopoulou A, Jenkinson PM, Tsakiris M, et al: Mirror-view reverses somatoparaphrenia: dissociation between first- and third-person perspectives on body ownership. Neuropsychologia 49(14):3946–3955, 2011 [Erratum in Neuropsychologia 50(9):2377, 2012] 22023911

Franklin GM, Nelson L: Environmental risk factors in multiple sclerosis: causes, triggers, and patient autonomy. Neurology 61(8):1032–1034, 2003 14581658

Fregni F, Santos CM, Myczkowski ML, et al: Repetitive transcranial magnetic stimulation is as effective as fluoxetine in the treatment of depression in patients with Parkinson's disease. J Neurol Neurosurg Psychiatry 75(8):1171–1174, 2004 15258224

Gainotti G, Azzoni A, Razzano C, et al: The Post-Stroke Depression Rating Scale: a test specifically devised to investigate affective disorders of stroke patients. J Clin Exp Neuropsychol 19(3):340–356, 1997 9268809

Gainotti G, Azzoni A, Marra C: Frequency, phenomenology and anatomical-clinical correlates of major post-stroke depression. Br J Psychiatry 175:163–167, 1999 10627800

Geda YE, Boeve BF, Negash S, et al: Neuropsychiatric features in 36 pathologically confirmed cases of corticobasal degeneration. J Neuropsychiatry Clin Neurosci 19(1):77–80, 2007 17308231

Gelauff J, Stone J, Edwards M, et al: The prognosis of functional (psychogenic) motor symptoms: a systematic review. J Neurol Neurosurg Psychiatry 85(2):220–226, 2013 24029543

George MS, Wassermann EM, Post RM: Transcranial magnetic stimulation: a neuropsychiatric tool for the 21st century. J Neuropsychiatry Clin Neurosci 8(4):373–382, 1996 9116472

Geyer HL, Bressman SB: The diagnosis of dystonia. Lancet Neurol 5(9):780–790, 2006 16914406

Ghaffar O, Feinstein A: The neuropsychiatry of multiple sclerosis: a review of recent developments. Curr Opin Psychiatry 20(3):278–285, 2007 17415083

Gill SJ, Lukmanji S, Fiest KM, et al: Depression screening tools in persons with epilepsy: a systematic review of validated tools. Epilepsia 58(5):695–705, 2017 28064446

Goldstein K: The Organism: A Holistic Approach to Biology Derived From Pathological Data in Man. New York, American Books, 1939

Goldstein MA, Harden CL: Epilepsy and anxiety. Epilepsy Behav 1(4):228–234, 2000 12609439

Goldstein LH, Mellers JDC: Ictal symptoms of anxiety, avoidance behaviour, and dissociation in patients with dissociative seizures. J Neurol Neurosurg Psychiatry 77(5):616–621, 2006 16614021

Goldstein LH, Mellers JDC: Psychologic treatment of functional neurologic disorders. Handb Clin Neurol 139:571–583, 2016 27719872

Goodarzi Z, Mele B, Guo S, et al: Guidelines for dementia or Parkinson's disease with depression or anxiety: a systematic review. BMC Neurol 16(1):244, 2016 27887589

Gorell JM, Rybicki BA, Johnson CC, et al: Smoking and Parkinson's disease: a dose-response relationship. Neurology 52(1):115–119, 1999 9921857

Grall-Bronnec M, Victorri-Vigneau C, Donnio Y, et al: Dopamine agonists and impulse control disorders: a complex association. Drug Saf 41(1):19–75, 2017 28861870

Graus F, Titulaer MJ, Balu R, et al: A clinical approach to diagnosis of autoimmune encephalitis. Lancet Neurol 15(4):391–404, 2016 26906964

Grimaldi-Bensouda L, Nordon C, Rossignol M, et al; PROTECT-WP6 study group: Antiepileptic drugs and risk of suicide attempts: a case-control study exploring the impact of underlying medical conditions. Pharmacoepidemiol Drug Saf 26(3):239–247, 2017 28052554

Gustafson Y, Olsson T, Asplund K, Hagg E: Acute confusional state (delirium) soon after stroke is associated with hypercortisolism. Cerebrovascular Diseases 3:33–38, 1993

Hackett ML, Anderson CS, House A, et al: Interventions for treating depression after stroke. Cochrane Database Syst Rev (4):CD003437, 2008 18843644

Hackett ML, Köhler S, O'Brien JT, et al: Neuropsychiatric outcomes of stroke. Lancet Neurol 13(5):525–534, 2014 24685278

Hallett M, Lang AE, Fahn S, et al: Psychogenic Movement Disorders. Philadelphia, PA, American Neurological Association and Lippincott Williams & Wilkins, 2005

Hallett M, Stone J, Carson A (eds): Functional Neurologic Disorders (Handbook of Neurology, Vol 139, 3rd Series, Aminoff MJ, Boller F, Swaab DJ, series eds). New York, Elsevier, 2016

Hama S, Yamashita H, Shigenobu M, et al: Depression or apathy and functional recovery after stroke. Int J Geriatr Psychiatry 22(10):1046–1051, 2007 17702056

Hamelsky SW, Lipton RB: Psychiatric comorbidity of migraine. Headache 46(9):1327–1333, 2006 17040330

Harper PS: Huntington's Disease. London, WB Saunders, 1991

Haussleiter IS, Brüne M, Juckel G: Psychopathology in multiple sclerosis: diagnosis, prevalence and treatment. Ther Adv Neurol Disorder 2(1):13–29, 2009 21180640

Headache Classification Committee of the International Headache Society: The International Classification of Headache Disorders, 3rd Edition. Cephalalgia 38(1):1–211, 2018 29368949. Available at: https://www.ichd-3.org/wp-content/uploads/2018/01/The-International-Classification-of-Headache-Disorders-3rd-Edition-2018.pdf. Accessed February 26, 2018.

Heaton RK, Nelson LM, Thompson DS, et al: Neuropsychological findings in relapsing-remitting and chronic-progressive multiple sclerosis. J Consult Clin Psychol 53(1):103–110, 1985 3980815

Hebb AO, Cusimano MD: Idiopathic normal pressure hydrocephalus: a systematic review of diagnosis and outcome. Neurosurgery 49(5):1166–1184, discussion 1184–1186, 2001 11846911

Henry JD, Beatty WW: Verbal fluency deficits in multiple sclerosis. Neuropsychologia 44(7):1166–1174, 2006 16293271

Hermann B, Seidenberg M: Epilepsy and cognition. Epilepsy Curr 7(1):1–6, 2007 17304341

Hesdorffer DC, Hauser WA, Annegers JF, et al: Major depression is a risk factor for seizures in older adults. Ann Neurol 47(2):246–249, 2000 10665498

Hind D, Cotter J, Thake A, et al: Cognitive behavioural therapy for the treatment of depression in people with multiple sclerosis: a systematic review and meta-analysis. BMC Psychiatry 14:5, 2014 24406031

Hirsch L, Jette N, Frolkis A, et al: The incidence of Parkinson's disease: a systematic review and meta-analysis. Neuroepidemiology 46(4):292–300, 2016 27105081

Hitiris N, Mohanraj R, Norrie J, et al: Predictors of pharmacoresistant epilepsy. Epilepsy Res 75(2–3):192–196, 2007 17628429

Hodges JR: Transient Amnesia: Clinical and Neuropsychological Aspects. London, WB Saunders, 1991

Hodges JR, Ward CD: Observations during transient global amnesia. A behavioural and neuropsychological study of five cases. Brain 112(Pt 3):595–620, 1989 2731023

Hoffmann S, Tittgemeyer M, von Cramon DY: Cognitive impairment in multiple sclerosis. Curr Opin Neurol 20(3):275–280, 2007 17495620

Hsieh S, Schubert S, Hoon C, et al: Validation of the Addenbrooke's Cognitive Examination III in frontotemporal dementia and Alzheimer's disease. Dement Geriatr Cogn Disord 36(3–4):242–250, 2013 23949210

Hyde TM, Ziegler JC, Weinberger DR: Psychiatric disturbances in metachromatic leukodystrophy. Insights into the neurobiology of psychosis. Arch Neurol 49(4):401–406, 1992 1532712

Ishikawa E, Yanaka K, Sugimoto K, et al: Reversible dementia in patients with chronic subdural hematomas. J Neurosurg 96(4):680–683, 2002 11990807

Israelsson H, Allard P, Eklund A, et al: Symptoms of depression are common in patients with idiopathic normal pressure hydrocephalus: the INPH-CRasH study. Neurosurgery 78(2):161–168, 2016 26528670

Jacobson RR, Lishman WA: Cortical and diencephalic lesions in Korsakoff's syndrome: a clinical and CT scan study. Psychol Med 20(1):63–75, 1990 2320699

Jalava M, Sillanpää M: Concurrent illnesses in adults with childhood-onset epilepsy: a population-based 35-year follow-up study. Epilepsia 37(12):1155–1163, 1996 8956846

James AC, Kaplan P, Lees A, et al: Schizophreniform psychosis and adrenomyeloneuropathy. J R Soc Med 77(10):882–884, 1984 6092633

Jehkonen M, Laihosalo M, Kettunen J: Anosognosia after stroke: assessment, occurrence, subtypes and impact on functional outcome reviewed. Acta Neurol Scand 114(5):293–306, 2006 17022776

Joffe RT, Lippert GP, Gray TA, et al: Mood disorder and multiple sclerosis. Arch Neurol 44(4):376–378, 1987 3827692

Johansson V, Lundholm C, Hillert J, et al: Multiple sclerosis and psychiatric disorders: comorbidity and sibling risk in a nationwide Swedish cohort. Mult Scler 20(14):1881–1891, 2014 25013151

Jones JE, Hermann BP, Barry JJ, et al: Clinical assessment of Axis I psychiatric morbidity in chronic epilepsy: a multicenter investigation. J Neuropsychiatry Clin Neurosci 17(2):172–179, 2005 15939970

Kanner AM: Depression and epilepsy: a new perspective on two closely related disorders. Epilepsy Curr 6(5):141–146, 2006 17260039

Kanner AM, Kozak AM, Frey M: The use of sertraline in patients with epilepsy: is it safe? Epilepsy Behav 1(2):100–105, 2000 12609138

Kasemsuk C, Oyama G, Hattori N: Management of impulse control disorders with deep brain stimulation: a double-edged sword. J Neurol Sci 374:63–68, 2017 28126343

Kianirad Y, Simuni T: Pimavanserin, a novel antipsychotic for management of Parkinson's disease psychosis. Expert Rev Clin Pharmacol 10(11):1161–1168, 2017 28817967

Kim JS, Choi-Kwon S: Poststroke depression and emotional incontinence: correlation with lesion location. Neurology 54(9):1805–1810, 2000 10802788

Kirkwood SC, Siemers E, Stout JC, et al: Longitudinal cognitive and motor changes among presymptomatic Huntington disease gene carriers. Arch Neurol 56(5):563–568, 1999 10328251

Knutsson E, Mårtensson A: Isokinetic measurements of muscle strength in hysterical paresis. Electroencephalogr Clin Neurophysiol 61(5):370–374, 1985 2412788

Kopelman MD: Rates of forgetting in Alzheimer-type dementia and Korsakoff's syndrome. Neuropsychologia 23(5):623–638, 1985 4058708

Kopelman MD, Stanhope N, Kingsley D: Retrograde amnesia in patients with diencephalic, temporal lobe or frontal lesions. Neuropsychologia 37(8):939–958, 1999 10426519

Korostil M, Feinstein A: Anxiety disorders and their clinical correlates in multiple sclerosis patients. Mult Scler 13(1):67–72, 2007 17294613

Kroenke K, Swindle R: Cognitive-behavioral therapy for somatization and symptom syndromes: a critical review of controlled clinical trials. Psychother Psychosom 69(4):205–215, 2000 10867588

Kuopio AM, Marttila RJ, Helenius H, et al: Changing epidemiology of Parkinson's disease in southwestern Finland. Neurology 52(2):302–308, 1999 9932948

LaFrance WC Jr, Baird GL, Barry JJ, et al; NES Treatment Trial (NEST-T) Consortium: Multicenter pilot treatment trial for psychogenic nonepileptic seizures: a randomized clinical trial. JAMA Psychiatry 71(9):997–1005, 2014 24989152

Lampl Y, Lorberboym M, Gilad R, et al: Auditory hallucinations in acute stroke. Behav Neurol 16(4):211–216, 2005 16518011

Langhorne P, Stott DJ, Robertson L, et al: Medical complications after stroke: a multicenter study. Stroke 31(6):1223–1229, 2000 10835436

Laurent C, Capron J, Quillerou B, et al: Steroid-responsive encephalopathy associated with autoimmune thyroiditis (SREAT): characteristics, treatment and outcome in 251 cases from the literature. Autoimmun Rev 15(12):1129–1133, 2016 27639840

Lazar RM, Marshall RS, Prell GD, et al: The experience of Wernicke's aphasia. Neurology 55(8):1222–1224, 2000 11071506

Leckman JF, Hardin MT, Riddle MA, et al: Clonidine treatment of Gilles de la Tourette's syndrome. Arch Gen Psychiatry 48(4):324–328, 1991 2009034

Lempert T, Bauer M, Schmidt D: Syncope: a videometric analysis of 56 episodes of transient cerebral hypoxia. Ann Neurol 36(2):233–237, 1994 8053660

Lennox BR, Palmer-Cooper EC, Pollak T, et al; PPiP study team: Prevalence and clinical characteristics of serum neuronal cell surface antibodies in first-episode psychosis: a case-control study. Lancet Psychiatry 4(1):42–48, 2017 27965002

Leo RJ: Movement disorders associated with the serotonin selective reuptake inhibitors. J Clin Psychiatry 57(10):449–454, 1996 8909330

Leo J, Lacasse J: Clinical trials of therapy versus medication: even in a tie, medication wins (letter). BMJ 338:b463, 2009

Leroi I, Michalon M: Treatment of the psychiatric manifestations of Huntington's disease: a review of the literature. Can J Psychiatry 43(9):933–940, 1998 9825166

Levy ML, Cummings JL, Fairbanks LA, et al: Apathy is not depression. J Neuropsychiatry Clin Neurosci 10(3):314–319, 1998 9706539

Lincoln NB, Flannaghan T, Sutcliffe L, et al: Evaluation of cognitive behavioural treatment for depression after stroke: a pilot study. Clin Rehabil 11(2):114–122, 1997 9199863

Lindesay J: Phobic disorders in the elderly. Br J Psychiatry 159:531–541, 1991 1751864

Lishman WA: Organic Psychiatry: The Psychological Consequences of Cerebral Disorder, 3rd Edition. Oxford, UK, Blackwell Science, 1997

Luc QN, Querubin J: Clinical management of dystonia in childhood. Paediatr Drugs 19(5):447–461, 2017 28620849

Lynch SG, Kroencke DC, Denney DR: The relationship between disability and depression in multiple sclerosis: the role of uncertainty, coping, and hope. Mult Scler 7(6):411–416, 2001 11795464

Mair WGP, Warrington EK, Weiskrantz L: Memory disorder in Korsakoff's psychosis: a neuro-pathological and neuropsychological investigation of two cases. Brain 102(4):749–783, 1979 116710

Manchanda R, Miller H, McLachlan RS: Post-ictal psychosis after right temporal lobectomy. J Neurol Neurosurg Psychiatry 56(3):277–279, 1993 8459245

Maraganore DM, Lees AJ, Marsden CD: Complex stereotypies after right putaminal infarction: a case report. Mov Disord 6(4):358–361, 1991 1758457

Marsh L: Depression and Parkinson's disease: current knowledge. Curr Neurol Neurosci Rep 13(12):409, 2013 24190780

Marson AG, Al-Kharusi AM, Alwaidh M, et al; SANAD Study group: The SANAD study of effectiveness of carbamazepine, gabapentin, lamotrigine, oxcarbazepine, or topiramate for treatment of partial epilepsy: an unblinded randomised controlled trial. Lancet 369(9566):1000–1015, 2007 17382827

Martino D, Dale RC, Gilbert DL, et al: Immunopathogenic mechanisms in Tourette syndrome: a critical review. Mov Disord 24(9):1267–1279, 2009 19353683

Mayes AR, Meudell PR, Mann D, et al: Location of lesions in Korsakoff's syndrome: neuropsy-chological and neuropathological data on two patients. Cortex 24(3):367–388, 1988 3191722

McDonald WI, Compston A, Edan G, et al: Recommended diagnostic criteria for multiple scle-rosis: guidelines from the International Panel on the diagnosis of multiple sclerosis. Ann Neurol 50(1):121–127, 2001 11456302

McEwen B: Stressful experience, brain and emotions: developmental genetic and hormonal in-fluences, in The Cognitive Neurosciences. Edited by Gazzaniga MS. Cambridge, MA, MIT Press, 1996, pp 1117–1135

McGonigal A, Oto M, Russell AJ, et al: Outpatient video EEG recording in the diagnosis of non-epileptic seizures: a randomised controlled trial of simple suggestion techniques. J Neurol Neurosurg Psychiatry 72(4):549–551, 2002 11909925

McKeon GL, Robinson GA, Ryan AE, et al: Cognitive outcomes following anti-N-methyl-D-aspartate receptor encephalitis: a systematic review. J Clin Exp Neuropsychol 6:1–19, 2017 28585453

McManus J, Pathansali R, Hassan H, et al: The course of delirium in acute stroke. Age Ageing 38(4):385–389, 2009a 19383773

McManus J, Pathansali R, Hassan H, et al: The evaluation of delirium post-stroke. Int J Geriatr Psychiatry 24(11):1251–1256, 2009b 19388034

Mead GE, Hsieh CF, Lee R, et al: Selective serotonin reuptake inhibitors (SSRIs) for stroke re-covery. Cochrane Database Syst Rev (11):CD009286, 2012 23152272

Meijer KA, Eijlers AJC, Douw L, et al: Increased connectivity of hub networks and cognitive impairment in multiple sclerosis. Neurology 88(22):2107–2114, 2017 28468841

Mendez MF: Huntington's disease: update and review of neuropsychiatric aspects. Int J Psy-chiatry Med 24(3):189–208, 1994 7890478

Meudell P, Mayes AR: Normal and abnormal forgetting: some comments on the human amne-sic syndrome, in Normality and Pathology in Cognitive Functions. Edited by Willis AW. London, Academic Press, 1982, pp 203–238

Mijajlović DD, Pavlović A, Brainin M, et al: Post-stroke dementia—a comprehensive review. BMC Med 15(1):11, 2017 28095900

Mohr DC, Cox D, Epstein L, et al: Teaching patients to self-inject: pilot study of a treatment for injection anxiety and phobia in multiple sclerosis patients prescribed injectable medications. J Behav Ther Exp Psychiatry 33(1):39–47, 2002 12389798

Morgante L, Colosimo C, Antonini A, et al; PRIAMO Study Group: Psychosis associated to Parkinson's disease in the early stages: relevance of cognitive decline and depression. J Neurol Neurosurg Psychiatry 83(1):76–82, 2012 21836035

Mostert JP, Admiraal-Behloul F, Hoogduin JM, et al: Effects of fluoxetine on disease activity in relapsing multiple sclerosis: a double-blind, placebo-controlled, exploratory study. J Neurol Neurosurg Psychiatry 79(9):1027–1031, 2008 18450787

Mula M, Trimble MR, Yuen A, et al: Psychiatric adverse events during levetiracetam therapy. Neurology 61(5):704–706, 2003 12963770

Murphy R, O'Donoghue S, Counihan T, et al: Neuropsychiatric syndromes of multiple sclerosis. J Neurol Neurosurg Psychiatry 88(8):697–708, 2017 28285265

Nance MA: Genetic counseling and testing for Huntington's disease: a historical review. Am J Med Genet B Neuropsychiatr Genet 174(1):75–92, 2017 27174011

Neilley LK, Goodin DS, Goodkin DE, et al: Side effect profile of interferon beta-1b in MS: results of an open label trial. Neurology 46(2):552–554, 1996 8614531

Newman EJ, Grosset DG, Kennedy PG: The parkinsonism-hyperpyrexia syndrome. Neurocrit Care 10(1):136–140, 2009 18712508

Niccolai C, Goretti B, Amato MP: Disease modifying treatments and symptomatic drugs for cognitive impairment in multiple sclerosis: where do we stand? Multiple Sclerosis and Demyelinating Disorders 2(1):8, 2017

Nielsen G, Ricciardi L, Demartini B, et al: Outcomes of a 5-day physiotherapy programme for functional (psychogenic) motor disorders. J Neurol 262(3):674–681, 2015 25557282

Nielsen G, Buszewicz M, Stevenson F, et al: Randomised feasibility study of physiotherapy for patients with functional motor symptoms. J Neurol Neurosurg Psychiatry 88(6):484–490, 2016 27694498

Nighoghossian N, Zeng L, Derex L, et al: Warning compulsive behavior preceding acute ischemic stroke. Eur Neurol 56(1):39–40, 2006 16914930

Ó Donnchadha S, Burke T, Bramham J, et al: Symptom overlap in anxiety and multiple sclerosis. Mult Scler 19(10):1349–1354, 2013 23413298

Okun MS, Weintraub D: Should impulse control disorders and dopamine dysregulation syndrome be indications for deep brain stimulation and intestinal levodopa? Mov Disord 28(14):1915–1919, 2013 24243803

Olanow CW, Watts RL, Koller WC: An algorithm (decision tree) for the management of Parkinson's disease (2001): treatment guidelines. Neurology 56 (11, suppl 5):S1–S88, 2001 11402154

Oostrom KJ, Smeets-Schouten A, Kruitwagen CL, et al; Dutch Study Group of Epilepsy in Childhood: Not only a matter of epilepsy: early problems of cognition and behavior in children with "epilepsy only"—a prospective, longitudinal, controlled study starting at diagnosis. Pediatrics 112(6 Pt 1):1338–1344, 2003 14654607

Oribe E, Amini R, Nissenbaum E, et al: Serum prolactin concentrations are elevated after syncope. Neurology 47(1):60–62, 1996 8710125

Pact V, Giduz T: Mirtazapine treats resting tremor, essential tremor, and levodopa-induced dyskinesias. Neurology 53(5):1154, 1999 10496290

Palmieri A, Abrahams S, Sorarù G, et al: Emotional lability in MND: relationship to cognition and psychopathology and impact on caregivers. J Neurol Sci 278(1–2):16–20, 2009 19103449

Papapetropoulos S, Katzen H, Schrag A, et al: A questionnaire-based (UM-PDHQ) study of hallucinations in Parkinson's disease. BMC Neurol 20:8–21, 2008 18570642

Pareés I, Kojovic M, Pires C, et al: Physical precipitating factors in functional movement disorders. J Neurol Sci 338(1–2):174–177, 2014 24439198

Patten SB, Francis G, Metz LM, et al: The relationship between depression and interferon beta-1a therapy in patients with multiple sclerosis. Mult Scler 11(2):175–181, 2005a 15794391

Patten SB, Svenson LW, Metz LM: Psychotic disorders in MS: population-based evidence of an association. Neurology 65(7):1123–1125, 2005b 16217073

Paulsen JS, Nehl C, Hoth KF, et al: Depression and stages of Huntington's disease. J Neuropsychiatry Clin Neurosci 17(4):496–502, 2005 16387989

Paulsen JS, Long JD, Ross CA, et al; PREDICT-HD Investigators and Coordinators of the Huntington Study Group: Prediction of manifest Huntington's disease with clinical and imaging measures: a prospective observational study. Lancet Neurol 13(12):1193–1201, 2014 25453459

Pessiglione M, Seymour B, Flandin G, et al: Dopamine-dependent prediction errors underpin reward-seeking behaviour in humans. Nature 442(7106):1042–1045, 2006 16929307

Peterson KA, Savulich G, Jackson D, et al: The effect of shunt surgery on neuropsychological performance in normal pressure hydrocephalus: a systematic review and meta-analysis. J Neurol 263(8):1669–1677, 2016 27017344

Pfeil SA, Lynn DJ: Wilson's disease: copper unfettered. J Clin Gastroenterol 29(1):22–31, 1999 10405226

Pioro EP, Brooks BR, Cummings J, et al; Safety, Tolerability, and Efficacy Results Trial of AVP-923 in PBA Investigators: Dextromethorphan plus ultra low-dose quinidine reduces pseudobulbar affect. Ann Neurol 68(5):693–702, 2010 20839238

Planche V, Gibelin M, Cregut D, et al: Cognitive impairment in a population-based study of patients with multiple sclerosis: differences between late relapsing-remitting, secondary progressive and primary progressive multiple sclerosis. Eur J Neurol 23(2):282–289, 2016 25903918

Pohlmann-Eden B, Stefanou A, Wellhäusser H: Serum prolactate in syncope. Neurology 48(5):1477–1478, 1997 9153512

Pompili M, Di Cosimo D, Innamorati M, et al: Psychiatric comorbidity in patients with chronic daily headache and migraine: a selective overview including personality traits and suicide risk. J Headache Pain 10(4):283–290, 2009 19554418

Pondal M, Marras C, Miyasaki J, et al: Clinical features of dopamine agonist withdrawal syndrome in a movement disorders clinic. J Neurol Neurosurg Psychiatry 84(2):130–135, 2012 22933817

Popp RF, Fierlbeck AK, Knüttel H, et al: Daytime sleepiness versus fatigue in patients with multiple sclerosis: a systematic review on the Epworth sleepiness scale as an assessment tool. Sleep Med Rev 32:95–108, 2017 27107751

Postuma RB, Lang AE, Massicotte-Marquez J, et al: Potential early markers of Parkinson disease in idiopathic REM sleep behavior disorder. Neurology 66(6):845–851, 2006 16567700

Postuma RB, Gagnon JF, Bertrand JA, et al: Parkinson risk in idiopathic REM sleep behavior disorder: preparing for neuroprotective trials. Neurology 84(11):1104–1113, 2015 25681454

Price A, Rayner L, Okon-Rocha E, et al: Antidepressants for the treatment of depression in neurological disorders: a systematic review and meta-analysis of randomised controlled trials. J Neurol Neurosurg Psychiatry 82(8):914–923, 2011 21558287

Privitera MD, Welty TE, Ficker DM, Welge J: Vagus nerve stimulation for partial seizures. Cochrane Database Syst Rev (1):CD002896, 2002 11869641

Pujari S, Kharkar S, Metellus P, et al: Normal pressure hydrocephalus: long-term outcome after shunt surgery. J Neurol Neurosurg Psychiatry 79(11):1282–1286, 2008 18356257

Rabinstein AA, Shulman LM: Management of behavioral and psychiatric problems in Parkinson's disease. Parkinsonism Relat Disord 7(1):41–50, 2000 11008195

Rahkonen T, Mäkelä H, Paanila S, et al: Delirium in elderly people without severe predisposing disorders: etiology and 1-year prognosis after discharge. Int Psychogeriatr 12(4):473–481, 2000 11263714

Ramasubbu R: Denial of illness and depression in stroke (letter). Stroke 25(1):226–227, 1994 8266375

Rao SM: Neuropsychology of multiple sclerosis: a critical review. J Clin Exp Neuropsychol 8(5):503–542, 1986 3805250

Rao SM, Leo GJ, Bernardin L, et al: Cognitive dysfunction in multiple sclerosis, I: frequency, patterns, and prediction. Neurology 41(5):685–691, 1991 2027484

Reitz C, Bos MJ, Hofman A, et al: Prestroke cognitive performance, incident stroke, and risk of dementia: the Rotterdam Study. Stroke 39(1):36–41, 2008 18006863

Reuber M, Elger CE: Psychogenic nonepileptic seizures: review and update. Epilepsy Behav 4(3):205–216, 2003 12791321

Reuber M, Fernández G, Bauer J, et al: Diagnostic delay in psychogenic nonepileptic seizures. Neurology 58(3):493–495, 2002 11839862

Richard IH, McDermott MP, Kurlan R, et al; SAD-PD Study Group: A randomized, double-blind, placebo-controlled trial of antidepressants in Parkinson disease. Neurology 78(16):1229–1236, 2012 22496199

Rinne JO, Lee MS, Thompson PD, et al: Corticobasal degeneration. A clinical study of 36 cases. Brain 117(Pt 5):1183–1196, 1994 7953598

Robinson RG, Arndt S: Incomplete financial disclosure in a study of escitalopram and problem-solving therapy for prevention of poststroke depression. JAMA 301(10):1023–1024, 2009 19278945

Robinson RG, Penningworth PW: Clinical trials of medication versus therapy: even in a tie, medication wins. BMJ 338:b463, 2009. Available at: http://www.bmj.com/rapid-response/2011/11/02/clinical-trials-therapy-versus-medication-even-tie-medication-wins. Accessed November 8, 2017.

Robinson RG, Jorge RE, Moser DJ, et al: Escitalopram and problem-solving therapy for prevention of poststroke depression: a randomized controlled trial. JAMA 299(20):2391–2400, 2008 18505948

Rocha FL, Murad MG, Stumpf BP, et al: Antidepressants for depression in Parkinson's disease: systematic review and meta-analysis. J Psychopharmacol 27(5):417–423, 2013 23427193

Rodrigo Escalona P, Adair JC, Roberts BB, et al: Obsessive-compulsive disorder following bilateral globus pallidus infarction. Biol Psychiatry 42(5):410–412, 1997 9276081

Rog DJ, Nurmikko TJ, Friede T, et al: Randomized, controlled trial of cannabis-based medicine in central pain in multiple sclerosis. Neurology 65(6):812–819, 2005 16186518

Rohrer JD, Isaacs AM, Mizielinska S, et al: C9orf72 expansions in frontotemporal dementia and amyotrophic lateral sclerosis. Lancet Neurol 14(3):291–301, 2015 25638642

Rosenblatt A, Ranen NG, Nance MA, et al: A Physician's Guide to the Management of Huntington's Disease, 2nd Edition. New York, Huntington's Disease Society of America, 1999

Rossi S, Mataluni G, Codecà C, et al: Effects of levetiracetam on chronic pain in multiple sclerosis: results of a pilot, randomized, placebo-controlled study. Eur J Neurol 16(3):360–366, 2009 19364364

Rovaris M, Comi G, Filippi M: MRI markers of destructive pathology in multiple sclerosis-related cognitive dysfunction. J Neurol Sci 245(1–2):111–116, 2006 16626748

Ruffmann C, Bogliun G, Beghi E: Epileptogenic drugs: a systematic review. Expert Rev Neurother 6(4):575–589, 2006 16623656

Sadovnick AD, Remick RA, Allen J, et al: Depression and multiple sclerosis. Neurology 46(3):628–632, 1996 8618657

Samkoff LM, Daras M, Tuchman AJ, et al: Amelioration of refractory dysesthetic limb pain in multiple sclerosis by gabapentin. Neurology 49(1):304–305, 1997 9222213

Sbardella E, Petsas N, Tona F, et al: Assessing the correlation between grey and white matter damage with motor and cognitive impairment in multiple sclerosis patients. PLoS One 8(5):e63250, 2013 23696802

Schacter DL: Implicit memory: history and current status. Journal of Experimental Psychology: Learning, Memory, and Cognition 13(3):501–518, 1987

Schippling S, O'Connor P, Knappertz V, et al: Incidence and course of depression in multiple sclerosis in the multinational BEYOND trial. J Neurol 263(7):1418–1426, 2016 27177997

Schott JM: Limbic encephalitis: a clinician's guide. Practical Neurology 6(3):143–153, 2006

Schrag A, Trimble M, Quinn N, Bhatia K: The syndrome of fixed dystonia: an evaluation of 103 patients. Brain 127(Pt 10):2360–2372, 2004 15342362

Scott AJ, Sharpe L, Hunt C, et al: Anxiety and depressive disorders in people with epilepsy: a meta-analysis. Epilepsia 58(6):973–982, 2017 28470748

Servello D, Zekaj E, Saleh C, et al: Sixteen years of deep brain stimulation in Tourette's syndrome: a critical review. J Neurosurg Sci 60(2):218–229, 2016 26788742

Sethi KD: Clinical aspects of Parkinson disease. Curr Opin Neurol 15(4):457–460, 2002 12151843

Shanmugiah A, Sinha S, Taly AB, et al: Psychiatric manifestations in Wilson's disease: a cross-sectional analysis. J Neuropsychiatry Clin Neurosci 20(1):81–85, 2008 18305288

Sharpe M, Carson A: "Unexplained" somatic symptoms, functional syndromes, and somatization: do we need a paradigm shift? Ann Intern Med 134(9 Pt 2):926–930, 2001 11346330

Sharpe M, Stone J, Hibberd C, et al: Neurology out-patients with symptoms unexplained by disease: illness beliefs and financial benefits predict 1-year outcome. Psychol Med 40(4):689–698, 2010 19627646

Sharpe M, Walker J, Williams C, et al: Guided self-help for functional (psychogenic) symptoms: a randomized controlled efficacy trial. Neurology 77(6):564–572, 2011 21795652

Sheng AZ, Shen Q, Cordato D, et al: Delirium within three days of stroke in a cohort of elderly patients. J Am Geriatr Soc 54(8):1192–1198, 2006 16913984

Shi Q, Presutti R, Selchen D, et al: Delirium in acute stroke: a systematic review and meta-analysis. Stroke 43(3):645–649, 2012 22267831

Shin S, Lee JE, Hong JY, et al: Neuroanatomical substrates of visual hallucinations in patients with non-demented Parkinson's disease. J Neurol Neurosurg Psychiatry 83(12):1155–1161, 2012 22933812

Shotbolt P, Samuel M, David A: Quetiapine in the treatment of psychosis in Parkinson's disease. Ther Adv Neurol Disorder 3(6):339–350, 2010 21179595

Shprecher D, Schwalb J, Kurlan R: Normal pressure hydrocephalus: diagnosis and treatment. Curr Neurol Neurosci Rep 8(5):371–376, 2008 18713572

Sijens PE, Mostert JP, Irwan R, et al: Impact of fluoxetine on the human brain in multiple sclerosis as quantified by proton magnetic resonance spectroscopy and diffusion tensor imaging. Psychiatry Res 164(3):274–282, 2008 19017554

Spencer SS: The relative contributions of MRI, SPECT, and PET imaging in epilepsy (Original Text). Epilepsia 35 (suppl 6):S72–S89, 1994 8206016

Spencer S, Huh L: Outcomes of epilepsy surgery in adults and children. Lancet Neurol 7(6):525–537, 2008 18485316

Stadelmann C, Albert M, Wegner C, et al: Cortical pathology in multiple sclerosis. Curr Opin Neurol 21(3):229–234, 2008 18451703

Starkstein SE: Mood disorders after stroke, in Cerebrovascular Disease. Edited by Grinsberg M, Bogousslavsky J. Oxford, UK, Blackwell Science, 1998, pp 131–138

Starkstein SE, Robinson RG: Affective disorders and cerebral vascular disease. Br J Psychiatry 154:170–182, 1989 2673474

Starkstein SE, Pearlson GD, Boston J, et al: Mania after brain injury. A controlled study of causative factors. Arch Neurol 44(10):1069–1073, 1987 3632381

Starkstein SE, Berthier ML, Fedoroff P, et al: Anosognosia and major depression in 2 patients with cerebrovascular lesions. Neurology 40(9):1380–1382, 1990 2392222

Starkstein SE, Fedoroff JP, Price TR, et al: Catastrophic reaction after cerebrovascular lesions: frequency, correlates, and validation of a scale. J Neuropsychiatry Clin Neurosci 5(2):189–194, 1993 8508037

Steur EN: Increase of Parkinson disability after fluoxetine medication. Neurology 43(1):211–213, 1993 8423889

Stillhard G, Landis T, Schiess R, et al: Bitemporal hypoperfusion in transient global amnesia: 99m-Tc-HM-PAO SPECT and neuropsychological findings during and after an attack. J Neurol Neurosurg Psychiatry 53(4):339–342, 1990 2341849

Stone VE, Baron-Cohen S, Knight RT: Frontal lobe contributions to theory of mind. J Cogn Neurosci 10(5):640–656, 1998 9802997

Stone J, Zeman A, Sharpe M: Functional weakness and sensory disturbance. J Neurol Neurosurg Psychiatry 73(3):241–245, 2002 12185152

Stone J, Binzer M, Sharpe M: Illness beliefs and locus of control: a comparison of patients with pseudoseizures and epilepsy. J Psychosom Res 57(6):541–547, 2004 15596160

Stone J, Carson A, Sharpe M: Functional symptoms and signs in neurology: assessment and diagnosis. J Neurol Neurosurg Psychiatry 76 (suppl 1):i2–i12, 2005a 15718217

Stone J, Smyth R, Carson A, et al: Systematic review of misdiagnosis of conversion symptoms and "hysteria." BMJ 331(7523):989, 2005b 16223792

Stone J, Smyth R, Carson A, et al: La belle indifférence in conversion symptoms and hysteria: systematic review. Br J Psychiatry 188:204–209, 2006 16507959

Stone J, Carson A, Aditya H, et al: The role of physical injury in motor and sensory conversion symptoms: a systematic and narrative review. J Psychosom Res 66(5):383–390, 2009 19379954

Stone J, Reuber M, Carson A: Functional symptoms in neurology: mimics and chameleons. Pract Neurol 13(2):104–113, 2013 23468561

Stone J, Hoeritzauer I, Brown K, et al: Therapeutic sedation for functional (psychogenic) neurological symptoms. J Psychosom Res 76(2):165–168, 2014 24439694

Stone J, Carson A, Hallett M: Explanation as treatment for functional neurologic disorders. Handb Clin Neurol 139:543–553, 2016 27719870

Sullivan EV, Pfefferbaum A: Neuroimaging of the Wernicke-Korsakoff syndrome. Alcohol Alcohol 44(2):155–165, 2009 19066199

Sweet RA, Mulsant BH, Gupta B, et al: Duration of neuroleptic treatment and prevalence of tardive dyskinesia in late life. Arch Gen Psychiatry 52(6):478–486, 1995 7771918

Syed TU, Arozullah AM, Suciu GP, et al: Do observer and self-reports of ictal eye closure predict psychogenic nonepileptic seizures? Epilepsia 49(5):898–904, 2008 18070093

Tabrizi SJ, Scahill RI, Durr A, et al; TRACK-HD Investigators: Biological and clinical changes in premanifest and early stage Huntington's disease in the TRACK-HD study: the 12-month longitudinal analysis. Lancet Neurol 10(1):31–42, 2011 21130037

Tabrizi SJ, Scahill RI, Owen G, et al; TRACK-HD Investigators: Predictors of phenotypic progression and disease onset in premanifest and early stage Huntington's disease in the TRACK-HD study: analysis of 36-month observational data. Lancet Neurol 12(7):637–649, 2013 23664844

Tanner CM, Aston DA: Epidemiology of Parkinson's disease and akinetic syndromes. Curr Opin Neurol 13(4):427–430, 2000 10970060

Termsarasab P, Thammongkolchai T, Frucht SJ: Medical treatment of dystonia. J Clin Mov Disord 3:19, 2016 28031858

Tesei S, Antonini A, Canesi M, et al: Tolerability of paroxetine in Parkinson's disease: a prospective study. Mov Disord 15(5):986–989, 2000 11009210

Thompson AJ: Symptomatic treatment in multiple sclerosis. Curr Opin Neurol 11(4):305–309, 1998 9725075

Titulaer MJ, McCracken L, Gabilondo I, et al: Treatment and prognostic factors for long-term outcome in patients with anti-NMDA receptor encephalitis: an observational cohort study. Lancet Neurol 12(2):157–165, 2013 23290630

Trapp BD, Peterson J, Ransohoff RM, et al: Axonal transection in the lesions of multiple sclerosis. N Engl J Med 338(5):278–285, 1998 9445407

Uher T, Vaneckova M, Sormani MP, et al: Identification of multiple sclerosis patients at highest risk of cognitive impairment using an integrated brain magnetic resonance imaging assessment approach. Eur J Neurol 24(2):292–301, 2017 27873386

U.S. Department of Health and Human Services, Food and Drug Administration, Center for Evaluation and Research, et al: Statistical review and evaluation: antiepileptic drugs and suicidality. May 23, 2008. Available at: https://www.fda.gov/ohrms/dockets/ac/08/briefing/2008-4372b1-01-FDA.pdf. Accessed October 9, 2017.

van Dalen JW, Moll van Charante EP, Nederkoorn PJ, et al: Poststroke apathy. Stroke 44(3):851–860, 2013 23362076

van den Akker LE, Beckerman H, Collette EH, et al: Effectiveness of cognitive behavioral therapy for the treatment of fatigue in patients with multiple sclerosis: a systematic review and meta-analysis. J Psychosom Res 90:33–42, 2016 27772557

van Duijn E, Kingma EM, van der Mast RC: Psychopathology in verified Huntington's disease gene carriers. J Neuropsychiatry Clin Neurosci 19(4):441–448, 2007 18070848

Veazey C, Cook KF, Stanley M, et al: Telephone-administered cognitive behavioral therapy: a case study of anxiety and depression in Parkinson's disease. J Clin Psychol Med Settings 16(3):243–253, 2009 19404724

Victor M, Adams RD, Collins GH: The Wernicke-Korsakoff syndrome. Philadelphia, PA, FA Davis, 1971

Vighetto A, Aimard G, Confavreux C, et al: [Anatomo-clinical study of a case of topographic confabulation (or delusion)] (in French). Cortex 16(3):501–507, 1980 7214934

Vonsattel JPG, DiFiglia M: Huntington disease. J Neuropathol Exp Neurol 57(5):369–384, 1998 9596408

Voon V, Potenza MN, Thomsen T: Medication-related impulse control and repetitive behaviors in Parkinson's disease. Curr Opin Neurol 20(4):484–492, 2007 17620886

Warlow C, van Gijn J, Dennis M, et al: Stroke: Practical Management, 3rd Edition. Oxford, UK, Blackwell Publishing, 2008

Weatherall MW: Chronic daily headache. Pract Neurol 7(4):212–221, 2007 17636136

Weier K, Penner IK, Magon S, et al: Cerebellar abnormalities contribute to disability including cognitive impairment in multiple sclerosis. PLoS One 9(1):e86916, 2014 24466290

Weigartz P, Seidenberg M, Woodard A, et al: Co-morbid psychiatric disorder in chronic epilepsy: recognition and etiology of depression. Neurology 53 (5 suppl 2):S3–S8, 1999 10496228

Weintraub D, Siderowf AD, Potenza MN, et al: Association of dopamine agonist use with impulse control disorders in Parkinson disease. Arch Neurol 63(7):969–973, 2006 16831966

Wilhelm S, Deckersbach T, Coffey BJ, et al: Habit reversal versus supportive psychotherapy for Tourette's disorder: a randomized controlled trial. Am J Psychiatry 160(6):1175–1177, 2003 12777279

Williams DT, Lafaver K, Carson A, et al: Inpatient treatment for functional neurologic disorders. Handb Clin Neurol 139:631–641, 2016 27719878

Williams LS, Kroenke K, Bakas T, et al: Care management of poststroke depression: a randomized, controlled trial. Stroke 38(3):998–1003, 2007 17303771

Wintermark M, Ko NU, Smith WS, et al: Vasospasm after subarachnoid hemorrhage: utility of perfusion CT and CT angiography on diagnosis and management. AJNR Am J Neuroradiol 27(1):26–34, 2006 16418351

Witjas T, Kaphan E, Azulay JP, et al: Nonmotor fluctuations in Parkinson's disease: frequent and disabling. Neurology 59(3):408–413, 2002 12177375

Wolters ECH, Berendse HW: Management of psychosis in Parkinson's disease. Curr Opin Neurol 14(4):499–504, 2001 11470967

Yang TT, Wang L, Deng XY, Yu G: Pharmacological treatments for fatigue in patients with multiple sclerosis: a systematic review and meta-analysis. J Neurol Sci 380:256–261, 2017 28870581

Zakzanis KK: The subcortical dementia of Huntington's disease. J Clin Exp Neuropsychol 20(4):565–578, 1998 9892059

Zandi MS, Irani SR, Lang B, et al: Disease-relevant autoantibodies in first episode schizophrenia. J Neurol 258(4):686–688, 2011 20972895

Zappacosta B, Monza D, Meoni C, et al: Psychiatric symptoms do not correlate with cognitive decline, motor symptoms, or CAG repeat length in Huntington's disease. Arch Neurol 53(6):493–497, 1996 8660149

Zeman A, Butler C: Transient epileptic amnesia. Curr Opin Neurol 23(6):610–616, 2010 20885322

Zeman AZ, Boniface SJ, Hodges JR: Transient epileptic amnesia: a description of the clinical and neuropsychological features in 10 cases and a review of the literature. J Neurol Neurosurg Psychiatry 64(4):435–443, 1998 9576532

Zhang J, Xu CY, Liu J: Meta-analysis on the prevalence of REM sleep behavior disorder symptoms in Parkinson's disease. BMC Neurol 17(1):23, 2017 28160778

Zinn S, Bosworth HB, Hoenig HM, et al: Executive function deficits in acute stroke. Arch Phys Med Rehabil 88(2):173–180, 2007 17270514

Ziv I, Djaldetti R, Zoldan Y, et al: Diagnosis of "non-organic" limb paresis by a novel objective motor assessment: the quantitative Hoover's test. J Neurol 245(12):797–802, 1998 9840352

CHAPTER 31

Obstetrics and Gynecology

Donna E. Stewart, C.M., M.D., FRCPC

Simone N. Vigod, M.D., M.Sc., FRCPC

The specialty of obstetrics and gynecology deals with intensely emotional issues, including sexuality, menstruation, fertility, abortion, pregnancy, menopause, and other related topics. Psychiatrists can play a unique role in enhancing care provided by obstetricians and gynecologists, who usually receive little training in mental health care.

A complete understanding of women's mental health must consider the psychosocial context of their lives and reproductive factors across their life span, including social determinants of health such as gender, culture, environment, education, social support networks, employment, economic stability, and exposure to violence.

This chapter reviews a variety of topics related to both obstetrics and gynecology and psychiatry from biological, psychological, and social perspectives, including gender identity, fertility, contraception, sterilization, hysterectomy, abortion (both spontaneous and induced), chronic pelvic pain, premenstrual mood disturbance, pregnancy and the postpartum period, menopause, and urinary incontinence. Eating disorders are covered in Chapter 13, "Eating Disorders," and gynecological cancers are discussed in Chapter 22, "Oncology." It is beyond the scope of this chapter to address global variations in social context, presentations, and medical care.

Gender Identity

The first question about a fetus or newborn is whether it is a boy or girl, a determination made on the basis of the external genitalia as seen via ultrasound or direct visualization at birth. Ambiguous genitalia cause consternation; physicians and parents must decide whether to live with the ambiguity or assign the child to one gender or the other. Some believe that gender assignment should be made and carried out as early as possible so that the child can grow up with a clear gender, and others think that the child should be left as born and allowed to make a personal gender assignment when of age (Reiner 2002). Reproductive organs are the first defining feature of each human being, and gender remains a core aspect of identity throughout life. Sex hormones influence not only physical development and a host of physiological functions but also brain structure and activity. Environmental factors influence developing anatomy and ongoing physiology. A lifelong active interplay occurs among genetics, anatomy, physiology, environmental and social influences, and individual psychology.

The term *sex* refers to narrowly defined biological characteristics. The term *gender* includes social roles and an individual's sense of femininity or masculinity. Some evidence indicates that children are aware of their sexual organs and identity as early as toddlerhood. As puberty approaches in females, the sense of gender identity is powerfully reinforced and reshaped by society and by physical changes: the development of breasts and pubic hair and the onset of menstruation. In some cultures, girls are told at menarche that they are now women. With menarche comes fertility and the possibility that sexual activity will lead to pregnancy. Although girls can be sexually abused at any age, the possibility of rape is more overt after puberty, and vulnerability to attack becomes part of gender identity. The possibility of pregnancy can be at once a worry and a wish. Some young women may feel that they are not truly women until they have experienced heterosexual intercourse or until they have borne a child.

Girls who are sexually attracted to other girls face a crisis in gender identity because society expects them to date, form relationships, and engage in sexual activity with males. Sexual minorities such as lesbian, gay, bisexual, transsexual, queer, and questioning individuals may face special challenges (Subhrajit 2014). These individuals may be reluctant to seek health care because they fear or have experienced disapproval and misunderstanding, and as a result they may suffer adverse health outcomes. Psychiatrists can help gynecologists and primary care physicians to phrase questions about sexual orientation and activity in nonjudgmental terms.

Infertility

A common definition of infertility is 12 months of appropriately timed unprotected intercourse that does not result in conception (World Health Organization 2017b). However, a shorter time (6 months) is often used in women older than 35 years because the nature of fertility at this age makes it desirable to initiate diagnosis and treatment as soon as possible. The World Health Organization (2017b) has estimated that 1 in 4 couples experiences some type of fertility problem over the course of their reproductive lives. A study of 190 countries and territories (Mascarenhas et al. 2012) found differing rates of primary and secondary infertility, with 48.5 million couples affected by infertility worldwide. Although infertility rates did not increase between 1990 and 2010, more couples were seeking treatment for infertility at the later date (Mascarenhas et al. 2012). Estimates from the Centers for Disease Control and Prevention (2016) indicate that 12.5% of women ages 15–44 years have impaired fertility and that 11.3% have ever used infertility services. Social stigma, cost, availability, and emotional factors may reduce access to fertility treatments (Rich and Domar 2016).

Although women are often "blamed" for infertility, as much as 40% of infertility may be attributable to multiple causes (i.e., a combination of multiple male and female factors), and up to 10% of the time, the etiology remains completely unexplained. Historically, infertility that could not be explained on an organic basis was thought to be "psychogenic," related to ambivalence about becoming a parent, unconscious repudiation of femininity and motherhood, unconscious fears and conflict about sex, and wishes to remain dependent. However, these themes were based on psychoanalytic case reports and have been shown to be present in women with no trouble conceiving. Thus, the focus of research on the relationship between mental health and fertility has shifted toward exploration of the biological, psychological, and social factors that mediate psychiatric illness or psychological distress in couples with infertility. This research suggests that the relationship between fertility and mental health is complex. Practitioners must take into account the stresses of infertility itself, with the associated investigations and treatment, as well as how psychiatric morbidity may influence fertility and the outcomes of fertility treatments (Rooney and Domar 2016).

Scope of Psychiatric Illness Affecting Couples With Infertility

Infertility is experienced as stressful, with 50% of women and 15% of men undergoing infertility diagnosis or treatment ranking it the most stressful event of their lives (Freeman et al. 1985). Although some studies show that women with infertility are distressed but do not meet criteria for a major psychiatric disorder, others reveal rates of major depressive disorder (MDD) in infertile women that reach 40%, with anxiety disorders reaching 20% (Chen et al. 2004). Also, there are sex differences in the scope of psychiatric illness, with men reporting more symptoms of anxiety and depression than men in the general population, but far less than their female counterparts (Volgsten et al. 2008).

Factors Mediating Psychiatric Illness in Couples With Infertility

Biological factors related to infertility that may affect mental health include the cause and duration of infertility, as well as the effects of fertility treatment. There is evidence that the difference in psychological profile between fertile and infertile couples increases with infertility duration (Baldur-Felskov et al. 2013). Interestingly, men show greater distress and guilt when the infertility is attributable to male-factor etiology, but women are equally distressed regardless of the cause (Volgsten et al. 2010). Although the reasons for this difference have not been investigated, this may be a reflection of the association of fertility with virility, the social expectation on women for conception and delivery of a baby, and the pervasive shame associated with infertility.

Assisted reproductive technologies include in vitro fertilization (IVF), zygote intrafallopian tube transfer (ZIFT), gamete intrafallopian tube transfer (GIFT), intracytoplasmic sperm injection (ICST), donor eggs or sperm, and previously frozen embryos. Surrogate pregnancies or gestational carriers may also be used. A recent study showed that many claims made by fertility clinics about the benefits of treatments beyond standard in vitro fertilization procedures are costly and not backed up by evidence, often raising false hopes (Spencer et al. 2016). Each technology has its own success rate and psychological issues associated with it.

Becoming a parent is experienced as a developmental need for many women. Some women experience anger, a sense of loss of control, and reduced self-esteem when they are unable to conceive. Guilt may manifest with respect to being the cause of the infertility (e.g., older age because of choice to establish a career, prior sexually transmitted infection) or from upsetting spouses and disappointing families. Important social factors include gender roles, marital expectations, and familial and societal attitudes. When fertility treatments are unsuccessful, many couples (especially women) have trouble stopping treatment, and some may resort to unproven methods in desperation. Both infertility and perinatal loss are associated with lower quality of life, marital discord, MDD, anxiety disorders, and posttraumatic stress disorder (PTSD) (Bhat and Byatt 2016).

Fertility treatments themselves may have adverse effects on mental health. Interventions can be time-consuming, expensive, embarrassing, and invasive. The psychological effects, particularly mood alterations, of fertility-enhancing drugs are underappreciated. Careful attention should be paid to the potential contribution of recent changes in drug regimens to recent-onset psychiatric symptoms such as depression, anxiety, mania, and psychosis. Progesterone is often used for luteal phase abnormalities of the endometrium and can cause depression, insomnia, and somnolence. Clomiphene induces follicle-stimulating hormone (FSH) and has been associated with anxiety, insomnia, and psychosis (related to ongoing treatment or upon discontinuation of treatment) (Burns 2007; Seeman 2015).

Both hormone-stimulated intrauterine insemination (IUI) and IVF are associated with multiple gestations, which often cause maternal and fetal problems. Maternal complications include significant increases in cardiac morbidity, hematological morbidity, amniotic fluid embolus, pre-eclampsia, obstetric intervention, hysterectomy, and hemorrhage. Preterm birth is very common in multiple gestations and may be associated with cerebral palsy and other long-term infant sequelae that may cause psychological stress to the whole family (Walker et al. 2004). Limiting in vitro fertilization to only one or two embryos reduces the risk of multiple gestations and their associated maternal and infant health risks (Centers for Disease Control and Prevention 2017; Monteleone et al. 2016; National Institute for Health and Care Excellence 2014).

Effect of Psychiatric Illness on Fertility

Psychiatric illness and lifestyle may impact fertility directly through mechanisms related to chronic stress, altered immune responses, and hormonal changes, as well as indirectly through changes in behaviors such as smoking, alcohol use, poor nutrition, and lack of exercise (Rooney and Domar 2014). Eating disorders (anorexia nervosa, bulimia nervosa, obesity) are all associated with infertility. Restrictive or purging eating behaviors are often undisclosed and result in subfecundity and poor pregnancy outcomes (Assens et al. 2015).

It is also important to consider the impact of psychotropic medications on fertility. For example, selective serotonin reuptake inhibitors (SSRIs) have been shown to be associated with a small but increased risk of early miscarriage and postpartum hemorrhage (Hanley et al. 2016), valproic acid is associated with polycystic ovarian syndrome (see Chapter 21, "Endocrine and Metabolic Disorders"), and many antipsychotic medications are associated with anovulation due to hyperprolactinemia (Joffe 2007).

Psychosocial Assessment in Infertility Patients

Although it is not common practice to refer all couples with infertility for a mental health assessment, the stressful nature of infertility diagnosis and treatment is becoming more widely appreciated. Normally intimate and private behaviors are asked about, subjected to strict timing, and brought into the clinical arena. Careful inquiry should be made regarding any psychiatric side effects of fertility-enhancing drugs, particularly alterations in mood (Seeman 2015).

Some have suggested that current levels of distress and coping strategies should be assessed in couples before initiating infertility treatment to enhance their ability to cope with infertility and the associated medical investigations and procedures. Counseling is sometimes recommended in couples considering donor eggs or sperm or surrogacy. The goal of mental health evaluation is to identify and treat any comorbid psychiatric disorders, to prepare the couple for infertility treatments, to raise emotional and ethical issues that the couple may not have considered, and to offer support and coping strategies. Individual and group interventions are often helpful in providing mutual support, information, and coping techniques (Domar et al. 2015).

Contraception

Despite contraceptive information and care being widely available in the Western world, half of the pregnancies in North America each year are unintended, and one-third of births in the United States are classified as unwanted or mistimed. Contraceptive choices and use are affected by knowledge and misinformation, by women's comfort with their own sexuality and genitalia, by the preferences of sexual partners, by social custom, and by access to medical care. Many women are ill-informed about contraception (Picardo et al. 2003).

Psychodynamics and psychiatric conditions can interfere with a woman's use of a contraceptive technique. Pregnancy may be sought, consciously or unconsciously, as a proof of fertility and womanhood. Contraception, because it requires planning, requires acknowledgment of future sexual activity. For example, because of views about sex outside of marriage or cultural sanctions, some unmarried women may only engage in sexual intercourse when "swept away" by a romantic situation (and are thus unprepared to prevent pregnancy). Some women may feel uncomfortable about touching their own genitalia, as some contraceptive methods require. Many women have limited knowledge about their own anatomy, are too anxious to absorb the information in a hurried office or clinic visit, and are too embarrassed to ask for information to be repeated (Sanders et al. 2003). In a review of 16 studies that examined reasons for unprotected intercourse in adult women, Ayoola et al. (2007) found that reasons for unprotected intercourse included perceived inconvenience; unexpected/unplanned sex; ambivalence about pregnancy; problems using, acquiring, or storing the contraceptive method; lack of knowledge or misinformation (e.g., low perceived risk of getting pregnant, belief that contraception reduces pleasure or makes sex unnatural); and unwanted side effects from oral contraception. Other problems included access to contraception (e.g., problems getting appointments, cost, preferred method not being available), lack of continuity in care providers, and lack of privacy at contraceptive clinics. Alcohol use disorder, particularly binge drinking (the rates of which are rising in young women), may also be a contributing factor. Mental illness, particularly comorbid substance use disorders, was found to be associated with reduced contraceptive adherence and continuation in American women veterans (Callegari et al. 2015). Negative mood has also been found to be a risk factor for potentially health-threatening decisions about sexuality (e.g., not using contraceptives) (Velten et al. 2016).

Unplanned pregnancy is by no means always the result of the factors described above. Contraceptive methods do fail. Forced or unwanted sex is also a reason for unprotected intercourse, and gender and relationship power differentials play a major role in the use of contraception. Some women are sexually assaulted, bullied, or cajoled into unprotected sexual intercourse (Rickert et al. 2002). Ayoola et al. (2007) found that interpersonal reasons for unprotected sex were often partner-related (partner did not want to use contraception, fear of negative reaction from partner) or attributable to the influence of social custom. In a U.S. study of women at risk for sexually transmitted infections, a male partner's unwillingness to use condoms increased the odds of intercourse without barrier contraception by 4.1 (95% confidence interval [CI]=2.3–6.9) (Peipert et al. 2007). In a large sample of New Zealand women, those who experienced intimate partner violence were more likely to have a partner who had either refused to use condoms or tried to prevent the woman from using contraception (Fanslow et al. 2008). Despite these facts, it is women who are often blamed, both in societal and in medical contexts, for becoming pregnant at the wrong time or with the wrong partner. The resultant sense of shame and powerlessness can contribute to psychiatric symptoms and, paradoxically, can leave them more vulnerable to future unplanned pregnancies.

New Developments in Contraception

Newer developments in contraception have important psychosocial implications. For example, some forms of emergency contraception consist of higher doses of oral contraceptives taken after unprotected intercourse. Although more effective the earlier they are taken, they can be effective in preventing pregnancy up to 5 days after unprotected intercourse. Emergency contraception can be obtained at family planning clinics, some physicians' offices, hospital emergency departments, or pharmacies. A recent study of women's preferences about obtaining emergency contraception found that women were more likely to use services perceived as sympathetic, nonjudgmental, and protective of privacy (Seston et al. 2007). Women who are young, especially those who are poor or from certain cultural groups, may be uninformed, embarrassed, unaware of their level of risk for pregnancy, worried about side effects of emergency contraception, and concerned about negative responses from others (Shoveller et al. 2007). In the United States, England, Australia, Canada, and some other countries, emergency contraception is available without a prescription (U.S. Food and Drug Administration 2016b). Levonorgestrel (Plan B) has subsequently been found to be more effective than the older Yuzpe regimen (Leung et al. 2016). More recently, ulipristal acetate, a selective progesterone receptor modulator, was found to have reasonable tolerability and effectiveness in preventing pregnancy in women who presented for emergency contraceptives up to 120 hours (5 days) after unprotected intercourse. Ulipristal was at least as effective as levonorgestrel within the first 72 hours after unprotected intercourse, and it may be more effective than levonorgestrel when used between 72 hours and 120 hours after unprotected intercourse (Richardson and Maltz 2012). A copper-bearing intrauterine device inserted within 5 days of unprotected intercourse is at least as effective as forms of emergency contraception (World Health Organization 2017a). A Cochrane review of advance provision of emergency contraception found that this practice did not lead to increased rates of sexually transmitted infections (odds ratio [OR]=0.99; 95% CI=0.73–1.34), increased frequency of unprotected intercourse, or changes in contraceptive methods (Polis et al. 2007).

Hormonal implants and transdermal contraceptive patches have been developed to reduce the likelihood of contraceptive failure due to inconsistent use of the oral contraceptive pill or barrier contraceptive methods. They can also be used to treat dysmenorrhea and menorrhagia. However, continuous hormonal contraception does cause amenorrhea, an effect that may have psychosocial implications for women who hold beliefs about menstruation being necessary for cleansing and confirmation of femininity (Glasier et al. 2003). Hormonal implants may also cause a decrease in bone density that is reversible when the implant is removed. A Danish national prospective cohort study in more than 1 million women found that use of hormonal contraceptives (including combined oral contraceptives, progesterone-only pill, norelgestromin patch, vaginal ring, and levonorgestrel intrauterine system) was associated with a subsequent diagnosis of depression. Depression was most common within the first 6 months after starting a hormonal contraceptive, and in adolescent girls (Skovlund et al. 2016).

Management

Inquiries about sexual behavior and protection from unwanted consequences should be part of every medical and psychiatric history. Patients may be so accustomed to their birth control pills or injections that they fail to report them when asked what medications they are taking. Clinicians must ask about these contraceptives specifically in order to assess not only their adequacy but also the potential for drug–drug interactions. The major pathway of metabolism for both the estrogen and progesterone components of hormonal contraception is through cytochrome P450 (CYP) 3A4 (Oesterheld et al. 2008). Psychotropic medications that induce CYP3A4, thus reducing the efficacy of hormonal contraception, include phenobarbital, oxcarbazepine, carbamazepine, topiramate (at dosages >200 mg/day), modafinil, and St. John's wort. Oral contraceptives can also inhibit the oxidation of various psychiatric medications via CYP1A2, 2B6, 2C19, and 3A4. This can result in increased levels of benzodiazepines and tricyclic antidepressants (TCAs). Levels of valproate and lamotrigine can also be increased by oral contraceptives.

In summary, access to care and adequate information about contraception is essential. Certain groups, such as women with severe and persistent psychiatric illness, adolescents, and recent immigrants, may have increased vulnerability to some of the factors cited above and have been shown to use contraceptive methods suboptimally (Gelberg et al. 2002; Vieira da Silva Magalhães et al. 2009; Whitaker and Gilliam 2008). Atypical antipsychotics, other than risperidone, do not impair fertility as much as older antipsychotics and may result in unwanted pregnancies in women being treated for psychotic illnesses. Therefore, attention to contraceptive knowledge and use in these groups is of vital importance.

Sterilization

Sterilization is the most commonly used method of contraception in the world for women ages 15–49 years who are married or in ongoing heterosexual relationships, with the highest rates in less developed countries (United Nations 2007). It is intended to be a permanent solution to unwanted fertility, although some tubal ligations are reversible. A psychiatrist may be asked to consult when a young nulliparous woman, or a patient with low intelligence or a mental illness, desires to be sterilized. Assessment of capacity to provide informed consent to treatment is essential, highlighted by state laws enacted in the wake of past involuntary sterilization of individuals with low intelligence or mental illness. It may be appropriate for guardians to consent to sterilization procedures for severely cognitively impaired or developmentally delayed adult women who are unable to cope with the hygienic aspects of menstruation, are victimized by male predators, become pregnant, and are entirely unable to cope with the stresses of birth and parenting. However, mental illnesses cannot be equated with incapacity to make treatment decisions. Women may have psychotic symptoms, or a history of them, that interfere with capacity, but they also may make well-informed decisions not to have children, or more children, precisely because they recognize that their illness would interfere with their parenting. When there is uncertainty, a longitudinal assessment is appropriate. For example, the psychiatrist may ask the patient to return in a few months. If she is mature, not acutely psychotic, and persistent in her desire for sterilization, she may be as appropriate a candidate for the procedure as a woman without diagnosed psychiatric illness.

Poststerilization regret is usually reported as affecting fewer than 5% of those who undergo the procedure. Risk factors include age younger than 30 years (Curtis et al. 2006), depression (Becner et al. 2015), marital conflict over sterilization or changes in marital partnerships (Jamieson et al. 2002), death of a child (Machado et al. 2005), and no male child in some cultures (Malhotra et al. 2007). Sexual satisfaction does not appear to be affected (Peterson 2008). The provision of clear information about the nature, effectiveness, risks, and benefits of the procedure is a crucial factor in patient satisfaction. In general, most women experience sterilization as empowering and feel they can effectively exercise control over their sexuality and fertility (Brault et al. 2016).

Hysterectomy

Hysterectomy, the surgical removal of the uterus, is one of the most common surgical procedures performed on North American women. Rates have fallen over the past decade (Wright et al. 2013). Hysterectomy rates in the United States are between two and five times higher than those in European countries, although significant rate variations occur over small areas in most countries. These variations appear to depend on women's socioeconomic class, race/ethnicity, education level, and religion, as well as on physician practices, reimbursement schedules, and availability of newer technologies (Stewart et al. 2002).

Hysterectomy may be total or subtotal (i.e., the cervix is left intact) and also may be combined with removal of the fallopian tubes and ovaries (bilateral salpingo-oophorectomy [BSO]). Although vaginal hysterectomy is associated with lower mortality and shorter lengths of hospital stay, abdominal hysterectomy still remains a common hysterectomy procedure. Laparoscopic hysterectomy and robotic and mini-laparotomy surgeries are increasingly being used for benign conditions (Smorgick et al. 2014). A small proportion of hysterectomies are performed to treat malignancies or catastrophic hemorrhage, but the vast majority are elective procedures performed primarily to improve quality of life in women with abnormal uterine bleeding, fibroids, uterine prolapse, chronic pelvic pain, or endometriosis. The mean age of women undergoing hysterectomy is the mid-40s, or an average of 6–7 years before the mean age of natural menopause, when some of these problems (abnormal uterine bleeding, fibroids) spontaneously resolve. However, hysterectomy is the treatment of choice for certain gynecological conditions. The predicted advantage must be carefully weighed against the risks of surgery and other treatment alternatives, such as watchful waiting, hormonal therapy, myomectomy and endometrial ablation (Wright et al. 2013).

Information Needs and Decision-Making Preferences

Well-informed women who have been involved in decision making about the need for and type of hysterectomy have the best outcomes (Stewart et al. 2002). Women's decision making regarding discretionary hysterectomy (i.e., not for treatment of malignancy) is influenced by their age, socioeconomic status, education, desire for fertility, sexual orientation, ethnicity, and symptom severity. The influence of family, friends, and partners as well as health care professionals also plays a major role (Graham et al. 2008). Women who require hysterectomy for the treatment of malignancies are understandably focused more on the cancer, its overall treatment, and its prognosis.

Psychological and Sexual Outcomes

A 2005 review of the literature on psychological and sexual outcomes after hysterectomy located more than 100 studies (Flory et al. 2005). Although the methodological quality of many of the studies was poor, the authors concluded that whereas psychosexual and psychosocial effects were minimal overall, a subgroup of women (10%–20%) reported sexual dysfunction, depressive symptoms, and/or impaired body image. However, a more recent narrative review found that most sexual disorders improved after hysterectomy for benign uterine disease, and most patients who were sexually active before surgery had the same or better sexual functioning after surgery (Danesh et al. 2015).

Risk factors for poor outcome appear to be related to preoperative pain, sexual dysfunction, and psychiatric morbidity. A study of 228 hysterectomy patients who underwent elective abdominal, laparoscopic, or robotic surgery found no difference in satisfaction, well-being, or dyspareunia scores among the three groups (Schiff et al. 2015). Hartmann et al. (2004) reported that women with preoperative pain and depression had less improvement after hysterectomy than women without pain and depression preoperatively. Women with substantiated diagnoses and clear indications for hysterectomy have better physical and psychological outcomes than do women with less defined symptoms and indicators such as chronic pelvic pain.

Role of the Psychiatrist

There may be a role for psychiatrists in assessing mood, anxiety, understanding, and feelings about sexuality and fertility in vulnerable women undergoing hysterectomy. For the informed, psychologically healthy woman with a specific gynecological condition that has failed to respond to other treatment options, hysterectomy may offer an improved quality of life. However, for women with premorbid depression, anxiety, or personality disorders, especially if accompanied by ambivalence about sexuality, fertility, or the procedure, hysterectomy may fail to ameliorate, or may even exacerbate, preexisting symptoms. It is important to consider that premenopausal women undergoing hysterectomy with BSO have to confront the onset of sudden surgical menopause if estrogen therapy is not begun shortly after surgery. Even women whose ovaries were not removed may experience sudden menopause due to impaired blood supply to the ovaries. This sudden hormonal change may result in vasomotor symptoms, sleep loss, and depression, especially in vulnerable women with a history of depression associated with reproductive events. Therefore, psychiatrists should ascertain the hormonal status of women with sudden mood changes following hysterectomy and consider short-term hormonal treatment as well as antidepressants. Psychiatrists who assess women undergoing hysterectomy should evaluate their understanding of the procedure, attitudes toward fertility and sexuality, and experience and expectations of surgery, as well as psychiatric history. The appropriate treatment, whether psychotherapy, hormones, or psychotropics, will, as always, depend on the individual woman.

Abortion

Spontaneous Abortion

Abortion can be spontaneous (miscarriage) or induced (usually just termed *abortion*). Approximately 15%–20% of recognized pregnancies end in spontaneous abortion, with the majority occurring in the first trimester of pregnancy. Spontaneous abortion generally evokes feelings of failure and loss. A woman's body has failed to perform one of its basic functions; she has failed to produce a child for her partner and parents; she has expelled her own potential child; and she may have conceived an embryo with genetic anomalies (Friedman and Gath 1989). Spontaneous abortion, like a stillbirth or neonatal death, may precipitate complicated grief, depression, or PTSD (Engelhard et al. 2003; Kulathilaka et al. 2016). The psychological sequelae of miscarriage will be to some extent dependent on individual psychological factors, psychiatric history, and prior experiences with loss; there are also elements unique to spontaneous abortion. Women report that the failure of society in general and of friends and family to acknowledge their loss is painful and complicates the grieving process. People often say, "There must have been something wrong with the baby," or "You can just get pregnant again." There are no ceremonies to mark the occasion. Friends and co-workers tend to avoid the subject and to expect the woman to recover within days or weeks, but grief may last for months. Women may experience feelings of guilt if they believe that something they did (e.g., intercourse, exercise), ingested (e.g., coffee, drugs), or consented to (e.g., amniocentesis, fertility treatment) caused or contributed to the miscarriage. Women with repeated miscarriages are at greater risk of psychological sequelae. Gestational age and the degree to which a woman perceives the fetus as "real" have been shown to be associated with the nature and intensity of grief. The perception of the reality of the pregnancy increases when women have seen the fetus via ultrasonography or when they can feel fetal movement (both more likely with increased gestational age). It is important to note that although women are at higher risk of psychological reactions following miscarriage than men, their male partners can and do experience psychological sequelae, sometimes expressed as overinvolvement with work or sports.

Health care providers may have difficulty addressing the emotional effect of spontaneous abortion. They feel helpless to prevent it, and it is generally not associated with serious medical or obstetric complications. Psychiatrists can help them to understand and tolerate their patients' feelings and to appreciate the benefits of simply allowing patients to express them. Health care providers should be aware that emotional recovery, depending on the circumstances, can take months, and they need to know when and how to make the diagnosis of complicated grief. It is often helpful to meet with the patient weeks after the event to go over the medical findings, if any; the prognosis; and the state of the woman's recovery.

The loss of pregnancy through miscarriage or stillbirth is associated with an increase in anxiety and depression during a subsequent pregnancy. Data suggest that fears related to miscarriage may have a negative impact on pregnancy and intimate relationships (Haghparast et al. 2016). Although patients are frequently counseled to wait 6 months or a year after such a loss, they often conceive as soon as possible, especially if they feel that the fertility clock is ticking. There is evidence to suggest that medical counseling, either alone or combined with psychological counseling, can reduce a woman's distress with respect to grief, self-blame, and worry (Nikcević et al. 2007).

Induced Abortion

Psychiatric Sequelae

Nearly half of pregnancies in American women in 2011 were unintended, and 40% of these were terminated by induced abortion (Guttmacher Institute 2017). In 2014, 12% of U.S. abortions were in teenagers, and more than 50% were in women in their 20s; 59% of women who received abortions already had at least one child. More than 60% of abortions occurred within the first 8 weeks of pregnancy. Approximately-one half of abortions in 2014 were in women living below the poverty line, and 51% were in women who had used a contraceptive method (e.g., condom, hormonal) during the month they conceived (Guttmacher Institute 2017).

Approximately 926,200 surgical abortions (14.6 per 1,000 women ages 15–44 years) were performed in 2014, down from 1.06 million (16.9 per 1,000) in 2011 (Guttmacher Institute 2017). Abortion rates have been steadily falling since 1973, when abortion became legal; better access to medical abortion or decreasing access to surgical abortions may explain these declines. Mifepristone (medical abortion) is a safe alternative to surgical abortion during the first trimester and was approved for use by the U.S. Food and Drug Administration (FDA) in September 2000 (U.S. Food and Drug Administration 2001). In March 2016, the FDA updated the label for mifepristone to allow patients to take lower doses and make fewer provider visits, and also to allow its use for abortions up to the tenth gestational week (U.S. Food and Drug Administration 2016a). These revisions should result in further improvements in access to abortion (Guttmacher Institute 2017). First-trimester surgical abortion is a safe procedure that causes a minimal risk (less than 0.05%) of complications that may need hospital care. There does not appear to be a difference in psychological outcome based on the type of abortion (i.e., medical or surgical) that a woman undergoes, although many women prefer the privacy of medical abortion (Ashok et al. 2005).

Psychiatrists are seldom consulted about abortion and abortion decisions, and no evidence shows that formal mental health consultation is routinely necessary. The psychiatric ramifications of abortion have been a matter of some debate, but the findings are clear once methodological confounds are taken into account (Steinberg et al. 2012). Unbiased reviews of the literature indicate that self-limited feelings of guilt and sadness are common after abortion, although the predominant reaction is one of relief, and new episodes of psychiatric illness are rare (Charles et al. 2008). Although most research has examined factors associated with postabortion psychological health, research that follows women from before to after abortion consistently finds that depressive, anxiety, and stress symptoms are highest just before an abortion compared with any time afterward. A study of 353 women seeking abortions found that childhood and partner adversities, reproductive coercion, and abortion stigma were associated with negative mental health symptoms before abortion (Steinberg et al. 2016).

The National Comorbidity Survey Replication Study showed that women seeking abortion had more prior psychiatric disorders than did women in the childbirth group ($P<0.001$). After accounting for confounding factors, however, abortion was not a statistically significant predictor of subsequent anxiety, mood, impulse-control, or eating disorders or suicidal ideation (Steinberg et al. 2014). Similarly, women who received an abortion were at no higher risk of PTSD, depression, or anxiety than were women who were denied an abortion (Biggs et al. 2015, 2016). A U.S. longitudinal cohort study observed 956 women semiannually for 5 years. Eight days after seeking an abortion, women who were denied an abortion reported significantly more anxiety symptoms and lower self-esteem and life satisfaction—but similar levels of depression—compared with women who received an abortion; outcomes for both groups either improved or remained steady over time. Abortion denial may initially be associated with psychological harm to women, and findings do not support restricting abortion on the basis that it harms women's mental health (Biggs et al. 2017). In fact, studies have shown that women's quality of life improves during the period extending from before to after an early abortion (Westhoff et al. 2003). The best outcomes prevail when women are able to make autonomous, supported choices about their pregnancies. When women seek, but are denied, abortion, the resulting children have significantly poorer outcomes than do their siblings or matched control subjects (Kubicka et al. 2002).

Antiabortion groups and writers claim that abortion is associated with a higher risk of serious psychiatric disorders and suicide than is childbirth (Reardon et al. 2003; Thorp et al. 2003). These publications fail to address the circumstances of and reasons for abortion. Sometimes they confound common self-limited feelings of loss and guilt with diagnosable depression. Women often have abortions because they have been abandoned by the men who impregnated them, because those men threaten to leave if they continue the pregnancy, because the pregnancy is the result of rape or incest, because they are poor and overburdened with other responsibilities, or because they do not have the resources—educational, financial, emotional, or social—to provide adequate parenting. They may simply not want to be a parent. Preexisting serious psychiatric illness makes some women more vulnerable to unwanted pregnancy and less able to parent. A Danish population–based cohort study compared women with a record of one or more psychiatric admissions at least 9 months before a first-time, first-trimester abortion or childbirth. The risk of readmission was similar before and after abortion, in contrast to a marked increase in risk of postpartum readmission (Munk-Olsen et al. 2012).

Risk Factors for Psychological Difficulties After Abortion

Not surprisingly, coercion, lack of social support, poverty, rape, incest, and preexisting psychiatric illness are associated with increased risk for psychological difficulties following, but not causally related to, abortion. American women who belong to religious faiths opposed to abortion choose abortion as often as, or more often than, those who do not (Jerman et al. 2016). Demonstrators or fear of terrorism at an abortion facility may exacerbate patient stress, and the attitudes and behaviors of medical personnel during the abortion procedure have a significant impact on a patient's experience (Slade et al. 2001).

The delay of abortion into the second trimester, or later, is most often secondary to denial of pregnancy, difficulties with access, or the diagnosis of a serious fetal defect, each of which increases the risk for negative postabortion reactions. The discovery of a fetal defect in a wanted pregnancy or the need to abort because of serious illness in the mother arouses the same sense of failure and loss as a miscarriage, with the added concern that one is carrying a genetic anomaly or is physically unable to bear a child. Consultation may be sought when a woman or family cannot decide, or manifests overwhelming anxiety, when facing an abortion decision under these circumstances (Zlotogora 2002). It is essential that caregivers communicate hope, respect, and compassion to all women seeking abortion, but especially those with a fetal anomaly (Asplin et al. 2014). Continuing a pregnancy and relinquishing the child for adoption impose a psychological burden as well.

Minors and Abortion

A study of underage girls who underwent abortion or childbirth found shared risk factors of early-onset behavioral and emotional disorders, a history of foster care, and low socioeconomic status. Novel risk factors for induced abortions in adolescents were severe substance use disorder and adverse maternal reproductive history (Leppälahti et al. 2016). The effect of abortion on minors, and their ability to make decisions about abortion, is another area of controversy. The vast majority of pregnant minors choose to involve their parents in the abortion decision. No evidence shows that young women who believe that it is not safe or wise to inform their parents derive benefit from being forced to do so. Term pregnancy and delivery pose greater medical and psychological risks for adolescents than do abortions (Dailard and Richardson 2005). Arguments that minors are too immature to elect abortion overlook the fact that these same minors, if their pregnancies are not terminated, will soon be mothers with responsibility for infants. In a study of inner-city girls who obtained pregnancy tests at a school clinic, girls who had abortions had better outcomes compared with those who carried their pregnancies to term and even compared with those whose pregnancy test results were negative. This does not imply that the abortion improved these teens' mental health; rather, it may indicate that the inability to determine whether one is pregnant is associated with other psychosocial problems. Marriage of the pregnant teenager to the father of the baby does not improve outcome and may even worsen it (Zabin et al. 1989).

Chronic Pelvic Pain

Chronic pelvic pain is nonmenstrual pelvic pain of 6 or more months' duration that is severe enough to cause functional disability or require medical or surgical treatment (Howard 2003). It is a relatively common and significant disorder of women, with an estimated prevalence of 3.8% in adult women (Zondervan et al. 1999). Chronic pelvic pain may lead to disability, suffering, loss of employment, sexual dysfunction, marital discord and divorce, and overall decline in quality of life (Howard 2003).

Etiology of Chronic Pelvic Pain

Despite the severity and frequency of chronic pelvic pain, its etiology is often difficult to discern. Disorders of the reproductive, gastrointestinal, urological, musculoskeletal, and neurological systems may be associated with chronic pelvic pain. In many cases, however, the pain is related to a combination of physical and psychological factors, such as endometriosis, adhesions, interstitial cystitis, irritable bowel syndrome, myofascial pain, fibromyalgia, depression, anxiety, somatization, and past abusive experiences (Bryant et al. 2016; Dalpiaz et al. 2008; Suskind et al. 2013). Endometriosis and pelvic adhesive disease are responsible for most cases of chronic pelvic pain with organic findings, but a significant number of patients have no obvious etiology for their pain at laparoscopy (Gelbaya and El-Halwagy 2001). As with other chronic syndromes, especially those with ambiguous etiology, the biopsychosocial model offers the best way of integrating physical causes of pain with psychological and social factors (Speer et al. 2016). Chapter 34, "Pain," provides a discussion of the gate-control theory of pain, as well as an alternative theory, the diathesis–stress model; the latter might explain why a disproportionate number of patients with chronic pelvic pain report histories of physical and sexual abuse (Gelbaya and El-Halwagy 2001).

Psychological Factors Associated With Chronic Pelvic Pain

The relation of chronic pelvic pain to psychological state or personality style has received great attention. Cognitive-behavioral and psychophysiological theories have moved increasingly toward supporting more complex, multicausal views of chronic pelvic pain. A systematic review evaluating the literature on factors predisposing women to chronic or recurrent pelvic pain (Latthe et al. 2006) identified psychological variables that appear to be consistently associated. Both cyclic (i.e., dysmenorrhea) and noncyclic pelvic pain are associated with anxiety, depression, and history of physical and sexual assault. Although very few of these studies were designed in a way to separate psychological predictors of chronic pelvic pain from psychological sequelae, it is clear that chronic pelvic pain is a long-standing condition and women experiencing it are at greater risk of low self-esteem, depression or anxiety, low marital satisfaction and sexual dysfunction, and somatic symptoms (Weijenborg et al. 2007).

Management of Chronic Pelvic Pain

A multidisciplinary, multifocal approach to chronic pelvic pain, individualized for each woman, is essential (Dalpiaz et al. 2008; Gunter 2003), with special attention to the therapeutic relationship. Goals of management include improving function, restoring quality of life, and maintaining even small gains in treatment. First-line management includes a combination of physical therapy, nonnarcotic analgesics, and psychological support. Focused psychotherapy may be useful to address issues such as cognitive styles, pain self-efficacy, current conflicts, past sexual and physical abuse, current domestic violence, substance abuse, and sexual and marital dysfunction (Bryant et al. 2016). Phases of treatment include education, skills acquisition, behavior modification, and maintenance. Special techniques may increase the patient's coping ability and sense of control; such techniques include muscle relaxation, deep breathing and imagery, and cognitive-behavioral techniques to identify and address maladaptive thoughts. Because patients with chronic pelvic pain frequently limit their activity to avoid possible pain, activity programs can be initiated to decrease disability behaviors. Additional interventions might include medical therapies (e.g., antidepressants, ovarian cycle suppression), biofeedback, and surgical procedures.

Endometriosis

Endometriosis is defined as the presence of hormonally responsive endometrial tissue outside the uterine cavity. The precise pathogenesis is not clearly established but likely involves retrograde menstruation with seeding of endometrial glands in the dependent part of the pelvis. Endometriosis may affect sexual functioning, marital relations, and work performance (Culley et al. 2013; Pluchino et al. 2016). The mean age of women at diagnosis of endometriosis ranges from 25 to 30 years. This condition is often asymptomatic but is also found in association with dysmenorrhea, dyspareunia, infertility, chronic pelvic or back pain, and rectal discomfort. The pain from the disorder is often cyclic, although it can be constant. The gold standard for diagnosis and staging of endometriosis is laparoscopy; however, the intensity of pain and discomfort does not correlate well with the severity of the disease at laparoscopy (Lu and Ory 1995).

Management

Endometriosis can be treated by watchful waiting, medical or surgical management, or a combination of the latter two. Current treatment regimens with hormones or gonadotropin-releasing hormone (GnRH) agonists and other drugs attempt to create states of pseudo-pregnancy, pseudomenopause, or chronic anovulation. Nonsteroidal anti-inflammatory drugs (NSAIDs) are widely used for pain. Surgical treatments vary from conservative removal of endometrial implants to total abdominal hysterectomy with BSO. Implants have been shown to recur in up to 28% of patients within 18 months and up to 40% after 9 years of follow-up. However, there is some evidence that perioperative medical management with GnRH agonists may improve outcomes and increase time to recurrence of symptoms (Yeung et al. 2009). Although conservative surgical treatment is widely used to enhance fertility, its efficacy for endometriosis-associated infertility is uncertain.

Role of the Psychiatrist

Because endometriosis is often chronic, and its contribution to chronic pelvic pain is sometimes uncertain, psychiatric opinion may be sought. A systematic review of studies examining the association between endometriosis and psychiatric symptoms (total $N=999$ endometriosis patients) found that 56.4% of patients met the criteria for a psychiatric disorder, although causality was not estimated and may be bidirectional (Pope et al. 2015). However, treatment of any underlying psychiatric disorders or psychological issues is important to outcomes (Friedl et al. 2015). Depression occurs commonly in cases where endometriosis is accompanied by chronic pain, dyspareunia, or infertility. Depressive symptoms may be associated with GnRH agonist treatment. SSRIs appear to be significantly helpful in the treatment of mood symptoms during the course of GnRH agonist therapy (Warnock et al. 2000).

Vulvodynia

Vulvodynia is chronic burning, stinging, or pain in the vulva in the absence of objective clinical or laboratory findings. Vulvodynia is divided into two entities: 1) vulvar vestibulitis, which is restricted burning and pain in the vestibular region that is elicited by touch, and 2) dysesthetic vulvodynia, which is burning or pain not limited to the vestibule, which may occur without touch or pressure. A population-based National Institutes of Health study found that approximately 16% of women reported lower genital tract discomfort persisting for 3 months or longer (Edwards 2003), although a later national health survey estimated much lower rates for vulvodynia, with a current prevalence of 3.8% for chronic vulvar pain for at least 6 months (Arnold et al. 2007). Variability in disease definition may account for these discordant findings.

The etiology of vulvodynia is unknown, and previously suspected agents such as subclinical yeast infections and human papillomavirus have been discounted. Many women with vulvodynia also have comorbid disorders, such as interstitial cystitis, headaches, fibromyalgia, and irritable bowel syndrome, as well as clinical depression.

Psychiatrists may be asked to assess the role of psychosexual factors and depression in women with vulvodynia. One study of 80 women being treated for vulvodynia reported that more than 50% of the sample showed anxiety and more than 50% had a depressive disorder (Tribó et al. 2008). A study of 1,795 American women found that those with depression or PTSD had a 1.5- to 2-fold increased likelihood of having vulvodynia (Iglesias-Rios et al. 2015). Multidisciplinary teams and cognitive-behavioral therapy (CBT) should be considered in treatment. One review concluded that distress in women with vulvodynia is related to the woman's sense of sexual identity and is impacted by social influences related to expectations of femininity (Cantin-Drouin et al. 2008). Antidepressants and anticonvulsants used in other chronic pain syndromes may be helpful, although there is very little evidence to provide guidance (Brown et al. 2008; Harris et al. 2007; Meltzer-Brody et al. 2009; Reed et al. 2006).

Pregnancy

The entire range of psychiatric disorders occurs during pregnancy, and some conditions are unique to pregnancy. Their treatment is discussed later in this chapter.

Epidemiology of Psychiatric Disorders Occurring During Pregnancy

Depression

The prevalence of depression in pregnancy has been estimated at approximately 10%, which is similar to depression prevalence in age-matched nonpregnant women. However, the signs and symptoms of depression must be carefully distinguished from the sleep, appetite, and energy changes often characteristic of pregnancy as well as from the signs and symptoms of thyroid dysfunction, anemia, or other medical disorders related to pregnancy. Risk factors for depression during pregnancy include a past history of depression and major life stressors, especially intimate partner violence, as well as low socioeconomic status and low levels of social support (Vigod et al. 2016). Risk for relapse on discontinuation of maintenance medication varies depending on the severity of the previous illness. In a prospective observational study of 201 women with a history of MDD (more than 75% of whom had a history of at least three episodes of depression), women who discontinued medication had a greater risk of relapse (68% vs. 26%) than did women who continued antidepressants in pregnancy (Cohen et al. 2006a). In contrast, in a prospective study of 778 women in which women with milder illness were included, only 16% relapsed during pregnancy, with no significant difference between those who continued and those who discontinued maintenance antidepressants (Yonkers et al. 2011).

Anxiety, Obsessive-Compulsive, and Trauma- and Stressor-Related Disorders

Because maternal symptoms of anxiety during pregnancy may be associated with adverse fetal and developmental outcomes, there has been increased attention to the course and impact of anxiety and related disorders in pregnancy (Ding et al. 2014). A recent systematic review of 102 studies incorporating 221,974 women from 34 countries found that the prevalence of any anxiety disorder during pregnancy was 15.6%, and that rates appeared to be highest in low- and middle-income countries (Dennis et al. 2017). There is little evidence that pregnancy is a high-risk time for new-onset psychiatric disorders, and the course of preexisting anxiety disorders during pregnancy appears to be variable (Goodman et al. 2014). However, an older systematic review of peripartum anxiety disorders (including DSM-IV [American Psychiatric Association 1994] obsessive-compulsive disorder [OCD] and PTSD) identified five studies indicating that as many as 40% of childbearing OCD outpatients have onset during pregnancy (Ross and McLean 2006). Although the finding of an underlying medical etiology is uncommon, new-onset anxiety symptoms should be investigated because of the consequences of missing a medical etiology (e.g., hyperthyroidism) or medication side effect. It should be noted that a subset of women do present with situational anxiety and/or specific fears about the upcoming labor and delivery (tokophobia) (Demšar et al. 2018). When the source of the anxiety is identified, it can be addressed by providing prenatal education about delivery, making plans to avoid the frightening aspects of care in the coming delivery, and teaching the patient behavioral self-management techniques.

Bipolar Disorder

Women with preexisting bipolar disorder may be at particularly high risk of relapse during pregnancy. In a clinical study of more than 1,000 women with bipolar disorder, the overall risk of a mood episode in pregnancy was 23%, with major depressive episodes being the most common, although manic, hypomanic, and mixed episodes were prevalent among those with bipolar I disorder (13.1%) (Viguera et al. 2011). Younger women with a history of previous postpartum episodes appeared to be at greatest risk of relapse. A smaller earlier study ($N=81$) showed that women who discontinued medication proximate to pregnancy, especially those who discontinued abruptly, were at increased risk of relapse and spent more time being ill than did those who continued maintenance medication (Viguera et al. 2007b). There may be a subgroup of women with stable disease who are able to discontinue mood stabilizers, at least during pregnancy (although risk of relapse postpartum without medication is greater) (Larsen and Saric 2016).

Psychotic Disorders

Because almost all women with psychotic disorders have been deinstitutionalized, and most newer antipsychotics do not impair fertility, fertility rates among women with psychotic disorders have been rising (Vigod et al. 2012). Pregnancy does not ameliorate—and may exacerbate—psychotic symptoms (Vigod and Ross 2010). In a retrospective population-based cohort study in Canada, women with schizophrenia ($n=1,391$), in comparison with women without diagnosed mental illness ($n=432,358$), had a higher risk of obstetric complications (e.g., pre-eclampsia), and their neonates were at greater risk of being born preterm, small for gestational age, or large for gestational age (Vigod et al. 2014). Psychotic episodes during pregnancy may be characterized by delusions that the fetus is evil or dangerous, leading the pregnant woman to stab herself in the abdomen or engage in other self-destructive behaviors. Alternatively, psychotic denial of pregnancy can lead to poor antenatal care and/or impair a woman's ability to recognize and react appropriately to the signs and symptoms of labor. Antipsychotic medication is a foundation of treatment, although electroconvulsive therapy (ECT) for acute affective psychotic episodes can be effective and is reasonably safe for the fetus (Anderson and Reti 2009). Special consideration must be given to the use of restraints for agitated pregnant patients to avoid compression of the vena cava (Solari et al. 2009).

Prenatal assessment and treatment can mitigate custody disputes after the infant is born. Serious psychiatric illness, if treated, can be compatible with successful mothering. The psychiatrist, obstetrician, and pediatrician, working together with the patient, family, and social agencies, can plan and make provision for the infant's needs. Psychiatrists may be called on to assist in the assessment of competency to parent an infant. In circumstances in which it is clear that a mother will not be able to care for her child, such as when the woman's other children have been taken into state custody for their protection, the psychiatrist can help the patient come to terms with the painful separation that will occur.

Alcohol and Substance Abuse

Alcohol and/or substance use disorders in a pregnant patient warrant heightened concern. Standing by while a woman's behavior puts her fetus at risk is painful for prenatal care professionals. The most serious and well-documented result of alcohol abuse during pregnancy is fetal alcohol syndrome (see Chapter 32, "Pediatrics"). Recent studies point to an increase in incidence of neonatal abstinence syndrome in infants born to women with opioid use disorders, and there is concern about the long-term implications of exposed children (Brandt and Finnegan 2017). Many or most pregnant women with alcohol or substance use disorders will accept treatment if it is practical (e.g., providing child care) and humane. Evidence indicates that the threat of coercion and punishment leads women to avoid seeking prenatal care altogether, obviating any opportunity to treat them and improve the fetus's intrauterine environment (see also Chapter 16, "Substance-Related Disorders," and Chapter 2, "Legal and Ethical Issues").

Goals for the treatment of substance-using pregnant women involve motivational enhancement and harm reduction. Clinicians should offer appropriate treatment for the substance use disorder (e.g., methadone maintenance for opioid dependence) and treat comorbid medical or psychiatric disorders. The safety of patient behaviors should be monitored throughout pregnancy and the postpartum period, and child and family services should be involved for risk reduction and facilitation of competent parenting behaviors as needed. A multidisciplinary long-term treatment plan is important, particularly for women returning to environments where they are at high risk of relapse.

Personality Disorders

Women with severe personality disorders may present with risky behaviors that raise concerns about fetal safety. It may also be challenging for prenatal providers to manage some of the interpersonal conflicts in which some of these patients excel. Psychiatrists may be helpful in assessing risk, explaining useful de-escalation strategies, emphasizing consistency in management, and providing ongoing support to staff and the patient.

Issues Unique to Pregnancy

Denial of Pregnancy

Some women go into full-term labor without having recognized, or their families having recognized, that they are pregnant. Many such patients are not psychotic, but some are women with schizophrenia who are delusional in denying pregnancy (Solari 2010). Older patients may report that they thought pregnancy was impossible at their age and therefore attributed their amenorrhea to menopause and the sensations of fetal movement to digestive problems. For some patients, preconscious or unconscious fears of the consequences of pregnancy are so terrifying that they keep its signs and symptoms out of awareness. They wear loose-fitting clothing and go about their usual activities. Sometimes these cases come to psychiatric attention only when the new mother kills the infant after birth. Therefore, these young women end up in the penal—rather than the mental health care—system, and there has been relatively little opportunity to work with them and their families to learn more about the dynamics of these situations. The estimated incidence of denial in pregnancy is about 1 case per 475 births (Jenkins et al. 2011). Risk factors for denial of pregnancy have been studied, but Wessel et al. (2007) concluded that women with denial of pregnancy are varied and were unable to define a "typology" of women at risk.

Pseudocyesis

At the other end of the spectrum is the patient who is convinced she is pregnant when she is not, referred to as *pseudocyesis.* The patient ceases to have menstrual periods. Her abdomen grows, and her cervix may show signs of pregnancy. Some patients with the delusion that they are pregnant are psychotic, but that is not the case in classic pseudocyesis. Patients with pseudocyesis are a heterogeneous group, and they have no other signs or symptoms of frank psychiatric disorder (Seeman 2014). They declare an expected date of delivery and move the date forward when delivery does not ensue. Their conviction may or may not be swayed by ultrasonographic evidence or physical examination. For unknown reasons, the incidence of this condition is decreasing. Frequent antecedents are pregnancy loss, infertility, isolation, naïveté, and a belief that childbearing is a woman's crucial role. It may be important to differentiate pseudocyesis from menstrual irregularity and lactation secondary to hyperprolactinemia in women taking antipsychotic medication. Case reports indicate that the symptoms of hyperprolactinemia may contribute to delusional beliefs about pregnancy in women with schizophrenia (Ahuja et al. 2008).

Hyperemesis

Pernicious vomiting in pregnancy was once thought to be the result of unconscious rejection of the pregnancy. Hyperemesis, which can result in dehydration and electrolyte imbalance and may require hospitalization and intravenous treatment, certainly could induce ambivalence about a pregnancy in a woman who had been very pleased at the prospect of becoming a mother, but no scientific evidence indicates that ambivalence induces the vomiting. Hyperemesis is no longer considered a psychiatric disorder. Mental health intervention can, however, help the patient and family cope until the condition resolves. In a survey of 808 women with hyperemesis, 83% reported negative psychosocial consequences, including socioeconomic stress (e.g., job loss), attitude changes like fear regarding future pregnancies, and psychiatric symptoms like feelings of depression and anxiety, which for some continued postpartum (Poursharif et al. 2008). There are several case reports of severe hyperemesis gravidarum resulting in Wernicke-Korsakoff encephalopathy. Treatment is usually with standard antiemetics, but mirtazapine may be helpful in treatment-resistant cases (Guclu et al. 2005).

Postpartum Psychiatric Issues

Perinatal Death

Stillbirth and neonatal death provoke much the same reactions as do losses earlier in pregnancy (as discussed earlier in this chapter), with the added stresses of full-term labor and delivery and the probability that many practical provisions for the expected infant have been made. Clinical practice in dealing with the bereaved and disappointed parents has varied over time. It is probably best to offer parents the opportunity to see or not to see the stillborn infant and to allow them to decide. Many bereaved parents report that their grief is exacerbated by the failure of friends and relatives to acknowledge the loss. For some, naming the baby and having a funeral service, with or without a burial, are helpful rituals.

When the cause of fetal or neonatal death is not clear, an autopsy or other tests may be performed. The results will not be immediately available. The obstetrician, pathologist, geneticist, and psychiatrist may want to meet with the parents some weeks later to convey the results, answer questions, observe the grieving process, and determine whether additional supports are necessary. Stillbirth increases the risk of PTSD, anxiety, and depression in a subsequent pregnancy, for both men and women (Turton et al. 2006). One study found these sequelae generally resolve within 1 year after the birth of a subsequent healthy child (Turton et al. 2001). In a subsequent pregnancy, premature birth or the stress of complicated, or even normal, labor can precipitate posttraumatic stress symptoms related to the previous perinatal death (Söderquist et al. 2009; Zaers et al. 2008).

Postpartum Psychiatric Disorders

"Baby Blues"

Within days after birth, 50%–80% of women experience significantly heightened emotional lability. Symptoms typically include tearfulness, mild irritability, and some anxiety, but none of the other signs or symptoms of depression are present, nor do the symptoms impair functioning. Symptoms tend to abate within 2–4 weeks after delivery. Clinicians should offer reassurance and continue to reassess postpartum women for progression to depression or other psychiatric disorders. About 25% of women with baby blues will not improve within 10 days and will progress to postpartum depression.

Postpartum Depression

Postpartum depression (PPD) occurs in up to 10%–15% of mothers. Some cases of PPD are simply continuations of antepartum depression. Symptoms can begin anytime from days to months after birth but generally appear later than "baby blues" and range from 4 weeks to 12 months postpartum. The diagnostic process can be complicated by the similarity of symptoms of the aftermath of delivery and the stresses of caring for a newborn and the signs and symptoms of depression. New mothers are often tired, sleepless, distracted, and preoccupied with infant care rather than the enjoyment of previous pursuits. Their meal schedules and sleep are disrupted. It is useful to ask whether the mother can sleep when the baby sleeps. Anxiety accompanies PPD in a large proportion of cases, as both a major symptom feature and as comorbid anxiety disorders (Falah-Hassani et al. 2017).

Risk factors for PPD include previous depression, especially previous PPD; complications of birth; and poor social supports. Newly immigrant women, who often have poor social supports, are at higher risk (Stewart and Vigod 2016; Stewart et al. 2008). Endocrine factors also play a major role; some women are particularly vulnerable to rapid changes in hormone levels across the life span. Some authors have proposed that there is a reproductive "subtype" of depression (Payne et al. 2009), and genetic factors may also play a role (Couto et al. 2015). Because women with thyroid auto-antibodies have an increased risk for postpartum depression (Dama et al. 2016), thyroid function should be assessed when a woman presents with new-onset depressive illness.

The thought content of a woman with PPD centers on mothering (e.g., ruminating that she is not a good mother and that her infant is suffering as a result). Sometimes the woman becomes obsessed with thoughts of harm coming to the infant and vividly imagines his or her injury or death. These ruminations are found both in women with OCD and in those with other psychiatric illnesses (e.g., MDD). There are no reports of women harming their infants solely as a result of obsessional thinking. Most women realize that these thoughts are unreasonable and go to great lengths to avoid harming their infants. However, obsessions must be differentiated from postpartum psychosis, where women are out of touch with reality and are not aware that their thoughts are unreasonable. Reassurance of eventual recovery is crucial. One of the fears of women with PPD, and their families, is that the depression is the first sign of a condition that will result in self-harm or infanticide. Relatives may be tempted to take over care of the infant of a depressed mother to allow her to rest and recuperate. This can be counterproductive, exacerbating her sense of failure and deprivation. It is preferable for them to help the mother with household tasks, allow her to care for the infant, and reinforce her sense of maternal adequacy.

Although obstetricians have become more aware of and responsive to PPD as a result of notorious cases in the media and educational initiatives by a variety of professional and advocacy organizations, they may not be in the optimal position to identify it. Women are discharged from the hospital within a day or two after delivery, with a rather cursory follow-up visit 4–6 weeks later. Obstetric clinicians should be encouraged to increase their contacts with and availability to new mothers. A simple query about depressed mood is often successful in identifying cases (Wisner et al. 2002). In England, the National Institute for Clinical Excellence recommends that all pregnant and postpartum women be screened with the PHQ-2 (the first two questions from the Patient Health Questionnaire–9), with a positive answer to either question triggering further evaluation (Howard et al. 2014). After the birth, the specialist women see most often is the pediatrician. There have been attempts, with mixed success, to convince pediatricians to be vigilant for maternal PPD. Several validated scales are available for screening: the Edinburgh Postnatal Depression Scale (Matthey et al. 2003) is the best known. The efficacy and effectiveness of screening for PPD are controversial (especially if good systems are not available for referral and treatment). Researchers in Hong Kong determined that screening should be delayed for several days after delivery to ensure accuracy (Lee et al. 2003), although earlier assessments have been found to be accurate in North America (Dennis 2003). Screening in an inner-city population in New York uncovered far more cases than had been anticipated (Morris-Rush et al. 2003).

Postpartum Psychosis

Postpartum psychosis is characterized by extreme agitation, delirium, confusion, sleeplessness, and hallucinations and/or delusions. Onset can be sudden and usually occurs between days 3 and 14 postpartum, with 90% of episodes occurring within 4 weeks of delivery (Harlow et al. 2007). The overall incidence of postpartum psychosis is estimated at 0.1%–0.2% and appears to have been stable for more than a century and among cultures. A Swedish population-based study found that 40% of women who were hospitalized for psychosis or bipolar disorder during pregnancy were rehospitalized in the postpartum period (Harlow et al. 2007). Only a fraction of these women will go on to attempt suicide or infanticide (Brockington 2017), but the risk and the stakes are high enough to warrant considering postpartum psychosis as a medical emergency and hospitalizing the patient, at least for a period of observation.

Many experts believe that most episodes of postpartum psychosis are bipolar disorder (Bergink et al. 2016). The risk of postpartum relapse of bipolar disorder is about 35%; these relapses can be acute and severe (Wesseloo et al. 2016). If pregnant women with bipolar disorder discontinue medication, there should be a plan for immediate medication resumption at delivery to lower the risk of recurrence.

Trials and media coverage of cases of infanticide disclose major misunderstandings about the state and motivation of the perpetrators. Most often, the mother in these cases has command hallucinations or delusions and/or is suicidal and does not wish to leave the child behind but wants to be reunited with him or her in Heaven. Appleby et al. (1998) reported that the risk of suicide in the first postnatal year is "increased 70-fold" in women hospitalized for a postpartum psychiatric disorder. In some countries, there has been a very proactive stance toward the identification and treatment of women who are at particularly high risk of developing severe mental illness postpartum. For example, in England, the National Institute for Clinical Excellence has issued guidelines that all health authorities in England are meant to implement (Howard et al. 2014).

Custody

Psychiatric illness in and of itself does not rule out the possibility of adequate mothering. For general evaluation, and for the legal and medical records, when the question of custody arises, it is useful to perform a regular mental status examination. What are most important, however, are the parenting knowledge, attitudes, and behaviors of the newly delivered patient. Has she been able to arrange adequate accommodations for herself and the infant? How does she plan to feed the infant? Does she know approximately how often a newborn must be fed and its diaper changed? Does she have delusions about the infant?

Observation of mother–infant interaction is key. It is very difficult to predict how a person will behave with an infant in the absence of the infant. The postpartum staff should allow the mother as much observed time with the infant as possible and note how the mother responds to the infant's cries and other needs, whether she can feed the infant and change his or her diapers, and how she relates to the infant overall. New mothers without psychiatric disorders can be tired and overwhelmed; expectations should be realistic.

Custody decisions can be life-or-death decisions. Removing a child from his or her mother, unless a well-disposed and capable relative can take over his or her care, exposes the child to the possibility of a lifetime in transient foster care. Allowing a severely ill mother to retain custody exposes the child to possible abuse and neglect. Interactions with child protective services can be problematic. Depending on current resources and recent scandals, child protective services may take a child into custody without giving the mother a chance to show her ability to parent, or they may refuse to intervene with a dangerously psychotic mother because the infant has not yet been harmed. Often, the most appropriate approach, when available, is the provision of home help and/or visiting nurse services, which provide both support and further opportunities for observation of the parenting and the condition of the infant. Having a mental illness does not diminish, and may exacerbate, the grief and rage of a mother whose child is taken away.

Legal aspects of maternal competency are discussed in Chapter 2, "Legal and Ethical Issues."

Treatment in Pregnancy and Lactation

Untreated depression during pregnancy or the postpartum period is associated with increased morbidity in the mother and her offspring. Potential complications in pregnancy and at delivery include increased risk of poor prenatal care, substance use during pregnancy, preterm birth, and low birth weight (Grigoriadis et al. 2013b). Women with depression in pregnancy are at high risk for postpartum depression and for impaired mother–infant interactions that have been associated with poor developmental and emotional outcomes in the offspring (Stein et al. 2014). Unfortunately, depression is undertreated during pregnancy, with fewer than 20% of women seeking treatment (Byatt et al. 2016).

No risk-free solution exists for treating mental illness during pregnancy and lactation, and a risk–benefit decision must be made in the face of imprecise data. Psychotherapy is indicated as acute therapy for mild to moderate illness. A recent systematic review of 29 trials in more than 2,000 patients found evidence that CBT and interpersonal therapy (IPT) each have a moderate treatment effect (van Ravesteyn et al. 2017). Psychotherapeutic treatments are also effective for postpartum depression (Miniati et al. 2014; Sockol 2015). However, psychotherapy may not be adequate if a woman has severe depression. Also, even in mild to moderate depression, psychotherapy may not improve depression for several weeks to months, leaving the mother and fetus (or even infant) exposed to the effects of untreated depression during that time. Psychotherapy alone is not an effective treatment for more severe mental illnesses such as bipolar or psychotic disorders.

When medications are used in pregnancy, there are additional considerations. Changes in drug metabolism and extracellular fluid volume during pregnancy may require dosage adjustment. For example, an increase in the usual dosage of lithium carbonate may be required during the second and third trimesters to achieve therapeutic serum levels, with a decrease postpartum. (See also Chapter 36, "Psychopharmacology," for a discussion of pharmacotherapy during pregnancy.)

Antidepressant Medication

Because antidepressant medications cross the placental barrier, patients and prescribing physicians are concerned about the safety of antidepressant exposure for the developing fetus. Most research on antidepressant safety has been with SSRIs and, to a lesser extent, serotonin–norepinephrine reuptake inhibitors (SNRIs). In most regards, the data are reassuring.

Antidepressants appear to be associated with little to no risk for spontaneous abortion (miscarriage) above that of depression-exposed pregnancies; the most reassuring data are with SSRI exposure (Ross et al. 2013). Antidepressant use in pregnancy does not appear to be associated with an increased risk of serious neonatal complications, or of stillbirth or fetal death (Jimenez-Solem et al. 2013; Stephansson et al. 2013). The highest-quality studies conducted to date suggest that SSRI exposure does not appear to increase the risk of hypertensive disorders of pregnancy. Although a U.S. study of 100,942 pregnant women with depression found no increased risk of preeclampsia from use of SSRIs during pregnancy, SNRIs (adjusted relative risk [RR]=1.52; 95% CI=1.26–1.83) and TCAs (adjusted RR=1.62; 95% CI=1.23–2.12) were each associated with increased risk. Given a baseline preeclampsia risk of 2%–3%, these RRs would translate to a possible rate of 3%–4.5% for women using SNRIs or TCAs in pregnancy (Palmsten et al. 2013b). It also appears that serotonergic antidepressants are associated with at least some increased risk of postpartum hemorrhage, although the absolute loss of blood volume is relatively small, with differences of less than 100 mL between antidepressant users and nonusers (Palmsten et al. 2013a).

Antidepressant use in pregnancy does not appear to be associated with an overall increased risk for congenital malformations. Some studies have suggested that it may be associated with a small absolute increased risk for specific cardiac defects (especially with paroxetine), but more recent rigorous studies do not support this interpretation. A U.S. study of more than 65,000 antidepressant exposures in pregnancy had sufficient sample size to explore specific antidepressants in a well-conducted propensity-matched analysis; this study found no association between antidepressant exposure in pregnancy and any type of cardiac malformation for paroxetine, sertraline, fluoxetine, TCAs, SNRIs, bupropion, or other antidepressants (Huybrechts et al. 2014). It appears that antidepressant use in pregnancy may be associated with both preterm birth and low birth weight. However, the magnitude of the effect, if it is real, appears to be small. A meta-analysis reported mean differences in gestational age and birth weight of −0.45 (95% CI: −0.64 to −0.25; 15 studies) and −74 g (95% CI: −117 to −31; 20 studies), respectively, between mothers who were exposed to any antidepressant and those who were not exposed to antidepressants (Ross et al. 2013).

Persistent pulmonary hypertension of the newborn is a rare but potentially fatal condition, with a background rate of about 1.2 per 1,000 births. Some studies have suggested that antidepressant exposure in the early third trimester of pregnancy may be associated with an increased risk. One well-conducted study of 11,014 pregnancies exposed to an SSRI after the 20th gestational week found an adjusted OR (aOR) of 2.1 (95% CI: 1.5 to 3.0), although this represented an increase from 1.2 to 3 per 1,000 births; risk was similar across SSRI types (Kieler et al. 2012). However, a more recent study with 102,179 SSRI exposures and 26,771 non-SSRI antidepressant exposures found that whereas risks were increased from 2.1 per 1,000 births in unexposed pregnancies to 3.2 per 1,000 and 2.9 per 1,000 in SSRI and non-SSRI antidepressant–exposed pregnancies, respectively, the associations were not statistically significant after analyses were restricted to women with depression only and comprehensively adjusted for confounders (aOR: 1.10, 95% CI: 0.94 to 1.29 for SSRIs; aOR: 1.02, 95% CI: 0.77 to 1.35 for non-SSRIs) (Huybrechts et al. 2015).

A poor neonatal adaptation syndrome (PNAS) has been described in association with late-pregnancy exposure to most antidepressants. PNAS can include a variety of neonatal neurobehavioral symptoms, such as respiratory distress, tremors, jitteriness, irritability, sleep disturbances, poor muscle tone, weak or absent cry, hypoglycemia, and seizures, among others. In a recent systematic review (Grigoriadis et al. 2013a), the pooled OR of PNAS was 5.07 (95% CI: 3.25 to 7.90; 8 studies), and risks of respiratory distress and tremors specifically were elevated. Symptoms were variably defined across studies, resulting in absolute risk estimates ranging from 5% to 85%. Furthermore, the severity of this syndrome is likely to be low. Another meta-analysis (Ross et al. 2013) found that the mean Apgar score was 0.2 point lower for antidepressant-exposed versus unexposed infants (14 studies), and a study of more than 6,000 infants exposed to antidepressants found the absolute risk for seizure to be 7 per 1,000 exposed pregnancies (Hayes et al. 2012). Reported rates of neonatal seizures in the general population range from 3 to 5 cases per 1,000 births, but rates are up to 10 times higher in preterm infants (Vasudevan and Levene 2013).

Some research has focused on long-term child outcomes, where it is difficult to disentangle the effects of antenatal antidepressant exposure from potential shared maternal–child genetic susceptibility and postnatal environmental influences such as maternal depression. Based on data from small studies, there may be some motor delay with antenatal exposure to antidepressants, but these effects do not usually warrant clinical attention on their own (Handal et al. 2016). Any effects on intelligence, language, and behavior are also likely to be subtle (Oberlander and Vigod 2016). Sibling-controlled studies, which are useful for isolating the potential confounding effects of genetics and environment, generally show similar risks for neurodevelopmental and child psychiatric disorders between exposed and unexposed siblings (Brown et al. 2017; Sujan et al. 2017).

In all cases, the small absolute risks associated with antidepressant use in pregnancy must be weighed against the risk of not treating depression. None of the treatment alternatives comes without risk of undesirable outcomes, and there is ongoing scientific uncertainty about risks and benefits of treatment. An additional layer of complexity is that a woman is making this decision not only for her own health but also for the health and development of her unborn child. Vigod et al. (2016) presented a clinical decision-making model to assist both clinicians and patients in making optimal clinical decisions about treatment of depression during pregnancy. The model guides the reader through the presentation of treatment options, including the risks of both untreated depression and antidepressant treatment during pregnancy. Physicians can then help the patient come to a decision about treatment based on the patient's values, perceptions of risk, and capacity to consent to treatment. Consideration should also be given to whether a woman has adequate support to make this complex decision.

Other Psychotropic Medications

A long-standing debate has existed regarding whether benzodiazepine use in pregnancy is associated with cleft lip or cleft palate; however, rigorously controlled studies do not support this assertion (Enato et al. 2011). Data are emerging to suggest that most second-generation antipsychotics are reasonably low-risk in pregnancy; high-potency antipsychotics, such as haloperidol, have been in use longer and are also considered to be reasonably low-risk (Tosato et al. 2017). Early reports warned of congenital heart disease in infants exposed in utero to lithium carbonate, but subsequent analyses have shown these risks to be only slightly greater than those in the general population (Altshuler et al. 1996). Other mood stabilizers, such as carbamazepine and valproic acid, are associated with greater teratogenicity than lithium (Stewart and Robinson 2001). A study of antiepileptic drugs found that fetal exposure to valproate (although not carbamazepine or lamotrigine) was related to poorer cognitive development at age 3 years in children of mothers with epilepsy (Meador et al. 2009). For women with unstable bipolar disorder, it is reasonable to continue lithium throughout pregnancy while carefully monitoring serum levels. Divided doses may be safer than once-daily dosing. An ultrasound during the first trimester can identify possible congenital cardiac malformations. Dosage should be reduced after delivery to avoid lithium toxicity in the early postpartum period.

Breast-Feeding and Psychotropic Medications

The use of psychotropic medications by breast-feeding women remains controversial. The amount of drug present in breast milk is small but is extremely variable over time, even in the same woman. No controlled studies of the effects of psychotropic medication during breast-feeding exist, but reviews provide further guidance (Stewart and Vigod 2016). In general, it appears relatively safe for depressed women to take antidepressants and antipsychotics while breast-feeding full-term and healthy babies. Fewer data are available for premature infants or newer antidepressants and antipsychotics. However, a systematic review of the literature on antipsychotics in breast-feeding advises that clozapine is not recommended due to risk of blood abnormalities and that olanzapine may increase the risk of extrapyramidal side effects in the infant (Gentile 2008). Lithium has been considered to be contraindicated while breast-feeding due to concerns about neonatal toxicity from passage of lithium into the breast milk. However, given lithium's unparalleled clinical efficacy, some experts are revisiting its postpartum use for certain women who wish to breast-feed. A study measuring lithium levels in 10 breast-fed infants of mothers found that breast milk levels were low and well tolerated. There were no adverse effects on the infants, but these results should be interpreted with caution, and infants should be monitored closely if lithium is used during lactation (Viguera et al. 2007a).

No adverse effects from the use of carbamazepine, valproate, or lamotrigine have been reported. However, serum concentrations of lamotrigine were 30% of maternal levels in one study, and Yonkers et al. (2004) recommend that such infants be monitored for rash if lamotrigine is used. Decisions about the care of women with a history of bipolar illness must be made on a case-by-case basis given the high risk of recurrence of bipolar disorder in the postpartum period (Viguera et al. 2007b).

Because new information on the use of drugs during pregnancy and lactation is frequently published, clinicians are advised to consult the most recent references in making risk–benefit decisions. The clinician must be cognizant that untreated mental illness in pregnancy and the postpartum period also poses risks to the woman and the developing fetus and newborn child. If difficulties with the breast-feeding process or lack of sleep are aggravating psychiatric symptoms, clinicians should support a woman's choice not to breast-feed. Decisions about specific medication dosages and breast-feeding should be made in consultation with the woman (and partner, if appropriate) and other health care providers (such as obstetricians and pediatricians), and discussions should be carefully documented in the patient's chart.

Classification of Drugs

The previous FDA five-letter system of pregnancy risk categories presented in prescription drug labeling—which ranged from A (no risk) through B, C, D, and X (contraindicated)—has been replaced with the Pregnancy and Lactation Labeling Rule (PLLR; U.S. Food and Drug Administration 2014). The PLLR establishes standards about the inclusion of narrative information related to the safety and use of medications in pregnancy and lactation in prescription medications. There are now three sections in the FDA labeling: 1) pregnancy, 2) lactation, and 3) females and males of reproductive potential. The latter section will provide information on the relation between drug therapies and pregnancy testing, contraception, and fertility. Each section includes information on potential risks in animals and humans, as well as clinical considerations regarding pharmacokinetics specific to pregnancy and/or lactation. This information cannot dictate clinical care; all data must be interpreted on a case-by-case basis and weighed against risks of other treatment options.

Electroconvulsive Therapy

ECT is generally regarded as a safe and effective treatment for severe depression, affective psychosis, and catatonia in pregnancy and the puerperium. ECT is underused and should be considered in emergency situations in which the safety of the mother, fetus, or child is jeopardized; to avoid first-trimester exposure to teratogenic drugs; and in patients who are refractory to psychotropics or who have previously had successful treatment with ECT (Stewart and Vigod 2016). ECT for acute affective psychotic episodes can be effective and is relatively safe for the fetus (Anderson and Reti 2009; see also Chapter 38, "Electroconvulsive Therapy and Other Brain Stimulation Therapies"). Newer physical treatments for depression, such as vagal nerve stimulation, deep brain stimulation, and transcranial magnetic stimulation, have not been adequately studied in pregnant women (Felipe and Ferrão 2016).

Premenstrual Psychiatric Symptoms: Premenstrual Syndrome and Premenstrual Dysphoric Disorder

The study of premenstrual symptoms poses unique methodological challenges. Many women, if asked, report premenstrual mood, behavior, and somatic changes. There is a strong cultural belief that the menstrual cycle is associated with such negative changes. In addition, both women and men attribute unpleasant or problematic feelings and behaviors to the menstrual cycle regardless of whether they are related. Most women presenting for care of premenstrual symptoms, when assessed with prospective ratings and careful diagnostic interviews, have symptoms completely unrelated to their menstrual cycles (American Psychiatric Association 2013). Nevertheless, premenstrual syndrome (PMS) and premenstrual dysphoric disorder (PMDD) remain popular attributions and diagnoses among women themselves, their families, and physicians. More commonly, women may experience premenstrual worsening of mood and anxiety disorders.

Etiology

Many attempts have been made, over decades, to identify circulating levels of reproductive hormones to account for mood symptoms occurring in concert with reproductive events and cycles. The reality is probably more complex than linear effects of hormone levels on mood. It would seem that some women are particularly sensitive not to specific levels but rather to changes in the levels of reproductive hormones. It has been reported for some time that women who report premenstrual symptoms are more likely to experience postpartum depression and may be predisposed to perimenopausal mood symptoms as well (Payne et al. 2007). Lending biological support to this hypothesis, Huo et al. (2007) reported that the risk of PMDD is associated with genetic variation in the estrogen receptor alpha gene, possibly representing abnormal estrogen signaling during the luteal phase of the menstrual cycle. This may lead to PMDD symptoms via estrogen's effects on serotonin, norepinephrine, gamma-aminobutyric acid (GABA), allopregnanolone, and various endorphins.

Diagnosis

Currently, premenstrual psychiatric symptoms are conceptualized and treated as part of the mood disorder spectrum. Although as many as 75% of women report mild premenstrual mood changes, approximately 2% of women report severe premenstrual mood symptoms that significantly impair their functioning. Experts, and the framers of DSM, have attempted to distinguish normative mood variations from symptoms worthy of medical attention by publishing research criteria for PMDD. For many years, the study of premenstrual psychiatric symptoms was complicated by the lack of a specific and uniform definition—for example, more than 100 physical, emotional, and cognitive signs and symptoms have been attributed to PMS (Janowsky et al. 2002). In DSM-5 (American Psychiatric Association 2013), PMDD was promoted from a research diagnosis to a full diagnosis under Depressive Disorders (Table 31–1).

TABLE 31–1.   DSM-5 diagnostic criteria for premenstrual dysphoric disorder

A. In the majority of menstrual cycles, at least five symptoms must be present in the final week before the onset of menses, start to improve within a few days after the onset of menses, and become minimal or absent in the week postmenses.

B. One (or more) of the following symptoms must be present:
   1. Marked affective lability (e.g., mood swings; feeling suddenly sad or tearful, or increased sensitivity to rejection).
   2. Marked irritability or anger or increased interpersonal conflicts.
   3. Marked depressed mood, feelings of hopelessness, or self-deprecating thoughts.
   4. Marked anxiety, tension, and/or feelings of being keyed up or on edge.

C. One (or more) of the following symptoms must additionally be present, to reach a total of five symptoms when combined with symptoms from Criterion B above:
   1. Decreased interest in usual activities (e.g., work, school, friends, hobbies).
   2. Subjective difficulty in concentration.
   3. Lethargy, easy fatigability, or marked lack of energy.
   4. Marked change in appetite; overeating; or specific food cravings.
   5. Hypersomnia or insomnia.
   6. A sense of being overwhelmed or out of control.
   7. Physical symptoms such as breast tenderness or swelling, joint or muscle pain, a sensation of "bloating," or weight gain.

Note: The symptoms in Criteria A–C must have been met for most menstrual cycles that occurred in the preceding year.

D. The symptoms are associated with clinically significant distress or interference with work, school, usual social activities, or relationships with others (e.g., avoidance of social activities; decreased productivity and efficiency at work, school, or home).

E. The disturbance is not merely an exacerbation of the symptoms of another disorder, such as major depressive disorder, panic disorder, persistent depressive disorder (dysthymia), or a personality disorder (although it may co-occur with any of these disorders).

F. Criterion A should be confirmed by prospective daily ratings during at least two symptomatic cycles. (**Note:** The diagnosis may be made provisionally prior to this confirmation.)

G. The symptoms are not attributable to the physiological effects of a substance (e.g., a drug of abuse, a medication, other treatment) or another medical condition (e.g., hyperthyroidism).

Source.   Reprinted from American Psychiatric Association: *Diagnostic and Statistical Manual of Mental Disorders,* 5th Edition, Arlington, VA, American Psychiatric Association, 2013, pp. 171–172. Copyright 2013, American Psychiatric Association. Used with permission.

Given the tendency to retrospectively overattribute symptoms to the menstrual cycle, prospective daily ratings and careful evaluation for other psychiatric disorders are essential (Landén and Eriksson 2003; Lane and Francis 2003).

The possibility of cyclical changes in symptoms and/or treatment response in all diagnostic categories should be considered in all menstruating women, or at least in those whose diagnoses or treatment responses are puzzling or unsatisfactory (Lande and Karamchandani 2002).

Psychosocial Effects

Another controversial aspect of PMDD is the severity or effect of the symptoms. The DSM-5 definition specifies a significant negative effect on life functioning. It has been difficult to specify the distinction between PMS and PMDD in this regard (Smith et al. 2003). Preexisting beliefs about work effect may color the findings in studies that use self-reports. A large study of randomly selected members of a health maintenance organization found that women with PMDD reported decreased work productivity as compared with women with milder premenstrual symptoms, but women with PMDD also reported lower productivity than the others in the follicular phase after the onset of menses, when their PMDD symptoms, according to the definition, should have been absent. This study did not produce significant evidence that premenstrual symptoms, regardless of their level of severity, caused women to stay in bed, reduce their hours at work, or decrease their activities at home or school (Chawla et al. 2002).

Management

No specific empirically supported treatments for PMS are available, but several approaches have proved helpful for both the symptoms and the patients' general health (Ismaili et al. 2016). These include taking vitamins (especially B vitamins), reducing or eliminating caffeine and nicotine, exercising, and using stress reduction techniques. Like other disorders in the mood spectrum, PMDD is well treated with SSRIs and SNRIs (Ismaili et al. 2016). For reasons still poorly understood, although SSRIs generally require 2–4 weeks for therapeutic effectiveness in depression, they are reported to be effective for PMDD when used only in the premenstrual phase. Perhaps because of the lack of continued administration, there is no discontinuation syndrome when SSRIs are used in this manner. A recent Cochrane meta-analysis confirmed the effectiveness of either luteal-phase or continuous dosing of the SSRIs fluoxetine, paroxetine, sertraline, fluvoxamine, and citalopram and the highly serotonergic TCA clomipramine (Marjoribanks et al. 2013). Evidence does indicate that symptoms recur rapidly when luteal-phase treatment is discontinued.

Exogenous hormones have not been traditionally effective for the treatment of PMDD. However, on the basis of randomized controlled trial evidence, the FDA has approved a combination of ethinyl estradiol and drospirenone for the treatment of PMDD (Lopez et al. 2012). It is thought that the anti-androgen and anti-mineralocorticoid properties of drospirenone account for its efficacy (as compared to traditional oral contraceptive pills). This indication has been limited to women who desire to take an oral contraceptive to prevent pregnancy, likely because the potential for adverse effects (e.g., deep vein thrombosis, pulmonary embolism) exceeds that of the SSRIs.

Perimenopause and Menopause

The average age at menopause in North American and European women is 51 years, although the entire period of transition may extend over several years. By definition, menopause is said to have occurred after 12 months of amenorrhea, and perimenopause is that period of time leading up to menopause but before 12 consecutive months of amenorrhea. During the perimenopause, the ovarian follicles gradually decline with age, estradiol and inhibin production by the ovary decreases, and FSH and luteinizing hormone levels rise (through loss of feedback inhibition). These changes are orchestrated through the hypothalamic-pituitary-ovarian axis, and cyclic variability often occurs throughout the transitional period. The perimenopause may be asymptomatic, but 70%–90% of women will experience some vasomotor symptoms consisting of hot flashes and night sweats. In addition, some women will experience palpitations, dizziness, fatigue, headaches, insomnia, joint pains, and paresthesias. Women also may complain of lack of concentration and loss of memory during the transitional period, but because men also complain of these symptoms, distinguishing them from normal aging is difficult.

The association of psychiatric symptoms with the perimenopause has traditionally been controversial. However, in a U.S. longitudinal prospective cohort study of premenopausal women with no lifetime diagnosis of MDD, women entering perimenopause had 1.8 times increased odds of developing depression compared with women who remained premenopausal (after adjustment for age and history of negative life events) (Cohen et al. 2006b). A 10-year follow-up of a population-based cohort of premenopausal women without depression or hot flashes at baseline found that 40% reported both symptoms during the study interval and that depressed mood was more likely to precede hot flashes (RR=2.1, 95% CI=1.5–2.9) (Freeman et al. 2009). Whether psychiatric symptoms are caused by hormonal changes, sociocultural factors, or psychological factors remains uncertain. Biological factors include estrogen shifts, whereas socio-cultural theories focus on the importance of role changes in parenting, marriage, sex, and work. In addition, attitudes toward aging and female roles vary by culture. A consistent finding is that women with lower socioeconomic status and education report more perimenopausal symptoms. Psychological theories focus on stress during the perimenopausal years as a result of diminished personal and family health, socioeconomic status, family and work changes, other losses, retirement, illness, and death (Avis 2003). In addition, one study has shown that a lifetime history of MDD may be associated with an early decline in ovarian function and earlier menopause (Harlow et al. 2003). Similar to depression in women at other stages of life, perimenopausal depression is accompanied by significant decreases in social support and quality of life and increases in disability (Wariso et al. 2017). Women with bipolar disorder may be at increased risk of perimenopausal depression, although not necessarily mania (Marsh et al. 2008).

The incidence of depression in women mirrors estrogen shifts across the life cycle: at puberty, premenopause, postpartum, and perimenopause (Stahl 2001). This has led to studies to determine whether estrogen therapy in perimenopause can alleviate symptoms of clinical depression. Two small randomized controlled trials found that estradiol was a well-tolerated and effective treatment for perimenopausal depression (Schmidt et al. 2000; Soares et al. 2001), but this finding has not been replicated.

Although estrogen appears to have a salutary effect on depression in some perimenopausal women, in contrast, progesterone and progestins are known to cause dizziness, drowsiness, and sedation in many women and may be associated with negative moods (Björn et al. 2000). Progestins are primarily used in women with an intact uterus to prevent an increase in endometrial cancer caused by unopposed estrogen therapy.

One small pilot placebo-controlled trial found estrogen effective when added to augment partial antidepressant response (Morgan et al. 2005). Further studies of estrogen and selective estrogen receptor modulators as psychotropic augmentation agents are needed.

Moreover, the role of estrogen in psychiatric disorders is not limited to depression. Work by Kulkarni et al. (2001), Seeman (2002), and others has shown a worsening in preexisting schizophrenia and other psychoses associated with decreases in estradiol during perimenopause and beyond. Interestingly, some patients appear to respond to estrogen as augmentation of antipsychotic drugs.

Of concern, however, were results from the U.S. Women's Health Initiative (WHI) study indicating that estrogen–progesterone therapy was associated with an increased risk of breast cancer, cardiovascular disease (Rossouw et al. 2002), cognitive dysfunction, and dementia (Rapp et al. 2003; Shumaker et al. 2003). The estrogen-only arm of the WHI was also prematurely terminated in 2004 when estrogen monotherapy was found to be associated with increased rates of stroke, dementia, and mild cognitive impairment (but not breast cancer) (Anderson et al. 2004). However, most of the women in this arm of the study were older than 60 years, rather than perimenopausal.

Emerging evidence may change practice, but at present, estrogen is useful to control severe vasomotor symptoms and vaginal dryness, with current FDA guidelines recommending use of the smallest dosage for the shortest time possible. Systematic reviews and meta-analyses of nonhormonal therapies for menopausal hot flashes concluded that there is evidence for SSRIs, SNRIs, clonidine, and gabapentin, although the efficacy of these treatments is less than that of estrogen. Results were mixed with respect to the efficacy of isoflavone extracts (Toulis et al. 2009).

In conclusion, the role of estrogen in treating mood, cognition, and psychosis, and as a psychotropic augmentation agent, requires further adequately powered randomized controlled trials. Personal, social, and physical factors always should be considered in assessing the individual woman, and psychotherapy may be helpful in navigating the many transitions at midlife.

Urinary Incontinence

Urinary incontinence, the involuntary loss of urine, affects up to 23% of adults, with a prevalence in women that is twice that in men (Minassian et al. 2008). Urinary incontinence affects the physical, psychological, social, and economic well-being of individuals and their families and imposes a considerable economic burden. Despite the increasing availability of effective treatments for urinary incontinence, many women do not seek help because they are embarrassed or ashamed or believe that this problem is a part of normal aging. A Canadian population-based survey found that only 32% of women with urinary incontinence sought help from a physician, while 40% reported a significant impact of urinary incontinence on their quality of life (Vigod and Stewart 2007).

Etiology and Classification

The etiology of urinary incontinence is multifactorial and may be caused by impairment of the lower urinary tract or the nervous system or by various external factors.

There are several subtypes of incontinence, but the most common are 1) stress incontinence (the involuntary loss of urine due to an increase in intra-abdominal pressure, such as coughing, laughing, or exercise); 2) urge incontinence (the involuntary loss of urine preceded by a strong urge to void whether or not the bladder is full); and 3) mixed incontinence (Minassian et al. 2008).

Psychosocial Effects

Urinary incontinence may affect quality of life, sexual function, and mood. Studies have found that incontinence has a major negative effect on quality of life for women and for couples (Lim et al. 2016). A population-based cross-sectional study of nearly 6,000 American women between the ages of 50 and 69 years found that 16% reported mild, moderate, or severe incontinence. A Canadian population-based cross-sectional study of 69,003 women found that the 12-month prevalence of MDD was 15.5% in women with urinary incontinence, compared with 9.9% in women without urinary incontinence. In this study, women with comorbid depression and urinary incontinence reported substantially worse quality of life than women with either condition alone (Vigod and Stewart 2006).

Role of the Psychiatrist

Given the high prevalence of incontinence, particularly in middle-aged and older women, and women's frequent reluctance to disclose their symptoms, psychiatrists may wish to tactfully ask about urinary problems, as well as comorbid psychiatric conditions and adjustment problems. TCAs and duloxetine are useful treatments for stress urinary incontinence, particularly in women who have concurrent depression, although side effects may limit their utility for some women (Maund et al. 2017). Other treatments that have been used for urinary incontinence with variable effects include behavioral training (with or without biofeedback), pelvic floor exercises, other drug therapies, intrapelvic devices such as pessaries, and surgical procedures (Leone Roberti Maggiore et al. 2017; Riemsma et al. 2017).

Psychosomatic Obstetrics/Gynecology and Men

Although a woman's significant other may be female or male, published studies of relationships' effects on obstetric and gynecological events have been conducted only in heterosexual couples. Virtually every study of the psychosocial aspects of an obstetric and gynecological event or treatment indicates that the attitude of the male partner is a major determinant of outcome. Women turn to their significant others for reaffirmation of their worthiness if infertile, for reaffirmation of their femininity after hysterectomy, and for help in deciding whether to take psychotropic medications while pregnant and whether to breast-feed or bottle-feed. Failure to achieve consensus on such decisions can cause serious long-term repercussions, as when a child is born with problems after (although not necessarily because of) the use of psychotropic medication during the mother's pregnancy, and the child's father blames the mother.

Fathers, brothers, sons, male partners, and husbands can be deeply affected by the obstetric and gynecological experiences of the women they care about, but they may feel uncomfortable, ignored, and excluded when their female loved ones are receiving care. Sometimes, one of the most useful interventions a psychiatric consultant can perform is to facilitate communication between the partners.

Conclusion

Obstetricians and gynecologists are busy practitioners, challenged to deal with both specialized technological developments and primary care and burdened by the likelihood of lawsuits. Despite the intense emotional aspects of much of their clinical work, obstetricians and gynecologists have relatively little training in or time to address psychiatric problems. Some obstetricians and gynecologists, however, are very interested in the psychosocial aspects of their work, and collaboration with these physicians offers promising opportunities for psychiatrists. The scope of psychosomatic medicine in obstetrics and gynecology includes psychopathological aspects of normal reproductive events, psychiatric aspects of obstetric and gynecological diseases and treatments, and psychiatric conditions specific to women's reproductive health. Gender-based medicine, which intersects psychosomatic obstetrics and gynecology at many points, is an exciting and promising area of research and clinical practice. Myriad opportunities exist for providing practical assistance to obstetricians and gynecologists as well as the women who are their patients, for educating fellow psychiatrists about developments in obstetrics and gynecology, and for conducting basic and clinical research.

References

Ahuja N, Moorhead S, Lloyd AJ, et al: Antipsychotic-induced hyperprolactinemia and delusion of pregnancy. Psychosomatics 49(2):163–167, 2008 18354070

Altshuler LL, Cohen L, Szuba MP, et al: Pharmacologic management of psychiatric illness during pregnancy: dilemmas and guidelines. Am J Psychiatry 153(5):592–606, 1996 8615404

American Psychiatric Association: Diagnostic and Statistical Manual of Mental Disorders, 4th Edition, Revised. Washington, DC, American Psychiatric Association, 1994

American Psychiatric Association: Diagnostic and Statistical Manual of Mental Disorders, 5th Edition. Arlington, VA, American Psychiatric Association, 2013

Anderson EL, Reti IM: ECT in pregnancy: a review of the literature from 1941 to 2007. Psychosom Med 71(2):235–242, 2009 19073751

Anderson GL, Limacher M, Assaf AR, et al; Women's Health Initiative Steering Committee: Effects of conjugated equine estrogen in postmenopausal women with hysterectomy: the Women's Health Initiative randomized controlled trial. JAMA 291(14):1701–1712, 2004 15082697

Appleby L, Mortensen PB, Faragher EB: Suicide and other causes of mortality after postpartum psychiatric admission. Br J Psychiatry 173:209–211, 1998 9926095

Arnold LD, Bachmann GA, Rosen R, et al: Assessment of vulvodynia symptoms in a sample of US women: a prevalence survey with a nested case control study. Am J Obstet Gynecol 196(2):128.e1–128.e6, 2007 17306651

Ashok PW, Hamoda H, Flett GMM, et al: Psychological sequelae of medical and surgical abortion at 10–13 weeks gestation. Acta Obstet Gynecol Scand 84(8):761–766, 2005 16026402

Asplin N, Wessel H, Marions L, et al: Pregnancy termination due to fetal anomaly: women's reactions, satisfaction and experiences of care. Midwifery 30(6):620–627, 2014 24269148

Assens M, Ebdrup NH, Pinborg A, et al: Assisted reproductive technology treatment in women with severe eating disorders: a national cohort study. Acta Obstet Gynecol Scand 94(11):1254–1261, 2015 26249555

Avis NE: Depression during the menopausal transition. Psychol Women Q 27(2):91–100, 2003

Ayoola AB, Nettleman M, Brewer J: Reasons for unprotected intercourse in adult women. J Womens Health (Larchmt) 16(3):302–310, 2007 17439376

Baldur-Felskov B, Kjaer SK, Albieri V, et al: Psychiatric disorders in women with fertility problems: results from a large Danish register-based cohort study. Hum Reprod 28(3):683–690, 2013 23223399

Becner A, Turkanović AB, But I: Regret following female sterilization in Slovenia. Int J Gynaecol Obstet 130(1):45–48, 2015 25916963

Berglink V, Rasgon N, Wisner KL: Postpartum psychosis: madness, mania, and melancholia in motherhood. Am J Psychiatry 173(12):1179–1188, 2016 27609245

Bhat A, Byatt N: Infertility and perinatal loss: when the bough breaks. Curr Psychiatry Rep 18(3):31, 2016 26847216

Biggs MA, Neuhaus JM, Foster DG: Mental health diagnoses 3 years after receiving or being denied an abortion in the United States. Am J Public Health 105(12):2557–2563, 2015 26469674

Biggs MA, Rowland B, McCulloch CE, et al: Does abortion increase women's risk for post-traumatic stress? Findings from a prospective longitudinal cohort study. BMJ Open 6(2):e009698, 2016 26832431

Biggs MA, Upadhyay UD, McCulloch CE, et al: Women's mental health and well-being 5 years after receiving or being denied an abortion. JAMA Psychiatry 74(2):169–178, 2017 27973641

Björn I, Bixo M, Nöjd KS, et al: Negative mood changes during hormone replacement therapy: a comparison between two progestogens. Am J Obstet Gynecol 183(6):1419–1426, 2000 11120505

Brandt L, Finnegan LP: Neonatal abstinence syndrome: where are we, and where do we go from here? Curr Opin Psychiatry 30(4):268–274, 2017 28426544

Brault MA, Schensul SL, Singh R, et al: Multilevel perspectives on female sterilization in low-income communities in Mumbai, India. Qual Health Res 26(11):1550–1560, 2016 26078329

Brockington I: Suicide and filicide in postpartum psychosis. Arch Women Ment Health 20(1):63–69, 2017 27778148

Brown CS, Franks AS, Wan J, et al: Citalopram in the treatment of women with chronic pelvic pain: an open-label trial. J Reprod Med 53(3):191–195, 2008 18441724

Brown HK, Ray JG, Wilton AS, et al: Association between serotonergic antidepressant use during pregnancy and autism spectrum disorder in children. JAMA 317(15):1544–1552, 2017 28418480

Bryant C, Cockburn R, Plante A-F, et al: The psychological profile of women presenting to a multidisciplinary clinic for chronic pelvic pain: high levels of psychological dysfunction and implications for practice. J Pain Res 9:1049–1056, 2016 27895510

Burns LH: Psychiatric aspects of infertility and infertility treatments. Psychiatr Clin North Am 30(4):689–716, 2007 17938041

Byatt N, Xiao RS, Dinh KH, et al: Mental health care use in relation to depressive symptoms among pregnant women in the USA. Arch Women Ment Health 19(1):187–191, 2016 25846018

Callegari LS, Zhao X, Nelson KM, et al: Contraceptive adherence among women Veterans with mental illness and substance use disorder. Contraception 91(5):386–392, 2015 25636807

Cantin-Drouin M, Damant D, Turcotte D: [Review of the literature on the psychoemotional reality of women with vulvodynia: difficulties met and strategies developed.] [Article in French] Pain Res Manag 13(3):255–263, 2008 18592063

Centers for Disease Control and Prevention: FastStats—infertility. July 2016. Available at: http://www.cdc.gov/nchs/fastats/infertility.htm. Accessed May 31, 2017.

Centers for Disease Control and Prevention: Single embryo transfer. Assisted Reproductive Technology (ART), Reproductive Health, CDC. February 2017. Available at: http://www.cdc.gov/art/patientresources/transfer.html. Accessed May 31, 2017.

Charles VE, Polis CB, Sridhara SK, et al: Abortion and long-term mental health outcomes: a systematic review of the evidence. Contraception 78(6):436–450, 2008 19014789

Chawla A, Swindle R, Long S, et al: Premenstrual dysphoric disorder: is there an economic burden of illness? Med Care 40(11):1101–1112, 2002 12409855

Chen TH, Chang SP, Tsai CF, et al: Prevalence of depressive and anxiety disorders in an assisted reproductive technique clinic. Hum Reprod 19(10):2313–2318, 2004 15242992

Cohen LS, Altshuler LL, Harlow BL, et al: Relapse of major depression during pregnancy in women who maintain or discontinue antidepressant treatment. JAMA 295(5):499–507, 2006a 16449615

Cohen LS, Soares CN, Vitonis AF, et al: Risk for new onset of depression during the menopausal transition: the Harvard study of moods and cycles. Arch Gen Psychiatry 63(4):385–390, 2006b 16585467

Couto TC, Brancaglion MY, Alvim-Soares A, et al: Postpartum depression: a systematic review of the genetics involved. World J Psychiatry 5(1):103–111, 2015 25815259

Culley L, Law C, Hudson N, et al: The social and psychological impact of endometriosis on women's lives: a critical narrative review. Hum Reprod Update 19(6):625–639, 2013 23884896

Curtis KM, Mohllajee AP, Peterson HB: Regret following female sterilization at a young age: a systematic review. Contraception 73(2):205–210, 2006 16413851

Dailard C, Richardson CT: Teenagers' access to confidential reproductive health services. The Guttmacher Report on Public Policy, 2005. Available at: https://www.guttmacher.org/sites/default/files/article_files/gr080406.pdf. Accessed May 31, 2017.

Dalpiaz O, Kerschbaumer A, Mitterberger M, et al: Chronic pelvic pain in women: still a challenge. BJU Int 102(9):1061–1065, 2008 18540938

Dama M, Steiner M, Lieshout RV: Thyroid peroxidase autoantibodies and perinatal depression risk: a systematic review. J Affect Disord 198:108–121, 2016 27011366

Danesh M, Hamzehgardeshi Z, Moosazadeh M, et al: The effect of hysterectomy on women's sexual function: a narrative review. Med Arh 69(6):387–392, 2015 26843731

Demšar K, Svetina M, Verdenik I, et al: Tokophobia (fear of childbirth): prevalence and risk factors. J Perinat Med 46(2):151–154, 2018 28379837

Dennis CL: The effect of peer support on postpartum depression: a pilot randomized controlled trial. Can J Psychiatry 48(2):115–124, 2003 12655910

Dennis CL, Falah-Hassani K, Shiri R: Prevalence of antenatal and postnatal anxiety: systematic review and meta-analysis. Br J Psychiatry 210(5):315–323, 2017 28302701

Ding XX, Wu YL, Xu SJ, et al: Maternal anxiety during pregnancy and adverse birth outcomes: a systematic review and meta-analysis of prospective cohort studies. J Affect Disord 159:103–110, 2014 24679397

Domar AD, Gross J, Rooney K, et al: Exploratory randomized trial on the effect of a brief psychological intervention on emotions, quality of life, discontinuation, and pregnancy rates in in vitro fertilization patients. Fertil Steril 104(2):440.e7–451.e7, 2015 26072382

Edwards L: New concepts in vulvodynia. Am J Obstet Gynecol 189 (3 suppl):S24–S30, 2003 14532900

Enato E, Moretti M, Koren G: The fetal safety of benzodiazepines: an updated meta-analysis. J Obstet Gynaecol Can 33(1):46–48, 2011 21272436

Engelhard IM, van den Hout MA, Kindt M, et al: Peritraumatic dissociation and posttraumatic stress after pregnancy loss: a prospective study. Behav Res Ther 41(1):67–78, 2003 12488120

Falah-Hassani K, Shiri R, Dennis CL: The prevalence of antenatal and postnatal co-morbid anxiety and depression: a meta-analysis. Psychol Med April 17:1–13, 2017 28414017

Fanslow J, Whitehead A, Silva M, et al: Contraceptive use and associations with intimate partner violence among a population-based sample of New Zealand women. Aust N Z J Obstet Gynaecol 48(1):83–89, 2008 18275577

Felipe RM, Ferrão YA: Transcranial magnetic stimulation for treatment of major depression during pregnancy: a review. Trends Psychiatry Psychother 38(4):190–197, 2016 28076639

Flory N, Bissonnette F, Binik YM: Psychosocial effects of hysterectomy: literature review. J Psychosom Res 59(3):117–129, 2005 16198184

Freeman EW, Boxer AS, Rickels K, et al: Psychological evaluation and support in a program of in vitro fertilization and embryo transfer. Fertil Steril 43(1):48–53, 1985 3965315

Freeman EW, Sammel MD, Lin H: Temporal associations of hot flashes and depression in the transition to menopause. Menopause 16(4):728–734, 2009 19188849

Friedl F, Riedl D, Fessler S, et al: Impact of endometriosis on quality of life, anxiety, and depression: an Austrian perspective. Arch Gynecol Obstet 292(6):1393–1399, 2015 26112356

Friedman T, Gath D: The psychiatric consequences of spontaneous abortion. Br J Psychiatry 155:810–813, 1989 2620207

Gelbaya TA, El-Halwagy HE: Focus on primary care: chronic pelvic pain in women. Obstet Gynecol Surv 56(12):757–764, 2001 11753178

Gelberg L, Leake B, Lu MC, et al: Chronically homeless women's perceived deterrents to contraception. Perspect Sex Reprod Health 34(6):278–285, 2002 12558090

Gentile S: Infant safety with antipsychotic therapy in breast-feeding: a systematic review. J Clin Psychiatry 69(4):666–673, 2008 18370569

Glasier AF, Smith KB, van der Spuy ZM, et al: Amenorrhea associated with contraception—an international study on acceptability. Contraception 67(1):1–8, 2003 12521650

Goodman JH, Chenausky KL, Freeman MP: Anxiety disorders during pregnancy: a systematic review. J Clin Psychiatry 75(10):e1153–e1184, 2014 25373126

Graham M, James EL, Keleher H: Predictors of hysterectomy as a treatment for menstrual symptoms. Womens Health Issues 18(4):319–327, 2008 18590884

Grigoriadis S, VonderPorten EH, Mamisashvili L, et al: The effect of prenatal antidepressant exposure on neonatal adaptation: a systematic review and meta-analysis. J Clin Psychiatry 74(4):e309–e320, 2013a 23656856

Grigoriadis S, VonderPorten EH, Mamisashvili L, et al: The impact of maternal depression during pregnancy on perinatal outcomes: a systematic review and meta-analysis. J Clin Psychiatry 74(4):e321–e341, 2013b 23656857

Guclu S, Gol M, Dogan E, et al: Mirtazapine use in resistant hyperemesis gravidarum: report of three cases and review of the literature. Arch Gynecol Obstet 272(4):298–300, 2005 16007504

Gunter J: Chronic pelvic pain: an integrated approach to diagnosis and treatment. Obstet Gynecol Surv 58(9):615–623, 2003 12972837

Guttmacher Institute: Induced abortion in the United States (fact sheet). January 2017. Available at: https://www.guttmacher.org/fact-sheet/induced-abortion-united-states. Accessed June 1, 2017.

Haghparast E, Faramarzi M, Hassanzadeh R: Psychiatric symptoms and pregnancy distress in subsequent pregnancy after spontaneous abortion history. Pak J Med Sci 32(5):1097–1101, 2016 27882001

Handal M, Skurtveit S, Furu K, et al: Motor development in children prenatally exposed to selective serotonin reuptake inhibitors: a large population-based pregnancy cohort study. BJOG 123(12):1908–1917, 2016 26374234

Hanley GE, Smolina K, Mintzes B, et al: Postpartum hemorrhage and use of serotonin reuptake inhibitor antidepressants in pregnancy. Obstet Gynecol 127(3):553–561, 2016 26855096

Harlow BL, Wise LA, Otto MW, et al: Depression and its influence on reproductive endocrine and menstrual cycle markers associated with perimenopause: the Harvard Study of Moods and Cycles. Arch Gen Psychiatry 60(1):29–36, 2003 12511170

Harlow BL, Vitonis AF, Sparen P, et al: Incidence of hospitalization for postpartum psychotic and bipolar episodes in women with and without prior prepregnancy or prenatal psychiatric hospitalizations. Arch Gen Psychiatry 64(1):42–48, 2007 17199053

Harris G, Horowitz B, Borgida A: Evaluation of gabapentin in the treatment of generalized vulvodynia, unprovoked. J Reprod Med 52(2):103–106, 2007 17393770

Hartmann KE, Ma C, Lamvu GM, et al: Quality of life and sexual function after hysterectomy in women with preoperative pain and depression. Obstet Gynecol 104(4):701–709, 2004 15458889

Hayes RM, Wu P, Shelton RC, et al: Maternal antidepressant use and adverse outcomes: a cohort study of 228,876 pregnancies. Am J Obstet Gynecol 207(1):49.e1–49.e9, 2012 22727349

Howard FM: Chronic pelvic pain. Obstet Gynecol 101(3):594–611, 2003 12636968

Howard LM, Megnin-Viggars O, Symington I, et al: Antenatal and postnatal mental health: summary of updated NICE guidance. BMJ 349:g7394, 2014 25523903

Huo L, Straub RE, Roca C, et al: Risk for premenstrual dysphoric disorder is associated with genetic variation in ESR1, the estrogen receptor alpha gene. Biol Psychiatry 62(8):925–933, 2007 17599809

Huybrechts KF, Palmsten K, Avorn J, et al: Antidepressant use in pregnancy and the risk of cardiac defects. N Engl J Med 370(25):2397–2407, 2014 24941178

Huybrechts KF, Bateman BT, Palmsten K, et al: Antidepressant use late in pregnancy and risk of persistent pulmonary hypertension of the newborn. JAMA 313(21):2142–2151, 2015 26034955

Iglesias-Rios L, Harlow SD, Reed BD: Depression and posttraumatic stress disorder among women with vulvodynia: evidence from the population-based woman to woman health study. J Womens Health (Larchmt) 24(7):557–562, 2015 25950702

Ismaili E, Walsh S, O'Brien PM, et al; Consensus Group of the International Society for Premenstrual Disorders: Fourth consensus of the International Society for Premenstrual Disorders (ISPMD): auditable standards for diagnosis and management of premenstrual disorder. Arch Women Ment Health 19(6):953–958, 2016 27378473

Jamieson DJ, Kaufman SCC, Costello C, et al; US Collaborative Review of Sterilization Working Group: A comparison of women's regret after vasectomy versus tubal sterilization. Obstet Gynecol 99(6):1073–1079, 2002 12052602

Janowsky DS, Rausch JL, Davis JM: Historical studies of premenstrual tension up to 30 years ago: implications for future research. Curr Psychiatry Rep 4(6):411–418, 2002 12441020

Jenkins A, Millar S, Robins J: Denial of pregnancy: a literature review and discussion of ethical and legal issues. J R Soc Med 104(7):286–291, 2011 21725094

Jerman J, Jones RK, Onda T: Characteristics of U.S. abortion patients in 2014 and changes since 2008. New York, Guttmacher Institute, 2016. Available at: https://www.guttmacher.org/report/characteristicsus-abortion-patients-2014. Accessed June 1, 2017.

Jimenez-Solem E, Andersen JT, Petersen M, et al: SSRI use during pregnancy and risk of stillbirth and neonatal mortality. Am J Psychiatry 170(3):299–304, 2013 23361562

Joffe H: Reproductive biology and psychotropic treatments in premenopausal women with bipolar disorder. J Clin Psychiatry 68 (suppl 9):10–15, 2007 17764379

Kieler H, Artama M, Engeland A, et al: Selective serotonin reuptake inhibitors during pregnancy and risk of persistent pulmonary hypertension in the newborn: population based cohort study from the five Nordic countries. BMJ 344:d8012, 2012 22240235

Kubicka L, Roth Z, Dytrych Z, et al: The mental health of adults born of unwanted pregnancies, their siblings, and matched controls: a 35-year follow-up study from Prague, Czech Republic. J Nerv Ment Dis 190(10):653–662, 2002 12409858

Kulathilaka S, Hanwella R, de Silva VA: Depressive disorder and grief following spontaneous abortion. BMC Psychiatry 16:100, 2016 27071969

Kulkarni J, Riedel A, de Castella AR, et al: Estrogen—a potential treatment for schizophrenia. Schizophr Res 48(1):137–144, 2001 11278160

Lande RG, Karamchandani V: Chronic mental illness and the menstrual cycle. J Am Osteopath Assoc 102(12):655–659, 2002 12501982

Landén M, Eriksson E: How does premenstrual dysphoric disorder relate to depression and anxiety disorders? Depress Anxiety 17(3):122–129, 2003 12768646

Lane T, Francis A: Premenstrual symptomatology, locus of control, anxiety and depression in women with normal menstrual cycles. Arch Women Ment Health 6(2):127–138, 2003 12720063

Larsen ER, Saric K: Pregnancy and bipolar disorder: the risk of recurrence when discontinuing treatment with mood stabilisers. A systematic review. Acta Neuropsychiatr 17:1–8, 2016 27852343

Latthe P, Mignini L, Gray R, et al: Factors predisposing women to chronic pelvic pain: systematic review. BMJ 332(7544):749–755, 2006 16484239

Lee DT, Yip AS, Chan SS, et al: Postdelivery screening for postpartum depression. Psychosom Med 65(3):357–361, 2003 12764207

Leone Roberti Maggiore U, Finazzi Agro E, Soligo M, et al: Long-term outcomes of TOT and TVT procedures for the treatment of female stress urinary incontinence: a systematic review and meta-analysis. Int Urogynecol J 28(8):1119–1130, 2017 28213797

Leppälahti S, Heikinheimo O, Paananen R, et al: Determinants of underage induced abortion—the 1987 Finnish Birth Cohort study. Acta Obstet Gynecol Scand 95(5):572–579, 2016 26915819

Leung VWY, Soon JA, Lynd LD, et al: Population-based evaluation of the effectiveness of two regimens for emergency contraception. Int J Gynaecol Obstet 133(3):342–346, 2016 26969148

Lim R, Liong ML, Leong WS, et al: Effect of stress urinary incontinence on the sexual function of couples and the quality of life of patients. J Urol 196(1):153–158, 2016 26812304

Lopez LM, Kaptein AA, Helmerhorst FM: Oral contraceptives containing drospirenone for premenstrual syndrome. Cochrane Database Syst Rev (2):CD006586, 2012 22336820

Lu PY, Ory SJ: Endometriosis: current management. Mayo Clin Proc 70(5):453–463, 1995 7731255

Machado KM, Ludermir AB, da Costa AM: Changes in family structure and regret following tubal sterilization. Cad Saude Publica 21(6):1768–1777, 2005 16410861

Malhotra N, Chanana C, Garg P: Post-sterilization regrets in Indian women. Indian J Med Sci 61(4):186–191, 2007 17401255

Marjoribanks J, Brown J, O'Brien PM, et al: Selective serotonin reuptake inhibitors for premenstrual syndrome. Cochrane Database Syst Rev (6):CD001396, 2013 23744611

Marsh WK, Templeton A, Ketter TA, et al: Increased frequency of depressive episodes during the menopausal transition in women with bipolar disorder: preliminary report. J Psychiatr Res 42(3):247–251, 2008 17266987

Mascarenhas MN, Flaxman SR, Boerma T, et al: National, regional, and global trends in infertility prevalences since 1990: a systematic analysis of 277 health surveys. PLoS Med 9(12):e1001356, 2012 23271957

Matthey S, Barnett B, White T: The Edinburgh Postnatal Depression Scale. Br J Psychiatry 182:368–370, author reply 368, 2003 12668422

Maund E, Guski LS, Gotzsche PC: Considering benefits and harms of duloxetine for treatment of stress urinary incontinence: a meta-analysis of clinical study reports. CMAJ 189(5):E194–E203, 2017 28246265

Meador KJ, Baker GA, Browning N, et al; NEAD Study Group: Cognitive function at 3 years of age after fetal exposure to antiepileptic drugs. N Engl J Med 360(16):1597–1605, 2009 19369666

Meltzer-Brody SE, Zolnoun D, Steege JF, et al: Open-label trial of lamotrigine focusing on efficacy in vulvodynia. J Reprod Med 54(3):171–178, 2009 19370903

Minassian VA, Stewart WF, Wood GC: Urinary incontinence in women: variation in prevalence estimates and risk factors. Obstet Gynecol 111(2 Pt 1):324–331, 2008 18238969

Miniati M, Callari A, Calugi S, et al: Interpersonal psychotherapy for postpartum depression: a systematic review. Arch Women Ment Health 17(4):257–268, 2014 24957781

Monteleone PAA, Mirisola RJ, Gonçalves SP, et al: Outcomes of elective cryopreserved single or double embryo transfers following failure to conceive after fresh single embryo transfer. Reprod Biomed Online 33(2):161–167, 2016 27317130

Morgan ML, Cook IA, Rapkin AJ, et al: Estrogen augmentation of antidepressants in perimenopausal depression: a pilot study. J Clin Psychiatry 66(6):774–780, 2005 15960574

Morris-Rush JK, Freda MC, Bernstein PS: Screening for postpartum depression in an inner-city population. Am J Obstet Gynecol 188(5):1217–1219, 2003 12748483

Munk-Olsen T, Laursen TM, Pedersen CB, et al: First-time first-trimester induced abortion and risk of readmission to a psychiatric hospital in women with a history of treated mental disorder. Arch Gen Psychiatry 69(2):159–165, 2012 22310504

National Institute for Health and Care Excellence: Fertility problems. Quality statement 8: number of embryos transferred. October 2014. Available at: https://www.nice.org.uk/guidance/qs73/chapter/Quality-statement-8-Number-of-embryos-transferred. Accessed June 1, 2017.

Nikcević AV, Kuczmierczyk AR, Nicolaides KH: The influence of medical and psychological interventions on women's distress after miscarriage. J Psychosom Res 63(3):283–290, 2007 17719366

Oberlander TF, Vigod SN: Developmental effects of prenatal selective serotonin reuptake inhibitor exposure in perspective: are we comparing apples to apples? J Am Acad Child Adolesc Psychiatry 55(5):351–352, 2016 27126845

Oesterheld JR, Cozza K, Sandson NB: Oral contraceptives. Psychosomatics 49(2):168–175, 2008 18354071

Palmsten K, Hernandez-Diaz S, Huybrechts KF, et al: Use of antidepressants near delivery and risk of postpartum hemorrhage: cohort study of low income women in the United States. BMJ 347:f4877, 2013a 23965506

Palmsten K, Huybrechts KF, Michels KB, et al: Antidepressant use and risk for preeclampsia. Epidemiology 24(5):682–691, 2013b 23873072

Payne JL, Roy PS, Murphy-Eberenz K, et al: Reproductive cycle-associated mood symptoms in women with major depression and bipolar disorder. J Affect Disord 99(1–3):221–229, 2007 17011632

Payne JL, Palmer JT, Joffe H: A reproductive subtype of depression: conceptualizing models and moving toward etiology. Harv Rev Psychiatry 17(2):72–86, 2009 19373617

Peipert JF, Lapane KL, Allsworth JE, et al: Women at risk for sexually transmitted diseases: correlates of intercourse without barrier contraception. Am J Obstet Gynecol 197(5):474.e1–474.e8, 2007 17714677

Peterson HB: Sterilization. Obstet Gynecol 111(1):189–203, 2008 18165410

Picardo CM, Nichols M, Edelman A, et al: Women's knowledge and sources of information on the risks and benefits of oral contraception. J Am Med Womens Assoc (1972) 58(2):112–116, 2003 12744425

Pluchino N, Wenger J-M, Petignat P, et al: Sexual function in endometriosis patients and their partners: effect of the disease and consequences of treatment. Hum Reprod Update 22(6):762–774, 2016 27591248

Polis CB, Schaffer K, Blanchard K, et al: Advance provision of emergency contraception for pregnancy prevention (full review). Cochrane Database Syst Rev (2):CD005497, 2007 17443596

Pope CJ, Sharma V, Sharma S, et al: A systematic review of the association between psychiatric disturbances and endometriosis. J Obstet Gynaecol Can 37(11):1006–1015, 2015 26629721

Poursharif B, Korst LM, Fejzo MS, et al: The psychosocial burden of hyperemesis gravidarum. J Perinatol 28(3):176–181, 2008 18059463

Rapp SR, Espeland MA, Shumaker SA, et al; WHIMS Investigators: Effect of estrogen plus progestin on global cognitive function in postmenopausal women: the Women's Health Initiative Memory Study: a randomized controlled trial. JAMA 289(20):2663–2672, 2003 12771113

Reardon DC, Cougle JR, Rue VM, et al: Psychiatric admissions of low-income women following abortion and childbirth. CMAJ 168(10):1253–1256, 2003 12743066

Reed BD, Caron AM, Gorenflo DW, et al: Treatment of vulvodynia with tricyclic antidepressants: efficacy and associated factors. J Low Genit Tract Dis 10(4):245–251, 2006 17012991

Reiner WG: Gender identity and sex assignment: a reappraisal for the 21st century. Adv Exp Med Biol 511:175–189; discussion 189–197, 2002 12575762

Rich CW, Domar AD: Addressing the emotional barriers to access to reproductive care. Fertil Steril 105(5):1124–1127, 2016 27054306

Richardson AR, Maltz FN: Ulipristal acetate: review of the efficacy and safety of a newly approved agent for emergency contraception. Clin Ther 34(1):24–36, 2012 22154199

Rickert VI, Wiemann CM, Harrykissoon SD, et al: The relationship among demographics, reproductive characteristics, and intimate partner violence. Am J Obstet Gynecol 187(4):1002–1007, 2002 12388996

Riemsma R, Hagen S, Kirschner-Hermanns R, et al: Can incontinence be cured? A systematic review of cure rates. BMC Med 15(1):63, 2017 28335792

Rooney KL, Domar AD: The impact of lifestyle behaviors on infertility treatment outcome. Curr Opin Obstet Gynecol 26(3):181–185, 2014 24752004

Rooney KL, Domar AD: The impact of stress on fertility treatment. Curr Opin Obstet Gynecol 28(3):198–201, 2016 26907091

Ross LE, McLean LM: Anxiety disorders during pregnancy and the postpartum period: a systematic review. J Clin Psychiatry 67(8):1285–1298, 2006 16965210

Ross LE, Grigoriadis S, Mamisashvili L, et al: Selected pregnancy and delivery outcomes after exposure to antidepressant medication: a systematic review and meta-analysis. JAMA Psychiatry 70(4):436–443, 2013 23446732

Rossouw JE, Anderson GL, Prentice RL, et al; Writing Group for the Women's Health Initiative Investigators: Risks and benefits of estrogen plus progestin in healthy postmenopausal women: principal results From the Women's Health Initiative randomized controlled trial. JAMA 288(3):321–333, 2002 12117397

Sanders SA, Graham CA, Yarber WL, et al: Condom use errors and problems among young women who put condoms on their male partners. J Am Med Womens Assoc (1972) 58(2):95–98, 2003 12744422

Schiff L, Wegienka G, Sangha R, et al: Is cervix removal associated with patient-centered outcomes of pain, dyspareunia, well-being and satisfaction after laparoscopic hysterectomy? Arch Gynecol Obstet 291(2):371–376, 2015 25145555

Schmidt PJ, Nieman L, Danaceau MA, et al: Estrogen replacement in perimenopause-related depression: a preliminary report. Am J Obstet Gynecol 183(2):414–420, 2000 10942479

Seeman MV: Does menopause intensify symptoms in schizophrenia? in Psychiatric Illness in Women: Emerging Treatments and Research. Edited by Lewis-Hall F, Williams TS, Panetta J, et al. Washington, DC, American Psychiatric Publishing, 2002, pp 239–248

Seeman MV: Pseudocyesis, delusional pregnancy, and psychosis: the birth of a delusion. World J Clin Cases 2(8):338–344, 2014 25133144

Seeman MV: Transient psychosis in women on clomiphene, bromocriptine, domperidone and related endocrine drugs. Gynecol Endocrinol 31(10):751–754, 2015 26291819

Seston EM, Elliott RA, Noyce PR, et al: Women's preferences for the provision of emergency hormonal contraception services. Pharm World Sci 29(3):183–189, 2007 17279450

Shoveller J, Chabot C, Soon JA, et al: Identifying barriers to emergency contraception use among young women from various sociocultural groups in British Columbia, Canada. Perspect Sex Reprod Health 39(1):13–20, 2007 17355377

Shumaker SA, Legault C, Rapp SR, et al; WHIMS Investigators: Estrogen plus progestin and the incidence of dementia and mild cognitive impairment in postmenopausal women: the Women's Health Initiative Memory Study: a randomized controlled trial. JAMA 289(20):2651–2662, 2003 12771112

Skovlund CW, Mørch LS, Kessing LV, et al: Association of hormonal contraception with depression. JAMA Psychiatry 73(11):1154–1162, 2016 27680324

Slade P, Heke S, Fletcher J, et al: Termination of pregnancy: patients' perceptions of care. J Fam Plann Reprod Health Care 27(2):72–77, 2001 12457515

Smith MJ, Schmidt PJ, Rubinow DR: Operationalizing DSM-IV criteria for PMDD: selecting symptomatic and asymptomatic cycles for research. J Psychiatr Res 37(1):75–83, 2003 12482472

Smorgick N, Patzkowsky KE, Hoffman MR, et al: The increasing use of robot-assisted approach for hysterectomy results in decreasing rates of abdominal hysterectomy and traditional laparoscopic hysterectomy. Arch Gynecol Obstet 289(1):101–105, 2014 23839534

Soares CN, Almeida OP, Joffe H, et al: Efficacy of estradiol for the treatment of depressive disorders in perimenopausal women: a double-blind, randomized, placebo-controlled trial. Arch Gen Psychiatry 58(6):529–534, 2001 11386980

Sockol LE: A systematic review of the efficacy of cognitive behavioral therapy for treating and preventing perinatal depression. J Affect Disord 177:7–21, 2015 25743368

Söderquist J, Wijma B, Thorbert G, et al: Risk factors in pregnancy for post-traumatic stress and depression after childbirth. BJOG 116(5):672–680, 2009 19220236

Solari H: Psychotic denial of pregnancy. Curr Womens Health Rev 6(1):22–27, 2010

Solari H, Dickson KE, Miller L: Understanding and treating women with schizophrenia during pregnancy and postpartum—Motherisk Update 2008. Can J Clin Pharmacol 16(1):e23–e32, 2009 19164844

Speer LM, Mushkbar S, Erbele T: Chronic pelvic pain in women. Am Fam Physician 93(5):380–387, 2016 26926975

Spencer EA, Mahtani KR, Goldacre B, et al: Claims for fertility interventions: a systematic assessment of statements on UK fertility centre websites. BMJ Open 6(11):e013940, 2016 27890866

Stahl SM: Effects of estrogen on the central nervous system. J Clin Psychiatry 62(5):317–318, 2001 11411810

Stein A, Pearson RM, Goodman SH, et al: Effects of perinatal mental disorders on the fetus and child. Lancet 384(9956):1800–1819, 2014 25455250

Steinberg JR, Trussell J, Hall KS, et al: Fatal flaws in a recent meta-analysis on abortion and mental health. Contraception 86(5):430–437, 2012 22579105

Steinberg JR, McCulloch CE, Adler NE: Abortion and mental health: findings from the National Comorbidity Survey-Replication. Obstet Gynecol 123(2 Pt 1):263–270, 2014 24402590

Steinberg JR, Tschann JM, Furgerson D, et al: Psychosocial factors and pre-abortion psychological health: the significance of stigma. Soc Sci Med 150:67–75, 2016 26735332

Stephansson O, Kieler H, Haglund B, et al: Selective serotonin reuptake inhibitors during pregnancy and risk of stillbirth and infant mortality. JAMA 309(1):48–54, 2013 23280224

Stewart DE, Robinson G: Psychotropic drugs and electroconvulsive therapy during pregnancy and lactation, in Psychological Aspects of Women's Health Care: The Interface Between Psychiatry and Obstetrics and Gynecology, 2nd Edition. Edited by Stotland N, Stewart D. Washington, DC, American Psychiatric Press, 2001, pp 67–93

Stewart DE, Vigod S: Postpartum depression. N Engl J Med 375(22):2177–2186, 2016 27959754

Stewart DE, Leyland N, Shime J, et al: Achieving Best Practices in the Use of Hysterectomy: Report of Ontario's Expert Panel on Best Practices in the Use of Hysterectomy. Toronto, ON, Canada, Ontario Women's Health Council, 2002

Stewart DE, Gagnon A, Saucier JF, et al: Postpartum depression symptoms in newcomers. Can J Psychiatry 53(2):121–124, 2008 18357931

Subhrajit C: Problems faced by LGBT people in the mainstream society: some recommendations. International Journal of Interdisciplinary and Multidisciplinary Studies 1(5):317–331, 2014

Sujan AC, Rickert ME, Oberg AS, et al: Associations of maternal antidepressant use during the first trimester of pregnancy with preterm birth, small for gestational age, autism spectrum disorder, and attention-deficit/hyperactivity disorder in offspring. JAMA 317(15):1553–1562, 2017 28418479

Suskind AM, Berry SH, Suttorp MJ, et al: Health-related quality of life in patients with interstitial cystitis/bladder pain syndrome and frequently associated comorbidities. Qual Life Res 22(7):1537–1541, 2013 23054497

Thorp JM Jr, Hartmann KE, Shadigian E: Long-term physical and psychological health consequences of induced abortion: review of the evidence. Obstet Gynecol Surv 58(1):67–79, 2003 12544786

Tosato S, Albert U, Tomassi S, et al: A systematized review of atypical antipsychotics in pregnant women: balancing between risks of untreated illness and risks of drug-related adverse effects. J Clin Psychiatry 78(5):e477–e489, 2017 28297592

Toulis KA, Tzellos T, Kouvelas D, et al: Gabapentin for the treatment of hot flashes in women with natural or tamoxifen-induced menopause: a systematic review and meta-analysis. Clin Ther 31(2):221–235, 2009 19302896

Tribó MJ, Andión O, Ros S, et al: Clinical characteristics and psychopathological profile of patients with vulvodynia: an observational and descriptive study. Dermatology 216(1):24–30, 2008 18032895

Turton P, Hughes P, Evans CD, et al: Incidence, correlates and predictors of post-traumatic stress disorder in the pregnancy after stillbirth. Br J Psychiatry 178:556–560, 2001 11388974

Turton P, Badenhorst W, Hughes P, et al: Psychological impact of stillbirth on fathers in the subsequent pregnancy and puerperium. Br J Psychiatry 188:165–172, 2006 16449705

United Nations: World contraceptive use, 2007. United Nations, Department of Economic and Social Affairs, Population Division, November 2007. Available at: http://www.un.org/esa/population/publications/contraceptive2007/contraceptive_2007_table.pdf. Accessed June 1, 2017.

U.S. Food and Drug Administration: Drug approval package. Mifeprex (Mifepristone) NDA#20687. June 18, 2001. Available at: https://www.accessdata.fda.gov/drugsatfda_docs/nda/2000/20687_mifepristone.cfm. Accessed June 1, 2017.

U.S. Food and Drug Administration: Pregnancy and Lactation Labeling (Drugs) Final Rule. December 3, 2014. Available at: https://www.fda.gov/drugs/developmentapprovalprocess/developmentresources/labeling/ucm093307.htm. Accessed October 4, 2017.

U.S. Food and Drug Administration: Mifeprex (mifepristone) information. March 30, 2016a. Available at: https://www.fda.gov/Drugs/DrugSafety/ucm111323.htm. Accessed June 1, 2017.

U.S. Food and Drug Administration: Plan B (0.75 mg levonorgestrel) and plan B one-step (1.5 mg levonorgestrel) tablets information. May 2016b. Available at: http://www.fda.gov/Drugs/DrugSafety/PostmarketDrugSafetyInformationforPatientsandProviders/UCM109775. Accessed June 1, 2017.

van Ravesteyn LM, Lambregtse-van den Berg MP, Hoogendijk WJ, et al: Interventions to treat mental disorders during pregnancy: a systematic review and multiple treatment meta-analysis. PLoS One 12(3):e0173397, 2017 28358808

Vasudevan C, Levene M: Epidemiology and aetiology of neonatal seizures. Semin Fetal Neonatal Med 18(4):185–191, 2013 23746578

Velten J, Scholten S, Graham CA, et al: Unprotected intercourse and one-night stands: impact of sexual excitation, sexual inhibition, and atypical sexual arousal patterns on risky sexual behaviors in women. J Sex Med 13:361–373, 2016 26803457

Vieira da Silva Magalhães P, Kapczinski F, Kauer-Sant'Anna M: Use of contraceptive methods among women treated for bipolar disorder. Arch Women Ment Health 12(3):183–185, 2009 19277844

Vigod SN, Stewart DE: Major depression in female urinary incontinence. Psychosomatics 47(2):147–151, 2006 16508027

Vigod SN, Stewart DE: Treatment patterns in Canadian women with urinary incontinence: a need to improve case identification. J Womens Health (Larchmt) 16(5):707–712, 2007 17627406

Vigod SN, Ross LE: Epidemiology of psychotic symptoms during pregnancy and postpartum in women with schizophrenia. Curr Womens Health Rev 6:17–21, 2010

Vigod SN, Seeman MV, Ray JG, et al: Temporal trends in general and age-specific fertility rates among women with schizophrenia (1996–2009): a population-based study in Ontario, Canada. Schizophr Res 139(1–3):169–175, 2012 22658526

Vigod SN, Kurdyak PA, Dennis CL, et al: Maternal and newborn outcomes among women with schizophrenia: a retrospective population-based cohort study. BJOG 121(5):566–574, 2014 24443970

Vigod SN, Wilson CA, Howard LM: Depression in pregnancy. BMJ 352:i1547, 2016 27013603

Viguera AC, Newport DJ, Ritchie J, et al: Lithium in breast milk and nursing infants: clinical implications. Am J Psychiatry 164(2):342–345, 2007a 17267800

Viguera AC, Whitfield T, Baldessarini RJ, et al: Risk of recurrence in women with bipolar disorder during pregnancy: prospective study of mood stabilizer discontinuation. Am J Psychiatry 164(12):1817–1824; quiz 1923, 2007b 1805636

Viguera AC, Tondo L, Koukopoulos AE, et al: Episodes of mood disorders in 2,252 pregnancies and postpartum periods. Am J Psychiatry 168(11):1179–1185, 2011 21799064

Volgsten H, Skoog Svanberg A, Ekselius L, et al: Prevalence of psychiatric disorders in infertile women and men undergoing in vitro fertilization treatment. Hum Reprod 23(9):2056–2063, 2008 18583334

Volgsten H, Skoog Svanberg A, Ekselius L, et al: Risk factors for psychiatric disorders in infertile women and men undergoing in vitro fertilization treatment. Fertil Steril 93(4):1088–1096, 2010 19118826

Walker MC, Murphy KE, Pan S, et al: Adverse maternal outcomes in multifetal pregnancies. BJOG 111(11):1294–1296, 2004 15521878

Wariso BA, Guerrieri GM, Thompson K, et al: Depression during the menopause transition: impact on quality of life, social adjustment, and disability. Arch Women Ment Health 20(2):273–282, 2017 28000061

Warnock JK, Bundren JC, Morris DW: Depressive mood symptoms associated with ovarian suppression. Fertil Steril 74(5):984–986, 2000 11056245

Weijenborg PTM, Greeven A, Dekker FW, et al: Clinical course of chronic pelvic pain in women. Pain 132 (suppl 1):S117–S123, 2007 17689866

Wessel J, Gauruder-Burmester A, Gerlinger C: Denial of pregnancy—characteristics of women at risk. Acta Obstet Gynecol Scand 86(5):542–546, 2007 17464581

Wesseloo R, Kamperman AM, Munk-Olsen T, et al: Risk of postpartum relapse in bipolar disorder and postpartum psychosis: a systematic review and meta-analysis. Am J Psychiatry 173(2):117–127, 2016 26514657

Westhoff C, Picardo L, Morrow E: Quality of life following early medical or surgical abortion. Contraception 67(1):41–47, 2003 12521657

Whitaker AK, Gilliam M: Contraceptive care for adolescents. Clin Obstet Gynecol 51(2):268–280, 2008 18463458

Wisner KL, Parry BL, Piontek CM: Clinical practice. Postpartum depression. N Engl J Med 347(3):194–199, 2002 12124409

World Health Organization: Media centre: Emergency contraception (fact sheet). Updated June 2017a. Available at: http://www.who.int/mediacentre/factsheets/fs244/en/. Accessed June 1, 2017.

World Health Organization: Sexual and reproductive health: infertility definitions and terminology. 2017b. Available at: http://www.who.int/reproductivehealth/topics/infertility/definitions/en/. Accessed June 1, 2017.

Wright JD, Herzog TJ, Tsui J, et al: Nationwide trends in the performance of inpatient hysterectomy in the United States. Obstet Gynecol 122(2 Pt 1):233–241, 2013 23969789

Yeung PP Jr, Shwayder J, Pasic RP: Laparoscopic management of endometriosis: comprehensive review of best evidence. J Minim Invasive Gynecol 16(3):269–281, 2009 19423059

Yonkers KA, Wisner KL, Stowe Z, et al: Management of bipolar disorder during pregnancy and the postpartum period. Am J Psychiatry 161(4):608–620, 2004 15056503

Yonkers KA, Gotman N, Smith MV, et al: Does antidepressant use attenuate the risk of a major depressive episode in pregnancy? Epidemiology 22(6):848–854, 2011 21900825

Zabin LS, Hirsch MB, Emerson MR: When urban adolescents choose abortion: effects on education, psychological status and subsequent pregnancy. Fam Plann Perspect 21(6):248–255, 1989 2620716

Zaers S, Waschke M, Ehlert U: Depressive symptoms and symptoms of post-traumatic stress disorder in women after childbirth. J Psychosom Obstet Gynaecol 29(1):61–71, 2008 18266166

Zlotogora J: Parental decisions to abort or continue a pregnancy with an abnormal finding after an invasive prenatal test. Prenat Diagn 22(12):1102–1106, 2002 12454966

Zondervan KT, Yudkin PL, Vessey MP, et al: Patterns of diagnosis and referral in women consulting for chronic pelvic pain in UK primary care. Br J Obstet Gynaecol 106(11):1156–1161, 1999 10549960

CHAPTER 32

Pediatrics

Natacha D. Emerson, Ph.D.

Brenda Bursch, Ph.D.

Margaret L. Stuber, M.D.

In this chapter, we provide a brief overview of the major issues in psychiatric or psychological consultation to pediatrics. Many of the issues addressed in pediatrics are similar to those seen with adults. However, because the relative importance of development and of the family is sufficiently different in pediatrics, these issues should be considered at the start of any evaluation, and they infuse every intervention and recommendation.

General Principles in Evaluation and Management

Children's Developmental Understanding of Illness and Their Bodies

Children's conceptions about their bodies vary widely and are influenced by their experiences. However, in general, children appear to follow a developmental path of understanding their bodies that roughly corresponds to Piaget's stages of cognitive development. *Sensorimotor children* (birth to approximately 2 years) are largely preverbal and do not have the capacity to create narratives to explain their experiences. Their perception of their body and of illness is therefore primarily built on sensory experiences and does not involve any formal reasoning. *Preoperational children* (approximately 2–7 years) also understand through perception, but they are able to use words and some very basic concepts of cause and effect. They tend to be most aware of parts of the body that they can directly sense, such as bones and heart (which they can feel) and blood (which they have seen come out of their bodies). However, they do not have a clear sense of cause and effect and are therefore inclined to see events that are temporally related as causally related. They also have no real sense of organs but conceptualize blood and food as going into or coming out of their body as though the body were itself the container. This leads to many humorous but confusing assumptions and misunderstandings. *Concrete operational children* (approximately 7–11 years) are able to apply logic to their perceptions in a more integrative manner. However, the logic is quite literal or concrete and allows for only one cause for an effect. They tend to be eager to learn factual information about the body and illness but will have difficulty with any concepts that require abstract reasoning. *Formal operational children* (≥11 years) are able to use a level of abstract reasoning that allows discussion of systems rather than simple organs and can incorporate multiple causations of illness. It should not be assumed, however, that all adolescents approach the understanding of illness and their body at this level of cognition. In fact, most adults function at this level of thought only in areas of their own expertise, if at all.

As with all areas of cognition, education and experience make a difference. Children who have a medical problem (or who have a friend or family member with a medical history) may know more about the body and its functioning than do other children. However, children also will often be able to repeat what they hear without any real understanding of what it means. It is always important to assess children's level of understanding by asking them to explain in their own words or give their own version of why something is happening. This can alert providers to misunderstandings or fears that could influence adherence to treatment.

Family Systems

No pediatric patient can be considered in isolation from his or her family. Parents are the legal decision makers for the child and thus are involved in all aspects of care. Children look to their parents to understand the world. It is partially from their reactions to the illness and treatment that the child determines how dangerous the illness is and how to respond (Cousino and Hazen 2013). Given that heightened parental stress has been shown to predict poorer psychological adjustment in children with chronic illness (Cousino and Hazen 2013), addressing parental fear, helplessness, anger, or withdrawal is also helpful for their children.

Psychiatric Issues

Psychological Responses to Illness

Overview

Chronic illness in childhood is associated with a greater risk of emotional problems that can extend into adulthood (Secinti et al. 2017). Thus, the effective prevention or treatment of the emotional sequelae of childhood illness can have long-term benefits. For example, 20%–50% of pediatric solid transplant recipients experience significant psychological distress (Annunziato et al. 2012). Likewise, children with seizure disorders have been found to be at significantly higher risk of developing depression than normative peers, with prevalence estimates ranging from 12% to 40%, depending on diagnostic tool and demographic covariates (Reilly et al. 2011). Even children undergoing a surgical procedure as minor as a tonsillectomy may be at risk of distress. A study by Broekman et al. (2010) found that patients scheduled for such procedures had more behavioral and emotional problems than normative peers before their appointments, and up to one-quarter of children experienced an exacerbation of these psychological symptoms after the surgery, indicating that even isolated, routine conditions and treatments may place children at risk for lower well-being. Finally, the effects of pediatric illness may also be delayed. Subgroups of childhood cancer survivors have been found to have both chronic psychological distress and "sleeper effect" increases in psychological symptoms decades after the initial diagnosis (Brinkman et al. 2013).

An area of increasing clinical focus is illness- or treatment-related (iatrogenic) posttraumatic stress symptoms in children who undergo medical procedures and/or have life-threatening conditions. Several risk factors have been identified as increasing vulnerability for iatrogenic medical trauma symptoms. Davydow et al. (2010) found that premorbid psychopathology, female gender, younger age, developmental problems, and maternal negative life events increased the risk of psychiatric problems in pediatric survivors of critical illnesses. Other studies have highlighted the importance of peritraumatic factors as well. Having psychological or behavioral problems at the time of the trauma, a higher heart rate, and beliefs about the trauma being serious or life-threatening all increased the risk of initial symptom development (Brosbe et al. 2011). Once these preliminary symptoms developed, children's beliefs about their symptoms, use of thought suppression as a coping technique, and previous parental posttraumatic stress disorder (PTSD) further predisposed youth to developing acute stress disorder (Brosbe et al. 2011). While many of these cases focus on acute trauma reactions rather than full-fledged PTSD, these peritraumatic symptoms appear to predict decrements in functioning, quality of life (QoL), and psychological well-being well into adulthood (Agorastos et al. 2014).

Parents of children who are critically ill may be especially vulnerable to posttraumatic reactions. Although incidence estimates vary, rates of diagnosable PTSD in parents of children receiving intensive care may be as high as 21%, with rates of posttraumatic stress symptoms nearing 84% (Davidson et al. 2012; Nelson and Gold 2012). Lower education, previous psychopathology, unmarried status, and prior exposure to stressful life events seem to predict parental PTSD secondary to child trauma (Bronner et al. 2010; Davidson et al. 2012). Environmental factors are also important. Parents whose children's illness is unexpected or requires more acute care are at higher risk of PTSD (Davidson et al. 2012). System factors also matter, such that parents who report feeling uninformed or as though they have not received the expected help or information from medical staff are at higher risk of secondary trauma reactions (Davidson et al. 2012).

Social support appears to be a key element in psychological adjustment to illness. Pediatric patients often feel undesirably different from healthy peers; they may be bothered by their medical regimen, be disadvantaged academically due to missing school or experiencing adverse sequelae from their illness or its treatment, and be unable to participate in extracurricular activities or to benefit from the same social independence as normative peers (Compas et al. 2012; Pinquart 2013; Pinquart and Shen 2011). These vulnerabilities, which may explain some of the variance in increased risk of both depression (Pinquart and Shen 2011) and low self-esteem (Pinquart 2013), may be reduced by strengthening psychosocial support. Research on interventions aimed at reducing the psychosocial burden of chronic illness indicate that programs that integrate the family have more sustainable effects than do programs targeting the individual (Carr 2014; Janicke et al. 2014). Likewise, inclusion of a peer component in interventions for pediatric chronic illness shows promise (Distelberg et al. 2018). Support for parents of medically ill children is equally important, given that parental mental illness has been shown to negatively influence both the psychological and the physical well-being of children. One study found that children with asthma whose parents suffered from depression or anxiety had worse pulmonary function and poorer asthma control (Feldman et al. 2013; van Oers et al. 2014). Providing parents with social support, problem-solving and communication tools, and psychoeducation about the impact of illness may help reduce parental psychological distress and improve child and family well-being (van Oers et al. 2014).

In some cases, psychological distress and behavior problems can be directly caused by the illness or its treatment. For example, mood disorders and anxiety are relatively common manifestations of central nervous system (CNS) pediatric systemic lupus erythematosus (Knight et al. 2015). Attention and concentration problems have been observed as side effects of chemotherapy (Pierson et al. 2016) and of immunosuppressant drugs given after transplantation (Martínez-Sanchis et al. 2011). Preschool children with hypoglycemia may demonstrate behavioral changes such as irritability, agitation, quietness, and tantrums (Ly et al. 2014). Use of steroids for inflammatory conditions can have a significant negative effect on mood and behavior (Drozdowicz and Bostwick 2014; Miloh et al. 2017).

Screening and Prevention

Because psychological adjustment problems appear to be relatively common, it is recommended that children who are chronically ill, acutely ill, or injured be screened by pediatricians or other professionals for depression, anxiety, and behavioral disturbance (Brown and Wissow 2010). Preventive programs are indicated for some pediatric inpatient services in which anxiety and depression are common. For example, in highly painful conditions, such as pediatric burns, in which significant emotional distress is the norm, anxiety treatment is best built in along with pain management (Damanhuri and Enoch 2014). Some evidence indicates that this may help prevent development of PTSD (Birur et al. 2017). In conditions with high mortality, consistent psychosocial support should be available from the start.

Treatment Considerations

Treatment studies targeting the psychiatric symptoms of medically ill children are rare, but are increasing. Generally, treatment for anxiety that persists after normal adjustment and comfort are addressed is similar to that provided for anxiety in general psychiatric practice: cognitive-behavioral therapy (CBT) (Bennett et al. 2015; Hofmann et al. 2012; Rapp et al. 2013; Reynolds et al. 2012) and the use of selective serotonin reuptake inhibitors (SSRIs) (Strawn et al. 2015). Individual behavioral techniques, such as exposure and systematic desensitization, can be effective for patients with simple phobias such as needle phobia or food aversion. More extensive cognitive-behavioral treatment that addresses anxiety across many dimensions (including somatic, cognitive, and behavior problems) is indicated for children with complex anxiety disorders (Rapp et al. 2013). A combination of CBT and an SSRI has been shown to be more effective than a single-strategy approach (Wehry et al. 2015).

Hospitalized and chronically ill children often experience symptoms seen in depression. Depressed or irritable mood, diminished interest or pleasure in activities, significant weight loss or change in appetite, insomnia or hypersomnia, psychomotor agitation or retardation, and fatigue or loss of energy may be secondary either to the medical condition or to prolonged separation from friends and family. Careful evaluation regarding the timing and severity of such symptoms will aid the clinician in making appropriate treatment decisions. Feelings of worthlessness or inappropriate guilt, diminished ability to think or concentrate, or thoughts of suicide may indicate an intent to self-harm. Assessment of these symptoms should include inquiries about suicidal fantasies or actions, what the child thinks would happen if suicide were attempted or achieved, previous experiences with suicidal behavior, circumstances at the time of the suicidal behavior, motivations for suicide, experiences of death, and family and environmental situations. Questions should be tailored to the developmental level of the child (Caplan and Bursch 2013), and screening instruments should be validated for use with youth (Horowitz et al. 2014). Adolescents with suicidal intent and plan, family history of suicide, comorbid psychiatric disorder, intractable pain, persistent insomnia, lack of social support, inadequate coping skills, recent improvement in depressive symptoms, or impulsivity are at heightened risk of suicide (Glenn and Nock 2014; Horowitz et al. 2014).

While supportive and cognitive-behavioral interventions can lead to significant improvements in depressive symptoms (Gledhill and Hodes 2011; Hofmann et al. 2012), the combination of psychotherapy with an SSRI may prove optimal. For some adolescents, the thoughts about suicide provide an important source of control in the face of an unknown and uncontrollable illness course. Addressing the lack of perceived control, isolation, and distressing physical symptoms should be a top priority. Use of antidepressant medication in suicidal adolescents and young adults should be monitored closely, given the small chance of an increase in suicidal ideation.

In medically ill youth, citalopram, escitalopram, and sertraline should be considered as first-line in the treatment of depression. These SSRIs are efficacious and tolerable for children with complex medical problems and are the least likely SSRIs to have drug interactions (Bursch and Forgey 2013). They may also be helpful in the treatment of anxiety and iatrogenic medical trauma symptoms (Bursch and Forgey 2013). Second-line, both risperidone and quetiapine have proven to be effective for more severe anxiety and trauma symptoms (Bursch and Forgey 2013). Low dosages of benzodiazepines are frequently prescribed by pediatricians for acute anxiety and agitation in the hospital, because they can have a more immediate effect than SSRIs. However, benzodiazepines increase the risk of delirium, agitated (i.e., paradoxical) reactions, and/or posttraumatic stress symptoms, and therefore should be avoided whenever possible (Bursch and Forgey 2013). Psychiatric consultants can offer alternatives, including antipsychotics, when an immediate response is needed.

Interventions for Invasive Procedures

Consistent with the literature suggesting that avoidant coping is a major predictor of anxiety and depression in pediatric oncology patients (Compas et al. 2014; Wu et al. 2013), one area of intervention that has been extensively researched is preparation for the many invasive procedures children experience during cancer treatment. Cognitive-behavioral techniques, including imagery, relaxation, distraction, modeling, desensitization, and positive reinforcement, are well established as effective (Richter et al. 2015; Uman et al. 2013). Although all children have some distress with painful procedures, some are more sensitive to pain and have differential responses to psychological interventions for procedural distress (Racine et al. 2016). Child psychopathology, difficult temperament, previous pain events, and parent (or family) stress, temperament, reactions to child behavior, and anticipation of child distress have all been shown to predict more sensitivity to pain (Racine et al. 2016). Although multiple psychological and physical interventions have been established for reducing pain during procedures, integration of pharmacological interventions has proven useful in cases of children with severe distress (Cramton and Gruchala 2012; Neuhäuser et al. 2010). Topical anesthetic cream has been used with some success to alleviate the pain of venipuncture or the topical pain of other superficial procedures with pediatric oncology patients, if administered with sufficient time for it to become effective (M.L. Schmitz et al. 2015). Analgosedation—the combination of pain relief and sedation—is recommended over sedation alone to reduce the risk of subsequent posttraumatic symptoms (Neuhäuser et al. 2010). Interventions designed to enhance communication with pediatric cancer patients have been developed but not rigorously assessed. In general, youths with cancer may benefit from informational interventions, support related to procedures, and involvement in decision-making about their health to facilitate adjustment to illness (Coyne et al. 2016; Feenstra et al. 2014).

Adherence

The term *adherence* is generally used to describe the extent to which a patient's health behavior is consistent with medical recommendations. Defined as such, adherence includes not only taking medications and attending clinic appointments but also engaging in recommended diet, exercise, and other lifestyle behaviors such as smoking abstinence and sunscreen use (Ahmed and Aslani 2014). Adherence is a difficult construct to study and measure, given that health behaviors vary across medical conditions and illness severity levels. Variables known to moderate adherence include self-efficacy, degree of concordance between patient and provider, and culturally mediated differences in the understanding of an illness's cause, course, and treatment (Ahmed and Aslani 2014). Overall, chronic illness literature estimates that at least 50% of pediatric patients are nonadherent to their prescribed treatment regimen (Duncan et al. 2014). Nonadherence is linked to increased health care spending, emergency room visits, hospitalizations, exacerbations in morbidity, and premature mortality (McGrady and Hommel 2013; Oliva et al. 2013; Simon et al. 2011).

Predictors of nonadherence include age, socioeconomic status, length and complexity of treatment, miscommunication between families and physicians, and family factors such as daily stress and parental beliefs about the illness (Dawood et al. 2010). Paralleling recognized racial disparities in access to and use of health care, ethnic disparities in adherence and adherence-related prognosis have been established (Connelly et al. 2015; Shemesh et al. 2014). Discordant beliefs held by families and doctors about an illness's cause and its proper treatment appear to be more important than health literacy when examining adherence (Ahmed and Aslani 2014). Based on studies in adults, parents' sense of trust in physicians and their beliefs about doctors' cultural competence may predict adherence (Gaston 2013; Jones et al. 2012; Wall et al.

2013). Finally, comorbid psychopathology is associated with nonadherence across many pediatric patient populations, including youth with asthma, diabetes, organ transplants, and inflammatory bowel disease (Bitsko et al. 2014; Butwicka et al. 2016; Delamater et al. 2014; Gray et al. 2012; Kahana et al. 2008b; McCormick King et al. 2014).

Approaches used to increase adherence among pediatric patients and their families generally fall into three categories: 1) educational (written and verbal instructions), 2) organizational (simplification of regimens, improved access, increased supervision), and 3) behavioral (reminders, incentives, and self-monitoring) (Graves et al. 2010). In a meta-analysis of 70 studies examining psychological interventions for chronically ill youths, Kahana et al. (2008a) found medium effect sizes for behavioral and multiple-strategy interventions and a small effect size for education alone. One interesting study found that treating liver transplant recipients for PTSD improved their adherence to medication (Shemesh et al. 2000). Since the Kahana et al. (2008a) meta-analysis, subsequent studies that have used multicomponent approaches to target adherence (i.e., using both educational and behavioral strategies) have continued to show higher success rates and larger effect sizes than ones that used only one approach to target noncompliance (Duncan et al. 2014; Graves et al. 2010). Relatedly, a second meta-analysis of interventions for children with chronic illness concluded that successful intervention programs not only increased adherence but also improved health outcomes longitudinally (Graves et al. 2010).

Death, Dying, and Bereavement

One of the most emotionally difficult issues for anyone to cope with is the death of a child (van der Geest et al. 2014). Because of the tremendous advances in medicine and the seeming unfairness of death in childhood, pediatricians and families often resist making the transition from an emphasis on cure to a focus on comfort care. The psychiatric consultant may be called when disagreement occurs within the team or between the team and the child and/or family about whether this point has been reached or about how this transition is to be approached. Sometimes these differences are the result of cultural or philosophical differences. Clinicians who believe that life is to be pursued at all costs may have trouble understanding the feelings of other clinicians who feel that the child is being needlessly subjected to painful interventions. Families who are deeply religious and remain hopeful for a miracle may lead the medical team to request a psychiatric consult to address the family's "denial." Family members who wish to protect the child may feel that it is best to withhold information about disease prognosis or other potentially upsetting information. A dying child or adolescent might wish to be sedated to feel comfortable, whereas the family may want him or her to remain alert; or vice versa. The psychiatric consultant can facilitate these often highly emotionally charged discussions to allow all involved to understand one another well enough to plan together for the care of the child.

A variety of emotional responses may be seen in terminally ill children and should be anticipated in conversations with parents. Children and adolescents may manifest confusion and loss with negative, oppositional, aggressive, or emotional acting out, or with apathy and withdrawal from family and friends. They may talk about death or carry on conversations with someone who has died or with God. They may seem to know when they are going to die or "take a trip." What may initially appear to be confusion or delirium may actually be an attempt to communicate through a metaphor (Callanan and Kelley 2012). The consultant should encourage such conversations and support the staff and parents to help them tolerate these attempts of the child to cope with the process of dying. Play therapy or art therapy may be particularly helpful for younger children and for older children who prefer nonverbal modalities. In some cases, children will choose to address unfinished business, such as saying good-bye, making amends, being absolved of perceived transgressions, planning their memorial service, or deciding who gets particular belongings (Judd 2014). One study in parents of children who died of cancer found that both dying children and their parents benefited from a family-centered approach to advance care planning that included tools to help patients express their fears, hopes, and final preferences and to help parents initiate difficult discussions about prognosis, expectations, and treatment discontinuation (Lyon et al. 2013). Helping parents have such discussions may also improve the long-term well-being of bereaved parents by helping to reduce the guilt and regret that parents often report after their child dies (Goldman et al. 2012). Another study found that parents who gave higher ratings related to continuity of care and communication with the medical team reported lower levels of long-term parental grief after their child died (van der Geest et al. 2014).

Environmental interventions can relieve many physical discomforts. Interventions to improve communication and understanding can relieve many emotional discomforts and fears. If such interventions are not sufficient to resolve distressing symptoms, medications should be considered. It is important to recognize that children and parents vary in their preferences for sedation and tolerance of symptoms. For a more thorough review of emotional and physical symptom management, see the chapter by Forgey and Bursch (2014) and the book by Marcdante and Kliegman (2015). For a more thorough review on the topic of talking to children about death, refer to the chapter by Caplan and Bursch (2013).

Finally, careful preparation and support are necessary if a family is to take a child home to die. Many palliative interventions for symptom management can be initiated well before a transition to hospice care is considered. While it is sometimes best for the child to die at home, some families do not feel that such a plan would be best for the child and/or for other family members. Parents typically need emotional and technical support as well as respite services. Siblings will need age-appropriate information and emotional support.

Psychiatric Disorders

Delirium

Pediatric delirium (see Chapter 4, "Delirium") has received little clinical and research attention compared with adult delirium (Schieveld and Janssen 2014; Smith et al. 2011, 2013). It is estimated that at least 30% of critically ill children experience delirium (Smith et al. 2013), although this may be an underestimation given that hypoactive delirium is commonly underdiagnosed (Smith et al. 2011). As in adults, critically ill children can develop delirium with hyperactive, hypoactive, mixed, or veiled presentations (Bursch and Forgey 2013; Smith et al. 2013). Across the life span, delirium may sometimes present with psychotic symptoms (Smith et al. 2013). Several features, however, are considered unique or more common to pediatric populations, including labile affect, inconsolability, signs of autonomic dysregulation, and purposeless actions (Smith et al. 2013). Given the wide range of symptoms and presentations in pediatric delirium, reasons for psychiatric consultation requests can vary widely, from agitation and oppositionality to unexplained lethargy, depression, or confusion.

Failure to recognize pediatric delirium may have important repercussions. Although outcome studies in children are sparse, studies in adults have found that delirium independently predicts prolonged mechanical ventilation, longer hospitalizations, and higher mortality, as well as cognitive impairment (Smith et al. 2011; Traube et al. 2017). Research has also shown that children with delirium may fare worse than adults (Smith et al. 2013) and that children with hypoactive delirium may have poorer prognoses than children with other delirium types (Smith et al. 2011).

Some pediatric intensive care units (ICUs) have recently begun initiatives to conduct universal delirium screening (Simone et al. 2017). Both the Pediatric Confusion Assessment Method for the ICU (pCAM-ICU; Smith et al. 2011) and the Cornell Assessment of Pediatric Delirium (CAP-D; Silver et al. 2012) have been validated in inpatient medical settings and show good specificity and sensitivity (Smith et al. 2013). The CAP-D may be especially helpful for use in detecting hypoactive delirium and for use in young and/or developmentally delayed children (Schieveld and Janssen 2014; Smith et al. 2013). Given that both of these screening tools rely on examiner observation and interactions with the patient, supplemental chart review is also recommended.

Support and orienting cues by nursing staff and family members can be helpful in reducing the fear and confusion (Turkel and Hanft 2014). These include the presence of familiar objects, photographs, and people who can reassure and orient the child, as well as age-appropriate clocks, calendars, or signs. Education can help the parents understand what is happening, reduce their distress, and help them to respond supportively to the child rather than with irritation or fear. Treatment with atypical antipsychotics appears to be safe and effective (Herrera and Falcone 2015; Joyce et al. 2015; Turkel et al. 2012). Turkel and Hanft (2014) recommend using olanzapine (given its oral disintegrating tablet form), risperidone (for younger patients, since the drug can be given in very small doses and also comes in multiple forms), or quetiapine (for delirium with insomnia). Of note, avoiding or weaning off benzodiazepines is recommended, as this class of drugs appears to exacerbate delirium (Herrera and Falcone 2015; Schieveld and Janssen 2014; Vet et al. 2016) and to increase the risk of subsequent PTSD (Forgey and Bursch 2013).

Delirium risk may be further attenuated through regulation of sleep (Herrera and Falcone 2015). Melatonin, given its effectiveness and benign side-effect profile, may be considered for regulating the sleep–wake cycle in children (Herrera and Falcone 2015). Behavioral interventions aimed at establishing and maintaining diurnal routines so as to minimize insomnia-related delirium exacerbations are also recommended (Turkel et al. 2012). Finally, a number of drugs (dexmedetomidine, ketamine, clonidine, and propofol) have shown promise in reducing the likelihood of delirium emergence postoperatively, although more research is needed to establish the safety and efficacy profiles of these drugs in critically ill youth (Herrera and Falcone 2015).

Factitious Disorders

Illness Falsification

Factitious disorders are defined as the intentional falsification of physical or psychological signs or symptoms to satisfy a psychological need. *Factitious disorder imposed on self* refers to self-directed falsification behaviors, and *factitious disorder imposed on another* refers to falsification behaviors directed at another human or animal. *Malingering* denotes the intentional falsification of one's own physical or psychological signs or symptoms to achieve external gain or to avoid unwanted responsibilities or outcomes. Illness falsification can include exaggeration, fabrication, simulation, and induction. Exaggeration is embellishment of a true symptom or problem. Fabrications are false statements about the medical history or symptoms. Simulation can include the alteration of records, medical test procedures, or symptoms to incorrectly suggest a problem. Induction involves directly causing a problem or worsening a preexisting problem.

Little research has been conducted on the topic of illness falsification behaviors exhibited by children and adolescents (see Chapter 12, "Deception Syndromes: Factitious Disorders and Malingering"). The literature suggests that adult factitious disorder may have origins in childhood for some individuals (Libow 2002), and that some children and adolescents who falsify illness in themselves may have had earlier experiences as a victim of illness falsification or as a recipient of caregiver reinforcement for illness falsification. The child victim experience, including feelings of powerlessness, chronic lack of control, and disappointment in the medical care system, is a possible dynamic in the future development of illness falsification.

The Libow (2000) literature review of cases of child and adolescent patients who falsified illness identified 42 published cases, in which the mean age of patients was 13.9 years (range: 8–18 years). Most patients were female (71%), with the gender imbalance greater among older children. Patients engaged in false symptom reporting and induction, including self-inflicted injections, bruising, and ingestions. The most commonly falsified conditions were fevers, ketoacidosis, purpura, and infections. The average duration of the falsifications before detection was about 16 months. Many patients admitted to their deceptions when confronted, and some had positive outcomes at follow-up. The children were described as bland, depressed, and fascinated with health care.

Child Victims of Illness Falsification Imposed on Another

Child victims of illness falsification can experience significant psychological problems during childhood, including feelings of helplessness, self-doubt, and poor self-esteem; self-destructive ideation; eating disorders; behavioral growth problems; nightmares; and school concentration problems (Bools et al. 1993; Libow 1995; Porter et al. 1994). Adult survivors describe emotional difficulties, including suicidal feelings, anxiety, depression, low self-esteem, intense rage reactions, and PTSD symptoms (Libow 1995).

Ayoub (2002) presented longitudinal data on a sample of 40 children found by courts to be victims of illness falsification. The findings indicated that child victims frequently develop serious psychiatric symptoms that vary depending on the child's developmental age, the length and intensity of the child's exposure, and the current degree of protection and support. She found that PTSD and oppositional disorders are significant sequelae, as are patterns of reality distortion, poor self-esteem, and attachment difficulties. Although these children can superficially appear socially skilled and well adjusted, they often struggle with basic relationships. Lying is common, as is manipulative illness behavior and sadistic behavior toward other children. Many remain trauma-reactive and experience cyclical anger, depression, and oppositionality. Children who fared best were separated from their biological parents and remained in a single protected placement or had an abuser who admitted to the abuse and worked over a period of years toward reunification (Ayoub 2002).

In terms of treatment for victims of illness falsification, efforts should be made to normalize the child's life as much as possible, including health, socialization, activities of daily living, and school attendance. Worrisome psychiatric or behavioral symptoms, both internalizing and externalizing, should be addressed using evidence-based approaches. Additionally, youth should be supported in their efforts to understand and grieve their past as they are confronted with the reality of improved health.

Feeding Disorders

Food Refusal, Selectivity, and Phobias

Feeding problems and eating disturbances in toddlers and young school-age children are common (see also Chapter 13, "Eating Disorders"); their prevalence is estimated as 25%–45% in typically developing children and as high as 80% in children with developmental disabilities (Bryant-Waugh et al. 2010). Most of these disturbances are transient and can be easily addressed with parent training, education about nutrition or normal child development, child–caregiver interaction advice, and suggestions for food preparation and presentation. However, severe eating disturbances requiring more aggressive treatment occur in 3%–10% of young children and are most common in children with other physical or developmental problems (Sharp et al. 2010). These children are at risk of aspiration, malnutrition, invasive medical procedures, hospitalizations, limitations in normal functioning and development, liver failure, and death. In fact, 1%–5% of pediatric hospitalizations are attributed to failure to thrive (Nationwide Children's Hospital 2017; also see section "Failure to Thrive" below). The most recent DSM introduced a new diagnosis, avoidant/restrictive food intake disorder, defined as a maladaptive eating or feeding pattern (not attributable to a concurrent medical condition or traditional eating disorder) that results in significant concerns including weight loss, impaired growth or nutritional deficiency, dependence on enteral feeding or nutritional supplements, or interference with psychosocial functioning (American Psychiatric Association 2013).

Physical factors that can impair normal eating include anatomical abnormalities, sensory perceptual impairments, oral motor dysfunction, and chronic medical problems (e.g., reflux, short gut syndrome, inflammatory bowel disease, hepatic or pancreatic disease, cancer). Other contributing factors can include the pairing of eating with an aversive experience (posttraumatic feeding disorders), inadvertent caregiver reinforcement of progressively more selective food choices, or a lack of normal early feeding experiences. As many as 80% of feeding problems are considered to have a significant behavioral component (Bryant-Waugh et al. 2010; Sharp et al. 2010).

Feeding disorders can be classified into three categories: eating too little, eating a restricted number of foods (e.g., picky eating), and displaying a fear of eating (e.g., phobia of novel foods or fear of the sensations associated with feeding) (Kerzner et al. 2015). In regard to the latter, feeding-associated phobias can be assessed via interview and/or by observing fear or anxiety behaviors on food presentation (Kerzner et al. 2015). Treatment goals for such cases are centered on reducing anxiety in both patient and feeder through reassurance and through appraisal and treatment of causes of discomfort (Kerzner et al. 2015). Munk and Repp (1994) developed methods for assessing feeding problems in individuals with severe cognitive and physical disabilities that allow categorization of individual feeding patterns based on responses to repeated presentation of food.

In regard to interventions for eating problems not caused by anxiety disorders, research on feeding disorder treatments is difficult to synthesize because of differing methodologies, lack of comparison groups, and discrepancies in type and length of treatment (Lukens and Silverman 2014). Whenever possible, treatment should be multidisciplinary and should incorporate behavioral techniques. Behaviorally focused treatment provided in inpatient or day treatment settings show the best outcomes (Lukens and Silverman 2014). Moreover, although behavioral observation of a meal in clinic has long been considered the gold standard of feeding assessment, some have argued that this approach is 1) not consistently feasible given the time needed for such an observation, and 2) not necessarily generalizable to the home environment in which the majority of feeding occurs (Sharp et al. 2013). In general, food aversion and oral motor dysfunction can be treated by a skilled mental health care clinician, speech pathologist, or occupational therapist. Effective behavioral interventions include contingency management with positive reinforcement for appropriate feeding and ignoring or guiding for inappropriate responses. Desensitization techniques can be effectively used to address phobias or altered sensory processing. Although no research has directly examined the use of psychotropic medications in treating food refusal, selectivity, or phobias, it may be valuable to consider use of such medications in children with eating disturbances associated with anxiety disorders.

Failure to Thrive

Children whose current weight or rate of weight gain is significantly below that of other children of similar age and sex are diagnosed with failure to thrive (FTT). Although FTT is generally categorized as resulting from either organic (medical) or nonorganic (relational) causes, it is helpful to think of FTT as a presenting symptom with varied and potentially multiple biopsychosocial causes, especially given that a clear etiology is absent in the majority of cases (Cole and Lanham 2011). For instance, parents might have a poor understanding of feeding techniques or might improperly prepare formula; mothers may also have an inadequate supply of breast milk. Biological contributors to FTT include defects in food assimilation, excessive loss of ingested calories, increased energy requirements, and prenatal insults; environmental contributors include economic or emotional deprivation.

Cole and Lanham (2011) recommend classifying FTT into three categories: inadequate caloric intake, inadequate caloric absorption, and excessive caloric expenditure. Most cases of FTT fall into the category of inadequate caloric intake and are thought to be highly influenced by family factors, including unresponsive parenting or caregiving (Black and Aboud 2011), inadequate knowledge about feeding and nutrition, and financial difficulties (Cole and Lanham 2011). In fact, Black and Aboud's (2011) review of parenting differences in FTT revealed that strained parent–child relationships may explain much of the variance in this problematic feeding dynamic. Unresponsive parenting/caregiving is characterized by a lack of reciprocity between feeder and eater due to controlling caregiver behaviors (controlling/pressuring), controlling eater behavior (indulgence), or lack of reciprocity owing to emotional detachment between the two parties. A disturbed feeding dynamic may have long-lasting consequences because it can further derail the attachment relationship between parent and child and subsequently disrupt the child's hunger cues and his or her developing sense of competence and autonomy (Black and Aboud 2011). Given the likelihood of a fractured bond between parent and child and the increased likelihood that children with FTT are abused, child neglect and abuse must always be part of the FTT assessment (Cole and Lanham 2011).

Recent research has expanded its focus to include psychosocial factors other than disturbed family dynamics. For example, parents who lack proper education about parenting and child development and who are under significant stress, characteristics that are overrepresented in low-income samples, are at increased risk of having a child with FTT (Black and Aboud 2011). Other psychosocial contributors to FTT may include consumption of a particular food in excess (e.g., food fads) or parent anxiety inadvertently leading to FTT. Classic teaching has been that etiology can be determined by the child's ability to gain weight in the hospital, with a psychosocial etiology presumed if the child gains weight under these conditions. However, some FTT children who have an inadequate caregiver will still lose weight in the hospital if they are separated from the caregiver or otherwise stressed by the hospitalization. Longitudinal studies of former FTT children reveal an increased risk of learning or behavioral difficulties and deficits in IQ (Jaffe 2011). However, these studies have historically examined the most severely affected children and therefore those likeliest to also suffer from negative consequences (Jaffe 2011).

The goal of treatment is to provide the medical, psychiatric, social, and environmental resources needed to promote satisfactory growth and reduce risk factors that increase the likelihood of weight faltering (Black et al. 2016; Cole and Lanham 2011). Given the breadth of systems to target, a multidisciplinary approach to treatment is recommended. Children with feeding skills deficits or maladaptive behavior related to food are likely to benefit from behavioral interventions. Primary caregivers might require specific psychiatric assessment and treatment. Interventions targeting the child–parent relationship, sometimes including in-home intervention, can be effective for selected families (Black et al. 2016). Interventions targeting the socioeconomic burdens of the family can be critical. In some cases of inadequate parenting, foster care is required while the parent receives needed financial assistance, parent training and/or psychiatric care. In such cases, the return to home should be closely monitored and based on the parents' demonstrated ability and resources to care adequately for their child.

Pica

Pica is defined as eating nonnutritious, nonfood substances on a regular basis (over a period of at least 1 month) (Hartmann et al. 2012). It is most frequently comorbid with the psychiatric diagnoses of intellectual development disorder, autism spectrum disorder, obsessive-compulsive and related disorders, and schizophrenia (Hartmann et al. 2012); it is also commonly seen in children with zinc or iron deficiencies (O'Callaghan and Gold 2012; Paoletti et al. 2014). Pica can also be associated with trichotillomania and with excoriation disorder, typically with the hair or skin ingested (Frey et al. 2005). Pica has a high prevalence in children with sickle cell disease, with preliminary studies suggesting that 30%–55% engage in this behavior (Ivascu et al. 2001; Lemanek et al. 2002), most often those who are younger and have lower hemoglobin levels (Aloni et al. 2015).

Mouthing and occasional eating of nonnutritious, nonfood substances are considered normal in children younger than 3 years. Young children with pica are most likely to eat sand, bugs, paint, plaster, paper, or other items within reach. Adolescents are more likely to eat clay, soil, paper, or similar substances. Pica can be a conditioned behavior, an indication of distress or environmental neglect, or evidence of a vitamin or mineral deficiency.

Children with pica often go undiagnosed until ingestion requires medical treatment (Kelly et al. 2014). Although research on psychosocial correlates of pica is rare, family factors are thought to be important to the development and maintenance of the disorder (O'Callaghan and Gold 2012), and one case report has linked the disorder to self-harm (Žganjer et al. 2011). Medical assessment includes screening for ingestion of toxic substances and evaluation for possible nutritional deficits. Children with pica are at increased risk of elevated lead levels. An evaluation and treatment plan to reduce psychosocial stress are also clearly important.

Rumination

Rumination refers to the effortless regurgitation of recently ingested food into the mouth. The behavior, which can be voluntary or involuntary, may develop as a conditioned response after an illness, present as a sign of general distress, or develop as a form of self-stimulation or self-soothing. It is most commonly seen in infants and the developmentally disabled but also occurs in children and adolescents with otherwise normal functioning (Kessing et al. 2014).

Individuals who engage in rumination may go years without diagnosis and can be misdiagnosed as having bulimia nervosa, gastroesophageal reflux disease, or upper gastrointestinal motility disorders such as gastroparesis (Rajindrajith et al. 2012). They may also undergo extensive, costly, and invasive medical testing before diagnosis. Complications most often include dental erosions, halitosis, weight loss, bloating, abdominal pain, and electrolyte disturbances (Rajindrajith et al. 2012). A large percentage of pediatric patients have comorbid physical and/or psychological problems, with significant disability (Rajindrajith et al. 2012). Youth who engage in rumination behaviors are more likely to be described as perfectionistic and are at higher risk of developing depression and anxiety (Kelly et al. 2014). There is also overlap with bulimia nervosa, although patients with bulimia do not re-swallow food, and their purging behavior is self-induced rather than spontaneous (Hyams et al. 2016).

Rumination syndrome is a clinical diagnosis based on symptoms that (following appropriate medical evaluation) cannot be attributed to another medical condition or to an eating disorder (Hyams et al. 2016). Rumination is most often diagnosed by clinical interview. Patients of age to self-report symptoms generally indicate that symptoms start effortlessly, during or shortly after meals, sans nausea, and the regurgitation taste is often described as pleasant (Kessing et al. 2014). If patients or families are unable to self-disclose symptoms to make the diagnosis, antroduodenal manometric evaluation demonstrating the typical R-wave pattern during regurgitation after meals may aid in confirming the diagnosis (Green et al. 2011).

In cases of rumination associated with environmental neglect, the primary caregiver–child relationship and possible psychiatric disturbance in the primary caregiver should be evaluated and addressed. In regard to treatment, although experimental trials are lacking, explanation of the syndrome and its mechanisms by an experienced clinician is warranted (Kessing et al. 2014). Habit reversal using diaphragmatic breathing or chewing gum as the competing response may also be effective in older children and adolescents (Chial et al. 2003). In one study of 54 adolescents who were followed up 10 months after treatment, provision of supportive therapy and diaphragmatic breathing resulted in improvement in 56% of cases and complete cessation of the behavior in an additional 30% (Chial et al. 2003). In cases of severe rumination syndrome, in which patients may be at risk of dehydration and malnutrition, enteral tube feedings or parenteral nutrition are sometimes employed. As an alternative to this invasive approach, Green et al. (2011) have proposed that patients with severe rumination should be treated as inpatients by a multidisciplinary team using a behavioral approach (Green et al. 2011). Rumination in the presence of other psychosocial problems or psychiatric disorders in the child or primary caregiver may require additional therapeutic interventions.

Autism Spectrum Disorder

Autism spectrum disorder (ASD) encompasses neurodevelopmental disorders characterized by social communication deficits and restricted and repetitive behaviors and interests (American Psychiatric Association 2013; Volkmar et al. 2014). Given the prevalence of and comorbidities associated with ASD, along with the additional coping challenges faced by these patients, one would expect to regularly encounter pediatric inpatients with ASD or ASD traits. ASD may be associated with known genetic conditions (e.g., fragile X syndrome, Rett syndrome), learning disorders and intellectual disabilities, and psychiatric comorbidities such as attention-deficit/hyperactivity disorder (ADHD) and anxiety (American Psychiatric Association 2013; Levy et al. 2010; Volkmar et al. 2014). The steep rise in prevalence of ASD, including a 78% surge in ASD diagnoses between the years 2002 and 2008 (Centers for Disease Control and Prevention 2014b), further increases the likelihood that ASD will be encountered in pediatric practice. The Centers for Disease Control and Prevention (CDC) estimated that 1 in 68 children, and 1 in every 42 boys, has an ASD (Centers for Disease Control and Prevention 2014b). Common medical presentations include seizures, gastrointestinal symptoms (weight loss or gain, nausea, vomiting, constipation, diarrhea due to unusual eating habits, abnormal sensory signaling, or underlying gastrointestinal problems), injuries (due to self-injurious behavior, sensory signaling problems, physical altercations, lack of fear, inattentiveness, or clumsiness), pain or other sensory abnormalities, and substance use disorders. Additional reasons for psychiatric consultation might include requests for evaluation and recommendations regarding difficulty coping with hospitalization or illness, nonadherence, capacity to refuse treatment, or pretransplantation evaluations.

If patients have not yet received a diagnosis, it can be extremely helpful to children with ASD and their parents to learn of their diagnosis and to be educated about the children's specific strengths, weaknesses, and needs. For hospitalized children with ASD, beneficial strategies include carefully preparing them for procedures and daily routines, allowing them time to adjust to unexpected changes, minimizing the number of staff involved with their care, and carefully managing distressing sensory stimuli. Extra effort may be required to communicate with a child with ASD and to learn how a specific child senses and communicates pain or other symptoms. Resources have now been developed to help staff support children with ASD in emergency (Al Sharif and Ratnapalan 2016), surgical (Thompson and Tielsch-Goddard 2014), and inpatient medical settings (Pratt et al. 2012).

Chronic Somatic Symptoms

Children and adolescents often report persistent physical concerns and associated functional disabilities that do not correspond to an identifiable underlying illness or medical condition (Hinton and Kirk 2016). Examples can include disabling headaches, chronic nausea or vomiting, dizziness, fibromyalgia, chronic fatigue, functional abdominal pain, irritable bowel syndrome, myofascial pain, chest pain or palpitations, conversion paralysis, and nonepileptic seizures (Heruti et al. 2002; Hinton and Kirk 2016; Lee et al. 2012; Plioplys et al. 2007; Vila et al. 2009). When somatic symptoms, of known or unknown etiology, are associated with significant distress and impairment, as well as excessive and disproportionate thoughts, feelings, and behaviors regarding those symptoms, the individual may meet DSM-5 criteria for somatic symptom disorder (American Psychiatric Association 2013).

Historically, disability and symptoms in excess of what would be expected given the amount of "organic" pathology were considered psychogenic. In such circumstances, children and families were sometimes informed by well-meaning clinicians that the symptoms had no physiological basis, with the intended or unintended suggestion that the children were fabricating the symptoms. Advances in research, as well as clinical experience, suggest that it is misleading and confusing to families to dichotomize symptoms as organic or nonorganic, because all symptoms are associated with neurosensory changes and influenced by psychosocial factors. Maintaining the organic versus nonorganic dichotomy can lead to unnecessary tests and treatments or to an unhelpful lack of empathy. Consequently, it is helpful to remember, and to communicate to families, that experiences of somatic symptoms are the result of an integration of biological processes, psychological and developmental factors, and social context (Williams and Zahka 2017). Whereas DSM-IV (American Psychiatric Association 2000) criteria for somatoform disorders emphasized the concept of medically unexplained symptoms, DSM-5 criteria abandoned that emphasis, instead focusing on the degree to which patients' thoughts, feelings, and behaviors about their somatic symptoms are disproportionate or excessive (American Psychiatric Association 2013).

Psychiatric assessment is geared toward identifying psychiatric symptoms, behavioral reinforcements, and psychosocial stressors that could be exacerbating the symptoms. Common comorbid findings include anxiety disorders (most frequently generalized anxiety disorder), alexithymia, depression, unsuspected learning disorders (in high-achieving children), developmental or communication disorders, social problems, physical or emotional trauma, family illness, chronic stress, and family distress (Williams and Zahka 2017).

The family and treatment team often worry about missing a life-threatening problem or a diagnosis that could be remedied within a traditional biomedical model. This fear is particularly strong when the patient has significant distress about the symptoms. The treatment team must believe that a reasonable evaluation has been completed so that they can clearly communicate to the family that no further evaluation is indicated to understand and treat the problem. A rehabilitation approach can improve independent and normal functioning, enhance coping and self-efficacy, and serve to prevent secondary disabilities (Williams and Zahka 2017). Functioning, rather than symptoms, should be tracked to determine whether progress is being made. As functioning, coping skills, and self-efficacy improve, symptoms and the distress related to the symptoms often remit.

Specific treatment plans target the biological, psychological, and social factors that are exacerbating or maintaining the symptoms and disability. Treatment techniques designed to target underlying sensory signaling mechanisms and specific symptoms can include cognitive-behavioral strategies (e.g., psychotherapy, hypnosis, biofeedback, or meditation), behavioral techniques, family interventions, physical interventions (e.g., massage, yoga, acupuncture, transcutaneous electrical nerve stimulation [TENS], physical therapy, heat and cold therapies, occupational therapy), sleep hygiene, and pharmacological interventions (Eccleston et al. 2014; Katholi et al. 2014; Kundu and Berman 2007; Logan et al. 2012; Reilly et al. 2013; Rutten et al. 2013; Williams and Zahka 2017). In general, interventions that promote active coping are preferred over those that require passive dependency.

Most of the currently used pharmacological strategies are extrapolated from adult trials without evidence of efficacy in children. Classes of medications to consider include tricyclic antidepressants (TCAs) or anticonvulsants for neuropathic pain or irritable bowel syndrome; SSRIs for symptoms of functional abdominal pain, anxiety, or depression; muscle relaxants for myofascial pain; and low-dose antipsychotics (especially those with low potency) for acute anxiety, multiple somatic symptoms with significant distress, and chronic nausea (Bursch 2006; Campo et al. 2004; Mathew et al. 2014; Weissmann and Uziel 2016). Benzodiazepines sometimes elicit paradoxical reactions in those children who are hypervigilant to their bodies and concerned about losing control. Blocks, trigger point injections, epidurals, and other invasive assessments and treatments that further stimulate the CNS can sometimes exacerbate the problem. Evidence-based treatments should be used whenever available.

Specific Medical Disorders

Oncology

In 2014, more than 15,000 children in the United States were expected to receive a diagnosis of cancer, and nearly 2,000 were expected to die from the illness (American Cancer Society 2014). Although cancer is the disease most frequently causing death among U.S. children ages 1–14 years, it is rare. Leukemias and CNS cancers are the two most common cancer types among children. Because of improved treatment approaches, survival rates have improved dramatically since 1975. However, many children do experience both short- and longer-term treatment side effects.

It is of interest that children with cancer, in comparison with healthy schoolchildren or children with asthma, have been found to report fewer symptoms of depression and to more often rely on repression and avoidant coping (Phipps et al. 2001). An explanation for this observation was proposed by Erickson and Steiner (2000), who found that coping styles among long-term pediatric cancer survivors were shaped by traumatic avoidance. Congruent with this finding, research now supports the conceptualization of cancer diagnosis and its treatment as being potentially traumatic, highlighting the importance of addressing these experiences early in order to prevent long-term psychological disturbance (Kazak et al. 2007; Mullins et al. 2014). A study of 6,542 childhood cancer survivors and 368 of their siblings found a fourfold greater risk of PTSD in the cancer survivors compared with the siblings (Stuber et al. 2010). More intensive cancer treatment increased the risk of later PTSD (Stuber et al. 2010; see the earlier section in this chapter, "Interventions for Invasive Procedures"). In a review of family-based programs, Meyler et al. (2010) found that both universal-level (i.e., skills-based, preventive, and supportive interventions) and targeted-level (CBT or family therapy for families experiencing significant difficulties) interventions had clinical utility. Sahler et al. (2013) found improvements in problem-solving skills, mood, anxiety, and posttraumatic stress in mothers of children with cancer who completed Bright IDEAS, a problem-solving skills-training intervention.

Cystic Fibrosis

Cystic fibrosis (CF) affects approximately 30,000 individuals in the United States (Cohen and Prince 2012) and is the most common hereditary disease in Caucasian children. A defective gene causes the body to produce a thick, sticky mucus that clogs the lungs and leads to life-threatening lung infections. These secretions also obstruct the pancreas, preventing digestive enzymes from reaching the intestines. CF occurs in approximately 1 of every 3,400 births, with about 1,000 new cases diagnosed each year. More than 75% of patients are diagnosed by the age of 2 years; the median age of survival is close to 40 years of age.

Although patients with CF have a variety of symptoms—including persistent coughing; wheezing or shortness of breath; excessive appetite but poor weight gain; and greasy, bulky stools, pulmonary disease is considered to be the most challenging problem and the most important determinant of QoL and longevity (Cohen and Prince 2012). Treatment of CF depends on the stage of the disease and the organs involved. Clearing mucus from the lungs is part of the daily CF treatment regimen; this entails vigorous clapping on the back and chest. Although the life expectancy of patients with CF has increased in recent decades, management of CF still requires a complex, time-consuming regimen that places patients at risk of nonadherence and its medical and psychological sequelae (Quittner et al. 2016). CF lung-clearing regimens consume an average of 2–4 hours daily, making it one of the most taxing chronic illnesses to manage (Quittner et al. 2016). Moreover, although people with CF can lead remarkably normal lives and maintain hope with the possibilities of gene therapy and organ transplantation in the event of severe deterioration, 85% of those with CF will die as a direct result of the disease (Quittner et al. 2016).

Besides medical treatment, CF also requires lifestyle alterations to mitigate disease activity. Given that malnutrition has been shown to lead to poorer growth, delayed puberty, impaired respiratory function, reduced exercise tolerance, and increased risk of infection, increased calorie and fat intake may reduce symptom severity and improve outcomes (Yen et al. 2013). In fact, optimizing nutrition has been linked to improved pulmonary function and survival rates (Yen et al. 2013). A high-calorie, fat-unrestricted diet is recommended (Yen et al. 2013). Despite the importance of diet, however, dietary adherence is poor, especially among adolescent patients (Simon et al. 2011). Nonadherence may be particularly problematic for female patients, who are at higher risk of health decline and early mortality (Simon et al. 2011).

Despite the high disease burden, most patients and parents report a good QoL. Psychopathology prevalence estimates are based on relatively small samples, with estimates of mood and anxiety disorders as high as 29% for patients and 35% for caregivers (Smith et al. 2010). Anxiety appears to be most prevalent and is associated with improved adherence (White et al. 2009). On the other hand, depression is associated with decreased lung function and more frequent CF exacerbations (Ploessl et al. 2014), lower body mass index (BMI) (Snell et al. 2014), and worse adherence (Hilliard et al. 2015). Epidemiological studies of CF demonstrate high comorbidity between depression and anxiety (Quittner et al. 2016). Quittner et al. (2016) developed recommendations for standardization of screening and treatment of psychiatric symptoms in CF patients that include 1) screening patients with the Patient Health Questionnaire 9-item scale (PHQ-9) and the Generalized Anxiety Disorder 7-item scale (GAD-7) for depression and anxiety, respectively; and 2) providing psychoeducation and guidance for patients who have mild elevations in scores and evidence-based psychotherapy (e.g., CBT) for those who have moderate or higher elevations in scores. Finally, given that both adherence and health status are partially predicted by parental psychosocial variables (Ernst et al. 2010), family-centered approaches should also be considered.

Asthma

Asthma is the most common serious pediatric chronic illness, frequently responsible for missed school days and hospitalizations (American Lung Association 2010). Both prevalence and morbidity are rising, despite better pharmacological treatments (Baïz and Annesi-Maesano 2012). Comorbid psychiatric disorders may reduce asthma treatment compliance, impair daily functioning, or have a direct effect on autonomic reactions and pulmonary function (Boulet et al. 2012). The literature contains some contradictory findings about the prevalences and types of comorbid psychiatric problems; however, it appears that internalizing disorders are common in patients with asthma, with prevalence estimates varying from 5% to 43% (Booster et al. 2016). Although some researchers have proposed that shared mechanisms underlying both asthma and psychiatric disorders explain their association with each other, others have suggested that psychiatric comorbidity may simply reflect the degree of asthma disease severity. For instance, Letitre et al. (2014) found that in comparison with matched healthy control children, children with well-controlled asthma did not have higher rates of anxiety, depression, and poor self-esteem. These researchers also found a correlation between poorly controlled asthma and higher rates of depression and anxiety symptoms, suggesting that disease burden may explain the increased prevalence of psychological distress associated with asthma.

Nevertheless, disease severity and burden likely do not explain all of the shared variance between psychiatric illnesses and asthma. Instead, authors have suggested that immunological, endocrine, and peripheral nervous system dysfunctions common to both asthma and psychiatric disorders may explain the association (Brehm et al. 2015; Thabrew et al. 2017). To begin with, the symptoms of asthma may naturally predispose patients to worry, given that losing one's breath is naturally anxiety-provoking (Thabrew et al. 2017). Likewise, an inflammatory allergic response may release cytokines and other mediators that cause fatigue, trouble concentrating, and irritability, often interpretable as depressive symptoms. Panic symptoms are also common, again understandable given that physiological responses associated with strong emotions may trigger wheezing. One possible explanation for the association between panic and asthma is that panic acts as an asphyxia alarm system that is triggered by central chemoreceptors monitoring partial pressure of carbon dioxide in arterial blood ($PaCO_2$). Children with a genetic vulnerability to panic disorder who also have periodic increases in $PaCO_2$ from asthma exacerbations may thus have panic attacks triggered by asthma attacks. Left undiagnosed and untreated, this anxiety can develop into panic disorder. Indeed, prospective epidemiological studies indicate that the primary risk factor for development of panic disorder in young adulthood is a history of childhood asthma (Goodwin et al. 2003). The heightened risk is likely also impacted by the interaction of both environmental and genetic factors. One study found that high levels of child and household stress and expression of a susceptibility gene for PTSD and anxiety were associated with asthma morbidity (Brehm et al. 2015). Yet another reason for increased comorbidity is the fact that most asthma medications (e.g., steroids, beta-agonists) are known to cause psychiatric symptoms.

Asthma may also predispose children to ADHD. A recent meta-analysis revealed that children with atopic disorders had a 30%–50% greater chance of developing ADHD than normative peers (van der Schans et al. 2017). Similar to comorbidity with depression and anxiety, children with asthma may be prone to developing ADHD due to shared genetic and environmental factors. In fact, pathophysiological effects of asthma, including increased inflammatory cytokines and psychological stress, may interfere with the maturation of prefrontal cortex regions that are affected in ADHD (Buske-Kirschbaum et al. 2013).

Genetic, familial, or pathophysiological etiologies notwithstanding, psychological disorders must be aggressively treated because of their impact on health status and QoL. Children and adolescents with asthma and psychological disorders have been shown to have worse health status and health outcomes than those with asthma alone (Feldman et al. 2013; Peters and Fritz 2011). Pediatric asthma patients reporting more than one psychiatric condition or those reporting poor asthma control and co-occurring anxiety or depression had the lowest QoL ratings, suggesting that psychological distress may be additive in its effects on health (Sundbom et al. 2016).

Clinicians seeing children with asthma should assess for 1) psychosocial disruption and psychiatric symptoms, especially symptoms of anxiety and depression (including medical trauma); 2) the likelihood of nonadherence; 3) the ability to perceive symptoms; and 4) the presence of vocal cord dysfunction (see subsection below). Asthma can increase family burden, and having depressed primary caregivers increases the risk of poorer treatment adherence. Electronic monitoring of adherence with inhaled medications helps determine how much nonadherence is undermining outcome. Having patients guess their peak flow or rate their symptoms before spirometry or after a methacholine challenge is one way to assess whether these patients are accurate perceivers. Patients who have difficulty with symptom perception (either under- or overperceiving symptoms) can be trained to use objective assessment methods, such as peak flow meters. Asthma education has been found to be associated with improved adherence and better health outcomes (Cabana et al. 2014; Dalcin et al. 2011).

Pharmacological and psychological treatments for medically ill children with psychosocial difficulties are largely applicable to those with asthma. Although more research is needed, psychosocial interventions that teach behavioral strategies to parents appear to be more successful than those that rely solely on asthma education (Clarke and Calam 2012). With regard to pharmacological treatment, antidepressants generally appear to be safe and effective for the treatment of depression and anxiety, with SSRIs considered first-line medications (Wamboldt et al. 1997). There is no contraindication to use of antipsychotics, and they may be particularly indicated for steroid-induced psychosis. Theophylline increases lithium clearance, requiring that levels of both drugs be monitored (Oruch et al. 2014).

Vocal Cord Dysfunction

Vocal cord dysfunction (VCD)—also known as periodic occurrence of laryngeal obstruction (POLO)—can mimic asthma and commonly occurs comorbidly with asthma. VCD is a condition caused be involuntary paradoxical adduction of the vocal cords during the inspiratory phase of the respiratory cycle, manifesting primarily as noisy breathing and dyspnea, and often accompanied by cough, chest or throat tightness, changes in voice, and anxiety (Christopher and Morris 2010; Guglani et al. 2014). The condition is often not improved by asthma medications. Clinicians can assess for VCD by asking patients where they feel short of breath and if they have throat tightness. A flow-volume loop can be helpful in showing VCD, especially on the inspiratory part of the loop. Definitive diagnosis of VCD is made by visualization of adducted cords during an acute episode via laryngoscopy. Provocation of symptoms during laryngoscopy has been achieved with methacholine, histamine, or exercise challenges. VCD patients tend to have psychiatric comorbidities, including anxiety and depression. The primary treatments for VCD are speech therapy, psychotherapy, biofeedback, and hypnotherapy geared toward increasing awareness and control of breathing and throat muscles (Christopher and Morris 2010; Guglani et al. 2014).

Childhood Obesity

Genetic factors may account for as much as 70% of the variability in human body weight (Albuquerque et al. 2015). Despite alarming increases in the prevalence of childhood obesity in the United States over the past quarter-century, the prevalence has plateaued in the last 10 years, with no significant changes between 2003–2004 and 2011–2012 (Ogden et al. 2014). Children and adolescents are considered obese if they have a BMI greater than or equal to the 95th percentile for age and sex, and they are considered overweight if their BMI is between the 85th and the 95th percentile (Ogden et al. 2014). Data from the 2011–2012 National Health and Nutrition Examination

Survey indicated that approximately 17% of U.S. youth are obese (Ogden et al. 2014). These findings can be compared with the 5% obesity reported in a similar study conducted between 1976 and 1980 (Troiano et al. 1995). This dramatic increase in obesity has been attributed to the proliferation of inexpensive, calorie-rich foods that are quickly and readily available in the United States and the increased number of hours children spend in sedentary activities, such as watching television and playing computer games (Han et al. 2010). Similar increases in childhood obesity have been documented in most industrialized countries and many urban areas of low-income countries, including a two- to threefold increase in prevalence in Australia, Brazil, Canada, Chile, Finland, France, Germany, Greece, Japan, and the United Kingdom (Han et al. 2010). Of note, the leveling-off of the prevalence growth in the United States has been attributed to concerted public health efforts such as more federal regulations on food and packaging, detailed medical recommendations, and CDC-funded state- and community-level interventions (Ogden et al. 2014).

The effect of obesity is both immediate and long-lasting. Children and adolescents with a BMI at or above the 95th percentile have been found to have significantly reduced health-related QoL and self-esteem (Griffiths et al. 2010). The immediate health risks of childhood obesity include cardiovascular problems (insulin resistance; elevated inflammatory cytokines; and vascular, arterial, and endothelial dysfunction) leading to nearly 1 in 5 obese children having dyslipidemia, hypertension, or hyperinsulinemia (Kelly et al. 2013). Other immediate health consequences of obesity in childhood include metabolic risks, obstructive sleep apnea, nonalcoholic fatty liver disease, musculoskeletal problems, psychosocial problems, and disordered eating (Kelly et al. 2013). Obese children are likely to become obese adults (Rooney et al. 2011) and to suffer from several physical comorbidities as adults, including metabolic and sleep problems, asthma, and dental health issues, as well as internalizing and externalizing psychological disorders (Pulgarón 2013).

Interventions for pediatric obesity span pharmacological, surgical, exercise-based, and psychosocial approaches. A meta-analysis of 61 trials determined that short-term medications, including sibutramine and orlistat, were effective in reducing BMI among overweight children and adolescents (McGovern et al. 2008). Interventions focused on physical activity have a moderate treatment effect on body fat but not BMI (McGovern et al. 2008). Short-term changes in weight status have been demonstrated with combined lifestyle interventions, with preliminary evidence also showing a longer-term effect (McGovern et al. 2008). Other meta-analyses have concluded that lifestyle interventions are generally effective in reducing weight and improving cardiovascular health in overweight/obese youths, with significant improvement seen in the treatment group compared with control groups (Ho et al. 2012). Given the significant influence of eating and lifestyle choices on obesity and the importance of family factors in enabling change, researchers are increasingly conducting studies of family-based behavioral programs. Family interventions generally consist of encouraging families to modify their dietary intake, physical activity habits, or both (Janicke et al. 2014). A meta-analysis of behavioral family interventions that focused on three key components—dietary intake, increased physical activity, and behavioral strategies—found that multicomponent programs demonstrated medium effect sizes both at the end of the study and at follow-up, showing promise for long-term change in affected families (Janicke et al. 2014). Among interventions designed to prevent pediatric obesity, a meta-analysis by Wang et al. (2015) compared single-component versus multi-component programs in school, home, and community settings. Strong effects were found for physical activity–only interventions delivered in schools with a home component and for combined diet–physical activity interventions delivered in schools with *both* home *and* community components. Medium effects were found for diet-only or physical activity–only interventions delivered in schools, combined diet–physical activity interventions delivered in schools with *either* a home *or* a community component, and combined diet–physical activity interventions delivered in the community with a school component. Evidence was less promising for combined interventions delivered in the childcare or home setting (Wang et al. 2015).

Bariatric surgery for obese adolescents remains controversial. On the one hand, surgery may have adverse effects on the growth and development of patients who have not reached physical maturity. On the other hand, this early intervention may also prevent the onset of the many aforementioned adverse health outcomes related to obesity (Paulus et al. 2015). A meta-analysis of surgical interventions for adolescents identified sustained and clinically significant BMI reductions for both laparoscopic adjustable gastric banding (LAGB) and Roux-en-Y gastric bypass (RYGB), the two most commonly used surgical procedures (Wang et al. 2015). Although RYBG shows the best outcomes in terms of sustained weight loss, complications such as growth deficiencies were more frequent and severe with RYBG than with LAGB (Wang et al. 2015). Given the likelihood that adolescents will not adhere to diet and other instructions, the potential interference with growth, the challenges of obtaining true informed consent from adolescents, and the lack of information on long-term consequences of these procedures, surgical interventions should be reserved for patients who have significant complications from their obesity and who have not responded to more conventional interventions, with RYBG recommended only for the most seriously affected adolescents (Black et al. 2013; Wang et al. 2015) (see also Chapter 28, "Surgery").

Sickle Cell Disease

The sickle cell gene for hemoglobin is the most common inherited blood condition in the United States, with an estimated 72,000 people affected. Although the average life span of people with sickle cell disease (SCD) has significantly increased in past decades, life expectancy is still 20–30 years shorter due to complications related to vascular occlusion (Yawn et al. 2014). Symptoms do not usually appear until late in the first year of life and may include fever; swelling of the hands and feet; pain in the chest, abdomen, limbs, and joints; nosebleeds; and frequent upper respiratory infections. Pain is the most common complaint after infancy, as are the added problems of anemia, fatigue, irritability, and jaundice. Children and adolescents may experience delayed puberty, severe joint pain, progressive anemia, leg sores, gum disease, long-term damage to major organs, stroke, and acute chest syndrome. A compromised spleen can cause increased susceptibility to infections. Current treatments for SCD are designed to prolong life and improve QoL, although they appear to be underused (Yawn et al. 2014). Specifically, both hydroxyurea therapy and long-term blood transfusions are recommended as disease-modifying treatments (Yawn et al. 2014). In children specifically, daily oral prophylactic penicillin use is recommended until 5 years of age to reduce the risk of invasive pneumococcal disease. Annual transcranial Doppler examinations are also recommended to screen for hypertension, retinopathy, and stroke (Yawn et al. 2014). Cure rates in excess of 80% have been achieved in children who undergo blood or marrow transplant with a human leukocyte antigen–matched sibling as the donor (Bolaños-Meade and Brodsky 2014).

Sickle cell crises are acute pain episodes that are usually followed by periods of remission and a relatively normal life. Some patients have few crises, others need to be frequently hospitalized, and still others have clusters of severe attacks with long intermittent remissions. Daily pain is reported by 10% of pediatric patients. Undertreatment of pain may predispose SCD patients to chronic pain and should thus be aggressively treated from the first crisis (Ballas et al. 2012). The risk of a crisis is increased by anything that boosts the body's oxygen requirement (e.g., illness, physical stress, high altitudes). The first day of the crisis is usually the worst, with sharp, intense, and throbbing pain in the arms, legs, and back. Shortness of breath, bone pain, and abdominal pain are also common. Hepatomegaly can cause pain, nausea, low-grade fever, and jaundice. Males may experience priapism. Acute chest syndrome can be life-threatening.

Stroke is a common complication and cause of death among sickle cell patients. For every 10 pediatric patients, 1 will experience a stroke and another 3 will experience a silent cerebral infarction (Yawn et al. 2014). These events predispose patients to neuropsychological impairment and future cerebral events, making a strong case for the use of the two disease-modifying therapies described above (Yawn et al. 2014) as well as for blood or marrow transplant (Dalle 2013). Compared with healthy control subjects, pediatric patients with SCD show decrements in working memory, central executive function, processing/rehearsal speed (Smith and Schatz 2016), and visuomotor performance (Hijmans et al. 2011), although the extent of these impairments depends on complications of the disease. Although stroke certainly exacerbates neuropsychological deficits, SCD patients with no significant cerebral history have also shown deficits in cognitive performance. Increased cytokine levels and the subsequent chronic inflammatory response may explain some of the variance in cognitive deficits (Andreotti et al. 2015). Memory impairments may also be related to chronic anemia-related and acute stroke-related hypoxia (Iampietro et al. 2014). Some progress in cognitive rehabilitation has been made to address cognitive deficits among children with SCD who have had a stroke (King et al. 2008).

Compared with youth in the general population, children and adolescents with SCD are at higher risk of developing comorbid psychiatric disorders—in particular, internalizing disorders such as depression and anxiety (Benton et al. 2011). Besides the toll that chronic pain takes, psychosocial and familial factors may also increase vulnerability. A study by Ünal et al. (2011) revealed that children with SCD were more likely to suffer from anxiety and depression than normative peers, a vulnerability predicted both by the number of pain crises and by the psychological well-being of their mothers. Patients with SCD may also fare worse than peers with other chronic illnesses (Benton et al. 2011). In fact, as many as 50% of pediatric patients with SCD have a co-occurring psychiatric condition. In addition to internalizing symptoms, behavioral disorders such as ADHD and oppositional defiant disorder are more common among children with SCD and may reflect sequelae from ischemic events (Benton et al. 2011; O'Callaghan and Gold 2012). Finally, the association between pica and iron deficiency likely explains the high prevalence of pica in SCD (Ivascu et al. 2001; O'Callaghan and Gold 2012).

Psychiatric assessment should assess for 1) psychosocial disruption or psychiatric symptoms, especially related to pica, anxiety, and depression; 2) school or social problems that could reflect subtle neurocognitive problems; and 3) chronic pain. Pharmacological and psychological treatments with efficacy to treat psychiatric disorders in children are applicable to those with sickle cell anemia. Problems with academic or social functioning might be assessed via neurocognitive testing and addressed within the school system with an individualized educational program (IEP). Pain associated with vascular crises is most commonly managed pharmacologically through the combination of rehydration with anti-inflammatories, analgesics, and vasodilators (Ballas et al. 2012). Chronic and acute pediatric SCD pain also can be reduced with behavioral, psychological, or physical interventions used in other chronic pain patients (Palermo et al. 2010; see also Chapter 23, "Hematology").

Renal Disease

Each year 20,000 children are born with kidney abnormalities, and 4,500 children require dialysis for renal failure. Incidence of pediatric chronic kidney disease (CKD) has increased in recent years, with notable socioeconomic and racial disparities (Gulati 2015). Whereas pediatric renal disease is still predominantly caused by congenital anomalies or hereditary disease (Kaspar et al. 2016), the increased incidence of CKD in low-income and minority children calls attention to the growing impact of nonorganic etiologies on kidney disease.

Seventy percent of children with CKD will progress to end-stage renal disease (ESRD) by age 20 years (Gulati 2015). With the exception of very young children, youth with CKD have a much higher 5-year survival probability than do adults. Children with ESRD on dialysis have a 5-year survival rate of 89%, with death most commonly attributed to cardiopulmonary malfunction or infection (Kaspar et al. 2016). The basic principles of treatment of ESRD are similar in adults and children (see Chapter 20, "Renal Disease"). However, attention to dialysis adequacy, control of osteodystrophy, nutrition, and correction of anemia are crucial in children because these factors can influence growth, cognitive development, and school performance (Warady et al. 2014).

Patients with CKD are at risk of a variety of medical conditions, namely metabolic acidosis and renal osteodystrophy, cardiovascular disease, and anemia. In pediatrics specifically, patients are especially vulnerable to urological problems and renal dysplasia. One study found CKD-associated anemia to be associated with worse QoL and neurocognitive ability (Wong et al. 2012). It has not yet been determined whether monitoring for and treating these complications aggressively can reduce negative effects and alter outcomes (Kaspar et al. 2016).

Pediatric patients with CKD—particularly those with higher illness severity—have more psychosocial problems than do healthy children (Kaspar et al. 2016; Marciano et al. 2011; Moreira et al. 2015). As the disease progresses, CKD is inevitably associated with functional impairment and alterations in daily routines and QoL of pediatric patients, paving the way for psychosocial difficulties (Moreira et al. 2015). Psychological well-being is also affected by high rates of mortality and frequent needs for hospitalization (Moreira et al. 2015). Although Varni et al. (2007) originally reported that patients with CKD fared better than peers with other chronic conditions, other researchers have found that youth with CKD are just as vulnerable to developing adjustment disorders, depressive symptoms, anxiety, and cognitive impairment (Moreira et al. 2015). In fact, even less physically ill children with CKD appear to have increased difficulties with school adjustment and more feelings of loneliness (Kaspar et al. 2016; Moreira et al. 2015).

Although children who receive a transplant have a fourfold higher survival rate than those on dialysis (Kaspar et al. 2016), findings regarding differences in psychosocial outcomes of patients by treatment type are mixed, with some studies showing that transplant recipients fare better than those on dialysis, and others reporting the opposite (Marciano et al. 2011). According to the latest statistics from the United Network for Organ Sharing (OPTN) as of March 2017 (U.S. Department of Health and Human Services 2017a), 996 children were waiting for a kidney transplant, including 3 younger than 1 year, 194 in the 1- to 5-year-old age group, 94 in the 6- to 10-year-old group, and 530 in the 11- to 17-year-old group. Median wait time for patients younger than 18 years was nearly 2 years. More than 12,000 pediatric renal transplants are performed each year (U.S. Department of Health and Human Services 2017b), with most transplanted kidneys coming from cadavers. At least 30% of pediatric renal transplant patients report difficulty adhering to medical recommendations (Dobbels et al. 2010). Adverse consequences of nonadherence include medical complications and hospitalizations, higher health care costs and family stress, and increased risk of graft loss (Dobbels et al. 2010; McCormick King et al. 2014). Special attention should be paid to patients entering the teenage years, given that puberty is associated with deterioration of kidney function (Kaspar et al. 2016) as well as a higher prevalence of nonadherence (Dobbels et al. 2010).

Clinicians conducting mental health evaluations of children with renal disease should consider the potential effects of cognitive deficits, adaptation difficulties, and family strain on social and academic functioning as well as on adherence. As with all pediatric patients, it is essential to evaluate and address stress and distress in families of patients with renal disease as part of a larger treatment approach. Given the link between emotional well-being and adherence to posttransplantation regimens (McCormick King et al. 2014), evaluations should include depression and anxiety screening. Recommendations related to the use of psychotropic medication must be extrapolated from adult studies (see Chapter 20, "Renal Disease").

Diabetes

Affecting approximately 200,000 youth in the United States (Centers for Disease Control and Prevention 2014a), juvenile-onset diabetes mellitus saw a 21% jump in incidence between 2001 and 2009 (Dabelea et al. 2014).

Development of type 1 diabetes mellitus (T1DM) has been linked to cognitive dysfunction throughout the life span (Nunley et al. 2015). A meta-analysis conducted by Gaudieri et al. (2008) determined that childhood-onset T1DM was associated with slightly lower overall cognitive abilities, with particular decrements in verbal and visual learning, memory, attention, and executive functioning. The effects of the disease continue well into adulthood. Middle-aged adults with childhood-onset T1DM have been shown to be five times as likely to have clinically relevant cognitive impairment, a relationship predicted by rates of chronic hyperglycemia and extent of microvascular disease (Nunley et al. 2015).

The physiological changes of puberty can lead to increased insulin resistance, which may explain the particularly steep rise in incidence of T1DM that occurs in adolescence and early adulthood (Dabelea et al. 2014). In addition, the importance of peer acceptance and the withdrawal of parental supervision with the normal developmental focus on identity and autonomy lead to significant adherence problems during adolescence (Rausch et al. 2012). Poor control of diabetes has been repeatedly confirmed with HbA$_{1c}$. Besides older age, other variables identified as predictors of poor metabolic control and increased diabetes-related complications include lower parental monitoring and help with diabetes management, lower self-control and functional autonomy (King et al. 2012), longer diabetes duration, minority status, having unmarried caregivers, and using injected insulin versus continuous subcutaneous insulin infusion (Hilliard et al. 2013).

Psychiatric comorbidity in T1DM is a major issue for psychiatric consultants to pediatrics. Some moodiness and feelings of isolation and of loss or grief, as well as mild anxiety about the future, are to be expected as normal responses to diabetes. Psychiatric disorders may be more prevalent in adolescents and young adults with diabetes, with rates as high as 42% in some studies (Fritsch et al. 2010). Whereas depression and anxiety are the disorders most commonly associated with diabetes, eating disorders may be elevated in young women (Fritsch et al. 2010). The importance of screening for mental health problems is highlighted by the established link between mood problems and poorer glycemic control (Fritsch et al. 2010) and lower diabetes-related QoL (Hanna et al. 2014). Increased incidence of depression and anxiety is not limited to older children. A study of young children with T1DM found that they were more likely to show abnormal emotional and behavioral symptoms compared with age-matched normative peers, regardless of demographic or illness covariates, suggesting an early link between diabetes and psychological health (Zenlea et al. 2014).

Treatment of comorbid psychiatric disorders with medications requires careful monitoring, because most antidepressant, mood stabilizer, and atypical antipsychotic medications may affect appetite, weight, and/or glucose tolerance. Meta-analytic studies indicate that youths exposed to antipsychotics have a significantly elevated risk of developing type 2 diabetes mellitus in comparison with psychiatric control subjects not receiving antipsychotics (Galling et al. 2016). Nevertheless, prompt psychiatric evaluation and treatment are also important, given that mental health symptoms may moderate the incidence of diabetes (N. Schmitz et al. 2016).

The effectiveness of psychosocial interventions for children with diabetes may vary on a number of factors, including focus (adherence vs. HbA$_{1c}$), child developmental level and illness duration, and modality (individual vs. family-based programs) (Carr 2014). Programs should be tailored to the child's age and illness stage. Newly diagnosed children may benefit from family-based psychoeducation, whereas adolescents learning to negotiate the responsibility of self-management may respond to skills-based programs that target communication and problem solving with parents (Farrell et al. 2002). In general, meta-analytic studies indicate that interventions targeting family dynamics seem to be more successful than those focused on behavioral coaching alone (Hood et al. 2010). Outcome research on psychosocial programs for youth with poorly controlled diabetes is complicated by methodological issues (Christie and Channon 2014; Pillay et al. 2015; Powell et al. 2014). For instance, HbA_{1c} may not change until 2–3 months after a program ends (Pillay et al. 2015), and because many programs fail to follow participants long-term, findings on effect sizes have historically been limited to measurements of the change between pre- and post-program HbA_{1c} (Pillay et al. 2015). Studies of motivational interviewing, commonly used for adolescents with diabetes (Christie and Channon 2014), have also demonstrated that programs targeting adherence are more effective than those focused solely on glycemic outcomes (Powell et al. 2014).

Cardiac Disease

Congenital Heart Defects and Disease

Congenital heart defects (CHDs) and disease include patent ductus arteriosus, atrial septal defects, and ventricular septal defects. About 40,000 children are born with a heart defect each year, and most can benefit from surgery. Acquired heart diseases that develop during childhood include Kawasaki disease, rheumatic fever, and infective endocarditis.

Illness severity (as measured by cardiac medication use) has been positively associated with more parent-reported behavioral problems (Spijkerboer et al. 2010). By contrast, use of palliative procedures before surgery (i.e., palliative use of a shunt, pulmonary banding, aortic stenosis, and other procedures designed to minimize surgical side effects) has been negatively related to behavioral symptoms at follow-up (Spijkerboer et al. 2010). Studying preschool-aged patients with CHDs, Brosig et al. (2017) found that children did not significantly differ from normative peers except for mild decrements in fine motor skills and adaptive functioning. However, Schaefer et al. (2013) found that adolescents with CHDs had lower perceptual reasoning and working memory and lower IQs, yet typical psychological adjustment and QoL. Potentially explaining these discrepant findings, the adverse effects of CHDs, as manifested by higher prevalence of developmental delays and long-term neuropsychological deficits, may become more evident in middle and late childhood as school and social demands increase and reveal decrements in functioning that previously were not apparent (Latal 2016; Mussatto et al. 2014).

Heart Transplant Recipients

Uzark et al. (2012) compared the QoL among pediatric heart transplant recipients with that among children and adolescents who underwent conventional cardiac surgery and children who had no health problems. Although most transplant recipients generally rated their QoL as "good," self- and proxy-reported QoL ratings among transplant recipients were significantly lower than those among healthy children for both physical and psychosocial well-being, with one-third of children reporting significant psychosocial impairment. Differences in QoL between transplant and surgery patients were not statistically significant; however, transplant recipients reported fewer symptoms than did patients with moderate or severe heart disease, a difference that may be related to the corrective nature of transplantation (Uzark et al. 2012). DeMaso et al. (2004) similarly found that among the 15 patients they studied, most (73%) had good psychological functioning after their heart transplant. The researchers found no association between medical severity and posttransplantation psychological functioning, but they did identify a significant association between family functioning and posttransplantation emotional adjustment (for the first 2 years after transplant) that was not detected prior to the transplant. Relaxation and imagery techniques have been used successfully in pediatric patients undergoing routine endomyocardial biopsy after heart transplantation (Bullock and Shaddy 1993). A review of the literature related to cognition found that children and adolescents generally perform normally on measures of cognitive functioning posttransplantation, although a complicated transplantation course (e.g., caused by infection or rejection) may increase the risk of cognitive difficulties (Todaro et al. 2000). In terms of compliance with medical regimens, Oliva et al. (2013) found medication adherence to be relatively high, with only 9% of children reporting an episode of nonadherence to immunosuppressants. The authors highlighted that more than two-thirds of nonadherence episodes occurred after the age of 12 years. Besides adolescence itself predicting noncompliance, African American race, Medicaid insurance, and need for a ventilator or ventricular assist device before transplant all increased the risk of nonadherence. Notably, nonadherence-contingent risk of death was 26% at year 1 posttransplant and 33% at year 2 (Oliva et al. 2013).

Chest Pain

Chest pain as a presenting symptom in a previously healthy child is not as ominous a symptom as it is in an adult because in a child it is rarely a sign of underlying cardiac disease; 99% of pediatric patients referred to cardiology for this symptom have normal echocardiograms (Sert et al. 2013). Common non-cardiac-related causes of chest pain include musculoskeletal, idiopathic, and psychological disorders (Sert et al. 2013). Somatic presentations of psychological distress are more fully discussed in the section "Chronic Somatic Symptoms" earlier in this chapter.

Psychotropic Medications

Most psychoactive medications prescribed for children younger than 12 years old are not specifically approved by the U.S. Food and Drug Administration (FDA) for use in children. In 1999, the American Heart Association (AHA) (Gutgesell et al. 1999) published recommendations for the use of psychotropic medications in children. They concluded that stimulants cause increases in heart rate and blood pressure that are typically clinically insignificant. In 2011, the FDA restated their prior conclusion that there is no increased risk of sudden death in healthy patients taking stimulants for ADHD, but cautioned about use of stimulants and atomoxetine in children who have "serious heart problems, or for whom an increase in blood pressure or heart rate would be problematic" (U.S. Food and Drug Administration 2011). More recently, Aggarwal et al. (2016) reevaluated the recommendations outlined by the AHA and FDA. Along with reiterating prior findings that there is no increased incidence of sudden cardiac death with the use of stimulants despite their association with minimal increases in heart rate and blood pressure (as also echoed by Cooper et al. (2011), the authors concluded that routine electrocardiograms (ECGs) prior to stimulant initiation are not indicated. They also indicated that ECGs may increase anxiety in families and postpone treatment initiation (Aggarwal et al. 2016). Other recommendations for use of psychotropic medications in pediatric patients with cardiac disease include a thorough evaluation of family history before treatment initiation; prompt evaluation of children who report palpitations, chest pain, syncope, or any other paroxysmal cardiac event while on stimulants; close monitoring of all patients with tachycardia, hypertension, chest pain, or palpitations; and evaluation by a pediatric cardiologist for pediatric patients with cardiac conditions or positive family histories (Aggarwal et al. 2016).

In children as in adults, cardiac disease carries an increased risk of QTc prolongation and torsade de pointes. Some psychotropic medications can themselves increase the QT interval, and other medications can cause it to be increased by inhibiting the metabolism of other QTc-prolonging drugs. Nevertheless, investigators have concluded that the benefits of antipsychotics (Jensen et al. 2015) and antidepressants (Uchida et al. 2015) in pediatrics generally outweigh the risks, especially given that both classes of drugs are not associated with prolonged QTc at the dosages typically prescribed for children (Jensen et al. 2015; Uchida et al. 2015). Psychiatric consultants may be required to alert pediatricians about the use of other QTc-prolonging agents, such as methadone, if QTc concerns are raised as a reason to discontinue a psychotropic medication.

Fetal Alcohol Spectrum Disorders

Prenatal alcohol exposure is one of the leading preventable causes of congenital neurological impairment, affecting as many as 2%–5% of children in the United States and Western Europe (May et al. 2014), with severe lifelong consequences for affected individuals. The effects of prenatal alcohol exposure are much broader than were initially recognized; the most deleterious impacts are on brain development and on neurocognitive and behavioral functioning. Current prevalence estimates indicate that as many as 7 children per 1,000 qualify for a full-fledged fetal alcohol syndrome (FAS) diagnosis, while as many as 5 in 100 children meet criteria for fetal alcohol spectrum disorder (FASD), an umbrella term identifying the range of outcomes from gestational alcohol exposure, including children with FAS (the most severe form), those who meet some but not all criteria for FAS, and those with alcohol-related neurodevelopmental disorder (ARND) (Pei et al. 2011; Riley et al. 2011).

Although the four commonly used diagnostic schemas developed for FAS and FASD—the 4-digit code (Astley and Clarren 2000), the National Task Force/CDC (Bertrand et al. 2004, 2005), the Canadian Guidelines (Chudley et al. 2005), and the Revised Institute of Medicine (Hoyme et al. 2005)—differ on some points, they all agree that FAS reflects three broad symptom clusters: facial anomalies, growth deficiencies, and CNS dysfunction (Riley et al. 2011). Facial anomalies most frequently described in individuals with FAS include short palpebral fissures and abnormalities in the premaxillary zone, including a thin vermilion and smooth philtrum (Riley et al. 2011). Growth deficiencies are characterized as growth or weight in the bottom 10th percentile or demonstrating disproportion in height versus weight measurements (Riley et al. 2011). CNS involvement reflects a variety of symptoms, including small head circumference, abnormalities in brain structures, evidence of neurological dysfunction, and cognitive deficits (Riley et al. 2011). Diminished intellectual capacity may be more specifically observed as lower verbal IQ, working memory, executive functioning, and general and conceptual ability, as well as high rates of ADHD, behavioral and adaptive problems, poor academic achievement, social skills deficits, and delays in motor and language development (Mattson et al. 2011; May et al. 2014; Riley et al. 2011). In regard to ADHD, some research suggests that children with FAS and comorbid ADHD demonstrate fewer problems with sustained attention than do those with pure ADHD, yet more difficulties in visuospatial skills, information encoding, and problem-solving flexibility (Pei et al. 2011). If diagnostic criteria for FAS or FASD are met, maternal alcohol use does not need to be confirmed to establish a diagnosis (Riley et al. 2011). Likewise, diagnosis is also permissible in the absence of demarcated facial abnormalities (Riley et al. 2011).

Conclusion

While some psychiatric issues in pediatrics are similar to those seen in adults, several key differences distinguish the two. One, conceptualizations and treatment plans must take into account a child's developmental stage. Two, given the importance of family factors in the development, maintenance, and prognosis of psychiatric issues, a patient's family should always be considered when conceptualizing psychosocial difficulties, identifying strengths and challenges, defining treatment targets, and attempting to resolve contextual stressors relevant to both patient and family.

Both clinical practice and evidence-based research also inform us of the importance of multimodal approaches to the treatment of psychiatric issues in pediatrics. These should inevitably incorporate sensitive evaluation and screening, psychotherapeutic services for patient and family, and, as needed, pharmacotherapy. Current scientific knowledge points to the efficacy, utility, and practicality of skills-based cognitive-behavioral strategies. In terms of pharmacotherapy, clinicians working with medically ill children should consider drugs that are least likely to have adverse events for physically compromised youth, with SSRIs being considered first line for their tolerability and efficacy. Together, the combination of careful evaluation, psychotherapeutic support, and psychotropic medications provides clinicians with the necessary tools to mitigate the impact of psychiatric concerns in pediatrics.

References

Aggarwal V, Aggarwal A, Khan D: Electrocardiogram before starting stimulant medications: to order or not? Cardiol Young 26(1):216–219, 2016 26278960
Agorastos A, Pittman JO, Angkaw AC, et al; Marine Resiliency Study Team: The cumulative effect of different childhood trauma types on self-reported symptoms of adult male depression and PTSD, substance abuse and health-related quality of life in a large active-duty military cohort. J Psychiatr Res 58:46–54, 2014 25139009
Ahmed R, Aslani P: What is patient adherence? A terminology overview. Int J Clin Pharm 36(1):4–7, 2014 24104760
Albuquerque D, Stice E, Rodríguez-López R, et al: Current review of genetics of human obesity: from molecular mechanisms to an evolutionary perspective. Mol Genet Genomics 290(4):1191–1221, 2015 25749980
Aloni MN, Lecerf P, Lê PQ, et al: Is pica under-reported in children with sickle cell disease? A pilot study in a Belgian cohort. Hematology 20(7):429–432, 2015 25494639

Al Sharif S, Ratnapalan S: Managing children with autism spectrum disorders in emergency departments. Pediatr Emerg Care 32(2):101–103, 2016 26835567

American Cancer Society: Cancer facts and figures 2014. American Cancer Society, 2014. Available at: https://www.cancer.org/research/cancer-facts-statistics/all-cancer-facts-figures/cancer-facts-figures-2014.html. Accessed June 1, 2017.

American Lung Association: Asthma. American Lung Association, 2010. Available at: http://www.lung.org/lung-health-and-diseases/lung-disease-lookup/asthma/. Accessed June 1, 2017.

American Psychiatric Association: Diagnostic and Statistical Manual of Mental Disorders, 4th Edition, Text Revision. Arlington, VA, American Psychiatric Association, 2000

American Psychiatric Association: Diagnostic and Statistical Manual of Mental Disorders, 5th Edition. Arlington, VA, American Psychiatric Association, 2013

Andreotti C, King AA, Macy E, et al: The association of cytokine levels with cognitive function in children with sickle cell disease and normal MRI studies of the brain. J Child Neurol 30(10):1349–1353, 2015 25512362

Annunziato RA, Jerson B, Seidel J, et al: The psychosocial challenges of solid organ transplant recipients during childhood. Pediatr Transplant 16(7):803–811, 2012 22738295

Astley S, Clarren SK: Diagnosing the full spectrum of fetal alcohol-exposed individuals: introducing the 4-digit diagnostic code. Alcohol Alcohol 35(4):400–410, 2000 10906009

Ayoub CC: Munchausen by proxy: child placement and emotional health. Presented at the 14th International Congress for the Prevention of Child Abuse and Neglect, Denver, CO, July 7–10, 2002

Baïz N, Annesi-Maesano I: Is the asthma epidemic still ascending? Clin Chest Med 33(3):419–429, 2012 22929092

Ballas SK, Gupta K, Adams-Graves P: Sickle cell pain: a critical reappraisal. Blood 120(18):3647–3656, 2012 22923496

Bennett S, Shafran R, Coughtrey A, et al: Psychological interventions for mental health disorders in children with chronic physical illness: a systematic review. Arch Dis Child 100(4):308–316, 2015 25784736

Benton TD, Boyd R, Ifeagwu J, et al: Psychiatric diagnosis in adolescents with sickle cell disease: a preliminary report. Curr Psychiatry Rep 13(2):111–115, 2011 21312010

Bertrand J, Floyd RL, Weber MK, et al: Fetal alcohol syndrome: guidelines for referral and diagnosis. Atlanta, GA, Centers for Disease Control and Prevention, 2004. Available at: http://www.cdc.gov/ncbddd/fasd/documents/FAS_guidelines_accessible.pdf. Accessed July 23, 2017.

Bertrand J, Floyd RL, Weber MK; Fetal Alcohol Syndrome Prevention Team, Division of Birth Defects and Developmental Disabilities, National Center on Birth Defects and Developmental Disabilities, Centers for Disease Control and Prevention (CDC): Guidelines for identifying and referring persons with fetal alcohol syndrome. MMWR Recomm Rep 54(RR–11):1–14, 2005 16251866

Birur B, Moore NC, Davis LL, et al: An evidence-based review of early intervention and prevention of posttraumatic stress disorder. Community Ment Health J 53(2):183–201, 2017 27470261

Bitsko MJ, Everhart RS, Rubin BK: The adolescent with asthma. Paediatr Respir Rev 15(2):146–153, 2014 23972334

Black JA, White B, Viner RM, et al: Bariatric surgery for obese children and adolescents: a systematic review and meta-analysis. Obes Rev 14(8):634–644, 2013 23577666

Black MM, Aboud FE: Responsive feeding is embedded in a theoretical framework of responsive parenting. J Nutr 141(3):490–494, 2011 21270366

Black MM, Tilton N, Bento S, et al: Recovery in young children with weight faltering: child and household risk factors. J Pediatr 170:301–306, 2016 26687578

Bolaños-Meade J, Brodsky RA: Blood and marrow transplantation for sickle cell disease: is less more? Blood Rev 28(6):243–248, 2014 25217413

Bools CN, Neale BA, Meadow SR: Follow up of victims of fabricated illness (Munchausen syndrome by proxy). Arch Dis Child 69(6):625–630, 1993 8285772

Booster GD, Oland AA, Bender BG: Psychosocial factors in severe pediatric asthma. Immunol Allergy Clin North Am 36(3):449–460, 2016 27401618

Boulet LP, Vervloet D, Magar Y, et al: Adherence: the goal to control asthma. Clin Chest Med 33(3):405–417, 2012 22929091

Brehm JM, Ramratnam SK, Tse SM, et al: Stress and bronchodilator response in children with asthma. Am J Respir Crit Care Med 192(1):47–56, 2015 25918834

Brinkman TM, Zhu L, Zeltzer LK, et al: Longitudinal patterns of psychological distress in adult survivors of childhood cancer. Br J Cancer 109(5):1373–1381, 2013 23880828

Broekman BF, Olff M, Tan FM, et al: The psychological impact of an adenoidectomy and adeno-tonsillectomy on young children. Int J Pediatr Otorhinolaryngol 74(1):37–42, 2010 19910058

Bronner MB, Peek N, Knoester H, et al: Course and predictors of posttraumatic stress disorder in parents after pediatric intensive care treatment of their child. J Pediatr Psychol 35(9):966–974, 2010 20150338

Brosbe MS, Hoefling K, Faust J: Predicting posttraumatic stress following pediatric injury: a systematic review. J Pediatr Psychol 36(6):718–729, 2011 21262743

Brosig CL, Bear L, Allen S, et al: Preschool neurodevelopmental outcomes in children with congenital heart disease. J Pediatr 183:80–86.e1, 2017 28081891

Brown JD, Wissow LS: Screening to identify mental health problems in pediatric primary care: considerations for practice. Int J Psychiatry Med 40(1):1–19, 2010 20565041

Bryant-Waugh R, Markham L, Kreipe RE, et al: Feeding and eating disorders in childhood. Int J Eat Disord 43(2):98–111, 2010 20063374

Bullock EA, Shaddy RE: Relaxation and imagery techniques without sedation during right ventricular endomyocardial biopsy in pediatric heart transplant patients. J Heart Lung Transplant 12(1 Pt 1):59–62, 1993 8443203

Bursch B: Somatization disorders, in Comprehensive Handbook of Personality and Psychopathology, Vol III: Child Psychopathology. Edited by Hersen M, Thomas JC (Ammerman RT, volume editor). New York, Wiley, 2006, pp 403–421

Bursch B, Forgey M: Psychopharmacology for medically ill adolescents. Curr Psychiatry Rep 15(10):395, 2013 23963629

Buske-Kirschbaum A, Schmitt J, Plessow F, et al: Psychoendocrine and psychoneuroimmunological mechanisms in the comorbidity of atopic eczema and attention deficit/hyperactivity disorder. Psychoneuroendocrinology 38(1):12–23, 2013 23141851

Butwicka A, Fendler W, Zalepa A, et al: Psychiatric disorders and health-related quality of life in children with type 1 diabetes mellitus. Psychosomatics 57(2):185–193, 2016 26774893

Cabana MD, Slish KK, Evans D, et al: Impact of physician asthma care education on patient outcomes. Health Educ Behav 41(5):509–517, 2014 25270176

Callanan M, Kelley P: Final Gifts: Understanding the Special Awareness, Needs, and Communications of the Dying. New York, Simon & Schuster, 2012

Campo JV, Perel J, Lucas A, et al: Citalopram treatment of pediatric recurrent abdominal pain and comorbid internalizing disorders: an exploratory study. J Am Acad Child Adolesc Psychiatry 43(10):1234–1242, 2004 15381890

Caplan R, Bursch B: How Many More Questions? Techniques for Clinical Interviews of Young Medically Ill Children. New York, Oxford University Press, 2013

Carr A: The evidence base for family therapy and systemic interventions for child-focused problems. J Fam Ther 36(2):107–157, 2014

Centers for Disease Control and Prevention: National Diabetes Statistics Report, 2014a. Available at: https://www.cdc.gov/diabetes/data/statistics/2014statisticsreport.html. Accessed June 1, 2017.

Centers for Disease Control and Prevention: Prevalence of autism spectrum disorder among children aged 8 years-autism and developmental disabilities monitoring network, 11 sites, United States, 2010. MMWR Surveill Summ 63(2):6–21, 2014b 24670961

Chial HJ, Camilleri M, Williams DE, et al: Rumination syndrome in children and adolescents: diagnosis, treatment, and prognosis. Pediatrics 111(1):158–162, 2003 12509570

Christie D, Channon S: The potential for motivational interviewing to improve outcomes in the management of diabetes and obesity in paediatric and adult populations: a clinical review. Diabetes Obes Metab 16(5):381–387, 2014 23927612

Christopher KL, Morris MJ: Vocal cord dysfunction, paradoxic vocal fold motion, or laryngomalacia? Our understanding requires an interdisciplinary approach. Otolaryngol Clin North Am 43(1):43–66, 2010 20172256

Chudley AE, Conry J, Cook JL, et al; Public Health Agency of Canada's National Advisory Committee on Fetal Alcohol Spectrum Disorder: Fetal alcohol spectrum disorder: Canadian guidelines for diagnosis. CMAJ 172 (5 suppl):S1–S21, 2005 15738468

Clarke SA, Calam R: The effectiveness of psychosocial interventions designed to improve health-related quality of life (HRQOL) amongst asthmatic children and their families: a systematic review. Qual Life Res 21(5):747–764, 2012 21901377

Cohen TS, Prince A: Cystic fibrosis: a mucosal immunodeficiency syndrome. Nat Med 18(4):509–519, 2012 22481418

Cole SZ, Lanham JS: Failure to thrive: an update. Am Fam Physician 83(7):829–834, 2011 21524049

Compas BE, Jaser SS, Dunn MJ, et al: Coping with chronic illness in childhood and adolescence. Annu Rev Clin Psychol 8:455–480, 2012 22224836

Compas BE, Desjardins L, Vannatta K, et al: Children and adolescents coping with cancer: self- and parent reports of coping and anxiety/depression. Health Psychol 33(8):853–861, 2014 25068455

Connelly J, Pilch N, Oliver M, et al: Prediction of medication non-adherence and associated outcomes in pediatric kidney transplant recipients. Pediatr Transplant 19(5):555–562, 2015 25917112

Cooper WO, Habel LA, Sox CM, et al: ADHD drugs and serious cardiovascular events in children and young adults. N Engl J Med 365(20):1896–1904, 2011 22043968

Cousino MK, Hazen RA: Parenting stress among caregivers of children with chronic illness: a systematic review. J Pediatr Psychol 38(8):809–828, 2013 23843630

Coyne I, O'Mathúna DP, Gibson F, et al: Interventions for promoting participation in shared decision-making for children with cancer. Cochrane Database Syst Rev (11):CD008970, 2016 27898175

Cramton RE, Gruchala NE: Managing procedural pain in pediatric patients. Curr Opin Pediatr 24(4):530–538, 2012 22732639

Dabelea D, Mayer-Davis EJ, Saydah S, et al; SEARCH for Diabetes in Youth Study: Prevalence of type 1 and type 2 diabetes among children and adolescents from 2001 to 2009. JAMA 311(17):1778–1786, 2014 24794371

Dalcin PdeT, Grutcki DM, Laporte PP, et al: Impact of a short-term educational intervention on adherence to asthma treatment and on asthma control. J Bras Pneumol 37(1):19–27, 2011 21390428

Dalle JH: Hematopoietic stem cell transplantation in SCD. C R Biol 336(3):148–151, 2013 23643397

Damanhuri N, Enoch S: Assessment and non-pharmacological management of pain in children with burns, in The Handbook of Behavioral Medicine. Edited by Mostofsky DI. New York, Wiley, 2014, pp 143–154

Davidson JE, Jones C, Bienvenu OJ: Family response to critical illness: postintensive care syndrome—family. Crit Care Med 40(2):618–624, 2012 22080636

Davydow DS, Richardson LP, Zatzick DF, et al: Psychiatric morbidity in pediatric critical illness survivors: a comprehensive review of the literature. Arch Pediatr Adolesc Med 164(4):377–385, 2010 20368492

Dawood OT, Izham M, Ibrahim M, et al: Medication compliance among children. World J Pediatr 6(3):200–202, 2010 20706818

Delamater AM, de Wit M, McDarby V, et al; International Society for Pediatric and Adolescent Diabetes: ISPAD Clinical Practice Consensus Guidelines 2014. Psychological care of children and adolescents with type 1 diabetes. Pediatr Diabetes 15 (suppl 20):232–244, 2014 25182317

DeMaso DR, Douglas Kelley S, Bastardi H, et al: The longitudinal impact of psychological functioning, medical severity, and family functioning in pediatric heart transplantation. J Heart Lung Transplant 23(4):473–480, 2004 15063408

Distelberg B, Tapanes D, Emerson ND, et al: Prospective pilot study of the Mastering Each New Direction psychosocial family systems program for pediatric chronic illness. Fam Proc 57(1):83–99, 2018 28299791

Dobbels F, Ruppar T, De Geest S, et al: Adherence to the immunosuppressive regimen in pediatric kidney transplant recipients: a systematic review. Pediatr Transplant 14(5):603–613, 2010 20214741

Drozdowicz LB, Bostwick JM: Psychiatric adverse effects of pediatric corticosteroid use. Mayo Clin Proc 89(6):817–834, 2014 24943696

Duncan CL, Mentrikoski JM, Wu YP, et al: Practice-based approach to assessing and treating non-adherence in pediatric regimens. Clin Pract Pediatr Psychol 2(3):322–336, 2014 25506046

Eccleston C, Palermo TM, Williams AC, et al: Psychological therapies for the management of chronic and recurrent pain in children and adolescents. Cochrane Database Syst Rev (5):CD003968, 2014 24796681

Erickson SJ, Steiner H: Trauma spectrum adaptation: somatic symptoms in long-term pediatric cancer survivors. Psychosomatics 41(4):339–346, 2000 10906356

Ernst MM, Johnson MC, Stark LJ: Developmental and psychosocial issues in cystic fibrosis. Child Adolesc Psychiatr Clin N Am 19(2):263–283, viii, 2010 20478499

Farrell E, Cullen R, Carr A: Prevention of adjustment problems in children with diabetes, in Prevention: What Works With Children and Adolescents? A Critical Review of Psychological Prevention Programmes for Children, Adolescents, and their Families. Edited by Carr A. London, Routledge, 2002, pp 249–266

Feenstra B, Boland L, Lawson ML, et al: Interventions to support children's engagement in health-related decisions: a systematic review. BMC Pediatr 14:109, 2014 24758566

Feldman JM, Steinberg D, Kutner H, et al: Perception of pulmonary function and asthma control: the differential role of child versus caregiver anxiety and depression. J Pediatr Psychol 38(10):1091–1100, 2013 23873703

Forgey M, Bursch B: Assessment and management of pediatric iatrogenic medical trauma. Curr Psychiatry Rep 15(2):340, 2013 23307562

Forgey M, Bursch B: Psychopharmacology in palliative care and oncology: childhood and adolescence, in Psychopharmacology in Oncology and Palliative Care. Edited by Grassi L, Riba M. New York, Springer, 2014, pp 331–348

Frey AS, McKee M, King RA, et al: Hair apparent: Rapunzel syndrome. Am J Psychiatry 162(2):242–248, 2005 15677585

Fritsch SL, Overton MW, Robbins DR: The interface of child mental health and juvenile diabetes mellitus. Child Adolesc Psychiatr Clin N Am 19(2):335–352, ix, 2010 20478503

Galling B, Roldán A, Nielsen RE, et al: Type 2 diabetes mellitus in youth exposed to antipsychotics: a systematic review and meta-analysis. JAMA Psychiatry 73(3):247–259, 2016 26792761

Gaston GB: African-Americans' perceptions of health care provider cultural competence that promote HIV medical self-care and antiretroviral medication adherence. AIDS Care 25(9):1159–1165, 2013 23356569

Gaudieri PA, Chen R, Greer TF, et al: Cognitive function in children with type 1 diabetes: a meta-analysis. Diabetes Care 31(9):1892–1897, 2008 18753668

Gledhill J, Hodes M: The treatment of adolescents with depression. CML Psychiatry 22(3):1–7, 2011

Glenn CR, Nock MK: Improving the prediction of suicidal behavior in youth. International Journal of Behavioral Consultation and Therapy 9(3):7–10, 2014 PMCID: PMC4557617

Goldman A, Hain R, Liben S: Oxford Textbook of Palliative Care for Children. New York, Oxford University Press, 2012

Goodwin RD, Pine DS, Hoven CW: Asthma and panic attacks among youth in the community. J Asthma 40(2):139–145, 2003 12765315

Graves MM, Roberts MC, Rapoff M, et al: The efficacy of adherence interventions for chronically ill children: a meta-analytic review. J Pediatr Psychol 35(4):368–382, 2010 19710248

Gray WN, Denson LA, Baldassano RN, et al: Treatment adherence in adolescents with inflammatory bowel disease: the collective impact of barriers to adherence and anxiety/depressive symptoms. J Pediatr Psychol 37(3):282–291, 2012 22080456

Green AD, Alioto A, Mousa H, et al: Severe pediatric rumination syndrome: successful interdisciplinary inpatient management. J Pediatr Gastroenterol Nutr 52(4):414–418, 2011 21407115

Griffiths LJ, Parsons TJ, Hill AJ: Self-esteem and quality of life in obese children and adolescents: a systematic review. Int J Pediatr Obes 5(4):282–304, 2010 20210677

Guglani L, Atkinson S, Hosanagar A, et al: A systematic review of psychological interventions for adult and pediatric patients with vocal cord dysfunction. Front Pediatr 2:82, 2014 25152871

Gulati S: Chronic kidney disease in children. 2015. Available at: http://emedicine.medscape.com/article/984358-overview. Accessed June 1, 2017.

Gutgesell H, Atkins D, Barst R, et al: AHA Scientific Statement: cardiovascular monitoring of children and adolescents receiving psychotropic drugs. J Am Acad Child Adolesc Psychiatry 38(8):1047–1050, 1999 10434498

Han JC, Lawlor DA, Kimm SY: Childhood obesity. Lancet 375(9727):1737–1748, 2010 20451244

Hanna KM, Weaver MT, Slaven JE, et al: Diabetes-related quality of life and the demands and burdens of diabetes care among emerging adults with type 1 diabetes in the year after high school graduation. Res Nurs Health 37(5):399–408, 2014 25164122

Hartmann AS, Becker AE, Hampton C, Bryant-Waugh B: Pica and rumination disorder in DSM-5. Psychiatr Ann 42(11):426–430, 2012

Herrera M, Falcone T: Delirium in pediatric patients, in Pediatric Pathways: The Squeeze of Chiari Malformation. Edited by Wyllie E, Luciano M. Cleveland, IL, Cleveland Clinic Neurological Institute, 2015, pp 19–21

Heruti RJ, Levy A, Adunski A, et al: Conversion motor paralysis disorder: overview and rehabilitation model. Spinal Cord 40(7):327–334, 2002 12080460

Hijmans CT, Fijnvandraat K, Grootenhuis MA, et al: Neurocognitive deficits in children with sickle cell disease: a comprehensive profile. Pediatr Blood Cancer 56(5):783–788, 2011 21370411

Hilliard ME, Wu YP, Rausch J, et al: Predictors of deteriorations in diabetes management and control in adolescents with type 1 diabetes. J Adolesc Health 52(1):28–34, 2013 23260831

Hilliard ME, Eakin MN, Borrelli B, et al: Medication beliefs mediate between depressive symptoms and medication adherence in cystic fibrosis. Health Psychol 34(5):496–504, 2015 25110847

Hinton D, Kirk S: Families' and healthcare professionals' perceptions of healthcare services for children and young people with medically unexplained symptoms: a narrative review of the literature. Health Soc Care Community 24(1):12–26, 2016 25684117

Ho M, Garnett SP, Baur L, et al: Effectiveness of lifestyle interventions in child obesity: systematic review with meta-analysis. Pediatrics 130(6):e1647–e1671, 2012 23166346

Hofmann SG, Asnaani A, Vonk IJ, et al: The efficacy of cognitive behavioral therapy: a review of meta-analyses. Cognit Ther Res 36(5):427–440, 2012 23459093

Hood KK, Rohan JM, Peterson CM, et al: Interventions with adherence-promoting components in pediatric type 1 diabetes: meta-analysis of their impact on glycemic control. Diabetes Care 33(7):1658–1664, 2010 20587726

Horowitz LM, Bridge JA, Pao M, et al: Screening youth for suicide risk in medical settings: time to ask questions. Am J Prev Med 47 (3 suppl 2):S170–S175, 2014 25145735

Hoyme HE, May PA, Kalberg WO, et al: A practical clinical approach to diagnosis of fetal alcohol spectrum disorders: clarification of the 1996 Institute of Medicine criteria. Pediatrics 115(1):39–47, 2005 15629980

Hyams JS, Di Lorenzo C, Saps M, et al: Functional disorders: children and adolescents. Gastroenterology S0016–5085(16):00181–00185, 2016 27144632

Iampietro M, Giovannetti T, Tarazi R: Hypoxia and inflammation in children with sickle cell disease: implications for hippocampal functioning and episodic memory. Neuropsychol Rev 24(2):252–265, 2014 24744195

Ivascu NS, Sarnaik S, McCrae J, et al: Characterization of pica prevalence among patients with sickle cell disease. Arch Pediatr Adolesc Med 155(11):1243–1247, 2001 11695934

Jaffe AC: Failure to thrive: current clinical concepts. Pediatr Rev 32(3):100–107, quiz 108, 2011 21364013

Janicke DM, Steele RG, Gayes LA, et al: Systematic review and meta-analysis of comprehensive behavioral family lifestyle interventions addressing pediatric obesity. J Pediatr Psychol 39(8):809–825, 2014 24824614

Jensen KG, Juul K, Fink-Jensen A, et al: Corrected QT changes during antipsychotic treatment of children and adolescents: a systematic review and meta-analysis of clinical trials. J Am Acad Child Adolesc Psychiatry 54(1):25–36, 2015 25524787

Jones DE, Carson KA, Bleich SN, et al: Patient trust in physicians and adoption of lifestyle behaviors to control high blood pressure. Patient Educ Couns 89(1):57–62, 2012 22770676

Joyce C, Witcher R, Herrup E, et al: Evaluation of the safety of quetiapine in treating delirium in critically ill children: a retrospective review. J Child Adolesc Psychopharmacol 25(9):666–670, 2015 26469214

Judd D: Give Sorrow Words: Working With a Dying Child. London, Karnac, 2014

Kahana S, Drotar D, Frazier T: Meta-analysis of psychological interventions to promote adherence to treatment in pediatric chronic health conditions. J Pediatr Psychol 33(6):590–611, 2008a 18192300

Kahana SY, Frazier TW, Drotar D: Preliminary quantitative investigation of predictors of treatment non-adherence in pediatric transplantation: a brief report. Pediatr Transplant 12(6):656–660, 2008b 18798360

Kaspar CD, Bholah R, Bunchman TE: A review of pediatric chronic kidney disease. Blood Purif 41(1–3):211–217, 2016 26766175

Katholi BR, Daghstani SS, Banez GA, et al: Noninvasive treatments for pediatric complex regional pain syndrome: a focused review. PM R 6(10):926–933, 2014 24780851

Kazak AE, Rourke MT, Alderfer MA, et al: Evidence-based assessment, intervention and psychosocial care in pediatric oncology: a blueprint for comprehensive services across treatment. J Pediatr Psychol 32(9):1099–1110, 2007 17626069

Kelly AS, Barlow SE, Rao G, et al: Severe obesity in children and adolescents: identification, associated health risks, and treatment approaches. A scientific statement from the American Heart Association. Circulation 128(15):1689–1712, 2013 24016455

Kelly NR, Shank LM, Bakalar JL, et al: Pediatric feeding and eating disorders: current state of diagnosis and treatment. Curr Psychiatry Rep 16(5):446, 2014 24643374

Kerzner B, Milano K, MacLean WC Jr, et al: A practical approach to classifying and managing feeding difficulties. Pediatrics 135(2):344–353, 2015 25560449

Kessing BF, Smout AJ, Bredenoord AJ: Current diagnosis and management of the rumination syndrome. J Clin Gastroenterol 48(6):478–483, 2014 24921208

King AA, DeBaun MR, White DA: Need for cognitive rehabilitation for children with sickle cell disease and strokes. Expert Rev Neurother 8(2):291–296, 2008 18271713

King PS, Berg CA, Butner J, et al: Longitudinal trajectories of metabolic control across adolescence: associations with parental involvement, adolescents' psychosocial maturity, and health care utilization. J Adolesc Health 50(5):491–496, 2012 22525113

Knight A, Weiss P, Morales K, et al: Identifying differences in risk factors for depression and anxiety in pediatric chronic disease: a matched cross-sectional study of youth with lupus/mixed connective tissue disease and their peers with diabetes. J Pediatr 167(6):1397.e1–1403.e1, 2015 26316371

Kundu A, Berman B: Acupuncture for pediatric pain and symptom management. Pediatr Clin North Am 54(6):885–889, x, 2007 18061782

Latal B: Neurodevelopmental outcomes of the child with congenital heart disease. Clin Perinatol 43(1):173–185, 2016 26876129

Lee LY, Abbott L, Mahlangu B, et al: The management of cyclic vomiting syndrome: a systematic review. Eur J Gastroenterol Hepatol 24(9):1001–1006, 2012 22634989

Lemanek KL, Brown RT, Amstrong FD, et al: Dysfunctional eating patterns and symptoms of pica in children and adolescents with sickle cell disease. Clin Pediatr (Phila) 41(7):493–500, 2002 12365311

Letitre SL, de Groot EP, Draaisma E, et al: Anxiety, depression and self-esteem in children with well-controlled asthma: case-control study. Arch Dis Child 99(8):744–748, 2014 24812302

Levy SE, Giarelli E, Lee LC, et al: Autism spectrum disorder and co-occurring developmental, psychiatric, and medical conditions among children in multiple populations of the United States. J Dev Behav Pediatr 31(4):267–275, 2010 20431403

Libow JA: Munchausen by proxy victims in adulthood: a first look. Child Abuse Negl 19(9):1131–1142, 1995 8528818

Libow JA: Child and adolescent illness falsification. Pediatrics 105(2):336–342, 2000 10654952

Libow JA: Beyond collusion: active illness falsification. Child Abuse Negl 26(5):525–536, 2002 12079088

Logan DE, Engle LB, Feinstein AB, et al: Ecological system influences in the treatment of pediatric chronic pain. Pain Res Manag 17(6):407–411, 2012 23248814

Lukens CT, Silverman AH: Systematic review of psychological interventions for pediatric feeding problems. J Pediatr Psychol 39(8):903–917, 2014 24934248

Ly TT, Maahs DM, Rewers A, et al; International Society for Pediatric and Adolescent Diabetes: ISPAD Clinical Practice Consensus Guidelines 2014. Assessment and management of hypoglycemia in children and adolescents with diabetes. Pediatr Diabetes 15 (suppl 20):180–192, 2014 25040141

Lyon ME, Jacobs S, Briggs L, et al: Family centered advance care planning for teens with cancer. JAMA Pediatr 167(5):460–467, 2013 23479062

Marcdante K, Kliegman RM: Nelson Essentials of Pediatrics, 7th Edition. New York, Elsevier Health Sciences, 2015

Marciano RC, Soares CM, Diniz JS, et al: Behavioral disorders and low quality of life in children and adolescents with chronic kidney disease. Pediatr Nephrol 26(2):281–290, 2011 21110044

Martínez-Sanchis S, Bernal MC, Montagud JV, et al: Effects of immunosuppressive drugs on the cognitive functioning of renal transplant recipients: a pilot study. J Clin Exp Neuropsychol 33(9):1016–1024, 2011 22082083

Mathew E, Kim E, Goldschneider KR: Pharmacological treatment of chronic non-cancer pain in pediatric patients. Paediatr Drugs 16(6):457–471, 2014 25304005

Mattson SN, Crocker N, Nguyen TT: Fetal alcohol spectrum disorders: neuropsychological and behavioral features. Neuropsychol Rev 21(2):81–101, 2011 21503685

May PA, Baete A, Russo J, et al: Prevalence and characteristics of fetal alcohol spectrum disorders. Pediatrics 134(5):855–866, 2014 25349310

McCormick King ML, Mee LL, Gutiérrez-Colina AM, et al: Emotional functioning, barriers, and medication adherence in pediatric transplant recipients. J Pediatr Psychol 39(3):283–293, 2014 24080552

McGovern L, Johnson JN, Paulo R, et al: Clinical review: treatment of pediatric obesity. A systematic review and meta-analysis of randomized trials. J Clin Endocrinol Metab 93(12):4600–4605, 2008 18782881

McGrady ME, Hommel KA: Medication adherence and health care utilization in pediatric chronic illness: a systematic review. Pediatrics 132(4):730–740, 2013 23999953

Meyler E, Guerin S, Kiernan G, et al: Review of family based psychosocial interventions for childhood cancer. J Pediatr Psychol 35(10):1116–1132, 2010 20444851

Miloh T, Barton A, Wheeler J, et al: Immunosuppression in pediatric liver transplant recipients: unique aspects. Liver Transpl 23(2):244–256, 2017 27874250

Moreira JM, Bouissou Morais Soares CM, Teixeira AL, et al: Anxiety, depression, resilience and quality of life in children and adolescents with pre-dialysis chronic kidney disease. Pediatr Nephrol 30(12):2153–2162, 2015 26210984

Mullins LL, Gillaspy SR, Molzon ES, Chaney JM: Parent and family interventions in pediatric psychology: clinical applications. Clin Pract Pediatr Psychol 2(3):281–293, 2014

Munk DD, Repp AC: Behavioral assessment of feeding problems of individuals with severe disabilities. J Appl Behav Anal 27(2):241–250, 1994 8063624

Mussatto KA, Hoffmann RG, Hoffman GM, et al: Risk and prevalence of developmental delay in young children with congenital heart disease. Pediatrics 133(3):e570–e577, 2014 24488746

Nationwide Children's Hospital: Feeding disorders. Gastroenterology, Hepatology, and Nutrition. 2017. Available at: http://www.nationwidechildrens.org/gi-feeding-disorders. Accessed June 1, 2017.

Nelson LP, Gold JI: Posttraumatic stress disorder in children and their parents following admission to the pediatric intensive care unit: a review. Pediatr Crit Care Med 13(3):338–347, 2012 21499173

Neuhäuser C, Wagner B, Heckmann M, et al: Analgesia and sedation for painful interventions in children and adolescents. Dtsch Arztebl Int 107(14):241–247, I–II, I, 2010 20436776

Nunley KA, Rosano C, Ryan CM, et al: Clinically relevant cognitive impairment in middle-aged adults with childhood-onset type 1 diabetes. Diabetes Care 38(9):1768–1776, 2015 26153270

O'Callaghan ET, Gold JI: Pica in children with sickle cell disease: two case reports. J Pediatr Nurs 27(6):e65–e70, 2012 22917881

Ogden CL, Carroll MD, Kit BK, et al: Prevalence of childhood and adult obesity in the United States, 2011–2012. JAMA 311(8):806–814, 2014 24570244

Oliva M, Singh TP, Gauvreau K, et al: Impact of medication non-adherence on survival after pediatric heart transplantation in the U.S.A. J Heart Lung Transplant 32(9):881–888, 2013 23755899

Oruch R, Elderbi MA, Khattab HA, et al: Lithium: a review of pharmacology, clinical uses, and toxicity. Eur J Pharmacol 740:464–473, 2014 24991789

Palermo TM, Eccleston C, Lewandowski AS, et al: Randomized controlled trials of psychological therapies for management of chronic pain in children and adolescents: an updated meta-analytic review. Pain 148(3):387–397, 2010 19910118

Paoletti G, Bogen DL, Ritchey AK: Severe iron-deficiency anemia still an issue in toddlers. Clin Pediatr (Phila) 53(14):1352–1358, 2014 24990367

Paulus GF, de Vaan LE, Verdam FJ, et al: Bariatric surgery in morbidly obese adolescents: a systematic review and meta-analysis. Obes Surg 25(5):860–878, 2015 25697125

Pei J, Denys K, Hughes J, Rasmussen C: Mental health issues in fetal alcohol spectrum disorder. J Ment Health 20(5):438–448, 2011 21780939

Peters TE, Fritz GK: Psychological considerations of the child with asthma. Pediatr Clin North Am 58(4):921–935, xi, 2011 21855714

Phipps S, Steele RG, Hall K, et al: Repressive adaptation in children with cancer: a replication and extension. Health Psychol 20(6):445–451, 2001 11714187

Pierson C, Waite E, Pyykkonen B: A meta-analysis of the neuropsychological effects of chemotherapy in the treatment of childhood cancer. Pediatr Blood Cancer 63(11):1998–2003, 2016 27463220

Pillay J, Armstrong MJ, Butalia S, et al: Behavioral programs for type 1 diabetes mellitus: a systematic review and meta-analysis. Ann Intern Med 163(11):836–847, 2015 26414020

Pinquart M: Self-esteem of children and adolescents with chronic illness: a meta-analysis. Child Care Health Dev 39(2):153–161, 2013 22712715

Pinquart M, Shen Y: Depressive symptoms in children and adolescents with chronic physical illness: an updated meta-analysis. J Pediatr Psychol 36(4):375–384, 2011 21088072

Plioplys S, Asato MR, Bursch B, et al: Multidisciplinary management of pediatric nonepileptic seizures. J Am Acad Child Adolesc Psychiatry 46(11):1491–1495, 2007 18049299

Ploessl C, Pettit RS, Donaldson J: Prevalence of depression and antidepressant therapy use in a pediatric cystic fibrosis population. Ann Pharmacother 48(4):488–493, 2014 24311728

Porter GE, Heitsch GM, Miller MD: Munchausen syndrome by proxy: unusual manifestations and disturbing sequelae. Child Abuse Negl 18(9):789–794, 1994 7528090

Powell PW, Hilliard ME, Anderson BJ: Motivational interviewing to promote adherence behaviors in pediatric type 1 diabetes. Curr Diab Rep 14(10):531, 2014 25142716

Pratt K, Baird G, Gringras P: Ensuring successful admission to hospital for young people with learning difficulties, autism and challenging behaviour: a continuous quality improvement and change management programme. Child Care Health Dev 38(6):789–797, 2012 22017703

Pulgarón ER: Childhood obesity: a review of increased risk for physical and psychological comorbidities. Clin Ther 35(1):A18–A32, 2013 23328273

Quittner AL, Abbott J, Georgiopoulos AM, et al; International Committee on Mental Health; EPOS Trial Study Group: International Committee on Mental Health in Cystic Fibrosis: Cystic Fibrosis Foundation and European Cystic Fibrosis Society consensus statements for screening and treating depression and anxiety. Thorax 71(1):26–34, 2016 26452630

Racine NM, Riddell RR, Khan M, et al: Systematic review: predisposing, precipitating, perpetuating, and present factors predicting anticipatory distress to painful medical procedures in children. J Pediatr Psychol 41(2):159–181, 2016 26338981

Rajindrajith S, Devanarayana NM, Crispus Perera BJ: Rumination syndrome in children and adolescents: a school survey assessing prevalence and symptomatology. BMC Gastroenterol 12(1):163, 2012 23157670

Rapp A, Dodds A, Walkup JT, Rynn M: Treatment of pediatric anxiety disorders. Ann N Y Acad Sci 1304:52–61, 2013 24279893

Rausch JR, Hood KK, Delamater A, et al: Changes in treatment adherence and glycemic control during the transition to adolescence in type 1 diabetes. Diabetes Care 35(6):1219–1224, 2012 22474040

Reilly C, Agnew R, Neville BG: Depression and anxiety in childhood epilepsy: a review. Seizure 20(8):589–597, 2011 21741277

Reilly C, Menlove L, Fenton V, Das KB: Psychogenic nonepileptic seizures in children: a review. Epilepsia 54(10):1715–1724, 2013 23944981

Reynolds S, Wilson C, Austin J, Hooper L: Effects of psychotherapy for anxiety in children and adolescents: a meta-analytic review. Clin Psychol Rev 32(4):251–262, 2012 22459788

Richter D, Koehler M, Friedrich M, et al: Psychosocial interventions for adolescents and young adult cancer patients: a systematic review and meta-analysis. Crit Rev Oncol Hematol 95(3):370–386, 2015 25922217

Riley EP, Infante MA, Warren KR: Fetal alcohol spectrum disorders: an overview. Neuropsychol Rev 21(2):73–80, 2011 21499711

Rooney BL, Mathiason MA, Schauberger CW: Predictors of obesity in childhood, adolescence, and adulthood in a birth cohort. Matern Child Health J 15(8):1166–1175, 2011 20927643

Rutten JM, Reitsma JB, Vlieger AM, et al: Gut-directed hypnotherapy for functional abdominal pain or irritable bowel syndrome in children: a systematic review. Arch Dis Child 98(4):252–257, 2013 23220208

Sahler OJ, Dolgin MJ, Phipps S, et al: Specificity of problem-solving skills training in mothers of children newly diagnosed with cancer: results of a multisite randomized clinical trial. J Clin Oncol 31(10):1329–1335, 2013 23358975

Schaefer C, von Rhein M, Knirsch W, et al: Neurodevelopmental outcome, psychological adjustment, and quality of life in adolescents with congenital heart disease. Dev Med Child Neurol 55(12):1143–1149, 2013 23937239

Schieveld JN, Janssen NJ: Delirium in the pediatric patient: on the growing awareness of its clinical interdisciplinary importance. JAMA Pediatr 168(7):595–596, 2014 24797545

Schmitz ML, Zempsky WT, Meyer JM: Safety and efficacy of a needle-free powder lidocaine delivery system in pediatric patients undergoing venipuncture or peripheral venous cannulation: randomized double-blind COMFORT-004 trial. Clin Ther 37(8):1761–1772, 2015 26164784

Schmitz N, Deschênes SS, Burns RJ, et al: Depression and risk of type 2 diabetes: the potential role of metabolic factors. Mol Psychiatry 21(12):1726–1732, 2016 26903269

Secinti E, Thompson EJ, Richards M, et al: Research review: childhood chronic physical illness and adult emotional health—a systematic review and meta-analysis. J Child Psychol Psychiatry 58(7):753–769, 2017 28449285

Sert A, Aypar E, Odabas D, et al: Clinical characteristics and causes of chest pain in 380 children referred to a paediatric cardiology unit. Cardiol Young 23(3):361–367, 2013 22874139

Sharp WG, Jaquess DL, Morton JF, et al: Pediatric feeding disorders: a quantitative synthesis of treatment outcomes. Clin Child Fam Psychol Rev 13(4):348–365, 2010 20844951

Sharp WG, Jaquess DL, Lukens CT: Multi-method assessment of feeding problems among children with autism spectrum disorders. Res Autism Spectr Disord 7(1):56–65, 2013

Shemesh E, Lurie S, Stuber ML, et al: A pilot study of posttraumatic stress and nonadherence in pediatric liver transplant recipients. Pediatrics 105(2):E29, 2000 10654989

Shemesh E, Kleinman LC, Howell EA, Annunziato R: Racial and economic disparities in transplant outcomes: the not-so-hidden morbidities. Liver Transpl 20(1):4–6, 2014 24288361

Silver G, Traube C, Kearney J, et al: Detecting pediatric delirium: development of a rapid observational assessment tool. Intensive Care Med 38(6):1025–1031, 2012 22407142

Simon SL, Duncan CL, Horky SC, et al: Body satisfaction, nutritional adherence, and quality of life in youth with cystic fibrosis. Pediatr Pulmonol 46(11):1085–1092, 2011 21626713

Simone S, Edwards S, Lardieri A, et al: Implementation of an ICU bundle: an interprofessional quality improvement project to enhance delirium management and monitor delirium prevalence in a single PICU. Pediatr Crit Care Med 18(6):531–540, 2017 28410275

Smith BA, Modi AC, Quittner AL, et al: Depressive symptoms in children with cystic fibrosis and parents and its effects on adherence to airway clearance. Pediatr Pulmonol 45(8):756–763, 2010 20597082

Smith HA, Boyd J, Fuchs DC, et al: Diagnosing delirium in critically ill children: validity and reliability of the Pediatric Confusion Assessment Method for the Intensive Care Unit. Crit Care Med 39(1):150–157, 2011 20959783

Smith HA, Brink E, Fuchs DC, et al: Pediatric delirium: monitoring and management in the pediatric intensive care unit. Pediatr Clin North Am 60(3):741–760, 2013 23639666

Smith KE, Schatz J: Working memory in children with neurocognitive effects from sickle cell disease: contributions of the central executive and processing speed. Dev Neuropsychol 41(4):231–244, 2016 27759435

Snell C, Fernandes S, Bujoreanu IS, et al: Depression, illness severity, and healthcare utilization in cystic fibrosis. Pediatr Pulmonol 49(12):1177–1181, 2014 24619910

Spijkerboer AW, De Koning WB, Duivenvoorden HJ, et al: Medical predictors for long-term behavioral and emotional outcomes in children and adolescents after invasive treatment of congenital heart disease. J Pediatr Surg 45(11):2146–2153, 2010 21034936

Strawn JR, Welge JA, Wehry AM, et al: Efficacy and tolerability of antidepressants in pediatric anxiety disorders: a systematic review and meta-analysis. Depress Anxiety 32(3):149–157, 2015 25449861

Stuber ML, Meeske KA, Krull KR, et al: Prevalence and predictors of posttraumatic stress disorder in adult survivors of childhood cancer. Pediatrics 125(5):e1124–e1134, 2010 20435702

Sundbom F, Malinovschi A, Lindberg E, et al: Effects of poor asthma control, insomnia, anxiety and depression on quality of life in young asthmatics. J Asthma 53(4):398–403, 2016 26666333

Thabrew H, Stasiak K, Hetrick SE, et al: Psychological therapies for anxiety and depression in children and adolescents with long-term physical conditions. Cochrane Database Syst Rev (1):CD012488, 2017

Thompson DG, Tielsch-Goddard A: Improving management of patients with autism spectrum disorder having scheduled surgery: optimizing practice. J Pediatr Health Care 28(5):394–403, 2014 24287372

Todaro JF, Fennell EB, Sears SF, et al: Review: cognitive and psychological outcomes in pediatric heart transplantation. J Pediatr Psychol 25(8):567–576, 2000 11085760

Traube C, Silver G, Gerber LM, et al: Delirium and mortality in critically ill children: epidemiology and outcomes of pediatric delirium. Crit Care Med 45(5):891–898, 2017 28288026

Troiano RP, Flegal KM, Kuczmarski RJ, et al: Overweight prevalence and trends for children and adolescents. The National Health and Nutrition Examination Surveys, 1963 to 1991. Arch Pediatr Adolesc Med 149(10):1085–1091, 1995 7550810

Turkel SB, Hanft A: The pharmacologic management of delirium in children and adolescents. Paediatr Drugs 16(4):267–274, 2014 24898718

Turkel SB, Jacobson J, Munzig E, et al: Atypical antipsychotic medications to control symptoms of delirium in children and adolescents. J Child Adolesc Psychopharmacol 22(2):126–130, 2012 22364403

Uchida M, Spencer AE, Biederman J, et al: A systematic evaluation of the QTc interval and antidepressants in youth: an electronic health record study. J Dev Behav Pediatr 36(6):434–439, 2015 26154713

Uman LS, Birnie KA, Noel M, et al: Psychological interventions for needle-related procedural pain and distress in children and adolescents. Cochrane Database Syst Rev (10):CD005179, 2013 24108531

Ünal S, Toros F, Kütük MÖ, Uyanıker MG: Evaluation of the psychological problems in children with sickle cell anemia and their families. Pediatr Hematol Oncol 28(4):321–328, 2011 21345077

U.S. Department of Health and Human Services: Organ Procurement and Transplantation Network (OPTN): Kidney competing risk median waiting time to deceased donor transplant for registrations listed: 2003–2014. Based on OPTN data as of March 16, 2017a. Available at: https://optn.transplant.hrsa.gov/data/view-data-reports/national-data/#. Accessed March 16, 2017.

U.S. Department of Health and Human Services: Organ Procurement and Transplantation Network (OPTN): Transplants in the U.S. by Recipient Age. Current U.S. Waiting List. Based on OPTN data as of March 16, 2017b. Available at: http://optn.transplant.hrsa.gov/data/. Accessed March 16, 2017.

U.S. Food and Drug Administration: Drug Safety Communication: Safety Review Update of Medications used to treat attention-deficit/hyperactivity disorder (ADHD) in children and young adults. November 1, 2011. Available at: https://www.fda.gov/Drugs/DrugSafety/ucm277770.htm. Accessed June 1, 2017.

Uzark K, Griffin L, Rodriguez R, et al: Quality of life in pediatric heart transplant recipients: a comparison with children with and without heart disease. J Heart Lung Transplant 31(6):571–578, 2012 22381209

van der Geest IM, Darlington AS, Streng IC, et al: Parents' experiences of pediatric palliative care and the impact on long-term parental grief. J Pain Symptom Manage 47(6):1043–1053, 2014 24120185

van der Schans J, Çiçek R, de Vries TW, et al: Association of atopic diseases and attention-deficit/hyperactivity disorder: a systematic review and meta-analyses. Neurosci Biobehav Rev 74(Pt A):139–148, 2017 28111269

van Oers HA, Haverman L, Limperg PF, et al: Anxiety and depression in mothers and fathers of a chronically ill child. Matern Child Health J 18(8):1993–2002, 2014 24791971

Varni JW, Limbers CA, Burwinkle TM: Impaired health-related quality of life in children and adolescents with chronic conditions: a comparative analysis of 10 disease clusters and 33 disease categories/severities utilizing the PedsQL 4.0 Generic Core Scales. Health Qual Life Outcomes 5(1):43, 2007 17634123

Vet NJ, de Wildt SN, Verlaat CW, et al; Stichting Kinder Intensive Care (Dutch collaborative PICU research network): Short-term health-related quality of life of critically ill children following daily sedation interruption. Pediatr Crit Care Med 17(11):e513–e520, 2016 27662565

Vila M, Kramer T, Hickey N, et al: Assessment of somatic symptoms in British secondary school children using the Children's Somatization Inventory (CSI). J Pediatr Psychol 34(9):989–998, 2009 19223276

Volkmar FR, Rogers S, Paul R, et al: Handbook of Autism and Pervasive Developmental Disorders, 4th Edition. Hoboken, NJ, Wiley, 2014

Wall W, Tucker CM, Roncoroni J, et al: Patients' perceived cultural sensitivity of health care office staff and its association with patients' health care satisfaction and treatment adherence. J Health Care Poor Underserved 24(4):1586–1598, 2013 24185154

Wamboldt MZ, Yancey AG Jr, Roesler TA: Cardiovascular effects of tricyclic antidepressants in childhood asthma: a case series and review. J Child Adolesc Psychopharmacol 7(1):45–64, 1997 9192541

Wang Y, Cai L, Wu Y, et al: What childhood obesity prevention programmes work? A systematic review and meta-analysis. Obes Rev 16(7):547–565, 2015 25893796

Warady BA, Neu AM, Schaefer F: Optimal care of the infant, child, and adolescent on dialysis: 2014 update. Am J Kidney Dis 64(1):128–142, 2014 24717681

Wehry AM, Beesdo-Baum K, Hennelly MM, et al: Assessment and treatment of anxiety disorders in children and adolescents. Curr Psychiatry Rep 17(7):52, 2015 25980507

Weissmann R, Uziel Y: Pediatric complex regional pain syndrome: a review. Pediatr Rheumatol Online J 14(1):29, 2016 27130211

White T, Miller J, Smith GL, et al: Adherence and psychopathology in children and adolescents with cystic fibrosis. Eur Child Adolesc Psychiatry 18(2):96–104, 2009 18807223

Williams SE, Zahka NE: Treating Somatic Symptoms in Children and Adolescents (Guilford Child and Adolescent Practitioner Series). New York, Guilford, 2017

Wong CJ, Moxey-Mims M, Jerry-Fluker J, et al: CKiD (CKD in children) prospective cohort study: a review of current findings. Am J Kidney Dis 60(6):1002–1011, 2012 23022429

Wu LM, Sheen JM, Shu HL, et al: Predictors of anxiety and resilience in adolescents undergoing cancer treatment. J Adv Nurs 69(1):158–166, 2013 22489627

Yawn BP, Buchanan GR, Afenyi-Annan AN, et al: Management of sickle cell disease: summary of the 2014 evidence-based report by expert panel members. JAMA 312(10):1033–1048, 2014 25203083

Yen EH, Quinton H, Borowitz D: Better nutritional status in early childhood is associated with improved clinical outcomes and survival in patients with cystic fibrosis. J Pediatr 162(3):530–535.e1, 2013 23062247

Zenlea IS, Mednick L, Rein J, et al: Routine behavioral and mental health screening in young children with type 1 diabetes mellitus. Pediatr Diabetes 15(5):384–388, 2014 24274235

Žganjer V, Žganjer M, Cizmić A, et al: Suicide attempt by swallowing sponge or pica disorder: a case report. Acta Med (Hradec Kralove) 54(2):91–93, 2011 21842726

CHAPTER 33

Physical Medicine and Rehabilitation

Jesse R. Fann, M.D., M.P.H.

Richard Kennedy, M.D.

Charles H. Bombardier, Ph.D.

The focus of physical medicine and rehabilitation, or *rehabilitation medicine,* is helping people reach the fullest physical, psychological, social, vocational, and educational potential consistent with their physiological or anatomical impairment, environmental limitations, and desires and life plans. Patients in the rehabilitation setting are highly diverse, and their problems range from acute to chronic and can involve nearly any organ system. Rehabilitation can take place in outpatient, inpatient, extended-care, and in-home programs and includes both prevention and treatment. Maximizing independence is central to the goal of optimizing quality of life.

Rehabilitation is generally a multidisciplinary or interdisciplinary effort. Rehabilitation medicine physicians (physiatrists) usually lead the team of other specialized professionals, including physical therapists, occupational therapists, speech pathologists, clinical psychologists and neuropsychologists, vocational rehabilitation counselors, recreation therapists, social workers, and nurses. Rehabilitation programs often have a dedicated psychologist on staff whose job is to conduct psychological and neuropsychological assessments; provide counseling to patients and families; oversee behavioral programs; and generally assist staff in the management of cognitive, behavioral, affective, and social aspects of rehabilitation.

Psychiatrists have an increasing role in the care of patients in the rehabilitation setting. As advances in medical care have increased survival in many conditions that previously were fatal, many rehabilitation opportunities and challenges have emerged that did not previously exist. Data from the 2016 National Health Interview Survey suggest that among civilian noninstitutionalized persons in the U.S. population, approximately 13% (43 million) have a limitation in usual activities because of one or more chronic health conditions (Lucas and Benson 2018).

The World Health Organization emphasizes "components of health" in the *International Classification of Functioning, Disability and Health* (ICF; World Health Organization 2001). The ICF conceptually differentiates health and health-related components of the disabling process at the levels of 1) *body structures* (anatomical parts of the body, such as organs, limbs, and their components) and *functions* (physiological functions of body systems, including psychological functions) and 2) *activities* (execution of a task or an action by an individual) and *participation* (involvement in a life situation—i.e., the "lived experience" of people). *Impairments* are defined as problems in body function or structure, such as a significant deviation or loss, and focus on *activity limitations* rather than disabilities and *participation limitations* rather than handicaps. Environmental and personal factors interact with a health condition to restore functioning or create a disability, depending on whether the factor is a facilitator or barrier. Figure 33–1 illustrates the interactive and dynamic dimensions of this model. The ICF places the burdens of all diseases and health conditions, including mental illness, on an equal footing. Psychosocial factors can cause impairment and limit activities and participation in many ways, thus affording opportunities for multifaceted psychosocial interventions in the rehabilitation setting.

In this chapter, we focus on the psychiatric issues encountered in the treatment of traumatic brain injury (TBI) and spinal cord injury (SCI), two common and highly complex rehabilitation challenges with aspects that may require psychiatric intervention. Although many of the other disorders encountered in the rehabilitation setting are covered in other chapters of this text, many of the principles discussed in this chapter also apply to them.

Traumatic Brain Injury

Epidemiology

TBI is a significant problem from both an individual and a public health perspective. An estimated 2.8 million Americans sustain a TBI each year; of these, approximately 282,000 are hospitalized and survive, and 2.5 million are treated and released from an emergency department (Taylor et al. 2017). These figures likely underestimate the incidence of TBI as a result of underreporting of milder injuries (Bazarian et al. 2006; Coronado et al. 2012) According to data from hospitalized individuals, at least 5.3 million persons in the United States, or about 2% of the population, live with disabilities resulting from TBI (Thurman et al. 1999). Although about 75% of TBIs are mild in severity, many people experience long-term somatic and psychiatric symptoms that may lead to disability (Langlois et al. 2006). TBI is often referred to as the *invisible epidemic*, because TBI-related disabilities are not readily visible to the general public.

With improvements in medical care, TBI mortality declined 17% from 1995 to 2009 (Coronado et al. 2012), leading to more long-term morbidity and disability. Decreases in TBI mortality also have been seen in military injuries because of advances in body armor (Okie 2005). The age groups with the highest incidence of TBI are 0- to 4-year-olds (mostly from falls), 15- to 24-year-olds (mostly from motor vehicle accidents), and persons 65 years and older (mostly from falls). Although TBI is often conceptualized as primarily occurring in young adult males as a result of accidents, the grow-

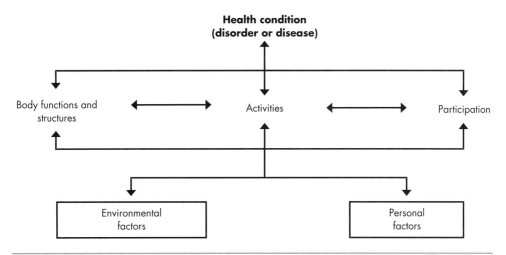

FIGURE 33–1. Interactions between components of health as defined in the *International Classification of Functioning, Disability and Health.*

Source. Reprinted from World Health Organization: *International Classification of Functioning, Disability and Health: ICF.* Geneva, World Health Organization, 2001. Used with permission.

ing elderly population has led to a steady increase in the age of individuals experiencing TBI, and falls have surpassed motor vehicle accidents as the leading cause of injury (Roozenbeek et al. 2013).

Early studies differentiated between military and civilian injuries, with injuries to military personnel outside of combat zones (which constitute the majority of TBI in the military; Armistead-Jehle et al. 2017; Defense and Veterans Brain Injury Center 2017) more closely resembling the latter than the former (Lanska 2009). TBI sustained during combat was noted in these studies to predominantly involve posterior injuries to the occipital and parietal lobes, whereas civilian TBI was noted to predominantly involve anterior injuries to the frontal and temporal lobes. The incidence of penetrating TBI was higher among military personnel than among civilians. However, blast injuries are now the predominant cause of injury among personnel in combat zones, and some experts categorize these injuries as being distinct from both penetrating and nonpenetrating injuries in civilians (Armistead-Jehle et al. 2017). However, studies to date have shown few differences between blast-related and non-blast-related injuries on cognitive and psychological outcomes (Armistead-Jehle et al. 2017). The demographics of those injured in current military operations reflect the overall demographics of those deployed, with a younger population (younger than 30 years) and an even higher percentage of males (Schwab et al. 2017).

TBI is associated with significant disability, and the societal burden is particularly prominent among younger individuals. Most studies report that only 30%–40% of individuals with TBI are able to return to work (Wehman et al. 2017), and approximately 43% of individuals hospitalized for TBI have long-term disability (Selassie et al. 2008). In the United States in 2013, direct and indirect costs of TBI totaled an estimated $63.4–$79.1 billion (Ma et al. 2014). Figures show that the direct medical costs of TBI range from $9.1 to $14.6 billion (Coronado et al. 2012). About 65% of TBI-related costs are accrued among survivors. Statistics for 2013 estimated that TBI-related missed work days, reduced productivity, and disability cost approximately $64.7 billion (Ma et al. 2014). Similar results have been reported among the military for recent conflicts, with an estimated total cost of $600–$900 million in the first year after diagnosis of TBI (Tanielian and Jaycox 2008). Long-term disability has primarily been attributed to psychiatric disorders and to behavior problems such as irritability (Gould et al. 2011; Sabaz et al. 2014).

Finally, self-reported TBI appears to be more frequent among psychiatric inpatients compared with the general population, with excess rates of 70%–94% (Fann et al. 2002; Liao et al. 2012). Thus, many psychiatrists will be involved at some level in the care of individuals with TBI.

Definition and Severity Classification

DSM-5 (American Psychiatric Association 2013), unlike previous DSM editions, provides explicit criteria for TBI, which is defined as an impact to the head or other mechanisms of rapid movement or displacement of the brain within the skull, with one or more of the following: 1) loss of consciousness (LOC); 2) posttraumatic amnesia (PTA); 3) disorientation and confusion; or 4) neurological signs, such as neuroimaging demonstrating injury, a new onset of seizures, a marked worsening of a preexisting seizure disorder, visual field cuts, anosmia, or hemiparesis. DSM-5 also provides thresholds for rating injury severity as *mild* (LOC less than 30 minutes and/or PTA duration of less than 24 hours, associated with Glasgow Coma Scale [GCS; Jennett and Bond 1975] scores of 13–15 at 30 minutes postinjury), *moderate* (LOC of 0.5–24 hours and/or PTA of 1–7 days, with GCS scores of 9–12 at 30 minutes postinjury), or *severe* (LOC greater than 24 hours and/or PTA greater than 7 days, with GCS scores of 3–8 at 30 minutes postinjury). Unfortunately, these variables can be difficult to determine in the trauma setting, making TBI ascertainment and severity classification problematic. The DSM-5 classification of mild TBI is consistent with the widely used American Congress of Rehabilitation Medicine definition (Kay et al. 1993). Patients with a GCS score of 13–15 and imaging evidence of intracranial pathology have outcomes more similar to those of moderate TBI and are often labeled as having *complicated mild injuries* (Williams et al. 1990), although this term is not part of the DSM-5 classification.

Pathophysiology

There has been considerable progress in understanding the pathophysiology of TBI in recent years. The physical forces in TBI initiate mechanical and chemical changes that lead to neurological dysfunction. These changes are divided into *primary damage,* which occurs at the moment of injury, and *secondary damage,* which is initiated at injury but evolves over time (Hawryluk and Bullock 2016). The latter is subdivided into direct injury, occurring within the neuron itself, and indirect injury, occurring outside the neuron but affecting its function. However, this distinction is becoming blurred as research shows that the effects of primary damage are not confined to the time of injury.

Primary damage consists of injuries such as skull fractures, brain contusions and lacerations, and intracranial hemorrhage. Because these occur at the time of injury, the key treatment is prevention. *Diffuse axonal injury* is the predominant mechanism of injury in most cases of TBI (McGinn and Povlishock 2016). Diffuse axonal injury was originally thought to be due to shearing forces at the time of injury resulting in temporary or permanent disruption of axonal function. It is now known that diffuse axonal injury results from progressive neuronal dysfunction leading to axonal disconnection, which can evolve over a period of 24–72 hours after injury. Although this delayed response makes diffuse axonal injury potentially responsive to pharmacological intervention, no currently used therapeutic modality is known to consistently influence its progression (Smith et al. 2013).

Direct secondary injury occurs via neurochemical changes evolving over time after the mechanical disruption of neuronal pathways (McGinn and Povlishock 2016). The acute phase of this process has been well described, with a rapid increase in excitatory glutamate levels occurring within minutes of injury. Excessive glutamate in turn leads to release of intracellular calcium, which contributes to neuronal damage through activation of calpains and caspases, generation of reactive oxygen and nitrogen species, and mitochondrial impairment. These neurochemical changes are accompanied by a global increase in glucose metabolism lasting for several days postinjury. TBI also triggers a proinflammatory state through activation of microglial immune cells in the central nervous system (CNS) and infiltration of peripheral immune cells, which release a variety of inflammatory signals.

The neurochemical changes in the subacute phase of TBI show a dramatic reversal of acute processes. Cerebral metabolism and function of many neurotransmitters, including glutamate, acetylcholine, dopamine, and norepinephrine, become depressed (Sun and Feng 2014); given the prominence of these neurotransmitters in psychiatric disorders, these alterations would potentially account for cognitive and neurobehavioral deficits in TBI. These changes are accompanied by global reductions in glucose metabolism that persists for weeks to months and parallels the course of recovery (McGinn and Povlishock 2016). Research in animal models of TBI has successfully identified pharmacotherapies to reduce behavioral and histological complications (Vink 2018). However, clinical investigations of such agents have been disappointing (Hawryluk and Bullock 2016). Interventions explored include anticholinergics, cholinomimetics, anti-inflammatory agents, calcium channel blockers, free radical scavengers, glutamate antagonists, and hypothermia.

Psychiatric Disorders in Traumatic Brain Injury

Although useful data have been collected regarding the epidemiology of psychiatric disorders after TBI, the numbers of studies and subjects for many disorders remain small. Recent studies have provided rigorous evaluation of subjects, using structured clinical interviews to assess current and past psychopathology in representative samples followed immediately after injury, which addresses limitations (reviewed by van Reekum et al. 2000) of many earlier studies. Assessments should be based on multiple sources of information, because individuals with TBI may lack insight into, and not report, their deficits. Psychiatrists may give greater weight to the reports of family and treating clinicians for this reason. However, family ratings may be influenced by other factors, including caregiver personality characteristics (McKinlay et al. 1981). Similarly, the clinician's emotional response to the patient may interfere with accurate assessment of deficits (Heilbronner et al. 1989). In addition to these general concerns, there may be differences in the presentation and phenomenology of specific disorders in the context of TBI.

The development of psychiatric disorders involves a complex interplay between premorbid biological and psychological factors, postinjury biological changes, and psychosocial and environmental factors. The role of many risk factors has yet to be well elucidated, and many risk factors are specific to a given disorder. A recent meta-analysis (Scholten et al. 2016) compiled risk factors for the development of psychiatric sequelae in general, and mood and anxiety disorders in particular. Risk factors for DSM-IV (American Psychiatric Association 1994) Axis I psychiatric disorders included previous history of psychiatric disorders (including substance use disorders), more severe injury, female sex, and unemployment. The evidence was inconsistent for age, time postinjury, and hospital length of stay. Fann et al. (2004) have suggested that moderate to severe TBI may be associated with higher initial risk for psychiatric problems, whereas mild TBI and prior psychiatric illness may increase the risk for more persistent psychiatric problems. They hypothesized that psychiatric symptoms that arise immediately after TBI may be etiologically related to the neurophysiological effects of the injury, consistent with the early relation between TBI severity and psychiatric risk, whereas other factors, such as psychological vulnerability, self-awareness of deficits, social influences, and secondary gain, may play roles over time, particularly in individuals with prior psychiatric illness and prior injury.

The role of TBI in the etiology of psychiatric disorders after TBI may have significant implications for prognosis and treatment, as well as medicolegal ramifications (van Reekum et al. 2001). Although several psychiatric disorders are common after TBI (Perry et al. 2016), establishing a causal link between TBI and these disorders remains difficult (Rogers and Read 2007; van Reekum et al. 2000). TBI disrupts neuronal systems involved in mood and behavior; other possible associations include the following: 1) the psychiatric disorder increases the risk for TBI (Fann et al. 2002); 2) the risks for both TBI and the psychiatric disorder are due to a common third factor, such as substance use disorder; and 3) a postinjury condition, such as pain or change in social status, contributes to the psychiatric disorder. There is also a lack of specificity—TBI has been postulated to cause a variety of psychiatric disorders and conditions rather than a single specific syndrome. Assigning TBI as the definitive cause of psychiatric disturbances in most instances is not possible under current evidence.

Major and Mild Neurocognitive Disorder

In DSM-5, most of the consequences of TBI are categorized under the framework of major and mild neurocognitive disorder (NCD). With the exception of delirium, the diagnosis of NCD incorporates all acquired cognitive disorders from the DSM-IV-TR (American Psychiatric Association 2000) diagnostic category Delirium, Dementia, and Amnestic and Other Cognitive Disorders. The primary difference between the two diagnoses is that of severity. Major NCD requires substantial cognitive impairment, defined as two or more standard deviations on a quantifiable clinical assessment, such as neuropsychological testing; and interference with independence in everyday activities. By contrast, mild NCD requires modest cognitive impairment, defined as one to two standard deviations on a quantifiable clinical assessment. Mild NCD by definition does not interfere with independence in everyday activities, although increased effort or compensatory strategies may be required to maintain independence. For a diagnosis of major or mild NCD due to TBI, DSM-5 requires that the cognitive deficits develop immediately after TBI (as defined in the earlier subsection

"Definition and Severity Classification") or immediately after recovery of consciousness (for those who experience LOC). Cognitive deficits are also required to persist past the postinjury period, a detail that differentiates NCD from delirium. DSM-5 specifically notes that the severity of NCD does not necessarily correspond to the severity of TBI injury, so mild TBI does not preclude more severe cognitive deficits.

Much effort has been devoted to characterizing the cognitive deficits that occur after TBI. Some researchers have suggested that deficits can be divided into four time periods (Rao and Lyketsos 2000). The first is the period of LOC that results from the injury. After emerging from unconsciousness, many individuals enter the second period, a phase characterized by fluctuations in cognition and behavior, which some have described as "posttraumatic delirium." The third period involves a rapid recovery of cognitive function, which plateaus over time, leading to the fourth period of persisting cognitive deficits. TBI is associated with deficits in multiple domains, including impaired memory, language deficits, reduced attention and concentration, slowed information processing, and executive dysfunction (Rabinowitz and Levin 2014).

Although TBI is associated with an acute decrement in cognitive function that typically improves over time, recovery is very individualized, and no universally applicable description of the recovery process exists. Rao and Lyketsos (2000) offered the following general timeline: the first two periods of recovery will last from a few days to a month, the third period will last 6–12 months, and the fourth period will last beyond 12–24 months. Such guidelines are more characteristic of moderate to severe injuries. By definition, individuals with mild TBI will have LOC of less than 30 minutes, with many having none at all (Kay et al. 1993). It is also estimated that 80%–85% of patients with uncomplicated mild TBI will recover to baseline status within 3–6 months and not enter the fourth phase of permanent deficits (Belanger and Vanderploeg 2005). Even among individuals with moderate to severe TBI, some recovery of cognitive function may occur 2 years or more after injury, although the gains are typically small (Millis et al. 2001). A few patients may experience decline late in the course of recovery, perhaps caused by depression or other factors.

Descriptions of the period of recovery from TBI vary in the rehabilitation literature. One classical term is *posttraumatic amnesia,* which occurs "from injury until recovery of full consciousness and the return of ongoing memory" (Grant and Alves 1987). This time frame includes the first two periods described in the previous paragraph and can potentially extend into the third. Stuss et al. (1999) advocated use of the term *posttraumatic confusion* because the deficits after TBI are not purely amnestic, but this term has not gained widespread use. Another common term for the period of recovery after TBI is *posttraumatic agitation,* which is characterized by "excesses of behavior that include some combination of aggression, akathisia, disinhibition, and/or emotional lability" (Sandel and Mysiw 1996, p. 619). This description would correspond closely to the second period described in the previous paragraph. Unfortunately, this terminology does not correspond exactly to DSM-5 psychiatric diagnoses. The terms *delirium, posttraumatic amnesia,* and *posttraumatic agitation* refer to conditions that share many common features but are not synonymous (Nakase-Thompson et al. 2004; Thompson et al. 2001). Most definitions of posttraumatic amnesia would be consistent with a period of delirium followed by an amnestic phase (Trzepacz et al. 2011). The term *posttraumatic confusion* more closely resembles the diagnosis of delirium but still omits certain features, such as mood and perceptual disturbances. *Posttraumatic agitation* is defined by some experts as a subtype of delirium, yet others have noted that agitation may resolve while the confusional state persists (van der Naalt et al. 2000). The diagnosis of NCD would apply to the long-term diffuse cognitive deficits seen after TBI. These longer-term outcomes would correspond to the fourth period described in the previous paragraph and potentially the third period when the recovery process is slow. Compelling evidence now exists for the association between TBI and long-term risk of dementia, including Alzheimer's disease. The risk is heightened as the number and severity of TBIs increase (Fann et al. 2018).

For NCD, severity of injury is consistently associated with the degree and duration of cognitive impairments. The extent of impairment is also influenced by premorbid intellectual abilities as well as by the time after injury at which the patient is assessed (Dikmen et al. 1995; Kreutzer et al. 1993). The cognitive domains affected will vary for each patient. Patients with TBI also may be at increased risk for developing dementia from other causes, such as Alzheimer's disease (Perry et al. 2016).

Postconcussive Syndrome

The diagnosis of postconcussive syndrome (PCS) has been a source of wide controversy, and some experts have called for it to be discarded (Silver 2014). It is important to differentiate postconcussive *symptoms* from postconcussive *syndrome.* The symptoms of PCS are nonspecific and include disturbances such as headache, dizziness, irritability, fatigue, and insomnia. Indeed, several studies have documented high base rates of postconcussive symptoms among individuals without TBI, often at rates similar to those with mild TBI (Broshek et al. 2015). Standardized diagnostic criteria for PCS have been published in ICD-10 (World Health Organization 1992) and are listed in Table 33–1. The symptoms of PCS are extremely common after mild TBI, with 80%–100% of patients experiencing one or more symptoms in the immediate postinjury period (Levin et al. 1987b); however, only a minority will have multiple symptoms consistent with an ICD-10 diagnosis of PCS. Several studies have shown that the majority of individuals with mild TBI have complete recovery over a period of days to weeks (Broshek et al. 2015; McCrea et al. 2009).

Whereas DSM-IV-TR listed provisional criteria for postconcussional disorder, DSM-5 incorporates these symptoms under the "with behavioral disturbance" modifier for major NCD due to traumatic brain injury. For reasons that are not clearly explained, DSM-5 does not allow use of the "with behavioral disturbance" modifier for mild NCD due to TBI. Additionally, although the behavioral disturbances modifier can be applied to postconcussive symptoms, the modifier also captures other neurobehavioral changes, such as agitation and aggression (see section "Anger, Agitation, and Aggression" later in chapter), that cause significant impairment but may not fit into a specific diagnosis. Unfortunately, this new nomenclature in DSM-5 may also lead to some uncertainty as to whether to apply the behavioral disturbances modifier or to diagnose a psychiatric disorder due to TBI, particularly for postconcussive symptoms that persist beyond the acute injury period. Postconcussive symptoms overlap with multiple psychiatric illnesses, including major depressive disorder (MDD), posttraumatic stress disorder (PTSD), and somatic symptom disorder (Mittenberg and Strauman 2000). Although DSM-5 does not specifically address this issue, experts have recommended that a psychiatric disorder due to TBI be diagnosed concurrently with NCD due to TBI when criteria for the former are met (Wortzel and

TABLE 33–1. **ICD-10 criteria for postconcussive syndrome**

A. History of head trauma with loss of consciousness precedes symptom onset by maximum of 4 weeks.

B. Symptoms in three or more of the following symptom categories:
1. Headache, dizziness, malaise, fatigue, noise intolerance
2. Irritability, depression, anxiety, emotional lability
3. Subjective concentration, memory, or intellectual difficulties without neuropsychological evidence of marked impairment
4. Insomnia
5. Reduced alcohol tolerance
6. Preoccupation with above symptoms and fear of brain damage with hypochondriacal concern and adoption of sick role

Source. From World Health Organization: *International Statistical Classification of Diseases and Related Health Problems,* 10th Edition. Geneva, Switzerland, World Health Organization, 1992a. Used with permission.

Arciniegas 2014). NCD due to TBI with behavioral disturbances would be diagnosed for subthreshold symptoms that cause impairment.

Although there is no universal agreement on the length of time that symptoms must persist in order to be considered "prolonged," the course of recovery after mild TBI may be considered to be prolonged when the individual experiences multiple postconcussive symptoms lasting more than 3–12 months (Cassidy et al. 2014). Persistent symptoms after concussion are significantly influenced by factors other than the TBI itself (Quinn et al. 2018). In one large study, years of education, preinjury psychiatric disorders, and prior TBI were the strongest predictors of 6-month postconcussive symptoms (Cnossen et al. 2017b). A systematic review on the prognosis after mild TBI (Carroll et al. 2004) reported that risk factors for persistent symptoms were primarily psychosocial: depression, posttraumatic stress, negative injury perceptions, poor expectations for recovery, emotional distress, anxiety, and litigation. However, it should be noted that few individuals involved in litigation have improvement in postconcussive symptoms after settlement (King 2003). Individuals with persistent symptoms after concussion also demonstrate significant cognitive deficits that exceed what would be expected on the basis of the severity of injury (Dean and Sterr 2013). This discrepancy suggests that individuals with persistent symptoms after concussion differ in significant respects from most individuals with TBI, with factors other than the injury itself playing a significant role.

Depression

Several studies have used structured interviews to determine rates of depression after TBI. Osborn et al. (2014) conducted a meta-analysis of 93 studies examining the prevalence of clinically diagnosed depression (MDD/dysthymia) and self-reports of depression in adult patients with TBI. The authors identified 31 studies (representing a total of 5,678 subjects) that used a structured clinical interview to diagnose MDD or dysthymia according to DSM criteria, and data from these studies were combined to yield an overall depression prevalence rate of 27%, with a range of 9%–67% across individual studies. The prevalence of MDD/dysthymia was higher (at 38%) when self-report measures were used, a finding that underscores the need to apply validated criteria in making a definitive diagnosis. Prevalence rates were also higher when self-administered scales were completed by mail rather than by telephone. Fann et al. (2005) found that the Patient Health Questionnaire–9 (PHQ-9) was highly correlated with the Structured Clinical Interview for DSM-IV (SCID) diagnosis of depression and other measures of depressive symptoms. Use of the criteria of at least five PHQ-9 symptoms being present for at least several days over the past 2 weeks, with at least one symptom being depressed mood or anhedonia, showed excellent operating characteristics, with a sensitivity of 93% and a specificity of 89% for MDD diagnosed by SCID. Therefore, the PHQ-9 can be used as a brief and valid screening tool for MDD.

Cnossen et al. (2017a) conducted a meta-analysis of risk factors for MDD following TBI, encompassing 17 studies that used a structured clinical interview for diagnosis. Significant risk factors that emerged were female gender, preinjury history of depression, and postinjury unemployment. Severity of injury at admission was inversely related to risk of depression, with individuals with an admission GCS in the mild to moderate range being more likely to develop MDD; however, severity at admission was assessed in only 2 of the studies. By contrast, there was no association between risk of MDD and injury severity at later time points (assessed using the GCS score or PTA duration). Age, education, and marital status were not predictive of depression. A preinjury history of psychiatric disorders other than depression, alcohol abuse, or substance abuse was not a significant risk factor. Additionally, race, socioeconomic status, preinjury unemployment, family history of psychiatric disorders, computed tomography abnormalities, and involvement in litigation were not associated with an increased risk of depression, although this finding must be interpreted cautiously because of the small number of studies that assessed these risk factors.

Early studies of MDD among individuals with TBI showed high rates of vegetative symptoms that exceeded the rates of depression. Although these investigations did not include structured psychiatric assessments, the findings raised concern about the validity of using physical symptoms in the diagnosis of depression after TBI. The "inclusive," "etiological," "substitutive," and "exclusive" approaches used in medically ill populations (Cohen-Cole and Stoudemire 1987) have similar advantages and disadvantages in the TBI population. Cook et al. (2011) examined the rates of somatic symptoms in TBI by comparing PHQ-9 responses from 3,000 outpatients in primary care with responses from 365 inpatients admitted with moderate to severe TBI. They used item response theory to demonstrate that no differential item functioning existed, indicating that the items on the PHQ-9 performed similarly in the two groups. Thus, it appears that the diagnosis of MDD can be accurately made with DSM criteria in patients with brain injury.

The course of MDD that develops after TBI has been well described (Bombardier et al. 2010). In their meta-analysis, Osborn et al. (2014) reported that prevalence rates for combined MDD and dysthymia were 21% at 6 months or less, 27% at 6 months to 2 years, 43% at 2–5 years, and 22% beyond 5 years. Although these percentages show that the onset of depression may be delayed after the occurrence of TBI in a significant number of individuals, they do not necessarily indicate the course for individual patients. Hart et al. (2012) conducted a longitudinal study of DSM-IV-defined MDD and minor (subsyndromal) depression among 1,089 subjects in the Traumatic Brain Injury Model Systems program. Of patients with no depression at year 1, 17% developed minor depression and 9% developed MDD by year 2. For patients with MDD at year 1, 55% continued to have MDD at year 2, 22% had minor depression, and 23% remitted. Thus, the course of MDD after TBI is quite variable; although most individuals without depression in the first year remain depression-free at follow-up, 26% will develop symptoms. Similarly, the majority of individuals with MDD early in the postinjury period will continue to have MDD at follow-up, but a substantial percentage will experience lessening or remission of symptoms.

Mania

The prevalence of bipolar disorder after TBI is difficult to determine because most reports have consisted of single cases or small case series, with few using structured interviews. A bipolar disorder prevalence of 2% in a population of 100 adults with TBI was reported by Hibbard et al. (1998), with all cases occurring after TBI. Jorge et al. (1993c) reported that 9% (6 out of 66) of their subjects met DSM-III-R (American Psychiatric Association 1987) criteria for a manic episode at some point during the year after injury. By contrast, in a study by Fann et al. (1995), none of the subjects developed bipolar disorder. Thus, although TBI may increase the risk of developing bipolar disorder, it appears to be a relatively rare consequence of injury.

Phenomenologically, all forms of bipolar disorder, including bipolar I, bipolar II, and rapid-cycling variants, have been reported in TBI populations (McAllister 1992). One study examining onset of mania after TBI suggested that patients are more likely to present with irritable than with euphoric mood (Shukla et al. 1987). Shukla et al. (1987) observed that mania after TBI was associated with posttraumatic seizures but not with a family history of bipolar disorder. Jorge et al. (1993c) noted that mania after TBI was significantly related to basopolar temporal lesions but was not associated with type or severity of TBI, degree of physical or intellectual impairment, family or personal history of psychiatric illness, or posttraumatic epilepsy. Of the six patients who developed mania after TBI, five experienced onset within 3 months after injury, and episodes lasted only about 2 months (Jorge et al. 1993c). These limited data suggest that episodes of bipolar disorder may occur soon after TBI. The duration of mania was relatively brief, although patients may have subsyndromal disturbances after mania resolves.

Posttraumatic Stress Disorder

Early opinion was that PTSD could not develop after TBI; investigators argued that LOC or PTA would prevent patients from having reexperiencing and avoidance because memories were not encoded (Harvey et al. 2003). However, multiple studies with structured assessments of PTSD have yielded different results. Carlson et al. (2011) conducted a systematic review of PTSD following TBI, with a specific focus on mild TBI. Across 34 studies, the prevalence of PTSD after any TBI ranged from 0% to 70%. Among the largest studies, the rates of PTSD were 32%–66% among patients with military-related trauma and 14%–56% among those with nonmilitary trauma. Among the 20 studies examining mild TBI, prevalence of PTSD ranged from 0% to 89%, with the largest studies reporting rates of 33%–39% for military-related trauma and 12%–27% for nonmilitary trauma. Overall, the evidence indicates that PTSD is a common occurrence after TBI, although there is wide variation in the estimates. The rates may be lower for more severe injuries with PTA, but a substantial proportion of patients across all injury severities will develop PTSD.

Cnossen et al. (2017a) reviewed risk factors for development of PTSD after TBI, identifying 12 studies that used structured clinical assessments in civilian populations. There was no association between PTSD and injury severity measured by the GCS, whereas shorter duration of PTA (another measure of injury severity) was associated with increased risk of PTSD. Individuals with memory of the traumatic event were more than five times more likely to develop PTSD than those without such memory. A diagnosis of acute stress disorder, or early PTSD symptoms, at 1 month were associated with increased risk of PTSD at 6 and 12 months, but preinjury psychiatric history was not significant. Similarly, age, gender, and educational level did not emerge as significant predictors. Finally, individuals with TBI who do not recall their injury may still develop PTSD around traumatic experiences during hospitalization (O'Donnell et al. 2010).

The criteria for PTSD underwent several changes in DSM-5 that may have a modest effect on the diagnosis of PTSD after TBI (Bryant 2011). The subjective requirement that the individual experience intense fear, helplessness, or horror in response to exposure to the traumatic event, which many individuals with TBI may not experience because of impaired consciousness, has been eliminated. The avoidance criteria have been split into separate criteria for active avoidance and for numbing and passive avoidance. The latter may raise issues in the differential diagnosis because symptoms of withdrawal and apathy can occur in TBI independent of PTSD (Bryant 2011). Similarly, the criteria for negative alterations in cognition and emotions have been expanded to include symptoms such as irritability or aggression, which are not uncommon after TBI and may complicate differential diagnosis. Careful adherence to the diagnostic criteria is required to avoid misdiagnosis of PTSD in the TBI population. Use of DSM-5 criteria may yield slightly lower prevalence estimates of PTSD than use of DSM-IV-TR criteria (Kilpatrick et al. 2013), but the prevalence under the new criteria has not been specifically investigated in patients with TBI (Kilpatrick et al. 2013).

Anxiety Disorders and Obsessive-Compulsive Disorder

Anxiety disorders are common following TBI. In a recent meta-analysis, Scholten et al. (2016) reported pooled prevalence rates of 6.9% for generalized anxiety disorder, 5.0% for panic disorder, 9.2% for agoraphobia, 5.7% for social phobia, and 2.6% for DSM-IV obsessive-compulsive disorder in the first year after injury. The prevalence of generalized anxiety disorder increased over time, with a pooled prevalence of 13.5% after the first year of injury. There were insufficient studies to estimate the prevalence of other anxiety disorders beyond the first year.

Risk factors for anxiety disorders after TBI have not been well studied. However, Hart et al. (2016), in a study assessing anxiety (using the 7-item Generalized Anxiety Disorder Scale [GAD-7]) in 1,838 patients with moderate to severe TBI, found that significant levels of anxiety were associated with middle age (between the ages of 31 and 60 years), black race, lower socioeconomic status, preinjury mental health problems, and previous TBI, although these risk factors could not be attributed to a specific type of anxiety disorder.

Psychosis

Relatively few studies have examined the prevalence of psychosis after TBI. Fujii and Ahmed (2014) reported prevalence rates of 0.9%–9.8%. They divided psychosis due to TBI into delusional disorder (characterized by delusions only) and schizophrenia-like psychosis (with both hallucinations and delusions). The latter has been reported more frequently than the former in the literature, but rates for each are difficult to determine. Psychosis due to TBI shares some phenomenology with idiopathic psychotic disorders; however, negative symptoms are relatively uncommon in psychosis after TBI. Delayed onset of symptoms, often 4–5 years after injury, is common, although establishing that psychotic symptoms are the physiological consequences of TBI can be challenging (Fujii and Ahmed 2014).

Risk factors for psychosis after TBI are similarly understudied. Malaspina et al. (2001) suggested a synergistic relation between schizophrenia and TBI, in which familial factors among schizophrenic patients and their relatives increases the risk of TBI, and the presence of TBI further increases the risk of schizophrenia in those with genetic vulnerability. The risk of psychosis after TBI is not strongly related to injury severity (Fujii and Ahmed 2014), although increased risk has been associated with pre-existing cognitive impairment, male gender, and a history of childhood TBI (Fujii and Ahmed 2001; Fujii and Fujii 2012). Among individuals with post-TBI psychosis, electroencephalogram (EEG) abnormalities (especially in the temporal lobe) were common, and rates of seizures were much higher than estimated rates of seizures after TBI in general (Fujii and Ahmed 2001; Fujii and Fujii 2012). Lesions (predominantly in the frontal and temporal lobes) were also frequently found in this population.

Anger, Aggression, and Agitation

Many patients with TBI have difficulty with emotional and behavioral dyscontrol (Arciniegas and Wortzel 2014), often described in the TBI literature as *posttraumatic agitation* (Sandel and Mysiw 1996). However, *agitation* is a poorly defined term with little consistency across studies (Yudofsky et al. 1997). Although there are several scales that reliably characterize agitation (Castaño Monsalve et al. 2014), these are rarely applied in clinical practice (Fugate et al. 1997). For this reason, reported prevalence rates of agitation following TBI have ranged from 11% to 70% of individuals admitted to inpatient rehabilitation with moderate to severe injury (Stéfan et al. 2016).

More severe behavioral dyscontrol is often characterized as *aggression*, a term that is also poorly defined (Kim et al. 2007). Although aggression may be a symptom of many disorders, aggression attributed to TBI often has certain characteristic features (Yudofsky et al. 1990). Such behavior is *nonreflective,* occurring without any premeditation or planning, and *nonpurposeful,* achieving no particular goals for the individual. It is also *reactive,* triggered by a stimulus, but often a stimulus that would not normally provoke a strong reaction. Aggression after TBI is *periodic*, occurring at intervals with relatively calm behavior in between, and *explosive,* occurring without a prodromal buildup. Finally, it is *ego-dystonic*, creating a great deal of distress for the patient. This classic presentation likely represents only a small proportion of aggression occurring after TBI; unplanned aggression toward a specific individual in response to a perceived threat, which is more difficult to attribute to the TBI itself, is a more common pattern (Wortzel and Arciniegas 2013). Reported rates of aggression after moderate to severe TBI have ranged from 25% to 39% (Stéfan et al. 2016).

The lack of precise definitions of agitation and aggression in the literature makes identification of risk factors difficult. Agitation is more likely to occur with lower cognitive function, comorbid infection, and use of certain sedating medications; there is no association of agitation with premorbid psychiatric (mood) disorders (Bogner et al. 2015). Risk of aggression is increased with a premorbid history of impulsive aggression, frontal lobe lesions, and preinjury history of substance abuse; evidence on cognitive function and socioeconomic status as risk factors is inconclusive (Kim et al. 2007). For these risk factors, it is often difficult to ascertain whether the aggression is a direct result of TBI, premorbid character pathology, or both (Kim 2002).

Little is known about the course of agitation or aggression after TBI. However, in a review of the literature, Silver et al. (2011) noted that 31%–71% of individuals with severe TBI exhibited these behaviors during long-term follow-up periods ranging from 1 to 15 years. Similarly, Baguley et al. (2006) noted that approximately 25% of inpatient rehabilitation patients with TBI showed aggression at 6, 24, and 60 months postinjury. Greater depressive symptomatology and younger age at injury were the most significant predictors of later aggression. A retrospective chart review of 80 patients who underwent rehabilitation following TBI (Nott et al. 2006) found that agitation was present at discharge in 70% and persisted for a mean of 23.9 days. Agitation was found to be associated with longer durations of PTA, increased lengths of stay, and greater cognitive impairment. Thus, it appears that agitation and aggression may be chronic problems that are not confined to the early stage of recovery. This trajectory would be expected for such behaviors that predate the injury; it is currently unclear whether agitation and aggression directly resulting from TBI follow this same chronic course.

Substance Use Disorders

Substance abuse and dependence are of great concern in the TBI population, both at the time of injury and afterward. Substance use disorders not only are highly prevalent and often the underlying cause of injury but also may adversely affect outcomes (Niemeier et al. 2016; West 2011). Alcohol intoxication at the time of injury may influence initial injury severity; however, preinjury alcohol abuse does not necessarily predict poorer postinjury cognitive functioning (Unsworth and Mathias 2017). Systematic review of the literature has shown that 44%–79% of patients with TBI had a history of significant alcohol-related problems before injury (West 2011) and that 37%–51% were intoxicated at the time of injury (Parry-Jones et al. 2006). Furthermore, 10%–44% of individuals with TBI had a preinjury history of illicit drug use (West 2011). In one study, 37.7% had a positive toxicology screen at the time of injury for one or more illicit drugs (23.7% for marijuana, 13.2% for cocaine, 8.8% for amphetamines) (Bombardier et al. 2002).

Studies using structured interviews to identify substance use disorder in patients with TBI have reported DSM-IV substance abuse prevalence rates of 8%–28% (Alway et al. 2016; Ashman et al. 2004), with up to 12.5% of cases involving new onset after TBI (Alway et al. 2016). Timing of assessment and differences in diagnostic criteria, as well as whether patients were unselected or from referral populations, likely explain some of these variations. Substance misuse declines after TBI, but this initial decrease in alcohol use may subsequently reverse as time after injury increases. Alway et al. (2016) reported that the prevalence of substance abuse dropped (from 38.5% preinjury) to 15.8% in the first year after injury; rose to 17.8% in the second year; dropped again to 9.6% in year 3; and thereafter remained fairly stable, at 10.3% in year 4 and 11.8% in year 5. Risk factors for postinjury substance misuse include male gender, history of legal problems related to substance abuse, substance abuse problems among family or friends, postinjury diagnosis of depression, younger age, and less severe injuries (Ponsford et al. 2007; Taylor et al. 2003).

Sleep Disorders

Sleep disturbances are a common component of many neuropsychiatric disorders occurring after TBI, including delirium, MDD, bipolar disorder, PTSD, anxiety disorders, and PCS. TBI also may have significant effects on sleep architecture that are independent of these illnesses, by altering the levels of several neurotransmitters involved in the regulation of sleep. The prevalence of sleep disturbance after TBI is high: Mathias and Alvaro (2012), in a meta-analysis of 21 studies, estimated that 50% of patients with TBI had some form of sleep disturbance, and that 25%–29% had a diagnosable sleep disorder, such as sleep apnea. In at least some cases, evidence suggested that the sleep disorder predated the TBI, raising the possibility that the sleep disorder increased the risk for TBI rather than vice versa. Mathias and Alvaro also noted several deficiencies in existing studies, including poor descriptions of comorbid physical and psychological conditions that may contribute to sleep disturbances, inadequate information about TBI severity and injury location, and lack of long-term studies (Mathias and Alvaro 2012).

Psychological Aspects of Traumatic Brain Injury

In addition to the defined DSM-5 psychiatric disorders, TBI is associated with psychological challenges that may not fit into specific diagnostic categories. Four areas of importance are neurological injury and resultant cognitive deficits, the psychological meaning of deficits and their effect on the patient, psychological factors that exist independently of TBI, and the broader social context (Lewis 1991).

Deficits due to neurological impairment may have a direct effect on psychological functioning. Impaired self-awareness is common after TBI, with 30%–97% of TBI patients showing some degree of impairment (Smeets et al. 2012). Impaired self-awareness may be global in nature or restricted to specific domains, such as physical, cognitive, or emotional/behavioral (Hart et al. 2009). However, impaired self-awareness is generally measured by comparing patients' reports with those of family members or rehabilitation providers, which may be biased by respondent characteristics such as depressed mood (Richardson et al. 2015). Comparing patient reports with neuropsychological test results can eliminate much of this subjectivity but may not allow the consultant to gauge the accuracy of patient self-reports of real-world functioning (Heaton and Pendleton 1981). Although validated instruments for measuring impaired self-awareness exist (Smeets et al. 2012), such instruments are rarely employed in clinical practice, even though providers describe self-awareness as an important contributor to rehabilitation outcomes (Winkens et al. 2014).

Impaired awareness has both neurological and psychological dimensions. At one extreme is anosognosia, wherein the person has no awareness of neurological impairments (Prigatano 1999). At the other extreme is defensive denial, which represents the person's attempt to cope with overwhelming anxiety associated with neurological impairment by minimizing the implications of the impairment. Apparent impaired awareness also can be the result of moderate to severe memory impairment that prevents the person from consolidating and acting on new information about his or her condition. Phenomenologically, decreased awareness might appear the same regardless of cause, but the cause of the impairment has significant treatment implications. Interventions designed to address denial and other forms of decreased awareness resulting from psychological causes may be ineffective when the decreased awareness is due to neurological dysfunction that cannot be reversed.

Psychological defenses and adaptations used by the individual prior to TBI are also important. In many cases, patients will continue to use previously learned defenses. However, in some instances, coping mechanisms used before the injury may no longer be available because of the degree of neurocognitive impairment, leading to considerable distress for the patient. Many behavioral traits are exacerbated by TBI rather than developing de novo after injury (Prigatano 1999). Depending on the degree of disturbance, such alterations would be diagnosed in DSM-5 as either neurocognitive disorder with behavioral disturbance or personality change due to TBI.

Finally, as is the case with many other chronic illnesses, TBI has a significant effect on family and social functioning. Approximately 60%–70% of individuals with TBI are unable to return to regular work without supportive services, and this loss of their former role as breadwinners causes significant distress, as well as placing considerable burdens on other members of the family system (Wehman et al. 2017). In general, neurobehavioral disturbances in the TBI patient are the most important source of stress for families (Tam et al. 2015), but this effect can be buffered by good social support and strong coping skills, as well as good preinjury family functioning (Baker et al. 2017). Family members are at significantly increased risk for psychological distress, particularly anxiety and depressive symptoms, although few studies have studied psychiatric disorders diagnosed according to DSM-5 (Ennis et al. 2013). Caregivers may experience problems such as unemployment or financial loss, placing additional stresses on the patient and family (Hall et al. 1994). Sexual dysfunction after TBI places further stress on intimate relationships, and partners may be uncomfortable with the dual role of caregiver (parent-like) and sexual partner (spouse) (Sander et al. 2016). Separation and divorce are common among individuals with TBI, although it is not clear that rates of marital breakdown are elevated in the TBI population compared with the general population (Godwin et al. 2011).

Spinal Cord Injury

Epidemiology

SCI results from trauma to the spinal cord, causing dysfunction in motor, sensory, and/or autonomic functioning. Approximately 276,281 people with SCI were predicted to be living in the United States in 2014 (DeVivo 2012). The annual incidence of SCI is stable and estimated to be 53 cases per 1 million population in the United States (Jain et al. 2015). Individuals who sustain SCIs are predominantly males (70.7%) and young (half are between the ages of 16 and 30 years) (DeVivo 2012). However, age-stratified incidence rates from 1993 to 2012 revealed a declining trend for individuals younger than 45 years and increasing incidence among those 65 years or older (Jain et al. 2015). The most common causes of SCI are motor vehicle crashes (31.0%), unintentional falls (40.4%), and firearm injuries (5.5%) (Jain et al. 2015).

Early survival rates and overall life expectancy for persons with SCI have improved significantly over the past 35 years. However, life expectancy in these persons remains below that in the general population, especially for those with more severe injuries who are older than 60 years. Leading causes of death are heart disease (19%); external causes such as accidents, suicide, and violence (18%); respiratory illness, especially pneumonia (18%); and septicemia (10%) (DeVivo et al. 1999). Deaths from suicide after SCI have decreased since the 1970s, from 91 cases per 100,000 person-years in 1973–1979 to 46 cases per 100,000 person-years in 1990–1999 (Cao et al. 2014). However, the 3.0 standardized mortality ratio calculated for 1990–1999 demonstrates that suicide rates in persons with SCI are still significantly higher than rates in the general population (Cao et al. 2014).

Severity Classification

Tetraplegia (or quadriplegia) denotes SCI that affects all four limbs, whereas *paraplegia* denotes injuries that affect only the lower extremities. SCI usually is described in terms of the level and the completeness of injury. *Level of injury* refers to the most caudal segment with normal motor or sensory function. Neurological level of injury (NLI) may vary on the right and the left side, and segments also may be partially innervated. More than half of all SCIs (55.7%) result in tetraplegia. Injury severity is most commonly classified according to the American Spinal Injury Association Impairment Scale (AIS; Table 33–2). Approximately half (48.7%) of all SCIs are considered to be AIS-A, or *complete* (DeVivo 2012). Of individuals admitted to inpatient rehabilitation with an AIS-A SCI, only 7.1% are expected to improve to the point of having functional motor recovery below the NLI at 1 year (Marino et al. 2011). In contrast, those admitted with an AIS-B (sensory incomplete) injury have about a 36.8% chance of regaining functional motor abilities below the NLI, and those admitted with an AIS-C (motor incomplete) injury have an 82.5% chance of regaining functional motor ability below the NLI (Marino et al. 2011).

Acute Management and Management of Secondary Complications

Emergency management of SCI involves immobilizing the spine as well as ensuring an open airway, breathing, and circulation. Despite limited evidence supporting this practice, medical staff at some sites routinely administer intravenous methylprednisolone within 8 hours of injury to minimize swelling and secondary injury within the spinal canal (Evaniew et al. 2016). Unstable spine fractures may require surgical decompression and stabilization. Various orthoses are used to stabilize the spine after surgery, typically for 3 months.

Key aspects of postsurgical care include respiratory management and prevention of pneumonia, management of orthostatic hypotension associated with blood pooling in the lower extremities, and prevention of deep venous thrombosis and pulmonary embolism. Neurogenic bladder and bowel management begins with indwelling or intermittent catheterization and establishment of a regular bowel regimen. After injury, heterotopic ossification may cause loss of range of motion. Spinal reflexes are initially depressed during the period of "spinal shock" but may become hyperactive

TABLE 33–2.   **American Spinal Injury Association Impairment Scale**

A.   **Complete**—No sensory or motor function is preserved in the sacral segments S4–S5.

B.   **Sensory incomplete**—Sensory but not motor function is preserved below the neurological level of injury (NLI) and includes the sacral segments S4–S5, *and* no motor function is preserved more than three levels below the motor level on either side of the body.

C.   **Motor incomplete**—Motor function is preserved below the NLI, and more than half of key muscles below the NLI have a muscle grade less than 3 (i.e., grades 0–2; active movement against gravity). There must be voluntary anal sphincter contraction or some sparing of sensory and/or motor function in the sacral segments S4–S5.

D.   **Motor incomplete**—Motor function is preserved below the NLI, and at least half of key muscles below the NLI have a muscle grade greater than or equal to 3.

E.   **Normal**—Patient had prior deficits, but sensory and motor functions are now normal.

Source.   From Kirshblum SC, Burns SP, Biering-Sorensen F, et al.: "International Standards for Neurological Classification of Spinal Cord Injury (Revised 2011)." *Journal of Spinal Cord Medicine* 34(6):535–546, 2011. Used with permission.

during the first 6 months after injury. Daily range of motion and static muscle stretching are used to reduce spasticity and prevent contractures, in conjunction with medications such as baclofen, diazepam, and clonidine.

Chronic pain is a common problem; 25% of patients with SCI complain of severe pain, and 44% report that pain interferes with daily activities (Staas et al. 1998). SCI-related pain is classified as above, at, or below the lesion level and as either nociceptive or neuropathic (Bryce et al. 2007). Between 30% and 34% of patients also sustain mild TBI, 11%–16% experience moderate TBI, and 6%–10% have severe TBI (Hagen et al. 2010; Macciocchi et al. 2008).

Among patients with recent SCI, 10%–60% may have cognitive impairment (Davidoff et al. 1992). Cognitive deficits may be attributable to a variety of factors, including preinjury learning disabilities, substance abuse, and TBI sustained at the time of SCI. Treatment noncompliance, anger, and agitation may be signs of comorbid TBI. *Autonomic dysreflexia,* a severe complication that can occur in people whose SCIs are rostral to the midthoracic level, involves a sympathetic discharge uninhibited by descending neural control that is most often triggered by a noxious stimulus below the NLI. Immediate steps must be taken to control the resulting hypertension (which may be life-threatening) and to identify and reverse the triggering stimulus. The most common secondary medical complications during the first year postinjury are urinary tract infections (62%), autonomic dysreflexia (43%), and pressure ulcers (41%) (Stillman et al. 2017).

Acute Rehabilitation

Patients are usually transferred to specialized rehabilitation programs once they are medically stable and capable of participating in therapies for at least 3 hours per day. Inpatient rehabilitation typically focuses on education, physical training, strengthening, and basic skill building needed to return to maximal functional independence for living in the community. Individuals with paraplegia are usually expected to be able to function and live independently once their rehabilitation is complete (Consortium for Spinal Cord Medicine 1999). Those with low cervical lesions (C7–C8) should be independent in most functional tasks. Depending on their neurological level, people with higher cervical lesions require different degrees of assistance for activities of daily living, such as bladder and bowel management regimens, bathing, dressing, eating, and transferring to and from a wheelchair. Whatever the level of injury, persons with SCI are expected to be independent in guiding others to care for them in areas they cannot perform on their own.

Psychosocial Outcomes of Spinal Cord Injury

Following discharge from acute rehabilitation, 91% of people with SCI are discharged to a home environment (Eastwood et al. 1999). Approximately 35% of people with SCI have paid employment after injury, compared with 79% employment in the general population (Ottomanelli and Lind 2009). People with SCI tend to report lower subjective quality of life (QOL) compared with persons without disabilities (Barker et al. 2009). QOL was found to be unrelated to NLI or injury severity and only weakly related to physical impairment (Barker et al. 2009). Instead, QOL was correlated with the ability to carry out day-to-day tasks and to participate in school, work, or other community activities; freedom from depression and greater health competence also had a strong impact on QOL (Barker et al. 2009; Mortenson et al. 2010). As a result, QOL can be higher than expected in people with very severe injuries. For example, 88% of those with ventilator-dependent C1–C4 tetraplegia say that they are "glad to be alive" (Hall et al. 1999).

Psychosocial adjustment to SCI can be viewed from multiple perspectives. Researchers have generally disputed the notion that people with SCI go through traditional "stages of grief" (Wortman and Silver 1989). Instead, the modal response to SCI is resilience and an absence of psychopathology (Bonanno et al. 2012). Recent research has identified adjustment trajectories in people with SCI that are similar to those in people who are exposed to other forms of trauma or loss. A relatively large European cohort study (N=233) that measured depression and anxiety at four time points during the first 2 years after SCI found that a minority of patients were persistently depressed over this period (10.7%) or developed late depression (9.8%) (Bonanno et al. 2012). About 13% of the cohort were depressed early but recovered, and the majority (66.1%) had stable low or no depressive symptoms. Compared with patients who appraised SCI as a threat or coped through social reliance and behavioral disengagement, patients who appraised SCI as a challenge or coped through acceptance and "fighting spirit" were less likely to be in one of the depression trajectories (Bonanno et al. 2012). A U.S. cohort study in 168 consecutive admissions to inpatient rehabilitation for acute SCI confirmed that resilience (stable low depression) was the most likely trajectory during the first year after SCI (63.8% of cohort), whereas a trajectory of persistent high depression was much less common (7.1%) (Bombardier et al. 2016). A preinjury history of MDD, early depression, and pronounced grief symptoms predicted a persistent depressive trajectory (Bombardier et al. 2016).

On the other hand, the emotional experience of some people with SCI appears to involve specific symptoms of grief, such as yearning for the way things were; feeling emotionally numb; avoiding reminders of the loss; and feeling stunned, shocked, or dazed (Klyce et al. 2015). Although DSM-5 does not recognize grief as a distinct diagnostic entity, these symptoms are present in people with SCI and are distinct from symptoms of depression (Klyce et al. 2015). Grief symptoms can be normal and self-limited or persistent and disabling. In our opinion, the dual-process model of grief effectively captures the oscillation of grief-related symptoms and thus offers a useful heuristic that may help clinicians to conceptualize the adjustment process facing these patients (Stroebe and Schut 1999).

One clinical implication of the above-described research is that, consistent with DSM-5, MDD following SCI should be diagnosed and treated, not conflated with grief or viewed as a normal response to catastrophic injury. Most people are resilient and experience manageable grief symptoms and low levels of depression that resolve naturally. Preinjury psychiatric history as well as how the person appraises and copes with injury may influence psychological responses to injury and present potential targets for treatment.

Psychiatric Disorders in Spinal Cord Injury

Depressive Disorders

MDD is probably the most common psychiatric disorder after SCI, with a point prevalence of 20%–43% during inpatient rehabilitation and 25%–30% in persons living in the community (Craig et al. 2009). As noted in the previous subsection ("Psychosocial Outcomes of Spinal Cord Injury"), longitudinal research suggests that a fraction (7.1%–10.7%) of persons are persistently depressed during the first 1–2 years after injury (Bombardier et al. 2016; Bonanno et al. 2012). A more recent prospective study, which used a diagnostic interview (Mini-International Neuropsychiatric Interview [MINI]) and DSM-5 criteria to determine the presence of psychiatric disorders in a cohort of 88 adults with SCI, found MDD in 10.3% during inpatient rehabilitation, 8.6% at discharge from rehabilitation, and 14.1% at 6 months after discharge (Craig et al. 2015). A significant minority of patients with SCI may experience chronic or recurrent depression for years; in one study, rates of probable MDD remained elevated (24%) almost 10 years after injury (Krause et al. 2000).

Depression is a significant and disabling problem for persons with SCI. Depression is associated with longer lengths of hospital stay and fewer functional improvements (Malec and Neimeyer 1983) as well as less functional independence and mobility at discharge (Umlauf and Frank 1983). Depression is associated with the occurrence of pressure sores and urinary tract infections (Herrick et al. 1994), poorer self-appraised health (Bombardier et al. 2004), less leisure activity (Elliott and Shewchuk 1995), poorer community mobility and social integration, and fewer meaningful social pursuits (Fuhrer et al. 1993; MacDonald et al. 1987). Persons with SCI and significant depression spend more days in bed and fewer days outside the home, require greater use of paid personal care, and incur higher medical expenses (Tate et al. 1994). Symptoms consistent with depression, such as documented expressions of despondency, hopelessness, shame, and apathy, are the variables most predictive of suicide 1–9 years after SCI (Charlifue and Gerhart 1991). Probable MDD predicts all-cause mortality after SCI (Krause et al. 2008).

Despite the high prevalence and adverse impact of depression after SCI, depression is undertreated. A multisite survey of 947 community-residing people with SCI found that among those with probable MDD ($n=223$), the percentages currently receiving any antidepressant treatment and guideline-level antidepressant treatment were 29% and 11%, respectively, and the percentages having received any psychotherapy and guideline-level psychotherapy over the past 3 months were 11% and 6% (Fann et al. 2011).

Posttraumatic Stress Disorder and Anxiety Disorders

Relatively few studies have examined PTSD or anxiety disorders after SCI. Estimates of current PTSD range from 1% to 22% in patients with SCI (Craig et al. 2015; Kennedy and Evans 2001; Radnitz et al. 1998). Rates of PTSD may be lower among persons with tetraplegia (2%) compared with those with paraplegia (22%) (Radnitz et al. 1998), possibly because of diminished psychophysiological arousal in higher-level injuries (Kennedy and Duff 2001). Veterans, persons previously exposed to violence, and those with limited social support may be at higher risk of PTSD (Kennedy and Duff 2001).

Current generalized anxiety disorder is identified in 3.4%, 4.9%, and 4.2% of people with SCI during inpatient rehabilitation, after discharge, and at 6 months postdischarge, respectively (Craig et al. 2015). Anxiety trajectories over the first 2 years after SCI reveal three patterns: stable low anxiety (57.5%), improved anxiety (by 1 year post-SCI, 29.6%), and delayed anxiety (peaking at 1 year, 12.8%) (Craig et al. 2015). Anxiety is associated with lower QOL (Budh and Osteråker 2007).

Substance Use Disorders

High rates of alcohol and drug abuse problems are found among trauma patients generally and SCI patients specifically. Current DSM-IV alcohol dependence or abuse was found in 10.3%, 7.4%, and 8.6% of SCI survivors during inpatient rehabilitation, after discharge, and 6 months postdischarge, respectively (Craig et al. 2015). Current DSM-IV drug abuse or dependence was found in 2.3%, 1.2%, and 7.0% of patients at the same three time points. In a study of 139 patients with recent SCI admitted to an inpatient rehabilitation unit, approximately 23% met criteria for alcohol intoxication at the time of injury, and 37.9% screened positive for a lifetime history of significant alcohol-related problems (Stroud et al. 2011). On the basis of self-report and toxicology results (available for 76 patients), 33%–44% were using illicit drugs around the time of their injury (Stroud et al. 2011).

Compared with preinjury substance use, substance abuse after SCI may be more harmful because of its association with poorer health maintenance behaviors (Krause 1992), including measures to prevent pressure ulcers (Tate et al. 2004). Acute SCI rehabilitation represents a potential "teachable moment" for patients with a history of alcohol use disorders to initiate changes in their drinking behavior. In a study of individuals with recent SCI undergoing inpatient rehabilitation, 71% of those with at-risk drinking reported that they were either considering changes in alcohol use or already taking action, and 41% reported interest in treatment or Alcoholics Anonymous (Stroud et al. 2011).

Sexual Dysfunction

Sexuality is often a major concern after SCI, and aspects of sexual functioning may be impaired. However, there are many ways to express sexuality and therefore many ways to cope with the dysfunction caused by SCI. Sexual desire, activity, and pleasure tend to decrease after SCI for both women and men, but most people remain interested in sexual activity.

Vaginal lubrication and orgasm may be affected in women with SCI. Women with complete upper-motor lesions affecting the sacral segments are likely to have vaginal lubrication from reflexive but not psychogenic mechanisms (Sipski et al. 1995). Women with incomplete upper motor lesions affecting the sacral segments retain the capacity for reflex lubrication but will have psychogenic lubrication only if they have intact pinprick sensation in the T11–L2 thoracic and lumbar dermatomes. Women with incomplete lower-motor lesions affecting the sacral segments are expected to achieve psychogenic lubrication in 25% of cases but will have no reflex lubrication. Decreased lubrication in females can be managed by water-based lubricants. A laboratory study reported that about 50% of women with SCI were able to experience orgasm, and this ability was not significantly related to level or completeness of neurological injury. Longer stimulation, greater sexual knowledge, and higher sexual drive were associated with higher rates of orgasm (Sipski et al. 1995).

Women with SCI remain fertile once menses resume. However, pregnancy and delivery can be complicated by increased risk of urinary tract infections, autonomic dysreflexia, changes in respiratory functioning, and biomechanical issues (e.g., wheelchair positioning) (Consortium for Spinal Cord Medicine 2010). These potential complications should not present a barrier to childbearing and can be managed successfully through consultation with an SCI specialist.

In men, SCI can affect erections, ejaculation, orgasm, and fertility. Approximately 70% of men with SCI recover some degree of erectile function (Sipski and Alexander 1997). Psychogenic erection is dependent on the integrity of the hypogastric plexus, which includes both the T11–L2 segments and the sacral plexus, and can be elicited by sexual thoughts or feelings (Sipski and Alexander 1997). Reflex erection ability is dependent on the parasympathetic reflex arc in the sacral segments (S2–S4) and can be elicited by direct stimulation of the penis or other erogenous areas. Among males with SCI, 38%–47% report achieving orgasm, which may be experienced as similar to or different from preinjury experiences (Sipski and Alexander 1997). Males with complete lesions affecting the S4–S5 level and no bulbocavernosis and anal wink reflex are unlikely to experience physiological orgasm (Consortium for Spinal Cord Medicine 2010). Depending on injury level and severity, ejaculation may be anterograde or retrograde, into the bladder. Men (and women) who lack sensation in the genital region may experience sexual pleasure, arousal, and possibly orgasm through stimulation of body areas such as the head, neck, face, ears, chest, abdomen, back, arms, hands, and toes, as well as other regions (especially in "transition zones" where sensation stops and starts) (Consortium for Spinal Cord Medicine 2010).

Numerous treatments are available for sexual dysfunction related to SCI (Consortium for Spinal Cord Medicine 2010). The first-line treatments for erectile dysfunction are sildenafil and other phosphodiesterase type 5 (PDE5) inhibitors (Lombardi et al. 2009). Large increases in rates of successful intercourse can be achieved with the use of PDE5 inhibitors. Ejaculation and orgasm rates also improve. All PDE5 inhibitors appear to be safe, with the caveat that most studies have been short term. Second-line treatments include vacuum erection devices, pharmacological penile injections, and penile implants. Ejaculatory dysfunction and related infertility are treated with vibratory or electroejaculation procedures in conjunction with intrauterine insemination, in vitro fertilization, or intracytoplasmic sperm injection, depending on sperm quality and motility, which can be diminished after SCI (Amador et al. 2000).

Regarding sexual enjoyment, patients can benefit from many standard counseling strategies adapted for people with SCI, such as enhancing communication skills, teaching sensate focus exercises, addressing sexual performance anxiety, and generally dispelling common counterproductive beliefs about sexual relationships (Consortium for Spinal Cord Medicine 2010). Although it is important to broach the topics of sexuality and fertility while the person is undergoing acute rehabilitation, studies indicate that during this time many patients rate other rehabilitation concerns as more important and may prefer to postpone discussions about sexual concerns until after the acute rehabilitation phase (Hanson and Franklin 1976).

Psychological and Neuropsychological Testing

Personality assessment among persons with SCI has received justifiable criticism related to negative bias, overreliance on measures designed only to detect pathology, and attribution of behavior to intrapsychic rather than situational or environmental factors (Elliott and Umlauf 1995). Measures such as the Minnesota Multiphasic Personality Inventory and the Hopkins Symptom Checklist–90 should be interpreted cautiously and with the aid of norms correcting for disability-related factors (Barncord and Wanlass 2000). Nonpathological measures such as the NEO Personality Inventory (NEO PI), the 16 Personality Factors Questionnaire (16PF), and the Myers-Briggs Type Indicator may be more appropriate tests of personality functioning in this population (Elliott and Shewchuk 1995). Standardized testing does reveal that certain personality characteristics are more prominent among individuals with SCI than among people in the uninjured population. Patients with SCI are likely to have a strong physical orientation, difficulty expressing emotion, a preference for working with things rather than people, and a dislike of intellectual or academic pursuits (Rohe and Krause 1998). Neuropsychological evaluation that documents areas of cognitive impairment and strength can be critical in guiding treatment and vocational rehabilitation, especially in the subgroup of patients with suspected comorbid TBI.

Treatment of Psychiatric Disorders in Traumatic Brain Injury and Spinal Cord Injury

General Principles

A patient's specific physical (e.g., spasticity) and cognitive (e.g., defects in executive functions) impairments must be considered in designing a treatment plan for psychiatric disorders in the rehabilitation setting. A detailed understanding of the patient's physical and psychological stage in rehabilitation and functional goals will help in choosing the most appropriate psychopharmacological or psychotherapeutic treatment modality. Consulting with other members of the multidisciplinary rehabilitation team will provide clues as to the patient's motivation and treatment limitations. Knowledge of the patient's current functional, social, and vocational status is required to tailor the psychiatric treatment to specific practical needs and limitations. For example, initial treatment with an activating antidepressant in a fatigued, cognitively impaired, depressed TBI patient who is not participating optimally in physical therapy may be more appropriate than attempting to engage the patient in cognitive-behavioral therapy (CBT).

Once rapport with the patient has been established, it is helpful to discuss the events that led up to the patient's impairment (e.g., the circumstances of the car crash that led to the TBI, the stroke that led to the left-sided hemiparesis) in order to explore the psychodynamic significance of these events. For example, patients will often blame themselves for their predicament, with such self-attribution leading to guilt and depression. By contrast, patients may not associate their psychiatric symptoms with their physical impairment, which may affect readiness for psychotherapy.

Interviewing the patient's family, friends, and caregivers can provide critical information about the patient's past and present mental states. How patients handled prior losses and health problems can provide clues as to how resilient they will be during rehabilitation. Moreover, patients may report different symptoms from those observed by people close to them. For example, a patient often focuses on physical and cognitive deficits, whereas family members may consider the patient's behavioral changes as being more disabling. Patients often report significantly less frequent symptoms of depression, aggression, and memory and attention problems on self-ratings compared with ratings by their significant others (Hart et al. 2003). Close communication with family members and caregivers can provide critical information about the progress of psychiatric treatment.

Because SCI may result in marked weight loss, alterations in appetite and sleep, and reduced energy and activity, diagnosing depression can be complicated. However, vegetative symptoms should not be dismissed, because altered psychomotor activity, appetite change, and sleep disturbance are predictive of MDD (Clay et al. 1995). Core symptoms of depression in people with physical disabilities such as arthritis and SCI are worthlessness or self-blame, depressed mood, and suicidal ideation (Frank et al. 1992). The patient's own experience and interpretation of the vegetative symptoms can aid the diagnostic process.

As discussed earlier in regard to TBI and SCI, the phenomenological presentation of psychiatric symptoms in rehabilitation patients may differ from the phenomenological presentation of symptoms that arise de novo or in other medical settings. Although psychopathology based on DSM-5 criteria should be thoroughly explored, psychiatric symptoms that do not meet DSM diagnostic criteria but that still give rise to significant functional impairment are common in the rehabilitation setting (e.g., a depressed TBI patient who has only four depressive symptoms but shows apathy that affects his or her level of functioning, or a severely anxious SCI patient with few autonomic symptoms). These syndromes, or symptom clusters, may nonetheless warrant close monitoring and treatment to maximize patient functioning. Therefore, in addition to monitoring and documenting psychiatric signs and symptoms, functional status should be monitored closely as an indicator of overall progress.

Consistent with the rehabilitation process's basic tenet of working toward realistic and measurable goals, psychiatric interventions should begin with defining treatment end points according to measurable outcomes. Examples of useful measures include the PHQ-9 (Spitzer et al. 1999) and the GAD-7 (Spitzer et al. 2006) for depression and anxiety, the Brief Symptom Inventory for general distress (Meachen et al. 2008), the Neurobehavioral Rating Scale (Levin et al. 1987a) for behavior and cognition, the Rivermead Post-Concussion Symptoms Questionnaire (King et al. 1995) for postconcussive symptoms, the Overt Agitation Severity Scale (Yudofsky et al. 1997) for severe agitation, and the Participation Assessment with Recombined Tools—Objective 17 (Whiteneck et al. 2011) for community participation. Improved participation in rehabilitation therapies, which may be the outcome of most concern for the referring physician, can be monitored with the Pittsburgh Rehabilitation Participation Scale (Lenze et al. 2004).

Realistic expectations, including the possibility of incomplete remission of symptoms, must be conveyed at the outset of treatment so that the patient, who is already frustrated with the often slow and arduous rehabilitation process, does not become even more discouraged or overwhelmed if some symptoms persist. In a survey of 16,403 community-dwelling elderly and disabled Medicare beneficiaries, those with disabilities reported poor communication and lack of thorough treatment as negative aspects of their care (Iezzoni et al. 2003). Because patients may have strong preexisting preferences for specific treatment approaches (Fann et al. 2009b, 2013), adequate time must be spent in providing education about evidence-based approaches. Collaboration with rehabilitation psychologists and counselors can provide significant depth of assessment and breadth of intervention. Psychiatrist attendance at rehabilitation team meetings is often a valuable and efficient way of communicating and coordinating needs and treatment. Because patients likely are already feeling overwhelmed about their situation, framing the psychiatric consultation and intervention as a modality similar to, for example, occupational or speech therapy that can help them achieve rehabilitation goals during a period of intense stress and adaptation can quickly put patients at ease. Often, appropriately applied treatments may not have been given ample time to work. This problem may be exacerbated by imposed pressures on rehabilitation centers to work within predetermined payment structures and lengths of stay based on medical diagnoses.

Treatment of psychiatric problems in the rehabilitation setting typically warrants a combination of pharmacological and psychosocial interventions. Because treatments for most chronic diseases are covered in other chapters, the following treatment recommendations focus on TBI and SCI.

Psychopharmacology

Psychotropic medications are used frequently in the rehabilitation setting (Hammond et al. 2015a). Potential medication side effects should be explained to the patient and caregivers, because unanticipated symptoms caused by medications may be incorrectly viewed as a sign that the underlying physical condition is worsening. For example, urinary retention from an anticholinergic drug may signal to the patient with SCI that the spinal lesion is progressing.

Several common physiological changes in SCI (Table 33–3), often more pronounced in tetraplegia than in paraplegia, can affect the pharmacokinetics and tolerability of many psychotropic medications. Medications that can cause weight gain, constipation, dry mouth, orthostatic hypotension, or sexual dysfunction may exacerbate already present pathophysiology. Medications that are sedating are of particular concern in TBI and SCI because they may impair mobility and cognition, increase the risk of pressure sores, and interfere with rehabilitation. Sedation is a frequent problem, because many patients with TBI and SCI are taking multiple CNS depressants, such as anticonvulsants, muscle relaxants, and opioids.

TABLE 33–3.   **Physiological changes commonly associated with spinal cord injury**

Increased body fat and glucose intolerance

Decreased gastrointestinal motility

Reduced cardiac output

Anemia

Orthostatic hypotension

Bradyarrhythmia

Decreased blood flow to skeletal muscle

Venous thrombosis

Osteoporosis

Because individuals with TBI or SCI are often more susceptible to sedative, extrapyramidal, anticholinergic, epileptogenic, and spasticity effects of medications, psychotropic dosages should be started at lower-than-standard levels and be increased slowly. Despite the need for caution, some patients may ultimately require full standard dosages.

Neuropsychiatric polypharmacy is common in patients with TBI and should be examined critically. When multiple psychotropics are needed, they should be initiated one at a time when possible, to accurately determine the therapeutic and adverse effects of each medication. This recommendation may be difficult to follow if patients' behavior endangers them or staff or significantly impairs rehabilitation, but it usually will prove beneficial in the long term.

Because few randomized, placebo-controlled studies have examined pharmacotherapy for psychiatric conditions in TBI and SCI populations, many of the following recommendations are based on case series and expert consensus (Barker-Collo et al. 2013; Fann et al. 2009a; Guillamondegui et al. 2011; Warden et al. 2006) or are extrapolated from findings in other neurological populations. Heterogeneous study populations, including those varying in time elapsed since injury, confound the interpretation of study results. When TBI or SCI occurs in the context of a preexisting psychiatric illness, it is logical to continue a previously effective medication regimen, but previously absent side effects may emerge that require changes in dosages and/or drugs.

Electroconvulsive therapy may be considered for refractory depression (Martino et al. 2008), mania, and prolonged posttraumatic delirium and agitation. However, efforts should be made to lessen cognitive dysfunction in TBI patients (e.g., by using high-dose unilateral electrode placement or twice-weekly treatment frequency), and caution should be exercised in treating patients with SCI who may have unstable spinal columns. Preliminary findings from studies of low-intensity magnetic field exposure (Baker-Price and Persinger 2003), neurofeedback (May et al. 2013), and transcranial magnetic stimulation (Fitzgerald et al. 2011) for improving mood after TBI have been reported and require further study.

Depression, Apathy, and Fatigue

Because of their favorable side-effect profile, selective serotonin reuptake inhibitors (SSRIs) usually are the first-line antidepressants for patients with TBI. SSRIs should be started at about half their usual starting dosage and increased slowly. SSRI-induced akathisia sometimes can be mistaken for TBI-related agitation. For patients at high risk of nonadherence (e.g., because of cognitive impairment), fluoxetine should be considered because of its lower risk for withdrawal symptoms.

A meta-analysis of nine studies examining three tricyclic antidepressants (TCAs) and four SSRIs (Salter et al. 2016) demonstrated that on the basis of within-group comparisons, pharmacological treatment of post-TBI depression is associated with significant improvement in depressive symptoms. On the basis of available data from two randomized controlled trials (RCTs) included in the meta-analysis and a subsequent placebo-controlled trial (Fann et al. 2017), there is insufficient evidence to establish definitively the superiority of antidepressant treatment over placebo response or natural recovery alone or to determine demographic and clinical predictors of treatment response.

Two RCTs have examined the usefulness of sertraline 50–100 mg/day in the prevention of MDD following TBI (Jorge et al. 2016; Novack et al. 2009). Although these studies suggest some benefit for this prophylactic strategy in the short term, the long-term benefits have yet to be determined, particularly when balanced against the potential for side effects among patients receiving sertraline treatment who are not depressed.

SSRIs are likely efficacious in patients with SCI; however, no RCTs in this population have been conducted, and these agents may increase the risk of spasticity (Stolp-Smith and Wainberg 1999).

Although not yet systematically studied, serotonin–norepinephrine reuptake inhibitors (SNRIs) are likely safe and effective in patients with TBI. The largest antidepressant RCT to date in persons with SCI ($N=133$) compared venlafaxine extended release with placebo and found venlafaxine to be superior in reducing core depressive symptoms, SCI-related disability, and nociceptive pain (Fann et al. 2015a; Richards et al. 2015). Venlafaxine may also improve voiding in SCI patients with urinary retention (Inghilleri et al. 2005).

Compared with the literature on tolerability and safety of SSRIs after TBI, findings for TCAs and monoamine oxidase inhibitors (MAOIs) are less consistent (Saran 1985; Wroblewski et al. 1996). Because of the potentially problematic adverse effects of TCAs and MAOIs (e.g., sedation, hypotension, anticholinergic effects) in patients with CNS impairment, and because of the narrow therapeutic index of these medications (which can lead to inadvertent overdose in patients with cognitive impairment), they should be used with extreme caution in patients with TBI. Autonomic dysfunction in patients with SCI makes them more vulnerable to TCA-related anticholinergic and orthostatic side effects. TCAs may also carry an increased risk of spasticity and autonomic dysreflexia in patients with SCI (Cardenas et al. 2002). If a TCA is chosen, nortriptyline or desipramine may cause the fewest side effects.

Mirtazapine, nefazodone, and trazodone may prove to be too sedating for some patients, particularly those who have cognitive impairment or gait instability, but if insomnia is a major problem, these drugs may be helpful.

Some data suggest that certain antidepressants, especially TCAs and bupropion, are associated with an increased risk of seizures, a particular concern following severe TBI (Wroblewski et al. 1990). However, if the drugs are titrated cautiously, most patients will not experience increased seizures, particularly if they are taking an anticonvulsant.

The symptoms of apathy and fatigue, which are commonly associated with CNS impairment, can occur either concomitantly with or independently of depression and are often mistaken for primary depression. For apathy and fatigue, medications that augment dopaminergic activity appear to be the most useful (Marin et al. 1995). Methylphenidate and dextroamphetamine are generally safe at standard dosages (e.g., methylphenidate 10–30 mg/day in divided doses) (Alban et al. 2004) and have been used successfully to enhance participation in rehabilitation. Psychostimulants also have been shown in case series and double-blind studies to be effective in improving some aspects of mood, mental speed, attention, and behavior, although improvement was not always sustained long term (Whyte et al. 2004; Willmott and Ponsford 2009). Dextroamphetamine may exacerbate dystonia and dyskinesia in some cases. Therapeutic use of psychostimulants in the medically ill rarely leads to abuse in patients without a personal or family history of substance use disorders, but substance misuse is overrepresented in the TBI and SCI populations.

Modafinil has been efficacious in treating fatigue in patients with multiple sclerosis (Niepel et al. 2013; Zifko et al. 2002) and excessive daytime sleepiness in patients with TBI (Teitelman 2001). Bupropion (Marin et al. 1995) and dopamine agonists such as amantadine (Kraus et al. 2005; Sawyer et al. 2008), bromocriptine (McDowell et al. 1998), and levodopa/carbidopa (Lal et al. 1988) have been used to treat apathy states, fatigue, and cognitive impairment. Bupropion's stimulating properties may be of particular benefit in fatigued or apathetic depressed patients. Stimulants and dopamine agonists can increase the risk of delirium and psychosis and thus should be used with caution in more vulnerable patients. Amantadine has been associated with an increased risk of seizures, but psychostimulants and bromocriptine do not appear to lower the seizure threshold at typical dosages.

Another secondary benefit of some antidepressants in TBI and SCI is their analgesic properties (see also Chapter 34, "Pain"). The TCA amitriptyline has been found to improve SCI-related neuropathic pain in the context of comorbid depressive symptomatology (Rintala et al. 2007). SNRIs may be effective in treating a variety of pain syndromes, including neuropathic pain; however, venlafaxine XR was found to be effective for nociceptive pain, but not for neuropathic pain, in one RCT in SCI patients (Richards et al. 2015).

Mania

For mania following TBI, lithium, mood-stabilizing anticonvulsants (valproic acid, carbamazepine), and typical and atypical antipsychotics all have been used successfully (Oster et al. 2007; Warden et al. 2006). Electroconvulsive therapy can be used as a second-line modality. Dikmen et al. (2000) have shown that valproic acid is well tolerated after TBI, but lithium and carbamazepine have been associated with neurocognitive adverse effects. Lithium has a narrow therapeutic window and can lower the seizure threshold; therefore, caution is required when lithium is used in TBI patients, whose cognitive impairment may lead to poor adherence or inadvertent overdosage. Although serum blood levels of valproic acid and carbamazepine are helpful in monitoring adherence and absorption, dosing should be guided primarily by therapeutic response and side effects. Possible roles for other anticonvulsants in secondary mania are reviewed in Chapter 9, "Psychosis, Mania, and Catatonia." The role of antipsychotics for post-TBI mania has not yet been studied.

Anxiety

Benzodiazepines are the treatment of choice for acute anxiety in TBI, but they should be used initially at lower dosages because of their propensity to exacerbate or cause cognitive impairment and oversedation. The high prevalence of substance use disorders in patients with TBI and SCI adds to the risk from benzodiazepines and may contraindicate their use in some patients. Although few studies have been conducted in patients with TBI, SSRIs, SNRIs, and TCAs also may be effective for anxiety, particularly in the context of comorbid depression. SSRIs have been found to be effective in reducing mood lability after brain injury (Warden et al. 2006), although this effect may take as long as their antidepressant effects. Valproic acid, gabapentin, and pregabalin may be of benefit, especially in patients with concomitant mood lability or seizures (Pande et al. 1999, 2000). Buspirone is another option for generalized anxiety symptoms. Antipsychotics should not be used as a first-line treatment for anxiety after TBI; rather, these agents should be reserved for patients with psychotic symptoms. When antipsychotic medications are indicated, quetiapine and olanzapine may be the most useful for anxiety and sleep.

Sleep Disorders

Treatment of sleep problems in patients with TBI and SCI ideally should be based on diagnosis of a specific sleep disorder. Sleep apnea is fairly common in TBI (Viola-Saltzman and Musleh (2016) and SCI (Chiodo et al. 2016), and nocturnal periodic leg movements are frequent in SCI (Proserpio et al. 2015). Insomnia often is associated with depression, anxiety, and pain after acute TBI, so treatment of these comorbid conditions is important. Minimal data exist on pharmacological treatment of insomnia or other sleep disorders in patients with TBI or SCI, but trazodone is widely used for middle or late insomnia, and hypnotics are used by as many as 20% of TBI patients (Worthington and Melia 2006). Cognitive effects from sedative-hypnotics and orthostatic hypotension from trazodone may be particularly problematic in the rehabilitation setting, however. Antihistamines such as diphenhydramine should be avoided because of their anticholinergic properties. (See Chapter 14, "Sleep Disorders," for discussion of diagnosis and treatment of sleep disorders.)

Anger, Aggression, and Agitation

Anger, aggression, and agitation are common following TBI and can occur in isolation or as part of delirium or other psychiatric disorders (see Chapter 6, "Aggression and Violence"). The published literature regarding treatment of anger, aggression, and agitation is often not diagnostically specific and consists largely of case reports, case series, and reviews (Fleminger et al. 2006; Levy et al. 2005; Plantier et al. 2016).

Treatment can be divided into acute treatment, in which the goal is timely management of behavior to prevent injury to self or others, and chronic treatment, in which the goal is long-term management and prevention. Many agents require from 2 to 8 weeks to attain full effectiveness. It is important to keep in mind that medications that worsen cognition or sedation can actually worsen confusion and may therefore worsen agitation during the confusional state of PTA after TBI. Because the effects of medications in patients with TBI can be unpredictable, and because medication side effects may actually potentiate behavior problems (e.g., akathisia from antipsychotics), it can be beneficial to systematically eliminate certain medications, including those that were initially prescribed to treat behavioral dyscontrol. The rationale for such a practice is that some patients have a natural course of recovery, and medication efficacy and patient needs may decrease over time.

The benzodiazepines offer rapid sedation that may be useful in the acute setting; however, in patients with TBI, benzodiazepines also have a high potential for neurocognitive effects, such as mental slowing, amnesia, disinhibition, and impaired balance. For this reason, low doses of a short-acting agent, such as lorazepam 1–2 mg orally or parenterally, should be used initially and increased incrementally as needed. If agitation is frequent, a longer-acting agent, such as clonazepam 0.5–1.0 mg two or three times a day, may be used for short durations. The combination of haloperidol and low-dose lorazepam (e.g., 0.5–1.0 mg) may offer a synergistic calming effect for some acutely agitated patients.

Evidence for the efficacy of atypical antipsychotics in treating acute aggression and agitation in TBI patients is still emerging (Scott et al. 2009), as well as in other neurological syndromes (Meehan et al. 2002). The typical antipsychotics, given orally or intramuscularly, also may be useful in the acute setting (Stanislav and Childs 2000), but the elevated risks of extrapyramidal and anticholinergic effects in TBI patients must be considered. Studies in animals have suggested that chronic use of haloperidol and other dopamine 2 D_2 receptor–blocking antipsychotics may impede neuronal and cognitive recovery (Hoffman et al. 2008; Phelps et al. 2015).

Antipsychotics for chronic agitation ideally should be reserved for situations when aggression occurs concomitantly with psychotic symptoms (Kim and Bijlani 2006). Clozapine's use in patients with TBI is limited by its seizure risk, although it has been found to be effective for chronic aggression (Kraus and Sheitman 2005).

Serotonergic antidepressants may be helpful in treating agitation and aggression in TBI populations. In 8-week nonrandomized trials with sertraline, Fann et al. (2000) showed that improved depression was associated with improved anger and aggression scores in patients with mild TBI, whereas Kant et al. (1998) found that improvements in aggression were independent of depression scores. One rationale for the use of antidepressants is the observation that serotonin and norepinephrine levels are reduced in the cerebrospinal fluid of agitated patients with brain injury (van Woerkom et al. 1977). Antidepressants and dextromethorphan/quinidine are also effective in treating emotional incontinence, such as pathological crying or laughing (Hammond et al. 2016; Nahas et al. 1998). Buspirone has demonstrated some efficacy for agitation in patients with TBI and other neurological disorders (Stanislav et al. 1994) and can be particularly useful when anxiety also is present.

Among the anticonvulsants, carbamazepine (Azouvi et al. 1999) and valproic acid (Lindenmayer and Kotsaftis 2000) have been the most extensively studied in the treatment of behavioral dyscontrol after TBI. Although evidence of seizures or epileptiform activity on EEG is a strong indication for anticonvulsant use in the agitated patient, these agents also have shown benefit in patients without EEG abnormalities. Oxcarbazepine, gabapentin, lamotrigine, and topiramate also may be efficacious, although data on these agents are more limited, and paradoxical agitation and cognitive dysfunction are potential risks (Pachet et al. 2003; Tatum et al. 2001). When anticonvulsants are used for behavioral control, serum levels may need to be higher than those required for seizure prophylaxis. According to case reports, lithium is also an effective mood stabilizer and has antiaggression properties in patients with TBI.

When anger, aggression, or agitation occurs without signs of other psychiatric syndromes, β-blockers should be considered. Placebo-controlled studies have shown their efficacy in treating agitation in patients with TBI (Fleminger et al. 2006). Dosages of propranolol in the range of 160–320 mg/day may be needed in some patients. Bradycardia and hypotension are potential side effects; contraindications to β-blocker treatment include asthma, chronic obstructive pulmonary disease, type 1 diabetes mellitus, congestive heart failure, persistent angina, significant peripheral vascular disease, and hyperthyroidism. Pindolol is less likely than other β-blockers to cause bradycardia.

Stimulants and dopamine agonists have also been used to treat anger and irritability after TBI (Lee et al. 2005). Although one 6-week placebo-controlled trial found that methylphenidate significantly reduced anger in a cohort of young adult men who had sustained a TBI an average of 27 months earlier (Mooney and Haas 1993), stimulants should be used with caution in agitated TBI patients because of the risks of exacerbating agitation and psychosis and of abuse. Amantadine is well tolerated and was found in an RCT to decrease patient-rated—but not observer-rated—irritability as well as aggression after acute TBI (Hammond et al. 2015b, 2017).

Psychosis

Because of the increased susceptibility of patients with TBI to experiencing anticholinergic and extrapyramidal side effects and of patients with SCI to experiencing problematic anticholinergic sequelae, the newer-generation atypical antipsychotics are the drugs of first choice for psychotic symptoms that emerge after TBI or SCI (Chew and Zafonte 2009) (see also Chapter 9, "Psychosis, Mania, and Catatonia"). Controlled trials are needed to compare the efficacy and tolerability of various antipsychotics in this population.

Cognitive Impairment

Few RCTs are available to guide selection of pharmacotherapies to enhance cognitive recovery following TBI; most data are derived from theoretical or animal models or case reports (Diaz-Arrastia et al. 2014; Dougall et al. 2015). Removing agents that may impair cognition is an important first step. Writer and Schillerstrom's (2009) review of the literature concluded that the greatest amount of evidence supported the treatment of attentional impairment with stimulants, memory impairment with stimulants and cholinesterase inhibitors, and executive impairment with stimulant and nonstimulant dopamine-enhancing agents.

Dopaminergic agents such as amantadine and bromocriptine may improve executive function (Warden et al. 2006). Because of the negative impact of depression on cognition, treating depression may improve cognitive performance. In addition, growth hormone deficiency should be considered as a contributor to cognitive dysfunction in patients with TBI; hormone replacement therapy may be indicated in these cases (Moreau et al. 2013). Acetylcholinesterase inhibitors enhance cholinergic activity and may improve cognition. The noradrenergic agents most commonly used to enhance cognition, perhaps by improving arousal, attention, and awareness, are the psychostimulant methylphenidate (Lee et al. 2005; Whyte et al. 2004) and atomoxetine, both of which also have dopaminergic effects. Modafinil also may show some benefit. Other promising agents being investigated include opioid antagonists, neuropeptides such as cerebrolysin, and monoamine stabilizers.

Psychological Treatment

Traumatic Brain Injury

A widely accepted model of psychological effects of TBI distinguishes among symptoms that represent *reactions to the effects of TBI* (e.g., depression, anxiety, irritability, anger, hopelessness, helplessness, social withdrawal, distrust, phobias), symptoms that are *neurologically based* (e.g., affective lability, impulsivity, agitation, paranoia, unawareness), and symptoms that *reflect long-standing personality traits* (e.g., obsessiveness, antisocial behavior, work attitude, social connectedness, dependence, entitlement) (Prigatano 1986). Although the genesis of symptoms can be multifactorial, it is useful to consider the potential contributions of all three of these factors to observed problem behaviors. Prigatano (1986) argued that reactive problems may be most amenable to psychotherapy, whereas neurologically mediated symptoms may require multimodal interventions that also target underlying cognitive impairment. Characterological problems may require making coordinated changes in environmental contingencies and working with families or caregivers.

Although psychotherapy is considered an important aspect of brain injury rehabilitation, there are few controlled studies in persons with TBI and little guidance on the indications for psychotherapeutic interventions. A systematic review of the literature on psychotherapeutic and rehabilitation interventions for depression after TBI (Fann et al. 2009a) suggested that cognitive-behavioral approaches, particularly holistic treatment programs for TBI that include activity scheduling and increasing positive interaction with the environment, may improve mood along with functional outcomes and productivity. The most recent systematic review on nonpharmacological interventions for depression in TBI, covering the literature up to early 2015, found only four RCTs testing psychotherapeutic interventions, and all had been completed within the previous 4 years (Gertler et al. 2015). Because many participants improved without intervention, study methodology differed greatly, and effect sizes for the interventions were small, no recommendations for specific treatments were offered.

Compared with psychological interventions used in non-TBI populations, such interventions for people with TBI are more likely to require the involvement of family members or caregivers to help cue follow-through and generalization to real-world situations. Psychotherapy has been used with selected patients to foster insight in comprehensive postacute neurorehabilitation programs (Prigatano and Ben-Yishay 1999). Insight-focused psychotherapy often begins by providing the patient with a simple model to explain what has happened. These explanations and coping strategies provided in psychotherapy must be rehearsed repeatedly until they are automatic. Group therapy may be used to foster more insight through feedback from peers.

Lessons learned from recent clinical trials of CBT in patients with TBI include the suggestions that 1) the behavioral-activation strategies typically used during the first 8 weeks of treatment, such as scheduling pleasant events and decreasing avoidance behaviors, are more effective than the cognitive therapy components used later in treatment, such as identifying negative thoughts; and 2) telephone-based CBT is equally acceptable as in-person CBT (Fann et al. 2015b). With the use of accommodations for patients with cognitive limitations, treatment effects did not differ by TBI severity or level of cognitive impairment. Booster sessions delivered after the end of formal treatment appear particularly important for establishing and maintaining gains (Ponsford et al. 2016).

It is important for therapists to try to match therapy approaches to the cognitive and physical limitations of patients. Findings reported by Fann et al. (2015b) suggest that a behavioral activation approach may be particularly useful for people with TBI, including those with significant cognitive impairment, who are able to increase their activity levels and exposure to reinforcing events. Available evidence suggests that the simpler components of CBT—including relaxation training (for patients with anxiety) and simple self-affirming statements that may be rehearsed at difficult times—may also be helpful for patients with TBI. There is mounting evidence that CBT strategies for acute and chronic posttraumatic stress are effective in patients with a history of TBI (Bryant et al. 2003; Walter et al. 2014; Wolf et al. 2015).

"Third-wave" therapies, including mindfulness-based psychotherapies, have not been fully tested in patients with TBI. One small study using a wait-list control showed that a 10-week course of mindfulness-based stress reduction resulted in significant reductions in symptoms on some, but not all, depression measures (Bédard et al. 2014).

Telephone-based problem-solving therapy was successful in reducing emotional distress—including depression, anxiety, and PTSD symptoms—in recently deployed military service members with mild TBI (Bell et al. 2017). CBT has been proposed as a promising treatment for persistent postconcussion symptoms because it is well suited to addressing maladaptive symptom attributions while combating avoidance and activity restriction, which can prolong recovery. One such treatment was shown to reduce anxiety and fatigue in a randomized wait-list controlled trial (Potter et al. 2016), although emotional distress remained unchanged.

One small RCT of a psychoeducational individual treatment for anger following acquired brain injury (Medd and Tate 2000) and two uncontrolled studies of group treatment have reported mixed but generally positive results (O'Leary 2000; Walker et al. 2010). As is true of many psychotherapeutic treatments, the mix of specific ingredients differs across studies, making conclusions about "active ingredients" difficult.

In an RCT in persons with chronic anger and irritability following moderate to severe TBI, Hart et al. (2017) compared Anger Self-Management Training (ASMT)—an eight-session psychoeducational treatment protocol consisting of education about anger and its links to brain injury; identification and self-monitoring of anger signals; and alternative responses for dealing with problematic situations—with a structurally equivalent educational control group condition. Compared with the control subjects, subjects who received ASMT showed greater improvements in self- and significant other–reported anger but not in outward expression of anger.

Therapies for impaired awareness have included several different strategies. Mildly impaired patients may benefit from information about the effects of brain injury coupled with test data and observations about the specific ways that their injuries have affected their thinking, including limited awareness. Basic cognitive compensatory strategies should be used to help patients attend to, understand, and recall this information. Family, friends, or caregivers should be included in these educational processes. With more severe or persistent problems, treatment may include more comprehensive, coordinated, and real-time feedback about impairments, such as via videotaping. Experiential learning paradigms can be used; in these exercises, the person is asked to predict how well he or she will perform on a given test and is reinforced for successively improving the accuracy of his or her predictions. Staff should minimize the potential for shame or humiliation that may occur with failures. When adaptive denial is present, staff may benefit from information about how such denial helps the person psychologically. Staff may be inclined to confront the denial, not realizing the value of defensive denial in helping the patient to manage anxiety and maintain a sense of self-efficacy.

Cognitive rehabilitation refers to teaching patients skills they can use to mitigate the severity and impact of brain injury–related cognitive impairment. The science of cognitive rehabilitation has advanced significantly in recent years. An international team of experts in cognitive rehabilitation (known as INCOG) published a series of evidence-based guidelines on assessing and managing cognitive impairments following TBI (Bayley et al. 2014). The guidelines on managing PTA and delirium after TBI are among the weakest and are limited to expert opinion recommendations that clinicians use valid measures to conduct serial assessments and avoid the use of antipsychotic medications (Ponsford et al. 2014b). On the basis of multiple RCTs, training in metacognitive strategies and dual tasking is recommended for attention impairments, and methylphenidate (0.3 mg/kg in divided doses) is recommended for slow speed of information processing (Ponsford et al. 2014a). Similarly, there is a substantial evidence base to recommend internal learning strategies (e.g., visualization, retrieval practice, self-cueing) and external compensatory techniques (e.g., memory book, electronic reminders) for memory impairment (Velikonja et al. 2014). On the basis of experimental data, the INCOG group recommended metacognitive strategies (typically, self-monitoring and incorporation of feedback into planning), structured problem-solving rubrics, and corrective feedback to manage executive dysfunction and poor awareness (Tate et al. 2014). Finally, there is evidence to support the following recommendations for management of cognitive–communication disorders following TBI: 1) provide the opportunity to practice communication skills in real-life settings and situations; 2) provide education and training of communication partners; and 3) provide group-based interventions to address patient-identified goals for improving social communication deficits (Togher et al. 2014).

Limited high-quality research has been conducted on the comparative effectiveness of comprehensive rehabilitation programs. Among active-duty military personnel who sustained moderate to severe TBI, a home-based program of physical and mental exercises overseen by a nurse was as effective as standardized 8-week inpatient rehabilitation in terms of return to duty and other outcomes (Salazar et al. 2000). However, inpatient rehabilitation produced higher rates of return to duty (80%) compared with home rehabilitation (58%) among patients who had been unconscious for more than 1 hour. In another study, holistic rehabilitation—which emphasizes greater integration of cognitive, interpersonal, and functional interventions directed at self-regulation of cognitive and emotional processes, including metacognitive processes of self-appraisal, prediction, self-monitoring, and self-evaluation—was more effective than a standard multidisciplinary rehabilitation program in reducing cognitive and functional disability after TBI (Cicerone et al. 2000). Inpatient rehabilitation that focused on individualized cognitive skills training produced similar long-term outcomes but superior short-term outcomes compared with functional–experiential treatment that focused on performing real-life tasks in a group setting (Vanderploeg et al. 2008).

Spinal Cord Injury

Within SCI rehabilitation, mental health professionals are often called on to help manage psychological and physical distress, such as depression, anxiety, pain, and insomnia, as well as grief or adjustment to disability. The rehabilitation team may also request assistance to help motivate patients to adhere to rehabilitation therapies or to make health behavior changes.

The evidence base for treatment of psychological distress in persons with SCI is limited in terms of the number, size, and quality of studies published to date. Nevertheless, two meta-analyses of controlled trials and cohort studies concluded that cognitive-behavioral-type interventions hold promise for improving depression, QOL, assertiveness, and self-efficacy after SCI. Significant effects were found on short-term but not long-term psychological outcomes (Dorstyn et al. 2011; Mehta et al. 2011). A meta-analysis of telephone-delivered supportive, cognitive-behavioral, and motivational counseling found evidence suggesting that these interventions can improve sleep and pain in SCI (Dorstyn et al. 2013). An RCT of an automated telephone intervention in people with SCI or multiple sclerosis reported improvements in depression (Houlihan et al. 2013). A pilot RCT of a telephone-based peer-led intervention led to reductions in social role impairment and improvements in life satisfaction (Houlihan et al. 2017).

To our knowledge, few studies have applied modern grief theory to SCI-related loss, and there have been no trials of interventions designed to improve symptoms of grief or bereavement experienced by individuals with SCI (Klyce et al. 2015). Nevertheless, we think that theory and research from the larger grief literature can inform the management of adjustment to SCI. Stroebe and Schut (1999) described their dual-process model of grief, which posits that bereaved individuals normally oscillate between confronting and seeking respite from loss experiences. This model explains and normalizes the transient (healthy) denial shown by many people with SCI. Maciejewski et al. (2007) showed that grief indicators such as acceptance and disbelief occur simultaneously; that acceptance begins early and increases steadily over time; and that by 6 months postloss, disbelief, yearning, anger, and depression have all peaked. These findings suggest that if grief symptoms have not begun to subside after 6 months, specialized treatment may be indicated. One review of the treatment literature concluded that early interventions to prevent grief may not be effective and may even cause harm, whereas interventions that are delivered later and only when indicated are more likely to be effective (Neimeyer and Currier 2009). Finally, comparative effectiveness research has demonstrated that treatment of chronic grief with an intervention that includes education about the dual-process model, managing grief symptoms, resuming a meaningful life, and exposure-based therapy techniques is more effective than an active control condition of interpersonal therapy (Shear et al. 2005).

If we apply this model to the situation of a patient with a complete SCI who insists that she is going to walk again, the patient's denial reflects the loss-avoidance phase of the dual-process model and her understandable hope or wish for neurological recovery. The consultant can express tolerance of verbal denial, especially when the patient is not engaging in behavioral denial (e.g., refusing to learn adaptive strategies such as wheelchair use or self-catheterization). If verbal and behavioral denial co-occur and interfere with rehabilitation progress, more exposure-based interventions may be needed, such as education about the nature and extent of the injury (including radiographic evidence), the prognosis for recovery, and the limitations of current research seeking a cure for SCI.

Nonadherence to treatment, and the associated conflicts with staff, often triggers psychiatric consultation in the rehabilitation setting. Causes of nonadherence are varied and include depression, amotivational states due to concomitant TBI, antisocial personality traits, ongoing substance abuse, and unrealistic staff expectations. Several RCTs have tested strategies for improving adherence to skin-care regimens. Trials of motivational interviewing alone and motivational interviewing plus self-management training in veterans with SCI failed to reduce pressure ulcer recurrence (Guihan et al. 2007, 2014). However, an automated branching-logic telephone intervention based on the transtheoretical model and social learning theory did reduce the prevalence of pressure ulcers (Houlihan et al. 2013). A peer-led intervention that used brief action planning improved patient activation and resource utilization (Houlihan et al. 2017).

Treatment adherence is a function of the interactions among somatic, psychological, and environmental variables (Trieschmann 1988). Environmental factors may be particularly salient in cases of nonadherence. Once primary psychiatric disorders are ruled out, the consultant should look for issues—perhaps related to pain, withdrawal of social contact, or relinquishing a sense of control—that may lead patients to perceive medication adherence as unrewarding. In some cases, nonadherence may be inadvertently rewarded by engaging staff in negative social interactions, asserting independence, or avoiding unwanted responsibilities. Behavioral principles such as rewarding successive approximations, ignoring disability-inappropriate behaviors, initiating behavioral activation, using quota systems (gradual increases in behavioral expectations), and explicitly linking progress in rehabilitation to desired outcomes (such as earlier discharge) may improve adherence to treatment (Fordyce 1976).

Conclusion

As survival from TBI continues to improve and our understanding of the psychosocial factors in disability evolves, psychiatrists will have an increasing role in the rehabilitation setting. To provide comprehensive evaluation and treatment of TBI and SCI, psychiatrists must appreciate and address the multiple complex facets of these conditions, from the acute neurological injury and its attendant psychological trauma through the chronic neurological, medical, psychiatric, and social sequelae of the injury. The multidisciplinary rehabilitation setting affords an environment in which psychiatrists can use their pharmacological and psychotherapeutic skills in psychosomatic medicine to maximize the long-term functional potential of their patients.

References

Alban JP, Hopson MM, Ly V, et al: Effect of methylphenidate on vital signs and adverse effects in adults with traumatic brain injury. Am J Phys Med Rehabil 83(2):131–137, quiz 138–141, 167, 2004 14758299

Alway Y, Gould KR, Johnston L, et al: A prospective examination of Axis I psychiatric disorders in the first 5 years following moderate to severe traumatic brain injury. Psychol Med 46(6):1331–1341, 2016 26867715

Amador M, Lynne C, Brackett N: A Guide and Resource Directory to Male Fertility Following Spinal Cord Injury/Dysfunction: Miami Project to Cure Paralysis. Miami, FL, University of Miami, 2000

American Psychiatric Association: Diagnostic and Statistical Manual of Mental Disorders, 3rd Edition, Revised. Washington, DC, American Psychiatric Association, 1987

American Psychiatric Association: Diagnostic and Statistical Manual of Mental Disorders, 4th Edition. Washington, DC, American Psychiatric Association, 1994

American Psychiatric Association: Diagnostic and Statistical Manual of Mental Disorders, 4th Edition, Text Revision. Washington, DC, American Psychiatric Association, 2000

American Psychiatric Association: Diagnostic and Statistical Manual of Mental Disorders, 5th Edition. Arlington, VA, American Psychiatric Association, 2013

Arciniegas DB, Wortzel HS: Emotional and behavioral dyscontrol after traumatic brain injury. Psychiatr Clin North Am 37(1):31–53, 2014 24529422

Armistead-Jehle P, Soble JR, Cooper DB, et al: Unique aspects of traumatic brain injury in military and veteran populations. Phys Med Rehabil Clin N Am 28(2):323–337, 2017 28390516

Ashman TA, Schwartz ME, Cantor JB, et al: Screening for substance abuse in individuals with traumatic brain injury. Brain Inj 18(2):191–202, 2004 14660230

Azouvi P, Jokic C, Attal N, et al: Carbamazepine in agitation and aggressive behaviour following severe closed-head injury: results of an open trial. Brain Inj 13(10):797–804, 1999 10576463

Baguley IJ, Cooper J, Felmingham K: Aggressive behavior following traumatic brain injury: how common is common? J Head Trauma Rehabil 21(1):45–56, 2006 16456391

Baker A, Barker S, Sampson A, et al: Caregiver outcomes and interventions: a systematic scoping review of the traumatic brain injury and spinal cord injury literature. Clin Rehabil 31(1):45–60, 2017 27009058

Baker-Price L, Persinger MA: Intermittent burst-firing weak (1 microTesla) magnetic fields reduce psychometric depression in patients who sustained closed head injuries: a replication and electroencephalographic validation. Percept Mot Skills 96(3 Pt 1):965–974, 2003 12831278

Barker RN, Kendall MD, Amsters DI, et al: The relationship between quality of life and disability across the lifespan for people with spinal cord injury. Spinal Cord 47(2):149–155, 2009 18594553

Barker-Collo S, Starkey N, Theadom A: Treatment for depression following mild traumatic brain injury in adults: a meta-analysis. Brain Inj 27(10):1124–1133, 2013 23895287

Barncord SW, Wanlass RL: A correction procedure for the Minnesota Multiphasic Personality Inventory-2 for persons with spinal cord injury. Arch Phys Med Rehabil 81(9):1185–1190, 2000 10987160

Bayley MT, Tate R, Douglas JM, et al; INCOG Expert Panel: INCOG guidelines for cognitive rehabilitation following traumatic brain injury: methods and overview. J Head Trauma Rehabil 29(4):290–306, 2014 24984093

Bazarian JJ, Veazie P, Mookerjee S, et al: Accuracy of mild traumatic brain injury case ascertainment using ICD-9 codes. Acad Emerg Med 13(1):31–38, 2006 16365331

Bédard M, Felteau M, Marshall S, et al: Mindfulness-based cognitive therapy reduces symptoms of depression in people with a traumatic brain injury: results from a randomized controlled trial. J Head Trauma Rehabil 29(4):E13–E22, 2014 24052092

Belanger HG, Vanderploeg RD: The neuropsychological impact of sports-related concussion: a meta-analysis. J Int Neuropsychol Soc 11(4):345–357, 2005 16209414

Bell KR, Fann JR, Brockway JA, et al: Telephone problem solving for service members with mild traumatic brain injury: a randomized clinical trial. J Neurotrauma 34(2):313–321, 2017 27579992

Bogner J, Barrett RS, Hammond FM, et al: Predictors of agitated behavior during inpatient rehabilitation for traumatic brain injury. Arch Phys Med Rehabil 96 (8 suppl):S274.e4–S281.e4, 2015 26212403

Bombardier CH, Rimmele CT, Zintel H: The magnitude and correlates of alcohol and drug use before traumatic brain injury. Arch Phys Med Rehabil 83(12):1765–1773, 2002 12474184

Bombardier CH, Richards JS, Krause JS, et al: Symptoms of major depression in people with spinal cord injury: implications for screening. Arch Phys Med Rehabil 85(11):1749–1756, 2004 15520969

Bombardier CH, Fann JR, Temkin NR, et al: Rates of major depressive disorder and clinical outcomes following traumatic brain injury. JAMA 303(19):1938–1945, 2010 20483970

Bombardier CH, Adams LM, Fann JR, et al: Depression trajectories during the first year after spinal cord injury. Arch Phys Med Rehabil 97(2):196–203, 2016 26525525

Bonanno GA, Kennedy P, Galatzer-Levy IR, et al: Trajectories of resilience, depression, and anxiety following spinal cord injury. Rehabil Psychol 57(3):236–247, 2012 22946611

Broshek DK, De Marco AP, Freeman JR: A review of post-concussion syndrome and psychological factors associated with concussion. Brain Inj 29(2):228–237, 2015 25383595

Bryant R: Post-traumatic stress disorder vs traumatic brain injury. Dialogues Clin Neurosci 13(3):251–262, 2011 22034252

Bryant RA, Moulds M, Guthrie R, et al: Treating acute stress disorder following mild traumatic brain injury. Am J Psychiatry 160(3):585–587, 2003 12611847

Bryce TN, Budh CN, Cardenas DD, et al: Pain after spinal cord injury: an evidence-based review for clinical practice and research. Report of the National Institute on Disability and Rehabilitation Research Spinal Cord Injury Measures meeting. J Spinal Cord Med 30(5):421–440, 2007 18092558

Budh CN, Osteråker AL: Life satisfaction in individuals with a spinal cord injury and pain. Clin Rehabil 21(1):89–96, 2007 17213246

Cao Y, Massaro JF, Krause JS, et al: Suicide mortality after spinal cord injury in the United States: injury cohorts analysis. Arch Phys Med Rehabil 95(2):230–235, 2014 24161272

Cardenas DD, Warms CA, Turner JA, et al: Efficacy of amitriptyline for relief of pain in spinal cord injury: results of a randomized controlled trial. Pain 96(3):365–373, 2002 11973011

Carlson KF, Kehle SM, Meis LA, et al: Prevalence, assessment, and treatment of mild traumatic brain injury and posttraumatic stress disorder: a systematic review of the evidence. J Head Trauma Rehabil 26(2):103–115, 2011 20631631

Carroll LJ, Cassidy JD, Peloso PM, et al; WHO Collaborating Centre Task Force on Mild Traumatic Brain Injury: Prognosis for mild traumatic brain injury: results of the WHO Collaborating Centre Task Force on Mild Traumatic Brain Injury. J Rehabil Med (43 suppl):84–105, 2004 15083873

Cassidy JD, Cancelliere C, Carroll LJ, et al: Systematic review of self-reported prognosis in adults after mild traumatic brain injury: results of the International Collaboration on Mild Traumatic Brain Injury Prognosis. Arch Phys Med Rehabil 95 (3 suppl):S132–S151, 2014 24581902

Castaño Monsalve B, Laxe S, Bernabeu Guitart M, et al: Behavioral scales used in severe and moderate traumatic brain injury. NeuroRehabilitation 35(1):67–76, 2014 24990011

Centers for Disease Control and Prevention: National Center for Injury Prevention and Control: Traumatic Brain Injury in the United States: A Report to Congress. Atlanta, GA, Centers for Disease Control and Prevention, 2015

Charlifue SW, Gerhart KA: Behavioral and demographic predictors of suicide after traumatic spinal cord injury. Arch Phys Med Rehabil 72(7):488–492, 1991 2059121

Chew E, Zafonte RD: Pharmacological management of neurobehavioral disorders following traumatic brain injury—a state-of-the-art review. J Rehabil Res Dev 46(6):851–879, 2009 20104408

Chiodo AE, Sitrin RG, Bauman KA: Sleep disordered breathing in spinal cord injury: a systematic review. J Spinal Cord Med 39(4):374–382, 2016 27077573

Cicerone KD, Dahlberg C, Kalmar K, et al: Evidence-based cognitive rehabilitation: recommendations for clinical practice. Arch Phys Med Rehabil 81(12):1596–1615, 2000 11128897

Clay DL, Hagglund KJ, Frank RG, et al: Enhancing the accuracy of depression diagnosis in patients with spinal cord injury using Bayesian analysis. Rehabil Psychol 40(3):171–180, 1995

Cnossen MC, Scholten AC, Lingsma HF, et al: Predictors of major depression and posttraumatic stress disorder following traumatic brain injury: a systematic review and meta-analysis. J Neuropsychiatry Clin Neurosci 29(3):206–224, 2017a 28193126

Cnossen MC, Winkler EA, Yue JK, et al: Development of a prediction model for post-concussive symptoms following mild traumatic brain injury: a TRACK-TBI pilot study. J Neurotrauma March 27, 2017b [Epub ahead of print] 28343409

Cohen-Cole SA, Stoudemire A: Major depression and physical illness: special considerations in diagnosis and biologic treatment. Psychiatr Clin North Am 10(1):1–17, 1987 3554179

Consortium for Spinal Cord Medicine: Outcomes following spinal cord injury: a clinical practice guideline for health care professionals. Washington, DC, Paralyzed Veterans of America, July 1999. Available at: www.pva.org/media/pdf/CPG_outcomes%20following%20traumatic%20SCI.pdf. Accessed October 12, 2017.

Consortium for Spinal Cord Medicine: Sexuality and reproductive health in adults with spinal cord injury: a clinical practice guideline for health-care professionals. J Spinal Cord Med 33(3):281–336, 2010 20737805

Cook KF, Bombardier CH, Bamer AM, et al: Do somatic and cognitive symptoms of traumatic brain injury confound depression screening? Arch Phys Med Rehabil 92(5):818–823, 2011 21530731

Coronado VG, McGuire LC, Sarmiento K, et al: Trends in traumatic brain injury in the U.S. and the public health response: 1995–2009. J Safety Res 43(4):299–307, 2012 23127680

Craig A, Tran Y, Middleton J: Psychological morbidity and spinal cord injury: a systematic review. Spinal Cord 47(2):108–114, 2009 18779835

Craig A, Nicholson Perry K, Guest R, et al: Prospective study of the occurrence of psychological disorders and comorbidities after spinal cord injury. Arch Phys Med Rehabil 96(8):1426–1434, 2015 25778773

Davidoff GN, Roth EJ, Richards JS: Cognitive deficits in spinal cord injury: epidemiology and outcome. Arch Phys Med Rehabil 73(3):275–284, 1992 1543433

Dean PJA, Sterr A: Long-term effects of mild traumatic brain injury on cognitive performance. Front Hum Neurosci 7:30, 2013 23408228

Defense and Veterans Brain Injury Center: DoD worldwide numbers for TBI. Silver Spring, MD, Defense and Veterans Brain Injury Center, 2017. Available at: https://dvbic.dcoe.mil/dod-worldwide-numbers-tbi. Accessed October 12, 2017.

DeVivo MJ: Epidemiology of traumatic spinal cord injury: trends and future implications. Spinal Cord 50(5):365–372, 2012 22270188

DeVivo MJ, Krause JS, Lammertse DP: Recent trends in mortality and causes of death among persons with spinal cord injury. Arch Phys Med Rehabil 80(11):1411–1419, 1999 10569435

Diaz-Arrastia R, Kochanek PM, Bergold P, et al: Pharmacotherapy of traumatic brain injury: state of the science and the road forward: report of the Department of Defense Neurotrauma Pharmacology Workgroup. J Neurotrauma 31(2):135–158, 2014 23968241

Dikmen S, Machamer JE, Winn HR, et al: Neuropsychological outcome at 1-year post head injury. Neuropsychology 9(1):80–90, 1995

Dikmen SS, Machamer JE, Winn HR, et al: Neuropsychological effects of valproate in traumatic brain injury: a randomized trial. Neurology 54(4):895–902, 2000 10690983

Dorstyn D, Mathias J, Denson L: Efficacy of cognitive behavior therapy for the management of psychological outcomes following spinal cord injury: a meta-analysis. J Health Psychol 16(2):374–391, 2011 20978150

Dorstyn D, Mathias J, Denson L: Applications of telecounselling in spinal cord injury rehabilitation: a systematic review with effect sizes. Clin Rehabil 27(12):1072–1083, 2013 23823709

Dougall D, Poole N, Agrawal N: Pharmacotherapy for chronic cognitive impairment in traumatic brain injury. Cochrane Database Syst Rev (12):CD009221, 2015 26624881

Eastwood EA, Hagglund KJ, Ragnarsson KT, et al: Medical rehabilitation length of stay and outcomes for persons with traumatic spinal cord injury—1990–1997. Arch Phys Med Rehabil 80(11):1457–1463, 1999 10569441

Elliott T, Shewchuk R: Social support and leisure activities following severe physical disability: testing the mediating effects of depression. Basic and Applied Social Psychology 16(4):471–587, 1995

Elliott T, Umlauf R: Measurement of personality and psychopathology in acquired disability, in Psychological Assessment in Medical Rehabilitation Settings. Edited by Cushman L, Scherer M. Washington, DC, American Psychological Association, 1995, pp 325–358

Ennis N, Rosenbloom BN, Canzian S, et al: Depression and anxiety in parent versus spouse caregivers of adult patients with traumatic brain injury: a systematic review. Neuropsychol Rehabil 23(1):1–18, 2013 22897335

Evaniew N, Belley-Côté EP, Fallah N, et al: Methylprednisolone for the treatment of patients with acute spinal cord injuries: a systematic review and meta-analysis. J Neurotrauma 33(5):468–481, 2016 26529320

Fann JR, Katon WJ, Uomoto JM, et al: Psychiatric disorders and functional disability in outpatients with traumatic brain injuries. Am J Psychiatry 152(10):1493–1499, 1995 7573589

Fann JR, Uomoto JM, Katon WJ: Sertraline in the treatment of major depression following mild traumatic brain injury. J Neuropsychiatry Clin Neurosci 12(2):226–232, 2000 11001601

Fann JR, Leonetti A, Jaffe K, et al: Psychiatric illness and subsequent traumatic brain injury: a case control study. J Neurol Neurosurg Psychiatry 72(5):615–620, 2002 11971048

Fann JR, Burington B, Leonetti A, et al: Psychiatric illness following traumatic brain injury in an adult health maintenance organization population. Arch Gen Psychiatry 61(1):53–61, 2004 14706944

Fann JR, Bombardier CH, Dikmen S, et al: Validity of the Patient Health Questionnaire-9 in assessing depression following traumatic brain injury. J Head Trauma Rehabil 20(6):501–511, 2005 16304487

Fann JR, Hart T, Schomer KG: Treatment for depression after traumatic brain injury: a systematic review. J Neurotrauma 26(12):2383–2402, 2009a 19698070

Fann JR, Jones AL, Dikmen SS, et al: Depression treatment preferences after traumatic brain injury. J Head Trauma Rehabil 24(4):272–278, 2009b 19625866

Fann JR, Bombardier CH, Richards JS, et al; PRISMS Investigators: Depression after spinal cord injury: comorbidities, mental health service use, and adequacy of treatment. Arch Phys Med Rehabil 92(3):352–360, 2011 21255766

Fann JR, Crane DA, Graves DE, et al: Depression treatment preferences after acute traumatic spinal cord injury. Arch Phys Med Rehabil 94(12):2389–2395, 2013 23872078

Fann JR, Bombardier CH, Richards JS, et al; PRISMS Investigators: Venlafaxine extended-release for depression following spinal cord injury: a randomized clinical trial. JAMA Psychiatry 72(3):247–258, 2015a 25607727

Fann JR, Bombardier CH, Vannoy S, et al: Telephone and in-person cognitive behavioral therapy for major depression after traumatic brain injury: a randomized controlled trial. J Neurotrauma 32(1):45–57, 2015b 25072405

Fann JR, Bombardier CH, Temkin N, et al: Sertraline for major depression during the year following traumatic brain injury: a randomized controlled trial. J Head Trauma Rehabil 32(5):332–342, 2017 28520672

Fann JR, Ribe AR, Pedersen HS, et al: Long-term risk of dementia among people with traumatic brain injury in Denmark: a population-based observational cohort study. Lancet Psychiatry April 10, 2018 [Epub ahead of print] 29653873

Fitzgerald PB, Hoy KE, Maller JJ, et al: Transcranial magnetic stimulation for depression after a traumatic brain injury: a case study. J ECT 27(1):38–40, 2011 20938348

Fleminger S, Greenwood RJ, Oliver DL: Pharmacological management for agitation and aggression in people with acquired brain injury. Cochrane Database Syst Rev (4):CD003299, 2006 17054165

Fordyce WE: Behavioral Methods for Chronic Pain and Illness. St. Louis, MO, Mosby Year Book, 1976

Frank RG, Chaney JM, Clay DL, et al: Dysphoria: a major symptom factor in persons with disability or chronic illness. Psychiatry Res 43(3):231–241, 1992 1438622

Fugate LP, Spacek LA, Kresty LA, et al: Measurement and treatment of agitation following traumatic brain injury, II: a survey of the Brain Injury Special Interest Group of the American Academy of Physical Medicine and Rehabilitation. Arch Phys Med Rehabil 78(9):924–928, 1997 9305262

Fuhrer MJ, Rintala DH, Hart KA, et al: Depressive symptomatology in persons with spinal cord injury who reside in the community. Arch Phys Med Rehabil 74(3):255–260, 1993 8439251

Fujii DE, Ahmed I: Risk factors in psychosis secondary to traumatic brain injury. J Neuropsychiatry Clin Neurosci 13(1):61–69, 2001 11207331

Fujii DE, Ahmed I: Psychotic disorder caused by traumatic brain injury. Psychiatr Clin North Am 37(1):113–124, 2014 24529427

Fujii D, Fujii DC: Psychotic disorder due to traumatic brain injury: analysis of case studies in the literature. J Neuropsychiatry Clin Neurosci 24(3):278–289, 2012 23037642

Gertler P, Tate RL, Cameron ID: Non-pharmacological interventions for depression in adults and children with traumatic brain injury. Cochrane Database Syst Rev (12):CD009871, 2015 26663136

Godwin EE, Kreutzer JS, Arango-Lasprilla JC, et al: Marriage after brain injury: review, analysis, and research recommendations. J Head Trauma Rehabil 26(1):43–55, 2011 21209562

Gould KR, Ponsford JL, Johnston L, et al: Relationship between psychiatric disorders and 1-year psychosocial outcome following traumatic brain injury. J Head Trauma Rehabil 26(1):79–89, 2011 21209565

Grant I, Alves W: Psychiatric and psychosocial disturbances in head injury, in Neurobehavioral Recovery From Head Injury. Edited by Levin HS, Grafman J, Eisenberg HM. New York, Oxford University Press, 1987, pp 234–235

Guihan M, Garber SL, Bombardier CH, et al: Lessons learned while conducting research on prevention of pressure ulcers in veterans with spinal cord injury. Arch Phys Med Rehabil 88(7):858–861, 2007 17601465

Guihan M, Bombardier CH, Ehde DM, et al: Comparing multicomponent interventions to improve skin care behaviors and prevent recurrence in veterans hospitalized for severe pressure ulcers. Arch Phys Med Rehabil 95(7):1246.e3–1253.e3, 2014 24486242

Guillamondegui OD, Montgomery SA, Phibbs FT, et al: Traumatic Brain Injury and Depression: Comparative Effectiveness Reviews, No 25. Rockville, MD, Agency for Healthcare Research and Quality, 2011

Hagen EM, Eide GE, Rekand T, et al: Traumatic spinal cord injury and concomitant brain injury: a cohort study. Acta Neurol Scand Suppl 122(190):51–57, 2010 20586736

Hall KM, Karzmark P, Stevens M, et al: Family stressors in traumatic brain injury: a two-year follow-up. Arch Phys Med Rehabil 75(8):876–884, 1994 8053794

Hall KM, Knudsen ST, Wright J, et al: Follow-up study of individuals with high tetraplegia (C1-C4) 14 to 24 years postinjury. Arch Phys Med Rehabil 80(11):1507–1513, 1999 10569448

Hammond FM, Barrett RS, Shea T, et al: Psychotropic medication use during inpatient rehabilitation for traumatic brain injury. Arch Phys Med Rehabil 96 (8 suppl):S256.e14–S273.e14, 2015a 26212402

Hammond FM, Sherer M, Malec JF, et al; Amantadine Irritability Multisite Study Group: Amantadine effect on perceptions of irritability after traumatic brain injury: results of the amantadine irritability multisite study. J Neurotrauma 32(16):1230–1238, 2015b 25774566

Hammond FM, Alexander DN, Cutler AJ, et al: PRISM II: an open-label study to assess effectiveness of dextromethorphan/quinidine for pseudobulbar affect in patients with dementia, stroke or traumatic brain injury. BMC Neurol 16:89, 2016 27276999

Hammond FM, Malec JF, Zafonte RD, et al: Potential impact of amantadine on aggression in chronic traumatic brain injury. J Head Trauma Rehabil 32(5):308–318, 2017 28891908

Hanson RW, Franklin MR: Sexual loss in relation to other functional losses for spinal cord injured males. Arch Phys Med Rehabil 57(6):291–293, 1976 1275682

Hart T, Whyte J, Polansky M, et al: Concordance of patient and family report of neurobehavioral symptoms at 1 year after traumatic brain injury. Arch Phys Med Rehabil 84(2):204–213, 2003 12601651

Hart T, Seignourel PJ, Sherer M: A longitudinal study of awareness of deficit after moderate to severe traumatic brain injury. Neuropsychol Rehabil 19(2):161–176, 2009 18609008

Hart T, Hoffman JM, Pretz C, et al: A longitudinal study of major and minor depression following traumatic brain injury. Arch Phys Med Rehabil 93(8):1343–1349, 2012 22840833

Hart T, Fann JR, Chervoneva I, et al: Prevalence, risk factors, and correlates of anxiety at 1 year after moderate to severe traumatic brain injury. Arch Phys Med Rehabil 97(5):701–707, 2016 26707456

Hart T, Brockway JA, Maiuro RD, et al: Anger self-management training for chronic moderate to severe traumatic brain injury: results of a randomized controlled trial. J Head Trauma Rehabil 32(5):319–331, 2017 28520666

Harvey AG, Brewin CR, Jones C, et al: Coexistence of posttraumatic stress disorder and traumatic brain injury: towards a resolution of the paradox. J Int Neuropsychol Soc 9(4):663–676, 2003 12755178

Hawryluk GWJ, Bullock MR: Past, present, and future of traumatic brain injury research. Neurosurg Clin N Am 27(4):375–396, 2016 27637391

Heaton RK, Pendleton MG: Use of neuropsychological tests to predict adult patients' everyday functioning. J Consult Clin Psychol 49(6):807–821, 1981 7309951

Heilbronner RL, Roueche JR, Everson SA, Epler L: Comparing patient perspectives of disability and treatment effects with quality of participation in a post-acute brain injury rehabilitation programme. Brain Inj 3(4):387–395, 1989 2819318

Herrick S, Elliott T, Crow F: Social support and the prediction of health complications among persons with SCI. Rehabil Psychol 39:231–250, 1994

Hibbard MR, Uysal S, Kepler K, et al: Axis I psychopathology in individuals with traumatic brain injury. J Head Trauma Rehabil 13(4):24–39, 1998 9651237

Hoffman AN, Cheng JP, Zafonte RD, et al: Administration of haloperidol and risperidone after neurobehavioral testing hinders the recovery of traumatic brain injury-induced deficits. Life Sci 83(17–18):602–607, 2008 18801378

Houlihan BV, Jette A, Friedman RH, et al: A pilot study of a telehealth intervention for persons with spinal cord dysfunction. Spinal Cord 51(9):715–720, 2013 23752260

Houlihan BV, Brody M, Everhart-Skeels S, et al: Randomized trial of a peer-led, telephone-based empowerment intervention for persons with chronic spinal cord injury improves health self-management. Arch Phys Med Rehabil 98(6):1067.e1–1076.e1, 2017 28284835

Iezzoni LI, Davis RB, Soukup J, et al: Quality dimensions that most concern people with physical and sensory disabilities. Arch Intern Med 163(17):2085–2092, 2003 14504123

Inghilleri M, Conte A, Frasca V, et al: Venlafaxine and bladder function. Clin Neuropharmacol 28(6):270–273, 2005 16340381

Jain NB, Ayers GD, Peterson EN, et al: Traumatic spinal cord injury in the United States, 1993–2012. JAMA 313(22):2236–2243, 2015 26057284

Jennett B, Bond M: Assessment of outcome after severe brain damage. Lancet 1(7905):480–484, 1975 46957

Jorge RE, Robinson RG, Starkstein SE, et al: Secondary mania following traumatic brain injury. Am J Psychiatry 150(6):916–921, 1993c 8494069

Jorge RE, Acion L, Burin DI, et al: Sertraline for preventing mood disorders following traumatic brain injury: a randomized clinical trial. JAMA Psychiatry 73(10):1041–1047, 2016 27626622

Kant R, Smith-Seemiller L, Zeiler D: Treatment of aggression and irritability after head injury. Brain Inj 12(8):661–666, 1998 9724837

Kay T, Harrington DE, Adams R, et al; Mild Traumatic Brain Injury Committee of the Head Injury Interdisciplinary Special Interest Group of the American Congress of Rehabilitation Medicine: Definition of mild traumatic brain injury. J Head Trauma Rehabil 8(3):86–87, 1993

Kennedy P, Duff J: Post traumatic stress disorder and spinal cord injuries. Spinal Cord 39(1):1–10, 2001 11224007

Kennedy P, Evans MJ: Evaluation of post traumatic distress in the first 6 months following SCI. Spinal Cord 39(7):381–386, 2001 11464312

Kilpatrick DG, Resnick HS, Milanak ME, et al: National estimates of exposure to traumatic events and PTSD prevalence using DSM-IV and DSM-5 criteria. J Trauma Stress 26(5):537–547, 2013 24151000

Kim E: Agitation, aggression, and disinhibition syndromes after traumatic brain injury. NeuroRehabilitation 17(4):297–310, 2002 12547978

Kim E, Bijlani M: A pilot study of quetiapine treatment of aggression due to traumatic brain injury. J Neuropsychiatry Clin Neurosci 18(4):547–549, 2006 17135382

Kim E, Lauterbach EC, Reeve A, et al; ANPA Committee on Research: Neuropsychiatric complications of traumatic brain injury: a critical review of the literature (a report by the ANPA Committee on Research). J Neuropsychiatry Clin Neurosci 19(2):106–127, 2007 17431056

King NS: Post-concussion syndrome: clarity amid the controversy? Br J Psychiatry 183:276–278, 2003 14519601

King NS, Crawford S, Wenden FJ, et al: The Rivermead Post Concussion Symptoms Questionnaire: a measure of symptoms commonly experienced after head injury and its reliability. J Neurol 242(9):587–592, 1995 8551320

Klyce DW, Bombardier CH, Davis TJ, et al: Distinguishing grief from depression during acute recovery from spinal cord injury. Arch Phys Med Rehabil 96(8):1419–1425, 2015 25748144

Kraus JE, Sheitman BB: Clozapine reduces violent behavior in heterogeneous diagnostic groups. J Neuropsychiatry Clin Neurosci 17(1):36–44, 2005 15746481

Kraus MF, Smith GS, Butters M, et al: Effects of the dopaminergic agent and NMDA receptor antagonist amantadine on cognitive function, cerebral glucose metabolism and D2 receptor availability in chronic traumatic brain injury: a study using positron emission tomography (PET). Brain Inj 19(7):471–479, 2005 16134735

Krause J: Delivery of substance abuse services during spinal cord injury rehabilitation. NeuroRehabilitation 2(1):45–51, 1992

Krause JS, Kemp B, Coker J: Depression after spinal cord injury: relation to gender, ethnicity, aging, and socioeconomic indicators. Arch Phys Med Rehabil 81(8):1099–1109, 2000 10943762

Krause JS, Carter RE, Pickelsimer EE, et al: A prospective study of health and risk of mortality after spinal cord injury. Arch Phys Med Rehabil 89(8):1482–1491, 2008 18674984

Kreutzer JS, Gordon WA, Rosenthal M, et al: Neuropsychological characteristics of patients with brain injury: preliminary findings from a multicenter investigation. Journal of Head Trauma Rehabilitation 8(2):47–59, 1993

Lal S, Merbtiz CP, Grip JC: Modification of function in head-injured patients with Sinemet. Brain Inj 2(3):225–233, 1988 2458792

Langlois JA, Rutland-Brown W, Wald MM: The epidemiology and impact of traumatic brain injury: a brief overview. J Head Trauma Rehabil 21(5):375–378, 2006 16983222

Lanska DJ: Historical perspective: neurological advances from studies of war injuries and illnesses. Ann Neurol 66(4):444–459, 2009 19847911

Lee H, Kim SW, Kim JM, et al: Comparing effects of methylphenidate, sertraline and placebo on neuropsychiatric sequelae in patients with traumatic brain injury. Hum Psychopharmacol 20(2):97–104, 2005 15641125

Lenze EJ, Munin MC, Quear T, et al: The Pittsburgh Rehabilitation Participation Scale: reliability and validity of a clinician-rated measure of participation in acute rehabilitation. Arch Phys Med Rehabil 85(3):380–384, 2004 15031821

Levin HS, High WM, Goethe KE, et al: The neurobehavioural rating scale: assessment of the behavioural sequelae of head injury by the clinician. J Neurol Neurosurg Psychiatry 50(2):183–193, 1987a 3572433

Levin HS, Mattis S, Ruff RM, et al: Neurobehavioral outcome following minor head injury: a three-center study. J Neurosurg 66(2):234–243, 1987b 3806205

Levy M, Berson A, Cook T, et al: Treatment of agitation following traumatic brain injury: a review of the literature. NeuroRehabilitation 20(4):279–306, 2005 16403996

Lewis L: A framework for developing a psychotherapy treatment plan with brain-injured patients. J Head Trauma Rehabil 6(4):22–29, 1991

Liao C-C, Chiu W-T, Yeh C-C, et al: Risk and outcomes for traumatic brain injury in patients with mental disorders. J Neurol Neurosurg Psychiatry 83(12):1186–1192, 2012 22773855

Lindenmayer JP, Kotsaftis A: Use of sodium valproate in violent and aggressive behaviors: a critical review. J Clin Psychiatry 61(2):123–128, 2000 10732659

Lombardi G, Macchiarella A, Cecconi F, et al: Ten years of phosphodiesterase type 5 inhibitors in spinal cord injured patients. J Sex Med 6(5):1248–1258, 2009 19210710

Lucas JW, Benson V: Tables of Summary Health Statistics for the U.S. Population: 2016 National Health Interview Survey. National Center for Health Statistics. 2018. Available at: https://www.cdc.gov/nchs/nhis/SHS/tables.htm. Accessed April 30, 2018.

Ma VY, Chan L, Carruthers KJ: Incidence, prevalence, costs, and impact on disability of common conditions requiring rehabilitation in the United States: stroke, spinal cord injury, traumatic brain injury, multiple sclerosis, osteoarthritis, rheumatoid arthritis, limb loss, and back pain. Arch Phys Med Rehabil 95(5):986.e1–995.e1, 2014 24462839

Macciocchi S, Seel RT, Thompson N, et al: Spinal cord injury and co-occurring traumatic brain injury: assessment and incidence. Arch Phys Med Rehabil 89(7):1350–1357, 2008 18586138

MacDonald MR, Nielson WR, Cameron MG: Depression and activity patterns of spinal cord injured persons living in the community. Arch Phys Med Rehabil 68(6):339–343, 1987 3592945

Maciejewski PK, Zhang B, Block SD, et al: An empirical examination of the stage theory of grief. JAMA 297(7):716–723, 2007 17312291

Malaspina D, Goetz RR, Friedman JH, et al: Traumatic brain injury and schizophrenia in members of schizophrenia and bipolar disorder pedigrees. Am J Psychiatry 158(3):440–446, 2001 11229986

Malec J, Neimeyer R: Psychologic prediction of duration of inpatient spinal cord injury rehabilitation and performance of self-care. Arch Phys Med Rehabil 64(8):359–363, 1983 6882174

Marin RS, Fogel BS, Hawkins J, et al: Apathy: a treatable syndrome. J Neuropsychiatry Clin Neurosci 7(1):23–30, 1995 7711487

Marino RJ, Burns S, Graves DE, et al: Upper- and lower-extremity motor recovery after traumatic cervical spinal cord injury: an update from the national spinal cord injury database. Arch Phys Med Rehabil 92(3):369–375, 2011 21353821

Martino C, Krysko M, Petrides G, et al: Cognitive tolerability of electroconvulsive therapy in a patient with a history of traumatic brain injury. J ECT 24(1):92–95, 2008 18379342

Mathias JL, Alvaro PK: Prevalence of sleep disturbances, disorders, and problems following traumatic brain injury: a meta-analysis. Sleep Med 13(7):898–905, 2012 22705246

May G, Benson R, Balon R, et al: Neurofeedback and traumatic brain injury: a literature review. Ann Clin Psychiatry 25(4):289–296, 2013 24199220

McAllister TW: Neuropsychiatric sequelae of head injuries. Psychiatr Clin North Am 15(2):395–413, 1992 1603732

McCrea M, Iverson GL, McAllister TW, et al: An integrated review of recovery after mild traumatic brain injury (MTBI): implications for clinical management. Clin Neuropsychol 23(8):1368–1390, 2009 19882476

McDowell S, Whyte J, D'Esposito M: Differential effect of a dopaminergic agonist on prefrontal function in traumatic brain injury patients. Brain 121(Pt 6):1155–1164, 1998 9648550

McGinn MJ, Povlishock JT: Pathophysiology of traumatic brain injury. Neurosurg Clin N Am 27(4):397–407, 2016 27637392

McKinlay WW, Brooks DN, Bond MR, et al: The short-term outcome of severe blunt head injury as reported by relatives of the injured persons. J Neurol Neurosurg Psychiatry 44(6):527–533, 1981 7276967

Meachen SJ, Hanks RA, Millis SR, et al: The reliability and validity of the brief symptom inventory-18 in persons with traumatic brain injury. Arch Phys Med Rehabil 89(5):958–965, 2008 18452746

Medd J, Tate R: Evaluation of an anger management therapy programme following acquired brain injury: a preliminary study. Neuropsychol Rehabil 10(2):185–201, 2000

Meehan KM, Wang H, David SR, et al: Comparison of rapidly acting intramuscular olanzapine, lorazepam, and placebo: a double-blind, randomized study in acutely agitated patients with dementia. Neuropsychopharmacology 26(4):494–504, 2002 11927174

Mehta S, Orenczuk S, Hansen KT, et al; Spinal Cord Injury Rehabilitation Evidence Research Team: An evidence-based review of the effectiveness of cognitive behavioral therapy for psychosocial issues post-spinal cord injury. Rehabil Psychol 56(1):15–25, 2011 21401282

Millis SR, Rosenthal M, Novack TA, et al: Long-term neuropsychological outcome after traumatic brain injury. J Head Trauma Rehabil 16(4):343–355, 2001 11461657

Mittenberg W, Strauman S: Diagnosis of mild head injury and the postconcussion syndrome. J Head Trauma Rehabil 15(2):783–791, 2000 10739967

Mooney GF, Haas LJ: Effect of methylphenidate on brain injury-related anger. Arch Phys Med Rehabil 74(2):153–160, 1993 8431099

Moreau OK, Cortet-Rudelli C, Yollin E, et al: Growth hormone replacement therapy in patients with traumatic brain injury. J Neurotrauma 30(11):998–1006, 2013 23323993

Mortenson WB, Noreau L, Miller WC: The relationship between and predictors of quality of life after spinal cord injury at 3 and 15 months after discharge. Spinal Cord 48(1):73–79, 2010 19636329

Nahas Z, Arlinghaus KA, Kotrla KJ, et al: Rapid response of emotional incontinence to selective serotonin reuptake inhibitors. J Neuropsychiatry Clin Neurosci 10(4):453–455, 1998 9813792

Nakase-Thompson R, Sherer M, Yablon SA, et al: Acute confusion following traumatic brain injury. Brain Inj 18(2):131–142, 2004 14660226

Neimeyer RA, Currier JM: Grief therapy: evidence of efficacy and emerging directions. Current Directions in Psychological Science 18(6):352–356, 2009

Niemeier JP, Leininger SL, Whitney MP, et al: Does history of substance use disorder predict acute traumatic brain injury rehabilitation outcomes? NeuroRehabilitation 38(4):371–383, 2016 27061165

Niepel G, Bibani RH, Vilisaar J, et al: Association of a deficit of arousal with fatigue in multiple sclerosis: effect of modafinil. Neuropharmacology 64:380–388, 2013 22766394

Nott MT, Chapparo C, Baguley IJ: Agitation following traumatic brain injury: an Australian sample. Brain Inj 20(11):1175–1182, 2006 17123934

Novack TA, Banos JH, Brunner R, et al: Impact of early administration of sertraline on depressive symptoms in the first year after traumatic brain injury. J Neurotrauma 26(11):1921–1928, 2009 19929217

O'Donnell ML, Creamer M, Holmes ACN, et al: Posttraumatic stress disorder after injury: does admission to intensive care unit increase risk? J Trauma 69(3):627–632, 2010 20118816

Okie S: Traumatic brain injury in the war zone. N Engl J Med 352(20):2043–2047, 2005 15901856

O'Leary CA: Reducing aggression in adults with brain injuries. Behav Interv 15(3):205–216, 2000

Osborn AJ, Mathias JL, Fairweather-Schmidt AK: Depression following adult, non-penetrating traumatic brain injury: a meta-analysis examining methodological variables and sample characteristics. Neurosci Biobehav Rev 47:1–15, 2014 25038422

Oster TJ, Anderson CA, Filley CM, et al: Quetiapine for mania due to traumatic brain injury. CNS Spectr 12(10):764–769, 2007 17934381

Ottomanelli L, Lind L: Review of critical factors related to employment after spinal cord injury: implications for research and vocational services. J Spinal Cord Med 32(5):503–531, 2009 20025147

Pachet A, Friesen S, Winkelaar D, et al: Beneficial behavioural effects of lamotrigine in traumatic brain injury. Brain Inj 17(8):715–722, 2003 12850956

Pande AC, Davidson JR, Jefferson JW, et al: Treatment of social phobia with gabapentin: a placebo-controlled study. J Clin Psychopharmacol 19(4):341–348, 1999 10440462

Pande AC, Pollack MH, Crockatt J, et al: Placebo-controlled study of gabapentin treatment of panic disorder. J Clin Psychopharmacol 20(4):467–471, 2000 10917408

Parry-Jones BL, Vaughan FL, Miles Cox W: Traumatic brain injury and substance misuse: a systematic review of prevalence and outcomes research (1994–2004). Neuropsychol Rehabil 16(5):537–560, 2006 16952892

Perry DC, Sturm VE, Peterson MJ, et al: Association of traumatic brain injury with subsequent neurological and psychiatric disease: a meta-analysis. J Neurosurg 124(2):511–526, 2016 26315003

Phelps TI, Bondi CO, Ahmed RH, et al: Divergent long-term consequences of chronic treatment with haloperidol, risperidone, and bromocriptine on traumatic brain injury-induced cognitive deficits. J Neurotrauma 32(8):590–597, 2015 25275833

Plantier D, Luauté J; SOFMER group: Drugs for behavior disorders after traumatic brain injury: systematic review and expert consensus leading to French recommendations for good practice. Ann Phys Rehabil Med 59(1):42–57, 2016 26797170

Ponsford J, Whelan-Goodinson R, Bahar-Fuchs A: Alcohol and drug use following traumatic brain injury: a prospective study. Brain Inj 21(13–14):1385–1392, 2007 18066940

Ponsford J, Bayley M, Wiseman-Hakes C, et al; INCOG Expert Panel: INCOG recommendations for management of cognition following traumatic brain injury, part II: attention and information processing speed. J Head Trauma Rehabil 29(4):321–337, 2014a 24984095

Ponsford J, Janzen S, McIntyre A, et al; INCOG Expert Panel: INCOG recommendations for management of cognition following traumatic brain injury, part I: posttraumatic amnesia/delirium. J Head Trauma Rehabil 29(4):307–320, 2014b 24984094

Ponsford J, Lee NK, Wong D, et al: Efficacy of motivational interviewing and cognitive behavioral therapy for anxiety and depression symptoms following traumatic brain injury. Psychol Med 46(5):1079–1090, 2016 26708017

Potter SD, Brown RG, Fleminger S: Randomised, waiting list controlled trial of cognitive-behavioural therapy for persistent postconcussional symptoms after predominantly mild-moderate traumatic brain injury. J Neurol Neurosurg Psychiatry 87(10):1075–1083, 2016 27496149

Prigatano GP: Personality and psychosocial consequences of brain injury, in Neuropsychological Rehabilitation After Brain Injury. Edited by Prigatano GP, Fordyce DJ, Zeiner HK, et al. Baltimore, MD, Johns Hopkins University Press, 1986, pp 29–50

Prigatano GP: Principles of Neuropsychological Rehabilitation. New York, Oxford University Press, 1999

Prigatano GP, Ben-Yishay Y: Psychotherapy and psychotherapeutic interventions in brain injury rehabilitation, in Rehabilitation of the Adult and Child With Traumatic Brain Injury. Edited by Rosenthal M, Griffith ER, Kreutzer JS, et al. Philadelphia, PA, FA Davis, 1999, pp 271–283

Proserpio P, Lanza A, Sambusida K, et al: Sleep apnea and periodic leg movements in the first year after spinal cord injury. Sleep Med 16(1):59–66, 2015 25454844

Quinn DK, Mayer AR, Master CL, Fann JR: Prolonged postconcussive symptoms. Am J Psychiatry 175(2):103–111, 2018 29385828

Rabinowitz AR, Levin HS: Cognitive sequelae of traumatic brain injury. Psychiatr Clin North Am 37(1):1–11, 2014 24529420

Radnitz CL, Hsu L, Tirch DD, et al: A comparison of posttraumatic stress disorder in veterans with and without spinal cord injury. J Abnorm Psychol 107(4):676–680, 1998 9830255

Rao V, Lyketsos C: Neuropsychiatric sequelae of traumatic brain injury. Psychosomatics 41(2):95–103, 2000 10749946

Richards JS, Bombardier CH, Wilson CS, et al: Efficacy of venlafaxine XR for the treatment of pain in patients with spinal cord injury and major depression: a randomized, controlled trial. Arch Phys Med Rehabil 96(4):680–689, 2015 25527253

Richardson C, McKay A, Ponsford JL: Factors influencing self-awareness following traumatic brain injury. J Head Trauma Rehabil 30(2):E43–E54, 2015 24721809

Rintala DH, Holmes SA, Courtade D, et al: Comparison of the effectiveness of amitriptyline and gabapentin on chronic neuropathic pain in persons with spinal cord injury. Arch Phys Med Rehabil 88(12):1547–1560, 2007 18047869

Rogers JM, Read CA: Psychiatric comorbidity following traumatic brain injury. Brain Inj 21(13–14):1321–1333, 2007 18066935

Rohe DE, Krause JS: Stability of interests after severe physical disability: an 11-year longitudinal study. Journal of Vocational Behavior 52(1):45–58, 1998

Roozenbeek B, Maas AIR, Menon DK: Changing patterns in the epidemiology of traumatic brain injury. Nat Rev Neurol 9(4):231–236, 2013 23443846

Sabaz M, Simpson GK, Walker AJ, et al: Prevalence, comorbidities, and correlates of challenging behavior among community-dwelling adults with severe traumatic brain injury: a multicenter study. J Head Trauma Rehabil 29(2):E19–E30, 2014 23640541

Salazar AM, Warden DL, Schwab K, et al; Defense and Veterans Head Injury Program (DVHIP) Study Group: Cognitive rehabilitation for traumatic brain injury: a randomized trial. JAMA 283(23):3075–3081, 2000 10865301

Salter KL, McClure JA, Foley NC, et al: Pharmacotherapy for depression post traumatic brain injury: a meta-analysis. J Head Trauma Rehabil 31(4):E21–E32, 2016 26479398

Sandel ME, Mysiw WJ: The agitated brain injured patient, part I: definitions, differential diagnosis, and assessment. Arch Phys Med Rehabil 77(6):617–623, 1996 8831483

Sander AM, Maestas KL, Pappadis MR, et al; NIDILRR Traumatic Brain Injury Model Systems Module Project on Sexuality After TBI: Multicenter study of sexual functioning in spouses/partners of persons with traumatic brain injury. Arch Phys Med Rehabil 97(5):753–759, 2016 26845190

Saran AS: Depression after minor closed head injury: role of dexamethasone suppression test and antidepressants. J Clin Psychiatry 46(8):335–338, 1985 4019422

Sawyer E, Mauro LS, Ohlinger MJ: Amantadine enhancement of arousal and cognition after traumatic brain injury. Ann Pharmacother 42(2):247–252, 2008 18212258

Scholten AC, Haagsma JA, Cnossen MC, et al: Prevalence of and risk factors for anxiety and depressive disorders after traumatic brain injury: a systematic review. J Neurotrauma 33(22):1969–1994, 2016 26729611

Schwab K, Terrio HP, Brenner LA, et al: Epidemiology and prognosis of mild traumatic brain injury in returning soldiers: a cohort study. Neurology 88(16):1571–1579, 2017 28314862

Scott LK, Green R, McCarthy PJ, et al: Agitation and/or aggression after traumatic brain injury in the pediatric population treated with ziprasidone: clinical article. J Neurosurg Pediatr 3(6):484–487, 2009 19485732

Selassie AW, Zaloshnja E, Langlois JA, et al: Incidence of long-term disability following traumatic brain injury hospitalization, United States, 2003. J Head Trauma Rehabil 23(2):123–131, 2008 18362766

Shear K, Frank E, Houck PR, Reynolds CF 3rd: Treatment of complicated grief: a randomized controlled trial. JAMA 293(21):2601–2608, 2005 15928281

Shukla S, Cook BL, Mukherjee S, et al: Mania following head trauma. Am J Psychiatry 144(1):93–96, 1987 3799847

Silver JM: Neuropsychiatry of persistent symptoms after concussion. Psychiatr Clin North Am 37(1):91–102, 2014 24529425

Silver JM, Yudofsky SC, Anderson KE: Aggressive disorders, in Textbook of Traumatic Brain Injury. Edited by Silver JM, McAllister TW, Yudofsky SC. Washington, DC, American Psychiatric Press, 2011, pp 225–238

Sipski M, Alexander C: Sexual Function in People With Disabilities and Chronic Illness. Gaithersburg, MD, Aspen Publishers, 1997

Sipski ML, Alexander CJ, Rosen RC: Orgasm in women with spinal cord injuries: a laboratory-based assessment. Arch Phys Med Rehabil 76(12):1097–1102, 1995 8540784

Smeets SMJ, Ponds RWHM, Verhey FR, et al: Psychometric properties and feasibility of instruments used to assess awareness of deficits after acquired brain injury: a systematic review. J Head Trauma Rehabil 27(6):433–442, 2012 21897287

Smith DH, Hicks R, Povlishock JT: Therapy development for diffuse axonal injury. J Neurotrauma 30(5):307–323, 2013 23252624

Spitzer RL, Kroenke K, Williams JB: Validation and utility of a self-report version of PRIME-MD: the PHQ primary care study. Primary Care Evaluation of Mental Disorders. Patient Health Questionnaire. JAMA 282(18):1737–1744, 1999 10568646

Spitzer RL, Kroenke K, Williams JBW, et al: A brief measure for assessing generalized anxiety disorder: the GAD-7. Arch Intern Med 166(10):1092–1097, 2006 16717171

Staas W, Formal C, Freedman M, et al: Spinal cord injury and spinal cord injury medicine, in Rehabilitation Medicine: Principles and Practice. Edited by DeLisa J, Gans BM. Philadelphia, PA, Lippincott-Raven Publishers, 1998, pp 1259–1291

Stanislav SW, Childs A: Evaluating the usage of droperidol in acutely agitated persons with brain injury. Brain Inj 14(3):261–265, 2000 10759043

Stanislav SW, Fabre T, Crismon ML, et al: Buspirone's efficacy in organic-induced aggression. J Clin Psychopharmacol 14(2):126–130, 1994 8195453

Stéfan A, Mathé J-F; SOFMER group: What are the disruptive symptoms of behavioral disorders after traumatic brain injury? A systematic review leading to recommendations for good practices. Ann Phys Rehabil Med 59(1):5–17, 2016 26768944

Stillman MD, Barber J, Burns S, et al: Complications of spinal cord injury over the first year after discharge from inpatient rehabilitation. Arch Phys Med Rehabil 98(9):1800–1805, 2017 28115072

Stolp-Smith KA, Wainberg MC: Antidepressant exacerbation of spasticity. Arch Phys Med Rehabil 80(3):339–342, 1999 10084445

Stroebe M, Schut H: The dual process model of coping with bereavement: rationale and description. Death Stud 23(3):197–224, 1999 10848151

Stroud MW, Bombardier CH, Dyer JR, et al: Preinjury alcohol and drug use among persons with spinal cord injury: implications for rehabilitation. J Spinal Cord Med 34(5):461–472, 2011 22118253

Stuss DT, Binns MA, Carruth FG, et al: The acute period of recovery from traumatic brain injury: posttraumatic amnesia or posttraumatic confusional state? J Neurosurg 90(4):635–643, 1999 10193606

Sun Z-L, Feng D-F: Biomarkers of cognitive dysfunction in traumatic brain injury. J Neural Transm (Vienna) 121(1):79–90, 2014 23942913

Tam S, McKay A, Sloan S, et al: The experience of challenging behaviours following severe TBI: a family perspective. Brain Inj 29(7–8):813–821, 2015 25914927

Tanielian T, Jaycox LH (eds): Invisible Wounds of War: Psychological and Cognitive Injuries, Their Consequences, and Services to Assist Recovery. Santa Monica, CA, RAND Center for Military Health Policy Research, 2008

Tate DG, Stiers W, Daugherty J, et al: The effects of insurance benefits coverage on functional and psychosocial outcomes after spinal cord injury. Arch Phys Med Rehabil 75(4):407–414, 1994 8172500

Tate DG, Forchheimer MB, Krause JS, et al: Patterns of alcohol and substance use and abuse in persons with spinal cord injury: risk factors and correlates. Arch Phys Med Rehabil 85(11):1837–1847, 2004 15520979

Tate R, Kennedy M, Ponsford J, et al: INCOG recommendations for management of cognition following traumatic brain injury, part III: executive function and self-awareness. J Head Trauma Rehabil 29(4):338–352, 2014 24984096

Tatum WO4th, French JA, Faught E, et al; PADS Investigators. Post-marketing antiepileptic drug survey: Postmarketing experience with topiramate and cognition. Epilepsia 42(9):1134–1140, 2001 11580760

Taylor CA, Bell JM, Breiding MJ, Xu L: Traumatic brain injury–related emergency department visits, hospitalizations, and deaths—United States, 2007 and 2013. MMWR Surveill Summ 66(9):1–16, 2017 28301451

Taylor LA, Kreutzer JS, Demm SR, et al: Traumatic brain injury and substance abuse: a review and analysis of the literature. Neuropsychol Rehabil 13(1–2):165–188, 2003 21854333

Teitelman E: Off-label uses of modafinil (letter). Am J Psychiatry 158(8):1341, 2001 11481196

Thompson R, Sherer M, Yablon S, et al: Confusion following TBI: inspection of indices of delirium and amnesia (abstract). J Int Neuropsychol Soc 7(2):177, 2001

Thurman DJ, Alverson C, Dunn KA, et al: Traumatic brain injury in the United States: a public health perspective. J Head Trauma Rehabil 14(6):602–615, 1999 10671706

Togher L, Wiseman-Hakes C, Douglas J, et al; INCOG Expert Panel: INCOG recommendations for management of cognition following traumatic brain injury, part IV: cognitive communication. J Head Trauma Rehabil 29(4):353–368, 2014 24984097

Trieschmann RB: Spinal Cord Injuries: Psychological, Social and Vocational Rehabilitation. New York, Demos Publication, 1988

Trzepacz PT, Kean J, Kennedy RE: Delirium and posttraumatic confusion, in Textbook of Traumatic Brain Injury. Edited by Silver JM, McAllister TW, Yudofsky SC. Washington, DC, American Psychiatric Press, 2011, pp 145–171

Umlauf R, Frank RG: A cluster-analytic description of patient subgroups in the rehabilitation setting. Rehabilitation Psychology 28(3):157–167, 1983

Unsworth DJ, Mathias JL: Traumatic brain injury and alcohol/substance abuse: a Bayesian meta-analysis comparing the outcomes of people with and without a history of abuse. J Clin Exp Neuropsychol 39(6):547–562, 2017 27829310

van der Naalt J, van Zomeren AH, Sluiter WJ, et al: Acute behavioural disturbances related to imaging studies and outcome in mild-to-moderate head injury. Brain Inj 14(9):781–788, 2000 11030452

Vanderploeg RD, Schwab K, Walker WC, et al; Defense and Veterans Brain Injury Center Study Group: Rehabilitation of traumatic brain injury in active duty military personnel and veterans: Defense and Veterans Brain Injury Center randomized controlled trial of two rehabilitation approaches. Arch Phys Med Rehabil 89(12):2227–2238, 2008 19061734

van Reekum R, Cohen T, Wong J: Can traumatic brain injury cause psychiatric disorders? J Neuropsychiatry Clin Neurosci 12(3):316–327, 2000 10956565

van Reekum R, Streiner DL, Conn DK: Applying Bradford Hill's criteria for causation to neuropsychiatry: challenges and opportunities. J Neuropsychiatry Clin Neurosci 13(3):318–325, 2001 11514637

van Woerkom TC, Teelken AW, Minderhous JM: Difference in neurotransmitter metabolism in frontotemporal-lobe contusion and diffuse cerebral contusion. Lancet 1(8015):812–813, 1977 66617

Velikonja D, Tate R, Ponsford J, et al; INCOG Expert Panel: INCOG recommendations for management of cognition following traumatic brain injury, part V: memory. J Head Trauma Rehabil 29(4):369–386, 2014 24984098

Vink R: Large animal models of traumatic brain injury. J Neurosci Res 96(4):527–535, 2018 28500771

Viola-Saltzman M, Musleh C: Traumatic brain injury-induced sleep disorders. Neuropsychiatr Dis Treat 12:339–348, 2016 26929626

Walker AJ, Nott MT, Doyle M, et al: Effectiveness of a group anger management programme after severe traumatic brain injury. Brain Inj 24(3):517–524, 2010 20184408

Walter KH, Dickstein BD, Barnes SM, Chard KM: Comparing effectiveness of CPT to CPT-C among U.S. veterans in an interdisciplinary residential PTSD/TBI treatment program. J Trauma Stress 27(4):438–445, 2014 25158637

Warden DL, Gordon B, McAllister TW, et al; Neurobehavioral Guidelines Working Group: Guidelines for the pharmacologic treatment of neurobehavioral sequelae of traumatic brain injury. J Neurotrauma 23(10):1468–1501, 2006 17020483

Wehman PH, Targett PS, Avellone LE: Educational and vocational issues in traumatic brain injury. Phys Med Rehabil Clin N Am 28(2):351–362, 2017 28390518

West SL: Substance use among persons with traumatic brain injury: a review. NeuroRehabilitation 29(1):1–8, 2011 21876290

Whiteneck GG, Dijkers MP, Heinemann AW, et al: Development of the participation assessment with recombined tools-objective for use after traumatic brain injury. Arch Phys Med Rehabil 92(4):542–551, 2011 21367393

Whyte J, Hart T, Vaccaro M, et al: Effects of methylphenidate on attention deficits after traumatic brain injury: a multidimensional, randomized, controlled trial. Am J Phys Med Rehabil 83(6):401–420, 2004 15166683

Williams DH, Levin HS, Eisenberg HM: Mild head injury classification. Neurosurgery 27(3):422–428, 1990 2234336

Willmott C, Ponsford J: Efficacy of methylphenidate in the rehabilitation of attention following traumatic brain injury: a randomised, crossover, double blind, placebo controlled inpatient trial. J Neurol Neurosurg Psychiatry 80(5):552–557, 2009 19060022

Winkens I, Van Heugten CM, Visser-Meily JMA, et al: Impaired self-awareness after acquired brain injury: clinicians' ratings on its assessment and importance for rehabilitation. J Head Trauma Rehabil 29(2):153–156, 2014 23381019

Wolf GK, Kretzmer T, Crawford E, et al: Prolonged exposure therapy with veterans and active duty personnel diagnosed with PTSD and traumatic brain injury. J Trauma Stress 28(4):339–347, 2015 26201688

World Health Organization: International Statistical Classification of Diseases and Related Health Problems, 10th Revision. Geneva, World Health Organization, 1992

World Health Organization: International Classification of Functioning, Disability and Health: ICF. Geneva, Switzerland, World Health Organization, 2001

Worthington AD, Melia Y: Rehabilitation is compromised by arousal and sleep disorders: results of a survey of rehabilitation centres. Brain Inj 20(3):327–332, 2006 16537274

Wortman CB, Silver RC: The myths of coping with loss. J Consult Clin Psychol 57(3):349–357, 1989 2661609

Wortzel HS, Arciniegas DB: A forensic neuropsychiatric approach to traumatic brain injury, aggression, and suicide. J Am Acad Psychiatry Law 41(2):274–286, 2013 23771941

Wortzel HS, Arciniegas DB: The DSM-5 approach to the evaluation of traumatic brain injury and its neuropsychiatric sequelae. NeuroRehabilitation 34(4):613–623, 2014 24820171

Writer BW, Schillerstrom JE: Psychopharmacological treatment for cognitive impairment in survivors of traumatic brain injury: a critical review. J Neuropsychiatry Clin Neurosci 21(4):362–370, 2009 19996244

Wroblewski BA, McColgan K, Smith K, et al: The incidence of seizures during tricyclic antidepressant drug treatment in a brain-injured population. J Clin Psychopharmacol 10(2):124–128, 1990 2341586

Wroblewski BA, Joseph AB, Cornblatt RR: Antidepressant pharmacotherapy and the treatment of depression in patients with severe traumatic brain injury: a controlled, prospective study. J Clin Psychiatry 57(12):582–587, 1996 9010122

Yudofsky SC, Silver JM, Hales RE: Pharmacologic management of aggression in the elderly. J Clin Psychiatry 51 (suppl):22–28, discussion 29–32, 1990 1976621

Yudofsky SC, Kopecky HJ, Kunik M, et al: The Overt Agitation Severity Scale for the objective rating of agitation. J Neuropsychiatry Clin Neurosci 9(4):541–548, 1997 9447494

Zifko UA, Rupp M, Schwarz S, et al: Modafinil in treatment of fatigue in multiple sclerosis. Results of an open-label study. J Neurol 249(8):983–987, 2002 12195441

CHAPTER 34

Pain

J. Greg Hobelmann, M.D., M.P.H.
Michael R. Clark, M.D., M.P.H., M.B.A.

In this chapter, we first review definitions, assessment, and epidemiology of pain. We then discuss selected acute and chronic pain syndromes, followed by the major psychiatric comorbidities of chronic pain, including somatization, substance use, depression, anxiety, and other emotional states. Finally, we review treatments for pain, including medications, psychological therapies, and interdisciplinary programs.

Definitions

Pain is a complex experience that integrates affective, cognitive, and behavioral factors with an extensive neurobiology. Pain has been defined by the International Association for the Study of Pain as "an unpleasant sensory and emotional experience associated with actual or potential tissue damage, or described in terms of such damage" (Merskey 2007). This definition recognizes that pain may be experienced in the absence of tissue damage and is, therefore, a subjective experience. Many terms are used to describe different types of painful experiences (Table 34–1).

Pain is a subjective experience and is difficult to assess, especially in patients with terminal illnesses or significant cognitive impairment (Nikolaus 1997). Pain rating scales attempt to measure the severity and intensity of pain. Many factors can influence ratings, including disease states, mental disorders, distress, personality traits, and the meanings assigned to symptoms based on personal beliefs. A variety of verbal and behavioral assessment tools can be used for rating pain in elderly populations (Kaasalainen and Crook 2003).

TABLE 34–1.   **Definitions relating to pain sensations**

Type of pain	Description
Allodynia	Pain from a stimulus that does not normally provoke pain
Deafferentation pain	Pain resulting from loss of sensory input into the central nervous system
Dysesthesia	Unpleasant, abnormal sensation that can be spontaneous or evoked
Hyperalgesia	Increased response to a stimulus that is normally painful
Hyperesthesia	Abnormal increase in sensitivity to stimuli
Hypoesthesia	Abnormal decrease in sensitivity to stimuli
Neuropathic pain	Pain arising from a lesion or disease of the somatosensory system that is often accompanied by maladaptive changes in the nervous system
Nociception	Detection of tissue damage by transducers in skin and deeper structures and central propagation of this information via A delta and C fibers in the peripheral nerves
Paresthesia	Abnormal sensation, spontaneous or evoked, that is not unpleasant
Sensitization	Lowered threshold for pain and prolonged/enhanced response to stimulation

Source.   Adapted from Merskey et al. 1986.

Epidemiology

Pain is the number one reason that patients present to physicians and is the cause of considerable societal burden (Cherry et al. 2003). Prevalence estimates of chronic pain vary considerably because of varying definitions of chronic pain as well as a lack of patient databases for pain statistics (Henschke et al. 2015). However, a recent study used National Health Interview Survey data to calculate the point prevalence of *persistent pain,* defined as constant or frequent pain persisting for at least 3 months (Kennedy et al. 2014). Findings showed that about 19% of adults in the United States report persistent pain, with rates being higher among women, adults ages 60–69 years, adults who rated their health as fair to poor, adults who were overweight or obese, and adults who were hospitalized one or more times in the preceding year. Patients with chronic pain utilize about twice as many health care resources as the general population. In 2010, U.S. health care costs secondary to pain ranged from $560 billion to $635 billion (Gaskin and Richard 2012).

Acute Pain

The Joint Commission (formerly the Joint Commission on Accreditation of Healthcare Organizations) has implemented pain management standards for all patient encounters (Phillips and Joint Commission on Accreditation of Healthcare Organizations 2000). Acute pain is usually the result of trauma from a surgery, an injury, or an exacerbation of chronic disease, especially musculoskeletal conditions. Treatment is focused on controlling inflammation, preventing tissue destruction, and repairing injury, with more emphasis placed on pain relief to facilitate reaching these goals.

The approach to acute pain management usually will be successful with straightforward strategies such as relaxation, immobilization, analgesics (aspirin, acetaminophen, nonsteroidal anti-inflammatory drugs [NSAIDs], opioids), massage, and transcutaneous electrical nerve stimulation (Institute for Clinical Systems Improvement 2008). The absence of signs consistent with acute pain, such as elevated heart rate and blood pressure or diaphoresis, does not rule out the presence of pain. Acute pain management initiated as early as possible and focused on preventing occurrence and reemergence of pain may reduce dosage requirements for analgesics. Analgesics, especially opioids, should be prescribed only for pain relief (Manchikanti et al. 2012a, 2012b). Although analgesia may produce many benefits, other symptoms commonly coinciding with acute pain (e.g., insomnia, anxiety) should be managed separately from pain. Sleep deprivation and anxiety may intensify the sensation of pain and lead to increased requests for more medication. Alleviating anxiety and insomnia may reduce analgesic requirements.

In acute pain management, psychiatric consultation is requested when a patient requires more analgesia than expected or has a history of substance abuse. Patients with an active or recent history of opioid addiction and those receiving opioid agonist maintenance therapy usually have developed tolerance to opioids and when receiving short-acting opioids for acute pain management may require doses up to 50% higher than those required by opioid-naive patients (see Chapter 16, "Substance-Related Disorders"). Although it is important to monitor opioid use carefully in these patients, adequate treatment of acute pain is a priority. Inadequate dosing is significantly more common than abuse or diversion in these patients.

Psychiatric Comorbidity

Somatic Symptoms Related to Pain

When a medical cause for pain cannot be identified, many clinicians begin to seek psychological causes. The concept of pain "caused" by emotional factors first appeared in DSM-II (American Psychiatric Association 1968) under psychophysiological disorders, and DSM-III (American Psychiatric Association 1980) introduced psychogenic pain disorder, which in DSM-III-R (American Psychiatric Association 1987) was revised to somatoform pain disorder.

Prevalence estimates depend on the diagnostic criteria used to define the pain condition. For example, the DSM-III-R diagnosis of somatoform pain disorder had an estimated lifetime prevalence of 34% and a 6-month prevalence of 17% in the general population. The updated DSM-IV (American Psychiatric Association 1994) diagnosis of pain disorder included a new requirement for "significant distress or psychosocial impairment due to somatoform pain" that reduced the lifetime prevalence to 12% and the 6-month prevalence to 5%, with a female:male ratio of 2:1 (Grabe et al. 2003). The diagnosis pain disorder was eliminated in DSM-5 (American Psychiatric Association 2013), and a new diagnostic category, somatic symptom and related disorders, was introduced, along with its prototype, somatic symptom disorder (SSD). Criteria for SSD differed from those for the DSM-IV diagnosis of somatization disorder, with the most significant change being abolition of the distinction between medically explained and medically unexplained somatic complaints (for a detailed discussion, see Chapter 11, "Somatic Symptom Disorder and Illness Anxiety Disorder"). There is little research on SSD to date, because it was recently introduced in DSM-5.

Even when pain is the chief complaint, the experience of pain is influenced by psychological factors. Injured workers who developed DSM-III-R somatoform pain disorder had more sites of pain with spread of pain beyond the area of original injury, more opioid and benzodiazepine use, and greater involvement with compensation and litigation compared with workers who did not develop this disorder (Streltzer et al. 2000). Pain disorder was often equated with "psychogenic" pain that has no "real" cause. However, neuroimaging studies in patients with DSM-IV pain disorder showed significant decreases in gray matter density in prefrontal, cingulate, and insular cortexes, regions that are known to modulate the subjective experience of pain (Valet et al. 2009). Unfortunately, the diagnosis retains an inherent either/or dualism regarding psychological versus physical domains instead of pointing the way toward an appreciation of how those domains interrelate. Regardless of the etiology of pain, the physical and/or psychological distress resulting from pain can cause significant reductions in quality of life (QOL) (Rief and Martin 2014).

Whereas multiple pain complaints were typical in DSM-IV somatization disorder, patients with chronic pain rarely received this diagnosis. Rather, the somatization disorder diagnosis was more commonly given to patients with multiple painful and other somatic complaints (especially in primary care settings) who had high rates of symptom persistence and health care use (Jackson and Kroenke 2008). In DSM-5, such patients would be considered for a diagnosis of SSD. These patients are more likely to have catastrophic thinking, to believe that the cause of their pain is a mysterious medical disease, to have feelings of losing control, and to think that their physicians judge their pain to be imaginary (Jackson and Kroenke 2008). Patients with chronic pain and multiple somatic symptoms also are at risk of iatrogenic consequences such as excessive diagnostic tests, inappropriate medications, and unnecessary surgery. Overlap between SSD and related disorders and depressive or anxiety disorders is common. Patients with multiple somatic complaints that are not able to be medically explained experience significant functional disability and role impairment independent of psychiatric and medical comorbidity (Harris et al. 2009).

Substance Use Disorders

The prevalence of DSM-IV substance dependence or addiction in patients with chronic pain has been estimated to range from 3% to 48%, depending on the population sampled (Morasco et al. 2011). The essential criteria for a substance use disorder in patients with chronic pain include loss of control over the use of pain medication, excessive preoccupation with obtaining the medication despite adequate analgesia, and adverse consequences associated with the medication's use (Compton et al. 1998). The availability of opioids has risen exponentially over the past 25 years. The number of opioid prescriptions written annually has also increased dramatically, from 76 million in 1991 to 207 million in 2013, and a significant rise in opioid abuse has followed, including a major increase in heroin abuse over the past few years (Kanouse and Compton 2015). Americans represent less than 5% of the world's population but consume 80% of the global opioid supply, including 99% of the hydrocodone produced (Manchikanti and Singh 2008).

Aberrant medication-taking behaviors can be mistaken for addiction. Persistent pain can lead to an increased preoccupation with obtaining opioids, with the patient taking measures to ensure an adequate medication supply. Patients understandably fear the reemergence of pain and withdrawal symptoms that will occur if they run out of medication. Medication-seeking behavior may be the result of an anxious patient trying to maintain a previous level of pain control or improve on a partial but inadequate response to analgesics. However, rather than representing a true addiction, these actions may indicate pseudoaddiction arising from therapeutic dependence and current or potential undertreatment (Kirsh et al. 2002). The distinction between pseudoaddiction and true addiction is based on how the patient responds to adequate analgesic therapy—i.e., whether the behaviors abate and functioning improves, or, alternatively, the behaviors persist in the context of deteriorating function. However, empirical evidence supporting pseudoaddiction as a diagnosis distinct from addiction has not emerged, so clinicians should always maintain a high index of suspicion (Greene and Chambers 2015).

Patterns of nonadherence to or misuse of prescribed medications have complex associations with emotional distress, disability, perceived need for medication, and patients' concerns about addiction and excessive scrutiny of medication use by others (McCracken et al. 2006). These factors influence the risk of developing an addiction to prescribed medications. During the first 5 years after the onset of a chronic pain problem, patients are at increased risk for developing new substance use problems and disorders. The risk is highest among those with a history of substance use disorder or psychiatric comorbidity. Not infrequently, a history of substance abuse emerges only after the current misuse of medications has been identified, thus requiring physicians to monitor treatment closely.

Although patients exposed to long-term opioid therapy are at significant risk of developing addiction, they are at much higher risk of aberrant medication-taking behaviors and illicit drug use, reinforcing the need for risk screening and monitoring (Fishbain et al. 2008). Aberrant medication-taking behaviors occur in approximately 50% of patients with chronic pain receiving long-term opioid analgesic therapy, with even higher rates in patients with a history of substance abuse (Passik et al. 2006). Risk-prediction instruments such as the Screener and Opioid Assessment for Patients with Pain (SOAPP), the Opioid Risk Tool (ORT), and the Current Opioid Misuse Measure (COMM) offer valuable guidance but have significant limitations (Chou et al. 2009). Strategies to optimize outcomes and minimize abuse require careful analysis of the behaviors of both patients and physicians (Passik and Kirsh 2008).

From the opposite perspective, patients with substance use disorders have increased rates of chronic pain. Although it is true that opioid-dependent patients with chronic pain have relatively high rates of substance abuse (Peles et al. 2005; Rosenblum et al. 2003), they are at risk of stigmatization and undertreatment. Integrating care for chronic pain with innovative stepped-care models of substance abuse treatment would likely improve outcomes by bringing together both types of expertise (Bair et al. 2015; Haibach et al. 2014).

Depression

The relation between pain and depression is intimate and bidirectional. Physical symptoms are common in patients with major depressive disorder (MDD). Approximately 60% of patients with depression report pain symptoms at diagnosis. A study using World Health Organization research data from 14 countries on 5 continents found that 69% (range: 45%–95%) of patients with depression presented with only somatic symptoms, of which pain complaints were most common (Simon et al. 1999). It has been estimated that patients with depression have about a fourfold increase in the prevalence of pain conditions (Ohayon and Schatzberg 2003). Additionally, baseline depressive symptoms more accurately predict future pain and disability than do initial ratings of the actual pain (Schieir et al. 2009).

Individuals with chronic physical complaints have higher rates of lifetime MDD. Among patients presenting to clinics specializing in chronic pain, one-third to more than half met criteria for current MDD (Dersh et al. 2007; Rayner et al. 2016). Depression in patients with chronic pain is associated with greater pain intensity; more pain persistence; application for early retirement; and greater interference from pain, including more pain behaviors observed by others (Rayner et al. 2016). High levels of depression my worsen pain and pain-related disability (Lerman et al. 2015). Depression is a better predictor of disability than are pain intensity and duration. In a study of more than 15,000 employees who filed health claims, the cost of managing chronic conditions such as back problems was almost doubled when the employees had comorbid depression (Druss et al. 2000).

Most chronic pain conditions have been associated with an increased risk of suicide (Ilgen et al. 2013). In an Australian study in 1,514 individuals receiving prescribed opioids, 36.5% reported experiencing suicidal ideation in the past 12 months, and 16.4% reported a lifetime suicide attempt (Campbell et al. 2016). Patients with chronic pain complete suicide at two to three times the rate of people in the general population (Fishbain et al. 1991). Although other psychosocial variables play a role, it is depression that most consistently and strongly predicts suicidal ideation and behaviors in patients with chronic pain (Braden and Sullivan 2008). Pain is even more likely to be an independent risk factor for suicide in patients with headache or multiple types of pain (Ilgen et al. 2008).

Depression with comorbid chronic pain can be more resistant to treatment than depression without pain (Kroenke et al. 2008). Depression should be treated aggressively and not simply "understood" as an expected outcome of suffering with chronic pain. Pain often subsides with improvement in depressive symptoms, resulting in improvement in function and QOL. This effect is independent of the direct treatment of pain and may be explained by overlap between the neurobiology of pain and depression (Bair et al. 2003).

Anxiety Disorders and Posttraumatic Stress Disorder

Anxiety symptoms are present in almost half of patients with chronic pain. Up to 30% of these patients meet criteria for an anxiety disorder (e.g., generalized anxiety disorder, panic disorder, agoraphobia) or for posttraumatic stress disorder (PTSD) (Outcalt et al. 2015). PTSD is increasingly recognized as a comorbid condition with significant consequences for patients with medical illnesses, especially chronic pain disorders

(Liebschutz et al. 2007). PTSD has strong independent negative associations with pain, disability, psychological status, and QOL (Outcalt et al. 2015). A follow-up reassessment of people who had sustained a severe accident 3 years earlier found that PTSD symptoms and other psychological factors were stronger predictors of the development of chronic pain than were sociodemographic and accident-related variables (Jenewein et al. 2009). Conversely, anxiety symptoms and disorders are associated with high levels of somatic preoccupation and physical symptoms. In a study in 139 patients with panic disorder, almost two-thirds reported at least one current pain symptom (Schmidt et al. 2002). Pain was associated with higher levels of anxiety symptoms, panic frequency, and panic-related cognitive variables (e.g., anxiety sensitivity) (Schmidt et al. 2002). Patients with pain and comorbid anxiety have worse outcomes than do pain patients without an anxiety disorder (Jordan and Okifuji 2011).

Fear and Catastrophizing

Fear of pain, of movement, of reinjury, and of other negative consequences leads to avoidance of activities and promotes initiation and maintenance of chronic pain disability (Greenberg and Burns 2003). Restriction of activities can result in physiological changes, such as weight gain and muscle atrophy, and functional deterioration (Verbunt et al. 2003). This process is reinforced by low self-efficacy, catastrophic interpretations, and increased expectations of failure regarding attempts to engage in rehabilitation. The fear–avoidance model of musculoskeletal pain (Leeuw et al. 2007) incorporated elements such as pain severity, pain catastrophizing, hypervigilance to pain, pain-related fear, escape or avoidance behavior, disability, disuse, and individual vulnerabilities to explain the transition from acute to chronic low back pain (LBP). Pain-related fear and avoidance represent one of the most significant predictors of failure to return to work in patients with chronic LBP and are also predictive of poor adjustment to chronic pain (Hasenbring et al. 2001).

Catastrophic thinking can be described as the amplification of threatening information. Catastrophic thinking about pain interferes with patients' ability to remain involved in productive activities (Crombez et al. 1998). It intensifies the experience of pain and increases emotional distress and self-perceived disability (Sullivan et al. 2001). Although catastrophic thinking is often conceptualized as a psychological entity, Campbell and Edwards (2009) theorized that catastrophizing exerts biological effects that may account for some of its negative consequences. For example, a follow-up study of participants in a Dutch population-based questionnaire survey found that high levels of catastrophizing and fear of injury prospectively predicted disability due to new-onset LBP 6 months later (Picavet et al. 2002). Similarly, a systematic review found that catastrophizing was an independent risk factor for chronic pain after total knee arthroplasty (Burns et al. 2015). Pain-related catastrophizing has been shown to be a predictor of suicidal ideation independent of depressive symptoms and pain severity (Edwards et al. 2006).

Sleep Problems

There is ample evidence to suggest that pain and sleep are related, but the association between these two conditions is complex. The prevailing view has been that they are reciprocally related. However, emerging evidence from population-based longitudinal studies suggests that sleep problems may exert a greater influence on pain than pain does on sleep problems (Finan et al. 2013). A study examining associations between self-reported sleep measures (including sleep duration, sleep-onset latency, sleep efficiency, and frequency/severity of insomnia)—and pain sensitivity found that all parameters except sleep duration were significantly associated with reduced pain tolerance (Sivertsen et al. 2015). Further study is needed to guide clinical efforts to develop and improve treatments for chronic sleep disturbance in the setting of chronic pain.

Chronic Pain Conditions

Postherpetic Neuralgia

Postherpetic neuralgia (PHN) is defined as pain persisting or recurring at the site of shingles (herpes zoster) at least 3 months after the onset of the acute varicella zoster viral rash. PHN occurs in about 10% of patients with acute herpes zoster. More than half of patients older than 65 years with shingles develop PHN, and it is more likely to occur in patients with cancer, diabetes mellitus, systemic lupus erythematous, recent trauma, or severe immunosuppression (Forbes et al. 2016). It occurs in less than 6% of immunocompetent people, however (Johnson and Rice 2014). Other risk factors for PHN are longer duration of prodromal symptoms, greater acute pain and rash severity, sensory impairment, and psychological distress (Volpi et al. 2008). Most cases gradually improve over time, with only about 25% of patients with PHN experiencing pain at 1 year after diagnosis. Approximately 15% of referrals to pain clinics are for the treatment of PHN.

Although degeneration and destruction of motor and sensory fibers of the mixed dorsal root ganglion characterize acute varicella zoster, other neurological damage may include inflammation of the spinal cord, myelin disruption, axonal damage, and decreases in the number of nerve endings in the affected skin. Studies have suggested the role of both peripheral and central mechanisms resulting from the loss of large-caliber neurons and subsequent central sensitization or adrenergic receptor activation and alterations in C fiber activity (Truini et al. 2008). Approaches to management of PHN include prevention with vaccination or antiviral medication and treatment of resulting pain. Current guidelines recommend treating the pain in a hierarchical manner with anticonvulsants, tricyclic antidepressants (TCAs), and topical lidocaine as first-line agents (Mallick-Searle et al. 2016).

Peripheral Neuropathic Pain

The most common cause of painful peripheral neuropathy is diabetes mellitus (Veves et al. 2008; Zochodne 2008). Up to 90% of patients with diabetes will experience pain from diabetic neuropathy; risk factors include longer duration of illness and poor glycemic control (Schreiber et al. 2015). The pain of a peripheral neuropathy can range from constant burning to pain that is episodic, paroxysmal, and lancinating in quality (Mendell and Sahenk 2003). These phenomena are primarily the result of axonal degeneration and segmental demyelination (Tomlinson and Gardiner 2008). Diabetic peripheral neuropathic pain is a stronger predictor of depression than other diabetic complications (D'Amato et al. 2016). Patients with diabetic neuropathic pain who have depression or anxiety receive greater amounts of pain medication and have higher health care utilization (Boulanger et al. 2009). Often, a combination of treatment modalities with different mechanisms of action is required to manage the pain. Medication with proven efficacy include TCAs, serotonin–norepinephrine reuptake inhibitors (SNRIs), anticonvulsants, and topical lidocaine. Adjuvant treatments such as acupuncture, transcutaneous electrical nerve stimulation, cognitive-behavioral therapy (CBT), and neuromodulation have also demonstrated effectiveness (Rosenberg and Watson 2015).

Central Pain After Stroke or Spinal Cord Injury

Pain associated with central nervous system lesions is common after stroke (8%) or spinal cord trauma (60%–70%) (Finnerup 2008; Singer et al. 2017). Symptoms of spinal cord injury (SCI) pain or central poststroke pain are independent of sensory deficits and often are poorly localized, vary over time, and include allodynia (>50% of patients with central poststroke pain), hyperalgesia, dysesthesias, lancinating pain, and muscle and visceral pain. Pain is described as burning, aching, lacerating, or pricking. Radiological studies may reveal lesions in the thalamus, although other sites, such as the spinothalamic tracts, are often involved, especially in SCI (Hari et al. 2009). Excitatory amino acids are likely involved in the development of central sensitization associated with central pain, and the onset of pain can occur more than a month after the stroke, suggesting multiple processes (Hains and Waxman 2007; Hulsebosch et al. 2009; Oh and Seo 2015).

As a result of its complexity and symptom heterogeneity, central poststroke pain is difficult to treat, and there is no universal consensus regarding effective treatment (Mulla et al. 2015). Antidepressants, anticonvulsants, and opioids are used, often in combination (Seifert et al. 2013). For patients who are nonresponsive to medical management, motor cortex stimulation, deep-brain stimulation, and repetitive transcranial magnetic stimulation have been used (Hirabayashi et al. 2011).

Migraine and Chronic Daily Headache

Migraine

The International Headache Society has published guidelines for the classification of headache. Over the life span, 18% of women and 6% of men will experience migraine headaches, with peak incidence between the ages of 30 and 40 years (Lipton et al. 2007; Silberstein et al. 2007). Common migraine is a unilateral pulsatile headache that may be associated with other symptoms, such as nausea, vomiting, photophobia, and phonophobia. The classic form of migraine includes visual prodromal symptoms such as scintillating scotomata. Complicated migraine includes focal neurological signs such as cranial nerve palsies and is often described by the name of the primary deficit (e.g., hemiplegic, vestibular, or basilar migraine). Anxiety and depression are the psychiatric comorbidities most commonly associated with migraine, and anxiety is more robustly associated with increase in migraine risk than is depression. In addition, the physical symptoms of depression are more closely linked to migraine than are the emotional symptoms (Peres et al. 2017). The primary goals of migraine treatment are relieving pain, restoring function, and reducing headache frequency (Lipton and Silberstein 2015).

Evidence from placebo-controlled clinical trials supports the use of NSAIDs and triptans for acute treatment of migraine attacks, with propranolol, metoprolol, flunarizine, valproate, topiramate, and onabotulinumtoxinA (botulinum toxin A) recommended as the best prophylactic agents (Becker 2015; Mulleners and Chronicle 2008; Silberstein 2015). In general, calcium channel blockers, β-blockers, antidepressants, and anticonvulsants are the treatments of choice for more refractory migraine (Silberstein 2008). Behavioral treatments such as CBT and biofeedback or relaxation training are effective therapies (Carod-Artal 2014). A group-based multidisciplinary treatment for migraine consisting of stress management, supervised exercise, dietary education, and massage therapy significantly improved pain outcomes (i.e., self-perceived pain intensity, frequency, and duration) as well as functional status, QOL, depression, and pain-related disability (Lemstra et al. 2002).

Chronic Daily Headache

Chronic daily headache affects about 5% of the population and encompasses constant (transformed) migraine, medication-overuse headache, chronic tension-type headaches, new-onset daily persistent headache, and hemicrania continua (Dodick 2006). Individuals with chronic daily headache are more likely than those without daily headaches to overuse analgesics, leading to rebound headache; to have psychiatric comorbidity such as depression and anxiety; to report functional disability; and to experience stress-related headache exacerbations (Fernández-de-las-Peñas and Schoenen 2009). Chronic daily headache is difficult to manage and is often unresponsive to medication (Halker et al. 2011). Evidence from placebo-controlled clinical trials is sparse but supports the use of amitriptyline, gabapentin, tizanidine, mirtazapine, topiramate, memantine, and onabotulinumtoxinA (Dodick 2006). Various medications have been recommended, including serotonin agonists, serotonin antagonists, and α_2-adrenergic agonists. Combined medication and CBT are more effective than either treatment alone (Lipchik and Nash 2002).

Fibromyalgia

Fibromyalgia is a chronic pain syndrome characterized by widespread musculoskeletal pain in all four limbs and trunk, stiffness, and exaggerated tenderness. These symptoms are usually accompanied by poor sleep, cognitive difficulties, depression, and fatigue. There is little evidence to support theories of inflammatory, autoimmune, or infectious etiologies (Borchers and Gershwin 2015). Placebo-controlled trials have demonstrated the effectiveness of cyclobenzaprine, milnacipran, gabapentin, pregabalin, duloxetine, and tramadol in fibromyalgia (Crofford 2008). In addition to these medications, treatment should include education, patient support, physical therapy, nutrition, and exercise (Borchers and Gershwin 2015).

Fibromyalgia is discussed in detail in Chapter 25, "Chronic Fatigue and Fibromyalgia Syndromes."

Phantom Limb Pain

Pain in a body part that has been removed occurs in 40%–80% of amputees within a year of the amputation (Schley et al. 2008). *Phantom limb pain,* considered to be neuropathic and described as stabbing, throbbing, burning, or cramping, is more intense in the distal portion of the phantom limb. Any area of the body can manifest phantom pain; for example, phantom breast sensations and pain are common after mastectomy (Luo and Anderson 2016). Although TCAs, gabapentin, and carbamazepine are considered the first-line treatments for phantom pain, no controlled trials support their use. Newer antidepressants and anticonvulsants generally cause fewer side effects and may be more effective in treating phantom limb pain if patients can tolerate higher doses. In controlled studies, morphine, calcitonin, and ketamine have been shown to reduce phantom pain in the short term. Controlled trials have discredited anecdotal reports of the effectiveness of neural blockade and onabotulinumtoxinA (Alviar et al. 2016).

Complex Regional Pain Syndrome

Complex regional pain syndrome (CRPS; formerly called reflex sympathetic dystrophy and causalgia) represents an array of painful conditions characterized by ongoing spontaneous burning pain that is precipitated by a specific noxious trauma or cause of immobilization and often is associated with hyperalgesia or allodynia in response to cutaneous stimuli (Hsu 2009; Sharma et al. 2009). It occurs in about 7% of patients following limb fractures, limb surgeries, or other injuries (Bruehl 2015). Pain is regional but is not limited to a single peripheral nerve or dermatome. Edema, blood flow abnormalities, or sudomotor dysfunction is often evident in the pain region (Albazaz et al. 2008). Motor changes such as weakness, tremor, dystonia, and limitations in movement are common (Harden et al. 2007). Sympathetically maintained pain is present in most, but not all, cases (Gibbs et al. 2008). Patients with sympathetically maintained pain often report hyperalgesia to cold stimuli and temporary relief with sympathetic blockade (Pontell 2008). Patients with CRPS commonly have comorbid mood (46%), anxiety (27%), and substance use (14%) disorders, which are generally considered to be a consequence of chronic pain rather than its cause, when coupled with maladaptive personality traits and coping styles (Bruehl and Chung 2006). In addition, anxiety, pain-related fear, and disability have been associated with poorer outcomes in CRPS and should be considered as target variables for early treatment (Bean et al. 2015). Studies have also shown a relationship between CRPS and suicide risk. Significant risk factors for suicidal ideation in patients with CRPS include greater severity of pain, presence of depressive symptoms, and decreased functioning (Lee et al. 2014).

Pharmacotherapy for CRPS has showed limited benefit, and relatively few randomized controlled trials (RCTs) are available to guide treatment selection (Mackey and Feinberg 2007). Symptoms often improve with NSAIDs or corticosteroids in the acute, or inflammatory, stage of the disease. Evidence suggests efficacy for gabapentin, pregabalin, carbamazepine, TCAs, and opioids. RCTs of calcitonin and bisphosphonates in CRPS found reduced pain and improved joint mobility. Clinical trials of local anesthetic sympathetic blockade, once considered the gold standard therapy for CRPS, have been inconclusive (Sharma et al. 2006). Multidisciplinary care, which centers on functionally focused therapies, is recommended (Bruehl 2015).

Orofacial Pain

Trigeminal neuralgia (tic douloureux) is a chronic pain syndrome with a prevalence of 0.015% (Montano et al. 2015) characterized by severe, paroxysmal, recurrent, lancinating unilateral pain localized to the sensory distribution of cranial nerve V, most commonly involving the mandibular division (Obermann and Katsarava 2009; Prasad and Galetta 2009). Sensory or motor deficits are not usually present. Episodes of pain can be spontaneous or evoked by nonpainful stimuli to trigger zones, activities such as talking or chewing, or environmental conditions. Between episodes, patients are typically pain free. Uncontrolled pain with frequent or severe prolonged attacks increases the risk of insomnia, weight loss, social withdrawal, anxiety, and depression, including suicide (Wu et al. 2015).

Pharmacological treatment includes anticonvulsants, antidepressants, baclofen, mexiletine, lidocaine, and opioids (Bescós et al. 2015). Placebo-controlled trials have identified carbamazepine (number needed to treat of 1.8) as the first-line treatment, with oxcarbazepine and lamotrigine as additional options. Evidence is insufficient to recommend clonazepam, gabapentin, phenytoin, tizanidine, topical capsaicin, valproate, or onabotulinumtoxinA (Cruccu et al. 2008). Given the pathophysiological similarities between trigeminal neuralgia and PHN and painful peripheral neuropathies, other medications, such as TCAs and SNRIs, would be appropriate options to consider. When pharmacological treatments fail, a variety of surgical procedures may be undertaken (Al-Quliti 2015; Montano et al. 2015).

Temporomandibular disorder (TMD) is a general term referring to complaints involving the temporomandibular joint, muscles of mastication, and other orofacial musculoskeletal structures, often precipitated by jaw movement (e.g., opening the mouth or chewing). In contrast to the vague, diffuse pain of myalgia, temporomandibular joint dysfunction causes sharp, sudden, and intense pain with joint movement that is often localized to the preauricular area. Associated symptoms include feelings of muscle fatigue, weakness, and tightness as well as changes in bite (malocclusion) or in the ability to open or close the jaw. Joint sounds such as clicking, popping, and crepitation are common. TMD is often associated with psychological stress, but no evidence is available to compare the clinical effectiveness of usual treatment (occlusal splint therapy) versus psychological interventions (Roldán-Barraza et al. 2014). Treatment should initially be based on conservative and evidence-based therapeutic modalities, with more invasive interventions reserved for refractory pain (Dugashvili et al. 2013).

Burning mouth syndrome is covered in Chapter 19, "Gastrointestinal Disorders."

Low Back Pain

LBP is extremely common, with a lifetime risk greater than 80% (Patrick et al. 2016). It is the most expensive medical condition when lost productivity and health care costs are included (Deyo et al. 2009). Psychological factors, including distress, depressed mood, and multiple somatic symptoms that have not received an adequate medical explanation, are highly correlated with LBP and predict the transition from acute to chronic pain. The most powerful predictor of chronicity is poor functional status beyond 1 month of seeking treatment. In patients with chronic nonmalignant back pain, the presence of both economic (e.g., disability income) and social rewards (e.g., avoidance of onerous tasks) was associated with higher levels of disability and depression (Ciccone et al. 1999). The presence of a depressive disorder has been shown to increase the risk of developing musculoskeletal pain in general, and chronic LBP in particular (Pinheiro et al. 2016). Depression has been associated with a nearly fourfold increase in the likelihood of seeking treatment for new-onset LBP. Conversely, chronic LBP can increase the risk of developing psychopathology that affects outcome and treatment response (Dersh et al. 2007).

Treatment of chronic LBP has been pursued with multiple modalities alone and in combination (Deyo and Weinstein 2001). Recommendations for managing LBP emphasize patient education, short-term use of NSAIDS, physical therapy, back exercises, and behavioral therapy. Short-term opioid treatment should be used only for severe acute exacerbations (Dagenais et al. 2010). Few RCTs have evaluated the effectiveness of adjuvant treatment with anticonvulsants or antidepressants; although these agents can provide significant pain relief, they are also associated with side effects that may outweigh their benefits (Chung et al. 2013). Evidence indicates that surgery may be effective for a carefully selected group of patients with chronic LBP (Fritzell et al. 2001). Although treatments often produce symptom reduction, evidence for their ability to improve functional status—particularly with respect to returning to work—is conflicting (Staiger et al. 2003). The patient's perception of disability is a critical factor that must be addressed in order for treatment to succeed.

Treatment of Chronic Pain

Pharmacotherapy

Numerous medications are used in the treatment of chronic pain (Moulin et al. 2007). The pharmacological targets are mechanisms of peripheral and central nervous system sensitization, such as sodium and calcium channel upregulation, spinal hyperexcitability, descending modulation, and aberrant sympathetic–somatic nervous system interactions. Many classes of medication have been used alone or in combination, but no algorithm can provide a simple, straightforward approach to the complexities encountered during the treatment of chronic pain.

Opioids

Opioids reduce the sensory and affective components of pain by interacting with μ, δ, and κ opioid receptors located in both the peripheral and the central nervous systems. Controversy surrounds the long-term use of opioids for chronic nonmalignant pain because of concerns about long-term efficacy and safety, particularly the risk of tolerance, dependence, abuse, and fatal overdose (Noble et al. 2010). Studies of opioid efficacy generally last less than 18 months and are complicated by high rates of discontinuation due to adverse events or insufficient pain relief. Evidence suggests that the risk of serious side effects from opioids is dose dependent (Chou et al. 2015). Opioids should be slowly tapered to avoid withdrawal and should be completely discontinued if the risks (side effects, toxicities, aberrant drug-related behaviors) outweigh the objective benefits (analgesia, functional improvements).

Successful treatment with opioids requires the assessment and documentation of improvement in pain, function, and analgesia without adverse side effects or aberrant behaviors. Guidelines have been established for the use of opioids in chronic pain that help balance the beneficial effects against the unwanted adverse effects (Manchikanti et al. 2012a, 2012b). Appropriate patients are those with moderate or severe pain that has persisted for more than 3 months and that adversely affects functioning or QOL. Before initiating opioid therapy, additional factors—such as the patient's specific pain syndrome, response to other therapies, and potential for aberrant drug-related behaviors—should be considered (Ballantyne and LaForge 2007). A patient's suitability for long-term opioid therapy can be assessed with standardized questionnaires such as the ORT, the SOAPP, and the Diagnosis, Intractability, Risk, Efficacy (DIRE) assessment tool. Treatment outcomes, including adequacy of analgesia, performance of activities of daily living, adverse events, and potential aberrant drug-related behaviors, can be assessed with the Pain Assessment and Documentation Tool (PADT; Passik et al. 2004). The COMM instrument can be used to evaluate opioid-treated patients for concurrent signs or symptoms of intoxication, emotional volatility, poor response to medication, addiction, inappropriate health care use, and problematic medication behaviors.

Clinically available opioids include naturally occurring compounds (morphine and codeine), semisynthetic derivatives (hydromorphone, oxymorphone, hydrocodone, oxycodone, dihydrocodeine, and buprenorphine), and synthetic opioid analgesics (meperidine, fentanyl, methadone, tramadol, pentazocine, and propoxyphene). *Morphine,* because of its hydrophilicity, has poor oral bioavailability (22%–48%) as well as delayed central nervous system absorption and onset of action. This delay prolongs the analgesic effect of morphine relative to its plasma half-life, which reduces the potential for accumulation and toxicity with repeated dosing. *Oxycodone* has higher oral bioavailability (>60%), a faster onset of action, and more predictable plasma levels compared with morphine. Although its analgesic efficacy is similar to that of morphine, oxycodone releases less histamine and is less likely to cause hallucinations (Riley et al. 2008). *Hydrocodone* is similar to oxycodone, with rapid oral absorption and onset of analgesia. Hydrocodone is metabolized by *N*-demethylation to *hydromorphone,* which has properties similar to those of morphine but fewer side effects. *Fentanyl* is highly lipophilic, which allows for transdermal or transmucosal delivery; however, it is the most potent opioid and therefore is associated with greater risk of fatal overdose. The duration of action of transdermal preparations is up to 72 hours, but individual variability is considerable. Meperidine can cause seizures and an agitated delirium and is now rarely used to treat pain. Tramadol is a "semi-opioid" that weakly binds to opioid receptors and weakly inhibits the reuptake of serotonin and norepinephrine.

Methadone is notable for its association with injection drug addiction, low cost, high bioavailability, rapid onset of action, slow hepatic clearance, multiple receptor affinities, lack of neurotoxic metabolites, and incomplete cross-tolerance with other opioids. Compared with other opioids, methadone, due to its uniquely long half-life, carries a significantly greater risk of overdose because of the longer time needed for adaptation with oral use and greater variations in plasma half-life (15–120 hours) (Sandoval et al. 2005). Methadone is unique among opioids in its heightened propensity to cause QTc interval prolongation and torsades de pointes (Pani et al. 2013). The drug's extensive tissue distribution and prolonged half-life prevent withdrawal symptoms with once-daily dosing. However, methadone elimination is biphasic, and the more rapid elimination phase effectively limits the duration of analgesic effects to approximately 6 hours. Repeated dosing, with accumulation in tissue, may increase the duration of analgesia to 8–12 hours.

The most common side effect of long-term opioid therapy is decreased gastrointestinal motility, causing constipation, vomiting, and abdominal pain. Oral opioid agents differ in their propensity to cause these symptoms. Long-term opioid administration may lead to analgesic tolerance or opioid-induced hyperalgesia (Mitra 2008). When tolerance develops, coadministration of other analgesics, opioid rotation to a more potent agonist, or intermittent cessation of certain agents may restore analgesic effects (Dumas and Pollack 2008). Readers are referred to Chapter 16, "Substance-Related Disorders," for a more detailed discussion of treatment of pain in patients receiving methadone or buprenorphine maintenance treatment.

Antidepressants

The analgesic properties of antidepressants remain underappreciated (McCleane 2008). The TCAs and SNRIs, in particular, are effective treatments for many chronic pain syndromes, including diabetic neuropathy, PHN, central pain, poststroke pain, tension-type headache, migraine, and orofacial pain, but not for nonspecific LBP (Verdu et al. 2008). The analgesic effect of antidepressants is thought to be independent of their antidepressant effect and is mediated primarily by the blockade of norepinephrine and serotonin reuptake, thereby enhancing the activation of descending inhibitory neurons in the dorsal horn of the spinal cord (McCleane 2008; Micó et al. 2006). However, antidepressants may produce antinociceptive effects through a variety of pharmacological mechanisms, including modulation by monoamines; interactions with opioid systems; inhibition of ion channel activity; and inhibition of *N*-methyl-D-aspartate, histamine, and cholinergic receptors (Dick et al. 2007).

Tricyclic antidepressants.   Meta-analyses of RCTs have concluded that TCAs are the most effective agents for neuropathic pain and that they are also effective for headache syndromes (Finnerup et al. 2015). TCAs have been shown to effectively treat central poststroke pain, PHN, many types of painful polyneuropathies, and postmastectomy pain syndrome, but have not been shown to benefit SCI pain, phantom limb pain, or painful HIV neuropathy. The various TCAs are equally effective for pain, but secondary-amine TCAs (e.g., nortriptyline) are better tolerated than tertiary agents (e.g., amitriptyline) (Dworkin et al. 2007). In the treatment of pain, TCAs generally produce analgesia at lower dosages than those used to treat depression, with an earlier onset of effect (Rojas-Corrales et al. 2003). Lack of analgesic effects may be a result of inadequate dosing; therefore, careful titration guided by serum-level monitoring should be used to achieve optimal response. Chronic pain in PHN and diabetic peripheral neuropathy has been treated successfully with TCAs at average dosages of 100–250 mg/day (Max 1994). In contrast, a study using a U.S. health insurance claims database to examine TCA use for neuropathic pain in older patients (≥65 years) found that the average dosage was only 23 mg/day, suggesting unrealized potential for additional pain relief (Berger et al. 2006).

Serotonin–norepinephrine reuptake inhibitors.   Duloxetine, venlafaxine, desvenlafaxine, and milnacipran inhibit the presynaptic reuptake of serotonin, norepinephrine, and (to a lesser extent) dopamine. Although SNRIs are associated with fewer side effects and less toxicity than TCAs, they cannot be monitored with serum levels.

In placebo-controlled trials, venlafaxine significantly reduced neuropathic pain following breast cancer treatment (Tasmuth et al. 2002). It is effective in migraine prophylaxis (Dharmshaktu et al. 2012; Ozyalcin et al. 2005) and reduces allodynia and hyperalgesia in neuropathic pain (Yucel et al. 2005). Venlafaxine also may be effective for fibromyalgia (VanderWeide et al. 2015). Duloxetine has demonstrated analgesic efficacy both in preclinical models and in clinical populations including patients with fibromyalgia (Arnold et al. 2005), painful diabetic neuropathy (Wernicke et al. 2006), or osteoarthritis (Micca et al. 2013). A Cochrane review recommends duloxetine as an effective treatment for neuropathic pain (Lunn et al. 2014). The efficacy of duloxetine in painful diabetic neuropathy was greater in patients with more severe pain but was not related to the severity of diabetes or neuropathy (Ziegler et al. 2007). Patients with depression and painful somatic symptoms experienced relief when taking duloxetine, but the analgesic effects were independent of the drug's antidepressant actions (Perahia et al. 2006).

Selective serotonin reuptake inhibitors.   In clinical trials, the efficacy of selective serotonin reuptake inhibitors (SSRIs) in chronic pain syndromes has been inconsistent, especially in the treatment of neuropathic pain (Finnerup et al. 2005). A Cochrane review found SSRIs no more efficacious than placebo for migraine and less efficacious than TCAs for tension-type headache (Banzi et al. 2015). However, fluoxetine improved outcome measures (i.e., pain impact and severity) in women with fibromyalgia (Arnold et al. 2002) and was comparable to amitriptyline in significantly reducing rheumatoid arthritis pain (Rani et al. 1996). Citalopram improved abdominal pain in irritable bowel syndrome, and its therapeutic effects on pain were independent of its effects on anxiety and depression (Tack et al. 2006). Paroxetine and citalopram, but not fluoxetine, decreased the pain of diabetic peripheral neuropathy in some controlled studies (Goodnick 2001). In a study comparing gabapentin, paroxetine, and citalopram for painful diabetic peripheral neuropathy, the three agents had similar efficacy for pain, but patients reported better satisfaction, compliance, and mood with the SSRIs (Giannopoulos et al. 2007). Overall, SSRIs are not recommended as a first-line therapy for chronic pain but may be worth considering when comorbid depression is present.

Novel antidepressants.   Few controlled trials have examined the efficacy of novel antidepressants, such as mirtazapine, bupropion, trazodone, vortioxetine, and vilazodone, in pain syndromes, but their pharmacology suggests antinociceptive properties. In controlled trials, mirtazapine reduced the duration and intensity of chronic tension-type headaches (Bendtsen and Jensen 2004), and bupropion reduced pain intensity and interference of pain with QOL (Semenchuk et al. 2001). Trazodone can be useful in treating chronic pain, but sedation can hinder titration to the effective dose (Bossini et al. 2015). Vortioxetine and vilazodone are too new to have accumulated evidence of efficacy in treating pain.

Anticonvulsants

Anticonvulsants reduce pain by inhibiting excessive neuronal activity. They have shown efficacy in treating a variety of neuropathic pain syndromes, such as trigeminal neuralgia, diabetic neuropathy, and PHN, as well as in prevention of migraine recurrence (Seidel et al. 2013). Anticonvulsants have also demonstrated efficacy in neuropathic pain (number needed to treat ranging from ~2 to ~4), and are associated with better medication adherence compared with TCAs because they have fewer adverse effects (Finnerup et al. 2005).

First-generation anticonvulsants.   Phenytoin was first reported as a successful treatment for trigeminal neuralgia in 1942 (Bergouignan 1942). Carbamazepine is the most widely studied anticonvulsant in neuropathic pain (Wiffen et al. 2014a). Valproate is most commonly used for prophylaxis of migraine headaches, but it is also effective for neuropathic pain (Gill et al. 2014).

Second-generation anticonvulsants.   Second-generation anticonvulsants include gabapentin, pregabalin, lamotrigine, and topiramate. Pregabalin and gabapentin are effective for the treatment of painful diabetic neuropathy, PHN, fibromyalgia, postamputation phantom limb pain, and central neuropathic pain associated with SCI (Moore et al. 2014; Ogawa et al. 2016). In patients with PHN, flexible titration strategies result in fewer discontinuations, higher final dosages, and slightly better pain relief compared with fixed-dosage schedules (Stacey et al. 2008). Gabapentin and pregabalin are entirely renally excreted, so lower dosages must be used in patients with impaired renal function (Atalay et al. 2013).

Lamotrigine is effective in treating HIV-related neuropathy and central poststroke pain but has not shown efficacy in other neuropathic conditions (Wiffen and Rees 2007). Dosages greater than 300 mg/day were more effective than lower dosages in the treatment of painful diabetic neuropathy (Vinik et al. 2007). Topiramate offers the advantages of minimal hepatic metabolism and unchanged renal excretion, few drug interactions, a long half-life, and the unusual side effect of weight loss. Topiramate has shown efficacy in migraine prophylaxis and in treatment of chronic LBP and pain from lumbar radiculopathy and diabetic neuropathy; however, its benefits are not clearly established, and it can impair cognition (Wiffen et al. 2013a).

Other anticonvulsants.   Oxcarbazepine is a carbamazepine derivative with an improved safety and tolerability profile that is effective for the treatment of diabetic peripheral neuropathy but not other neuropathic pain (Zhou et al. 2013). Tiagabine, vigabatrin, retigabine, levetiracetam, and zonisamide are new anticonvulsants with a spectrum of pharmacological actions and antinociceptive effects in animal models, but few clinical studies exist to support their use as first-line therapy for chronic pain (Wiffen et al. 2013b, 2014b). Combinations of anticonvulsants with complementary mechanisms of action may increase effectiveness and decrease adverse effects of treatment, but this has not been clearly established.

Benzodiazepines

Benzodiazepines are commonly prescribed for insomnia, anxiety, and spasticity. Although there is some evidence that benzodiazepines have antihyperalgesic (reduction of increased sensitivity to pain) properties (Howard et al. 2014), their use in conjunction with opioids may be countertherapeutic (Gauntlett-Gilbert et al. 2016) and potentially dangerous: the combination of benzodiazepines with opioids in treatment of chronic pain significantly increases the risk of fatal overdose (Sun et al. 2017). Benzodiazepines cause sedation and cognitive impairment, especially in elderly and other vulnerable patients. In patients with chronic pain, benzodiazepines, but not opioids, were associated with reduced activity levels, increased rates of health care utilization and depression, and increased disability days (Ciccone et al. 2000).

Antipsychotics

Antipsychotics have been used in diabetic neuropathy, PHN, headache, facial pain, pain associated with AIDS and cancer, and musculoskeletal pain, with increasing evidence supporting their effectiveness, mainly as an add-on therapy to other agents (Fishbain et al. 2004; Seidel et al. 2013). However, a meta-analysis of 11 controlled trials concluded that the evidence was mixed regarding use of antipsychotics as add-on therapy in the treatment of painful conditions (Seidel et al. 2013). Compared with typical antipsychotics, atypical antipsychotics offer a broader therapeutic spectrum and lower rates of extrapyramidal side effects; however, these benefits have been offset by concerns about their adverse metabolic effects.

Local Anesthetics

Topical lidocaine has been approved for the treatment of PHN and does not produce significant serum levels (Khaliq et al. 2007), but the evidence to date in neuropathic pain is not strong (Derry et al. 2014). Oral mexiletine has been used for various types of neuropathic pain, but supportive evidence is lacking.

Capsaicin.   Capsaicin is derived from the chili pepper and has been used for centuries as a natural pain reliever. Although low-dose topical capsaicin has limited effectiveness in pain, high-dose capsaicin, when tolerated, has shown benefit in the treatment of chronic musculoskeletal pain and neuropathic pain (Smith and Brooks 2014). Topical capsaicin may also be useful for patients who are unresponsive or intolerant to other treatments (Mason et al. 2004).

Psychological Interventions

Cognitive-Behavioral Models

Psychological treatment for chronic pain was pioneered by Fordyce, who used an operant conditioning behavioral model (Fordyce et al. 1973). The behavioral approach focuses on understanding pain in a social context. The behavior of a patient with chronic pain not only influences and shapes the behaviors of others (including physicians) but also is reinforced and shaped by the behaviors of others. Behaviors signifying pain, such as facial expressions (grimacing), nonverbal utterances (moans), and body movements (guarding) have well-recognized features that define and differentiate them from behaviors associated with other states (Keogh 2014). The behavioral model assumes that if pain behaviors persist, pain and disability will likewise persist. In treatment, healthy behaviors are targeted for reinforcement to replace extinguished pain behaviors.

Since the initial applications of CBT to chronic pain, much research has established the importance of cognitive and behavioral processes in how individuals adapt to chronic pain (Ehde et al. 2014). The cognitive-behavioral model of chronic pain assumes that individual beliefs, attitudes, and expectations affect emotional and behavioral reactions to life experiences. Pain and the resultant pain behaviors are influenced by biomedical, psychological, and socioenvironmental variables.

If patients believe that pain, depression, and disability are inevitable and uncontrollable, then they will likely experience more negative affective responses, increased pain, and even more impaired physical and psychosocial functioning. The components of CBT, such as relaxation, guided imagery, biofeedback, meditation, hypnosis, motivational interviewing, external reinforcement, cognitive restructuring, and coping self-statement training, interrupt this cycle of disability. Patients are taught to become active participants in the management of their pain by using methods that minimize distressing thoughts and feelings. Regardless of the techniques used, the goals of CBT focus the patient on self-control and self-management to increase activity, independence, and resourcefulness. A recent review revealed that CBT reduced pain intensity in 43% of trials and that online and in-person formats had comparable efficacy (Knoerl et al. 2016). A Cochrane review concluded that CBT had significant but small effects on pain and disability and moderate effects on mood and catastrophizing (Williams et al. 2012). The benefits of CBT have been found to continue up to 6 months after the completion of active treatment sessions.

Pain beliefs.   In CBT, pain beliefs are conceptualized as the thoughts of an individual about his or her personal pain problem (Morley and Wilkinson 1995). Psychosocial dysfunction has been correlated with receiving overly solicitous responses from family, believing emotions are related to pain, and attributing the inability to function to pain (Jensen et al. 1994b). In contrast, although physical disability was correlated with beliefs about pain interfering with function, patients also endorsed the belief that pain signifies injury, and therefore that activity should be avoided. A change in perceived control over pain was the most significant predictor of beneficial effects of CBT for chronic TMD pain (Turner et al. 2007).

Cognitive variables derived from social learning theory that are relevant to chronic pain include self-efficacy, outcome expectancies, and locus of control (Solberg Nes et al. 2009). A self-efficacy expectancy is a belief about one's ability to perform a specific behavior, whereas an outcome expectancy is a belief about the consequences of performing a behavior. Individuals are thought to be more likely to engage in coping efforts they believe are within their capabilities and will result in a positive outcome. Patients with a variety of chronic pain syndromes who score higher on measures of self-efficacy or who have an internal locus of control report lower levels of pain, higher pain thresholds, increased exercise performance, and more positive coping efforts. Interestingly, physician expectations of pain relief were significant predictors of patient pain relief ratings, a finding that supports the important role of other persons in an individual's chronic pain experience.

Acceptance of chronic pain is a two-factor construct (activity engagement and pain willingness) associated with multiple domains of the experience of chronic pain. Acceptance of pain was found to be associated with reports of lower pain intensity, less pain-related anxiety and avoidance, less depression, less physical and psychosocial disability, more daily uptime, and better work status (McCracken 1998). Acceptance has been found to mediate the effects of catastrophizing on depression, avoidance, and functioning in patients with chronic pain (Vowles et al. 2008). A patient's acceptance of chronic pain predicts his or her adjustment to the illness and is independent of catastrophizing, coping skills, and pain-related beliefs and cognitions (Esteve et al. 2007; Vowles et al. 2007).

Coping strategies for pain.   *Coping* can be defined as "a person's cognitive and behavioral efforts to manage the internal and external demands of the person–environment transaction that is appraised as taxing or exceeding the person's resources"

(Folkman et al. 1986, p. 571). Coping strategies support the cognitive-behavioral model of chronic pain, whether active versus passive or adaptive versus maladaptive (Jensen 2009). However, patients who remain passive or who continue to use maladaptive coping strategies—such as catastrophizing, ignoring or reinterpreting pain sensations, or diverting attention from pain—have higher disability (Jensen et al. 1994a).

The effectiveness of particular coping strategies depends on many aspects of the patient's experience with pain. For example, reinterpreting pain sensations as not being signs of ongoing injury typically has been formulated as useful for reducing the effects of experimentally induced pain. However, focusing on pain and disability for greater periods of time, such as is needed in CBT, can be detrimental if it diverts patients from engaging in social activities and healthy behaviors. Catastrophic thinking about pain involves amplification of threatening somatic information and disruption of the attentional focus needed for patients to maintain involvement in productive rather than pain-related activities (Crombez et al. 1998). In one study, high levels of catastrophizing combined with lower levels of active pain coping predicted higher levels of depressive symptoms and disability (Buenaver et al. 2008). The use of adaptive coping skills decreased pain and disability when patients perceived an increase in the effectiveness of their new skills and reduced their use of maladaptive coping strategies such as catastrophic thinking.

Placebo Response

Placebos are arguably the most commonly prescribed drug across cultures and throughout history (Gold and Lichtenberg 2014). Placebo effects and patient responses to them are complex phenomena but are similar to the effects of and patient responses to active treatments (Kleinman et al. 1994). There is not a single placebo effect, but many effects (Benedetti 2006). Placebo analgesia is a biologically measurable phenomenon (Greene et al. 2009). In a clinical setting, it is difficult to separate "true" improvements from placebo responses. The expectations and previous experiences of both patients and physicians are well-established key mediators of placebo effects (Reicherts et al. 2016). How physicians communicate with patients influences the magnitude of placebo effects (Czerniak et al. 2016).

Historically, placebo interventions were a part of paternalistic medicine's treatment armamentarium (Kaptchuk 1998). In the era of RCTs, placebos may be used if informed consent is obtained. The clinical use of placebos without patients' knowledge is unethical (Gold and Lichtenberg 2014). Use of placebos to determine whether the patient's pain is "real" or to "cure" a psychogenic condition by replacing an analgesic with a "neutral" substance is dishonest, misleading, and counterproductive. A positive placebo response neither proves that the patient's pain is psychogenic nor shows that the patient would not benefit from an active treatment. Such an intervention also can result in loss of the patient's trust and render future treatment less effective.

Interdisciplinary Rehabilitation

Patients with chronic pain report lower levels of physical, psychological, and social well-being and greater impairments in health-related QOL compared with patients with almost all other medical conditions (O'Connor 2009). Interdisciplinary pain rehabilitation programs provide a full range of treatments for the most difficult pain syndromes within a framework of collaborative ongoing communication among team members, patients, and other interested parties (Stanos and Houle 2006).

Substantial evidence indicates that interdisciplinary pain rehabilitation programs improve functioning in several areas for patients with various chronic pain syndromes, even those with severe disability (Lake et al. 2009; van Wilgen et al. 2009). A recent Cochrane review concluded that for chronic LBP, interdisciplinary rehabilitation interventions were more effective than usual care and physical treatments in decreasing pain and disability (Kamper et al. 2015). The goal of treating chronic pain is to end disability and return people to work or other productive activities, and interdisciplinary interventions do show efficacy in returning patients to work (Norlund et al. 2009). Overall, evidence suggests that interdisciplinary programs allow early treatment and reduce unnecessary health costs (Malaty et al. 2014).

Conclusion

Chronic pain is a significant public health problem and is frustrating to everyone affected by it, especially patients, who may feel that health care has failed them. Psychiatrists as medical specialists should take an active role in the care of these patients because pharmacological and psychological treatments are now recognized as being effective in the management of chronic pain. Recent advances in the treatment of chronic pain include diagnosis and treatment of psychiatric comorbidity, application of psychiatric treatments to chronic pain, and development of interdisciplinary efforts to provide comprehensive health care to patients with disabling and refractory chronic pain syndromes. Specifically, the psychiatrist provides expertise in examining mental life and behavior as well as in understanding the individual person and the systems in which he or she interacts. Finally, psychiatrists can facilitate the integration of medical care delivery with mental health care and specialist care in a collaborative interdisciplinary environment.

References

Albazaz R, Wong YT, Homer-Vanniasinkam S: Complex regional pain syndrome: a review. Ann Vasc Surg 22(2):297–306, 2008 18346583

Al-Quliti KW: Update on neuropathic pain treatment for trigeminal neuralgia. The pharmacological and surgical options. Neurosciences (Riyadh) 20(2):107–114, 2015 25864062

Alviar MJ, Hale T, Dungca M: Pharmacologic interventions for treating phantom limb pain. Cochrane Database Syst Rev (10):CD006380, 2016 27737513

American Psychiatric Association: Diagnostic and Statistical Manual of Mental Disorders, 2nd Edition. Washington, DC, American Psychiatric Association, 1968

American Psychiatric Association: Diagnostic and Statistical Manual of Mental Disorders, 3rd Edition. Washington, DC, American Psychiatric Association, 1980

American Psychiatric Association: Diagnostic and Statistical Manual of Mental Disorders, 3rd Edition, Revised. Washington, DC, American Psychiatric Association, 1987

American Psychiatric Association: Diagnostic and Statistical Manual of Mental Disorders, 4th Edition. Washington, DC, American Psychiatric Association, 1994

American Psychiatric Association: Diagnostic and Statistical Manual of Mental Disorders, 5th Edition. Arlington, VA, American Psychiatric Association, 2013

Arnold LM, Hess EV, Hudson JI, et al: A randomized, placebo-controlled, double-blind, flexible-dose study of fluoxetine in the treatment of women with fibromyalgia. Am J Med 112(3):191–197, 2002 11893345

Arnold LM, Rosen A, Pritchett YL, et al: A randomized, double-blind, placebo-controlled trial of duloxetine in the treatment of women with fibromyalgia with or without major depressive disorder. Pain 119(1–3):5–15, 2005 16298061

Atalay H, Solak Y, Biyik Z, et al: Cross-over, open-label trial of the effects of gabapentin versus pregabalin on painful peripheral neuropathy and health-related quality of life in haemodialysis patients. Clin Drug Investig 33(6):401–408, 2013 23572323

Bair MJ, Robinson RL, Katon W, et al: Depression and pain comorbidity: a literature review. Arch Intern Med 163(20):2433–2445, 2003 14609780

Bair MJ, Ang D, Wu J, et al: Evaluation of stepped care for chronic pain (ESCAPE) in veterans of the Iraq and Afghanistan conflicts: a randomized clinical trial. JAMA Intern Med 175(5):682–689, 2015 25751701

Ballantyne JC, LaForge KS: Opioid dependence and addiction during opioid treatment of chronic pain. Pain 129(3):235–255, 2007 17482363

Banzi R, Cusi C, Randazzo C, et al: Selective serotonin reuptake inhibitors (SSRIs) and serotonin-norepinephrine reuptake inhibitors (SNRIs) for the prevention of tension-type headache in adults. Cochrane Database Syst Rev (5):CD011681, 2015 25931277

Bean DJ, Johnson MH, Heiss-Dunlop W, et al: Do psychological factors influence recovery from complex regional pain syndrome type 1? A prospective study. Pain 156(11):2310–2318, 2015 26133727

Becker WJ: Acute migraine treatment. Coninuum (Minneap Minn) 21(4, Headache):953–972, 2015 26252584

Bendtsen L, Jensen R: Mirtazapine is effective in the prophylactic treatment of chronic tension-type headache. Neurology 62(10):1706–1711, 2004 15159466

Benedetti F: Placebo analgesia. Neurol Sci 27 (suppl 2):S100–S102, 2006 16688609

Berger A, Dukes EM, Edelsberg J, et al: Use of tricyclic antidepressants in older patients with painful neuropathies. Eur J Clin Pharmacol 62(9):757–764, 2006 16802165

Bergouignan M: Cures heureuses de nevralgies faciales essentielles par le diphenyl-hydantoinate de soude. Rev Laryngol Otol Rhinol (Bord) 63:34–41, 1942

Bescós A, Pascual V, Escosa-Bage M, et al: Treatment of trigeminal neuralgia: an update and future prospects of percutaneous techniques [in Spanish]. Rev Neurol 61(3):114–124, 2015 26178516

Borchers AT, Gershwin ME: Fibromyalgia: a critical and comprehensive review. Clin Rev Allergy Immunol 49(2):100–151, 2015 26445775

Bossini L, Coluccia A, Casolaro I, et al: Off-label trazodone prescription: evidence, benefits and risks. Curr Pharm Des 21(23):3343–3351, 2015 26088119

Boulanger L, Zhao Y, Foster TS, et al: Impact of comorbid depression or anxiety on patterns of treatment and economic outcomes among patients with diabetic peripheral neuropathic pain. Curr Med Res Opin 25(7):1763–1773, 2009 19505204

Braden JB, Sullivan MD: Suicidal thoughts and behavior among adults with self-reported pain conditions in the national comorbidity survey replication. J Pain 9(12):1106–1115, 2008 19038772

Bruehl S: Complex regional pain syndrome. BMJ 351:h2730, 2015 26224572

Bruehl S, Chung OY: Psychological and behavioral aspects of complex regional pain syndrome management. Clin J Pain 22(5):430–437, 2006 16772797

Buenaver LF, Edwards RR, Smith MT, et al: Catastrophizing and pain-coping in young adults: associations with depressive symptoms and headache pain. J Pain 9(4):311–319, 2008 18165160

Burns LC, Ritvo SE, Ferguson MK, et al: Pain catastrophizing as a risk factor for chronic pain after total knee arthroplasty: a systematic review. J Pain Res 8:21–32, 2015 25609995

Campbell CM, Edwards RR: Mind-body interactions in pain: the neurophysiology of anxious and catastrophic pain-related thoughts. Transl Res 153(3):97–101, 2009 19218091

Campbell G, Bruno R, Darke S, et al: Prevalence and correlates of suicidal thoughts and suicide attempts in people prescribed pharmaceutical opioids for chronic pain. Clin J Pain 32(4):292–301, 2016 26295378

Carod-Artal FJ: Tackling chronic migraine: current perspectives. J Pain Res 7:185–194, 2014 24748814

Cherry DK, Burt CW, Woodwell DA: National Ambulatory Medical Care Survey: 2001 summary. Adv Data (337):1–44, 2003 12924075

Chou R, Fanciullo GJ, Fine PG, et al: Opioids for chronic noncancer pain: prediction and identification of aberrant drug-related behaviors: a review of the evidence for an American Pain Society and American Academy of Pain Medicine clinical practice guideline. J Pain 10(2):131–146, 2009 19187890

Chou R, Turner JA, Devine EB, et al: The effectiveness and risks of long-term opioid therapy for chronic pain: a systematic review for a National Institutes of Health Pathways to Prevention Workshop. Ann Intern Med 162(4):276–286, 2015 25581257

Chung JW, Zeng Y, Wong TK: Drug therapy for the treatment of chronic nonspecific low back pain: systematic review and meta-analysis. Pain Physician 16(6):E685–E704, 2013 24284847

Ciccone DS, Just N, Bandilla EB: A comparison of economic and social reward in patients with chronic nonmalignant back pain. Psychosom Med 61(4):552–563, 1999 10443765

Ciccone DS, Just N, Bandilla EB, et al: Psychological correlates of opioid use in patients with chronic nonmalignant pain: a preliminary test of the downhill spiral hypothesis. J Pain Symptom Manage 20(3):180–192, 2000 11018336

Compton P, Darakjian J, Miotto K: Screening for addiction in patients with chronic pain and "problematic" substance use: evaluation of a pilot assessment tool. J Pain Symptom Manage 16(6):355–363, 1998 9879160

Crofford LJ: Pain management in fibromyalgia. Curr Opin Rheumatol 20(3):246–250, 2008 18388513

Crombez G, Eccleston C, Baeyens F, et al: When somatic information threatens, catastrophic thinking enhances attentional interference. Pain 75(2–3):187–198, 1998 9583754

Cruccu G, Gronseth G, Alksne J, et al; American Academy of Neurology Society; European Federation of Neurological Society: AAN-EFNS guidelines on trigeminal neuralgia management. Eur J Neurol 15(10):1013–1028, 2008 18721143

Czerniak E, Beigon A, Ziv A, et al: Manipulating the placebo response in experimental pain by altering doctor's performance style. Front Psychol 7:874, 2016 27445878

Dagenais S, Tricco AC, Haldeman S: Synthesis of recommendations for the assessment and management of low back pain from recent clinical practice guidelines. Spine J 10(6):514–529, 2010 20494814

D'Amato C, Morganti R, Greco C, et al: Diabetic peripheral neuropathic pain is a stronger predictor of depression than other diabetic complications and comorbidities. Diab Vasc Dis Res 13(6):418–428, 2016 27334483

Derry S, Wiffen PJ, Moore RA, et al: Topical lidocaine for neuropathic pain in adults. Cochrane Database Syst Rev (7):CD010958, 2014 25058164

Dersh J, Mayer T, Theodore BR, et al: Do psychiatric disorders first appear preinjury or postinjury in chronic disabling occupational spinal disorders? Spine 32(9):1045–1051, 2007 17450081

Deyo RA, Weinstein JN: Low back pain. N Engl J Med 344(5):363–370, 2001 11172169

Deyo RA, Mirza SK, Turner JA, et al: Overtreating chronic back pain: time to back off? J Am Board Fam Med 22(1):62–68, 2009 19124635

Dharmshaktu P, Tayal V, Kalra BS: Efficacy of antidepressants as analgesics: a review. J Clin Pharmacol 52(1):6–17, 2012 21415285

Dick IE, Brochu RM, Purohit Y, et al: Sodium channel blockade may contribute to the analgesic efficacy of antidepressants. J Pain 8(4):315–324, 2007 17175203

Dodick DW: Clinical practice. Chronic daily headache. N Engl J Med 354(2):158–165, 2006 16407511

Druss BG, Rosenheck RA, Sledge WH: Health and disability costs of depressive illness in a major U.S. corporation. Am J Psychiatry 157(8):1274–1278, 2000 10910790

Dugashvili G, Menabde G, Janelidze M, et al: Temporomandibular joint disorder (review). Georgian Med News 215(215):17–21, 2013 23482357

Dumas EO, Pollack GM: Opioid tolerance development: a pharmacokinetic/pharmacodynamic perspective. AAPS J 10(4):537–551, 2008 18989788

Dworkin RH, O'Connor AB, Backonja M, et al: Pharmacologic management of neuropathic pain: evidence-based recommendations. Pain 132(3):237–251, 2007 17920770

Edwards RR, Smith MT, Kudel I, et al: Pain-related catastrophizing as a risk factor for suicidal ideation in chronic pain. Pain 126(1–3):272–279, 2006 16926068

Ehde DM, Dillworth TM, Turner JA: Cognitive-behavioral therapy for individuals with chronic pain: efficacy, innovations, and directions for research. Am Psychol 69(2):153–166, 2014 24547801

Esteve R, Ramírez-Maestre C, López-Marínez AE: Adjustment to chronic pain: the role of pain acceptance, coping strategies, and pain-related cognitions. Ann Behav Med 33(2):179–188, 2007 17447870

Fernández-de-las-Peñas C, Schoenen J: Chronic tension-type headache: what is new? Curr Opin Neurol 22(3):254–261, 2009 19300250

Finan PH, Goodin BR, Smith MT: The association of sleep and pain: an update and a path forward. J Pain 14(12):1539–1552, 2013 24290442

Finnerup NB: A review of central neuropathic pain states. Curr Opin Anaesthesiol 21(5):586–589, 2008 18784483

Finnerup NB, Otto M, McQuay HJ, et al: Algorithm for neuropathic pain treatment: an evidence based proposal. Pain 118(3):289–305, 2005 16213659

Finnerup NB, Attal N, Haroutounian S, et al: Pharmacotherapy for neuropathic pain in adults: a systematic review and meta-analysis. Lancet Neurol 14(2):162–173, 2015 25575710

Fishbain DA, Goldberg M, Rosomoff RS, et al: Completed suicide in chronic pain. Clin J Pain 7(1):29–36, 1991 1809412

Fishbain DA, Cutler RB, Lewis J, et al: Do the second-generation "atypical neuroleptics" have analgesic properties? A structured evidence-based review. Pain Med 5(4):359–365, 2004 15563321

Fishbain DA, Cole B, Lewis J, et al: What percentage of chronic nonmalignant pain patients exposed to chronic opioid analgesic therapy develop abuse/addiction and/or aberrant drug-related behaviors? A structured evidence-based review. Pain Med 9(4):444–459, 2008 18489635

Folkman S, Lazarus RS, Gruen RJ, et al: Appraisal, coping, health status, and psychological symptoms. J Pers Soc Psychol 50(3):571–579, 1986 3701593

Forbes HJ, Thomas SL, Smeeth L, et al: A systematic review and meta-analysis of risk factors for postherpetic neuralgia. Pain 157(1):30–54, 2016 26218719

Fordyce WE, Fowler RS Jr, Lehmann JF, et al: Operant conditioning in the treatment of chronic pain. Arch Phys Med Rehabil 54(9):399–408, 1973 4729785

Fritzell P, Hägg O, Wessberg P, Nordwall A; Swedish Lumbar Spine Study Group: Lumbar fusion versus nonsurgical treatment for chronic low back pain: a multicenter randomized controlled trial from the Swedish Lumbar Spine Study Group. Spine 26(23):2521–2532, discussion 2532–2534, 2001 11725230

Gaskin DJ, Richard P: The economic costs of pain in the United States. J Pain 13(8):715–724, 2012 22607834

Gauntlett-Gilbert J, Gavriloff D, Brook P: Benzodiazepines may be worse than opioids: negative medication effects in severe chronic pain. Clin J Pain 32(4):285–291, 2016 25968447

Giannopoulos S, Kosmidou M, Sarmas I, et al: Patient compliance with SSRIs and gabapentin in painful diabetic neuropathy. Clin J Pain 23(3):267–269, 2007 17314587

Gibbs GF, Drummond PD, Finch PM, et al: Unravelling the pathophysiology of complex regional pain syndrome: focus on sympathetically maintained pain. Clin Exp Pharmacol Physiol 35(7):717–724, 2008 18215185

Gill D, Derry S, Wiffen PJ, et al: Valproic acid and sodium valproate for neuropathic pain and fibromyalgia in adults. Cochrane Database Syst Rev (10):CD009183, 2014 21975791

Gold A, Lichtenberg P: The moral case for the clinical placebo. J Med Ethics 40(4):219–224, 2014 23750027

Goodnick PJ: Use of antidepressants in treatment of comorbid diabetes mellitus and depression as well as in diabetic neuropathy. Ann Clin Psychiatry 13(1):31–41, 2001 11465683

Grabe HJ, Meyer C, Hapke U, et al: Somatoform pain disorder in the general population. Psychother Psychosom 72(2):88–94, 2003 12601226

Greenberg J, Burns JW: Pain anxiety among chronic pain patients: specific phobia or manifestation of anxiety sensitivity? Behav Res Ther 41(2):223–240, 2003 12547382

Greene CS, Goddard G, Macaluso GM, et al: Topical review: placebo responses and therapeutic responses. How are they related? J Orofac Pain 23(2):93–107, 2009 19492534

Greene MS, Chambers RA: Pseudoaddiction: fact or fiction? An investigation of the medical literature. Curr Addict Rep 2(4):310–317, 2015 26550549

Haibach JP, Beehler GP, Dollar KM, et al: Moving toward integrated behavioral intervention for treating multimorbidity among chronic pain, depression, and substance-use disorders in primary care. Med Care 52(4):322–327, 2014 24556895

Hains BC, Waxman SG: Sodium channel expression and the molecular pathophysiology of pain after SCI. Prog Brain Res 161:195–203, 2007 17618978

Halker RB, Hastriter EV, Dodick DW: Chronic daily headache: an evidence-based and systematic approach to a challenging problem. Neurology 76(7) (suppl 2):S37–S43, 2011 21321350

Harden RN, Bruehl S, Stanton-Hicks M, et al: Proposed new diagnostic criteria for complex regional pain syndrome. Pain Med 8(4):326–331, 2007 17610454

Hari AR, Wydenkeller S, Dokladal P, et al: Enhanced recovery of human spinothalamic function is associated with central neuropathic pain after SCI. Exp Neurol 216(2):428–430, 2009 19162017

Harris AM, Orav EJ, Bates DW, et al: Somatization increases disability independent of comorbidity. J Gen Intern Med 24(2):155–161, 2009 19031038

Hasenbring M, Hallner D, Klasen B: Psychological mechanisms in the transition from acute to chronic pain: over- or underrated? [in German]. Schmerz 15(6):442–447, 2001 11793149

Henschke N, Kamper SJ, Maher CG: The epidemiology and economic consequences of pain. Mayo Clin Proc 90(1):139–147, 2015 25572198

Hirabayashi H, Kawata K, Hoshida T, et al: Neuromodulation therapy for neuropathic pain (recent advances in neuromodulation). Japanese Journal of Neurosurgery 20(2):93–102, 2011

Howard P, Twycross R, Shuster J, et al: Benzodiazepines. J Pain Symptom Manage 47(5):955–964, 2014 24681184

Hsu ES: Practical management of complex regional pain syndrome. Am J Ther 16(2):147–154, 2009 19300041

Hulsebosch CE, Hains BC, Crown ED, et al: Mechanisms of chronic central neuropathic pain after spinal cord injury. Brain Res Brain Res Rev 60(1):202–213, 2009 19154757

Ilgen MA, Zivin K, McCammon RJ, et al: Pain and suicidal thoughts, plans and attempts in the United States. Gen Hosp Psychiatry 30(6):521–527, 2008 19061678

Ilgen MA, Kleinberg F, Ignacio RV, et al: Noncancer pain conditions and risk of suicide. JAMA Psychiatry 70(7):692–697, 2013 23699975

Institute for Clinical Systems Improvement: Health Care Guideline: Assessment and Management of Acute Pain, 6th Edition. March 2008

Jackson JL, Kroenke K: Prevalence, impact, and prognosis of multisomatoform disorder in primary care: a 5-year follow-up study. Psychosom Med 70(4):430–434, 2008 18434494

Jenewein J, Moergeli H, Wittmann L, et al: Development of chronic pain following severe accidental injury: results of a 3-year follow-up study. J Psychosom Res 66(2):119–126, 2009 19154854

Jensen MP: Research on coping with chronic pain: the importance of active avoidance of inappropriate conclusions. Pain 147(1–3):3–4, 2009 19692180

Jensen MP, Turner JA, Romano JM: Correlates of improvement in multidisciplinary treatment of chronic pain. J Consult Clin Psychol 62(1):172–179, 1994a 8034820

Jensen MP, Turner JA, Romano JM, et al: Relationship of pain-specific beliefs to chronic pain adjustment. Pain 57(3):301–309, 1994b 7936708

Johnson RW, Rice AS: Clinical practice: postherpetic neuralgia. N Engl J Med 371(16):1526–1533, 2014 25317872

Jordan KD, Okifuji A: Anxiety disorders: differential diagnosis and their relationship to chronic pain. J Pain Palliat Care Pharmacother 25(3):231–245, 2011 21882977

Kaasalainen S, Crook J: A comparison of pain-assessment tools for use with elderly long-term-care residents. Can J Nurs Res 35(4):58–71, 2003 14746121

Kamper SJ, Apeldoorn AT, Chiarotto A, et al: Multidisciplinary biopsychosocial rehabilitation for chronic low back pain: Cochrane systematic review and meta-analysis. BMJ 350:h444, 2015 25694111

Kanouse AB, Compton P: The epidemic of prescription opioid abuse, the subsequent rising prevalence of heroin use, and the federal response. J Pain Palliat Care Pharmacother 29(2):102–114, 2015 26095479

Kaptchuk TJ: Powerful placebo: the dark side of the randomised controlled trial. Lancet 351(9117):1722–1725, 1998 9734904

Kennedy J, Roll JM, Schraudner T, et al: Prevalence of persistent pain in the U.S. adult population: new data from the 2010 national health interview survey. J Pain 15(10):979–984, 2014 25267013

Keogh E: Gender differences in the nonverbal communication of pain: a new direction for sex, gender, and pain research? Pain 155(10):1927–1931, 2014 24997352

Khaliq W, Alam S, Puri N: Topical lidocaine for the treatment of postherpetic neuralgia. Cochrane Database Syst Rev (2):CD004846, 2007 17443559

Kirsh KL, Whitcomb LA, Donaghy K, et al: Abuse and addiction issues in medically ill patients with pain: attempts at clarification of terms and empirical study. Clin J Pain 18 (4 suppl):S52–S60, 2002 12479254

Kleinman I, Brown P, Librach L: Placebo pain medication: ethical and practical considerations. Arch Fam Med 3(5):453–457, 1994 8032507

Knoerl R, Lavoie Smith EM, Weisberg J: Chronic pain and cognitive behavioral therapy: an integrative review. West J Nurs Res 38(5):596–628, 2016 26604219

Kroenke K, Shen J, Oxman TE, et al: Impact of pain on the outcomes of depression treatment: results from the RESPECT trial. Pain 134(1–2):209–215, 2008 18022319

Lake AE 3rd, Saper JR, Hamel RL: Comprehensive inpatient treatment of refractory chronic daily headache. Headache 49(4):555–562, 2009 19245391

Lee DH, Noh EC, Kim YC, et al: Risk factors for suicidal ideation among patients with complex regional pain syndrome. Psychiatry Investig 11(1):32–38, 2014 24605121

Leeuw M, Goossens ME, Linton SJ, et al: The fear-avoidance model of musculoskeletal pain: current state of scientific evidence. J Behav Med 30(1):77–94, 2007 17180640

Lemstra M, Stewart B, Olszynski WP: Effectiveness of multidisciplinary intervention in the treatment of migraine: a randomized clinical trial. Headache 42(9):845–854, 2002 12390609

Lerman SF, Rudich Z, Brill S, et al: Longitudinal associations between depression, anxiety, pain, and pain-related disability in chronic pain patients. Psychosom Med 77(3):333–341, 2015 25849129

Liebschutz J, Saitz R, Brower V, et al: PTSD in urban primary care: high prevalence and low physician recognition. J Gen Intern Med 22(6):719–726, 2007 17503105

Lipchik GL, Nash JM: Cognitive-behavioral issues in the treatment and management of chronic daily headache. Curr Pain Headache Rep 6(6):473–479, 2002 12413406

Lipton RB, Silberstein SD: Episodic and chronic migraine headache: breaking down barriers to optimal treatment and prevention. Headache 55 (suppl 2):103–122, quiz 123–126, 2015 25662743

Lipton RB, Bigal ME, Diamond M, et al; AMPP Advisory Group: Migraine prevalence, disease burden, and the need for preventive therapy. Neurology 68(5):343–349, 2007 17261680

Lunn MP, Hughes RA, Wiffen PJ: Duloxetine for treating painful neuropathy, chronic pain or fibromyalgia. Cochrane Database Syst Rev (1):CD007115, 2014 24385423

Luo Y, Anderson TA: Phantom limb pain: a review. Int Anesthesiol Clin 54(2):121–139, 2016 26967805

Mackey S, Feinberg S: Pharmacologic therapies for complex regional pain syndrome. Curr Pain Headache Rep 11(1):38–43, 2007 17214920

Malaty A, Sabharwal J, Lirette LS, et al: How to assess a new patient for a multidisciplinary chronic pain rehabilitation program: a review article. Ochsner J 14(1):96–100, 2014 24688340

Mallick-Searle T, Snodgrass B, Brant JM: Postherpetic neuralgia: epidemiology, pathophysiology, and pain management pharmacology. J Multidiscip Healthc 9:447–454, 2016 27703368

Manchikanti L, Singh A: Therapeutic opioids: a ten-year perspective on the complexities and complications of the escalating use, abuse, and nonmedical use of opioids. Pain Physician 11 (2 suppl):S63–S88, 2008 18443641

Manchikanti L, Abdi S, Atluri S, et al; American Society of Interventional Pain Physicians: American Society of Interventional Pain Physicians (ASIPP) guidelines for responsible opioid prescribing in chronic non-cancer pain, part I—evidence assessment. Pain Physician 15 (3 suppl):S1–S65, 2012a 22786448

Manchikanti L, Abdi S, Alturi S, et al; American Society of Interventional Pain Physicians: American Society of Interventional Pain Physicians (ASIPP) guidelines for responsible opioid prescribing in chronic non-cancer pain, part 2—guidance. Pain Physician 15 (3 suppl):S67–S116, 2012b 22786449

Mason L, Moore RA, Derry S, et al: Systematic review of topical capsaicin for the treatment of chronic pain. BMJ 328(7446):991, 2004 15033881

Max MB: Treatment of post-herpetic neuralgia: antidepressants. Ann Neurol 35 (suppl):S50–S53, 1994 8185299

McCleane G: Antidepressants as analgesics. CNS Drugs 22(2):139–156, 2008 18193925

McCracken LM: Learning to live with the pain: acceptance of pain predicts adjustment in persons with chronic pain. Pain 74(1):21–27, 1998 9514556

McCracken LM, Hoskins J, Eccleston C: Concerns about medication and medication use in chronic pain. J Pain 7(10):726–734, 2006 17018333

Mendell JR, Sahenk Z: Clinical practice. Painful sensory neuropathy. N Engl J Med 348(13):1243–1255, 2003 12660389

Merskey H: The taxonomy of pain. Med Clin North Am 91(1):13–20, vii, 2007 17164101

Merskey H, Lindblom U, Mumford JM, et al: Pain terms: a current list with definitions and notes on usage. Pain 24 (suppl 1):S215–S221, 1986

Micca JL, Ruff D, Ahl J, Wohlreich MM: Safety and efficacy of duloxetine treatment in older and younger patients with osteoarthritis knee pain: a post hoc, subgroup analysis of two randomized, placebo-controlled trials. BMC Musculoskelet Disord 14:137, 2013 23590727

Micó JA, Ardid D, Berrocoso E, et al: Antidepressants and pain. Trends Pharmacol Sci 27(7):348–354, 2006 16762426

Mitra S: Opioid-induced hyperalgesia: pathophysiology and clinical implications. J Opioid Manag 4(3):123–130, 2008 18717507

Montano N, Conforti G, Di Bonaventura R, et al: Advances in diagnosis and treatment of trigeminal neuralgia. Ther Clin Risk Manag 11:289–299, 2015 25750533

Moore RA, Wiffen PJ, Derry S, et al: Gabapentin for chronic neuropathic pain and fibromyalgia in adults. Cochrane Database Syst Rev (4):CD007938, 2014 24771480

Morasco BJ, Gritzner S, Lewis L, et al: Systematic review of prevalence, correlates, and treatment outcomes for chronic non-cancer pain in patients with comorbid substance use disorder. Pain 152(3):488–497, 2011 21185119

Morley S, Wilkinson L: The Pain Beliefs and Perceptions Inventory: a British replication. Pain 61(3):427–433, 1995 7478685

Moulin DE, Clark AJ, Gilron I, et al; Canadian Pain Society: Pharmacological management of chronic neuropathic pain: consensus statement and guidelines from the Canadian Pain Society. Pain Res Manag 12(1):13–21, 2007 17372630

Mulla SM, Wang L, Khokhar R, et al: Management of central poststroke pain: systematic review of randomized controlled trials. Stroke 46(10):2853–2860, 2015 26359361

Mulleners WM, Chronicle EP: Anticonvulsants in migraine prophylaxis: a Cochrane review. Cephalalgia 28(6):585–597, 2008 18454787

Nikolaus T: Assessment of chronic pain in elderly patients [in German]. Ther Umsch 54(6):340–344, 1997 9289872

Noble M, Treadwell JR, Tregear SJ, et al: Long-term opioid management for chronic noncancer pain. Cochrane Database Syst Rev (1):CD006605, 2010 20091598

Norlund A, Ropponen A, Alexanderson K: Multidisciplinary interventions: review of studies of return to work after rehabilitation for low back pain. J Rehabil Med 41(3):115–121, 2009 19229442

Obermann M, Katsarava Z: Update on trigeminal neuralgia. Expert Rev Neurother 9(3):323–329, 2009 19271941

O'Connor AB: Neuropathic pain: quality-of-life impact, costs and cost effectiveness of therapy. Pharmacoeconomics 27(2):95–112, 2009 19254044

Ogawa S, Arakawa A, Hayakawa K, et al: Pregabalin for neuropathic pain: why benefits could be expected for multiple conditions. Clin Drug Investig 36(11):877–888, 2016 27448285

Oh H, Seo W: A comprehensive review of central post-stroke pain. Pain Manag Nurs 16(5):804–818, 2015 25962545

Ohayon MM, Schatzberg AF: Using chronic pain to predict depressive morbidity in the general population. Arch Gen Psychiatry 60(1):39–47, 2003 12511171

Outcalt SD, Kroenke K, Krebs EE, et al: Chronic pain and comorbid mental health conditions: independent associations of posttraumatic stress disorder and depression with pain, disability, and quality of life. J Behav Med 38(3):535–543, 2015 25786741

Ozyalcin SN, Talu GK, Kiziltan E, et al: The efficacy and safety of venlafaxine in the prophylaxis of migraine. Headache 45(2):144–152, 2005 15705120

Pain-Topics.org: Pain Treatment Topics: Opioid Risk Management. 2010. Available at: www.pain-topics.org/opioid_rx/risk.php#AssessTools. Accessed October 14, 2017.

Pani PP, Trogu E, Maremmani I, et al: QTc interval screening for cardiac risk in methadone treatment of opioid dependence. Cochrane Database Syst Rev (6):CD008939 2013 23787716

Passik SD, Kirsh KL: The interface between pain and drug abuse and the evolution of strategies to optimize pain management while minimizing drug abuse. Exp Clin Psychopharmacol 16(5):400–404, 2008 18837636

Passik SD, Kirsh KL, Whitcomb L, et al: A new tool to assess and document pain outcomes in chronic pain patients receiving opioid therapy. Clin Ther 26(4):552–561, 2004 15189752

Passik SD, Kirsh KL, Donaghy KB, et al: Pain and aberrant drug-related behaviors in medically ill patients with and without histories of substance abuse. Clin J Pain 22(2):173–181, 2006 16428952

Patrick N, Emanski E, Knaub MA: Acute and chronic low back pain. Med Clin North Am 100(1):169–181, 2016 26614726

Peles E, Schreiber S, Gordon J, et al: Significantly higher methadone dose for methadone maintenance treatment (MMT) patients with chronic pain. Pain 113(3):340–346, 2005 15661442

Perahia DG, Pritchett YL, Desaiah D, et al: Efficacy of duloxetine in painful symptoms: an analgesic or antidepressant effect? Int Clin Psychopharmacol 21(6):311–317, 2006 17012978

Peres MFP, Mercante JPP, Tobo PR, et al: Anxiety and depression symptoms and migraine: a symptom-based approach research. J Headache Pain 18(1):37, 2017 28324317

Phillips DM; Joint Commission on Accreditation of Healthcare Organizations: JCAHO pain management standards are unveiled. JAMA 284(4):428–429, 2000 10904487

Picavet HS, Vlaeyen JW, Schouten JS: Pain catastrophizing and kinesiophobia: predictors of chronic low back pain. Am J Epidemiol 156(11):1028–1034, 2002 12446259

Pinheiro MB, Ferreira ML, Refshauge K, et al: Symptoms of depression as a prognostic factor for low back pain: a systematic review. Spine J 16(1):105–116, 2016 26523965

Pontell D: A clinical approach to complex regional pain syndrome. Clin Podiatr Med Surg 25(3):361–380, vi, 2008 18486850

Prasad S, Galetta S: Trigeminal neuralgia: historical notes and current concepts. Neurologist 15(2):87–94, 2009 19276786

Rani PU, Naidu MU, Prasad VB, et al: An evaluation of antidepressants in rheumatic pain conditions. Anesth Analg 83(2):371–375, 1996 8694321

Rayner L, Hotopf M, Petkova H, et al: Depression in patients with chronic pain attending a specialised pain treatment centre: prevalence and impact on health care costs. Pain 157(7):1472–1479, 2016 26963849

Reicherts P, Gerdes AB, Pauli P, et al: Psychological placebo and nocebo effects on pain rely on expectation and previous experience. J Pain 17(2):203–214, 2016 26523863

Rief W, Martin A: How to use the new DSM-5 somatic symptom disorder diagnosis in research and practice: a critical evaluation and a proposal for modifications. Annu Rev Clin Psychol 10:339–367, 2014 24387234

Riley J, Eisenberg E, Müller-Schwefe G, et al: Oxycodone: a review of its use in the management of pain. Curr Med Res Opin 24(1):175–192, 2008 18039433

Rojas-Corrales MO, Casas J, Moreno-Brea MR, et al: Antinociceptive effects of tricyclic antidepressants and their noradrenergic metabolites. Eur Neuropsychopharmacol 13(5):355–363, 2003 12957334

Roldán-Barraza C, Janko S, Villanueva J, et al: A systematic review and meta-analysis of usual treatment versus psychosocial interventions in the treatment of myofascial temporomandibular disorder pain. J Oral Facial Pain Headache 28(3):205–222, 2014 25068215

Rosenberg CJ, Watson JC: Treatment of painful diabetic peripheral neuropathy. Prosthet Orthot Int 39(1):17–28, 2015 25614498

Rosenblum A, Joseph H, Fong C, et al: Prevalence and characteristics of chronic pain among chemically dependent patients in methadone maintenance and residential treatment facilities. JAMA 289(18):2370–2378, 2003 12746360

Sandoval JA, Furlan AD, Mailis-Gagnon A: Oral methadone for chronic noncancer pain: a systematic literature review of reasons for administration, prescription patterns, effectiveness, and side effects. Clin J Pain 21(6):503–512, 2005 16215336

Schieir O, Thombs BD, Hudson M, et al: Symptoms of depression predict the trajectory of pain among patients with early inflammatory arthritis: a path analysis approach to assessing change. J Rheumatol 36(2):231–239, 2009 19132790

Schley MT, Wilms P, Toepfner S, et al: Painful and nonpainful phantom and stump sensations in acute traumatic amputees. J Trauma 65(4):858–864, 2008 18849803

Schmidt NB, Santiago HT, Trakowski JH, et al: Pain in patients with panic disorder: relation to symptoms, cognitive characteristics and treatment outcome. Pain Res Manag 7(3):134–141, 2002 12420022

Schreiber AK, Nones CF, Reis RC, et al: Diabetic neuropathic pain: physiopathology and treatment. World J Diabetes 6(3):432–444, 2015 25897354

Seidel S, Aigner M, Ossege M, et al: Antipsychotics for acute and chronic pain in adults. Cochrane Database Syst Rev (8):CD004844, 2013 23990266

Seifert CL, Mallar Chakravarty M, Sprenger T: The complexities of pain after stroke—a review with a focus on central post-stroke pain. Panminerva Med 55(1):1–10, 2013 23474660

Semenchuk MR, Sherman S, Davis B: Double-blind, randomized trial of bupropion SR for the treatment of neuropathic pain. Neurology 57(9):1583–1588, 2001 11706096

Sharma A, Williams K, Raja SN: Advances in treatment of complex regional pain syndrome: recent insights on a perplexing disease. Curr Opin Anaesthesiol 19(5):566–572, 2006 16960493

Sharma A, Agarwal S, Broatch J, et al: A Web-based cross-sectional epidemiological survey of complex regional pain syndrome. Reg Anesth Pain Med 34(2):110–115, 2009 19282709

Silberstein SD: Treatment recommendations for migraine. Nat Clin Pract Neurol 4(9):482–489, 2008 18665146

Silberstein SD: Preventive migraine treatment. Continuum (Minneap Minn) 21(4 Headache):973–989, 2015 26252585

Silberstein S, Loder E, Diamond S, et al; AMPP Advisory Group: Probable migraine in the United States: results of the American Migraine Prevalence and Prevention (AMPP) study. Cephalalgia 27(3):220–229, 2007 17263769

Simon GE, VonKorff M, Piccinelli M, et al: An international study of the relation between somatic symptoms and depression. N Engl J Med 341(18):1329–1335, 1999 10536124

Singer J, Conigliaro A, Spina E, et al: Central poststroke pain: a systematic review. Int J Stroke 12(4):343–355, 2017 28494691

Sivertsen B, Lallukka T, Petrie KJ, et al: Sleep and pain sensitivity in adults. Pain 156(8):1433–1439, 2015 25915149

Smith H, Brooks JR: Capsaicin-based therapies for pain control. Prog Drug Res 68:129–146, 2014 24941667

Solberg Nes L, Roach AR, Segerstrom SC: Executive functions, self-regulation, and chronic pain: a review. Ann Behav Med 37(2):173–183, 2009 19357933

Stacey BR, Barrett JA, Whalen E, et al: Pregabalin for postherpetic neuralgia: placebo-controlled trial of fixed and flexible dosing regimens on allodynia and time to onset of pain relief. J Pain 9(11):1006–1017, 2008 18640074

Staiger TO, Gaster B, Sullivan MD, et al: Systematic review of antidepressants in the treatment of chronic low back pain. Spine 28(22):2540–2545, 2003 14624092

Stanos S, Houle TT: Multidisciplinary and interdisciplinary management of chronic pain. Phys Med Rehabil Clin N Am 17(2):435–450, vii, 2006 16616276

Streltzer J, Eliashof BA, Kline AE, et al: Chronic pain disorder following physical injury. Psychosomatics 41(3):227–234, 2000 10849455

Sullivan MJ, Thorn B, Haythornthwaite JA, et al: Theoretical perspectives on the relation between catastrophizing and pain. Clin J Pain 17(1):52–64, 2001 11289089

Sun EC, Dixit A, Humphreys K, et al: Association between concurrent use of prescription opioids and benzodiazepines and overdose: retrospective analysis. BMJ 356:j760, 2017 28292769

Tack J, Broekaert D, Fischler B, et al: A controlled crossover study of the selective serotonin reuptake inhibitor citalopram in irritable bowel syndrome. Gut 55(8):1095–1103, 2006 16401691

Tasmuth T, Härtel B, Kalso E: Venlafaxine in neuropathic pain following treatment of breast cancer. Eur J Pain 6(1):17–24, 2002 11888224

Tomlinson DR, Gardiner NJ: Diabetic neuropathies: components of etiology. J Peripher Nerv Syst 13(2):112–121, 2008 18601656

Truini A, Galeotti F, Haanpaa M, et al: Pathophysiology of pain in postherpetic neuralgia: a clinical and neurophysiological study. Pain 140(3):405–410, 2008 18954941

Turner JA, Holtzman S, Mancl L: Mediators, moderators, and predictors of therapeutic change in cognitive-behavioral therapy for chronic pain. Pain 127(3):276–286, 2007 17071000

Valet M, Gündel H, Sprenger T, et al: Patients with pain disorder show gray-matter loss in pain-processing structures: a voxel-based morphometric study. Psychosom Med 71(1):49–56, 2009 19073757

VanderWeide LA, Smith SM, Trinkley KE: A systematic review of the efficacy of venlafaxine for the treatment of fibromyalgia. J Clin Pharm Ther 40(1):1–6, 2015 25294655

van Wilgen CP, Dijkstra PU, Versteegen GJ, et al: Chronic pain and severe disuse syndrome: long-term outcome of an inpatient multidisciplinary cognitive behavioural programme. J Rehabil Med 41(3):122–128, 2009 19229443

Verbunt JA, Seelen HA, Vlaeyen JW, et al: Disuse and deconditioning in chronic low back pain: concepts and hypotheses on contributing mechanisms. Eur J Pain 7(1):9–21, 2003 12527313

Verdu B, Decosterd I, Buclin T, et al: Antidepressants for the treatment of chronic pain. Drugs 68(18):2611–2632, 2008 19093703

Veves A, Backonja M, Malik RA: Painful diabetic neuropathy: epidemiology, natural history, early diagnosis, and treatment options. Pain Med 9(6):660–674, 2008 18828198

Vinik AI, Tuchman M, Safirstein B, et al: Lamotrigine for treatment of pain associated with diabetic neuropathy: results of two randomized, double-blind, placebo-controlled studies. Pain 128(1–2):169–179, 2007 17161535

Volpi A, Gatti A, Pica F, et al: Clinical and psychosocial correlates of post-herpetic neuralgia. J Med Virol 80(9):1646–1652, 2008 18649332

Vowles KE, McCracken LM, Eccleston C: Processes of change in treatment for chronic pain: the contributions of pain, acceptance, and catastrophizing. Eur J Pain 11(7):779–787, 2007 17303452

Vowles KE, McCracken LM, Eccleston C: Patient functioning and catastrophizing in chronic pain: the mediating effects of acceptance. Health Psychol 27(2S)(suppl):S136–S143, 2008 18377155

Wernicke JF, Pritchett YL, D'Souza DN, et al: A randomized controlled trial of duloxetine in diabetic peripheral neuropathic pain. Neurology 67(8):1411–1420, 2006 17060567

Wiffen PJ, Rees J: Lamotrigine for acute and chronic pain. Cochrane Database Syst Rev (2):CD006044, 2007 17443611

Wiffen PJ, Derry S, Lunn MP, et al: Topiramate for neuropathic pain and fibromyalgia in adults. Cochrane Database Sys Rev (8):CD008314, 2013a 23996081

Wiffen PJ, Derry S, Moore RA, et al: Antiepileptic drugs for neuropathic pain and fibromyalgia: an overview of Cochrane reviews. Cochrane Database Syst Rev (11):CD010567, 2013b 24217986

Wiffen PJ, Derry S, Moore RA: Carbamazepine for neuropathic pain and fibromyalgia in adults. Cochrane Database Sys Rev (4):CD005451, 2014a 24719027

Wiffen PJ, Derry S, Moore RA, Lunn MP: Levetiracetam for neuropathic pain in adults. Cochrane Database Syst Rev (7):CD010943, 2014b 25000215

Williams AC, Eccleston C, Morley S: Psychological therapies for the management of chronic pain (excluding headache) in adults. Cochrane Database Syst Rev (11):CD007407, 2012 23152245

Wu TH, Hu LY, Lu T, et al: Risk of psychiatric disorders following trigeminal neuralgia: a nationwide population-based retrospective cohort study. J Headache Pain 16:64, 2015 26174508

Yucel A, Ozyalcin S, Koknel TG, et al: The effect of venlafaxine on ongoing and experimentally induced pain in neuropathic pain patients: a double blind, placebo controlled study. Eur J Pain 9:407–416, 2005 15979021

Zhou M, Chen N, He L, et al: Oxcarbazepine for neuropathic pain. Cochrane Database Syst Rev (3):CD007963, 2013 23543558

Ziegler D, Pritchett YL, Wang F, et al: Impact of disease characteristics on the efficacy of duloxetine in diabetic peripheral neuropathic pain. Diabetes Care 30(3):664–669, 2007 17327338

Zochodne DW: Diabetic polyneuropathy: an update. Curr Opin Neurol 21(5):527–533, 2008 18769245

CHAPTER 35

Medical Toxicology

J. J. Rasimas, M.D., Ph.D.

Toxicology is the clinical specialty dedicated to caring for illnesses induced by exposure to exogenous compounds—that is, substances that are not naturally produced by the human body (also known as *xenobiotics*). This chapter focuses on the presentation, evaluation, and treatment of toxicology patients with particular relevance to psychiatric practice, including deliberate overdoses; surreptitious ingestions; accidental poisonings; environmental or occupational exposures to toxins causing neuropsychiatric symptoms; delirium; adverse drug reactions and interactions; and illnesses that represent feared or imagined toxic exposures.

As observed by Paracelsus, the first scientist of toxicology, any substance can be a medicine or a poison, depending on the dose (Deichmann et al. 1986). With very few exceptions, minimal exposures rarely produce progressive or persistent deficits. The level of medical acuity in toxic exposures can vary widely. The effects of toxins may be delayed after exposure, appearing abruptly and then progressing. This means that a diagnosis of poisoning may not be obvious on initial presentation, and seemingly stable patients may suddenly deteriorate and succumb to seizures, arrhythmias, or refractory hypotension (Hoffman et al. 2015). Therefore, psychiatrists need to know enough toxicology to make their own assessments, rather than always relying upon another physician's determination that a patient is "medically clear."

Since the brain is the organ most commonly affected by acute poisoning, any patient whose behavior, level of consciousness, or cognition is acutely disturbed should prompt concerns about toxicity (Maldonado 2008). Thus, many psychiatric consultations have the potential to be toxicologically relevant. Barriers to recognition of a toxic exposure include lack of awareness, deception by patients after intentional ingestion, physicians' failure to consider iatrogenic toxicity, and manifestations of the toxic exposure itself. The most important diagnostic factor in uncovering a toxic etiology is the clinician's consideration of its possibility.

Toxicology in Psychiatric Practice

The consulting psychiatrist is likely to encounter three categories of patients with possible toxic exposures, requiring different approaches:

1. The acutely presenting toxic patient, often with a purposeful ingestion or recreational drug misadventure
2. The neurobehaviorally disturbed hospital patient, sometimes with a mental illness history, whose symptoms may be toxically mediated
3. The subacutely or chronically afflicted outpatient about whom there is a question of toxin exposure versus somatic symptom disorder

Nearly 20% of Americans who die by their own hand accomplish suicide by ingesting toxic substances (Miniño et al. 2007). A patient whose intentional ingestion has not resulted in a substantial change in mental status may be at high risk because of ongoing self-injurious urges, complicating toxicological management (Rasimas et al. 2017). Early involvement of a psychiatric consultant can be valuable even in the critical-care phase of treatment (Rasimas and Carter 2016). General principles in the psychiatric management of the suicidal patient in medical settings are discussed in Chapter 8, "Suicidality."

A number of studies have highlighted the unreliability of patients' reports regarding the identities and amounts of what they ingest in overdose, although stated times of ingestion are typically more accurate and can help to guide management (Pohjola-Sintonen et al. 2000). Cognitive disorders can introduce additional complications, increasing the risk for medication errors that may lead to self-poisoning (irrespective of intent) and interfering with communication of a reliable history to inform toxicological care. The subjective data in any case must therefore always be considered in light of the vital signs, objective physical findings, and laboratory results. The pharmacokinetic profiles of the substances potentially involved define the assessment and monitoring process, as well as the duration of toxicity after a purposeful exposure (Figure 35–1). A short period of observation for a minimally symptomatic patient may be sufficient, but some substances—including extended-release, anticholinergic, and opioid medications—can produce delayed and/or prolonged toxicity.

Physical Examination

Clues evident on physical examination can be particularly helpful in identifying possible overdose or toxin exposure (Pizon et al. 2016). The most common early presentations of drug toxicity involve gastrointestinal (GI) symptoms and central nervous system (CNS)/autonomic nervous system signs. Withdrawal states manifest in these physiological systems as well—opioids with a clear-thinking, self-limited though uncomfortable syndrome; alcohol or sedatives with potentially life-threatening hemodynamic changes and delirium; and stimulants with a relatively anergic presentation characterized by hypoadrenergia, hunger, and dysphoria. Nystagmus is a nonspecific physical finding, but its new onset strongly suggests a toxic process. Although much

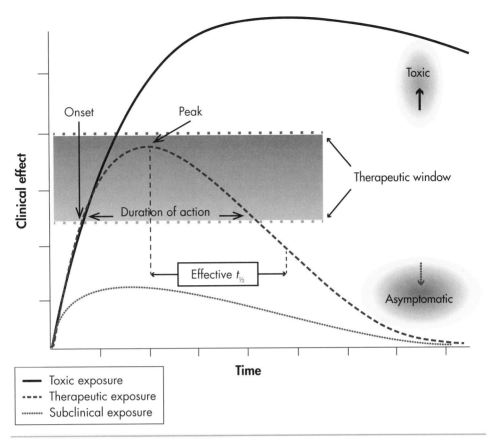

FIGURE 35–1. Pharmacokinetics relevant to a poisoning event.

Under circumstances of a single event of potentially toxic exposure, three parameters define the assessment and treatment process for each suspected substance of concern. *Time of onset* defines how long it will take after exposure to observe a clinical effect. *Time to peak effect* provides an estimate for the point of maximal physiological impact. *Effective half-life* ($t_{1/2}$) defines roughly how long acute consequences will persist if a threshold of clinical effect is crossed. Standard published values for each of these parameters are based on therapeutic dosing (*dashed-line curve*). The therapeutic window is bounded by the minimum dose necessary to produce an observable clinical effect and the maximum dose that can be tolerated without harm. The half-life of a substance is toxicologically irrelevant if a patient has passed the onset and peak times without manifesting any clinical effects (*dotted-line curve*). If an effect is observed but the peak is passed without toxic severity, then further passage of time will only yield a decrease in symptoms (*dashed-line curve*) until the duration of action ends with clearance of the substance below its minimum threshold of effect. Under circumstances of a toxic exposure, pharmacokinetics can be perturbed, with both a delay to peak effect and a lengthening of the effective half-life (*solid-line curve*). Substances that delay their own absorption, readily overwhelm clearance mechanisms, and/or have large volumes of distribution display abnormal toxicokinetics. Proper clinical observation will ensure against missing acuity in the overdose situation, because onset time will remain unchanged, and observable signs and symptoms will not only manifest on the expected timetable but then intensify and persist. In most situations involving toxicity, it will take at least two, and often three, effective half-lives for symptoms to decrease in intensity below the toxic threshold. This guiding principle of toxicokinetics outlines the necessary period of observation and expected duration of treatment, assuming no ongoing exposure and no end-organ damage has been sustained. Under circumstances of chronic exposure (purposeful, accidental, or iatrogenic), toxicity may persist due to high tissue burden and protracted elimination kinetics.

attention is paid to examination of the pupils, size and reactivity are highly variable, except in opioid toxicity, when they are almost always miotic. Cutaneous abnormalities may suggest specific toxins or indicate intravenous drug use. Muscle tone, motor signs, and deep tendon reflexes are also central to the examination. Unusual odors on the patient's breath, skin, clothing, vomitus, or nasogastric aspirate may also provide useful diagnostic clues (Table 35–1) (Goldfrank et al. 1982). The absence of such odors, however, should not be taken as evidence that suspected agents are not present.

Laboratory Testing

Patients in whom purposeful ingestion is suspected or known will often receive specific testing for acetaminophen and salicylate levels, because these are readily available, potentially lethal, frequently coingested drugs with nonspecific clinical presentations, and test results can be obtained rapidly to guide management (Hepler et al. 1986). Relevant concentrations of lithium and anticonvulsants, along with selected toxins such as carbon monoxide, can be assayed rapidly as well, when suspicion for these exposures warrants. Although the yield may be relatively low, some toxicologists recommend testing for lithium and valproate in all acutely presenting bipolar patients, since there is a delay in manifestation of symptoms after overdose, and early intervention can minimize toxicity. Serum levels for many other substances can be ordered, but intervention is typically required well before the results of quantitative testing become available (e.g., tricyclic antidepressants [TCAs]) (Boehnert and Lovejoy 1985).

Abnormalities in conventional laboratory tests such as electrolytes, renal function, and blood gas analysis can point to specific ingestions. Metabolic acidosis with an increased anion gap suggests the ingestion of methanol, ethylene glycol, paraldehyde, toluene, iron, isoniazid, nonsteroidal anti-inflammatory drugs (NSAIDs), or salicylates. The latter often produce a mixed acid–base picture, with coexisting respiratory alkalosis as well. An elevated measured serum osmolarity compared with a calculated osmolarity (i.e., osmolar gap) indicates the presence of a low-molecular-weight osmotically active compound, such as ethylene glycol, methanol, or isopropanol. Hypoglycemia is common in patients poisoned with one of these toxic alcohols or with isoniazid, acetaminophen, salicylates, propranolol, valproic acid, or sulfonylureas. Serum aminotransferase levels are useful, since they will be elevated in most cases of hepatotoxicity caused by medications. Rhabdomyolysis, indicated by elevated serum creatine phosphokinase and myoglobinuria, may be due to prolonged immobility after any overdose with CNS depressive effects (especially opioids), but it is also caused by compounds that impair cellular metabolism, produce muscle rigidity, precipitate seizures, and/or directly impair myocytes (e.g., ethanol, cholesterol modulators, strychnine, antipsychotics, antidepressants, dextromethorphan, stimulants, pesticides, botanicals, venoms) (Janković et al. 2013). Aspartate aminotransferase (AST) is present in myocytes, so elevated serum concentration of this "liver enzyme" out of proportion to alanine aminotransferase (ALT) levels should prompt further workup (Weibrecht et al. 2010), including examination of all major muscle groups for the possibility of compartment syndrome (Curry et al. 1989).

Decreased oxygen saturation of hemoglobin with a normal or increased arterial oxygen partial pressure is found in patients with carbon monoxide poisoning or in methemoglobinemia, which can be caused by metoclopramide, phenacetin, nitroglycerin, topical anesthetics, and some antimicrobials (e.g., dapsone). Noncardio-

TABLE 35–1. **Selected odors from toxic exposures**

Characteristic odor	Possible intoxicant
Bitter almonds/sweaty locker room	Cyanide
Burned rope	Cannabis, opium
Carrots	Water hemlock (cicutoxin)
Disinfectant	Phenol
Fruity	Ethanol, acetone, isopropyl alcohol, paraldehyde, nitrites, chlorinated hydrocarbons (e.g., chloroform)
Garlic	Arsenic, dimethyl sulfoxide (DMSO), organophosphates, white phosphorus, selenium, thallium
Glue	Toluene, xylene, organic solvents
Mothballs	Paradichlorobenzene, naphthalene, camphor
Acrid/pear-like	Chloral hydrate, paraldehyde
Violets	Turpentine (metabolites in the urine)
Rotten eggs	Disulfiram, hydrogen sulfide, sulfa drugs, stibine
Shoe polish	Nitrobenzene
Wintergreen	Methyl salicylate

genic pulmonary edema on a chest radiograph suggests opioid, cocaine, or salicylate toxicity (Schwartz 2015). Some drugs are radiopaque (e.g., heavy metals, phenothiazines, potassium, calcium, chlorinated hydrocarbons) and can occasionally be visualized within the GI tract on roentgenography, but abdominal X rays are rarely helpful in the evaluation of a poisoned patient except to monitor the decontamination of metals or body packets (Craig 2001; Schwartz 2015).

Toxicological Testing

In some cases, despite thorough evaluation, the specifics of a poisoning remain concealed. Toxicology testing may be helpful in confirming the clinical diagnosis. However, identifying all available toxins with a high degree of specificity and sensitivity is impossible because of limitations of time and expense. Instead, drug screening is sometimes performed. Standard urine drug screening is conducted using immunoassay techniques, offering the advantage of rapid turnaround time with detection of some commonly used and abused compounds. Urine screening utility is limited by relatively high false-negative and false-positive rates. Sensitivity for detection of benzodiazepines (notoriously low [Rainey 2015]) has, however, been improving in recent years as part of a general trend toward using rapid mass spectrometry techniques to identify previously hidden analytes (Jagerdeo and Schaff 2016; McMillin et al. 2015). Screening for compounds sharing the tricyclic structure of older antidepressants has been eliminated from most panels—an unfortunate development, in that a positive result can raise suspicion for a variety of deliriogenic anticholinergic agents. Novel substances of abuse (e.g., synthetic cannabinoids, cathinones, synthetic opioids) are not detected by standard screening panels.

Comprehensive toxicology screening may detect a wider range of analgesics, narcotics, psychotropics, and various other drugs but takes time to complete. The best chance to detect an unknown toxin is usually via assay of the urine, where drugs are excreted in concentrated form; testing concurrently drawn blood can be useful for quantitation to correlate drug levels with the clinical picture. It is important to note that negative results of comprehensive testing do not rule out a toxic state, because even many commonly ingested agents cannot be assayed, and because the gathering of bodily fluids may be mistimed. Even true-positive tests can be misleading, since drugs found on screening may not be those responsible for the patient's symptoms (Montague et al. 2001). Substances with a large volume of distribution and/or high fat solubility can be detected in urine for a long time after the last dose, but the clinical presentation may not be the result of those compounds. The history and physical examination (including an account of all available and administered medications before and during hospitalization) are therefore more important in the acute management of drug toxicity than is a comprehensive drug screen (Pohjola-Sintonen et al. 2000). Tandem chromatography–mass spectrometry testing is becoming more widely available in some hospital laboratories, with rapid turnaround times for a broader array of substances (Jagerdeo and Schaff 2016; Kong et al. 2017), but results still may not impact acute treatment (Christian et al. 2017). Assay development for novel synthetics always lags behind use and abuse trends. Toxicology screening and/or quantitation may be more useful in the outpatient setting when chronic exposure is suspected and symptoms are less severe, rather than in the acute hospital setting, where the demand for rapid intervention does not allow time for assays (Hiemke et al. 2011; Rainey 2015; Schütze and Schwarz 2016).

Principles of Acute Exposure Management

The three main goals in the acute phase of toxicological treatment are preventing further drug absorption, providing antidotal therapy, and hastening the elimination of an absorbed toxin. Sometimes toxic effects on patients' behavior can interfere with these goals. Rapid tranquilization with benzodiazepines can protect against injury, prevent seizures, and allow vital medical interventions to proceed. Antipsychotics are effective as well (Battaglia 2005) and may be less likely to exacerbate delirium, but their greater potential for adverse effects or interactions with unknown ingestants (e.g., precipitation of seizures, induction of arrhythmias) warrants caution in their use (Martel et al. 2005; Olson 2007). Physical restraints should be avoided but may occasionally be necessary to prevent patients from interfering with life-saving care (Rasimas and Carter 2016). If information is available to confirm the specifics of the poisoning, and if comorbid conditions and/or toxicities do not preclude its safe use, direct antidotal therapy should be instituted immediately. A list of antidotes for selected known exposures is provided in Table 35–2. Guidance is needed regarding these therapies, since their use is not required in all cases, and some carry a risk of adverse effects. Poison control centers and medical toxicologists can provide specific recommendations, especially for more esoteric or unfamiliar poisons and for management of multidrug ingestions with complex clinical courses.

Except for specific life-saving antidotes against certain toxins, many poisoned patients require only toxidrome recognition and removal of the offending agent with supportive therapy. A standard historical home remedy was gastric emptying by

TABLE 35–2. **Emergency antidotes for selected ingestions**

Toxin	Antidote
Acetaminophen	*N*-acetylcysteine (NAC)
Anticholinergics	Physostigmine
Benzodiazepines and nonbenzodiazepine hypnotics	Flumazenil
Beta-adrenergic blockers	Glucagon
Calcium channel blockers	Calcium, insulin + glucose
Cyanide, hydrogen sulfide	Hydroxocobalamin, sodium thiosulfate
Digitalis glycosides	Digoxin immune fab
Ethylene glycol, methanol	Fomepizole (preferred over ethanol)
Iron	Deferoxamine
Lead	Dimercaprol (BAL), calcium disodium versenate ($CaNa_2EDTA$), succimer (DMSA)
Opioids, alpha$_2$ agonists	Naloxone, nalmefene
Organophosphates and carbamates	Atropine, glycopyrrolate, pralidoxime
Sulfonylureas	Octreotide
Valproic acid	L-Carnitine

Note. BAL=British Anti-Lewisite (2,3-dimercaptopropanol); DMSA=dimercaptosuccinic acid; EDTA=ethylenediaminetetraacetic acid.

induction of emesis with ipecac. However, ipecac can sensitize the myocardium to arrhythmogenic effects of other ingested substances and also perpetuate bulimic behavior, so it is no longer recommended (American Academy of Pediatrics Committee on Injury, Violence, and Poison Prevention 2003). Inducing emesis does not improve toxin retrieval significantly when used in the emergency department, may cause aspiration, and may delay the effective use of more beneficial treatments such as activated charcoal and specific antidotes (Kulig et al. 1985).

Activated charcoal minimizes GI absorption of many toxins by adsorptive binding, producing better toxin recovery and fewer complications than emesis or gastric lavage. Therefore, it should be considered as the primary means of decontamination in most overdoses (Albertson et al. 1989). Use of activated charcoal is not recommended for ingestions of agents that do not adsorb to charcoal, such as ions, solvents, alcohols, and most metals (Table 35–3).

Activated charcoal may be beneficial when given early after an ingestion (most effective within 1 hour) and when used for an ingested drug that has delayed absorption, such as aspirin, anticholinergics, opioids, sustained-release medications, or drug packets in "body stuffers." For patients who present hours after a toxic ingestion, charcoal is usually ineffective. Furthermore, charcoal aspiration can occur, causing bronchospasm and pneumonitis (Givens et al. 1992). Use of activated charcoal should therefore be limited to conscious patients with an intact gag reflex, unless airway protection can be ensured via intubation before nasogastric administration in obtunded patients (Juurlink 2016). Activated charcoal administered in multiple doses enhances the serum clearance of certain medications (Table 35–4), taking advantage of enterohepatic recirculation and adsorption of drugs diffusing back across the GI mucosa

TABLE 35–3.   Toxins poorly adsorbed by activated charcoal

Ethanol, methanol, isopropanol, ethylene glycol	Iron
Acids	Heavy metals
Alkalis	Cyanide
Hydrocarbons	Borates
Lithium	Bromides

TABLE 35–4.   Toxins for which elimination is potentially enhanced by multiple-dose activated charcoal

Valproic acid	Theophylline, aminophylline
Phenobarbital	Digoxin, digitoxin
Carbamazepine	Cyclosporine
Phenytoin	Quinine
Salicylates	Dapsone

(American Academy of Clinical Toxicology and European Association of Poisons Centres and Clinical Toxicologists 1999; Smith and Howland 2015). Constipation progressing to ileus is a potential risk but is exceedingly rare (Dorrington et al. 2003).

In general, decontamination procedures should be used only when an ingestion is recent and potentially life-threatening and when such procedures can be performed without undue risk. Gastric decontamination does not generally improve outcomes in most overdose patients, even though it is still performed (Bond 2002). Whole-bowel irrigation with a polyethylene glycol solution may be useful in certain cases of massive, recent ingestion of medications with sustained release and delayed absorption (e.g., some calcium channel antagonists, extended-release lithium, and enteric-coated aspirin). It can aid in the clearance of other toxins, such as metals that are not well adsorbed by activated charcoal. Whole-bowel irrigation has also been used to aid in the evacuation of large pill fragments and drug packets from "body packers" (Tenenbein et al. 1997). Gastric lavage with the aim of removing unabsorbed compounds is rarely indicated and should be considered only when a patient is seen less than an hour after ingesting a highly toxic substance (e.g., calcium channel blocker, TCA, colchicine) and/or one that delays gastric emptying (e.g., opioid, anticholinergic) or forms concretions (Vale et al. 2004). It is contraindicated in alkali ingestions because of the increased risk of esophageal perforation. Some studies have shown an increase in adverse outcomes with the use of gastric lavage, including aspiration pneumonitis and prolonged intensive care (Merigian et al. 1990). Given the uncertain benefits of gastric lavage, patients who are otherwise asymptomatic should not be sedated and intubated for the sole purpose of performing this procedure (Vale et al. 2004).

To enhance elimination of an absorbed poison, the available procedures that have the greatest value are manipulation of urine pH, hemodialysis, and hemoperfusion. Again, these methods should be used only when the danger of the persisting poison likely exceeds that of removing it and when the method is known to be effective for that toxin. Alteration of urinary pH is effective in hastening elimination only if the toxin is cleared primarily by the kidneys. Diuresis does little to clear compounds that are highly protein-bound, highly lipid-soluble, or hepatically excreted. Alkalinization of the urine enhances elimination of weak acid compounds (3.0<pK<7.2), aspirin and phenobarbital being the most commonly overdosed drugs in this category. Elevation of urine pH is accomplished by adding sodium bicarbonate and potassium to intravenous fluids. In theory, weak bases (7.2<pK<9.8) such as phencyclidine and amphetamine can be eliminated more rapidly in acidified urine, but this course is almost never recommended. Acidosis (metabolic or respiratory) frequently accompanies severe overdoses, and therefore treatment with acidifying compounds risks worsening the clinical course (Olson 2007), especially in patients with underlying kidney or liver disease (Fortenberry and Mariscalco 2006).

In the setting of impaired renal function and/or overwhelming intoxication, extracorporeal therapies may effectively remove drugs that are minimally protein-bound, are highly water-soluble, or have a low volume of distribution. Lithium ions and small molecules such as methanol, ethylene glycol, salicylates, and phenobarbital rapidly diffuse across synthetic membranes and are therefore removed effectively by hemodialysis. Even compounds such as valproate (Ghannoum et al. 2015), carbamazepine (Ghannoum et al. 2014), and phenytoin (Anseeuw et al. 2016), which are protein-bound at therapeutic dosing ranges, may be removed to a clinically meaningful degree by hemodialysis in cases of toxicity with elevated free drug concentrations. Hypotension, hemolysis, hypoxemia, and arrhythmias can result from the procedure, but hemodialysis is still the most widely recommended and utilized modality (Ghannoum et al. 2016). Hemoperfusion has also been shown to be an effective method of extracting some drugs, including barbiturates, TCAs, theophylline, and aspirin. Although hemoperfusion is more expensive than hemodialysis, the facilities and skills necessary for hemoperfusion are essentially the same as those needed to perform hemodialysis. Potential complications include hypotension, thrombocytopenia, hypothermia, and hypocalcemia (Cutler et al. 1987); these risks often outweigh hemoperfusion's benefits. Continuous renal replacement therapy (CRRT) may be a reasonable alternative to hemodialysis or hemoperfusion in certain scenarios, although decreased risk of complications comes at the expense of efficiency (Mendonca et al. 2012).

Chelation therapy can also enhance elimination, and its evidence base—like that for the enhanced elimination techniques of hemodialysis and hemoperfusion—is largely confined to the acute setting. Metal chelators such as ethylenediaminetetraacetic acid (EDTA), dimercaptosuccinic acid (DMSA, or succimer), and 2,3-dimercaptopropanol (British Anti-Lewisite, or BAL) make it possible to quickly remove large amounts of lead (Goyer et al. 1995) or arsenic (Mückter et al. 1997) from the body. Coupling the use of a chelator to other elimination modalities such as activated charcoal, hemodialysis, or hemoperfusion can be lifesaving in some poisonings (e.g., thallium). The same is true for immunological therapies designed to bind up specific compounds such as digoxin, preventing them from exerting their toxic effects in tissues and allowing for their safe elimination.

Overdoses and Toxic Exposures

What follows is a survey of common overdoses and exposures not primarily involving psychotropic compounds; for further details on psychotropic medication and illicit drug toxicities, readers are referred to Chapter 36 ("Psychopharmacology") and Chapter 16 ("Substance-Related Disorders"), as well as to the "Toxidromes" section later in this chapter.

Acetaminophen

Acetaminophen is the pharmaceutical most frequently involved in overdose, given that it is both readily available and potentially lethal. Accidental poisoning is more common in young children and in the elderly, whereas almost all adolescents and adults with acute acetaminophen toxicity have intentionally harmed themselves. An acute overdose of as little as 15 g can cause toxicity in adults, and a single ingestion of 200 mg/kg can bring serious harm to children.

Hepatotoxicity is the primary concern and the target for medical intervention. Following oral ingestion, approximately 94% of the drug is metabolized to the glucuronide or sulfate conjugate, and about 2% is excreted unchanged in the urine. Neither the parent drug nor the conjugated forms are hepatotoxic. The remaining 4%, however, is metabolized primarily through cytochrome P450 (CYP) 2E1 and, to some extent, CYP3A4, to form a toxic metabolite, N-acetyl-p-benzoquinone imine (NAPQI). After therapeutic dosing, NAPQI is conjugated with normal hepatic stores of glutathione (GSH) to produce the nontoxic mercapturic acid, which is excreted in the urine. In the setting of a significant overdose, CYP2E1 metabolizes more acetaminophen, large amounts of NAPQI are formed, and the pool of GSH is rapidly depleted. Direct effects of excess NAPQI and liver failure can impact the functioning of other organ systems, including the kidneys, pancreas, and CNS.

Clinically, patients present with nausea, vomiting, and malaise within 24 hours of acute ingestion. Despite evolving liver injury (as reflected by elevations in hepatocellular enzymes and prolongation of prothrombin time), there can be a window of time when patients look and feel better. If they present for care at this stage, and clinicians fail to consider acetaminophen overdose because of the patient's benign appearance, the consequences can be fatal. Coagulation status declines and transaminase levels can exceed 10,000 IU/L before metabolic acidosis, jaundice, and encephalopathy herald fulminant hepatic failure.

Hence, it is vital to quickly identify patients with significant acetaminophen overdose and institute the antidote N-acetylcysteine (NAC) without delay. NAC repletes GSH stores to detoxify NAPQI and works as an antioxidant to prevent evolving toxicity until nondamaging metabolic pathways clear the parent drug. The need for treatment after a single oral overdose can be calculated based on a timed plasma acetaminophen level drawn at least 4 hours after ingestion (Rumack and Matthew 1975). The "treatment line" defined by this nomogram has been debated over time, with recommendations to move it both up and down based on new rounds of clinical research and experience (Bateman et al. 2014). Currently, a 4-hour level of 150 μg/mL defines a log-linear threshold for antidotal intervention in the United States, Australia, and New Zealand, whereas the United Kingdom uses a 100 μg/mL threshold; some other nations still do not typically treat overdoses in which 4-hour levels are below 200 μg/mL. The choice to treat only when a patient's serum acetaminophen concentration is "above the 200-line" may be made, in part, due to limited resource availability, even though this threshold is most consistent with the original data analysis defining toxicity risk (Prescott 1978). There remains disagreement about the dosing of NAC, with ongoing studies aimed at streamlining protocols and optimizing outcomes (Chiew et al. 2016).

Delay before presenting for antidotal therapy is the most important predictor of poor prognosis. Other risk factors generally relate to the propensity of a given individual to produce more of the toxic acetaminophen metabolite or to be less able to withstand its oxidative effects. Advanced age, states of malnutrition (e.g., anorexia nervosa), and active liver disease predispose patients to greater toxicity. Obesity is associated with higher levels of CYP2E1 activity. Chronic alcohol use also induces CYP2E1 and depletes GSH stores, thus increasing the risk of a poorer outcome. Alcohol co-ingestion at the time of overdose, however, can be slightly protective, since ethanol competes with acetaminophen for CYP2E1, thus decreasing production of the toxic NAPQI.

Salicylates

Toxicity from aspirin and other salicylates is a significant source of morbidity and mortality. Child-resistant packaging has decreased the incidence of aspirin ingestion in children, but intentional overdoses of this ubiquitous analgesic still cause adolescent and adult deaths. The diagnosis of salicylism is often delayed because its symptoms of fever, vomiting, and tachypnea may be attributed to other illnesses, including the disease for which the salicylate was taken.

Aspirin is absorbed rapidly from the upper small intestine under normal circumstances. In the setting of overdose, pylorospasm occurs and absorption is slowed; salicylate serum concentrations can increase for more than 24 hours after ingestion. At therapeutic doses, most salicylate is bound to plasma proteins, but in overdose, the amount of non-protein-bound drug increases, thereby increasing the potential for significant toxicity. Conditions that deplete albumin and other proteins (e.g., anorexia nervosa) predispose patients to a disproportionate risk of toxicity at a given plasma concentration (Alván et al. 1981). Salicylates are eliminated primarily through the kidneys via both glomerular filtration and tubular secretion.

The toxic pathophysiology of salicylism is complex. Metabolic acidosis results from several effects of salicylates, including uncoupled oxidative phosphorylation. Salicylates also produce hyperventilation secondary to direct stimulation of the CNS respiratory center, leading to respiratory alkalosis; unexplained hyperpnea should raise suspicion for aspirin overdose and not merely be attributed to anxiety. The classic acid–base presentation is a mixed one of anion-gap metabolic acidosis with a slight alkalemia driven by respiratory alkalosis (Gabow et al. 1978). Severe dehydration, electrolyte disturbances, and significant glycemic shifts can occur with salicylate toxicity as well.

The usual symptoms of acute toxicity include tinnitus, nausea, vomiting, dehydration, hyperpnea, hyperpyrexia, acute tubular necrosis, and oliguria, with progression to delirium, seizures, and coma. Other less common findings include bleeding, hemolysis, pulmonary edema, bronchospasm, and anaphylaxis. Reversible ototoxicity is directly related to unbound serum salicylate concentration. The onset of symptoms usually occurs within 1–2 hours of an acute ingestion but may be delayed 4–6 hours due to sustained-release preparations, pylorospasm, or formation of gastric concretions.

There is no direct antidote for salicylates, so management is aimed at preventing further absorption and increasing elimination; interventions include activated charcoal, fluid resuscitation with sodium bicarbonate solutions to promote alkaline diuresis, and hemodialysis (Proudfoot et al. 2004).

Nonsteroidal Anti-Inflammatory Drugs

Although much less toxic than salicylates, other NSAIDs are even more widely used in nonprescription products and therefore more frequently encountered in suicidal ingestions. Ibuprofen, naproxen, and ketoprofen exert both therapeutic and toxic effects through competitive, reversible inhibition of type 1 cyclooxygenase. Enzymatic selectivity with the type 2 cyclooxygenase inhibitors (celecoxib, meloxicam, rofecoxib, and valdecoxib) is lost at extremely high doses; therefore, these agents can produce similar toxic presentations in massive overdose.

After an acute ingestion, GI distress in the form of epigastric pain, nausea, and vomiting is virtually always present, and its absence makes toxicity unlikely (Hall et al. 1988). Metabolic acidosis with an elevated anion gap is common. In very large overdoses, confusion and depressed level of consciousness with progression to seizures, coma, and death can result (Halpern et al. 1993). In addition to supportive measures, aggressive intravenous fluid therapy is indicated to eliminate the drug more rapidly, resolve acidosis, and protect the kidneys from acute damage. Unless complications develop from CNS depression, most patients poisoned with NSAIDs survive without long-term consequences.

Carbon Monoxide

Carbon monoxide (CO) is a toxic gas that is essentially undetectable by human sensory modalities. Sources of exposure include combustion engine exhaust, smoke from fires, fuel stoves, and, to a lesser extent, cigarette smoke. Purposeful exposure to exhaust fumes or burning charcoal is a particularly lethal suicide method. The toxin binds to hemoglobin with 250 times greater affinity than does oxygen, thereby markedly reducing tissue oxygen delivery. Most patients experience nausea, headache, and dizziness. Psychosis, depression, mutism, amnesia, and delirium have all been reported as presenting symptoms. Syncope and coma follow more severe exposures. Cardiovascular toxicity progresses from dyspnea and angina to hypotension, myocardial infarction, and potentially lethal arrhythmia.

When a patient is thwarted during a suicide attempt, CO poisoning may be obvious. With a chronic or undifferentiated presentation in the absence of such a history, diagnosis can be challenging. Very few patients actually display classic cherry-red skin; most appear "shocky" and gray. Routine blood gas analysis and pulse oximetry fail to identify poisoning despite profound systemic hypoxia. Serum carboxyhemoglobin concentration is diagnostic and helps to guide therapy; it should be assayed without delay in any overdose patient found in a vehicle. Treatment with 100% oxygen is critically important, as it helps to address hypoxia and enhance elimination of the toxic gas. Hyperbaric oxygenation further speeds elimination of CO and may produce better outcomes in more severely poisoned patients. Persistently altered mental status with poor visuospatial functioning and signs of ataxia and apraxia are the most important indicators of the need for hyperbaric treatment (Weaver 2009). The potential for in utero toxicity due to avid binding interactions between CO and fetal hemoglobin lowers the threshold for more aggressive oxygen therapy in pregnant patients.

Survivors of severe CO poisoning are likely to have residual deficits from hypoxic injury to the CNS. Neuroimaging can reveal cerebral atrophy, periventricular white matter changes, and low-density lesions in the basal ganglia (Brown 2002). Neuropsychiatric sequelae may be present in up to one-half of patients and range from mild memory and concentration deficits to mood and personality changes, parkinsonism, and dense encephalopathy (Aslan et al. 2004; Ku et al. 2006; Lam et al. 2004). Patients have similar complaints after chronic exposure to low levels of carbon monoxide (Myers et al. 1998), but no studies have demonstrated objective neuropsychiatric effects in the absence of a severe, acute episode of poisoning.

Toxic Alcohols

A handful of liquids that are more acutely dangerous than ethanol are occasionally consumed as substitutes by persons with severe alcoholism. Sometimes children are drawn to the attractive colors and/or sweet tastes of such liquids. Frequently these agents are ingested with suicidal intent. Ethylene glycol is the primary ingredient in antifreeze. Propylene glycol is also found in antifreeze and as a diluent in parenteral formulations of lorazepam, diazepam, esmolol, and other medications, making continuous infusions a potential source of iatrogenic toxicity (Zar et al. 2007). Windshield washer fluid and fuel additives contain methanol. Isopropanol is found in rubbing alcohol. Like ethanol, all of these compounds are rapidly absorbed after oral ingestion, and their metabolism depends on alcohol dehydrogenase. It is the body's enzymatic handling of ethylene glycol, propylene glycol, and methanol that creates much of their toxicity.

The initial effects of toxic alcohols are similar to those of ethanol, with slurred speech, ataxia, and CNS depression that can progress to stupor and coma in severe overdose. Because rapid breakdown by alcohol dehydrogenase produces organic acids from both methanol (formic acid) and ethylene glycol (glycolic and oxalic acids), metabolic acidosis with an elevated anion gap is a key finding. Isopropanol is metabolized to acetone, so the result of this ingestion is CNS depression and ketosis (along with the characteristic fruity breath odor) without significant acidosis. The parent compounds and some of their breakdown products are also osmotically active, so an osmolar gap is present. Acidosis and the direct effects of the alcohols and their metabolites lead to end-organ damage, including nephrotoxicity with ethylene glycol and blindness with methanol. Methanol also can cause necrosis in the putamen, the result being an irreversible movement disorder resembling parkinsonism (Sefidbakht et al. 2007).

The mainstay of toxic alcohol treatment is inhibition of metabolism while hastening elimination. Inhibiting alcohol dehydrogenase is a critical intervention for patients with methanol or ethylene glycol poisoning (Barceloux et al. 1999, 2002), but in those with an isopropanol ingestion, such treatment only prolongs CNS effects without providing systemic protection from toxicity and is therefore not appropriate therapy. Fomepizole is the preferred antidote (Brent et al. 1999, 2001), but if any delay before provision of advanced hospital treatment is anticipated, oral doses of ethanol can be temporizing and potentially lifesaving (Jacobsen and McMartin 1997). Elimination of the toxic alcohols can be enhanced by hemodialysis if necessary.

Hydrocarbons and Inhalants

Like the toxic alcohols, hydrocarbons are found in commonly available products, most of them polishes, solvents, lubricants, and fuels. Oral ingestion typically reflects an accident in children or suicidal intent in adults, but fatal outcomes are rare unless aspiration into the lungs occurs. Several hydrocarbons are abused as inhalants; sniffing, huffing, and bagging these agents are all intended to produce a euphoric high. Psychiatric consequences of intentional or unintentional inhalation of hydrocarbons include mood disorders (e.g., affective lability, irritability, depression, mania), psychosis, insomnia, amnesia, confusion, and bizarre/violent behavior. Although purposeful solvent abuse was not documented until 1951, the history of accidental exposures with serious consequences is much older. In the nineteenth-century rubber industry, carbon disulfide toxicity caused mood and psychotic symptoms that resulted in suicides of factory workers (Hartman 1988). Neuropsychiatric impairment is a serious problem with other agents, such as trichloroethylene, methyl chloride, toluene, ethylene oxide, propane, acetone, and nitrous oxide. However, the magnitude and the duration of solvent exposure necessary to cause psychiatric problems remain controversial, as does the potential duration of CNS symptoms following cessation of use. Inhalant abusers have high rates of comorbid psychiatric disorders (Wu and Howard 2007). Many will show brain abnormalities on computed tomography or magnetic resonance imaging, including diffuse white matter changes, cerebral and cerebellar atrophy, callosal thinning, and damage to the basal ganglia (Brown 2002). With chronic abuse of sufficient dose and duration, such changes are often irreversible (Schaumburg 2000). Psychometric testing may delineate functional correlates of the anatomic pathology and help to guide rehabilitation (Filley et al. 1988). Neuropathies can also develop with chronic use and persist long after discontinuation. Large acute exposures may lead to ataxia, cranial nerve palsies, delirium, seizures, and coma. "Sudden sniffing death" can result from cardiac dysrhythmias, usually involving inhalation of fluorinated hydrocarbons (Kulig and Rumack 1981). The primary danger with oral ingestion of hydrocarbons and other solvents is aspiration, leading to chemical pneumonitis. Pneumonitis and associated respiratory compromise can occur merely with huffing, even when the solvent is not aspirated in liquid form.

The management of acute hydrocarbon ingestion is primarily symptomatic. Care of patients with chronic toxicity involves rehabilitative therapies, chemical dependency intervention, targeted psychopharmacology, and neuropsychiatric reassessment.

Pesticides

Agents used to kill animal, plant, and fungal pests have the potential to cause significant acute and chronic toxicity in humans. In the United States, exposures rarely cause death, but intentional ingestions of more toxic mixtures in Africa and the Indian subcontinent result in thousands of completed suicides every year (Gunnell et al. 2007). In the West, environmental toxicity causing more subtle, chronic somatic and neuropsychiatric manifestations is the major public health issue. Additionally, the use of some of these compounds in times of war has produced questions about whether they may have an etiological role in unexplained symptoms found in veterans (Brown 2007; see also "Gulf War Syndrome" section later in this chapter). The following subsections focus on selected pesticides most relevant to psychiatrists.

Strychnine

Strychnine is an alkaloid botanical derivative that was once marketed for therapeutic uses, but is now commercially available only as a laboratory reagent and in products used to kill small mammals and birds. It is, however, a fairly common adulterant in illicit drugs such as heroin, ecstasy, and cocaine (O'Callaghan et al. 1982). Strychnine is occasionally employed with suicidal or homicidal intent. It has been found in some Chinese and Cambodian herbal medicines designed to treat rheumatism and GI illness (Chan 2002; Katz et al. 1996). Strychnine toxicity causes rapid, widespread peripheral manifestations of neural excitation, including nystagmus, hyperreflexia, and severe generalized painful skeletal muscle contraction, often resulting in hyperthermia, rhabdomyolysis, renal failure, tonic respiratory paralysis, and death.

The myoclonus, *risus sardonicus,* and opisthotonic posturing of strychnine toxicity may be mistaken for seizures. The differential diagnosis also includes tetanus, serotonin syndrome, neuroleptic malignant syndrome, stimulant toxicity, and drug-induced dystonia. Patients have both metabolic and respiratory acidosis, as well as myoglobinuria and elevated levels of creatine phosphokinase and serum aminotransferases (Smith 1990). Patients who survive strychnine poisoning do not generally have long-term physical sequelae, but posttraumatic stress disorder (PTSD) may follow the harrowing conscious experience of physical symptoms.

Insecticides

There are a number of insecticides that produce toxicity in humans. Although resolution of even severe, acute exposure to many insecticides is expected to proceed without sequelae, chronic exposure is a well-documented source of morbidity that may be misattributed or remain medically unexplained. Case reports of low-level exposures suggest a range of chronic problems, including memory loss, peripheral neuropathy, and nonspecific dermatological findings (Roldan-Tapia et al. 2006).

Organophosphates are not only used to eliminate pests; some (sarin, tabun, and soman) have also been used in chemical warfare. In rural areas of Taiwan, China, and India, purposeful ingestion of organophosphates leads to many deaths every year (Wei and Chua 2008). Accidental exposure on the farm or in the garden, particularly for children, is also a significant source of toxicity. Medication errors or overdoses with carbamates (e.g., pyridostigmine, neostigmine) pose a similar danger. These substances all exert their effects through inhibition of acetylcholinesterase, resulting in characteristic manifestations of excess cholinergic activity (discussed in the "Toxidromes" section later in this chapter). Organophosphates, as a rule, more readily cross the blood–brain barrier than do carbamates (Gallo and Lawryk 1991), and are likely to produce seizures with progression to coma. Organophosphates are also deadlier if there is any delay in treatment, because their binding to the enzyme is irreversible and produces more severe, longer-lasting cholinergic toxicity (Gallo and Lawryk 1991).

Treatment first requires careful decontamination of skin and clothing to prevent further exposure to the patient (and health care providers), followed by specific antidotes. Atropine counteracts the effects of excessive vagal stimulation; multiple doses are usually necessary. Pralidoxime reactivates cholinesterase by dislodging the toxin from the active site (Wong et al. 2000). Patients who do recover from acute poisoning often suffer no sequelae, although delirium, mood changes, anxiety, and self-limited parkinsonian movements have been described, and some psychiatric symptoms can last for months after the event (Gershon and Shaw 1961; Rosenstock et al. 1990).

Chronic organophosphate toxicity usually arises from work-related exposure. Symptoms include blurred vision with miosis, nausea, diarrhea, diaphoresis, weakness, and other neurological complaints (Eddleston 2015). Pyramidal tract signs are sometimes found (Bhatt et al. 1999); data are mixed on the association between organophosphate exposure and the development of frank parkinsonism (Engel et al. 2001; Taylor et al. 1999). Peripheral neuropathy and CNS effects, including memory complaints, mood changes, and irritable or otherwise abnormal behavior, have also been reported secondary to chronic organophosphate exposure (Jamal 1997).

Other insecticides have been implicated in toxic syndromes with relatively low levels of exposure. Organic chlorines (e.g., dichlorodiphenyltrichloroethane [DDT]) all lower the seizure threshold (Ecobichon and Joy 1994). Some related compounds, such as the antihelminthic lindane, may adversely affect cognition and behavior, particularly in children, for whom this low-cost scabies treatment is most frequently prescribed. Chronic occupational exposure to chlordecone, a highly lipophilic insecticide, can cause diffuse tremors, ataxia, an exaggerated startle reflex, opsoclonus, weakness, weight loss, and metabolic liver injury (Faroon et al. 1995). Intentional overdose of N,N-diethyl-3-methylbenzamide (DEET), found commonly in commercial bug sprays, may cause seizures. Encephalopathy and seizures have been reported in young children with excessive skin exposure to DEET (Briassoulis et al. 2001).

Radiation

Ionizing radiation sources include nuclear weapons and reactors, natural elements (e.g., radon), and consumer products, as well as diagnostic and therapeutic isotopes. Ionizing radiation preferentially harms cells with high turnover rates, including those of the skin, immune system, pulmonary epithelium, and GI tract. In the CNS, radiation damage and necrosis can produce neurological dysfunction and mental status changes, although the mere stress from perceived or actual exposure to ionizing radiation can also result in psychiatric impairment. Symptoms of toxicity include depression, sleep disturbance, fatigue, memory problems, poor concentration, and (rarely) psychosis (Brown 2007). While sometimes necessary for cancer survival, cranial irradiation increases the risk of neuropsychiatric abnormalities, particularly in children (Anderson et al. 2004; Cole and Kamen 2006). However, not all cranial irradiation causes dysfunction, and in some cases, improvement in cognition results, depending on the location and type of neoplasm and the specifics of treatment (Lam et al. 2003; Torres et al. 2003). Ionizing radiation is a developmental teratogen, so high-level exposure of the fetus can cause intellectual disability.

Studies examining whether low levels of ionizing radiation cause neurocognitive dysfunction have been confounded by the frequently high levels of comorbid stress and unrelated illness and injury in those who are suspected of having sustained an exposure. Most long-term studies of radiation survivors conclude that survivors are at risk of mood and anxiety disorders, particularly the latter, because of lasting worries about health consequences of the exposure (Honda et al. 2002; Kawano et al. 2006; Yamada and Izumi 2002). Posttraumatic responses to the mere threat of irradiation after an accident or attack are significant, and psychiatric symptoms are commonly reported even when little or no energy has been released (Brown 2002). "Radiophobia" refers to psychological and functional somatic syndromes that reflect a stress response not due to the radiation itself (Pastel 2002; Pastel and Mulvaney 2001). Emotional and physical manifestations of anxiety typically accompany fears about cancer and other illnesses being caused by various exposures, ranging from nuclear power plants to natural sources to diagnostic radiography.

Non-ionizing radiation does not have the toxic potential outlined above, because of the low energy of electromagnetic frequencies (e.g., radar, microwaves, television signals, mobile telephone transmission). Nevertheless, there are patients with syndromic symptoms similar to those reported in idiopathic environmental intolerance (see "Blame-X Syndromes" section later in this chapter) who are "sensitive" to radiation in the electromagnetic range, and studies have shown that these patients demonstrate certain perceptual differences relative to age- and gender-matched control subjects (Landgrebe et al. 2008). Although clear causal relationship between exposure and symptoms is lacking (Feychting et al. 2005; Rubin et al. 2005), patients may be helped with psychological interventions such as cognitive-behavioral therapy (Hillert et al. 1998; Rubin et al. 2006).

Metals

Despite advances in preventing exposures, metal poisonings continue to cause serious illness, with frequent neuropsychiatric manifestations. The neurotoxic metals of greatest importance to psychosomatic practice are lead, arsenic, thallium, manganese, selenium, and mercury. Toxicity can occur from acute ingestion, but most cases result from chronic exposures with insidious development of vague physical symptoms and psychiatric manifestations. A general workup for neuropsychiatric symptoms suspected to be the result of metal toxicity includes a careful neurological and mental status examination, complete blood count, and screening assays of serum and urine for metals. Even though metals can be chelated, there is a limited role for this intervention in most chronic and/or low-level exposures; guiding patients away from potentially harmful treatments that lack an evidence base is important. Neuropsychological testing can help to delineate cognitive impairment and guide rehabilitation. Specific details about each element follow.

Lead

The syndrome resulting from lead poisoning was classically referred to as *plumbism*. Although acute symptomatic lead poisoning and plumbic encephalopathy are rare since the removal of lead from house paints and gasoline, lead toxicity remains a major problem, particularly in pediatrics, where it is still underdiagnosed. The fact that the major source of lead for children is old paint places inner-city residents at increased risk simply from the high metal content of dust in their homes (Chiodo et al. 2004; Reyes et al. 2006). Children are at greater risk from airborne exposures due to their higher respiratory rates compared with adults. Lead paint has a sweet flavor, and consumption of a single 1-g flake can exceed the permissible weekly intake for any individual (especially a small child) by many orders of magnitude. Some imported toys and low-cost jewelry decorated with lead-based paints can pose an ingestion risk (Weidenhamer and Clement 2007). Contamination of public water supplies has recently become a major concern as well (Hanna-Attisha et al. 2016).

Lead poisoning in adults results from occupational or environmental exposures to lead-based products (Anderson and Islam 2006). Removal of lead from gasoline has markedly reduced airborne emissions, and blood lead concentrations have correspondingly declined. However, indoor shooting ranges without adequate ventilation poison many Americans every year (Laidlaw et al. 2017), and hobbies such as stained glass and ceramics may introduce lead into household air and dust. Certain cosmetics traditionally used by Hindu and Muslim populations have extremely high concentrations of lead. Some Mexican folk remedies—such as azarcon and greta, used for GI disorders—contain large amounts of lead as well.

Lead interferes with normal development and function of the CNS. Elevated serum levels are associated with lower IQ, poor concentration, sleep problems, and mood dysregulation (Bellinger et al. 1987). With acute, progressive poisoning, headache, emesis, clumsiness, staggering, and drowsiness may presage the onset of encephalopathy, which may progress to convulsions, stupor, and coma (Wiley et al. 1995). Other systemic signs and symptoms can help to distinguish milder, chronic plumbism in the differential diagnosis. GI effects include crampy pain, anorexia, weight loss, nausea, and constipation. Lead also causes anemia, peripheral motor neuropathy, nephropathy, and adverse reproductive outcomes. The metal has a long half-life in neuronal tissue and is stored for an extremely long time in bone. Because the majority of total body lead is found in bone, and late-life demineralization allows the metal back into systemic circulation, early exposure has been proposed as a risk factor for Alzheimer's dementia (Shcherbatykh and Carpenter 2007). Conditions such as massive traumatic fracture, hyperthyroidism, and pregnancy can also remobilize lead, with the potential for toxicity to emerge in an adult or in a developing fetus.

An elevated whole-blood lead level is the most useful indicator of exposure. The threshold for acceptable lead levels was originally set at 60 µg/dL, but evidence of attributable risk with lesser exposures has led to steady reductions in this threshold, with the current acceptable level being 10 µg/dL. In the United States, more than 2% of children younger than 6 years have blood lead levels greater than 10 µg/dL (Woolf et al. 2007). Even in the absence of other physical symptoms, there is good evidence for toxic neuronal injury from levels below 10 µg/dL in the form of cognitive and behavioral impairment (Chiodo et al. 2004; Shannon 2003). Abnormalities in speech and language, attention, and classroom behavior also have been reported in relation to low-level lead exposure. A follow-up of lead-exposed but apparently asymptomatic subjects into young adulthood found that the high-lead group had a sevenfold increase in high school graduation failure and a sixfold increase in reading disabilities (Needleman et al. 1990). Behavioral dyscontrol and antisocial personality features are also more prevalent in lead-exposed cohorts in a dose–response relationship—higher blood lead levels in early childhood correlate with greater manifestations of delinquency as children age (Dietrich et al. 2001).

The cornerstone of lead toxicity treatment is identifying the source and terminating exposure. Chelation is important in cases of acute illness and does have a role when assayed levels are high (especially in children), but it is unlikely that chelation will benefit any patient whose blood level is lower than 10 µg/dL. Neuropsychiatric impairments may resolve slowly and incompletely, with a resulting need for rehabilitation, symptomatic psychopharmacology, and psychosocial and educational accommodations (Needleman 2006).

Arsenic

Arsenic is found in commercial, industrial, and pharmaceutical products, and a range of different exposures can result in toxicity. Poisoning may be unintentional, suicidal, homicidal, occupational, environmental, or iatrogenic (Hunt et al. 1999). Contaminated water, soil, and food are the primary sources of exposure for most people. Arsenic is also found in herbicides, fungicides, and pesticides. Arsenic trioxide is used to treat acute promyelocytic leukemia. Asian natural remedy preparations sometimes contain significant levels of arsenic (Saper et al. 2008). Inorganic arsenic is odorless and tasteless and is well absorbed by a variety of routes.

Acute oral poisoning produces nausea, vomiting, and severe diarrhea within minutes to hours (Schoolmeester and White 1980). Hypotension, tachyarrhythmias, and shock often follow. Delirium typically manifests early but can be delayed in onset by days. Peripheral neuropathy with severe dysesthesias and dermatological changes emerge within weeks of ingestion.

Low-level exposure to arsenic over time produces a different picture (Yoshida et al. 2004). Fatigue, anemia, leukopenia, skin hypopigmentation, and hyperkeratosis are common. Peripheral vascular insufficiency, including Raynaud's phenomenon, is observed. Patients suffer from noncirrhotic portal hypertension with elevated transaminases. Memory loss, cerebellar dysfunction, and mild cortical impairment are seen in adults with chronic exposure. Anxiety, irritability, and personality changes have also been reported (Brown 2007). Children show signs of intellectual disability.

Thallium

Poisoning with thallium is now uncommon, given that removal of depilatory and rodenticide compounds from the market has drastically reduced thallium's availability. It still occurs, however, from accidental exposures as well as homicide and suicide attempts (Rusyniak et al. 2002). Thallium is used in the manufacture of some jewelry. It may be ingested in herbal preparations and in adulterated illicit drugs such as heroin and cocaine (Insley et al. 1986; Questel et al. 1996; Schaumburg and Berger 1992). Occupational exposures are rare. Delirium, seizures, and respiratory failure mark the mortal trajectory after acute ingestion.

Chronic thallium toxicity should be suspected in patients when neuropsychiatric complaints (e.g., depression, irritability, paranoia, memory loss, confusion) are accompanied by alopecia, nail dystrophy, painful neuropathy, and GI disturbances (Bank 1980). Chorea and ophthalmoplegia are sometimes observed. CNS pathology includes cerebral and brain stem edema. Psychiatric symptoms may persist long after resolution of other toxic sequelae (Rusyniak et al. 2002). Diagnosis should be confirmed by 24-hour urine collection, given that single-specimen urinary excretion and serum levels of thallium are variable. In a case where poisoning is suspected but urinary assays are negative, hair or nail testing can reveal the diagnosis (as it may for arsenic).

Manganese

Manganese intoxication is usually the result of chronic occupational exposure in miners, metalworkers, and welders who inhale the metal. The earliest descriptions of poisoning in Chilean manganese miners in the early twentieth century outlined symptoms of uncontrollable affective expression with agitation and psychosis, and a similar syndrome is still recognized (Bouchard et al. 2007; Bowler et al. 2007). "Manganese madness" was the term used to describe the initial psychiatric syndrome of compulsive behavior, emotional lability, and hallucinations. Memory and concentration deficits are common. There is also a manganese-based fungicide that is suspected as a cause of chronic neuropsychiatric toxicity. Parkinsonism and other movement disorders frequently occur but usually do not manifest until psychiatric problems have been present for some time. In these cases, brain magnetic resonance imaging often identifies manganese deposition, especially in the basal ganglia (Bowler et al. 2006). Serum and urine assays can be performed, but results do not correlate with symptoms in chronic toxicity. Treatment for acute inhalation is supportive, and pharmacotherapy of chronic neuropsychiatric sequelae is frequently ineffective after manganese has damaged the brain (Bouchard et al. 2007).

Selenium

Selenium is an essential trace element that can cause toxicity at high doses, most commonly from exposure to industrial compounds or dietary supplements. Fatalities are usually the result of purposeful ingestion of selenous acid or selenium salts (Pentel et al. 1985). The acid (found most commonly in gun bluing solutions) causes corrosive injury to the upper GI tract, vomiting, diarrhea, hypotension, myopathy, renal impairment, respiratory failure, and progressive CNS depression (Köppel et al. 1986). Chronic selenosis results in fatigue, brittle hair and nails, and a variety of dermatological changes. Accumulation of selenium also causes hyperreflexia, paresthesias, irritability, depression, and anxiety (Holness et al. 1989).

Assays for whole-blood and erythrocyte concentrations of selenium are more reliable for confirming toxicity than serum levels (Barceloux 1999). Activated charcoal may be useful in acute ingestions, but no other treatments apart from supportive care have established efficacy. Reversing chronic selenosis depends primarily on identifying and removing the source of ongoing exposure. The antioxidants ascorbic acid and NAC may have some value in acute or chronic toxicity.

Mercury

Mercury is found in pharmaceuticals, folk medicines, laboratory and agricultural chemicals, industrial devices, and substituted alkyl compounds that accumulate in the bodies of large carnivorous fish. Toxicity from the metallic form of mercury is mediated through inhalational exposure, whereas organic mercury and its salts cause poisoning via ingestion.

Acute inhalation can cause severe chemical pneumonitis. Acute ingestion of mercury salts produces hemorrhagic gastroenteritis. It is more chronic exposure that gives rise to neuropsychiatric symptoms. Chronic inhalation can lead to a singular combination of personality changes, with shyness and withdrawal alternating with explosive, flushed-face irritability. This syndrome is known as *erethism.* Volatile mercury was once used to prepare fur for hats; erethism is the condition referenced by the epithet "mad as a hatter" (Brown 2002). Anxiety, mania, memory loss, and poor concentration have been reported with elemental mercury poisoning. Patients can also develop tremors and choreiform movements (Sue 2015).

The CNS is the primary site of toxicity with ingestion of organic mercury as well. Symptoms usually differ from those caused by inorganic mercury and include paresthesias, dysarthria, ataxia, and loss of vision and hearing (Winship 1986). Organic mercury compounds are also teratogenic, and fetal exposure can result in developmental disabilities and neurological impairment that mimics cerebral palsy. For this reason, pregnant and nursing women are advised to limit their intake of predatory fish (Mozaffarian and Rimm 2006).

Much attention has focused on the possibility that autism is caused by ethylmercury thiosalicylate (Thimerosal), a preservative used in childhood vaccines. Rigorous epidemiological studies have found no evidence to support a link between mercury in vaccines and autism (Parker et al. 2004) (see also Chapter 26, "Infectious Diseases"). Randomized controlled trials of chelation therapy for autism were halted in late 2008 because of safety concerns (Mitka 2008). There is also no evidence to suggest that the small amount of mercury in dental amalgam produces systemic toxicity that would warrant extraction of fillings or chelation therapy (Fung and Molvar 1992).

Over-the-Counter Remedies

Medicines available without a prescription are commonly used in supratherapeutic doses (both mistakenly and purposely) and are also ingested with suicidal intent. Cough and cold preparations are too often administered by parents and other childcare providers to induce sedation, even in the absence of allergic or infectious symptoms, occasionally with lethal consequences for young children (Dart et al. 2009). In addition to analgesics (discussed earlier in this chapter), some products contain a number of different potentially toxic compounds in combinations that can complicate diagnosis and treatment.

Dextromethorphan

Dextromethorphan is ubiquitous in cough and cold products. This antitussive is a synthetic analog of codeine that is frequently abused by adolescents (Baker and Borys 2002). Its potency in cough suppression is roughly equivalent to that of codeine, but it has very weak opioid activity, even in overdose. The drug primarily enhances serotonin activity via multiple mechanisms and, to a lesser degree, antagonizes glutamate receptors. These neurotransmitter alterations mediate both the desirable and the harmful effects of dextromethorphan. At low levels of intoxication, euphoria and hallucinosis can occur, along with dizziness, ataxia, nystagmus, and akathisia. Serotonin syndrome is common in large overdoses and also occurs at normal doses when the drug is taken with other serotonergic agents. More severe dextromethorphan poisoning induces seizures and CNS depression, with progression to respiratory failure and coma. The drug is efficiently bound by activated charcoal in the recent wake of an acute ingestion. Naloxone has been reported to improve mental status in some symptomatic cases (Schneider et al. 1991), but benzodiazepines, fluids, cooling, and supportive care (i.e., to treat serotonin syndrome and its sequelae) are the cornerstone of dextromethorphan overdose management (Chyka et al. 2007).

Decongestants and Related Drugs

Some sympathomimetic drugs are used to induce local and peripheral vasoconstriction, thereby acting as nasal decongestants. They can be found alone or in combination preparations for use in managing symptoms of upper respiratory infection and environmental allergies. The most commonly used drugs in this class are pseudoephedrine and phenylephrine, both of which are alpha-adrenergic agonists, with pseudo-ephedrine additionally exerting some beta-stimulatory activity (Johnson and Hricik 1993). Ephedrine also has more nonspecific adrenergic effects and is found in herbal preparations ingested recreationally, taken for energy enhancement, or used as adjuncts to fitness regimens (Nelson and Perrone 2000). Hypertension is the main toxic effect of acute concern with all of these agents, particularly in large overdose. However, they have psychiatric effects as well, including anxiety, irritability, euphoria, and insomnia; the presentation of acute and/or chronic abuse can resemble mania, with effects lasting considerably longer than the physical effects on hemodynamics (Dalton 1990; Lake et al. 1983). Survival of the acute phase of toxicity from these short-acting compounds without an adverse vascular event generally leads to full recovery.

Antihistamines

Histamine receptor antagonists are used for the treatment of allergies, motion sickness, and short-term insomnia. This discussion is confined to histamine-1 (H_1) receptor blockers, since the histamine-2 (H_2) blockers are relatively harmless, even in massive overdose (Illingworth and Jarvie 1979; Krenzelok et al. 1987). Accidental supratherapeutic ingestions occur (frequently in children), but toxicity from H_1 blockers is most commonly encountered either in elderly patients with delirium or in suicidal patients after intentional overdose with the most widely available and potentially toxic agent in the class, diphenhydramine. Doxylamine and hydroxyzine are also problematic in overdose. Newer H_1 blockers are more selective for peripheral H_1 receptors and correspondingly less toxic (Nolen 1997).

Acute intoxication presents as anticholinergic poisoning due to direct activity of these compounds on muscarinic receptors and the overlap of histaminergic and cholinergic neurotransmission pathways. Patients often have classic symptoms of flushed dry skin, tachycardia, impaired consciousness, hallucinations, and abnormal movements. Given that H_1 receptor activity is important in memory, attention, concentration, executive function, and regulation of the sleep–wake cycle, it is no surprise that antihistamines precipitate delirium. Slowing of GI motility may prolong absorption and the duration of toxicity from these otherwise short-acting agents. Seizures and rhabdomyolysis occur in serious overdose. Massive diphenhydramine ingestion can produce cardiac conduction disturbances and precipitate lethal arrhythmias secondary to sodium channel blockade (similar to TCA toxicity). Cardiotoxicity, as with TCAs, requires alkalinization of the serum using bicarbonate-containing intravenous fluids. The cholinesterase inhibitor physostigmine is an effective antidote for anticholinergic symptoms (Burns et al. 2000). In more severe poisonings, multiple doses of this short-acting remedy may be required. Use of physostigmine is discussed in more detail in the following section.

Toxidromes

Certain constellations of signs and symptoms, commonly called *toxidromes,* may suggest poisoning by a specific class of compounds (Table 35–5). The findings represent direct pharmacological effects of the agents in question, thus providing objective clinical data about the status of the patient and what has been ingested. Recognition of such patterns can be very helpful, but clinical pictures are not always obvious. It is important to seek historical information on all of the potential medications and substances to which a patient may have access and to attend well to the details of the presentation and evolving course, because polydrug overdoses and/or the effects of medical interventions may result in overlapping and confusing mixed syndromes. Nevertheless, recognition of the dominant features of particular classes of pharmacological toxicities can be a vital diagnostic and therapeutic starting point. Because every toxidrome discussed in this section may present with delirium, pattern recognition can help guide rational pharmacological intervention.

Anticholinergics

Anticholinergic delirium occurs frequently because many common medications and other xenobiotics have anticholinergic properties. It is a particularly prevalent problem in elderly medically ill individuals, who, on average, take more medications and are more sensitive to their adverse effects. A number of commonly used drugs not typically classified as anticholinergics (e.g., antipsychotics, muscle relaxants, antihypertensives) do possess some anticholinergic activity (Tune 2000). Anticholinergic toxicity in the CNS causes delirium, frequently with mumbling speech and carphology or floccillation—aimless "picking movements" of the fingers. Vivid visual hallucinosis and undressing behavior are not uncommon. Peripheral anticholinergic signs, although not always present in individuals with delirium, can include tachycardia, dry mouth, flushed skin, temperature elevation, mydriasis, ileus, and urinary retention (see Table 35–5). Duration and severity of CNS manifestations typically exceed those of peripheral effects (Tune 2001).

Most patients recover with removal of the offending agents and provision of supportive therapy, but delirium may last for well over 24 hours after an acute overdose of muscarinic antagonists, and considerably longer if medications that add to the problem continue to be administered. Physostigmine is a useful antidote that can rapidly resolve delirium. Because it has a short half-life, repeated weight-based doses (0.02 mg/kg given 0.5 mg/min IV) may be needed in severe anticholinergic toxicity. Extensive clinical experience has documented physostigmine's safety and utility in anticholinergic states induced by medications that can affect cardiac conduction (Rasimas et al. 2014; Schneir et al. 2003). Relative contraindications to the use of physostigmine include reactive airway disease, active parkinsonism, and atrioventricular blockade. Side effects of physostigmine include nausea, vomiting, diarrhea, and seizures; only excessive dosing would be expected to produce bronchospasm or significant bradycardia (Rasimas et al. 2014).

Cholinergics

The cholinergic syndrome is uncommon but is important to recognize, because lifesaving treatment is available. Cholinergic toxicity produces a "wet" patient (profuse sweating, sialorrhea, lacrimation, vomiting, diarrhea, urinary incontinence), as opposed to the anticholinergic syndrome, which typically causes the patient to be "dry." The CNS (e.g., seizures, coma) and skeletal muscles (e.g., weakness, fasciculations) can also be involved (see Table 35–5). Cholinergic excess is most frequently caused by accidental organophosphate or carbamate pesticide exposure, which may occur

TABLE 35–5.   Toxidromes: prominent clinical findings

Drug class	Examples	Clinical signs	Antidote
Anticholinergics	Atropine, antihistamines, scopolamine, antispasmodics, TCAs, phenothiazines, antiparkinsonian agents, jimsonweed	Agitation, hallucinations, picking movements, tachycardia, mydriasis, dry membranes, hyperthermia, decreased bowel sounds, urinary retention, flushed/dry skin	Physostigmine
Cholinergics	Organophosphates, carbamate insecticides, cholinesterase inhibitors	Hypersalivation, lacrimation, incontinence, gastrointestinal cramping, emesis, bradycardia, diaphoresis, miosis, pulmonary edema, weakness, paralysis, fasciculations	Atropine, glycopyrrolate, pralidoxime
Opioids	Oxycodone, hydrocodone, hydromorphone, propoxyphene, fentanyl, meperidine, morphine, codeine, heroin, methadone, buprenorphine, carfentanil	CNS and respiratory depression, miosis, bradycardia, hypotension, hypothermia, pulmonary edema, hyporeflexia	Naloxone, nalmefene
Sedative-hypnotics	Benzodiazepines, zolpidem, zaleplon, eszopiclone, barbiturates, ethanol, chloral hydrate, ethchlorvynol, meprobamate, various muscle relaxants	CNS depression, hyporeflexia, slow respirations, hypotension, hypothermia, bradycardia	Flumazenil (for some)
Sympathomimetics	Psychostimulants, amphetamines, pseudoephedrine, phenylephrine, ephedrine, cocaine, synthetic cathinones and other phenethylamines	Hypertension, tachycardia, arrhythmias, agitation, paranoia, hallucinations, mydriasis, nausea, vomiting, abdominal pain, piloerection	Benzodiazepines, alpha$_2$-adrenergic agonists, direct vasodilators

TABLE 35–5. Toxidromes: prominent clinical findings *(continued)*

Drug class	Examples	Clinical signs	Antidote
Neuroleptics	Typical and atypical antipsychotics, phenothiazine antiemetics	Hypotension, oculogyric crisis, trismus, dystonia, ataxia, parkinsonism, anticholinergic manifestations (some)	Physostigmine (for some)
Serotonergics	SSRIs, SNRIs, TCAs, MAOIs, buspirone, vortioxetine, tramadol, meperidine, fentanyl, dextromethorphan, sibutramine, phenethylamines and some synthetic cannabinoids	Akathisia, tremor, agitation, hyperthermia, hypertension, diaphoresis, hyperreflexia, clonus, lower extremity muscular hypertonicity, diarrhea	Benzodiazepines, alpha$_2$-adrenergic agonists, cyproheptadine[a]

Note. CNS=central nervous system; MAOIs=monoamine oxidase inhibitors; SNRIs=serotonin–norepinephrine reuptake inhibitors; SSRIs=selective serotonin reuptake inhibitors; TCAs=tricyclic antidepressants.
[a]Evidence supporting cyproheptadine's effectiveness in cases of severe serotonin toxicity is lacking (Isbister et al. 2007).

through unsuspected dermal contamination (Hodgson and Parkinson 1985). Such agents and other cholinesterase inhibitors used therapeutically for dementia can be employed in suicide attempts as well. Cholinergic effects are also the cause of toxicity from "nerve gases" such as sarin and from clitocybe and inocybe mushrooms. Recognition of the cholinergic syndrome should prompt the use of atropine and, in some cases of severe toxicity from selected agents, the cholinesterase regenerator pralidoxime (Eddleston et al. 2002; Syed et al. 2015).

Opioids

Toxicity from opioids progresses from analgesia to anesthetic CNS depression, coma, shock, and death. Respiratory depression is particularly pronounced with opioid overdose, and the tidal volume or respiratory rate can be diminished before decreases in blood pressure or pulse occur. Miosis is also characteristic (see Table 35–5) and is a fairly reliable finding in pure opioid toxicity (Sporer 1999). The diagnosis of opioid overdose is often confirmed by administration of naloxone or nalmefene in doses adequate to reverse the toxidrome (Hoffman and Goldfrank 1995). Naloxone has an elimination half-life of about 1 hour, whereas that of nalmefene is greater than 10 hours, making the latter μ-receptor antagonist potentially useful in the case of opioid toxicity from a long-acting drug (e.g., methadone) (Glass et al. 1994). In most patients, naloxone is the preferred agent, since a shorter-acting antidote allows for more careful titration without precipitation of withdrawal. In known chronic users of opioids, starting with a 0.04 mg intravenous dose of naloxone and carefully repeating this dose every 30 seconds until respiratory drive returns is a reasonable approach to avoid triggering dangerously agitated withdrawal (Hoffman et al. 2015). A dose of 0.4 mg is usually sufficient to restore adequate ventilation; higher doses merely increase the likelihood of agitated withdrawal without providing added benefit to neurological or respiratory status—unless the antidote is being employed to reverse high-affinity synthetic opioids (Nelson and Olsen 2015), in which case doses of 2 mg or more may be useful. Ongoing monitoring after antidote administration is vital, since cardiopulmonary symptoms are not reversed as durably as CNS depression, and life-threatening symptoms can recur.

Sedative-Hypnotics

Sedative-hypnotic agents can produce neurological depression similar to that produced by opioids, and are frequently coingested (or, unfortunately, coadministered in the hospital) to the point of toxicity. "Pure" gamma-aminobutyric acid (GABA)–ergic toxidromes can sometimes be distinguished on the basis of history, relatively preserved pulmonary function, and the absence of constricted pupils (see Table 35–5). When taken in sufficient doses, sedative-hypnotics cause general anesthesia, with a complete loss of awareness and reflex activity and, potentially, deterioration in cardiopulmonary function. However, the effect of benzodiazepines on heart rate and blood pressure is not nearly as profound as that of opioids. Reversal of this syndrome can be accomplished with the benzodiazepine antagonist flumazenil. In addition to its use in reversing toxicity from benzodiazepines and nonbenzodiazepine hypnotics (e.g., zolpidem, zaleplon, eszopiclone), flumazenil has shown some efficacy in overdoses of the centrally acting skeletal muscle relaxants baclofen, carisoprodol, and metaxalone (Kim

2007). However, flumazenil must be used with caution in the context of mixed overdoses that may include agents that are proarrhythmic or proconvulsant, given that GABA activity is protective against drug-induced arrhythmias and seizures (Seger 2004). Autonomic indices, along with examination of motor and reflex activity, guide proper patient selection (Rasimas et al. 2015). Then, so long as doses are kept low (0.5 mg) and are delivered over at least 30 seconds into a flowing intravenous line, side effects due to flumazenil (including benzodiazepine withdrawal) are generally avoided (Rasimas et al. 2015), although patients can emerge from sedation in a transient state of anxiety (Ngo et al. 2007). Flumazenil is short acting, so multiple doses may be necessary, and continued neurological and cardiopulmonary monitoring is vital.

Sympathomimetics

The sympathomimetic syndrome is usually seen after acute or chronic abuse of cocaine, amphetamines, synthetic designer drugs (e.g., cathinones), or decongestants (discussed earlier in the section "Decongestants and Related Drugs"). The clinical picture overlaps with that of serotonin syndrome, as these compounds have multiple neurotransmitter effects (Kehr et al. 2011). Signs of the sympathomimetic syndrome include agitation, tachycardia, hypertension, mydriasis, and piloerection (see Table 35–5). In contrast to anticholinergic poisoning, the skin is typically not dry, but the two toxidromes can be difficult to distinguish on clinical examination. Mild toxicity rarely leads to cardiac complications, but large sympathomimetic overdoses can produce arrhythmias, cardiovascular compromise, and shock. Patients may be psychotic, with intricate and paranoid delusions (Berman et al. 2009). Seizures are common, and the postictal state can contribute further to alterations in mental status. No specific antidotes exist, but benzodiazepines are the cornerstone of treatment because they attenuate catecholamine release, reduce hypertension, prevent seizures, and provide helpful sedation. Supreme agitation has been observed, with a need for potent, rapid-acting sedatives to prevent hyperthermia and acidosis from becoming lethal and to protect patients and emergency personnel from injury. Ketamine has been advocated as an option, but despite the critical advantage of shorter time to sedation, this catecholamine releaser may generate more complications than traditional sedatives in patients with "agitated delirium" caused by sympathomimetics (Cole et al. 2016; Sleigh et al. 2014). Central alpha$_2$ agonists (e.g., dexmedetomidine) may have a role in agitation management while providing desired sympatholysis (Lam et al. 2017). Beta-blockers should be used with caution because they may leave alpha-adrenergic stimulation unopposed; thus, direct vasodilators such as hydralazine, nitroprusside, or phentolamine are preferred for treatment of severe hypertension that does not respond to sedatives alone (Hoffman and Nelson 2016). Failure of confusion and agitation to resolve with physostigmine can help to distinguish this toxidrome and serotonin syndrome from anticholinergic delirium. Psychiatric sequelae from sympathomimetic toxicity can linger long after physical symptoms have resolved and may require antipsychotic medication (Berman et al. 2009).

Antipsychotics

Toxidromes involving psychotropic compounds that block dopaminergic transmission are discussed in depth in Chapter 36, "Psychopharmacology." These compounds were initially called "neuroleptics"—and continue to be known by this name in much of the toxicological literature—due to their slowing and restrictive impact on a range of neurological functions. While antidopaminergic effects may dominate adverse reactions with therapeutic use (see Table 35–5), many antipsychotic medications are highly anticholinergic in overdose, making physostigmine a potentially useful antidote. Neuroleptic malignant syndrome is an idiopathic extreme extrapyramidal reaction that results in severe muscle rigidity, rhabdomyolysis, hyperthermia, autonomic instability, and altered mental status; it requires discontinuation of antipsychotic medication and aggressive symptom-focused medical interventions. The varied and complex pharmacological effects of antipsychotic medications make supportive care after removal of the offending agent key to management in any case of toxicity.

Serotonergics

Serotonergic agents (sometimes in suicidal monoingestion or unintentional combined polypharmacy, but even more frequently with concomitant use of cocaine or other stimulants) can produce serotonin syndrome, characterized by neuromuscular symptoms, hyperthermia, and altered mental status. Classic signs of lower-extremity muscle rigidity, hyperreflexia, and especially ankle clonus, along with increased GI motility and diaphoresis, help to distinguish this potentially lethal toxidrome from anticholinergic poisoning (see Table 35–5). In addition to differences in precipitating medications, neuroleptic malignant syndrome does not cause GI symptoms and typically results in more generalized and severe muscle rigidity without hyperreflexia (Boyer and Shannon 2005; Caroff 2003). It is important to note, however, that the newest antipsychotic medications that function as partial agonists at both dopamine and serotonin receptors (i.e., aripiprazole, brexpiprazole, and cariprazine) can contribute to serotonin toxicity, produce confusing neuromuscular signs, and complicate the diagnostic picture. Serotonin toxicity demands removal of the offending agents and supportive care with fluids and cooling measures. It is also important that medications employed in supportive care do not exacerbate the syndrome; thus, fentanyl should be avoided in toxicology patients in whom serotonin excess is suspected (Pedavally et al. 2014). Benzodiazepines are the mainstay of pharmacological treatment. The oral antihistamine cyproheptadine has some antiserotonergic activity and may be useful for symptom management in cases of mild to moderate toxicity, but it has not been demonstrated to improve outcomes (see Table 35–5). Cyproheptadine may reduce symptoms but can only be administered orally, so severely affected patients are unable to benefit from it and instead require large doses of parenteral benzodiazepines, sometimes augmented by other sedatives (Isbister et al. 2007). As in sympathomimetic toxicity, there may be a role for alpha$_2$ agonists to target hyperautonomia and reduce the GABAergic treatment burden (Lam et al. 2017). Serotonin syndrome is discussed further in Chapter 36, "Psychopharmacology."

Gulf War Syndrome

Gulf War syndrome refers to the medically unexplained somatic symptoms of thousands of military and civilian personnel who served in conflicts in the Persian Gulf. Over 10% of returning troops have reported a variable host of symptoms, including rashes, GI upset, fatigue, muscle aches, paresthesias, headaches, memory impairment, concentration difficulties, irritability, and insomnia (Cohn et al. 2008). These presentations, however, do not constitute a toxidrome, for with the majority of the symptoms being subjective, nonspecific, and referable to multiple organ systems requiring multiple pharmacological mechanisms, the likelihood of a toxic etiology is quite low (Iversen et al. 2007; Kang et al. 2009). Similarities between the troops' presentations and those of troops returning from previous wars led some experts to conclude that Gulf War syndrome represents a complex reaction of psyche and soma to the many severe traumas of armed conflict (Iversen et al. 2007). While various toxic explanations continue to be raised because deployed military personnel were given pest repellents, antidotes, and vaccines (e.g., Nettleman 2015), no causal role for any of these compounds has been substantiated. Treatment is therefore not best accomplished using a disease model that anticipates identification of specific etiological agents. Since toxicological mechanisms neither explain the disability nor suggest interventions to address it, a population-based multidisciplinary biopsychosocial approach is advised (Engel et al. 2006). Proper formulation and intervention includes the recognition that PTSD almost always manifests somatic symptoms, and patients with Gulf War syndrome may be best treated using a model that acknowledges xenobiotic exposure as one aspect of the traumatizing experience that produces phases and stages of illness (McFarlane et al. 2017).

Blame-X Syndromes

In some cases, not only does the history fail to reveal a specific toxic exposure but the examination and laboratory testing also do not suggest that an exogenous substance is responsible for the patient's suffering. As exemplified by the Gulf War syndrome, there is a growing number of conditions in which a constellation of complaints is attributed to an exposure with lack of corresponding objective toxicological data. Some such conditions involve a single suspected exposure, while others involve concerns about repeated or continuous dosing from the environment. In many instances, specific agents have been investigated but have failed to meet causality standards, and in other instances, a toxic etiology seems plausible but no compounds have yet been identified. Although it is clear that psychiatric factors play a major role for many such patients, it is important to remember that the history of medicine is filled with illnesses viewed as psychogenic until physiological causes were elucidated.

A helpful framework for conceptualizing the emergence and evolution of these syndromes in the modern world was laid out by Dr. Alvan Feinstein, who referred to functional somatic presentations with external attributions as the Blame-X syndrome (Feinstein 2001). Availability of almost limitless diagnostic (including toxicological) testing contributes to medicalization of distress. On the basis of mere statistical probability, some abnormal results are bound to arise, even if they have nothing to do with a patient's complaints. There is then a tendency to abandon the demand for pathophysiological correlation of symptoms and objective findings. As a result, early suspicion and a corresponding desire for answers prompt the appellation of new diseases before etiologies have been rigorously established. Such Blame-X rendering of diagnoses can stand in the way of patients' functional recovery and also impede ongoing research that could properly elucidate underlying causes (Feinstein 2001). Three of these related syndromes involving toxicological issues are discussed below.

In all of these Blame-X syndromes involving medically unexplained symptoms, there is a broad psychiatric differential diagnostic spectrum, including somatic symptom, posttraumatic stress, obsessive-compulsive, psychotic, and factitious disorders, as well as health anxiety, abnormal illness behavior, and malingering. The longitudinal course of symptoms that are initially unexplained is variable and depends on a host of factors, including their nature and severity as well as the demographics of the population in which they arise (Carson et al. 2003; Crimlisk et al. 1998). Long-term complaints, especially those that wax and wane or worsen with time, are very unlikely to be toxicological in origin unless some ongoing exposure can be documented (Leikin et al. 2004).

Medication Sensitivity

Some patients have an extensive list of medication intolerances. The term *medication sensitivity* is being used here not to label a new syndrome, but rather to describe a characteristic complaint of patients commonly encountered in practice. It should be distinguished from *multiple chemical sensitivity,* a condition synonymous with idiopathic environmental intolerance (discussed in the following subsection), particularly with reference to individuals who are sensitive to odors and airborne substances. Because some patients have concerns about both therapeutics and environmental xenobiotics, the term *medication sensitivity* as used here refers to patient symptoms or experiences that are attributed specifically to medications.

The majority of drug allergy entries in medical charts are not indicative of true allergic reactions, but instead are presumed medication toxicities. Patients with extensive medication sensitivities may blame unrelated symptoms on a relatively benign medication given in the recent or remote past (Heller et al. 2015), but they lack objective physical or pathological findings. Most patients who seem to respond poorly to a number of drugs do not have elevated allergic sensitivity to antigenic challenge (Mitchell et al. 2000). Medication rechallenge studies, especially double-blind trials, that would help to document a starting point for further toxicological study of these patients are also lacking (Waddell 1993). Some of these drug reactions are "nocebo" responses—adverse effects that would occur even with placebo because of the patient's anticipatory anxiety and pessimistic expectation that a drug will produce unpleasant or harmful side effects (Amanzio et al. 2009). Although little research has been performed to better understand patients with extensive nonallergic medication intolerance, clinical experience indicates a high rate of psychiatric comorbidity (Black 2000) and also a higher frequency of medical complaints and contacts with medical services in general (Faasse et al. 2015). Assisting patients to seek relief from nonpharmacological therapies may represent the most important intervention in such cases.

Idiopathic Environmental Intolerance

Some patients report a constellation of symptoms that they ascribe to the toxic effects of one or more components of the external environment. Rather than identifying a medication as the precipitant of their symptoms, most patients in this category attribute their symptoms and impairments to ongoing exposures to various agents. *Idio-*

pathic environmental intolerance has also been labeled *multiple chemical sensitivity, environmental somatization syndrome, environmental allergy syndrome,* and, in earlier terms, *total allergy syndrome* or *twentieth-century disease* (the latter name emphasizing the suspected role of ecological threats from the modern industrialized world). Characteristics of the syndrome include 1) onset after an environmental exposure that may have produced minimal (or no) objective evidence of health effects; 2) symptoms that wax and wane, that may vary in response to stimuli, and that are referable to multiple organs and systems; and 3) lack of evidence of organ damage or of abnormal test results to account for symptoms (Fung 2004a).

Suspected toxins include construction materials, fabrics, food additives, drinking water, fumes, non-ionizing radiation, and agrochemicals. Symptoms are as varied as the causes and may include shortness of breath, palpitations, headaches, fatigue, insomnia, cough, nausea, diarrhea, constipation, paresthesias, muscle twitching, skeletal pain, bloating, and diaphoresis. An extensive review of the clinical science found no evidence of toxic or allergic mechanisms that might explain the symptoms (Hetherington and Battershill 2013). Hygienic factors should be considered but rarely contribute to an effective treatment plan unless an epidemic of exposure—and therefore, perhaps, a bona fide toxin—is suspected (Göthe et al. 1995).

Population-based research suggests that health anxiety of this type exists on a continuum, and that greater concern about the dangers of xenobiotics from modern life correlates with depression and lower functionality (Rief et al. 2012). Patients are not similar to those with major mood or psychotic illnesses (Weiss et al. 2017), but instead share features with those suffering from somatic symptom disorders (Bailer et al. 2005; Bornschein et al. 2002). In outpatient toxicology clinic studies, lack of objective physical findings in patients presenting with concerns about a single toxin correlate with negative chemical assay results and high degrees of maladaptive projection and somatization (Leikin et al. 2004; Zilker 2002). Malingering is not uncommon. On the other hand, formally diagnosed psychiatric illness does not fully account for the association between worries about the modern world being unhealthy and the experience of nonspecific physical symptoms (Baliatsas et al. 2015). At the extreme of severity, management of comorbid psychiatric illness is indicated and can provide a starting point for longer-term mental health intervention in this group of patients, who otherwise tend to flee from psychotherapeutic interventions. Treatment of idiopathic environmental intolerance should be directed toward minimizing external attributions and emphasizing functionality through behavioral and cognitive therapies (Staudenmayer 2000).

Sick Building Syndrome

Concerns about symptoms attributable to a particular indoor environment, usually the workplace, characterize the *sick building syndrome* (SBS). Patients frequently complain of lethargy, blocked nasal airways, dry throat, mucosal irritation, and headaches. Some feel chest tightness and dyspnea. Suspected toxins include insulation and other construction materials, residues from office products, and inadequately ventilated airborne contaminants, including fungal spores. In cases in which toxic precipitants are identified, susceptible individuals show elevated histamine release that appears to correlate with respiratory symptoms (Meggs 1994). When an underlying disease such as bronchitis, asthma, or hypersensitivity pneumonitis is discovered, targeted treatment can be effective. Although direct evidence of infectious disease or toxic exposure in individual patients is typically lacking, some studies have supported a possible role for mold species (Burge 2004; Cooley et al. 1998) or certain volatile compounds (Sahlberg et al. 2013) in buildings where prevalence rates are high. Other data do not support links between symptoms and either toxins (Glas et al. 2015) or airborne pathogens (Sahlberg et al. 2013; Straus et al. 2003). Treatment studies with antibiotics and antifungals have yet to yield benefit (Straus et al. 2003).

Some patients present with complaints of neuropsychiatric impairment claimed to be secondary to brain damage from mold exposure, but medical evaluations do not demonstrate any neuropathology. Malingering on neuropsychological testing of litigious individuals in this group is not uncommon (Stone et al. 2006). The prevalence of SBS is higher in women who have desk jobs involving computer work and who perform a substantial amount of photocopying (Skov et al. 1989). However, toxins in these specific environments have not been identified, and variable symptoms are found in similar workspaces. Psychosocial factors related to workplace stress and job satisfaction correlate with somatic symptoms but in limited controlled studies do not account for patient differences attributable to factors about the buildings themselves (Skov et al. 1989). Thus, some research supports the idea that sufferers of SBS are "canaries in coal mines"—having identified unhealthy workplaces in which attention to cleanliness, lighting, temperature, ventilation, and other aspects of the physical environment, in addition to psychosocial climate, has the best chance of decreasing illness burden (Abdel-Hamid et al. 2013). Staying away from the building in question does resolve many—but not all—cases of this illness (Fung 2004b), but this option is not available to many low-income sufferers of SBS, in whom low education, lack of employment, and dissatisfaction with housing may correlate with symptoms (Barmark 2015). Supportive mental health treatment to aid with management of associated stress and comorbid conditions is the only currently relevant psychiatric intervention.

Conclusion

A thorough history (often gathered from several sources) and physical examination are key to toxicological diagnosis. Medication toxicities are a frequent and commonly misdiagnosed problem in hospitalized patients. Many psychiatric patients misuse drugs with a variety of motivations and corresponding outcomes. Exposures to other poisons may be intentional or accidental, obvious or hidden, and may occur at home, in the workplace, or even in the hospital. The differential diagnosis of unexplained acute or chronic neuropsychiatric symptoms should include potential exposures to agents capable of causing CNS toxicity. Removal of the patient from sources of ongoing exposure and institution of appropriate treatment are required. Psychiatric consultation may uncover precipitating factors related to addiction, vulnerability, abuse, or malicious intent, with corresponding opportunities to make the acute hospital stay less traumatic and reduce the likelihood of recidivism (Rasimas and Carter 2016). In patients with functional impairment attributed to toxic reactions who have no demonstrable underlying toxic pathology, psychotherapeutic interventions, beginning with a supportive stance and an eye toward other etiological factors, can help to facilitate well-being and recovery.

References

Abdel-Hamid MA, A Hakim S, Elokda EE, Mostafa NS: Prevalence and risk factors of sick building syndrome among office workers. J Egypt Public Health Assoc 88(2):109–114, 2013 23963091

Albertson TE, Derlet RW, Foulke GE, et al: Superiority of activated charcoal alone compared with ipecac and activated charcoal in the treatment of acute toxic ingestions. Ann Emerg Med 18(1):56–59, 1989 2562913

Alván G, Bergman U, Gustafsson LL: High unbound fraction of salicylate in plasma during intoxication. Br J Clin Pharmacol 11(6):625–626, 1981 7272181

Amanzio M, Corazzini LL, Vase L, Benedetti F: A systematic review of adverse events in placebo groups of anti-migraine clinical trials. Pain 146(3):261–269, 2009 19781854

American Academy of Clinical Toxicology, European Association of Poisons Centres and Clinical Toxicologists: Position statement and practice guidelines on the use of multi-dose activated charcoal in the treatment of acute poisoning. J Toxicol Clin Toxicol 37:731–751, 1999 10584586

American Academy of Pediatrics Committee on Injury, Violence, and Poison Prevention: Poison treatment in the home: American Academy of Pediatrics Committee on Injury, Violence, and Poison Prevention. Pediatrics 112(5):1182–1185, 2003 14595067

Anderson HA, Islam KM: Trends in occupational and adult lead exposure in Wisconsin 1988–2005. WMJ 105(2):21–25, 2006 16628970

Anderson VA, Godber T, Smibert E, et al: Impairments of attention following treatment with cranial irradiation and chemotherapy in children. J Clin Exp Neuropsychol 26(5):684–697, 2004 15370390

Anseeuw K, Mowry JB, Burdmann EA, et al; EXTRIP Workgroup: Extracorporeal treatment in phenytoin poisoning: systematic review and recommendations from the EXTRIP (Extracorporeal Treatments in Poisoning) Workgroup. Am J Kidney Dis 67(2):187–197, 2016 26578149

Aslan S, Karcioglu O, Bilge F, et al: Post-interval syndrome after carbon monoxide poisoning. Vet Hum Toxicol 46(4):183–185, 2004 15303387

Bailer J, Witthöft M, Paul C, et al: Evidence for overlap between idiopathic environmental intolerance and somatoform disorders. Psychosom Med 67(6):921–929, 2005 16314597

Baker SD, Borys DJ: A possible trend suggesting increased abuse from Coricidin exposures reported to the Texas Poison Network: comparing 1998 to 1999. Vet Hum Toxicol 44(3):169–171, 2002 12046973

Baliatsas C, van Kamp I, Hooiveld M, et al: The relationship of modern health worries to non-specific physical symptoms and perceived environmental sensitivity: a study combining self-reported and general practice data. J Psychosom Res 79(5):355–361, 2015 26526308

Bank WJ: Thallium, in Experimental and Clinical Neurotoxicology. Edited by Spencer PS, Schaumburg HH. Baltimore, MD, Williams & Wilkins, 1980, pp 570–577

Barceloux DG: Selenium. J Toxicol Clin Toxicol 37(2):145–172, 1999 10382553

Barceloux DG, Krenzelok EP, Olson K, Watson W; Ad Hoc Committee: American Academy of Clinical Toxicology practice guidelines on the treatment of ethylene glycol poisoning. J Toxicol Clin Toxicol 37(5):537–560, 1999 10497633

Barceloux DG, Bond GR, Krenzelok EP, et al; American Academy of Clinical Toxicology Ad Hoc Committee on the Treatment Guidelines for Methanol Poisoning: American Academy of Clinical Toxicology practice guidelines on the treatment of methanol poisoning. J Toxicol Clin Toxicol 40(4):415–446, 2002 12216995

Barmark M: Social determinants of the sick building syndrome: exploring the interrelated effects of social position and psychosocial situation. Int J Environ Health Res 25(5):490–507, 2015 25424591

Bateman DN, Carroll R, Pettie J, et al: Effect of the UK's revised paracetamol poisoning management guidelines on admissions, adverse reactions and costs of treatment. Br J Clin Pharmacol 78(3):610–618, 2014 24666324

Battaglia J: Pharmacological management of acute agitation. Drugs 65(9):1207–1222, 2005 15916448

Bellinger D, Leviton A, Waternaux C, et al: Longitudinal analyses of prenatal and postnatal lead exposure and early cognitive development. N Engl J Med 316(17):1037–1043, 1987 3561456

Berman SM, Kuczenski R, McCracken JT, London ED: Potential adverse effects of amphetamine treatment on brain and behavior: a review. Mol Psychiatry 14(2):123–142, 2009 18698321

Bhatt MH, Elias MA, Mankodi AK: Acute and reversible parkinsonism due to organophosphate pesticide intoxication: five cases. Neurology 52(7):1467–1471, 1999 10227636

Black DW: The relationship of mental disorders and idiopathic environmental intolerance. Occup Med 15(3):557–570, 2000 10903550

Boehnert MT, Lovejoy FH Jr: Value of the QRS duration versus the serum drug level in predicting seizures and ventricular arrhythmias after an acute overdose of tricyclic antidepressants. N Engl J Med 313(8):474–479, 1985 4022081

Bond GR: The role of activated charcoal and gastric emptying in gastrointestinal decontamination: a state-of-the-art review. Ann Emerg Med 39(3):273–286, 2002 11867980

Bornschein S, Hausteiner C, Zilker T, Förstl H: Psychiatric and somatic disorders and multiple chemical sensitivity (MCS) in 264 "environmental patients." Psychol Med 32(8):1387–1394, 2002 12455937

Bouchard M, Mergler D, Baldwin M, et al: Neuropsychiatric symptoms and past manganese exposure in a ferro-alloy plant. Neurotoxicology 28(2):290–297, 2007 16962176

Bowler RM, Koller W, Schulz PE: Parkinsonism due to manganism in a welder: neurological and neuropsychological sequelae. Neurotoxicology 27(3):327–332, 2006 16457889

Bowler RM, Roels HA, Nakagawa S, et al: Dose-effect relationships between manganese exposure and neurological, neuropsychological and pulmonary function in confined space bridge welders. Occup Environ Med 64(3):167–177, 2007 17018581

Boyer EW, Shannon M: The serotonin syndrome. N Engl J Med 352(11):1112–1120, 2005 15784664

Brent J, McMartin K, Phillips S, et al; Methylpyrazole for Toxic Alcohols Study Group: Fomepizole for the treatment of ethylene glycol poisoning. N Engl J Med 340(11):832–838, 1999 10080845

Brent J, McMartin K, Phillips S, et al; Methylpyrazole for Toxic Alcohols Study Group: Fomepizole for the treatment of methanol poisoning. N Engl J Med 344(6):424–429, 2001 11172179

Briassoulis G, Narlioglou M, Hatzis T: Toxic encephalopathy associated with use of DEET insect repellents: a case analysis of its toxicity in children. Hum Exp Toxicol 20(1):8–14, 2001 11339626

Brown JS: Environmental and Chemical Toxins and Psychiatric Illness. Washington, DC, American Psychiatric Publishing, 2002

Brown JS Jr: Psychiatric issues in toxic exposures. Psychiatr Clin North Am 30(4):837–854, 2007 17938048

Burge PS: Sick building syndrome. Occup Environ Med 61(2):185–190, 2004 14739390

Burns MJ, Linden CH, Graudins A, et al: A comparison of physostigmine and benzodiazepines for the treatment of anticholinergic poisoning. Ann Emerg Med 35(4):374–381, 2000 10736125

Caroff SN: Neuroleptic malignant syndrome, in Neuroleptic Malignant Syndrome and Related Conditions, 2nd Edition. Edited by Mann SC, Caroff SN, Keck PE, et al. Washington, DC, American Psychiatric Publishing, 2003, pp 1–44

Carson AJ, Best S, Postma K, et al: The outcome of neurology outpatients with medically unexplained symptoms: a prospective cohort study. J Neurol Neurosurg Psychiatry 74(7):897–900, 2003 12810775

Chan TY: Herbal medicine causing likely strychnine poisoning. Hum Exp Toxicol 21(8):467–468, 2002 12412642

Chiew AL, Isbister GK, Duffull SB, Buckley NA: Evidence for the changing regimens of acetylcysteine. Br J Clin Pharmacol 81(3):471–481, 2016 26387650

Chiodo LM, Jacobson SW, Jacobson JL: Neurodevelopmental effects of postnatal lead exposure at very low levels. Neurotoxicol Teratol 26(3):359–371, 2004 15113598

Christian MR, Lowry JA, Algren DA, et al: Do rapid comprehensive urine drug screens change clinical management in children? Clin Toxicol (Phila) 55(9):977–980, 2017 28594290

Chyka PA, Erdman AR, Manoguerra AS, et al; American Association of Poison Control Centers: Dextromethorphan poisoning: an evidence-based consensus guideline for out-of-hospital management. Clin Toxicol (Phila) 45(6):662–677, 2007 17849242

Cohn S, Dyson C, Wessely S: Early accounts of Gulf War illness and the construction of narratives in UK service personnel. Soc Sci Med 67(11):1641–1649, 2008 18829146

Cole JB, Moore JC, Nystrom PC, et al: A prospective study of ketamine versus haloperidol for severe prehospital agitation. Clin Toxicol (Phila) 54(7):556–562, 2016 27102743

Cole PD, Kamen BA: Delayed neurotoxicity associated with therapy for children with acute lymphoblastic leukemia. Ment Retard Dev Disabil Res Rev 12(3):174–183, 2006 17061283

Cooley JD, Wong WC, Jumper CA, Straus DC: Correlation between the prevalence of certain fungi and sick building syndrome. Occup Environ Med 55(9):579–584, 1998 9861178

Craig SA: Radiology, in Clinical Toxicology. Edited by Ford M, Delaney K, Ling L, et al. Philadelphia, PA, WB Saunders, 2001, pp 61–72

Crimlisk HL, Bhatia K, Cope H, et al: Slater revisited: 6 year follow up study of patients with medically unexplained motor symptoms. BMJ 316(7131):582–586, 1998 9518908

Curry SC, Chang D, Connor D: Drug- and toxin-induced rhabdomyolysis. Ann Emerg Med 18(10):1068–1084, 1989 2679245

Cutler RE, Forland SC, Hammond PG, Evans JR: Extracorporeal removal of drugs and poisons by hemodialysis and hemoperfusion. Annu Rev Pharmacol Toxicol 27:169–191, 1987 3579241

Dalton R: Mixed bipolar disorder precipitated by pseudoephedrine hydrochloride. South Med J 83(1):64–65, 1990 2300837

Dart RC, Paul IM, Bond GR, et al: Pediatric fatalities associated with over the counter (nonprescription) cough and cold medications. Ann Emerg Med 53(4):411–417, 2009 19101060

Deichmann WB, Henschler D, Holmstedt B, Keil G: What is there that is not poison? A study of the Third Defense by Paracelsus. Arch Toxicol 58(4):207–213, 1986 3521542

Dietrich KN, Ris MD, Succop PA, et al: Early exposure to lead and juvenile delinquency. Neurotoxicol Teratol 23(6):511–518, 2001 11792521

Dorrington CL, Johnson DW, Brant R; Multiple Dose Activated Charcoal Complication Study Group: The frequency of complications associated with the use of multiple-dose activated charcoal. Ann Emerg Med 41(3):370–377, 2003 12605204

Ecobichon DJ, Joy RM: Pesticides and Neurological Diseases, 2nd Edition. Boca Raton, FL, CRC Press, 1994

Eddleston M: Insecticides: Organic phosphorous compounds and carbamates, in Goldfrank's Toxicologic Emergencies, 10th Edition. Edited by Hoffman RS, Howland MA, Lewin NA, et al. New York, McGraw-Hill, 2015, pp 1409–1424

Eddleston M, Szinicz L, Eyer P, Buckley N: Oximes in acute organophosphorus pesticide poisoning: a systematic review of clinical trials. QJM 95(5):275–283, 2002 11978898

Engel CC, Hyams KC, Scott K: Managing future Gulf War Syndromes: international lessons and new models of care. Philos Trans R Soc Lond B Biol Sci 361(1468):707–720, 2006 16687273

Engel LS, Checkoway H, Keifer MC, et al: Parkinsonism and occupational exposure to pesticides. Occup Environ Med 58(9):582–589, 2001 11511745

Faasse K, Grey A, Horne R, Petrie KJ: High perceived sensitivity to medicines is associated with higher medical care utilisation, increased symptom reporting and greater information-seeking about medication. Pharmacoepidemiol Drug Saf 24(6):592–599, 2015 25851232

Faroon O, Kueberuwa S, Smith L, DeRosa C: ATSDR evaluation of health effects of chemicals, II. Mirex and chlordecone: health effects, toxicokinetics, human exposure, and environmental fate. Toxicol Ind Health 11(6):1–203, 1995 8723616

Feinstein AR: The Blame-X syndrome: problems and lessons in nosology, spectrum, and etiology. J Clin Epidemiol 54(5):433–439, 2001 11337205

Feychting M, Ahlbom A, Kheifets L: EMF and health. Annu Rev Public Health 26:165–189, 2005 15760285

Filley CM, Franklin GM, Keaton RK, et al: White matter dementia: clinical disorders and implications. Neuropsychiatry, Neuropsychology, and Behavioral Neurology 1(4):239–254, 1988

Fortenberry JD, Mariscalco MM: General principles of poisoning management, in Oski's Pediatrics: Principles and Practice, 4th Edition. Edited by McMillan JA, Feigin RD, DeAngelis CD, et al. New York, Lippincott Williams & Wilkins, 2006, pp 747–753

Fung F: Multiple chemical sensitivity and idiopathic environmental intolerance, in Medical Toxicology, 3rd Edition. Edited by Dart RC, Caravate EM, McGuigan MA, et al. Philadelphia, PA, Lippincott Williams & Wilkins, 2004a, pp 98–101

Fung F: Sick building syndrome, in Medical Toxicology, 3rd Edition. Edited by Dart RC, Caravate EM, McGuigan MA, et al. Philadelphia, PA, Lippincott Williams & Wilkins, 2004b, pp 131–135

Fung YK, Molvar MP: Toxicity of mercury from dental environment and from amalgam restorations. J Toxicol Clin Toxicol 30(1):49–61, 1992 1542149

Gabow PA, Anderson RJ, Potts DE, Schrier RW: Acid-base disturbances in the salicylate-intoxicated adult. Arch Intern Med 138(10):1481–1484, 1978 708168

Gallo MA, Lawryk NJ: Organic phosphorous pesticides, in Handbook of Pesticide Toxicology. Edited by Hayes WJ, Laws ER. San Diego, CA, Academic Press, 1991, pp 917–1090

Gershon S, Shaw FH: Psychiatric sequelae of chronic exposure to organophosphorus insecticides. Lancet 1(7191):1371–1374, 1961 13704751

Ghannoum M, Yates C, Galvao TF, et al; EXTRIP Workgroup: Extracorporeal treatment for carbamazepine poisoning: systematic review and recommendations from the EXTRIP workgroup. Clin Toxicol (Phila) 52(10):993–1004, 2014 25355482

Ghannoum M, Laliberté M, Nolin TD, et al; EXTRIP Workgroup: Extracorporeal treatment for valproic acid poisoning: systematic review and recommendations from the EXTRIP workgroup. Clin Toxicol (Phila) 53(5):454–465, 2015 25950372

Ghannoum M, Lavergne V, Gosselin S, et al: Practice Trends in the Use of Extracorporeal Treatments for Poisoning in Four Countries. Semin Dial 29(1):71–80, 2016 26551956

Givens T, Holloway M, Wason S: Pulmonary aspiration of activated charcoal: a complication of its misuse in overdose management. Pediatr Emerg Care 8(3):137–140, 1992 1614903

Glas B, Stenberg B, Stenlund H, Sunesson AL: Exposure to formaldehyde, nitrogen dioxide, ozone, and terpenes among office workers and associations with reported symptoms. Int Arch Occup Environ Health 88(5):613–622, 2015 25274505

Glass PS, Jhaveri RM, Smith LR: Comparison of potency and duration of action of nalmefene and naloxone. Anesth Analg 78(3):536–541, 1994 8109774

Goldfrank L, Weisman R, Flomenbaum N: Teaching the recognition of odors. Ann Emerg Med 11(12):684–686, 1982 7149364

Göthe CJ, Molin C, Nilsson CG: The environmental somatization syndrome. Psychosomatics 36(1):1–11, 1995 7871128

Goyer RA, Cherian MG, Jones MM, Reigart JR: Role of chelating agents for prevention, intervention, and treatment of exposures to toxic metals. Environ Health Perspect 103(11):1048–1052, 1995 8605855

Gunnell D, Eddleston M, Phillips MR, Konradsen F: The global distribution of fatal pesticide self-poisoning: systematic review. BMC Public Health 7:357, 2007 18154668

Hall AH, Smolinske SC, Kulig KW, Rumack BH: Ibuprofen overdose—a prospective study. West J Med 148(6):653–656, 1988 3176471

Halpern SM, Fitzpatrick R, Volans GN: Ibuprofen toxicity. A review of adverse reactions and overdose. Adverse Drug React Toxicol Rev 12(2):107–128, 1993 8357944

Hanna-Attisha M, LaChance J, Sadler RC, Champney Schnepp A: Elevated blood lead levels in children associated with the Flint drinking water crisis: a spatial analysis of risk and public health response. Am J Public Health 106(2):283–290, 2016 26691115

Hartman DE: Neuropsychological Toxicology: Identification and Assessment of Human Neurotoxic Syndromes. New York, Pergamon, 1988

Heller MK, Chapman SC, Horne R: Beliefs about medication predict the misattribution of a common symptom as a medication side effect—evidence from an analogue online study. J Psychosom Res 79(6):519–529, 2015 26519128

Hepler BR, Sutheimer CA, Sunshine I: Role of the toxicology laboratory in the treatment of acute poisoning. Med Toxicol 1(1):61–75, 1986 3537616

Hetherington L, Battershill J: Review of evidence for a toxicological mechanism of idiopathic environmental intolerance. Hum Exp Toxicol 32(1):3–17, 2013 23060407

Hiemke C, Baumann P, Bergemann N, et al: AGNP consensus guidelines for therapeutic drug monitoring in psychiatry: update 2011. Pharmacopsychiatry 44(6):195–235, 2011 21969060

Hillert L, Kolmodin Hedman B, Dölling BF, Arnetz BB: Cognitive behavioural therapy for patients with electric sensitivity—a multidisciplinary approach in a controlled study. Psychother Psychosom 67(6):302–310, 1998 9817951

Hodgson MJ, Parkinson DK: Diagnosis of organophosphate intoxication. N Engl J Med 313(5):329, 1985 2409442

Hoffman RJ, Nelson LS: Sympathomimetic agents, in Critical Care Toxicology: Diagnosis and Management of the Critically Poisoned Patient. Edited by Brent J, Burkhart KK, Dargan P, et al. Switzerland, Springer International Publishing, 2016, pp 851–865

Hoffman RS, Goldfrank LR: The poisoned patient with altered consciousness. Controversies in the use of a "coma cocktail." JAMA 274(7):562–569, 1995 7629986

Hoffman RS, Howland MA, Lewin NA, et al: Principles of managing the acutely poisoned or overdosed patient, in Goldfrank's Toxicologic Emergencies, 10th Edition. Edited by Hoffman RS, Howland MA, Lewin NA, et al. New York, McGraw-Hill, 2015, pp 30–37

Holness DL, Taraschuk IG, Nethercott JR: Health status of copper refinery workers with specific reference to selenium exposure. Arch Environ Health 44(5):291–297, 1989 2684043

Honda S, Shibata Y, Mine M, et al: Mental health conditions among atomic bomb survivors in Nagasaki. Psychiatry Clin Neurosci 56(5):575–583, 2002 12193250

Hunt E, Hader SL, Files D, Corey GR: Arsenic poisoning seen at Duke Hospital, 1965–1998. N C Med J 60(2):70–74, 1999 10344130

Illingworth RN, Jarvie DR: Absence of toxicity in cimetidine overdosage. BMJ 1(6161):453–454, 1979 427404

Insley BM, Grufferman S, Ayliffe HE: Thallium poisoning in cocaine abusers. Am J Emerg Med 4(6):545–548, 1986 3778602

Isbister GK, Buckley NA, Whyte IM: Serotonin toxicity: a practical approach to diagnosis and treatment. Med J Aust 187(6):361–365, 2007 17874986

Iversen A, Chalder T, Wessely S: Gulf War Illness: lessons from medically unexplained symptoms. Clin Psychol Rev 27(7):842–854, 2007 17707114

Jacobsen D, McMartin KE: Antidotes for methanol and ethylene glycol poisoning. J Toxicol Clin Toxicol 35(2):127–143, 1997 9120880

Jagerdeo E, Schaff JE: Rapid screening for drugs of abuse in biological fluids by ultra high performance liquid chromatography/Orbitrap mass spectrometry. J Chromatogr B Analyt Technol Biomed Life Sci 1027:11–18, 2016 27236533

Jamal GA: Neurological syndromes of organophosphorus compounds. Adverse Drug React Toxicol Rev 16(3):133–170, 1997 9512762

Janković SR, Stosić JJ, Vucinić S, et al: Causes of rhabdomyolysis in acute poisonings. Vojnosanit Pregl 70(11):1039–1045, 2013 24397200

Johnson DA, Hricik JG: The pharmacology of alpha-adrenergic decongestants. Pharmacotherapy 13(6 Pt 2):110S–115S, discussion 143S–146S, 1993 7507588

Juurlink DN: Activated charcoal for acute overdose: a reappraisal. Br J Clin Pharmacol 81(3):482–487, 2016 26409027

Kang HK, Li B, Mahan CM, et al: Health of US veterans of 1991 Gulf War: a follow-up survey in 10 years. J Occup Environ Med 51(4):401–410, 2009 19322107

Katz J, Prescott K, Woolf AD: Strychnine poisoning from a Cambodian traditional remedy. Am J Emerg Med 14(5):475–477, 1996 8765115

Kawano N, Hirabayashi K, Matsuo M, et al: Human suffering effects of nuclear tests at Semi-palatinsk, Kazakhstan: established on the basis of questionnaire surveys. J Radiat Res (Tokyo) 47 (suppl A):A209–A217, 2006 16571939

Kehr J, Ichinose F, Yoshitake S, et al: Mephedrone, compared with MDMA (ecstasy) and amphetamine, rapidly increases both dopamine and 5-HT levels in nucleus accumbens of awake rats. Br J Pharmacol 164(8):1949–1958, 2011 21615721

Kim S: Skeletal muscle relaxants, in Poisoning and Drug Overdose, 5th Edition. Edited by Olson KR, Anderson IB, Benowitz NL, et al. New York, McGraw-Hill, 2007, pp 341–343

Kong TY, Kim JH, Kim JY, et al: Rapid analysis of drugs of abuse and their metabolites in human urine using dilute and shoot liquid chromatography-tandem mass spectrometry. Arch Pharm Res 40(2):180–196, 2017 27988881

Köppel C, Baudisch H, Beyer KH, et al: Fatal poisoning with selenium dioxide. J Toxicol Clin Toxicol 24(1):21–35, 1986 3701906

Krenzelok EP, Litovitz T, Lippold KP, McNally CF: Cimetidine toxicity: an assessment of 881 cases. Ann Emerg Med 16(11):1217–1221, 1987 3662179

Ku BD, Shin HY, Kim EJ, et al: Secondary mania in a patient with delayed anoxic encephalopathy after carbon monoxide intoxication. J Clin Neurosci 13(8):860–862, 2006 16935513

Kulig K, Rumack B: Hydrocarbon ingestion. Topics in Emergency Medicine 3:1–5, 1981

Kulig K, Bar-Or D, Cantrill SV, et al: Management of acutely poisoned patients without gastric emptying. Ann Emerg Med 14(6):562–567, 1985 2859819

Laidlaw MA, Filippelli G, Mielke H, et al: Lead exposure at firing ranges—a review. Environ Health 16(1):34, 2017 28376827

Lake CR, Tenglin R, Chernow B, Holloway HC: Psychomotor stimulant-induced mania in a genetically predisposed patient: a review of the literature and report of a case. J Clin Psychopharmacol 3(2):97–100, 1983 6341419

Lam LC, Leung SF, Chan YL: Progress of memory function after radiation therapy in patients with nasopharyngeal carcinoma. J Neuropsychiatry Clin Neurosci 15(1):90–97, 2003 12556578

Lam RP, Yip WL, Wan CK, Tsui MS: Dexmedetomidine use in the ED for control of methamphetamine-induced agitation. Am J Emerg Med 35(4):665.e1–665.e4, 2017 27842924

Lam SP, Fong SY, Kwok A, et al: Delayed neuropsychiatric impairment after carbon monoxide poisoning from burning charcoal. Hong Kong Med J 10(6):428–431, 2004 15591604

Landgrebe M, Frick U, Hauser S, et al: Cognitive and neurobiological alterations in electromagnetic hypersensitive patients: results of a case-control study. Psychol Med 38(12):1781–1791, 2008 18366821

Leikin JB, Mycyk MB, Bryant S, et al: Characteristics of patients with no underlying toxicologic syndrome evaluated in a toxicology clinic. J Toxicol Clin Toxicol 42(5):643–648, 2004 15462157

Maldonado JR: Delirium in the acute care setting: characteristics, diagnosis and treatment. Crit Care Clin 24(4):657–722, vii, 2008 18929939

Martel M, Sterzinger A, Miner J, et al: Management of acute undifferentiated agitation in the emergency department: a randomized double-blind trial of droperidol, ziprasidone, and midazolam. Acad Emerg Med 12(12):1167–1172, 2005 16282517

McFarlane AC, Lawrence-Wood E, Van Hooff M, et al: The need to take a staging approach to the biological mechanisms of PTSD and its treatment. Curr Psychiatry Rep 19(2):10, 2017 28168596

McMillin GA, Marin SJ, Johnson-Davis KL, et al: A hybrid approach to urine drug testing using high-resolution mass spectrometry and select immunoassays. Am J Clin Pathol 143(2):234–240, 2015 25596249

Meggs WJ: RADS and RUDS—the toxic induction of asthma and rhinitis. J Toxicol Clin Toxicol 32(5):487–501, 1994 7932908

Mendonca S, Gupta S, Gupta A: Extracorporeal management of poisonings. Saudi J Kidney Dis Transpl 23(1):1–7, 2012 22237210

Merigian KS, Woodard M, Hedges JR, et al: Prospective evaluation of gastric emptying in the self-poisoned patient. Am J Emerg Med 8(6):479–483, 1990 1977400

Miniño AM, Heron MP, Murphy SL, Kochanek KD; Centers for Disease Control and Prevention National Center for Health Statistics National Vital Statistics System: Deaths: final data for 2004. Natl Vital Stat Rep 55(19):1–119, 2007 17867520

Mitchell CS, Donnay A, Hoover DR, Margolick JB: Immunologic parameters of multiple chemical sensitivity. Occup Med 15(3):647–665, 2000 10903557

Mitka M: Chelation therapy trials halted. JAMA 300(19):2236, 2008 19017902

Montague RE, Grace RF, Lewis JH, Shenfield GM: Urine drug screens in overdose patients do not contribute to immediate clinical management. Ther Drug Monit 23(1):47–50, 2001 11206043

Mozaffarian D, Rimm EB: Fish intake, contaminants, and human health: evaluating the risks and the benefits. JAMA 296(15):1885–1899, 2006 17047219

Mückter H, Liebl B, Reichl FX, et al: Are we ready to replace dimercaprol (BAL) as an arsenic antidote? Hum Exp Toxicol 16(8):460–465, 1997 9292286

Myers RA, DeFazio A, Kelly MP: Chronic carbon monoxide exposure: a clinical syndrome detected by neuropsychological tests. J Clin Psychol 54(5):555–567, 1998 9696105

Needleman HL: Lead poisoning, in Oski's Pediatrics: Principles and Practice, 4th Edition. Edited by McMillan JA, Feigin RD, DeAngelis CD, et al. New York, Lippincott Williams & Wilkins, 2006, pp 767–772

Needleman HL, Schell A, Bellinger D, et al: The long-term effects of exposure to low doses of lead in childhood. An 11-year follow-up report. N Engl J Med 322(2):83–88, 1990 2294437

Nelson LS, Olsen D: Opioids, in Goldfrank's Toxicologic Emergencies, 10th Edition. Edited by Hoffman RS, Howland MA, Lewin NA, et al. New York, McGraw-Hill, 2015, pp 492–509

Nelson L, Perrone J: Herbal and alternative medicine. Emerg Med Clin North Am 18(4):709–722, 2000 11130934

Nettleman M: Gulf War illness: challenges persist. Trans Am Clin Climatol Assoc 126:237–247, 2015 26330683

Ngo AS, Anthony CR, Samuel M, et al: Should a benzodiazepine antagonist be used in unconscious patients presenting to the emergency department? Resuscitation 74(1):27–37, 2007 17306436

Nolen TM: Sedative effects of antihistamines: safety, performance, learning, and quality of life. Clin Ther 19(1):39–55, discussion 2–3, 1997 9083707

O'Callaghan WG, Joyce N, Counihan HE, et al: Unusual strychnine poisoning and its treatment: report of eight cases. Br Med J (Clin Res Ed) 285(6340):478, 1982 6809135

Olson KR: Emergency evaluation and treatment, in Poisoning and Drug Overdose, 5th Edition. Edited by Olson KR, Anderson IB, Benowitz NL, et al. New York, McGraw-Hill, 2007, pp 1–57

Parker SK, Schwartz B, Todd J, Pickering LK: Thimerosal-containing vaccines and autistic spectrum disorder: a critical review of published original data. Pediatrics 114(3):793–804, 2004 15342856

Pastel RH: Radiophobia: long-term psychological consequences of Chernobyl. Mil Med 167 (2 suppl):134–136, 2002 11873498

Pastel RH, Mulvaney J: Fear of radiation in U.S. military medical personnel. Mil Med 166 (12 suppl):80–82, 2001 11778447

Pedavally S, Fugate JE, Rabinstein AA: Serotonin syndrome in the intensive care unit: clinical presentations and precipitating medications. Neurocrit Care 21(1):108–113, 2014 24052457

Pentel P, Fletcher D, Jentzen J: Fatal acute selenium toxicity. J Forensic Sci 30(2):556–562, 1985 3998702

Pizon AF, Yanta JH, Swartzentruber GS: The Diagnostic Process in Medical Toxicology, in Critical Care Toxicology: Diagnosis and Management of the Critically Poisoned Patient. Edited by Brent J, Burkhart KK, Dargan P, et al. Switzerland, Springer International Publishing, 2016, pp 29–41

Pohjola-Sintonen S, Kivistö KT, Vuori E, et al: Identification of drugs ingested in acute poisoning: correlation of patient history with drug analyses. Ther Drug Monit 22(6):749–752, 2000 11128245

Prescott LF: The chief scientist reports… prevention of hepatic necrosis following paracetamol overdosage. Health Bull (Edinb) 36(4):204–212, 1978 669953

Proudfoot AT, Krenzelok EP, Vale JA: Position Paper on urine alkalinization. J Toxicol Clin Toxicol 42(1):1–26, 2004 15083932

Questel F, Dugarin J, Dally S: Thallium-contaminated heroin. Ann Intern Med 124(6):616, 1996 8597335

Rainey PM: Laboratory principles, in Goldfrank's Toxicologic Emergencies, 10th Edition. Edited by Hoffman RS, Howland MA, Lewin NA, et al. New York, McGraw-Hill, 2015, pp 62–75

Rasimas JJ, Carter GL: Psychiatric issues in the critically poisoned patient, in Critical Care Toxicology: Diagnosis and Management of the Critically Poisoned Patient. Edited by Brent J, Burkhart KK, Dargan P et al. Switzerland, Springer International Publishing, 2016, pp 117–157

Rasimas JJ, Sachdeva KK, Donovan JW: Revival of an antidote: bedside experience with physostigmine. Journal of the American Association for Emergency Psychiatry 12:5–24, 2014

Rasimas JJ, Kivovich V, Sachdeva K, et al: Antagonizing the errors of history: bedside experience with flumazenil. Journal of the American Association for Emergency Psychiatry 13:17–34, 2015

Rasimas JJ, Smolcic EE, Sinclair CM: Themes and trends in intentional self-poisoning: perspectives from critical care toxicology. Psychiatry Res 255:304–313, 2017 28601000

Reyes NL, Wong LY, MacRoy PM, et al: Identifying housing that poisons: a critical step in eliminating childhood lead poisoning. J Public Health Manag Pract 12(6):563–569, 2006 17041305

Rief W, Glaesmer H, Baehr V, et al: The relationship of modern health worries to depression, symptom reporting and quality of life in a general population survey. J Psychosom Res 72(4):318–320, 2012 22405228

Roldan-Tapia L, Nieto-Escamez FA, del Aguila EM, et al: Neuropsychological sequelae from acute poisoning and long-term exposure to carbamate and organophosphate pesticides. Neurotoxicol Teratol 28(6):694–703, 2006 17029710

Rosenstock L, Daniell W, Barnhart S, et al: Chronic neuropsychological sequelae of occupational exposure to organophosphate insecticides. Am J Ind Med 18(3):321–325, 1990 2220838

Rubin GJ, Das Munshi J, Wessely S: Electromagnetic hypersensitivity: a systematic review of provocation studies. Psychosom Med 67(2):224–232, 2005 15784787

Rubin GJ, Das Munshi J, Wessely S: A systematic review of treatments for electromagnetic hypersensitivity. Psychother Psychosom 75(1):12–18, 2006 16361870

Rumack BH, Matthew H: Acetaminophen poisoning and toxicity. Pediatrics 55(6):871–876, 1975 1134886

Rusyniak DE, Furbee RB, Kirk MA: Thallium and arsenic poisoning in a small Midwestern town. Ann Emerg Med 39(3):307–311, 2002 11867986

Sahlberg B, Gunnbjörnsdottir M, Soon A, et al: Airborne molds and bacteria, microbial volatile organic compounds (MVOC), plasticizers and formaldehyde in dwellings in three North European cities in relation to sick building syndrome (SBS). Sci Total Environ 444:433–440, 2013 23280302

Saper RB, Phillips RS, Sehgal A, et al: Lead, mercury, and arsenic in US- and Indian-manufactured Ayurvedic medicines sold via the Internet. JAMA 300(8):915–923, 2008 18728265

Schaumburg HH: Toluene, in Experimental and Clinical Neurotoxicology, 2nd Edition. Edited by Spencer PS, Schaumburg HH, Ludolph AC. New York, Oxford University Press, 2000, pp 1183–1189

Schaumburg HH, Berger A: Alopecia and sensory polyneuropathy from thallium in a Chinese herbal medication. JAMA 268(24):3430–3431, 1992 1334161

Schneider SM, Michelson EA, Boucek CD, Ilkhanipour K: Dextromethorphan poisoning reversed by naloxone. Am J Emerg Med 9(3):237–238, 1991 2018593

Schneir AB, Offerman SR, Ly BT, et al: Complications of diagnostic physostigmine administration to emergency department patients. Ann Emerg Med 42(1):14–19, 2003 12827117

Schoolmeester WL, White DR: Arsenic poisoning. South Med J 73(2):198–208, 1980 7355321

Schütze G, Schwarz MJ: Therapeutic drug monitoring for individualised risk reduction in psychopharmacotherapy. TTrAC Trends in Analytic Chemistry 84(Pt B):14–22, 2016

Schwartz DT: Diagnostic imaging, in Goldfrank's Toxicologic Emergencies, 10th Edition. Edited by Hoffman RS, Howland MA, Lewin NA, et al. New York, McGraw-Hill, 2015, pp 38–61

Sefidbakht S, Rasekhi AR, Kamali K, et al: Methanol poisoning: acute MR and CT findings in nine patients. Neuroradiology 49(5):427–435, 2007 17294234

Seger DL: Flumazenil—treatment or toxin. J Toxicol Clin Toxicol 42(2):209–216, 2004 15214628

Shannon M: Lead levels in children: how low must they go? Child Health Alert 21:1–2, 2003 12814089

Shcherbatykh I, Carpenter DO: The role of metals in the etiology of Alzheimer's disease. J Alzheimers Dis 11(2):191–205, 2007 17522444

Skov P, Valbjørn O, Pedersen BV; Danish Indoor Climate Study Group: Influence of personal characteristics, job-related factors and psychosocial factors on the sick building syndrome. Scand J Work Environ Health 15(4):286–295, 1989 2772583

Sleigh J, Harvey M, Voss L, Denny B: Ketamine—more mechanisms of action than just NMDA blockade. Trends in Anaesthesia and Critical Care 4(2–3):76–81, 2014

Smith BA: Strychnine poisoning. J Emerg Med 8(3):321–325, 1990 2197324

Smith SA, Howland MA: Activated charcoal, in Goldfrank's Toxicologic Emergencies, 10th Edition. Edited by Hoffman RS, Howland MA, Lewin NA, et al. New York, McGraw-Hill, 2015, pp 97–103

Sporer KA: Acute heroin overdose. Ann Intern Med 130(7):584–590, 1999 10189329

Staudenmayer H: Psychological treatment of psychogenic idiopathic environmental intolerance. Occup Med 15(3):627–646, 2000 10903556

Stone DC, Boone KB, Back-Madruga C, Lesser IM: Has the rolling uterus finally gathered moss? Somatization and malingering of cognitive deficit in six cases of "toxic mold" exposure. Clin Neuropsychol 20(4):766–785, 2006 16980261

Straus DC, Cooley JD, Wong WC, Jumper CA: Studies on the role of fungi in Sick Building Syndrome. Arch Environ Health 58(8):475–478, 2003 15259426

Sue Y: Mercury, in Goldfrank's Toxicologic Emergencies, 10th Edition. Edited by Hoffman RS, Howland MA, Lewin NA, et al. New York, McGraw-Hill, 2015, pp 1250–1258

Syed S, Gurcoo SA, Farooqui AK, et al: Is the World Health Organization-recommended dose of pralidoxime effective in the treatment of organophosphorus poisoning? A randomized, double-blinded and placebo-controlled trial. Saudi J Anaesth 9(1):49–54, 2015 25558199

Taylor CA, Saint-Hilaire MH, Cupples LA, et al: Environmental, medical, and family history risk factors for Parkinson's disease: a New England-based case control study. Am J Med Genet 88(6):742–749, 1999 10581500

Tenenbein M; American Academy of Clinical Toxicology; European Association of Poisons Centres and Clinical Toxicologists: Position statement: whole bowel irrigation. J Toxicol Clin Toxicol 35(7):753–762, 1997 9482429

Torres IJ, Mundt AJ, Sweeney PJ, et al: A longitudinal neuropsychological study of partial brain radiation in adults with brain tumors. Neurology 60(7):1113–1118, 2003 12682316

Tune LE: Serum anticholinergic activity levels and delirium in the elderly. Semin Clin Neuropsychiatry 5(2):149–153, 2000 10837103

Tune LE: Anticholinergic effects of medication in elderly patients. J Clin Psychiatry 62 (suppl 21):11–14, 2001 11584981

Vale JA, Kulig K; American Academy of Clinical Toxicology; European Association of Poisons Centres and Clinical Toxicologists: Position paper: gastric lavage. J Toxicol Clin Toxicol 42(7):933–943, 2004 15641639

Waddell WJ: The science of toxicology and its relevance to MCS. Regul Toxicol Pharmacol 18(1):13–22, 1993 8234914

Weaver LK: Clinical practice. Carbon monoxide poisoning. N Engl J Med 360(12):1217–1225, 2009 19297574

Wei KC, Chua HC: Suicide in Asia. Int Rev Psychiatry 20(5):434–440, 2008 19012128

Weibrecht K, Dayno M, Darling C, Bird SB: Liver aminotransferases are elevated with rhabdomyolysis in the absence of significant liver injury. J Med Toxicol 6(3):294–300, 2010 20407858

Weidenhamer JD, Clement ML: Widespread lead contamination of imported low-cost jewelry in the US. Chemosphere 67(5):961–965, 2007 17166553

Weiss EM, Singewald E, Baldus C, et al: Differences in psychological and somatic symptom cluster score profiles between subjects with Idiopathic environmental intolerance, major depression and schizophrenia. Psychiatry Res 249:187–194, 2017 28113122

Wiley J, Henretig F, Foster R: Status epilepticus and severe neurologic impairment from lead encephalopathy (poster). Journal of Toxicology: Clinical Toxicology 33(5):529–530, 1995

Winship KA: Organic mercury compounds and their toxicity. Adverse Drug React Acute Poisoning Rev 5(3):141–180, 1986 3538823

Wong L, Radic Z, Brüggemann RJ, et al: Mechanism of oxime reactivation of acetylcholinesterase analyzed by chirality and mutagenesis. Biochemistry 39(19):5750–5757, 2000 10801325

Woolf AD, Goldman R, Bellinger DC: Update on the clinical management of childhood lead poisoning. Pediatr Clin North Am 54(2):271–294, viii, 2007 17448360

Wu LT, Howard MO: Psychiatric disorders in inhalant users: results from The National Epidemiologic Survey on Alcohol and Related Conditions. Drug Alcohol Depend 88(2–3):146–155, 2007 17129683

Yamada M, Izumi S: Psychiatric sequelae in atomic bomb survivors in Hiroshima and Nagasaki two decades after the explosions. Soc Psychiatry Psychiatr Epidemiol 37(9):409–415, 2002 12242616

Yoshida T, Yamauchi H, Fan Sun G: Chronic health effects in people exposed to arsenic via the drinking water: dose-response relationships in review. Toxicol Appl Pharmacol 198(3):243–252, 2004 15276403

Zar T, Yusufzai I, Sullivan A, Graeber C: Acute kidney injury, hyperosmolality and metabolic acidosis associated with lorazepam. Nat Clin Pract Nephrol 3(9):515–520, 2007 17717564

Zilker T: Assessment of risks from environmental exposure: practical implications in clinical toxicology (abstract 55). Journal of Toxicology: Clinical Toxicology 40(3):296–297, 2002

PART IV

Treatment

CHAPTER 36

Psychopharmacology

James A. Owen, Ph.D.[†]

Ericka L. Crouse, Pharm.D., BCPP, BCGP

Cynthia K. Kirkwood, Pharm.D., BCPP

James L. Levenson, M.D.

Psychopharmacological interventions are an essential part of the management of medically ill persons; at least 35% of psychiatric consultations include recommendations for medication (Bronheim et al. 1998). Appropriate use of psychopharmacology in the medically ill requires careful consideration of the underlying medical illness, potential alterations to pharmacokinetics, drug–drug interactions, and contraindications. In this chapter we review basic psychopharmacological concepts, including pharmacokinetics and pharmacodynamics in the medically ill, adverse effects, toxicity, drug–drug interactions, and alternative routes of administration for each psychotropic drug class. Considerations for the use of psychotropic drugs in patients with major organ dysfunction are discussed. The use of complementary medicines, including herbal medicines and nonherbal dietary supplements, is also briefly reviewed.

Pharmacokinetics in the Medically Ill

Pharmacokinetics characterizes the rate and extent of drug absorption, distribution, metabolism, and excretion, thus determining the rate of drug delivery to, and concentration at, its sites of action. *Pharmacodynamics* determines the relationship between drug concentration and response for both therapeutic and adverse effects.

[†]James Owen, who authored this chapter in the first two editions of the *Textbook*, passed away prematurely on November 7, 2013. Dr. Owen's knowledge regarding psychopharmacology in the medically ill was encyclopedic, and his enthusiasm for teaching and disseminating it inspirational and infectious. He will be greatly missed.

Absorption

Drug absorption is influenced by the characteristics of the absorption site and the chemical properties of a drug. Specific site properties that may affect absorption include surface area, ambient pH, mucosal integrity and functioning, and local blood flow. Orally administered drugs absorbed through the gastrointestinal (GI) tract may be extensively altered by "first-pass" hepatic metabolism before entering the systemic circulation. Sublingual, intranasal, topical, and intramuscular administration of drugs minimizes this first-pass effect, and rectal administration may reduce the first-pass effect by 50%. Drug formulation, drug–drug interactions, gastric motility, and the characteristics of the absorptive surface all influence the *rate* of absorption, a key factor when rapid onset is desired. The *extent* of drug absorption, however, is more important with long-term administration. The *bioavailability* of a drug describes the rate and extent to which the drug ingredient is absorbed from the drug product and available for drug action. Intravenous drug delivery has 100% bioavailability.

Distribution

Systemic drug distribution is influenced by serum pH, blood flow, protein binding, lipid solubility, and the degree of ionization. Most drugs bind to proteins, either albumin or alpha$_1$ acid glycoprotein (AAGP), to a greater or lesser extent. Disease may alter the concentrations of serum proteins as well as binding affinities. For example, albumin binding is decreased in pregnancy and in a number of illnesses (e.g., cirrhosis, bacterial pneumonia, acute pancreatitis, renal failure, surgery, trauma). In contrast, some disease states, such as hypothyroidism, may increase protein binding. AAGP concentrations may increase in Crohn's disease, myocardial infarction, stress, surgery, and trauma.

Typically, acidic drugs (e.g., valproate, barbiturates) bind mostly to albumin, and more basic drugs (e.g., phenothiazines, tricyclic antidepressants, amphetamines, most benzodiazepines) bind to globulins. In general, only free (unbound to plasma proteins) drug is pharmacologically active. Decreases in protein binding increase the availability of the "free" drug for pharmacological action, metabolism, and excretion. Provided that metabolic and excretory processes are unchanged by disease, any changes to the protein binding of a drug are compensated by an increase in drug elimination (metabolism and excretion), resulting in little change in steady-state plasma concentrations of pharmacologically active free drug. However, although free drug levels may remain unchanged, changes in protein binding will reduce plasma levels of total drug (free+bound fractions). While of no consequence therapeutically, therapeutic drug monitoring that measures total drug levels could mislead the clinician by suggesting lower, possibly subtherapeutic, levels and might prompt a dosage increase with toxic effects. For this reason, use of therapeutic drug monitoring for dosage adjustment requires caution in pregnant patients or those with uremia, chronic hepatic disease, hypoalbuminemia, or a protein-binding drug interaction; clinical response to the drug, rather than laboratory-determined drug levels, should guide dosage.

Most diseases that affect protein binding also affect metabolism and excretion. In this case, disease-induced changes in free drug availability may have clinically significant consequences, especially for drugs with a low therapeutic index.

Volume of distribution is a function of a drug's lipid solubility and plasma- and tissue-binding properties. Most psychotropic drugs are lipophilic but are also extensively bound to plasma proteins. Volume of distribution is unpredictably altered by disease and is not useful in guiding dose adjustments for medically ill patients.

Metabolism (or Biotransformation) and Elimination

Biotransformation occurs throughout the body, with the greatest activity in the liver and gut wall. Most psychotropic drugs are eliminated by hepatic metabolism and renal excretion. Two phases of hepatic metabolism enable excretion by increasing drugs' water solubility. Phase I metabolism consists of oxidation (i.e., cytochrome P450 mono-oxygenase system), reduction, or hydrolysis, which prepares medications for excretion or further metabolism by phase II pathways. The monoamine oxidases (MAOs) are also considered part of phase I processes. Phase II metabolism consists of many conjugation pathways, the most common being glucuronidation, acetylation, and sulfation. Hepatic clearance may be limited by either the rate of delivery (i.e., hepatic blood flow) of the drug to the hepatic metabolizing enzymes or the intrinsic capacity of the enzymes to metabolize the substrate. Clinically significant decreases in hepatic blood flow occur only in severe cirrhosis. Hepatic disease may preferentially affect anatomic regions of the liver, thereby altering specific metabolic processes. For example, oxidative reactions are more concentrated in the pericentral regions affected by acute viral hepatitis or alcoholic liver disease. Disease affecting the periportal regions, such as chronic hepatitis (in the absence of cirrhosis), may spare some hepatic oxidative function. In addition, acute and chronic liver diseases generally spare glucuronide conjugation reactions. Metabolic reactions altering the intrinsic capacity of enzymes through inhibition and induction are discussed in the next section ("Drug–Drug Interactions").

The kidney's primary pharmacokinetic role is drug elimination. However, renal disease may affect absorption, distribution, and metabolism of drugs. Creatinine clearance is a more useful indicator of renal function than serum creatinine. Specific drugs and their use in renal failure are covered later in this chapter. In general, despite the complexity of pharmacokinetic changes in renal failure, most psychotropics, other than lithium, gabapentin, pregabalin, topiramate, memantine, paliperidone, paroxetine, desvenlafaxine, and venlafaxine, do not require drastic dosage adjustment (see Table 36–11 ["Dosage adjustment of psychotropic medications in renal insufficiency"] later in this chapter).

Disease processes, particularly those involving the GI tract, liver, heart, and kidneys, can alter absorption, distribution, metabolism, and elimination. Table 36–1 summarizes how disease in these organ systems may alter the pharmacokinetics of psychotropic medications.

Drug–Drug Interactions

Drug–drug interactions are pharmacodynamic or pharmacokinetic in nature. Pharmacodynamic interactions involve alterations in the pharmacological response to a drug, which may be additive, synergistic, or antagonistic. Pharmacokinetic interac-

TABLE 36–1.   Pharmacokinetics in the medically ill

Pharmacokinetic parameter	Potential factors	Clinical significance
Liver disease		

Absorption	Gastric acidity
	Gastric and intestinal motility
	Small intestine surface area (e.g., short gut)
	Enteric blood flow
	Reduced hepatic blood flow
	Portosystemic shunting
		Minimize GI side effects of psychotropics
		Liquid formulations may be better or more quickly
		  absorbed than solid drug formulations
		Motility, secretory, and enteric blood flow changes in
		  GI disease usually do not require dosage change
		Consider parenteral administration

Distribution	Alterations in liver blood flow
	Changes in plasma proteins
	  Albumin may fall
	  AAGP may rise
	  Decreases in binding affinities
	Fluid shifts (e.g., ascites)
		Reduce dose
		Serum levels of drugs (bound + free) may be misleading

Metabolism and excretion	Reduced hepatic blood flow Reduced intrinsic capacity of the enzymes	Clinically significant reductions only occur in severe cirrhosis
Renal disease		
Absorption	Ammonia buffering may raise gastric pH	Rarely clinically significant changes in pharmacokinetics Major exceptions—lithium and gabapentin

Distribution	Altered body water volume
	Reduced protein binding
		Exact prediction of pharmacokinetic changes in the
		  context of renal disease is impractical clinically
		Monitor drug levels more frequently, but interpretation
		  of blood levels is difficult
		Serum levels of drugs (bound + free) may be misleading

TABLE 36–1. Pharmacokinetics in the medically ill *(continued)*

Pharmacokinetic parameter	Potential factors	Clinical significance
Renal disease *(continued)*		
Metabolism and excretion	Reduced renal blood flow Glomerular function	Creatinine clearance is a useful indicator of renal function to guide dose adjustments Serum creatinine may be confounded by some diseases that affect creatinine metabolism Dialysis alters pharmacokinetics
Cardiac disease		
Absorption	Decreased perfusion of drug absorption sites Intestinal wall edema may reduce absorption Changes in autonomic activity may affect GI motility and cause vasoconstriction	Congestive heart failure may decrease absorption of drugs through the GI tract Intramuscular drug absorption may be decreased by vasoconstriction
Distribution	Changes in plasma proteins AAGP may rise Albumin may fall Volume of distribution is reduced Regional blood flow redistributions	Acute doses should be reduced by approximately 50% Intravenous infusions should be given at a slower rate to avoid toxicity
Metabolism and excretion	Reduced renal and hepatic blood flow	A 50% reduction in dosage for long-term drug administration should be considered

Note.   AAGP=alpha$_1$ acid glycoprotein; GI=gastrointestinal.

tions include altered absorption, distribution, metabolism, or excretion and often change drug levels.

Pharmacokinetic interactions are understood in terms of the actions of an interacting drug (a metabolic inhibitor or inducer) on a substrate drug. A *substrate* is an agent or a drug that is metabolized by an enzyme. An *inducer* is an agent or a drug that increases the activity of the metabolic enzyme, allowing for an increased rate of metabolism. Induction may decrease the amount of circulating parent drug and increase the number and amounts of metabolites produced. The clinical effect may be a loss or reduction in therapeutic efficacy or an increase in toxicity from metabolites. An *inhibitor* has the opposite effect, decreasing or blocking enzyme activity needed for the metabolism of other drugs. An enzyme inhibitor increases the concentration of any drug dependent on that enzyme for biotransformation, thereby prolonging the pharmacological effect or increasing toxicity.

The hepatic cytochrome P450 (CYP) enzyme system catalyzes most phase I reactions and is involved in most metabolic drug–drug interactions (refer to Owen and Crouse 2017; also see de Leon and Spina 2018; English et al. 2012; Spina et al. 2016). Three CYP enzyme families are important in humans: CYP1, CYP2, and CYP3. The families are divided into subfamilies identified by a capital letter (e.g., CYP3A), and the subfamilies are further divided into isozymes. The CYP enzymes responsible for psychotropic drug metabolism are primarily CYP1A2, 2C9, 2C19, 2D6, and 3A4. Because some of these enzymes exist in a polymorphic form, a small percentage of the population has one or more CYP enzymes with significantly altered activity. These individuals are identified as either poor or extensive metabolizers for that specific isozyme.

Phase II reactions are conjugation reactions in which the drug is coupled to water-soluble molecules to enhance its excretion. The most abundant phase II enzymes belong to the superfamily of uridine glucuronosyltransferases (UGTs). The UGT superfamily of enzymes is classified by a system similar to that for CYP enzymes. There are two clinically significant UGT subfamilies: 1A and 2B. As with the CYP system, there can be substrates, inhibitors, and inducers of UGT enzymes. For example, the benzodiazepines primarily metabolized by conjugation (i.e., oxazepam, lorazepam, and temazepam) are glucuronidated by UGT2B7. A number of nonsteroidal anti-inflammatory drugs (NSAIDs) are competitive inhibitors of UGT2B7. Phenobarbital, rifampin, and oral contraceptives appear to be inducers of UGT2B7.

A third system involved in drug elimination is P-glycoprotein. P-glycoprotein is an efflux transporter present in the gut, liver and biliary systems, gonads, kidneys, brain, and other organs. P-glycoproteins protect the body from harmful substances by transporting certain hydrophobic compounds out of the brain and other organs and into the gut, urine, and bile. The distribution and elimination of many clinically important therapeutic substances are altered by P-glycoproteins. P-glycoproteins in the gut limit absorption and significantly influence oral bioavailability and "first-pass" effects. P-glycoproteins in the blood–brain barrier contribute to the functional integrity of the barrier. As with the CYP and UGT enzyme systems, there are substrates, inhibitors, and inducers of the P-glycoprotein transporters. Administration of a P-glycoprotein inhibitor will increase oral bioavailability and central nervous system (CNS) access of a substrate drug, with opposite effects for an inducer. Many factors can alter P-glycoprotein function and influence P-glycoprotein–based interactions; these include genetic differences, gender, herbal supplements, foods, and hormones (Cozza et al. 2003).

General Principles

Prescribing in a polypharmacy environment, usually the norm in medically ill patients, requires vigilance regarding potential drug–drug interactions. With the constantly changing knowledge base and the development of new medications, it is not possible to memorize all potential psychotropic drug–drug interactions. Knowing a drug's metabolic pathways and the metabolic inhibitory or inductive effects of the co-administered drug enables us to predict its potential interactions. However, it should be remembered that drug concentration changes do not necessarily translate into clinically meaningful interactions. In patients taking multiple medications, it is preferable to avoid medications that significantly inhibit or induce CYP enzymes and to instead choose medications that are eliminated by multiple pathways and have a wide safety margin. In a polypharmacy environment, physicians should consult drug information resources to screen for clinically significant drug–drug interactions. Many computer systems used by pharmacists and physicians are equipped with a drug interaction checker. A useful summary table was recently published by Owen and Crouse (2017).

Identification of Potential Pharmacokinetic Interactions

Not all combinations of interacting drug with substrate will result in clinically significant interactions. For these interactions to be clinically relevant, the substrate must have certain characteristics. A *critical substrate* drug is a drug with a narrow therapeutic index and one primary CYP isozyme mediating its elimination. For example, aripiprazole is primarily metabolized by both CYP2D6 and CYP3A4 isozymes. The addition of a drug that is a potent CYP2D6 inhibitor, such as fluoxetine, will inhibit aripiprazole's metabolism. Without a compensatory reduction in aripiprazole dosage, aripiprazole levels will rise, and increased adverse effects or toxicity may result. On the other hand, the addition of a potent enzyme inducer, such as carbamazepine, will result in reduced levels and reduced efficacy of aripiprazole. It is recommended that concomitant use of carbamazepine with the long-acting injectable formulation of aripiprazole be avoided because of the inability to maintain therapeutic concentrations between injections (Otsuka 2017). Prescribing an inhibitor or inducer that interacts with a CYP isozyme other than CYP2D6 or CYP3A4 will have no significant effect on aripiprazole levels.

Metabolic drug–drug interactions are most likely to occur in three situations:

1. The addition of an interacting drug to a medication regimen containing a substrate drug at steady-state levels may alter substrate drug concentration. If the interacting drug is an inhibitor, substrate drug concentrations will rise as its elimination is reduced, and toxicity may result. Conversely, the addition of an enzyme inducer will increase elimination of the substrate, thereby lowering its concentration and therapeutic effect.
2. The withdrawal of an interacting drug from an established drug regimen containing a critical substrate drug (an often-overlooked cause of interaction). Previously, the substrate drug dosage will have been adjusted in the presence of the interacting drug to optimize therapeutic effect and minimize adverse effects. Withdrawal of an enzyme inhibitor will allow metabolism to return (increase) to normal levels, re-

sulting in lower levels and decreased therapeutic effect of the substrate drug. In contrast, removal of an enzyme inducer will increase substrate drug levels and may lead to drug toxicity as metabolism of the substrate decreases to a normal rate.
3. The addition of a critical substrate drug to a drug regimen containing an interacting drug can result in a clinically significant interaction if the substrate is dosed according to established guidelines. Most dosing guidelines do not account for the presence of a metabolic inhibitor or inducer and thus may lead to substrate concentrations that are, respectively, toxic or subtherapeutic. The prescribing information of newer approved medications contains recommendations for dosage adjustments when the medication is combined with a potent inducer or inhibitor.

Drug–drug interactions that affect renal drug elimination are clinically significant only if the parent drug or its active metabolite undergoes appreciable renal elimination. Changes in urine pH can modify the elimination of those compounds whose ratio of ionized/un-ionized forms is dramatically altered across the physiological range of urine pH (4.6–8.2) (i.e., the compound has a pKa within this pH range). Common drugs that alkalinize urine include antacids and carbonic anhydrase inhibitor diuretics. Un-ionized forms of drugs undergo greater glomerular resorption, whereas ionized drug forms are resorbed less and so have greater urinary excretion. For a basic drug such as amphetamine, alkalinization of urine increases the un-ionized fraction, enhancing resorption and thus prolonging activity. Other basic psychotropics, such as amitriptyline, imipramine, methadone, and memantine, may be similarly affected (Freudenthaler et al. 1998; Nilsson et al. 1982).

Side Effects and Toxicity of Major Psychotropic Drug Classes

Antidepressants

Antidepressants are used to treat mood, anxiety, eating, and some somatic symptom disorders as well as insomnia, enuresis, incontinence, headaches, and chronic pain.

Selective Serotonin Reuptake Inhibitors and Novel/Mixed-Action Agents

Adverse effects of selective serotonin reuptake inhibitors (SSRIs) and novel/mixed-action agents are common but are usually mild and dose-related and abate over time. However, serotonergic agents, especially when used in combination, can induce the potentially fatal serotonin syndrome (see "Serotonin Syndrome" later in this section).

Common short-term side effects with SSRIs and serotonin–norepinephrine reuptake inhibitors (SNRIs) include nausea, vomiting, anxiety, headache, sedation, tremors, and anorexia. Common long-term side effects include sexual dysfunction, dry mouth, sweating, impaired sleep, and potential weight gain. Milnacipran, an SNRI approved for depression in Europe and Japan and approved by the U.S. Food and Drug Administration (FDA) for fibromyalgia, is associated with constipation, flushing, sweating, vomiting, palpitations, increased heart rate and hypertension, and dry mouth (Allergan 2016), similar to other SNRIs. Trazodone and nefazodone do not disrupt sexual function or sleep. Trazodone causes sedation in 20%–50% of patients and is often used for its sedating properties. It also can cause priapism in rare cases. Trazodone and nefazodone can cause orthostatic hypotension, and nefazodone can cause hepatotoxicity.

Mirtazapine is associated with a high incidence of sedation, increased appetite, and weight gain (Merck 2016). Common adverse effects of bupropion include agitation, insomnia, anxiety, dry mouth, constipation, postural hypotension, and tachycardia. Nausea and vomiting are much less common with bupropion than with SSRIs (Vanderkooy et al. 2002). Patients treated with reboxetine (used only in Europe) often report dry mouth, insomnia, constipation, sweating, and hypotension (Andreoli et al. 2002).

Central nervous system effects. Bupropion causes a dose-related lowering of the seizure threshold and may precipitate seizures in susceptible patients receiving dosages above 450 mg/day. The incidence of seizure rises with increasing dosage of the immediate-release dosage form, from 0.1% at 100–300 mg/day, through 0.4% at 300–450 mg/day, to 2.3% at dosages over 600 mg/day (McEvoy 2017). Bupropion is contraindicated in persons with a seizure disorder, bulimia, or anorexia or in those at risk for alcohol or benzodiazepine withdrawal. The seizure risk reported for other antidepressants ranges from 0.04% for mirtazapine to 0.5% for clomipramine (Harden and Goldstein 2002; Rosenstein et al. 1993). Given that the annual incidence of first unprovoked seizure is 0.06% in the general population, seizure risk for patients taking most antidepressants is not elevated. However, it is clear that certain antidepressants, such as bupropion, clomipramine, maprotiline, and venlafaxine, are associated with greater seizure risk (Harden and Goldstein 2002; Whyte et al. 2003), although this risk is rarely significant except at toxic doses.

Potential side effects of SSRIs include extrapyramidal symptoms (EPS), likely resulting from serotonergic antagonism of dopaminergic pathways in the CNS. Tremor and akathisia are the most common. Certain patients appear to be at increased risk, such as the elderly and patients with the A1 allele of the dopamine D_2 receptor (DRD_2) gene Taq1A polymorphism (Hawthorne and Caley 2015; Hedenmalm et al. 2006).

Serotonin syndrome. Serotonin syndrome is an uncommon but potentially life-threatening complication of treatment with serotonergic agents. Overall, there is considerable heterogeneity in the reported clinical features of serotonin syndrome (Table 36–2), reflecting variation in its severity. The incidence of the syndrome is unknown, because there is no consensus on diagnostic criteria (Werneke et al. 2016). Virtually all medications that potentiate serotonergic neurotransmission in the CNS have been reported in association with serotonin syndrome. The antidepressant combinations most commonly implicated have been reversible and irreversible monoamine oxidase inhibitors (MAOIs) and tricyclic antidepressants (TCAs), MAOIs and SSRIs, and MAOIs and venlafaxine. Table 36–3 lists other serotonergic drugs.

The first operationalized criteria for serotonin syndrome were proposed by Sternbach (1991) but were found to have low specificity. The Hunter criteria have subsequently gained acceptance and are listed in Table 36–4 (Dunkley et al. 2003). A third set of criteria was proposed by Radomski et al. (2000). Unfortunately, there is poor agreement among these three criteria systems when applied for diagnosis (Werneke et al. 2016). Laboratory findings have not been commonly reported in cases of sero-

TABLE 36–2.   Clinical features of serotonin syndrome

Category	Clinical features
Mental status and behavioral	Delirium, confusion, agitation, anxiety, irritability, euphoria, dysphoria, restlessness
Neurological and motor	Ataxia/incoordination, tremor, muscle rigidity, myoclonus, hyperreflexia, clonus, seizures, trismus, teeth chattering
Gastrointestinal	Nausea, vomiting, diarrhea, hyperactive bowel sounds, incontinence
Autonomic nervous system	Hypertension, hypotension, tachycardia, diaphoresis, shivering, sialorrhea, mydriasis, tachypnea, pupillary dilation
Thermoregulation	Hyperthermia

Source.   Compiled in part from Haddad and Dursun 2008 and Boyer and Shannon 2005.

TABLE 36–3.   Drugs that potentiate serotonin in the central nervous system

Mechanism	Drug
Enhance serotonin synthesis	L-Tryptophan
Increase serotonin release	Cocaine, amphetamine, dextromethorphan, meperidine, fentanyl, MDMA (Ecstasy), lithium
Stimulate serotonin receptors	Buspirone, trazodone, nefazodone, vilazodone, ergot alkaloids
Inhibit serotonin catabolism	MAOIs, moclobemide, linezolid, tedizolid, isoniazid, procarbazine, methylene blue
Inhibit serotonin reuptake	SSRIs, SNRIs, mirtazapine, trazodone, nefazodone, vilazodone, vortioxetine, TCAs, tramadol, dextromethorphan, pentazocine, St. John's wort

Note.   MAOIs=monoamine oxidase inhibitors; MDMA=3,4-methylenedioxymethamphetamine; SNRIs=serotonin–norepinephrine reuptake inhibitors; SSRIs=selective serotonin reuptake inhibitors; TCAs=tricyclic antidepressants.

Source.   Compiled in part from Katus and Frucht 2016.

tonin syndrome, but some reports have noted metabolic acidosis, rhabdomyolysis with elevated creatine phosphokinase (CPK), serum hepatic transaminase elevations, and disseminated intravascular coagulopathy. The differential diagnosis includes CNS infection (e.g., encephalitis, meningitis), delirium tremens, poisoning with anticholinergic agents, neuroleptic malignant syndrome (NMS), and malignant hyperthermia. Differentiating serotonin syndrome from NMS can be very difficult in patients who are receiving both serotonergic and antipsychotic medications (see "Neuroleptic Malignant Syndrome" later in this chapter).

Serotonin syndrome is often self-limited and usually resolves quickly after discontinuation of serotonergic agents. Management includes the following basic principles: 1) discontinue all serotonergic agents; 2) provide supportive care; 3) control

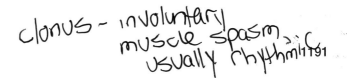
clonus - involuntary muscle spasm, usually rhythmic 1191

TABLE 36–4. **Diagnostic criteria for serotonin syndrome**

Use of a serotonergic agent

Plus any of the following symptoms:

Spontaneous clonus

Inducible clonus plus either agitation or diaphoresis

Tremor plus hyperreflexia

Muscle rigidity plus elevated body temperature plus either ocular clonus or inducible clonus

Exclude:

Infection, metabolic, endocrine, or toxic causes

Neuroleptic malignant syndrome

Delirium tremens

Malignant hyperthermia

Source. Compiled from Boyer and Shannon 2005; Dunkley et al. 2003.

agitation, autonomic instability, and hyperthermia; 4) consider administering anti-serotonergic agents; and 5) reassess the need for psychopharmacological therapy before reinstituting drug therapy (Boyer and Shannon 2005). Some patients will require admission to an intensive care unit, but most will show some improvement within 24 hours with supportive care alone. There are no specific antidotes available for the treatment of serotonin syndrome. The antihistamine cyproheptadine, which has serotonin antagonist properties, is the most commonly used treatment; however, evidence supporting its effectiveness is lacking. The recommended adult dose for cyproheptadine is 4–8 mg, and this dose may be repeated every 1–4 hours up to a maximum total daily dose of 32 mg. There is limited information on drug rechallenge in patients who have developed serotonin syndrome. General guidelines include reevaluating the necessity for drug therapy, considering a switch to a nonserotonergic medication, using single-drug therapy when serotonergic medications are required, and considering an extended (6-week) "serotonin drug–free" period before restarting a serotonergic agent (Mills 1997).

Autonomic and cardiovascular effects. The SSRIs and the novel/mixed-action antidepressants have a much safer cardiovascular profile than do the TCAs and MAOIs. In general, the SSRIs have little effect on blood pressure or cardiac conduction (Glassman et al. 2002). The SSRIs have in rare cases been reported to cause mild bradycardia in elderly patients with preexisting cardiac arrhythmias. Citalopram is the SSRI most likely to cause QTc prolongation (Beach et al. 2014; Vieweg et al. 2012). Although the FDA (U.S. Food and Drug Administration 2016b) mandated placement in the drug labeling of a warning against use of citalopram at dosages greater than 40 mg/day because of concerns about QTc prolongation, there is little evidence that higher dosages of citalopram are associated with increased risk of sudden cardiac death (Zivin et al. 2013).

The novel/mixed-action agents venlafaxine, desvenlafaxine, duloxetine, bupropion, nefazodone, mirtazapine, and reboxetine have little effect on cardiac conduction but may affect blood pressure or heart rate (Khawaja and Feinstein 2003; Pfizer 2016). Clinical trials of venlafaxine observed an average diastolic pressure increase of 7 mm Hg at dosages of more than 300 mg/day and clinically significant diastolic pressure increases (≥15 mm Hg) in 5.5% of patients taking the drug at dosages of more than 200 mg/day (Feighner 1995). Similar effects would be expected for desvenlafaxine. Duloxetine appears to be without clinically significant effects on heart rate, blood pressure, or QTc interval (Wernicke et al. 2007). Bupropion is reported to cause hypertension without affecting heart rate in some patients. In patients using transdermal nicotine, bupropion is associated with a 6.1% incidence of hypertension (Khawaja and Feinstein 2003). Reboxetine has also been associated with an increase in heart rate of 8–11 beats/minute (Fleishaker et al. 2001), but without any significant effect on electrocardiography (Andreoli et al. 2002). Trazodone lacks significant effects on cardiac conduction at therapeutic dosages but in rare cases and in overdose has been reported to cause ventricular ectopy and ventricular tachycardia. The most frequent cardiovascular adverse effect of trazodone is postural hypotension, which may be associated with syncope. Nefazodone is structurally related to trazodone but has a lower incidence of postural hypotension. Mirtazapine does not have significant effects on cardiac conduction, but because of its moderate alpha$_1$-antagonist activity, it has a 7% incidence of orthostatic hypotension (Khawaja and Feinstein 2003). Hypotension is observed in 10% of patients receiving reboxetine.

Gastrointestinal effects.   Nausea is the most common adverse effect associated with the serotonergic antidepressants. Nausea is most likely to occur in patients receiving fluvoxamine, venlafaxine, and duloxetine at a starting dosage of 60 mg/day (Detke et al. 2002). Other serotonergic antidepressants have a lower incidence of nausea. For patients experiencing significant nausea, mirtazapine should be considered over an SSRI.

Although most adverse GI effects of serotonergic antidepressants are dose related and generally decrease with continued treatment, severe side effects sometimes require antidepressant discontinuation. Minor elevations in transaminases are common with all antidepressants and are usually benign. Elevation of aspartate transaminase (AST) or alanine transaminase (ALT) levels of two to three times baseline or two times normal is significant, and any elevation of alkaline phosphatase (ALP) or bilirubin may be significant. Because of its potential to cause severe hepatotoxicity, nefazodone has been removed from the market in a number of countries, and it should not be used in patients with preexisting liver disease (Stewart 2002). The finding that duloxetine-related hepatotoxicity occurs in 1.1% of patients has prompted product monograph warnings (Eli Lilly 2016); however, a review of duloxetine hepatic safety found no increase in hepatotoxicity compared with other conventional antidepressants (McIntyre et al. 2008).

Hematological effects.   SSRIs are associated with a slightly increased risk of bleeding disorders, including GI bleeding (Papakostas 2010). This effect is discussed in the "Psychotropic Drug Use in the Medically Ill" section later in this chapter, as well as in Chapter 19 ("Gastrointestinal Disorders"), Chapter 23 ("Hematology"), and Chapter 28, ("Surgery").

Weight gain.   Many patients receiving antidepressants experience weight gain. Percentages of patients who gained ≥7% of their body weight over 1 year of treatment were highest for mirtazapine (26%); less for SSRIs (16%–19%); and similar to placebo (8%–12%) for bupropion, duloxetine (at dosages ≥60 mg/day), nefazodone, and venlafaxine. Paroxetine is more likely than other SSRIs to cause weight gain, whereas the weight-gain propensity of fluoxetine and escitalopram may be more similar to that of placebo (Papakostas 2010).

Syndrome of inappropriate antidiuretic hormone secretion.   In a review of the risk of syndrome of inappropriate antidiuretic hormone secretion (SIADH) in antidepressants, the risk was higher for SSRIs and venlafaxine compared with other antidepressants (De Picker et al. 2014). Elderly patients, especially those with concurrent diuretic use (especially thiazides), were found to be at higher risk of hyponatremia. Other reported risk factors for SSRI-induced hyponatremia were female sex, low baseline serum sodium, and chronic illness (Varela Piñón and Adán-Manes 2017).

Sexual dysfunction.   For a full discussion of the sexual side effects of psychotropic medication, see Chapter 15, "Sexual Dysfunctions."

Drug–drug interactions.   Many SSRIs (e.g., fluoxetine, fluvoxamine, paroxetine) and novel/mixed-action antidepressants are potent inhibitors of CYP isozymes and may significantly increase blood levels, and the potential for toxic effects, of other co-administered narrow-therapeutic-index medications metabolized by these enzymes (see English et al. 2012, Owen and Crouse 2017, and de Leon and Spina 2018 for listings of drug substrates for these enzymes). The combined use of multiple serotonergic drugs can induce serotonin syndrome (see Table 36–3 and "Serotonin Syndrome" subsection earlier in this chapter).

Serotonin discontinuation syndrome.   Abrupt discontinuation of SSRIs or SNRIs, especially those with short half-lives (e.g., fluvoxamine, paroxetine, venlafaxine), may give rise to a discontinuation syndrome characterized by a wide variety of symptoms, including psychiatric, neurological, and flulike (nausea, vomiting, sweats) symptoms, as well as sleep disturbances (Fava et al. 2015), usually resolving within 3 weeks. Some patients report electric shock–like sensations ("brain zaps") in the brain during withdrawal. Antidepressants should be withdrawn gradually. Discontinuation symptoms can lead to misdiagnosis and inappropriate treatment, particularly in patients with an active medical illness, and can also have negative effects on future medication adherence.

Toxicity/overdose.   In general, an overdose with SSRIs or SNRIs is considered less life-threatening than a TCA overdose. A review of 469 SSRI overdose admissions reported a 14% incidence of serotonin syndrome and a 1.9% incidence of seizure (Isbister et al. 2004). Citalopram and escitalopram have each been associated with QTc prolongation in overdose (Isbister et al. 2004; van Gorp et al. 2009); in the study by Isbister et al. (2004), 68% (65/96) of citalopram overdoses involved a QTc interval greater than 440 msec. In rare cases, venlafaxine and bupropion have also been linked to QTc prolongation in overdose (Jasiak and Bostwick 2014).

Tricyclic Antidepressants

TCAs are third-line treatments for depression because their adverse-effect profile is less benign than the profiles of SSRIs and novel/mixed-action agents. Death from TCA-induced cardiac conduction abnormalities is not uncommon in TCA overdose.

Many adverse effects of TCAs are attributable not to their effects on serotonin (5-HT) or norepinephrine reuptake inhibition but rather to their secondary pharmacological effects. TCAs are antagonists at histamine H_1, adrenergic alpha$_1$, and muscarinic receptors and have Type 1A antiarrhythmic (quinidine-like) effects. Adverse effects of TCAs include sedation, anticholinergic effects (dry mouth, dry eyes, constipation, urinary retention, decreased sweating, confusion, memory impairment, tachycardia, blurred vision), and postural hypotension. Tolerance to these effects usually develops over time. TCAs should not be given to individuals with closed-angle glaucoma, benign prostatic hypertrophy, or delirium. TCAs at or just above therapeutic plasma levels frequently cause prolongation of PR, QRS, and QTc intervals, but rarely to a clinically significant degree in patients without preexisting cardiac disease or conduction defects (Glassman 1984). TCAs can cause heart block, arrhythmias, palpitations, tachycardia, syncope, and heart failure and should be used with caution in patients who have preexisting cardiovascular disease or who are at risk of suicide.

Drug–drug interactions. The combination of TCAs and other drugs with sedating, hypotensive, antiarrhythmic, or seizure threshold–lowering properties may lead to additive toxicity. Concomitant use of TCAs and drugs with anticholinergic properties may cause an anticholinergic crisis characterized by delirium, hyperthermia (especially in hot environments), tachycardia, and paralytic ileus.

Coadministration of TCAs with MAOIs and other drugs with MAOI activity may precipitate serotonin syndrome or hyperpyretic crisis (hyperpyrexia, sweating, confusion, myoclonus, seizures, hypertension, and tachycardia), either of which may be fatal. The combination of serotonergic effects from cotherapy with some TCAs and SSRIs may precipitate serotonin syndrome.

TCAs are narrow-therapeutic-index drugs, each metabolized predominantly by either CYP2D6 or CYP3A4. Inhibitors of these enzymes can cause TCA toxicity by dramatically increasing TCA serum levels. Many agents, including certain SSRIs and novel/mixed-action antidepressants, are potent inhibitors of these CYP isozymes. Plasma levels of TCAs should be monitored if TCAs are coadministered with such inhibitors.

Toxicity/overdose. TCA overdose carries a risk of death from cardiac conduction abnormalities that result in malignant ventricular arrhythmias. Initial symptoms of a major overdose involve CNS stimulation, in part due to anticholinergic effects, and include hyperpyrexia, delirium, hypertension, hallucinations, seizure, agitation, hyperreflexia. The initial stimulation phase is typically followed by CNS depression, with drowsiness, areflexia, hypothermia, respiratory depression, severe hypotension, and coma. The risk of complications (death, seizures, ventricular arrhythmias) is high if the QRS interval exceeds 100 msec (Body et al. 2011).

Treatment for overdose includes removal of any unabsorbed medication from the stomach (gastric lavage or activated charcoal to reduce absorption), followed by supportive therapy and close monitoring (see Chapter 35, "Medical Toxicology"). In TCA overdose, the risk of aspiration should be considered prior to administration of activated charcoal (Body et al. 2011). Cardiac conduction abnormalities, arrhythmias, and hypotension may be treated with intravenous sodium bicarbonate to produce a serum pH of 7.45–7.55. Life-threatening anticholinergic effects may be managed with physostigmine in consultation with a poison control center if the patient is unresponsive to other therapies. Because of their large volumes of distribution and extensive protein binding, TCAs are not removed by dialysis.

TCA discontinuation syndrome. Abrupt discontinuation of TCAs may cause a discontinuation syndrome characterized by lethargy, headache, nightmares, insomnia, excess dreaming, and symptoms of cholinergic rebound, including nausea, vomiting, diarrhea, sweating, anxiety, and irritability (Haddad 2001). This syndrome can be avoided by gradual withdrawal.

Monoamine Oxidase Inhibitors

MAOIs, with the possible exception of moclobemide (not available in the United States), are last-line antidepressants because of their significant drug–drug interactions and the dietary restrictions that accompany their use. Moclobemide, a short-half-life reversible inhibitor of MAO-A, is less susceptible to dietary interactions provided that it is taken after meals. Common adverse effects of MAOIs include orthostatic hypotension, dizziness, headache, sedation, insomnia or hypersomnia, tremor, and hyperreflexia. Interactions between MAOIs and direct- or indirect-acting sympathomimetics or dopaminergic agonists may cause a hypertensive crisis. MAOIs may trigger serotonin syndrome when combined with other serotonergic medications. Moclobemide shares the potential to cause hypertensive crises and serotonin syndrome with the irreversible agents. MAOIs may greatly potentiate the hypotensive effects of antihypertensive agents, including diuretics. Selegiline, a semiselective MAO-B inhibitor, may also contribute to serotonin syndrome. At oral dosages greater than 10 mg/day, and transdermal strengths greater than 6 mg/day, tyramine dietary restrictions should be employed.

Toxicity/overdose. Symptoms of MAOI overdose are an extension of the normal adverse-effect profile. Treatment for overdose includes GI decontamination and supportive measures. Treatment for hypertensive crisis involves discontinuing the MAOI and slowly administering intravenous phentolamine (typical adult dose: 5 mg).

Mood Stabilizers/Anticonvulsants

Mood stabilizers are used in medically ill patients to treat primary and secondary mood disorders. Valproate, lamotrigine, carbamazepine, and oxcarbazepine are the most commonly used anticonvulsant mood stabilizers. In addition to their use in treating seizures, anticonvulsants are prescribed in the medically ill to manage headache, chronic pain, and alcohol withdrawal.

Lithium

Most individuals taking lithium experience some side effects, both acute (e.g., GI distress, tremor) and long term (e.g., polyuria and polydipsia, hypothyroidism, weight gain, impaired cognition, sedation, impaired coordination, edema, acne, hair loss), most of which are mild and dose related (Freeman and Freeman 2006; Livingstone and Rampes 2006; McEvoy 2017). Adverse effects of lithium can be minimized by reducing the dosage or decreasing the rate of absorption from the gut by administering the drug either in divided doses with meals or in a sustained-release dosage form.

Central nervous system effects. Headache, fatigue, hand tremor, and mild cognitive impairment are reported by up to 50% of patients beginning lithium treatment.

Hand tremor is usually benign and manifests as a fine, rapid intention tremor that resolves over time or can be managed by dosage reduction or use of low-dose beta-blockers. The tremor does not respond to antiparkinsonian drugs. Muscle weakness, fatigue, and ataxia are also common initial adverse effects of lithium that usually resolve (McEvoy 2017). Mild cognitive impairment may be experienced during the first 6–8 months of treatment; although rarely progressive, this impairment is the most common reason for medication nonadherence (Gitlin 2016).

Autonomic and cardiovascular effects.   Lithium causes benign reversible repolarization electrocardiographic changes—including T wave depression and inversion—in 20%–30% of patients (McEvoy 2017). Other cardiovascular effects of lithium include decreased heart rate, sinus node dysfunction, prolonged QTc interval, and arrhythmias (Burggraf 1997; van Noord et al. 2009).

Renal effects.   Lithium reduces renal response to antidiuretic hormone, resulting in polyuria and/or polydipsia initially in 30%–50% of patients and persisting in 10%–25%. Stopping lithium usually reverses this nephrogenic diabetes insipidus (McEvoy 2017). Apart from dry mouth, patients do not generally exhibit signs of dehydration. Management of polyuria may include changing to a single daily bedtime dose of lithium, decreasing the dosage, and/or administering amiloride (considered the treatment of choice) or thiazide diuretics. If thiazide diuretics are added, the lithium dosage should be reduced by 50% to compensate for thiazide-induced reduction of lithium excretion (McEvoy 2017). Use of amiloride does not require a reduction in lithium dosage (McEvoy 2017). Edema has been reported in patients with a high sodium intake (>170 mEq/day) and is responsive to reduction in sodium intake or spironolactone (Stancer and Kivi 1971).

The long-term effects of lithium on renal function are a subject of debate, with variable findings reported in recent retrospective and cohort studies (Levenson and Owen 2017; see also Chapter 20, "Renal Disease," for full discussion). Although long-term lithium treatment is the only well-established risk factor for lithium-induced nephropathy, other factors, such as age, previous episodes of lithium toxicity, and the presence of comorbid disorders, may also contribute. Lithium is so efficacious in bipolar disorder that the risk of renal dysfunction during long-term use is considered acceptable with appropriate monitoring of renal function.

Endocrine and metabolic effects.   Rates of hypothyroidism or changes in thyroid function vary widely, with prevalence rates as high as 47% in lithium-treated patients (Livingstone and Rampes 2006). Overt hypothyroidism has been reported to occur in 8%–19% of patients taking lithium, compared with a prevalence of 0.5%–1.8% in the general population. Subclinical hypothyroidism has been reported in up to 23% of patients receiving lithium therapy, compared with rates of up to 10.4% in the general population (Kleiner et al. 1999). Elevated thyroid-stimulating hormone (TSH) is present in approximately 30% of patients taking lithium for 6 months or longer, and progression to overt hypothyroidism (elevated TSH and low free thyroxine [T_4]) may occur in as many as 5%–10% of patients per year (Kleiner et al. 1999), with greater risk in thyroid antibody–positive individuals (Bocchetta et al. 2007). Thyroid function should be assessed before lithium is started and periodically during therapy. Hypothyroidism can be treated with levothyroxine and is not a contraindication to continuing lithium (Freeman and Freeman 2006; see also Chapter 21, "Endocrine and Metabolic Disorders"). Recognition of lithium-induced hypercalcemia associated with hyperparathyroidism is increasing, with reported incidence ranging from 6.3% to 50% (Livingstone and Rampes 2006).

Lithium-induced weight gain (>8% of baseline body weight) (Chengappa et al. 2002) is one of the most common reasons cited by patients for lithium nonadherence (Nemeroff 2003). Approximately 25% of lithium-treated patients will gain more than 4.5 kg (Nemeroff 2003). Weight gain may be a consequence of increased caloric intake secondary to consumption of high-calorie fluids in response to increased thirst (McEvoy 2017).

Dermatological effects. Dermatological adverse effects of lithium include dry skin, alopecia, acne, and psoriasis. Lithium-induced acne occurs in more than 30% of patients (Jafferany 2008). These effects usually respond to standard treatment (i.e., tretinoin or topical salicylic acid) and rarely require lithium discontinuation. Alopecia and exacerbation of psoriasis occur less frequently. Lithium-induced or -exacerbated psoriasis can be managed with standard treatments but may be less responsive to them (Jafferany 2008; see also Chapter 27, "Dermatology").

Drug–drug interactions. Lithium is almost entirely renally excreted, and most lithium filtered by the glomeruli is reabsorbed with sodium in the proximal tubule. Serum lithium levels are increased by thiazide diuretics, NSAIDs, angiotensin-converting enzyme (ACE) inhibitors, angiotensin receptor antagonists, sodium depletion, electrolyte abnormalities, and dehydration (Finley 2016). Symptoms of toxicity have been reported with addition of verapamil or diltiazem to lithium despite nonelevated concentrations. In patients who are elderly, medically ill, or on salt-restricted diets, loop diuretics may increase lithium toxicity; in other patient populations, loop diuretics may enhance elimination and reduce lithium levels. Carbonic anhydrase inhibitors, osmotic diuretics, methylxanthines, and caffeine reduce lithium levels, whereas potassium-sparing diuretics are considered to have no effect on lithium levels (Finley 2016). In medically ill persons, it is imperative to closely monitor for toxicity whenever medication changes are made.

Lithium is often used in combination with antipsychotics in bipolar disorder. Rare cases of severe neurotoxicity with this medication combination have been reported with both first-generation and second-generation antipsychotics. Whether the neurotoxicity associated with this combination represents a true adverse interaction remains controversial. In general, lithium can be safely combined with SSRIs; however, a handful of case reports from the early 1990s suggest that lithium in combination with other serotonin-enhancing drugs may precipitate serotonin syndrome (Finley 2016).

Toxicity/overdose. Toxicity increases markedly once serum lithium levels exceed 1.5 mEq/L, and serum levels greater than 2.0 mEq/L are dangerous. However, some patients experience toxicity at "therapeutic" levels. Symptoms of toxicity include nausea, vomiting, diarrhea, coarse tremor, blurred vision, impaired concentration, slurred speech, unsteady gait, weakness, confusion, and increased deep-tendon reflexes, and may progress to seizures, coma, cardiac arrhythmia, and possibly permanent neurological impairment as lithium levels increase (Gitlin 2016). Potentially irreversible complications can involve cerebellar dysfunction, including ataxia, dysarthria, and dysmetria (Gitlin 2016).

In mild toxicity, discontinuation of lithium may be sufficient. In moderate lithium toxicity, treatment involves volume resuscitation with normal sodium chloride (0.9% NaCl) solution to enhance renal elimination of lithium, as well as gastric lavage and/or whole-bowel irrigation with polyethylene glycol (for large amounts or controlled-release products). Lithium is not adsorbed by activated charcoal (Baird-Gunning et al. 2017; Gitlin 2016). In severe toxicity, extracorporeal treatment is recommended if the lithium level exceeds 4 mEq/L, if kidney impairment is present, or if symptoms of seizures, reduced consciousness, or life-threatening arrhythmias are present. Extracorporeal treatment is indicated if the lithium level exceeds 5 mEq/L, if confusion is present, or if the lithium level is expected to remain above 1 mEq/L after 36 hours (Decker et al. 2015). Hemodialysis is preferred over continuous renal replacement therapy (CRRT) and peritoneal dialysis. If hemodialysis is not available, CRRT may be an acceptable alternative (Baird-Gunning et al. 2017; Decker et al. 2015).

Anticonvulsants

Central nervous system effects.   The anticonvulsants valproate, carbamazepine, gabapentin, lamotrigine, oxcarbazepine, topiramate, tiagabine, zonisamide, and levetiracetam share a similar profile of CNS adverse effects. Sedation, ataxia, dizziness, muscle weakness, fatigue, and vision disturbances such as nystagmus and diplopia are common and often resolve with time, dosage reduction, or drug discontinuation. Studies of oxcarbazepine in epilepsy suggest that it has a lower rate of most adverse effects compared with carbamazepine (Schmidt and Elger 2004). Patients with a history of psychiatric disorders were more likely to experience psychiatric adverse effects with levetiracetam, including mood disorder (1%), psychosis (3%), and aggression (2%) (Mula et al. 2003). Brivaracetam appears to have a psychiatric adverse-effect profile similar to that of levetiracetam. Perampanel carries an FDA boxed warning regarding risk of psychiatric and behavioral adverse effects. Cognitive impairment is a common complication of anticonvulsant or lithium use but can also be a manifestation of bipolar disorder (Mago et al. 2014). Among anticonvulsants used in psychiatry, the incidence (lowest to highest) of cognitive adverse effects is as follows: gabapentin (7.3%), valproate (8.3%), lamotrigine (8.9%), carbamazepine (9.9%), levetiracetam (10.4%), oxcarbazepine (11.6%), phenytoin (14.6%), zonisamide (14.9%), topiramate (21.5%) (Arif et al. 2009). The incidence of adverse effects increases with anticonvulsant polypharmacy.

Gastrointestinal effects.   Symptoms of GI distress, including nausea, vomiting, dyspepsia, and diarrhea, are the most common adverse effects experienced with most anticonvulsants. These effects are often dose related and transient and can be minimized by giving the drug in divided doses, with meals, in delayed- or extended-release dosage forms, or with slow titration. GI effects appear less often with divalproex sodium than with valproate or sodium valproate. Transient elevations in liver enzymes occur with anticonvulsants (Anderson and Hakimian 2014). Significant changes in hepatic function are usually reversible with dosage reduction or discontinuation. However, fatal hepatotoxicity has been reported with valproate and carbamazepine. The risk of hepatic failure may be increased by combination therapy and comorbid hepatic disorders (Schmid et al. 2013). Valproate, carbamazepine, and lamotrigine have been infrequently associated with drug-induced pancreatitis (Zaccara et al.

2007). Hypersensitivity reactions can be associated with liver failure (Anderson and Hakimian 2014). See the subsection below on immunological effects for a discussion of the drug reaction with eosinophilia and systemic symptoms (DRESS) syndrome.

Hematological effects. Carbamazepine is associated with transient leukopenia and in rare cases may cause aplastic anemia or agranulocytosis. Thrombocytopenia has been reported to occur during the first 2 weeks of therapy and to resolve with discontinuation (Verrotti et al. 2014). If white blood cell (WBC) counts drop below 3.0×10^9/L in patients receiving carbamazepine, either the drug should be discontinued or the dosage should be reduced and WBC counts more frequently monitored. Carbamazepine should be discontinued in patients with WBC counts less than 2.0×10^9/L, or neutrophil counts less than 1.0×10^9/L. Clinicians should educate patients to report early signs of anemia, infection, or bleeding. Folic acid supplementation may reduce some carbamazepine-induced blood dyscrasias but requires further study (Verrotti et al. 2014).

Valproate-induced thrombocytopenia has been reported in 5%–60% of patients and is more common in children; this adverse effect is generally reversible with dosage reduction or drug discontinuation. Mild asymptomatic leukopenia and mild transient neutropenia have also been observed with valproate and were found to improve on discontinuation (Verrotti et al. 2014).

Hematological effects of lamotrigine are rare, with most cases involving leukopenia or neutropenia. Concomitant antiepileptic use or dosing that exceeds initial titration recommendations may be risk factors (Verrotti et al. 2014).

Renal effects. Carbamazepine and oxcarbazepine may cause SIADH, leading to hyponatremia and water intoxication. Hyponatremia is twice as likely with oxcarbazepine (29.9% of patients) as with carbamazepine (14.4%) (Dong et al. 2005) and is more common in the elderly (Van Amelsvoort et al. 1994). Some studies suggest that hyponatremia can be a dose-dependent adverse effect, and, therefore, that dosage reduction can improve sodium levels (Dong et al. 2005). (For further discussion of SIADH, see the "Antipsychotics" section later in this chapter.)

Endocrine and metabolic effects. Weight gain is a common factor in nonadherence (Mago et al. 2014; Nemeroff 2003; Velligan et al. 2009). Lithium and valproate are the mood stabilizers most likely to cause weight gain (Mago et al. 2014). Weight gain is especially a problem with valproate, which was associated with an average weight gain of >8% of baseline body weight over a period of 97 (±63) days (Chengappa et al. 2002). Valproate-treated patients may gain as much as 19.8 kg during treatment (Nemeroff 2003). Rates of weight gain associated with carbamazepine are lower than those associated with valproate or lithium (Nemeroff 2003). Lamotrigine has little effect on weight, whereas topiramate is associated with an average weight *loss* of 1.6–4.6 kg (Nemeroff 2003).

Topiramate inhibits carbonic anhydrase and can cause hyperchloremic, non–anion gap metabolic acidosis; in adult clinical trials, persistent reductions in serum bicarbonate occurred in 32% of patients, and serum bicarbonate levels were markedly low (<17 mEq/L) in up to 7%, depending on dosage (Janssen 2017). The incidence of a persistent reduction in serum bicarbonate is greater in pediatric patients (Janssen 2017). In pediatric clinical trials, persistent reductions in serum bicarbonate occurred in as many as 67% of patients, and serum bicarbonate levels were markedly low (<17 mEq/

L) in up to 11% (Janssen 2017). Conditions that increase risk of acidosis (e.g., renal disease, severe respiratory disorders, status epilepticus, diarrhea, ketogenic diet) may enhance the bicarbonate-lowering effects of topiramate (Janssen 2017).

Valproate can cause asymptomatic hyperammonemia and hyperammonemic encephalopathy. Routine ammonia-level monitoring is not recommended unless a patient is symptomatic. Women with bipolar disorder treated with valproate were more likely than non-valproate-treated bipolar patients to have polycystic ovarian syndrome (PCOS) (odds ratio [OR], 6.74; 95% confidence interval [CI], 1.66–27.32) (Zhang et al. 2016). The incidence of valproate-induced PCOS in bipolar disorder appears to be lower than the reported incidence in epilepsy (24.1% in a meta-analysis of 11 studies involving a total of 556 valproate-treated women with epilepsy [Hu et al. 2011]) (see Chapter 21).

Immunological effects.   Benign skin rashes occur in 5%–17% of patients receiving anticonvulsants; this side effect is most often associated with valproate, carbamazepine, and lamotrigine (Hirsch et al. 2006). However, serious and potentially fatal immune reactions to anticonvulsants are not uncommon. Incidence of the drug reaction with eosinophilia and systemic symptoms (DRESS) syndrome ranges from 1 in 1,000 to 1 in 10,000 exposures to drugs (Cacoub et al. 2011). Initial signs include rash (severe skin eruptions), fever, and internal organ involvement (Cacoub et al. 2011). DRESS has been reported most frequently with carbamazepine, followed by lamotrigine, and (more rarely) valproate (Anderson and Hakimian 2014; Cacoub et al. 2011). Stevens-Johnson syndrome and toxic epidermal necrolysis are severe and potentially fatal hypersensitivity cutaneous reactions that develop in 0.01% to 0.1% of new anticonvulsant users (Mockenhaupt et al. 2005). The highest risk occurs during the first 2 months of administration (Mockenhaupt et al. 2005). Death occurs in about 5%–10% of patients with Stevens-Johnson syndrome and in up to 45% of those with toxic epidermal necrolysis. Clinical trials suggest that about 25% of patients with hypersensitivity reactions to carbamazepine will also cross-react to oxcarbazepine (USPDI Editorial Board 2007). The onset of an anticonvulsant-induced rash requires prompt evaluation, with immediate drug discontinuation, especially if signs of a serious rash are present (see Chapter 27).

Drug–drug interactions.   Significant CYP isoenzyme induction occurs with carbamazepine (CYP1A2, CYP2C, and CYP 3A4), oxcarbazepine (CYP3A4), and valproate (CYP2C). Because valproate is highly bound to plasma proteins, it can significantly displace other highly protein-bound drugs. Valproate can also compete for hepatic glucuronidation (uridine 5'-diphosphate glucuronosyltransferase [UGT]) and inhibit elimination of drugs that primarily use this route of metabolism, such as lamotrigine and morphine. The carbapenem antibiotics (e.g., meropenem) can cause clinically significant reductions (approximately 60%) in valproic acid concentrations that lead to subtherapeutic levels within 24 hours of initiation. Reports suggest that despite compensatory increases in valproate dosage, valproate serum concentrations remained below therapeutic levels during the combined therapy period (C.C. Wu et al. 2016). Valproate concentrations returned to 90% of baseline within 7 days of discontinuing the carbapenem antibiotics (C.C. Wu et al. 2016).

Toxicity/overdose.   Symptoms of anticonvulsant overdose are often an extension of the usual adverse effects, including stupor, conduction disturbances, and hypotension. More severe complications include seizures, coma, respiratory depression, and blood dyscrasias (Lofton and Klein-Schwartz 2004; Schrettl et al. 2017). Treatment of overdose involves GI decontamination (i.e., activated charcoal) followed by supportive therapy. Hemodialysis is an effective means of enhancing drug elimination for valproate, gabapentin, pregabalin, topiramate, and levetiracetam. Limited data support use of L-arginine or L-carnitine to reduce ammonia levels in acute valproate overdose or hyperammonemia (Perrott et al. 2010; Schrettl et al. 2017).

Antipsychotics

Antipsychotics are used in medically ill populations to treat nearly all forms of psychosis, including psychosis secondary to general medical conditions, delirium, and dementia, and are less frequently used for nonspecific sedation, as adjuvants to analgesics, for hiccups (chlorpromazine), or for refractory nausea/vomiting.

Central Nervous System Effects

Acute extrapyramidal symptoms.   Acute EPS—akathisia, akinesia, and dystonia—occur in as many as 50%–75% of patients who take first-generation antipsychotics (FGAs) (Collaborative Working Group on Clinical Trial Evaluations 1998). High-potency FGAs (e.g., haloperidol) are associated with higher rates of EPS than are low-potency agents (e.g., chlorpromazine). Among the currently available second-generation antipsychotics (SGAs), the hierarchy of EPS risk (greater to lesser) is as follows: risperidone, lurasidone > ziprasidone, paliperidone ≥ asenapine > iloperidone > aripiprazole > olanzapine > quetiapine > clozapine (Citrome 2011; Gao et al. 2008; Leucht et al. 2013).

Most akathisia and acute dystonic reactions in the medically ill are caused by phenothiazine antiemetics (e.g., prochlorperazine) or metoclopramide, especially at high intravenous doses. When agitated medically ill patients are being treated with haloperidol, it can be very difficult to distinguish akathisia from the original target symptoms. It is also important to exclude other causes of restlessness that may mimic akathisia in medically ill patients, such as hypoglycemia, hypoxia, drug withdrawal, pain, electrolyte disturbances, iron deficiency, and restless legs syndrome. Severe dystonic reactions (e.g., opisthotonus) may be misdiagnosed as status epilepticus.

Chronic extrapyramidal symptoms.   Parkinsonian signs and tardive dyskinesia may occur with long-term use of antipsychotics, phenothiazine antiemetics, or metoclopramide. Bradykinesia may easily be missed in elderly or disabled medical patients.

Seizures.   Most antipsychotics lower the seizure threshold and increase seizure risk. Phenothiazines confer a dose-dependent seizure risk of 0.3%–1.2%, compared with a rate of first unprovoked seizure in the general population of about 23–61 per 100,000 person-years (Alldredge 1999; Porter and Chacko 2017). Most of the early case reports involved seizures with chlorpromazine (Alldredge 1999). Although there are no controlled comparative studies to allow an accurate assessment of relative seizure risk among the various agents, it appears that high-potency FGAs, aripiprazole, lurasidone, iloperidone, and risperidone (and likely paliperidone) are associated with the lowest risk of seizures; followed by quetiapine, and then olanzapine and low-potency FGAs, with an intermediate risk; and finally clozapine, with the highest risk (1% at 300 mg/day, increasing to 4.4% at >600 mg/day) (Alldredge 1999; Alper et al. 2007; Lertxundi et al. 2013; Williams and Park 2015).

Sedation. Sedation is the most common single side effect of antipsychotics, especially with the low-potency FGAs. Among the SGAs, the hierarchy of potential for sedation (greater to lesser) is as follows: clozapine > quetiapine, ziprasidone > olanzapine > asenapine > risperidone > lurasidone > aripiprazole, iloperidone, paliperidone, amisulpride (Citrome 2011; Leucht et al. 2013). Sedation is most prominent in the early stages of therapy, with some degree of tolerance developing over time.

Thermoregulation. Antipsychotics may interfere with temperature regulation; this effect is most often associated with the low-potency FGAs and the anticholinergic SGAs (e.g., olanzapine). Medically ill patients, especially elderly ones, are at particular risk because of their concomitant use of other anticholinergic drugs and their high rates of comorbid conditions predisposing to impaired thermoregulation (e.g., congestive heart failure, cerebrovascular disease). Depending on environmental exposure, drug-induced thermoregulation impairment may lead to either hyperthermia (heatstroke) or hypothermia (Kansagra et al. 2013; Kreuzer et al. 2012).

Neuroleptic malignant syndrome. NMS is a rare, potentially fatal idiosyncratic reaction to antipsychotics. NMS (or a similar syndrome) is also reported among patients with extrapyramidal disorders (e.g., Parkinson's disease) who have received antipsychotics or dopamine-depleting agents or who have had dopamine agonists (e.g., levodopa) abruptly withdrawn (Berman 2011). However, NMS is not specific to any one neuropsychiatric diagnosis, and it has been reported in non–psychiatrically ill individuals treated with other dopamine antagonists, such as metoclopramide or prochlorperazine (Berman 2011). Estimates of the incidence of NMS, once thought to be as high as 3.2%, are now (from more recent data) suggested to be 0.01%–0.02% (Berman 2011). Earlier mortality estimates exceeded 30%; however, with increased physician awareness and the use of SGAs, mortality has declined to around 10% (Berman 2011). Malnutrition, dehydration, iron deficiency, heat exposure, hyponatremia, and thyrotoxicosis appear to increase the risk for NMS (Berman 2011).

NMS generally develops over a 1- to 3-day period and lasts for 5–10 days after a nondepot antipsychotic is discontinued (and much longer with depot agents). The main clinical features of NMS are hyperthermia (>38°C), generalized muscle rigidity, mental status changes, and autonomic instability (Table 36–5). Temperature is greater than 38°C in the majority of cases and can exceed 40°C, predisposing patients to severe complications, including irreversible CNS and other organ damage. Muscle rigidity is often heterogeneous and can be either "lead-pipe" or cogwheeling. Signs of autonomic dysfunction include cardiac dysrhythmias, irregular blood pressure, and excessive sweating (see Table 36–5). Neurological dysfunction may consist of tremor, myoclonus, focal dystonias, dysphagia, dysarthria, opisthotonus, oculogyric crisis, and dyskinesias. Alterations in level of consciousness may range from decreased awareness to coma. CPK levels are always elevated in NMS as a result of muscle necrosis stemming from rigidity, hyperthermia, and ischemia. Elevated CPK levels are not proof of NMS, because they may result from agitation, use of physical restraints, or intramuscular injections. Extreme elevation in CPK levels (>100,000 U/L) constitutes rhabdomyolysis, which may be a consequence of NMS and/or other

---

TABLE 36–5. **Diagnostic criteria for neuroleptic malignant syndrome**

Use of dopamine-blocking agents or withdrawal of dopamine agonists within the past 72 hours

Antipsychotics

Antiemetics (phenothiazines, droperidol, metoclopramide)

Anti-Huntington's agents (tetrabenazine, deutetrabenazine)

Dopamine agonist withdrawal (levodopa)

Muscle rigidity

Generalized or localized (tongue, facial muscles), lead-pipe rigidity

Elevated creatine phosphokinase

Creatine phosphokinase 4 times the upper limit of normal

Hyperthermia

Hyperthermia to >38°C (orally) on 2 occasions

Altered level of consciousness

Mild confusion to coma

Level of consciousness fluctuating or decreased

Autonomic dysfunction

Hypertension, orthostatic hypotension, labile blood pressure, tachycardia, tachypnea, sialorrhea, diaphoresis, skin pallor, and urinary incontinence

---

Source. American Psychiatric Association 2013; Gurrera et al. 2011; Haddad and Dursun 2008; Levenson 1985.

---

causes in the medically ill (e.g., sepsis, shock, alcohol, medications). Serial CPK levels decline as NMS resolves. Leukocytosis with or without a left shift is common. Complications of NMS may include rhabdomyolysis, respiratory or renal failure, aspiration pneumonia, pulmonary embolus, deep vein thrombosis, electrolyte disturbances, and disseminated intravascular coagulopathy (Berman 2011; Pileggi and Cook 2016), as well as neuropsychiatric sequelae (Adityanjee et al. 2005). Other reported complications include cardiopulmonary failure, seizures, arrhythmias, myocardial infarction, and sepsis (Berman 2011).

The differential diagnosis of NMS is extensive (Table 36–6). Although most patients receiving antipsychotics who develop fever and rigidity will be found to have other conditions, the possibility of NMS should always be considered because of the importance of promptly halting antipsychotics. Many case reports describe physical exhaustion and dehydration prior to the onset of NMS (Strawn et al. 2007). Diagnosis may be guided by use of an NMS rating scale (Sachdev 2005). Several diagnostic criteria sets for NMS have been proposed, with the most recent developed through a formal international expert consensus process (Gurrera et al. 2011).

The main interventions in NMS are early diagnosis, prompt cessation of antipsychotic medications, and intensive supportive care (Minns and Clark 2012). Lithium and all other dopamine-blocking agents (see Table 36–5) should be discontinued. If the NMS has been triggered by withdrawal of a dopaminergic agent, the agent should be reinitiated as soon as possible. Aggressive hydration is often needed, and some cases may require bicarbonate loading to prevent kidney damage (Berman 2011).

TABLE 36–6.   Differential diagnosis of neuroleptic malignant syndrome

Differential diagnosis	Distinguishing clinical features
Serotonin syndrome	Occurs with combinations of drugs that increase serotonin transmission. Rapid onset over 24 hours; manifests as altered mental state, hyperreflexia, spontaneous or inducible clonus, autonomic instability. Nausea, vomiting, and diarrhea are common. Muscle rigidity is present only in very severe cases.
Malignant hyperthermia	Occurs after general anesthesia; familial.
Lethal catatonia	Symptoms similar to those of NMS, but occurs independently of AP exposure.
Heatstroke	Pyrexia, agitation, confusion, hypotension. Skin hot and dry; muscles flaccid; prior neuroleptic exposure may increase risk for heatstroke.
Severe EPS or Parkinson's disease	No fever, leukocytosis, or autonomic changes.
Central nervous system infection	Seizures more likely; abnormal CSF.
Allergic drug reaction	Rash, urticaria, wheezing, eosinophilia.
Toxic encephalopathy, lithium toxicity	No fever; low CPK.
Anticholinergic delirium	Dry skin, flaccid muscles, and low CPK.
Intoxication from drugs of abuse	Exposure to cocaine, amphetamines, MDMA, PCP, or synthetic cathinones. Hyperthermia, AMS, and autonomic instability common.
Systemic infection plus severe EPS	May appear identical to NMS.

Note.   AMS=altered mental status; AP=antipsychotic; CPK=creatine phosphokinase; CSF = cerebrospinal fluid; EPS=extrapyramidal symptoms: MDMA=methylenedioxymethamphetamine (Ecstasy); NMS=neuroleptic malignant syndrome; PCP=phencyclidine.

Source.   Compiled from Berman 2011; Haddad and Dursun 2008; Strawn et al. 2007.

Cooling blankets or ice packs should be used to treat hyperthermia (Berman 2011). No specific pharmacotherapies (e.g., benzodiazepines, dantrolene, bromocriptine, or amantadine) have been demonstrated to be superior to other measures (Strawn et al. 2007). Case reviews of pharmacotherapy in NMS have found outcomes varying from a beneficial effect from dantrolene or bromocriptine (Rosenberg and Green 1989; review of 67 cases) to a higher overall mortality or slower clinical recovery with dantrolene (Reulbach et al. 2007; review of 271 cases). Nonetheless, dantrolene and bromocriptine are frequently used; dantrolene's primary role is to treat extreme hyperthermia, rigidity, and hypermetabolism. Dantrolene should not be combined with calcium channel blockers because cardiovascular collapse may result (Berman 2011; Strawn et al. 2007). Most cases of NMS require initial treatment in a medical intensive care unit, and the patient should be transferred back to a psychiatric service only after he or she is medically stable. Among patients who recover from NMS, up to 30% may be at risk of NMS recurrence when rechallenged with an antipsychotic; however, for the majority of patients who require continued antipsychotic treatment, the medication can be cautiously reinstated with proper precautions (i.e., a least 2 weeks should be allowed to elapse after resolution of NMS before rechallenge) (Berman 2011; Haddad and Dursun 2008; Strawn et al. 2007). Additional information on NMS is available from the Malignant Hyperthermia Association of the United States (www.mhaus.org).

Autonomic and Cardiovascular Effects

Autonomic side effects result from cholinergic and alpha$_1$-adrenergic blockade, seen more frequently with low-potency FGAs. Among the SGAs, propensity to cause hypotension (from greatest risk to least risk) is as follows: clozapine > iloperidone > quetiapine > risperidone, paliperidone (estimated) > aripiprazole, asenapine, lurasidone, olanzapine, ziprasidone (Citrome 2011). Clozapine and quetiapine have been reported to cause tachycardia in 25% and 7% of cases, respectively. Tachycardia occurs in 5% of patients receiving risperidone or olanzapine, and in 2% of ziprasidone patients (Drici and Priori 2007). In 2017, an FDA warning was added to all antipsychotics regarding falls and fall-related injuries resulting from somnolence, orthostasis, and motor instability.

QTc prolongation and torsades de pointes.   A number of antipsychotics may be associated with QTc interval prolongation and risk for torsades de pointes. Sertindole was never marketed in the United States for this reason, but it is available in Europe with a restrictive label. Thioridazine and droperidol carry a black-box warning regarding dose-related QTc prolongation and risk for sudden death. Intravenous administration of haloperidol is associated with a higher risk of QTc prolongation than is oral use; risk of QTc prolongation and torsades de pointes associated with intravenous haloperidol is more similar to that of thioridazine (Beach et al. 2013). Among the various antipsychotic agents, the mean QTc interval prolongation (greatest to least) is as follows: thioridazine (36 msec) > ziprasidone (21 msec) > iloperidone with metabolic inhibition (19 msec) > quetiapine (15 msec) > paliperidone (12 msec) > risperidone (10 msec) > iloperidone without metabolic inhibition (9 msec) > olanzapine (6 msec) > oral haloperidol (5 msec) > asenapine (2–5 msec) > aripiprazole (< 1 msec) > lurasidone (negligible) (Beach et al. 2013; Citrome 2011; Leucht et al. 2013; Pfizer 2000, 2017; U.S. Food and Drug Administration 2003). Among patients taking thioridazine, 30% (9/30) had an increase in QTc interval of ≥60 msec, followed by 21% (7/33) of those taking ziprasidone, 11% (3/27) of those taking quetiapine, 5% (1/20) of those taking haloperidol, and approximately 4% of those taking olanzapine (1/26) or risperidone (1/28) (Pfizer 2000). A few subjects receiving thioridazine (10%) or ziprasidone (3%) had a QTc prolongation of 75 msec or greater (Pfizer 2000). Droperidol, pimozide, and sertindole have also been associated with QTc prolongation (Haddad and Anderson 2002).

Other cardiac side effects.   Potentially fatal myocarditis, cardiomyopathy, and heart failure have been reported with clozapine. Estimated rates of clozapine-associated myocarditis have ranged from 1 in 1,000 (most countries) to 1 in 100 (Australia) (Curto et al. 2016). The rate of clozapine-induced cardiomyopathy is approximately one-tenth the rate of clozapine-induced myocarditis (Curto et al. 2016). Most cases of clozapine-induced myocarditis develop during the first 2–3 months of therapy and may be accompanied by eosinophilia (Curto et al. 2016). Most cases of clozapine-induced cardiomyopathy appear later, within 6–9 months of beginning therapy (Curto et al. 2016); however, a review of case reports of cardiomyopathy suggested that the average time to symptom onset may be even longer (around 14 months) (Alawami et al. 2014). In the medical literature, estimated mortality rates associated with clozapine-induced cardiotoxicity range from 12.5% to 24% for myocarditis and from 10% to 30% for cardiomyopathy (Curto et al. 2016). Withdrawal of the drug might result in improvement of the cardiomyopathy. Clozapine rechallenge is generally discouraged in cases of myocarditis or cardiomyopathy (Alawami et al. 2014; Curto et al. 2016).

Endocrine and Metabolic Effects

For a full discussion of the endocrine and metabolic effects of antipsychotics, see Chapter 21.

Glucose tolerance.   Pharmacoepidemiological studies and case reports reveal an association between the use of various SGAs and hyperglycemia, new-onset type 2 diabetes, and occasionally ketoacidosis. These effects are not fully understood and are not solely explained by weight gain. Schizophrenia is itself a risk factor for type 2 diabetes regardless of treatment. A large retrospective study suggested that the risk of new-onset diabetes is greatest for clozapine and progressively decreases for olanzapine, quetiapine, and risperidone (E. A. Miller et al. 2005). A U.S. consensus statement concluded that hyperglycemia is associated with all marketed SGAs but is less common with aripiprazole and ziprasidone (American Diabetes Association et al. 2004). Diabetic ketoacidosis has been reported with olanzapine, clozapine, risperidone, quetiapine, and aripiprazole. The average time of symptom onset was 9 months after commencing treatment, with a range of 4 days to 4 years (Guenette et al. 2013). In more than one-third of cases, patients did not experience weight gain prior to the presentation of ketoacidosis.

Lipids.   Phenothiazines, but not butyrophenones, were long ago noted to elevate serum levels of cholesterol and triglycerides. Among SGAs, the risk of hyperlipidemia is highest with clozapine, olanzapine, and quetiapine, and lowest with risperidone, ziprasidone, aripiprazole, and lurasidone (Citrome 2011; Meyer and Koro 2004). Serum triglycerides usually peak in the first year of therapy.

Hyperprolactinemia.   Hyperprolactinemia is relatively common, especially with high-potency FGAs, risperidone, and paliperidone, and can result in amenorrhea or irregular menses, galactorrhea, gynecomastia, and sexual dysfunction. Osteoporosis can be a long-term consequence. Risperidone, paliperidone (Melkersson 2006), and amisulpride often elevate prolactin levels; clozapine, quetiapine, olanzapine, and ziprasidone are regarded as prolactin-sparing; and aripiprazole decreases prolactin levels (Haddad and Sharma 2007; Murray et al. 2017).

Weight gain.   All currently marketed antipsychotics (with the possible exceptions of haloperidol, ziprasidone, lurasidone, and aripiprazole) are associated with weight gain, which may increase health risks, stigmatization, nonadherence, impairment in quality of life, and social withdrawal. Among the SGAs, the relative propensity to cause weight gain (from greatest to least) is as follows: is olanzapine > clozapine >> iloperidone > quetiapine > risperidone, paliperidone >> asenapine > amisulpride >> aripiprazole > lurasidone > ziprasidone (Citrome 2011; Leucht et al. 2013; Murray et al. 2017). Consensus is lacking regarding which patients are more likely to gain weight on antipsychotics—those at normal weight at baseline or those who are already obese. A Metabolic Monitoring tool, incorporating current consensus guidelines for monitoring patients receiving SGAs and including forms for recording serial test results, is available from the Center for Quality Assessment and Improvement in Mental Health (www.cqaimh.org/pdf/tool_metabolic.pdf).

Syndrome of inappropriate antidiuretic hormone secretion. SIADH can occur with FGAs as well as SGAs (and also with some antidepressants and anticonvulsants). SIADH is characterized by a reduced ability to excrete water, resulting in extracellular dilution and hyponatremia. SIADH is distinguished from polydipsia (water intoxication) by urine osmolality, with relatively high urine osmolality in SIADH versus very low urine osmolality in polydipsia. Common symptoms include weakness, lethargy, headache, anorexia, and weight gain, and these may progress to confusion, convulsions, coma, and death.

Hematological Effects

Hematological side effects of antipsychotics include agranulocytosis, aplastic anemia, neutropenia, eosinophilia, and thrombocytopenia (Flanagan and Dunk 2008). Transient leukopenia and leukocytosis are not uncommon in the first few weeks of therapy and are usually not clinically significant. Agranulocytosis is the most common serious hematological side effect with clozapine, low-potency FGAs (<0.1%), and olanzapine. Prevalence rates for clozapine-induced agranulocytosis are 2%–3% for benign neutropenia (absolute neutrophil count [ANC] <1,500/mm^3) and 0.7% for severe, potentially fatal neutropenia (ANC <500/mm^3) (Li et al. 2018). Most cases of agranulocytosis occur during the first 6 months of therapy, with the highest risk during the first 6–18 weeks (Fitzsimons et al. 2005; Raja 2011). Clozapine is available through a distribution system that ensures monitoring of ANC according to a set schedule. Therapy interruption is recommended if ANC falls below 1,000/mm^3 in patients in the general population, or below 500/mm^3 in patients with benign ethnic neutropenia (Clozapine REMS 2017). Rechallenge may be considered if potential benefits outweigh risks. Further details on monitoring parameters are available from the Clozapine Risk Evaluation and Mitigation Strategy (REMS) program (Clozapine REMS 2017).

Hepatic and Pancreatic Effects

Liver function abnormalities during antipsychotic therapy have long been reported but seldom require drug discontinuation. Mild to moderate elevations in liver aminotransferases and alkaline phosphatase usually occur early in treatment and are unlikely to result in hepatic impairment. Cholestatic jaundice is an idiosyncratic reaction that in rare cases can occur with phenothiazines. Patients with significant antipsychotic-induced weight gain should be monitored for steatohepatitis (Slim et al. 2016). Antipsychotic-induced pancreatitis has been reported with clozapine, olanzapine, risperidone, aripiprazole, and ziprasidone (Silva et al. 2016; Tenner 2014).

Allergic, Dermatological, and Ophthalmological Effects

Dermatological adverse reactions include early allergic rashes, photosensitivity, and skin hyperpigmentation, especially with chlorpromazine. Pigmentary retinopathy has occurred in patients receiving thioridazine dosages higher than 800 mg/day. Ziprasidone has been associated with rash, urticaria, and rare cases of DRESS. Acute angle-closure glaucoma may occur in patients with a physiologically narrow anterior chamber angle who take anticholinergic medications.

Sexual Dysfunction

Antipsychotics may cause sexual dysfunction, an effect that in some cases is secondary to antipsychotic-induced hyperprolactinemia (see also Chapters 15 and 21).

Gastrointestinal and Respiratory Effects

Antipsychotics have been associated with esophageal dysmotility, dysphagia, and aspiration. A review of nonpsychiatric hospitalizations among clozapine-treated patients found that 32% of admissions were for pulmonary complaints (with more than half related to pneumonia) and 19.8% were for GI illness (primarily related to hypomotility) (Leung et al. 2017). Acute laryngeal dystonia and tardive respiratory dyskinesia are rare but potentially fatal consequences of antipsychotics.

Toxicity/Overdose

Overdoses with antipsychotics are common. Sedation and cardiovascular toxicity (tachycardia, mild hypotension, and QTc prolongation) are the most commonly reported presenting symptoms. Sedation usually occurs within 1–2 hours; however, it may be delayed with long-half-life agents (e.g., a delay of 9 hours with aripiprazole). QTc prolongation secondary to antipsychotic overdose is dose related and may be more common with amisulpride, ziprasidone, and thioridazine. Torsades de pointes has been reported in 7% of amisulpride overdoses. Overdoses of antipsychotics with antimuscarinic properties (i.e., clozapine, olanzapine) can result in antimuscarinic delirium (refer to subsection on TCA toxicity/overdose for management). Clozapine overdose has been associated with seizures. In rare cases, an antipsychotic overdose may result in NMS (Minns and Clark 2012).

Gastric emptying procedures are rarely necessary. Activated charcoal can be considered within 1 hour of ingestion. Whole-bowel irrigation may be considered in paliperidone overdose, given its sustained-release preparation. An electrocardiogram (ECG) should be obtained and cardiac monitoring initiated; electrolyte abnormalities should also be corrected (Minns and Clark 2012).

Drug–Drug Interactions

Most antipsychotics have sedating, hypotensive, anticholinergic, antiarrhythmic, and seizure threshold–lowering properties. Predictable drug interactions may occur when antipsychotics are combined with other drugs that also possess these properties. For example, antipsychotics may potentiate the sedative effects of other CNS depressants, and anticholinergic antipsychotics will have additive adverse effects with other anticholinergic drugs. Antipsychotics may greatly enhance the hypotensive effects of antihypertensive agents. Low-potency antipsychotics and ziprasidone should be avoided in patients receiving other drugs with type 1A antiarrhythmic properties.

Many antipsychotics, including aripiprazole, clozapine, olanzapine, risperidone, and asenapine, are prone to pharmacokinetic drug–drug interactions because of the limited number of CYP isozymes involved in their metabolism (see English et al.

2012; Owen and Crouse 2017; Spina et al. 2016). Increased adverse effects of CYP1A2 substrates (e.g., olanzapine, clozapine) may be experienced by newly admitted patients when they are no longer permitted to smoke.

Anxiolytics and Sedative-Hypnotics

Benzodiazepines have long been considered the cornerstone of pharmacotherapy for anxiety and insomnia. Alternatives include buspirone for anxiety; the nonbenzodiazepine hypnotics eszopiclone, zopiclone, zolpidem, and zaleplon; the melatonin agonist ramelteon; the antidepressant doxepin; and the orexin receptor antagonist suvorexant. These newer agents appear to have less tolerance and abuse potential and fewer adverse effects than benzodiazepines. Because of its association with rapid development of tolerance and dependence and fatalities on withdrawal, chloral hydrate is no longer FDA approved for use in the United States.

Benzodiazepines

Benzodiazepines commonly cause dose-related CNS adverse effects but rarely affect other organs, although in patients with cirrhosis they may precipitate hepatic encephalopathy.

Central nervous system effects.   Acute adverse CNS effects—including sedation, fatigue and weakness, ataxia, slurred speech, confusion, and memory impairment—are common, especially in older individuals and those who are medically ill. When benzodiazepines are used for the treatment of insomnia, long-half-life benzodiazepines are more likely to cause daytime sedation and cognitive impairment than short-half-life drugs. Benzodiazepine use is associated with an increased risk of falls and hip fractures. Elderly individuals and patients with brain injury are also susceptible to benzodiazepine-induced behavioral disinhibition manifesting as excitement, aggression, or paradoxical rage (Mancuso et al. 2004).

Physical tolerance often develops with long-term use of benzodiazepines, and some therapeutic effects (sedation but not anxiolysis) and adverse effects (e.g., sedation, psychomotor impairment) may diminish (O'Brien 2005). Although an increased risk of dementia with long-term benzodiazepine use has been reported (C.S. Wu et al. 2009), a more recent large case–control study found that benzodiazepine use was not associated with development of dementia (Imfeld et al. 2015). When the timing of benzodiazepine initiation was considered, individuals who started taking a benzodiazepine during the year before dementia diagnosis (presumably to manage anxiety and/or sleep disturbances) had increased odds of developing dementia, whereas those taking long-term benzodiazepines did not (Imfeld et al. 2015).

Respiratory effects.   Benzodiazepines decrease the central respiratory response to hypoxia but differ in their ability to cause respiratory depression (Guilleminault 1990), with long-acting agents such as flurazepam (Dolly and Block 1982) and nitrazepam (Sanger and Zivkovic 1992) having the most pronounced effects. Benzodiazepines can cause apnea} when used alone or in combination with other CNS depressants (most commonly alcohol) (Guilleminault 1990). The respiratory depressant effects of benzodiazepines may become clinically significant in individuals with pre-existing respiratory disorders, such as chronic obstructive pulmonary disease

(COPD) or sleep apnea, or in those with seizure disorders (which also can cause respiratory depression). Benzodiazepines should be used with caution in patients with compromised respiratory function or seizure disorder. Benzodiazepine use in patients with obstructive sleep apnea can be fatal (Dolly and Block 1982; see also Chapter 14, "Sleep Disorders").

Drug–drug interactions.   Additive CNS depressant effects, including respiratory depression, result from the combination of benzodiazepines and other CNS depressants, including alcohol. In 2016, the FDA issued a warning about the risk of respiratory depression, coma, and death with the concurrent use of benzodiazepines and opioids or opioid-containing products (U.S. Food and Drug Administration 2016a).

Many benzodiazepines, including alprazolam, bromazepam, clonazepam, diazepam, midazolam, and triazolam, undergo hepatic and intestinal metabolism mediated by CYP3A4. Significant inhibitors of CYP3A4 can reduce benzodiazepine elimination, whereas CYP3A4 inducers can increase their hepatic metabolism (see English et al. 2012; Owen and Crouse 2017). Oxazepam, lorazepam, and temazepam are eliminated primarily by conjugation and renal excretion and thus are preferred in patients with hepatic impairment.

Toxicity/overdose.   Benzodiazepines have a wide margin of safety; death from overdose is rare unless benzodiazepines are part of a multiple drug overdose. Overdose may result in sedation, ataxia, slurred speech, confusion, seizures, respiratory depression, and coma. Management involves supportive therapy and, if needed, mechanical ventilation.

Sudden discontinuation of benzodiazepines may result in severe withdrawal symptoms, including anxiety, agitation, dysphoria, anorexia, insomnia, sweating, vomiting, diarrhea, abdominal cramps, ataxia, psychosis, and seizures. The intensity of withdrawal symptoms is greater with higher dosages, prolonged treatment, abrupt discontinuation, and short-half-life benzodiazepines. Patients should be gradually withdrawn from benzodiazepines, especially those with a history of seizure disorder. Withdrawal from short-half-life agents can be facilitated by switching to a long-half-life agent before tapering.

Nonbenzodiazepine Hypnotics

Eszopiclone, zopiclone, zolpidem, and zaleplon are very-well-tolerated short-half-life hypnotics with very few dose-related adverse effects. Adverse effects of eszopiclone and zopiclone include bitter taste, dry mouth, difficulty rising in the morning, sleepiness, nausea, and nightmares (Allain et al. 1991; Najib 2006). Clinical trials of zaleplon reported adverse effects comparable to those seen with placebo (Hedner et al. 2000). Zolpidem's adverse effects include CNS (dizziness, drowsiness, and headache) and GI (nausea) effects (Krystal et al. 2008). Zolpidem use is associated with an increased risk of falls (Kolla et al. 2013). Tolerance to the hypnotic effects of these agents occurs less frequently than with benzodiazepines, but there are reports of withdrawal symptoms and abuse (Becker and Somiah 2015).

Ramelteon, a melatonin agonist FDA approved for sleep-onset insomnia, was demonstrated to have efficacy for insomnia, with no next-morning residual effects, an adverse-effect profile similar to that of placebo, and no withdrawal symptoms upon discontinuation, in a 6-month controlled clinical trial (Mayer et al. 2009).

Suvorexant, an orexin antagonist, has demonstrated efficacy for sleep latency and sleep maintenance. The most common adverse effect is somnolence. Although reports are rare, suvorexant can cause sleep paralysis, cataplexy, and hypnagogic and hypnopompic hallucinations. Use of suvorexant is contraindicated in patients with narcolepsy (Norman and Anderson 2016).

Low-dose doxepin, a potent histamine$_1$ receptor antagonist, is FDA approved for sleep-maintenance insomnia. Next-day somnolence has been reported with a 6-mg dose (Krystal et al. 2013).

Reports of complex sleep behaviors (e.g., sleep driving, sleep cooking, sleep eating, sleep conversations, sleep sex) in individuals taking these nonbenzodiazepine sedatives have prompted the FDA to require safety warnings. Such reports are rare, and the majority have been associated with zolpidem, the most widely used agent in this class (Dolder and Nelson 2008).

Respiratory effects. Unlike benzodiazepines, zolpidem, zopiclone, eszopiclone, and ramelteon at typical doses have no significant effects on respiratory drive and central control of breathing in patients with mild to moderate COPD (Girault et al. 1996; Muir et al. 1990; Sweetman et al. 2017). Suvorexant did not worsen sleep apnea when administered to patients with mild to moderate obstructive sleep apnea (Sun et al. 2016).

Drug–drug interactions. Ramelteon is oxidatively metabolized primarily by CYP1A2, with a much smaller contribution by CYP3A4. Fluvoxamine, a potent CYP1A2 inhibitor, has been reported to increase blood levels of ramelteon 70-fold and area under the curve (AUC) 190-fold (Takeda 2016). Ramelteon should not be used in combination with CYP1A2 inhibitors (e.g., fluvoxamine) or CYP1A2 inducers. Coadministration of ramelteon with strong CYP3A4 inhibitors (e.g., conazole antifungals, macrolide antibiotics, grapefruit juice) should also be avoided.

Suvorexant is primarily metabolized via CYP3A4 and to a minor extent through CYP1A2 and should be avoided in patients taking strong CYP3A4 inhibitors. A reduced starting dose of 5 mg is recommended for patients taking moderate CYP3A4 inhibitors (e.g., diltiazem) (Norman and Anderson 2016).

Toxicity/overdose. Fatal overdose of zolpidem is rare. A review of zolpidem ($n > 5,842$) and zaleplon ($n > 467$) overdoses identified two deaths with zolpidem and no fatalities with zaleplon (Forrester 2006). Symptoms of intentional overdose of zolpidem and zaleplon are similar and include drowsiness, slurred speech, ataxia, vomiting, and coma (Becker and Somiah 2015). Treatment is generally limited to supportive measures and, if appropriate, gastric lavage.

Fatal overdose with zopiclone has been reported but, as with zolpidem, appears rare (Bramness et al. 2001).

Buspirone

Buspirone is an anxiolytic with no effects on cognitive function or seizure threshold, little or no potential for physiological or psychological tolerance, and no abuse liability or withdrawal symptoms. Dizziness, drowsiness, nervousness, nausea, and headache are the most frequent adverse effects. Unlike benzodiazepines, buspirone does not potentiate the effects of alcohol or suppress respiration. Buspirone does not exhibit cross-tolerance with benzodiazepines and cannot be used to manage benzodiazepine withdrawal.

Drug–drug interactions.   Buspirone may in rare cases precipitate serotonin syndrome when used in combination with St. John's wort (Dannawi 2002) or SSRIs (Manos 2000), and it should not be combined with drugs possessing MAOI activity. Buspirone undergoes hepatic and intestinal metabolism mediated by CYP3A4. Secondary to first-pass metabolism, oral availability of buspirone is only about 5%. Coadministration with drugs that inhibit CYP3A4 (e.g., macrolide antibiotics, azole antifungals) can increase buspirone bioavailability 5- to 13-fold (Kivistö et al. 1997).

Toxicity/overdose.   No fatalities have been reported from buspirone overdose. Overdose symptoms include nausea, vomiting, drowsiness, miosis, and gastric distress. Treatment is primarily supportive. Immediate gastric lavage after acute ingestion has been recommended (McEvoy 2017) (but see Chapter 35 regarding risks of lavage).

Psychostimulants

Psychostimulants are used in the treatment of attention-deficit/hyperactivity disorder (ADHD), narcolepsy, depression, apathy, and analgesia augmentation in the medically ill. The well-established psychostimulant medications include methylphenidate, dexmethylphenidate, and amphetamines (a mixture of amphetamine salts; dextroamphetamine). Pemoline has been withdrawn from the market in many countries because of potentially fatal hepatotoxicity.

Newer compounds include atomoxetine (a specific norepinephrine reuptake inhibitor) and lisdexamfetamine (an amphetamine prodrug) for ADHD (Gibson et al. 2006), and modafinil and armodafinil for excessive sleepiness due to narcolepsy, shift work sleep disorder, and obstructive sleep apnea. Modafinil and armodafinil have demonstrated efficacy for excessive daytime sleepiness accompanying obstructive sleep apnea (Black and Hirshkowitz 2005; Roth et al. 2008). Modafinil improves fatigue and cognition accompanying multiple sclerosis (Lange et al. 2009).

Methylphenidate, Dexmethylphenidate, and Amphetamines

Common adverse effects of psychostimulants include CNS (insomnia, headache, nervousness, and social withdrawal) and GI (stomachache and anorexia) symptoms. Adverse effects are generally mild and diminish with continued treatment or with adjustment of dosage or dose timing. Lisdexamfetamine has a longer duration of action than dexamphetamine but otherwise has similar therapeutic and adverse effects (Cowles 2009).

Although psychostimulants may suppress appetite, this effect does not tend to occur at the low dosages used in medically ill patients (Masand et al. 1991). In healthy adults, methylphenidate ($\leq$30 mg/day) and dextroamphetamine ($\leq$15 mg/day) did not significantly alter heart rate or blood pressure (Martin et al. 1971). However, psychostimulants can cause elevations in heart rate and blood pressure, palpitations, hypertension, hypotension, and cardiac arrhythmias when taken at dosages higher than those routinely used in medically ill populations. In a review of methylphenidate in children with ADHD, the drug increased heart rate (by 3–10 beats/minute) and blood pressure (by 3.3–8.0 mm Hg systolic and 1.5–14.0 mm Hg diastolic) (Rapport and Moffitt 2002). Dexmethylphenidate and methylphenidate have similar therapeutic and adverse effects.

Drug–drug interactions. Psychostimulants may interact with sympathomimetics and MAOIs (including selegiline), resulting in headache, arrhythmias, hypertensive crisis, and hyperpyrexia. Psychostimulants should not be administered with MAOIs or within 14 days of their discontinuation. Despite the paucity of empirical evidence regarding TCA–stimulant metabolic interactions, warning statements are included in many drug manuals. One review of the effects of stimulants on the pharmacokinetics of desipramine in children found no statistically or clinically significant interaction regardless of age, gender, or type of stimulant (Cohen et al. 1999).

Higher dosages of psychostimulants may reduce the therapeutic effectiveness of antihypertensive medications. When psychostimulants are used concurrently with beta-blockers, the excessive alpha-adrenergic activity may cause hypertension, reflex bradycardia, and possible heart block.

Toxicity/overdose. Symptoms of psychostimulant overdose include cardiovascular (flushing, palpitations, hypertension, arrhythmias, and tachycardia), CNS (delirium, euphoria, hyperreflexia, and psychosis), and autonomic (hyperpyrexia and sweating) effects. Treatment is primarily supportive. Unabsorbed drug may be removed from the stomach (i.e., with activated charcoal). A short-acting sedative may be needed in patients with severe intoxication.

Modafinil, Armodafinil, and Atomoxetine

Modafinil, armodafinil (the active *R*-enantiomer of modafinil), and atomoxetine have adverse-effect profiles different from those of other psychostimulant drugs and do not have their same abuse potential. Modafinil's adverse effects include insomnia, nervousness, nausea, and rhinitis (McEvoy 2017). Palpitations, tachycardia, hypertension, and agitation have also been infrequently observed. Modafinil has been associated in rare cases with chest pain, palpitations, dyspnea, and transient ischemic T wave changes in association with mitral valve prolapse or left ventricular hypertrophy. Modafinil does not reduce appetite (Rugino and Copley 2001). Serious skin rash and possible Stevens-Johnson syndrome have been observed in modafinil trials and may occur with armodafinil (Cephalon 2017). Modafinil and armodafinil have similar therapeutic and adverse effects, and multiorgan hypersensitivity reactions are rarely reported (McEvoy 2017).

Atomoxetine side effects reported in clinical trials included insomnia, nausea, dry mouth, constipation, dizziness, decreased appetite, urinary hesitancy, sexual dysfunction, and palpitations (Adler et al. 2009; Eli Lilly 2017).

Drug–drug interactions. Atomoxetine is a potent inhibitor of CYP2D6 and is primarily eliminated through metabolism by CYP2D6. Atomoxetine may increase the toxicity of other coadministered narrow-therapeutic-index medications primarily metabolized by CYP2D6. Lower initial dosages should be used in patients who are poor CYP2D6 metabolizers or who are receiving strong CYP2D6 inhibitors (e.g., paroxetine, fluoxetine) (McEvoy 2017).

Modafinil and armodafinil are moderate inducers of CYP3A4 and moderate inhibitors of CYP2C19 (Darwish et al. 2008). Drug–drug interaction data for modafinil and armodafinil are limited. Clinical studies suggest that significant metabolic drug–drug interactions are most likely with compounds that undergo significant GI CYP3A4-

mediated first-pass metabolism, such as ethinylestradiol and triazolam (Robertson and Hellriegel 2003; Robertson et al. 2002).

Like other psychostimulants, atomoxetine, modafinil, and armodafinil should not be administered to patients receiving MAOIs or within 14 days of MAOI withdrawal.

Cognitive Enhancers

The currently approved treatments for dementia of the Alzheimer's type are the cholinesterase inhibitors donepezil, rivastigmine, and galantamine and the *N*-methyl-D-aspartate (NMDA) receptor antagonist memantine.

Cholinesterase Inhibitors

Cholinesterase inhibitors are generally well tolerated; most of their adverse effects are mild, dose related, and GI in nature (nausea, vomiting, and diarrhea). GI side effects can be minimized by slow dosage titration and administration with food. Adequate hydration reduces nausea. The procholinergic properties of these agents increase vagotonic and bronchoconstrictor effects; therefore, donepezil, rivastigmine, and galantamine should be used with caution in patients with cardiac conduction abnormalities or a history of asthma or COPD. Cholinesterase inhibitors have been associated with increased rates of syncope, bradycardia, and pacemaker placement (Gill et al. 2009). These agents have also been associated with anorexia. Agent-specific side effects include muscle cramps and insomnia with donepezil.

Drug–drug interactions.   Donepezil and galantamine are metabolized by CYP2D6 and CYP3A4 isozymes but are not associated with any clinically important CYP-mediated pharmacokinetic interactions. Rivastigmine is metabolized primarily by esterase-mediated hydrolysis and has been shown not to interact with CYP isozymes in vitro (Grossberg 2002).

Cholinesterase inhibitors have the potential to exacerbate the effects of other cholinesterase inhibitors (e.g., physostigmine) or cholinomimetic agents (e.g., bethanechol). Cholinesterase inhibitors prolong the duration of action of the depolarizing neuromuscular blocking agent succinylcholine (suxamethonium) by inhibiting metabolism of succinylcholine via plasma cholinesterase and increasing acetylcholine-mediated neuromuscular depolarization (Crowe and Collins 2003). By contrast, the cholinesterase inhibitor–mediated increase in acetylcholine levels antagonizes the actions of nondepolarizing neuromuscular blockers (e.g., atracurium) (Baruah et al. 2008). Cholinesterase inhibitors should be discontinued several weeks before surgery (Russell 2009).

Many prescription and nonprescription drugs possess anticholinergic activity that may impair cognitive function. In addition to drug classes commonly recognized as having anticholinergic effects, such as antiparkinsonian agents, antispasmodics, TCAs, low-potency antipsychotics, and antihistamines, many individual drugs also have these effects. The use of anticholinergic agents in patients with compromised cognitive function or delirium should be minimized. A partial listing of drugs with significant CNS anticholinergic effects is presented in Table 36–7. Drugs with anticholinergic properties may decrease the effect of cognitive enhancers. Conversely, cholinesterase inhibitors may have a countertherapeutic effect in patients receiving anticholinergic medications for medical conditions. In patients prescribed antipsychotic

TABLE 36–7. **Commonly used drugs with significant anticholinergic effects**

	Risk[a]		Risk[a]
Antidepressants		**Antipsychotics**	
Tertiary-amine TCAs	+++	Chlorpromazine	+++
Secondary-amine TCAs	++	Clozapine	+++
Mirtazapine	+	Haloperidol	+
Paroxetine	++	Olanzapine	++
Trazodone	+	Perphenazine	++
		Quetiapine	+
Antidiarrheals		Risperidone	+
Loperamide	++	Thioridazine	+++
		Ziprasidone	+
Antiemetics			
Metoclopramide	+	**Antispasmodics**	
Prochlorperazine	++	Atropine	+++
Promethazine	+++	Clidinium	+++
		Dicyclomine	+++
Antihistamines		Flavoxate	++
Brompheniramine	+++	Glycopyrrolate	++
Chlorpheniramine	++	Homatropine	+++
Cyproheptadine	++	Hyoscine	+++
Dimenhydrinate	+++	Hyoscyamine	+++
Diphenhydramine	+++	Methscopolamine	+++
Hydroxyzine	+++	Oxybutynin	+++
Meclizine	+++	Propantheline	++
		Scopolamine	+++
Antiparkinsonian agents		Tolterodine	++
Amantadine	++		
Benztropine	+++	**Mood stabilizers**	
Biperiden	+++	Lithium	+
Ethopropazine	+++		
Orphenadrine	+++	**Skeletal muscle relaxants**	
Pramipexole	+	Baclofen	++
Procyclidine	+++	Carisoprodol	+++
Selegiline	+	Chlorzoxazone	+++
Trihexyphenidyl	+++	Cyclobenzaprine	+++
		Metaxalone	+++
H$_2$ antagonists		Methocarbamol	+++
Cimetidine	++	Tizanidine	+++
Ranitidine	+		

[a]Risk of anticholinergic adverse effects at therapeutic dosages: +++=high; ++=medium; +=low. Risk is increased in the elderly and with multiple agents with anticholinergic activity.

Source. Compiled from Cancelli et al. 2009; Chew et al. 2008; McEvoy 2017; Rudolph et al. 2008.

medications, cholinesterase inhibitors can increase the risk of extrapyramidal adverse effects (Lexicomp 2017).

Overdose.   Overdose of cholinesterase inhibitors can cause a potentially fatal cholinergic crisis, with bradycardia, hypotension, muscle weakness, nausea, vomiting, respiratory depression, sialorrhea, diaphoresis, and seizures. Treatment is with atropine (1–2 mg intravenously, repeated as required) and supportive care.

NMDA Receptor Antagonist

in a meta-analysis of controlled long-term trials in patients with Alzheimer's disease, memantine was shown to be well tolerated, with an adverse-effect profile similar to that of placebo (Farlow et al. 2008). Memantine has no effect on respiration. It is primarily renally eliminated and requires reduced dosage in patients with moderate renal impairment.

Drug–drug interactions.   Memantine has no significant interactions with other drugs.

Alternative Routes of Administration

Psychotropic medications are usually delivered orally, but this may not represent the best administration route or even be possible for many medically ill patients. Oral administration of medications may be difficult in medically compromised populations, including patients with severe nausea or vomiting, dysphagia, severe malabsorption; unconscious or uncooperative patients; and patients unable to take medications by mouth. Alternative non-oral routes of administration include intravenous, intramuscular, subcutaneous, sublingual/buccal, rectal, topical or transdermal, and intranasal (Kaminsky et al. 2015).

The potential advantages of non-oral administration of psychotropics include guaranteeing compliance and providing options for those patients unable to take oral medications, as well as potential pharmacokinetic advantages associated with greater bioavailability, bypassing first-pass hepatic metabolism, and possible reductions in toxic metabolites or adverse effects. Intravenous delivery can be controlled from very rapid to slow infusion with 100% bioavailability and rapid drug distribution. Intramuscular administration provides fast absorption, avoidance of first-pass metabolism, and ensured compliance, but bioavailability is often less than 100% because of drug retention or metabolism by local tissues. Sublingual/buccal routes have rapid absorption and good bioavailability for small lipid-soluble drugs. Drugs absorbed sublingually avoid first-pass metabolism and may have fewer GI adverse effects. Significant sublingual/buccal absorption of oral liquids or oral disintegrating tablets cannot be assumed and must be evaluated on a drug-by-drug basis. Rectal absorption is often incomplete and erratic, but in comparison with oral administration, first-pass metabolism is reduced by about 50% (for a review, see van Hoogdalem et al. 1991a, 1991b). Transdermal drug delivery bypasses the gut, avoids first-pass metabolism, reduces GI adverse effects, and is unaffected by food intake. Continuous drug delivery from a transdermal patch produces fewer peak-to-trough fluctuations in drug levels compared with oral dosing and provides near-constant plasma drug levels, even for short-half-life drugs, over longer dosing intervals. The intranasal route has been suggested as the best alternative to parenteral injections for rapid systemic drug delivery. However, there are no approved intranasal formulations of psychotropic medications.

Medically ill patients in the intensive care setting often receive medications via nasogastric tube or percutaneous endoscopic gastrostomy tube. For medication administration via tubes, liquid forms are preferable when available. Some tablet formulations may be crushed and administered via tube. Some orally disintegrating tablets (i.e., olanzapine) may be dispersed in water or other suitable beverages and administered via tube. Extended-release or sustained-release formulations should not be crushed. The Institute for Safe Medication Practices (ISMP; www.ismp.org/Tools/) provides a list of medications that should not be crushed.

Many of the formulations discussed above are commercially available, although not necessarily in the United States or Canada. Customized formulations have been reported for a few agents. Caution is indicated when using a medication for which adequate studies of safety and efficacy with parenteral administration are lacking.

Antidepressants

Few antidepressants are available for parenteral administration. Intravenous clomipramine, amitriptyline, imipramine, maprotiline, doxepin, viloxazine, trazodone, and citalopram have been studied or widely used, mainly in Europe. None are currently available in the United States or Canada. Citalopram is the only SSRI available for parenteral administration. To date, open and double-blind randomized controlled trials (RCTs) have shown citalopram infusion followed by oral citalopram (Kasper and Müller-Spahn 2002) or escitalopram (Schmitt et al. 2006) to be effective and well tolerated for severe depression. However, the safety and efficacy of intravenous antidepressants in medically ill populations are uncertain because studies to date have been performed only in medically healthy patients.

No antidepressants are currently marketed in rectal preparations (e.g., enema, foam, or semisolid suppository formulations or gelatin capsules). However, several antidepressants, including trazodone, amitriptyline, imipramine, and clomipramine, have been compounded as rectal suppositories, with anecdotal reports of successful use in depression (Kaminsky et al. 2015; Koelle and Dimsdale 1998; Mirassou 1998). Therapeutic serum levels of doxepin were produced in three of four cancer patients following rectal insertion of oral capsules (Storey and Trumble 1992). The rectal bioavailability of fluoxetine oral capsules administered rectally was 15%, and this administration route was reasonably well tolerated in six healthy subjects (Kaminsky et al. 2015; Teter et al. 2005). With appropriate dosage adjustments, rectal administration of antidepressants may be feasible for patients who cannot take oral medications. Serum drug levels (if available) and clinical response should guide dosages.

The MAOI selegiline, available in a transdermal patch, is the only non-oral antidepressant formulation approved in the United States. The antidepressant dosage of oral selegiline requires dietary tyramine restriction because of clinically significant inhibition of intestinal MAO-A. By avoiding intestinal exposure to selegiline, transdermal administration reduces intestinal MAO-A inhibition and the need for dietary tyramine restrictions at dosages of 6 mg/day or less, as well as circumventing first-pass metabolism to provide higher plasma levels and reduced metabolite formation. An oral disintegrating tablet of selegiline, designed for buccal absorption, is approved in the United States for Parkinson's disease (Valeant 2017). There are no reports of its use for the treatment of depression.

Transdermal amitriptyline was reported to be well absorbed and effective in a case report (Kaminsky et al. 2015) but showed no significant systemic absorption in a small open trial (Lynch et al. 2005). This variability may be due to use of different transdermal formulations. Topical amitriptyline has also been used to treat neuropathic pain. Doxepin is commercially available as a topical cream for pruritus but has not been studied for depression (Kaminsky et al. 2015).

Sublingual administration of fluoxetine oral solution produced therapeutic plasma levels of fluoxetine plus norfluoxetine and improved depressive symptoms in two medically compromised patients with depression (Kaminsky et al. 2015).

Mirtazapine is available in an oral disintegrating tablet for gut absorption. In Canada, escitalopram is available in an orodispersible formulation for gut absorption. The extent of sublingual/buccal absorption from these formulations is unknown.

Anxiolytics and Sedative-Hypnotics

Internationally, many benzodiazepines are available in intravenous, intramuscular, rectal, sublingual, and intranasal preparations. Injectable forms of diazepam, lorazepam, and midazolam, and diazepam rectal gel, are marketed in the United States and Canada. Intravenous benzodiazepines are commonly used to treat status epilepticus or to calm severely agitated patients. Compared with diazepam, lorazepam has more predictable pharmacokinetics after intravenous administration. Midazolam is a short-acting, water-soluble benzodiazepine frequently used in preoperative sedation, induction and maintenance of anesthesia, anxiolysis, and the treatment of status epilepticus. Midazolam's onset of action following intravenous administration is usually within 1–5 minutes, and the action usually lasts less than 2 hours. Intravenous flunitrazepam, available in Europe and Japan, has been used for severe insomnia (Matsuo and Morita 2007) as well as for the treatment and prevention of alcohol withdrawal (Pycha et al. 1993). Intravenous benzodiazepine administration should always occur in a setting that offers ready access to personnel and equipment necessary for respiratory resuscitation.

Injectable forms of lorazepam, midazolam, and diazepam are available and may be administered intramuscularly. For behavioral emergencies, lorazepam is the preferred agent because it is readily absorbed and has no active metabolites. Midazolam is also rapidly absorbed after intramuscular administration, with an onset of action between 5 and 15 minutes. Intramuscular diazepam is not recommended because of its erratic absorption (Rey et al. 1999).

Sublingual benzodiazepines are often used to control anxiety in patients undergoing dental procedures. In Canada, lorazepam is marketed in a sublingual form, although most of the other benzodiazepines have been administered sublingually using commercial nonsublingual formulations (e.g., oral tablets, parenteral solutions) or custom preparations. Pharmacokinetic studies comparing sublingual administration of oral tablets with intramuscular administration suggest slightly slower sublingual drug absorption but similar bioavailability.

Rectal administration of benzodiazepines is useful for the acute management of seizures in children. Diazepam is available as a rectal gel for use when other routes are not readily available. Other benzodiazepines, such as clonazepam, triazolam, and midazolam, have also been administered rectally. Although rectal benzodiazepine absorption is rapid, it is not always reliable because rectal bioavailability is highly variable and the onset of action is delayed (Rey et al. 1999). Because lorazepam may be given intravenously, intramuscularly, or sublingually, there is little need for rectal administration of benzodiazepines in adults.

Benzodiazepines can also be administered intrathecally or intranasally. Intrathecal midazolam has been used principally for adjunctive pain management and has been found to be safe and effective in a variety of settings (Duncan et al. 2007). Although no benzodiazepines are commercially available in intranasal formulations, intranasal midazolam and lorazepam have been reported to be effective, with rapid absorption and high bioavailability (Björkman et al. 1997; Wermeling et al. 2006). Intranasal lorazepam has been used for anxiolysis and for termination of seizures. Intranasal lorazepam is approximately 80% bioavailable and reaches peak concentration within 30 minutes (Bailey et al. 2017).

Alternative formulations of zolpidem approved in the United States include a sublingual tablet and an oral spray. In a clinical study, the sublingual tablet produced significantly earlier sleep initiation than the oral preparation (Staner et al. 2010). The oral spray has been demonstrated to provide more rapid systemic absorption of zolpidem than the oral formulation (Magna Pharmaceuticals 2016).

Antipsychotics

Olanzapine, ziprasidone, chlorpromazine, fluphenazine, and haloperidol are available as short-acting intramuscular preparations. Haloperidol has been given intravenously and subcutaneously. Long-acting intramuscular depot formulations of aripiprazole, risperidone, olanzapine, paliperidone, haloperidol, and fluphenazine are available in the United States. In Canada, long-acting depot formulations of risperidone, fluphenazine, haloperidol, flupenthixol, pipotiazine, and zuclopenthixol are approved. Paliperidone is also available in the United States and Canada in a 3-month long-acting injectable.

Intravenous agents are usually reserved for treatment of acute agitation in which a rapid onset of effect is desirable. Although haloperidol is not approved by the FDA for intravenous use, it is often administered intravenously in medical inpatient settings, especially for management of delirium, aggression, or mania. The FDA recommends ECG monitoring for QT prolongation and arrhythmia if haloperidol is administered intravenously. High dosages of haloperidol (up to 1,000 mg/day) in patients with severe delirium have been reported to have minimal effects on heart rate, respiratory rate, blood pressure, and pulmonary artery pressure, with minimal EPS (Levenson 1995). If chlorpromazine is administered intravenously, it should be diluted and administered as a slow intravenous infusion not to exceed 1 mg/minute in adults or 0.5 mg/minute in children to reduce risk of hypotension (Lexicomp 2017). Droperidol is FDA approved for use as an intravenous anesthetic adjunct (but not for psychiatric conditions) but has been used for rapid tranquilization in acute medical settings.

Intramuscular antipsychotic formulations can be categorized on the basis of their pharmacokinetic features: short-acting preparations and long-acting depot preparations. Long-acting antipsychotics are typically used as antipsychotic maintenance treatment to optimize adherence and eliminate bioavailability problems. Short-acting antipsychotics are usually used in acute management of delirium, psychosis, mania, or aggression (see Chapter 4, "Delirium"; Chapter 6, "Aggression and Violence"; and Chapter 9, "Psychosis, Mania, and Catatonia"). Haloperidol is the most commonly used (and least costly) intramuscularly administered antipsychotic in medical settings. However, acute parenteral administration of high-potency antipsychotics is associated with a greater risk of adverse effects such as dystonia and other EPS. In patients with existing extrapyramidal disorders, an intramuscular antipsychotic other than haloperidol would be preferred. Parenteral administration of low-potency agents may cause more hypotension and lowered seizure threshold.

Intramuscular forms of SGAs are less likely than haloperidol to cause acute dystonia and akathisia (Currier and Medori 2006; Zimbroff 2008), but there has been less experience using these preparations in the medically ill, and they are more expensive. Haloperidol, but none of the SGAs, can be mixed with a benzodiazepine in the same syringe. Ziprasidone can be administered in conjunction with an intramuscular benzodiazepine but was designed to be given as monotherapy. Concurrent administration of intramuscular olanzapine with a parenteral benzodiazepine is not recommended because of the risk of excessive sedation, cardiorespiratory depression, and death (Marder et al. 2010). Intramuscular olanzapine should be used cautiously in patients intoxicated with alcohol. Ziprasidone (oral or intramuscular) is contraindicated in patients with QT prolongation or a recent myocardial infarction. Intramuscular ziprasidone has not been systematically studied in patients with significant hepatic or renal impairment. The excipient cyclodextrin in parenteral ziprasidone is renally cleared; therefore, this formulation should be administered cautiously in patients with renal impairment (Pfizer 2017). At this time, there are almost no data on intramuscular ziprasidone or olanzapine in the management of agitation in medically ill patients without an underlying psychiatric condition, so caution is advised.

Asenapine, the only antipsychotic available in a sublingual preparation, has poor oral absorption (<2%). Oral disintegrating tablets, designed to deliver drug for intestinal absorption, are available for aripiprazole, clozapine, olanzapine, and risperidone. In a study examining absorption of olanzapine solid oral dosage forms by different routes of administration in healthy volunteers, sublingual administration of the oral disintegrating tablet resulted in drug absorption that was similar in extent and rate to that of regular administration of this dosage form and faster than that of the standard oral tablet (Markowitz et al. 2006). Comparisons of sublingual versus buccal absorption of oral disintegrating tablets for other antipsychotics have not been reported. Because oral disintegrating tablets contain phenylalanine, this formulation should not be used in individuals with phenylketonuria.

Subcutaneous administration of haloperidol or methotrimeprazine (available in Canada and Europe) or fluphenazine (Health Canada–approved for subcutaneous administration) can be used to manage terminal restlessness or nausea/vomiting in palliative care patients. Loxapine has also been used subcutaneously in the palliative care setting. Most other phenothiazines are too irritating for subcutaneous injection.

Loxapine is approved for oral inhalation to manage acute agitation. This administration route achieves rapid absorption, with peak concentrations attained within approximately 2 minutes, but carries a risk of bronchospasm and is therefore contraindicated in persons with asthma, COPD, or other lung disease (Keating 2013).

In a small study (N=4 patients) comparing the pharmacokinetics of a 2.5-mg dose of haloperidol delivered intranasally versus intramuscularly or intravenously (over 15 minutes), intranasal administration achieved a peak concentration that was higher (9.8 ng/mL vs. 8.4 ng/mL) and occurred more rapidly (15 minutes vs. 37.5 minutes) than that achieved with intramuscular administration (J.L. Miller et al. 2008). Time to peak concentration for intranasal administration was similar to that for intravenous administration (also 15 minutes); however, intravenous administration achieved a higher peak concentration (23.3 ng/mL vs. 9.8 ng/mL). Two of the four patients reported mild to moderate nasal irritation (J.L. Miller et al. 2008). Further study is needed to guide recommendations regarding use of intranasal haloperidol.

Psychostimulants

Methylphenidate is available as a transdermal patch in the United States. The patch is worn for 9 hours but provides therapeutic effects through 12 hours. Duration of effect can be modified by early removal of the patch (Manos et al. 2007). A placebo-controlled comparison of transdermal methylphenidate and the osmotic-release oral capsule in children revealed similar treatment efficacy for the drugs but a higher incidence of tics and anorexia for transdermal methylphenidate (Findling et al. 2008). No clinical trials of transdermal methylphenidate in adults with serious medical illness have been published.

Although no other non-oral forms of psychostimulants are available, custom preparations have been described. Dextroamphetamine has been administered intravenously to human subjects in research but not in clinical populations (Ernst and Goldberg 2002). There is one published case report describing the use of 5-mg dextroamphetamine suppositories compounded by a pharmacy for treating depressed mood in a woman with a GI obstruction (Holmes et al. 1994).

Mood Stabilizers/Anticonvulsants

Mood stabilizers that have been administered intravenously include lithium carbonate and valproate. Parenteral lithium has rarely been used in the treatment of psychiatric disorders. Although it has been used for thyroid storm, renal and neurological toxicity prohibit its routine use. Lithium has also been administered in the dialysate in patients on continuous ambulatory peritoneal dialysis (Flynn et al. 1987). Lithium carbonate is not approved by the FDA for parenteral use, and there is not enough clinical experience or data to recommend its use by non-enteral routes.

Valproate is available in parenteral form in Europe and the United States (it was discontinued in Canada in 2004). Valproate is the only mood stabilizer to have an approved parenteral formulation with guidelines for use in acute bipolar disorder (Ghaleiha et al. 2014). The intravenous solution, prepared in dextrose, saline, or lactated Ringer's solution, should not be infused at a rate greater than 20 mg/minute, and the dosage should be reduced in elderly patients and in those with neurocognitive disorders. The infusion does not require cardiac monitoring and causes no significant risk of orthostatic hypotension (Norton 2001).

Several studies have reported that rectal administration of carbamazepine, lamotrigine, or topiramate provided acceptable bioavailability and tolerability. Carbamazepine has been rectally administered as a solution (Neuvonen and Tokola 1987) and as a crushed tablet in a gelatin capsule (Storey and Trumble 1992), attaining therapeutic blood levels in some, but not all, patients. Rectal formulations of lamotrigine and topiramate have been prepared from oral formulations. Whereas rectal lamotrigine had lower (by approximately 50%) bioavailability than oral lamotrigine, leading to lower drug levels and slower absorption (Birnbaum et al. 2001), rectal topiramate produced blood levels identical to those of oral topiramate (Conway et al. 2003). Provided that relative bioavailability is considered, rectal administration of an aqueous suspension of these tablets may be acceptable. Rectal absorption of other anticonvulsants, including oxcarbazepine and gabapentin, is not reliable (Clemens et al. 2007). Oxcarbazepine is available as an oral suspension that has been used rectally; however, mean bioavailability for the parent drug and its active metabolite achieved with rectal administration is only 10% of the bioavailability achieved with oral administration (Clemens et al. 2007).

Cholinesterase Inhibitors

Rivastigmine is the only cognitive enhancer available in a non-oral formulation (a transdermal patch). The rivastigmine patch is dosed daily and provides more stable plasma levels compared with the twice-daily oral capsules and the oral solution. The patch provides greater bioavailability but has slower absorption than the oral forms, resulting in peak drug levels that are 20% lower than those achieved with oral rivastigmine. The patch is associated with a lower incidence of nausea and vomiting (20% vs. 33% with the oral form) (Lefèvre et al. 2008). Donepezil is commercially available as an orally disintegrating tablet.

Complementary Medicines

In surveys, approximately 20% of U.S. adults report having used herbal medicines (natural products) and homeopathic treatments within the past year (Clarke et al. 2015), often without disclosing this use to their physicians. Many people assume that complementary medicines are "naturally" safe, and they may combine complementary and conventional therapies, believing that the combination will be more effective. The combined use of herbal and nonherbal drugs raises concerns about appropriate therapeutic use, contraindications, adverse effects, and drug–drug interactions of herbal and nonherbal drugs. Patients with chronic disease may be especially vulnerable to adverse effects from herbal medicines because of compromised organ function and polypharmacy with conventional agents.

The FDA Office of Dietary Supplement Programs (www.fda.gov/Food/Dietary Supplements/) and the Health Canada Office of Natural and Non-Prescription Health Products (www.canada.ca/en/health-canada/services/drugs-health-products/natural-non-prescription.html) provide a regulatory framework to encourage good manufacturing practices and adverse-effect reporting for natural health products. However, the FDA does not require efficacy or safety data for products marketed as dietary supplements.

The lack of government oversight and regulation has complicated attempts to assess the safety of herbal medicines. Manufacturers are not required to standardize the concentrations of active ingredients or even to identify them (Chandler 2000). Herbal preparations may contain several plant species used under a single name (Chandler 2000) and may be adulterated with unlisted pharmacological agents, pesticides, and heavy metals, including cadmium, lead, mercury, and arsenic (Saper et al. 2008). Drugs such as anti-inflammatory agents, steroids, diuretics, antihistamines, sildenafil-like compounds, and benzodiazepines may be intentionally added to herbal products for therapeutic effect (G.M. Miller and Stripp 2007; Wooltorton 2002a). Contraindications, major adverse effects, and significant drug–drug interactions for herbal medicines and nonherbal dietary supplements commonly used for neuropsychiatric symptoms are summarized in Table 36–8 and Table 36–9.

Psychotropic Drug Use in the Medically Ill

Psychosomatic medicine specialists routinely prescribe psychotropic medications— and advise other physicians regarding the use of such medications—in patients with multiple complex medical problems. As previously outlined in this chapter, safe prescribing of psychotropics in medically ill patients requires an understanding of disease-related changes in drug pharmacokinetics and pharmacodynamics, as well as attention to the many issues that arise during pharmacotherapeutic treatment in these vulnerable patients. In this section we summarize clinical recommendations for the use of psychotropic medications in specific medical/surgical populations.

Gastrointestinal Disorders

Hepatic Disease

Psychopharmacological concerns in patients with liver disease largely center on pharmacokinetic changes brought about by the disease (discussed earlier in this chapter in section "Pharmacokinetics in the Medically Ill"). Acute hepatitis usually does not require dosage alterations in psychotropics, but chronic hepatitis may require dosage adjustment, depending on the severity of liver dysfunction. In patients with cirrhosis, drug dosages will require significant modification. The severity of liver disease can be estimated using the Child–Pugh scoring system (see Chapter 19, "Gastrointestinal Disorders"). Moderate hepatic impairment is usually categorized as Child–Pugh class B (score of 7–9), whereas severe impairment is categorized as class C (score of 10–15). All plasma proteins are synthesized in the liver, so protein binding is altered in liver disease. The main clinical effect of chronically decreased protein binding is on the interpretation of blood levels (see discussion in the "Distribution" subsection under "Pharmacokinetics in the Medically Ill" at the beginning of this chapter). When prescribing hepatically metabolized psychotropic drugs to patients with impaired hepatic function, it is prudent to reduce the initial dosage and titrate more slowly, carefully monitor for clinical response and side effects, and choose drugs with a wide therapeutic index. Table 36–10 provides recommendations for dosing of extensively metabolized psychotropics in patients with hepatic disease.

Antidepressants. Most antidepressants undergo extensive phase I hepatic oxidative metabolism and should be dosed according to the recommendations described in Table 36–10 or the manufacturer's prescribing information. Anticholinergic TCAs may

TABLE 36–8.   Selected herbal medicines

Natural medicine/uses	Pharmacological effect(s)	Drug interactions	Precautions/comments
Black cohosh			
Menopausal symptoms	Has estrogen-like effects; may lower levels of luteinizing hormone	Avoid use with other hepatotoxic drugs	Contraindicated in pregnancy and lactation Avoid in women with estrogen-dependent tumors Hepatotoxicity Avoid during pregnancy Allergic contact dermatitis is common
Feverfew			
Migraine prophylaxis, arthritis	May inhibit platelet aggregation and prostaglandin synthesis	Anticoagulants, NSAIDs, SSRIs, and platelet inhibitors—increased bleeding risk	Withdrawal syndrome (anxiety, fatigue, joint ache) may occur on sudden discontinuation
Ginkgo biloba			
Ischemia associated with peripheral artery disease and vascular dementia	Improves peripheral and CNS blood flow and inhibits platelet activation factor	Anticoagulants, NSAIDs, SSRIs, platelet inhibitors—increased risk for bleeding disorders Anticonvulsant efficacy may be reduced	Intracerebral and intraocular hemorrhages have been reported; ginkgo may cause palpitations Seizures reported with high doses Discontinue at least 2 weeks before surgery

TABLE 36–8. Selected herbal medicines (continued)

Natural medicine/uses	Pharmacological effect(s)	Drug interactions	Precautions/comments
Ginseng			
Physical, mental, and sexual tonic, immunostimulant, and mood enhancer	Has estrogenic and hypoglycemic activity; inhibits platelet activation factor	Reduces the effects of antidiabetics, antihypertensives, anxiolytics, antidepressants, mood stabilizers, anti-estrogens, and immunosuppressants Anticoagulants, NSAIDs, SSRIs, platelet inhibitors—increases the risk of bleeding disorders Caffeine—additive stimulant effects Insulin—additive hypoglycemic effects	Avoid in patients with estrogen receptor–positive breast cancer May cause estrogen-related bleeding disorders (vaginal bleeding) and breast nodules, tachycardia, hypertension, nervousness, agitation, mania, and headache Long-term use may result in "ginseng abuse syndrome" (hypertension, nervousness, insomnia, skin eruptions, diarrhea, and tremor) Discontinue at least 7 days before surgery
Kava			
Mild anxiety, sleep disturbances	Modifies GABA receptors, affects calcium and sodium channels, inhibits MAO-B, and may inhibit reuptake of norepinephrine, and dopamine	CNS depressants—additive effects Kavalactones (the proposed active constituents of kava) inhibit major CYP enzymes and may cause interactions with concurrent medications	Dermopathy is common with heavy use Sale of kava has been banned in many countries because of several incidents of fatal hepatotoxicity Discontinue at least 2 weeks before surgery

TABLE 36–8.   Selected herbal medicines *(continued)*

Natural medicine/uses	Pharmacological effect(s)	Drug interactions	Precautions/comments
Ma huang (ephedra)			
Weight loss, obesity, athletic performance enhancement	Indirect sympathomimetic; contains ephedrine and pseudoephedrine which cause release of epinephrine and norepinephrine	Antihypertensives, beta-blockers, sedative-hypnotics, and anesthetics—reduced effects Caffeine—increased stimulant effects MAOIs—hypertensive crisis Pseudoephedrine and phenylpropanolamine—increased risk of hypertension and cardiovascular effects QT-prolonging drugs—increased risk of ventricular arrhythmias	Contraindicated in angina and pheochromocytoma Excessive sympathetic stimulation can lead to dizziness, headache, decreased appetite, GI distress, irregular heartbeat, tachycardia, hypertension, myocardial infarction, insomnia, flushing, seizures, stroke, and death FDA banned the sale of ephedra in 2004 following reports of ephedra-related deaths May cause mania and psychosis
St. John's wort			
Mild to moderate depression	Increases serotonin, norepinephrine, and dopamine activity and inhibits reuptake of GABA and glutamate	Tetracycline, piroxicam, and phenothiazines—increases risk of phototoxicity Serotonergic drugs—may induce serotonin syndrome and mania Induces CYP3A4, can interact with medications metabolized by CYP3A4 to lower drug levels and decrease therapeutic effect Digoxin, cyclosporine, and TCAs—reduced bioavailability and systemic exposure via P-gp induction	Causes GI upset, headaches, and dry mouth Photosensitizing properties may cause sun-induced skin rash, neuropathy, and possibly increased incidence of cataracts Discontinue at least 2 weeks before surgery

TABLE 36–8. Selected herbal medicines (continued)

Natural medicine/uses	Pharmacological effect(s)	Drug interactions	Precautions/comments
Valerian			
Insomnia, anxiety	Enhances GABA activity	CNS depressants—potentiates the sedative effects	Tolerance may develop and lead to withdrawal effects with abrupt discontinuation after prolonged high-dose use
			Withdrawal effects are similar to effects of benzodiazepine withdrawal
			Discontinue at least 2 weeks before surgery
Yohimbe			
Aphrodisiac, stimulant, erectile dysfunction	Alpha$_2$ antagonist with indirect sympathomimetic activity	Stimulants, MAOIs, and TCAs—exacerbates CNS and autonomic effects	Adverse effects include insomnia, anxiety, panic attacks, hallucinations, hypertension, tachycardia, nausea, and vomiting
			Avoid in patients with hypertension, sleep disorders, anxiety disorders, and psychosis
			Discontinue at least 2 weeks before surgery

Note. CNS=central nervous system; CYP=cytochrome P450; FDA=U.S. Food and Drug Administration; GABA=γ-aminobutyric acid; GI=gastrointestinal; MAO-B=monoamine oxidase–B; MAOI=monoamine oxidase inhibitor; NSAID=nonsteroidal anti-inflammatory drug; P-gp=P-glycoprotein; SSRI=selective serotonin reuptake inhibitor; TCA=tricyclic antidepressant.

Source. Compiled from Ang-Lee et al. 2001; Bent and Ko 2004; Brazier and Levine 2003; Chandler 2000; Ernst 2003; Ernst and Goldberg 2002; Gardiner et al. 2008; Gurley et al. 2008; Z. Hu et al. 2005; Mahady et al. 2008; Natural Medicines 2017; Ravindran et al. 2016; Sarris et al. 2011; Tracy and Kingston 2007.

TABLE 36–9.   Selected nonherbal supplements

Supplement/uses	Pharmacological effect(s)	Precautions/comments
DHEA (dehydroepiandrosterone)		
Depression, fibromyalgia, multiple sclerosis, osteoporosis, systemic lupus erythematosus, sexual dysfunction, dementia	Endogenous anabolic steroid that may undergo conversion in vivo to testosterone or androstenedione followed by conversion to estriol, estrone, and estradiol	May cause acne, weight gain, voice change, hirsutism, and menstrual irregularities in females and gynecomastia and prostatic hypertrophy in males Contraindicated in patients with liver dysfunction, prostate cancer, or hormone-dependent diseases such as estrogen-dependent breast cancer May inhibit CYP3A4
SAMe (S-adenosyl-L-methionine)		
Depression, osteoarthritis, cirrhosis, fibromyalgia	Principal endogenous methyl donor for methylation reactions; associated with increased turnover of serotonin and increased norepinephrine and dopamine levels	May cause nausea, vomiting, diarrhea, and insomnia May increase anxiety and restlessness in patients with depression, and mania and hypomania in patients with bipolar disorder Serotonin syndrome has been reported with increased risk in patients taking serotonergic drugs

Note.   CYP=cytochrome P450.

Source.   Compiled from Chandler 2000; Ernst 2003; Z. Hu et al. 2005; Natural Medicines 2017; Ravindran et al. 2016; Tracy and Kingston 2007.

TABLE 36–10. **Dosage adjustment of psychotropic medications in hepatic impairment (HI)**[a]

Antidepressants

MAOIs	Potentially hepatotoxic. Use is contraindicated in HI.
SSRIs	Decreased clearance and prolonged half-life. Initial dose should be reduced by 50%; subsequent incremental increases should be made at longer intervals than usual. Target dosages will be lower than usual.
TCAs	Potentially serious hepatic effects. No dosing guidelines.
Bupropion	Decreased clearance. Mild HI: use reduced dosage and/or dosing frequency. In moderate to severe HI, do not exceed 75 mg/day for IR tablets, or 100 mg/day (SR) or 150 mg every other day (SR and XL).
Desvenlafaxine	Primarily metabolized by conjugation. No adjustment in starting dose. Do not exceed 100 mg/day in moderate to severe HI.
Duloxetine	Reduced metabolism and elimination. Use is contraindicated in HI.
Mirtazapine, selegiline, trazodone	Exercise caution in HI. No dosing guidelines.
Nefazodone	May cause hepatic failure. Avoid use in patients with active liver disease.
Venlafaxine	Decreased clearance of venlafaxine and its active metabolite *O*-desmethylvenlafaxine. Dosage should be reduced by 50% in mild to moderate HI.

Second-generation antipsychotics

Asenapine, cariprazine	No dosage adjustment needed in mild to moderate HI. Use in severe HI not recommended.
Brexpiprazole	Reduced maximum dose in moderate to severe HI; 2 mg/day for MDD; 3 mg/day for schizophrenia.
Clozapine	Discontinue in patients with marked transaminase elevations or jaundice. No specific dosing guidelines, but dosage reduction may be necessary.
Iloperidone	Pharmacokinetics in mild or moderate HI unknown. Use in severe HI not recommended.
Lurasidone	Reduce initial dosage in HI. Maximum dosage is 80 mg/day in moderate HI and 40 mg/day in severe HI.
Olanzapine	Periodic assessment of LFTs is recommended.
Quetiapine	Clearance decreased 30%. For IR, start at 25 mg/day; increase by 25–50 mg/day; for XR, start at 50 mg/day; increase in 50-mg/day increments.

TABLE 36–10.   **Dosage adjustment of psychotropic medications in hepatic impairment (HI)[a] *(continued)***

Second-generation antipsychotics *(continued)*

Risperidone	Free fraction increased 35%. In severe HI, starting dosage and dose increments should not exceed 0.5 mg bid. Increases beyond 1.5 mg bid (3 mg/day) should be made at intervals of at least 1 week.
Ziprasidone	Increased half-life and serum level in mild to moderate HI. No dosage adjustments recommended.

First-generation antipsychotics

Haloperidol and others	All metabolized in the liver. No specific dosing recommendations. Phenothiazines (e.g., chlorpromazine, thioridazine) should be avoided. If nonphenothiazines are used, reduce dosage and titrate more slowly than usual.

Anxiolytic and sedative-hypnotic drugs

Alprazolam	Decreased metabolism and increased half-life. Reduce dosage by 50%. Avoid use in patients with cirrhosis.
Buspirone	Half-life prolonged; AUC increased 13-fold. Use in severe HI not recommended.
Chlordiazepoxide, clonazepam, diazepam, flurazepam, triazolam	Reduced clearance and prolonged half-life. Avoid use in HI if possible.
Lorazepam, oxazepam, temazepam	Metabolized by conjugation; clearance not affected. No dosage adjustment needed. Lorazepam is the preferred agent.
Ramelteon	Exposure increased 4-fold in mild HI and >10-fold in moderate HI. Use with caution in moderate HI. Use in severe HI not recommended.
Zaleplon, zolpidem	Reduced clearance. Maximum dose is 5 mg in mild to moderate HI. Use in severe HI not recommended.
Eszopiclone	No dosage adjustment needed for mild to moderate HI. In severe HI, exposure is doubled; recommend 1 mg initial dose with a maximum of 2 mg.
Zopiclone	Initial dose 3.75 mg in mild to moderate HI; may increase to 5 mg with caution. Use contraindicated in severe HI.

Mood stabilizers/anticonvulsants

Carbamazepine	Perform baseline LFTs and periodic evaluations during therapy. Discontinue for active liver disease or aggravation of liver dysfunction. No dosing guidelines available.
Lamotrigine	Reduce initial, escalation, and maintenance dosages by 50% in moderate HI and by 75% in severe HI.

(Tharwani et al. 2007; Zhang et al. 2013). Evidence for the safety and efficacy of newer antidepressants in patients with poststroke depression is lacking.

Antipsychotics. Concerns about an increased risk of cerebrovascular events (stroke, transient ischemic attack), including fatalities, were raised by an analysis of four placebo-controlled trials of risperidone in elderly patients with dementia-related psychosis (Health Canada 2002; Wooltorton 2002b). Further pharmacovigilance suggested that all SGAs were associated with an increased risk of cerebrovascular events, prompting Britain's Committee on Safety of Medicines in 2004 to recommend against use of SGAs in dementia patients. In 2005, the FDA ordered that all SGAs carry a black-box warning regarding an increased risk of death in elderly patients with dementia-related psychosis. Several subsequent studies suggested that all antipsychotics (both FGAs and SGAs) are associated with an increased risk of stroke in elderly patients, particularly those with dementia (Douglas and Smeeth 2008; Sacchetti et al. 2008). Recent meta-analyses paint a less clear picture, with two finding that FGAs—but not SGAs—are associated with an increased risk of cerebrovascular accidents (Hsu et al. 2017; Rao et al. 2016), and one confirming that SGAs are associated with risk (Ma et al. 2014).

Psychostimulants. Psychostimulants offer an alternative in treating poststroke depression, but poststroke patients may be more sensitive to their side effects. Hence, psychostimulants should be initiated at very low dosages and gradually increased as necessary (Masand and Tesar 1996).

Seizures

With the high rates of psychiatric comorbidity in seizure disorders, patients with these disorders are frequently prescribed psychotropic medications. Psychotropics that may lower the seizure threshold at normal dosages (antidepressants, antipsychotics) pose a risk primarily in patients with untreated (or undertreated) seizure disorder. In patients with seizure disorders, psychotropics associated with higher seizure risk, including high-dose bupropion, clozapine, and low-potency FGAs, should be avoided. One study of traumatic brain injury patients with posttraumatic seizures concluded that methylphenidate can be safely used even in those at high risk for seizures (Wroblewski et al. 1992).

Migraine Headache

Antidepressants. Many patients with migraine headache take triptans, which are potent $5\text{-HT}_{1B/1D}$ receptor agonists. Antidepressants are frequently prescribed for migraine prophylaxis (primarily TCAs and venlafaxine) or comorbid depression or anxiety. Cases of serotonin syndrome from antidepressant and triptan coadministration are quite rare. Triptan use does not contraindicate use of serotonergic antidepressants. The triptans vary widely in their potential for pharmacokinetic interactions (Dodick and Martin 2004). Some triptans, such as sumatriptan, rizatriptan, and zolmitriptan, are metabolized by MAO and should not be used during therapy with MAOIs (including selegiline) or within 2 weeks of MAOI discontinuation (McEvoy 2017). Other triptans are eliminated primarily through metabolism by CYP enzymes and/or are renally excreted and thus may be safer options in conjunction with MAOIs.

Parkinson's Disease

For additional discussion of use of medications in patients with Parkinson's disease, see Chapter 30.

Antidepressants.   Double-blind studies of imipramine, nortriptyline, desipramine, citalopram, and bupropion demonstrate antidepressant efficacy with no change in Parkinson's disease symptoms. The anticholinergic effects of TCAs may even be therapeutic for parkinsonism. There is a theoretical concern that serotonergic antidepressants could worsen motor symptoms of Parkinson's disease through serotonin-mediated inhibition of nigrostriatal dopamine release—this effect occurs rarely (Richard et al. 1999). In a retrospective analysis of patients with Parkinson's disease stabilized on levodopa, initiation of an SSRI was no more likely to result in a change in antiparkinsonian medication dosage than initiation of any other antidepressant class (Arbouw et al. 2007).

Mirtazapine may reduce tremor (Gordon et al. 2002). Selegiline, a highly selective MAO-B inhibitor at dosages used in the treatment of Parkinson's disease, is another antidepressant option, but it loses selectivity at the oral dosages required for antidepressant efficacy and so requires standard MAOI precautions.

Antipsychotics.   The major concern regarding antipsychotic use in Parkinson's disease is dopamine D_2 receptor blockade, especially with high-potency FGAs, which can worsen motor symptoms. Clozapine is the only SGA that has been demonstrated (in multiple controlled trials in patients with Parkinson's disease) to be effective against psychosis without aggravating the disease (for review, see Frieling et al. 2007), and it may even be beneficial in reducing tremor (Parkinson Study Group 1999). As reviewed by Frieling et al. (2007), quetiapine was well tolerated but failed to demonstrate efficacy in two placebo-controlled trials, and olanzapine was ineffective in improving psychotic symptoms and caused increased EPS in two controlled trials. Pimavanserin, a serotonin inverse agonist with no dopaminergic properties, recently received FDA approval for use in the treatment of Parkinson's disease psychosis (Bozymski et al. 2017). Pimavanserin does not worsen motor symptoms or cause hypotension in patients with Parkinson's disease.

Cholinesterase inhibitors.   Cholinesterase inhibitors are considered a promising alternative to antipsychotics in the treatment of psychosis in Parkinson's disease, although clinical trial evidence is limited and mixed regarding benefits (Burn et al. 2006; Ravina et al. 2005).

Dementia With Lewy Bodies

Antipsychotics.   Patients with dementia with Lewy bodies are sensitive to EPS from antipsychotics—an important consideration when antipsychotics are being prescribed for the treatment of hallucinations, delusions, and/or agitation in patients with dementia. No RCTs of antipsychotics in patients with dementia with Lewy bodies exist. Overall, SGAs are probably safer than FGAs but should be used at very low dosages.

Cholinesterase inhibitors.   Patients with Lewy body dementia typically present with cognitive, behavioral, and psychiatric symptoms. Cholinesterase inhibitors are considered by many to be first-line therapy for dementia with Lewy bodies. A meta-analysis of 17 studies suggested that cholinesterase inhibitors improve cognitive function, behavioral disturbances, and global functioning in Lewy body dementia without worsening motor function (Matsunaga et al. 2015).

Endocrine Disease
Diabetes Mellitus

Antidepressants.   SSRIs may be the preferred agents in patients with diabetes because of their minimal effects on glucose metabolism. However, in patients with both depression and diabetic neuropathic pain, SNRIs are preferred. First-line pharmacological treatments for diabetic neuropathic pain include TCAs, SNRIs, gabapentin, and pregabalin (Zin et al. 2008), which appear to be of comparable efficacy (Chou et al. 2009; Quilici et al. 2009). Compared with TCAs, duloxetine, venlafaxine, desvenlafaxine, and milnacipran cause fewer problematic side effects in diabetic individuals.

Antipsychotics.   For a comparison of agents' relative propensities to worsen diabetes, see the glucose tolerance subsection under "Antipsychotics" earlier in this chapter.

Respiratory Disease

For additional discussion of use of medications in patients with respiratory disease, see Chapter 18, "Lung Disease."

Antidepressants

Antidepressants generally do not cause problems in patients with respiratory disease. However, MAOIs are problematic in asthmatic patients because of the potential of these drugs to interact with sympathomimetic medications. Use of antidepressants with anticholinergic properties is of theoretical benefit because of their mild bronchodilator effect. Cyclic antidepressants, SSRIs, and other newer antidepressants have little to no effect on respiratory function.

Anxiolytics and sedative-hypnotics.   The respiratory depressant effects of all benzodiazepines are well established; most of these agents can significantly reduce the ventilatory response to hypoxia, which may precipitate respiratory failure in a patient with marginal respiratory reserve. Patients with moderate to severe COPD are at risk of carbon dioxide retention with long-acting benzodiazepines, even at relatively low dosages. However, benzodiazepines should not automatically be avoided in patients with COPD. Anxiety can reduce respiratory efficiency, and benzodiazepines may actually improve respiratory status in some patients, especially those with asthma or emphysema ("pink puffers") (Mitchell-Heggs et al. 1980). Patients with severe bronchitis ("blue bloaters") or severe restrictive lung disease are the most vulnerable to the adverse effects of benzodiazepines. Intermediate-acting agents (e.g., oxazepam, temazepam, lorazepam) have fewer respiratory depressant effects and are the benzodiazepines of first choice for anxiolysis in patients with COPD. For patients with severe COPD, baseline assessment of blood gases and pulmonary consultation may be necessary in deciding whether benzodiazepines are appropriate for use. Oximetry is likely adequate for ongoing monitoring of the patient's clinical status during benzodiazepine use unless the patient is a known CO_2 retainer, in which case blood gases are more appropriate. Benzodiazepines are contraindicated in most individuals with sleep apnea. Benzodiazepines should not be combined with opioids in patients with respiratory compromise.

Controlled trials with the short-acting nonbenzodiazepine hypnotics zopiclone, eszopiclone, zolpidem, and zaleplon suggest that these agents may be safely used in selected patients who have mild to moderate COPD without daytime hypercapnia. Zopiclone and zolpidem have been found to have no significant effects on ventilatory drive or central control of breathing in patients with mild to moderate COPD (Girault et al. 1996; Ranløv and Nielsen 1987). Zopiclone was studied in patients with upper-airway resistance syndrome and was demonstrated to have no adverse effects on sleep architecture, respiratory parameters during sleep, and daytime sleepiness (Lofaso et al. 1997). Ramelteon has been shown in controlled clinical trials to be safe in patients with mild to moderate COPD (Kryger et al. 2008) and with moderate to severe COPD (Kryger et al. 2009) without effects on arterial oxygen saturation. Further study is needed to better define the risk–benefit ratio of hypnotics in patients with COPD.

Buspirone is potentially a safer anxiolytic in pulmonary patients because it does not depress respiration in patients with COPD (Argyropoulou et al. 1993) or sleep apnea (Mendelson et al. 1991). A double-blind study of buspirone demonstrated no adverse effects of the drug on respiratory measures but also failed to show clinical benefit in patients with COPD (Singh et al. 1993).

Antipsychotics.   Antipsychotics may be helpful in pulmonary patients who are incapacitated by extreme panic and dyspnea that mutually exacerbate each other. Most FGAs and SGAs can be used in patients with chronic respiratory disease. Orally inhaled loxapine is contraindicated in patients with asthma or COPD; symptomatic bronchospasm occurred in 53.8% and 19.2% of patients, respectively, in two RCTs (Gross et al. 2014).

Cholinesterase inhibitors and memantine.   Because acetylcholine is a potent mediator of bronchoconstriction, cholinesterase inhibitors should be used with caution in patients with a history of asthma or COPD. Memantine has no effect on respiration and can be used safely in patients with COPD.

Cancer

For additional discussion of use of medications in patients with cancer, see Chapter 22, "Oncology."

Antidepressants

A large meta-analysis of 18 observational studies did not find an increased risk of breast cancer in women who used antidepressants (Eom et al. 2012). A recent prospective cohort study continued to find no association between risk of breast cancer and use of antidepressants (Brown et al. 2016). Antidepressant use was not associated with risk of ovarian cancer (C.S. Wu et al. 2015). SSRI use did not increase the risk of prostate cancer (Tamim et al. 2008) or colorectal cancer (Lee et al. 2017). Studies examining the relationship between antidepressant use and risk of lung cancer have reported conflicting findings (Boursi et al. 2015; Toh et al. 2007).

Antidepressants are often prescribed in cancer patients to treat pain, depression, or hot flashes. Tamoxifen is a prodrug requiring metabolism by CYP2D6 and CYP3A4 to its active form, endoxifen. Therefore, in women taking tamoxifen, antidepressants that inhibit CYP2D6 (e.g., fluoxetine, paroxetine, duloxetine, bupropion) should be avoided (McMichael et al. 2013).

Antipsychotics

Both increased and decreased rates of cancer in patients taking antipsychotics have been reported in epidemiological studies (Dalton et al. 2006; Mortensen 1987). No findings have been clearly replicated. Studies of antipsychotics that raise prolactin levels (e.g., risperidone, paliperidone, amisulpride, FGAs) have suggested that these agents may increase the risk of breast cancer (Wu Chou et al. 2017) but not of endometrial cancer (Klil-Drori et al. 2017); however, confounding factors may not have been controlled for in these studies. Although an association between risperidone and pituitary tumors was suggested in pharmacovigilance reviews, evidence has not confirmed this association (McCarren et al. 2012). Study evidence to date does not support avoidance of antipsychotic use based on concerns about cancer risk. Haloperidol and olanzapine have been used to treat chemotherapy-associated nausea and vomiting that are refractory to traditional therapies.

Anxiolytics, Mood Stabilizers/Anticonvulsants, and Hypnotics

Benzodiazepines (Pottegård et al. 2013), and the mood stabilizers lithium, valproate, and lamotrigine, are not associated with increased cancer risk. Despite reports from retrospective cohort studies of increased cancer risk with hypnotic use, methodological issues with confounding prevent conclusions regarding causality (Kripke et al. 2012; Sivertsen et al. 2015).

HIV/AIDS

See Chapter 26, "Infectious Diseases," as well as reviews by Gallego et al. (2012), Repetto and Petitto (2008), and Thompson et al. (2006), for guidance on the use of psychotropics in patients with HIV/AIDS.

Psychotropic Drug Use During Pregnancy and Breast-Feeding

For a full discussion of issues regarding medication use by pregnant or breast-feeding women, including consideration of the risks of withholding medication, see Chapter 31, "Obstetrics and Gynecology." Current information on drug use in pregnancy and breast-feeding is available through the Motherisk program (www.motherisk.org). Information handouts on medication use during pregnancy and breast-feeding are available from the Organization of Teratology Information Specialists (www.mothertobaby.org).

Conclusion

Rapid developments in medical care in general, and in psychopharmacology in particular, challenge clinicians to remain current on new agents, new indications for established agents, and potential pharmacokinetic and pharmacodynamic interactions in a polypharmacy environment (including over-the-counter and herbal preparations). In this chapter, the many key considerations relevant to the use of psychopharmacological agents in complex medically ill patients have been discussed. Detailed information on adverse effects, toxicities, drug–drug interactions, and alternative administration routes for each major psychotherapeutic drug class has been presented. Where possible, clinicians should use Internet resources to obtain the most up-to-date information. Many key online materials and data sources are cited in the References below, and their general use as a means of following developments in this area is encouraged.

References

Adinolfi LE, Nevola R, Rinaldi L, et al: Chronic hepatitis C virus infection and depression. Clin Liver Dis 21(3):517–534, 2017 28689590

Adityanjee SM, Sajatovic M, Munshi KR: Neuropsychiatric sequelae of neuroleptic malignant syndrome. Clin Neuropharmacol 28(4):197–204, 2005 16062103

Adler LA, Spencer T, Brown TE, et al: Once-daily atomoxetine for adult attention-deficit/hyperactivity disorder: a 6-month, double-blind trial. J Clin Psychopharmacol 29(1):44–50, 2009 19142107

Alawami M, Wasywich C, Cicovic A, et al: A systematic review of clozapine induced cardiomyopathy. Int J Cardiol 176(2):315–320, 2014 25131906

Allain H, Delahaye C, Le Coz F, et al: Postmarketing surveillance of zopiclone in insomnia: analysis of 20,513 cases. Sleep 14(5):408–413, 1991 1759093

Alldredge BK: Seizure risk associated with psychotropic drugs: clinical and pharmacokinetic considerations. Neurology 53(5) (suppl 2):S68–S75, 1999 10496236

Allergan: Savella (milnacipran) home page. 2016. Available at: http://www.savella.com. Accessed October 17, 2017.

Alper K, Schwartz KA, Kolts RL, et al: Seizure incidence in psychopharmacological clinical trials: an analysis of Food and Drug Administration (FDA) summary basis of approval reports. Biol Psychiatry 62(4):345–354, 2007 17223086

American Diabetes Association, American Psychiatric Association, American Association of Clinical Endocrinologists, et al: Consensus development conference on antipsychotics and obesity and diabetes. Diabetes Care 27:596–601, 2004 14747245

American Psychiatric Association: Diagnostic and Statistical Manual of Mental Disorders, 5th Edition. Arlington, VA, American Psychiatric Association, 2013

Anderson GD, Hakimian S: Pharmacokinetic of antiepileptic drugs in patients with hepatic or renal impairment. Clin Pharmacokinet 53(1):29–49, 2014 24122696

Andreoli V, Caillard V, Deo RS, et al: Reboxetine, a new noradrenaline selective antidepressant, is at least as effective as fluoxetine in the treatment of depression. J Clin Psychopharmacol 22(4):393–399, 2002 12172339

Ang-Lee MK, Moss J, Yuan C-S: Herbal medicines and perioperative care. JAMA 286(2):208–216, 2001 11448284

Arbouw ME, Movig KL, Neef C, et al: Influence of initial use of serotonergic antidepressants on antiparkinsonian drug use in levodopa-using patients. Eur J Clin Pharmacol 63(2):181–187, 2007 17200834

Argyropoulou P, Patakas D, Koukou A, et al: Buspirone effect on breathlessness and exercise performance in patients with chronic obstructive pulmonary disease. Respiration 60(4):216–220, 1993 8265878

Arif H, Buchsbaum R, Weintraub D, et al: Patient-reported cognitive side effects of antiepileptic drugs: predictors and comparison of all commonly used antiepileptic drugs. Epilepsy Behav 14(1):202–209, 2009 19010446

Asconapé JJ: Use of antiepileptic drugs in hepatic and renal disease. Handb Clin Neurol 119:417–432, 2014 24365310

Baghdady NT, Banik S, Swartz SA, et al: Psychotropic drugs and renal failure: translating the evidence for clinical practice. Adv Ther 26(4):404–424, 2009 19444657

Bailey AM, Baum RA, Horn K, et al: Review of intranasally administered medications for use in the emergency department. J Emerg Med 53(1):38–48, 2017 28259526

Baird-Gunning J, Lea-Henry T, Hoegberg LCG, et al: Lithium poisoning. J Intensive Care Med 32(4):249–263, 2017 27516079

Baruah J, Easby J, Kessell G: Effects of acetylcholinesterase inhibitor therapy for Alzheimer's disease on neuromuscular block. Br J Anaesth 100(3):420, 2008 18276655

Beach SR, Celano CM, Noseworthy PA, et al: QTc prolongation, torsades de pointes, and psychotropic medications. Psychosomatics 54(1):1–13, 2013 23295003

Beach SR, Kostis WJ, Celano CM, et al: Meta-analysis of selective serotonin reuptake inhibitor-associated QTc prolongation. J Clin Psychiatry 75(5):e441–e449, 2014 24922496

Becker PM, Somiah M: Non-benzodiazepine receptor agonists for insomnia. Sleep Med Clin 10(1):57–76, 2015 26055674

Bent S, Ko R: Commonly used herbal medicines in the United States: a review. Am J Med 116(7):478–485, 2004 15047038

Berman BD: Neuroleptic malignant syndrome: a review for neurohospitalists. Neurohospitalist 1(1):41–47, 2011 23983836

Birnbaum AK, Kriel RL, Im Y, et al: Relative bioavailability of lamotrigine chewable dispersible tablets administered rectally. Pharmacotherapy 21(2):158–162, 2001 11213851

Björkman S, Rigemar G, Idvall J: Pharmacokinetics of midazolam given as an intranasal spray to adult surgical patients. Br J Anaesth 79(5):575–580, 1997 9422893

Black JE, Hirshkowitz M: Modafinil for treatment of residual excessive sleepiness in nasal continuous positive airway pressure-treated obstructive sleep apnea/hypopnea syndrome. Sleep 28(4):464–471, 2005 16171291

Black JE, Hull SG, Tiller J, et al: The long-term tolerability and efficacy of armodafinil in patients with excessive sleepiness associated with treated obstructive sleep apnea, shift work disorder, or narcolepsy: an open-label extension study. J Clin Sleep Med 6(5):458–466, 2010 20957846

Bocchetta A, Cocco F, Velluzzi F, et al: Fifteen-year follow-up of thyroid function in lithium patients. J Endocrinol Invest 30(5):363–366, 2007 17598966

Body R, Bartram T, Azam F, et al: Guidelines in Emergency Medicine Network (GEMNet): guideline for the management of tricyclic antidepressant overdose. Emerg Med J 28(4):347–368, 2011 21436332

Boursi B, Lurie I, Mamtani R, et al: Anti-depressant therapy and cancer risk: a nested case-control study. Eur Neuropsychopharmacol 25(8):1147–1157, 2015 25934397

Boyer EW, Shannon M: The serotonin syndrome. N Engl J Med 352(11):1112–1120, 2005 15784664

Bozymski KM, Lowe DK, Pasternak KM, et al: Pimavanserin: a novel antipsychotic for Parkinson's disease psychosis. Ann Pharmacother 51(6):479–487, 2017 28375643

Bramness JG, Arnestad M, Karinen R, et al: Fatal overdose of zopiclone in an elderly woman with bronchogenic carcinoma. J Forensic Sci 46(5):1247–1249, 2001 11569575

Brazier NC, Levine MA: Drug-herb interaction among commonly used conventional medicines: a compendium for health care professionals. Am J Ther 10(3):163–169, 2003 12756423

Bronheim HE, Fulop G, Kunkel EJ, et al; The Academy of Psychosomatic Medicine: The Academy of Psychosomatic Medicine practice guidelines for psychiatric consultation in the general medical setting. Psychosomatics 39(4):S8–S30, 1998 9691717

Brown SB, Hankinson SE, Arcaro KF, et al: Depression, antidepressant use, and postmenopausal breast cancer risk. Cancer Epidemiol Biomarkers Prev 25(1):158–164, 2016 26578537

Burggraf GW: Are psychotropic drugs at therapeutic levels a concern for cardiologists? Can J Cardiol 13(1):75–80, 1997 9039069

Burn D, Emre M, McKeith I, et al: Effects of rivastigmine in patients with and without visual hallucinations in dementia associated with Parkinson's disease. Mov Disord 21(11):1899–1907, 2006 16960863

Cacoub P, Musette P, Descamps V, et al: The DRESS syndrome: a literature review. Am J Med 124(7):588–597, 2011 21592453

Cancelli I, Beltrame M, Gigli GL, et al: Drugs with anticholinergic properties: cognitive and neuropsychiatric side-effects in elderly patients. Neurol Sci 30(2):87–92, 2009 19229475

Cephalon: Nuvigil (armodafinil). 2017. Available at: http://www.nuvigil.com. Accessed October 17, 2017.

Chandler F (ed): Herbs: Everyday Reference for Health Professionals. Ottawa, ON, Canadian Pharmacist Association and Canadian Medical Association, 2000

Chengappa KN, Chalasani L, Brar JS, et al: Changes in body weight and body mass index among psychiatric patients receiving lithium, valproate, or topiramate: an open-label, nonrandomized chart review. Clin Ther 24(10):1576–1584, 2002 12462287

Chew ML, Mulsant BH, Pollock BG, et al: Anticholinergic activity of 107 medications commonly used by older adults. J Am Geriatr Soc 56(7):1333–1341, 2008 18510583

Chong SA, Mythily S, Mahendran R: Cardiac effects of psychotropic drugs. Ann Acad Med Singapore 30(6):625–631, 2001 11817292

Chou R, Carson S, Chan BK: Gabapentin versus tricyclic antidepressants for diabetic neuropathy and post-herpetic neuralgia: discrepancies between direct and indirect meta-analyses of randomized controlled trials. J Gen Intern Med 24(2):178–188, 2009 19089502

Citrome L: Iloperidone, asenapine, and lurasidone: a brief overview of 3 new second-generation antipsychotics. Postgrad Med 123(2):153–162, 2011 21474903

Clarke TC, Black LI, Stussman BJ, et al: Trends in the use of complementary health approaches among adults: United States, 2002–2012. National Health Statistics Reports, No 79. National Center for Health Statistics. 2015. Available at: https://www.cdc.gov/nchs/data/nhsr/nhsr079.pdf. Accessed October 17, 2017.

Clemens PL, Cloyd JC, Kriel RL, et al: Relative bioavailability, metabolism and tolerability of rectally administered oxcarbazepine suspension. Clin Drug Investig 27(4):243–250, 2007 17358096

Clozapine REMS: Clozapine risk evaluation and mitigation strategy. 2017. Available at: www.clozapinerems.com. Accessed October 17, 2017.

Cohen LG, Prince J, Biederman J, et al: Absence of effect of stimulants on the pharmacokinetics of desipramine in children. Pharmacotherapy 19(6):746–752, 1999 10391421

Cohen LM, Tessier EG, Germain MJ, et al: Update on psychotropic medication use in renal disease. Psychosomatics 45(1):34–48, 2004 14709759

Collaborative Working Group on Clinical Trial Evaluations: Assessment of EPS and tardive dyskinesia in clinical trials. J Clin Psychiatry 59 (suppl 12):23–27, 1998 9766616

Conway JM, Birnbaum AK, Kriel RL, et al: Relative bioavailability of topiramate administered rectally. Epilepsy Res 54(2–3):91–96, 2003 12837560

Cowles BJ: Lisdexamfetamine for treatment of attention-deficit/hyperactivity disorder. Ann Pharmacother 43(4):669–676, 2009 19318601

Cozza K, Armstrong S, Oesterheld J: Concise Guide to the Cytochrome P450 System: Drug Interaction Principles for Medical Practice. Washington, DC, American Psychiatric Publishing, 2003

Crone CC, Gabriel GM, DiMartini A: An overview of psychiatric issues in liver disease for the consultation-liaison psychiatrist. Psychosomatics 47(3):188–205, 2006 16684936

Crowe S, Collins L: Suxamethonium and donepezil: a cause of prolonged paralysis. Anesthesiology 98(2):574–575, 2003 12552219

Currier GW, Medori R: Orally versus intramuscularly administered antipsychotic drugs in psychiatric emergencies. J Psychiatr Pract 12(1):30–40, 2006 16432443

Curto M, Girardi N, Lionetto L, et al: Systematic review of clozapine cardiotoxicity. Curr Psychiatry Rep 18(7):68, 2016 27222142

Dalton SO, Johansen C, Poulsen AH, et al: Cancer risk among users of neuroleptic medication: a population-based cohort study. Br J Cancer 95(7):934–939, 2006 16926836

Dannawi M: Possible serotonin syndrome after combination of buspirone and St John's wort. J Psychopharmacol 16(4):401, 2002 12503845

Darwish M, Kirby M, Robertson P Jr, et al: Interaction profile of armodafinil with medications metabolized by cytochrome P450 enzymes 1A2, 3A4 and 2C19 in healthy subjects. Clin Pharmacokinet 47(1):61–74, 2008 18076219

DasGupta K, Jefferson JW: The use of lithium in the medically ill. Gen Hosp Psychiatry 12(2):83–97, 1990 2407615

Decker BS, Goldfarb DS, Dargan PI, et al; EXTRIP Workgroup: Extracorporeal treatment for lithium poisoning: systematic review and recommendations from the EXTRIP workgroup. Clin J Am Soc Nephrol 10(5):875–887, 2015 25583292

De Leon J, Spina E: Possible pharmacodynamic and pharmacokinetic drug-drug interactions that are likely to be clinically relevant and/or frequent in bipolar disorder. Curr Psychiatry Rep 20(3):17, 2018 29527636

De Picker L, Van Den Eede F, Dumont G, et al: Antidepressants and the risk of hyponatremia: a class-by-class review of literature. Psychosomatics 55(6):536–547, 2014 25262043

DeSanty KP, Amabile CM: Antidepressant-induced liver injury. Ann Pharmacother 41(7):1201–1211, 2007 17609231

Detke MJ, Lu Y, Goldstein DJ, et al: Duloxetine 60 mg once daily dosing versus placebo in the acute treatment of major depression. J Psychiatr Res 36(6):383–390, 2002 12393307

Dodick DW, Martin V: Triptans and CNS side-effects: pharmacokinetic and metabolic mechanisms. Cephalalgia 24(6):417–424, 2004 15154851

Dolder CR, Nelson MH: Hypnosedative-induced complex behaviours: incidence, mechanisms and management. CNS Drugs 22(12):1021–1036, 2008 18998740

Dolly FR, Block AJ: Effect of flurazepam on sleep-disordered breathing and nocturnal oxygen desaturation in asymptomatic subjects. Am J Med 73(2):239–243, 1982 7051825

Dong X, Leppik IE, White J, et al: Hyponatremia from oxcarbazepine and carbamazepine. Neurology 65(12):1976–1978, 2005 16380624

Douglas IJ, Smeeth L: Exposure to antipsychotics and risk of stroke: self controlled case series study. BMJ 337:a1227, 2008 18755769

Drici MD, Priori S: Cardiovascular risks of atypical antipsychotic drug treatment. Pharmacoepidemiol Drug Saf 16(8):882–890, 2007 17563919

Duncan MA, Savage J, Tucker AP: Prospective audit comparing intrathecal analgesia (incorporating midazolam) with epidural and intravenous analgesia after major open abdominal surgery. Anaesth Intensive Care 35(4):558–562, 2007 18020075

Dunkley EJ, Isbister GK, Sibbritt D, et al: The Hunter Serotonin Toxicity Criteria: simple and accurate diagnostic decision rules for serotonin toxicity. QJM 96(9):635–642, 2003 12925718

Eli Lilly: Zyprexa (olanzapine) home page. 2010. Available at: http://www.zyprexa.com. Accessed October 17, 2017.

Eli Lilly: Cymbalta (duloxetine) home page. 2016. Available at: http://www.cymbalta.com. Accessed October 17, 2017.

Eli Lilly: Strattera (atomoxetine) home page. 2017. Available at: http://www.strattera.com. Accessed October 17, 2017.

English BA, Dortch M, Ereshefsky L, et al: Clinically significant psychotropic drug-drug interactions in the primary care setting. Curr Psychiatry Rep 14(4):376–390, 2012 22707017. Available on PubMed Central (PMC) at: https://www.ncbi.nlm.nih.gov/pmc/articles/PMC4335312/. Accessed April 1, 2018.

Eom CS, Park SM, Cho KH: Use of antidepressants and the risk of breast cancer: a meta-analysis. Breast Cancer Res Treat 136(3):635–645, 2012 23139055

Ernst CL, Goldberg JF: The reproductive safety profile of mood stabilizers, atypical antipsychotics, and broad-spectrum psychotropics. J Clin Psychiatry 63 (suppl 4):42–55, 2002 11913676

Ernst E: Complementary medicine. Curr Opin Rheumatol 15(2):151–155, 2003 12598804

Eyler RF, Unruh ML, Quinn DK, et al: Psychotherapeutic agents in end-stage renal disease. Semin Dial 28(4):417–426, 2015 25857865

Farlow MR, Graham SM, Alva G: Memantine for the treatment of Alzheimer's disease: tolerability and safety data from clinical trials. Drug Saf 31(7):577–585, 2008 18558791

Fava GA, Gatti A, Belaise C, et al: Withdrawal symptoms after selective serotonin reuptake inhibitor discontinuation: a systematic review. Psychother Psychosom 84(2):72–81, 2015 25721705

Feighner JP: Cardiovascular safety in depressed patients: focus on venlafaxine. J Clin Psychiatry 56(12):574–579, 1995 8530334

Findling RL, Bukstein OG, Melmed RD, et al: A randomized, double-blind, placebo-controlled, parallel-group study of methylphenidate transdermal system in pediatric patients with attention-deficit/hyperactivity disorder. J Clin Psychiatry 69(1):149–159, 2008 18312050

Finley PR: Drug interactions with lithium: an update. Clin Pharmacokinet 55(8):925–941, 2016 26936045

Fitzsimons J, Berk M, Lambert T, et al: A review of clozapine safety. Expert Opin Drug Saf 4(4):731–744, 2005 16011451

Flanagan RJ, Dunk L: Haematological toxicity of drugs used in psychiatry. Hum Psychopharmacol 23 (suppl 1):27–41, 2008 18098216

Fleishaker JC, Francom SF, Herman BD, et al: Lack of effect of reboxetine on cardiac repolarization. Clin Pharmacol Ther 70(3):261–269, 2001 11557914

Flynn CT, Chandran PK, Taylor MJ, et al: Intraperitoneal lithium administration for bipolar affective disorder in a patient on continuous ambulatory peritoneal dialysis. Int J Artif Organs 10(2):105–107, 1987 3583425

Forrester MB: Comparison of zolpidem and zaleplon exposures in Texas, 1998–2004. J Toxicol Environ Health A 69(20):1883–1892, 2006 16952907

Freeman MP, Freeman SA: Lithium: clinical considerations in internal medicine. Am J Med 119(6):478–481, 2006 16750958

Freudenthaler S, Meineke I, Schreeb KH, et al: Influence of urine pH and urinary flow on the renal excretion of memantine. Br J Clin Pharmacol 46(6):541–546, 1998 9862242

Frieling H, Hillemacher T, Ziegenbein M, et al: Treating dopamimetic psychosis in Parkinson's disease: structured review and meta-analysis. Eur Neuropsychopharmacol 17(3):165–171, 2007 17070675

Gallego L, Barreiro P, López-Ibor JJ: Psychopharmacological treatments in HIV patients under antiretroviral therapy. AIDS Rev 14(2):101–111, 2012 22627606

Gallini A, Sommet A, Montastruc JL; French PharmacoVigilance Network: Does memantine induce bradycardia? A study in the French PharmacoVigilance Database. Pharmacoepidemiol Drug Saf 17(9):877–881, 2008 18500725

Gao K, Kemp DE, Ganocy SJ, et al: Antipsychotic-induced extrapyramidal side effects in bipolar disorder and schizophrenia: a systematic review. J Clin Psychopharmacol 28(2):203–209, 2008 18344731

Gardiner P, Phillips R, Shaughnessy AF: Herbal and dietary supplement—drug interactions in patients with chronic illnesses. Am Fam Physician 77(1):73–78, 2008 18236826

Gerstner T, Büsing D, Bell N, et al: Valproic acid-induced pancreatitis: 16 new cases and a review of the literature. J Gastroenterol 42(1):39–48, 2007 17322992

Ghaleiha A, Haghighi M, Sharifmehr M, et al: Oral loading of sodium valproate compared to intravenous loading and oral maintenance in acutely manic bipolar patients. Neuropsychobiology 70(1):29–35, 2014 25171133

Giardina EG, Johnson LL, Vita J, et al: Effect of imipramine and nortriptyline on left ventricular function and blood pressure in patients treated for arrhythmias. Am Heart J 109(5 Pt 1):992–998, 1985 3993532

Gibson AP, Bettinger TL, Patel NC, et al: Atomoxetine versus stimulants for treatment of attention deficit/hyperactivity disorder. Ann Pharmacother 40(6):1134–1142, 2006 16735655

Gill SS, Anderson GM, Fischer HD, et al: Syncope and its consequences in patients with dementia receiving cholinesterase inhibitors: a population-based cohort study. Arch Intern Med 169(9):867–873, 2009 19433698

Girault C, Muir JF, Mihaltan F, et al: Effects of repeated administration of zolpidem on sleep, diurnal and nocturnal respiratory function, vigilance, and physical performance in patients with COPD. Chest 110(5):1203–1211, 1996 8915222

Gitlin M: Lithium side effects and toxicity: prevalence and management strategies. Int J Bipolar Disord 4(1):27, 2016 27900734

Glassman AH: Cardiovascular effects of tricyclic antidepressants. Annu Rev Med 35:503–511, 1984 6372670

Glassman AH, O'Connor CM, Califf RM, et al; Sertraline Antidepressant Heart Attack Randomized Trial (SADHEART) Group: Sertraline treatment of major depression in patients with acute MI or unstable angina. JAMA 288(6):701–709, 2002 12169073

Gordon PH, Pullman SL, Louis ED, et al: Mirtazapine in parkinsonian tremor. Parkinsonism Relat Disord 9(2):125–126, 2002 12473405

Gross N, Greos LS, Meltzer EO, et al: Safety and tolerability of inhaled loxapine in subjects with asthma and chronic obstructive pulmonary disease—two randomized controlled trials. J Aerosol Med Pulm Drug Deliv 27(6):478–487, 2014 24745666

Grossberg GT: The ABC of Alzheimer's disease: behavioral symptoms and their treatment. Int Psychogeriatr 14 (suppl 1):27–49, 2002 12636179

Gubbins PO, Bertch KE: Drug absorption in gastrointestinal disease and surgery. Clinical pharmacokinetic and therapeutic implications. Clin Pharmacokinet 21(6):431–447, 1991 1782738

Guenette MD, Hahn M, Cohn TA, et al: Atypical antipsychotics and diabetic ketoacidosis: a review. Psychopharmacology (Berl) 226(1):1–12, 2013 23344556

Guilleminault C: Benzodiazepines, breathing, and sleep. Am J Med 88(3A):25S–28S, 1990 1968716

Gurley BJ, Swain A, Williams DK, et al: Gauging the clinical significance of P-glycoprotein-mediated herb-drug interactions: comparative effects of St. John's wort, Echinacea, clarithromycin, and rifampin on digoxin pharmacokinetics. Mol Nutr Food Res 52(7):772–779, 2008 18214850

Gurrera RJ, Caroff SN, Cohen A, et al: An international consensus study of neuroleptic malignant syndrome diagnostic criteria using the Delphi method. J Clin Psychiatry 72(9):1222–1228, 2011 21733489

Haddad PM: Antidepressant discontinuation syndromes. Drug Saf 24(3):183–197, 2001 11347722

Haddad PM, Anderson IM: Antipsychotic-related QTc prolongation, torsade de pointes and sudden death. Drugs 62(11):1649–1671, 2002 12109926

Haddad PM, Dursun SM: Neurological complications of psychiatric drugs: clinical features and management. Hum Psychopharmacol 23 (suppl 1):15–26, 2008 18098217

Haddad PM, Sharma SG: Adverse effects of atypical antipsychotics: differential risk and clinical implications. CNS Drugs 21(11):911–936, 2007 17927296

Harden CL, Goldstein MA: Mood disorders in patients with epilepsy: epidemiology and management. CNS Drugs 16(5):291–302, 2002 11994019

Hasnain M, Vieweg WV: QTc interval prolongation and torsade de pointes associated with second-generation antipsychotics and antidepressants: a comprehensive review. CNS Drugs 28(10):887–920, 2014 25168784

Hawthorne JM, Caley CF: Extrapyramidal reactions associated with serotonergic antidepressants. Ann Pharmacother 49(10):1136–1152, 2015 26185277

Health Canada: Important drug safety information: RISPERDAL (risperidone) and cerebrovascular adverse events in placebo-controlled dementia trials—Janssen-Ortho, October 11, 2002. Available at: http://healthycanadians.gc.ca/recall-alert-rappel-avis/hc-sc/2002/14720a-eng.php. Accessed March 30, 2018.

Hedenmalm K, Güzey C, Dahl ML, et al: Risk factors for extrapyramidal symptoms during treatment with selective serotonin reuptake inhibitors, including cytochrome P-450 enzyme, and serotonin and dopamine transporter and receptor polymorphisms. J Clin Psychopharmacol 26(2):192–197, 2006 16633151

Hedner J, Yaeche R, Emilien G, et al; The Zaleplon Clinical Investigator Study Group: Zaleplon shortens subjective sleep latency and improves subjective sleep quality in elderly patients with insomnia. Int J Geriatr Psychiatry 15(8):704–712, 2000 10960882

Heitmann J, Cassel W, Grote L, et al: Does short-term treatment with modafinil affect blood pressure in patients with obstructive sleep apnea? Clin Pharmacol Ther 65(3):328–335, 1999 10096265

Hirsch LJ, Weintraub DB, Buchsbaum R, et al: Predictors of lamotrigine-associated rash. Epilepsia 47(2):318–322, 2006 16499755

Holmes TF, Sabaawi M, Fragala MR: Psychostimulant suppository treatment for depression in the gravely ill. J Clin Psychiatry 55(6):265–266, 1994 8071285

Hsu WT, Esmaily-Fard A, Lai CC, et al: Antipsychotics and the risk of cerebrovascular accident: a systematic review and meta-analysis of observational studies. J Am Med Dir Assoc 18(8):692–699, 2017 28431909

Hu X, Wang J, Dong W, et al: A meta-analysis of polycystic ovary syndrome in women taking valproate for epilepsy. Epilepsy Res 97(1–2):73–82, 2011 21820873

Hu Z, Yang X, Ho PC, et al: Herb-drug interactions: a literature review. Drugs 65(9):1239–1282, 2005 15916450

Imfeld P, Bodmer M, Jick SS, Meier CR: Benzodiazepine use and risk of developing Alzheimer's disease or vascular dementia: a case-control analysis. Drug Saf 38(10):909–919, 2015 26123874

Isbister GK, Bowe SJ, Dawson A, et al: Relative toxicity of selective serotonin reuptake inhibitors (SSRIs) in overdose. J Toxicol Clin Toxicol 42(3):277–285, 2004 15362595

Jafferany M: Lithium and skin: dermatologic manifestations of lithium therapy. Int J Dermatol 47(11):1101–1111, 2008 18986438

Janssen: Topamax (topiramate), U.S. prescribing information. Revised June 2017. Available at: http://www.janssenlabels.com/package-insert/product-monograph/prescribing-information/TOPAMAX-pi.pdf. Accessed October 18, 2017.

Jasiak NM, Bostwick JR: Risk of QT/QTc prolongation among newer non-SSRI antidepressants. Ann Pharmacother 48(12):1620–1628, 2014 25204465

Kaminsky BM, Bostwick JR, Guthrie SK: Alternate routes of administration of antidepressant and antipsychotic medications. Ann Pharmacother 49(7):808–817, 2015 25907529

Kansagra A, Patel S, Wilcox SR: Prolonged hypothermia due to olanzapine in the setting of renal failure: a case report and review of the literature. Ther Adv Psychopharmacol 3(6):335–339, 2013 24294486

Kasper S, Müller-Spahn F: Intravenous antidepressant treatment: focus on citalopram. Eur Arch Psychiatry Clin Neurosci 252(3):105–109, 2002 12192466

Katus LE, Frucht SJ: Management of serotonin syndrome and neuroleptic malignant syndrome. Curr Treat Options Neurol 18(9):39, 2016 27469512

Keating GM: Loxapine inhalation powder: a review of its use in the acute treatment of agitation in patients with bipolar disorder or schizophrenia. CNS Drugs 27(6):479–489, 2013 23740380

Khawaja IS, Feinstein RE: Cardiovascular effects of selective serotonin reuptake inhibitors and other novel antidepressants. Heart Dis 5(2):153–160, 2003 12713682

Kivistö KT, Lamberg TS, Kantola T, Neuvonen PJ: Plasma buspirone concentrations are greatly increased by erythromycin and itraconazole. Clin Pharmacol Ther 62(3):348–354, 1997 9333111

Kleiner J, Altshuler L, Hendrick V, et al: Lithium-induced subclinical hypothyroidism: review of the literature and guidelines for treatment. J Clin Psychiatry 60(4):249–255, 1999 10221287

Klil-Drori AJ, Yin H, Abenhaim HA, et al: Prolactin-elevating antipsychotics and the risk of endometrial cancer. J Clin Psychiatry 78(6):714–719, 2017 28199787

Koelle JS, Dimsdale JE: Antidepressants for the virtually eviscerated patient: options instead of oral dosing. Psychosom Med 60(6):723–725, 1998 9847031

Kolla BP, Lovely JK, Mansukhani MP, et al: Zolpidem is independently associated with increased risk of inpatient falls. J Hosp Med 8(1):1–6, 2013 23165956

Kreuzer P, Landgrebe M, Wittmann M, et al: Hypothermia associated with antipsychotic drug use: a clinical case series and review of current literature. J Clin Pharmacol 52(7):1090–1097, 2012 21956608

Kripke DF, Langer RD, Kline LE: Hypnotics' association with mortality or cancer: a matched cohort study. BMJ Open 2(1):e000850, 2012 22371848

Kryger M, Wang-Weigand S, Zhang J, et al: Effect of ramelteon, a selective MT(1)/MT (2)-receptor agonist, on respiration during sleep in mild to moderate COPD. Sleep Breath 12(3):243–250, 2008 18060441

Kryger M, Roth T, Wang-Weigand S, et al: The effects of ramelteon on respiration during sleep in subjects with moderate to severe chronic obstructive pulmonary disease. Sleep Breath 13(1):79–84, 2009 18584227

Krystal AD, Erman M, Zammit GK, et al; ZOLONG Study Group: Long-term efficacy and safety of zolpidem extended-release 12.5 mg, administered 3 to 7 nights per week for 24 weeks, in patients with chronic primary insomnia: a 6-month, randomized, double-blind, placebo-controlled, parallel-group, multicenter study. Sleep 31(1):79–90, 2008 18220081

Krystal AD, Richelson E, Roth T: Review of the histamine system and the clinical effects of H$_1$ antagonists: basis for a new model for understanding the effects of insomnia medications. Sleep Med Rev 17(4):263–272, 2013 23357028

Lange R, Volkmer M, Heesen C, et al: Modafinil effects in multiple sclerosis patients with fatigue. J Neurol 256(4):645–650, 2009 19367356

Laursen SB, Leontiadis GI, Stanley AJ, et al: The use of selective serotonin receptor inhibitors (SSRIs) is not associated with increased risk of endoscopy-refractory bleeding, rebleeding or mortality in peptic ulcer bleeding. Aliment Pharmacol Ther 46(3):355–363, 2017 28543334

Lee HC, Chiu WC, Wang TN, et al: Antidepressants and colorectal cancer: a population-based nested case-control study. J Affect Disord 207:353–358, 2017 27744223

Lefèvre G, Pommier F, Sedek G, et al: Pharmacokinetics and bioavailability of the novel rivastigmine transdermal patch versus rivastigmine oral solution in healthy elderly subjects. J Clin Pharmacol 48(2):246–252, 2008 18199897

Lertxundi U, Hernandez R, Medrano J, et al: Antipsychotics and seizures: higher risk with atypicals? Seizure 22(2):141–143, 2013 23146619

Leucht S, Cipriani A, Spineli L, et al: Comparative efficacy and tolerability of 15 antipsychotic drugs in schizophrenia: a multiple-treatments meta-analysis. Lancet 382(9896):951–962, 2013 23810019

Leung J, Hasassri ME, Barreto JN, et al: Characterization of admission types in medically hospitalized patients prescribed clozapine. Psychosomatics 58(2):164–172, 2017 28153339

Levenson JL: Neuroleptic malignant syndrome. Am J Psychiatry 142(10):1137–1145, 1985 2863986

Levenson JL: High-dose intravenous haloperidol for agitated delirium following lung transplantation. Psychosomatics 36(1):66–68, 1995 7871137

Levenson JL, Owen JA: Renal and urological disorders, in Clinical Manual of Psychopharmacology in the Medically Ill, 2nd Edition. Edited by Levenson JL, Ferrando SJ. Arlington, VA, American Psychiatric Publishing, 2017, pp 195–232

Lexicomp: Lexi-Drugs Online. Wolters Kluwer Clinical Drug Information. 2017. Available at: https://online.lexi.com/lco/action/home.//online.lexi.com/lco/action/home. Accessed October 17, 2017.

Li KJ, Gurrera RJ, Delisi LE: Potentially fatal outcomes associated with clozapine. Schizophr Res March 1, 2018 [Epub ahead of print] 29503232

Livingstone C, Rampes H: Lithium: a review of its metabolic adverse effects. J Psychopharmacol 20(3):347–355, 2006 16174674

Lofaso F, Goldenberg F, Thebault C, et al: Effect of zopiclone on sleep, night-time ventilation, and daytime vigilance in upper airway resistance syndrome. Eur Respir J 10(11):2573–2577, 1997 9426097

Lofton AL, Klein-Schwartz W: Evaluation of lamotrigine toxicity reported to poison centers. Ann Pharmacother 38(11):1811–1815, 2004 15353576

Lynch ME, Clark AJ, Sawynok J, et al: Topical amitriptyline and ketamine in neuropathic pain syndromes: an open-label study. J Pain 6(10):644–649, 2005 16202956

Ma H, Huang Y, Cong Z, et al: The efficacy and safety of atypical antipsychotics for the treatment of dementia: a meta-analysis of randomized placebo-controlled trials. J Alzheimers Dis 42(3):915–937, 2014 25024323

Magna Pharmaceuticals: Zolpimist (zolpidem). 2016. Available at: http://myzolpimist.com/wp-content/uploads/2016/04/Zolpimist-PI-approved-final.pdf. Accessed March 24, 2018.

Mago R, Borra D, Mahajan R: Role of adverse effects in medication nonadherence in bipolar disorder. Harv Rev Psychiatry 22(6):363–366, 2014 25377611

Mahady GB, Low Dog T, Barrett ML, et al: United States Pharmacopeia review of the black cohosh case reports of hepatotoxicity. Menopause 15(4 Pt 1):628–638, 2008 18340277

Mancuso CE, Tanzi MG, Gabay M: Paradoxical reactions to benzodiazepines: literature review and treatment options. Pharmacotherapy 24(9):1177–1185, 2004 15460178

Manos GH: Possible serotonin syndrome associated with buspirone added to fluoxetine. Ann Pharmacother 34(7–8):871–874, 2000 10928399

Manos MJ, Tom-Revzon C, Bukstein OG, et al: Changes and challenges: managing ADHD in a fast-paced world. J Manag Care Pharm 13(9) (suppl B):S2–S13, quiz S14–S16, 2007 18062734

Marder SR, Sorsaburu S, Dunayevich E, et al: Case reports of postmarketing adverse event experiences with olanzapine intramuscular treatment in patients with agitation. J Clin Psychiatry 71(4):433–441, 2010 20156413

Markowitz JS, DeVane CL, Malcolm RJ, et al: Pharmacokinetics of olanzapine after single-dose oral administration of standard tablet versus normal and sublingual administration of an orally disintegrating tablet in normal volunteers. J Clin Pharmacol 46(2):164–171, 2006 16432268

Martin WR, Sloan JW, Sapira JD, et al: Physiologic, subjective, and behavioral effects of amphetamine, methamphetamine, ephedrine, phenmetrazine, and methylphenidate in man. Clin Pharmacol Ther 12(2):245–258, 1971 5554941

Masand PS, Tesar GE: Use of stimulants in the medically ill. Psychiatr Clin North Am 19(3):515–547, 1996 8856815

Masand P, Pickett P, Murray GB: Psychostimulants for secondary depression in medical illness. Psychosomatics 32(2):203–208, 1991 2027944

Matsunaga S, Kishi T, Yasue I, et al: Cholinesterase inhibitors for Lewy body disorders: a meta-analysis. Int J Neuropsychopharmacol 19(2):pyv086, 2015 26221005

Matsuo N, Morita T: Efficacy, safety, and cost effectiveness of intravenous midazolam and flunitrazepam for primary insomnia in terminally ill patients with cancer: a retrospective multicenter audit study. J Palliat Med 10(5):1054–1062, 2007 17985961

Mayer G, Wang-Weigand S, Roth-Schechter B, et al: Efficacy and safety of 6-month nightly ramelteon administration in adults with chronic primary insomnia. Sleep 32(3):351–360, 2009 19294955

McCarren M, Qiu H, Ziyadeh N, et al: Follow-up study of a pharmacovigilance signal: no evidence of increased risk with risperidone of pituitary tumor with mass effect. J Clin Psychopharmacol 32(6):743–749, 2012 23131882

McEvoy GE: American Hospital Formulary Service (AHFS) Drug Information 2017. Bethesda, MD, American Society of Health-System Pharmacists, 2017

McIntyre RS, Panjwani ZD, Nguyen HT, et al: The hepatic safety profile of duloxetine: a review. Expert Opin Drug Metab Toxicol 4(3):281–285, 2008 18363543

McMichael KS, Adams K, Breden Crouse EL: Tamoxifen and depression: drug interactions in breast cancer. Consult Pharm 28(9):584–591, 2013 24007891

Melkersson KI: Prolactin elevation of the antipsychotic risperidone is predominantly related to its 9-hydroxy metabolite. Hum Psychopharmacol 21(8):529–532, 2006 17094165

Mendelson WB, Maczaj M, Holt J: Buspirone administration to sleep apnea patients. J Clin Psychopharmacol 11(1):71–72, 1991 2040719

Merck: Remeron (mirtazapine). 2016. Available at: http://www.merck.com/product/usa/pi_circulars/r/remeron_soltab/remeron_soltab_pi.pdf. Accessed October 18, 2017.

Meyer JM, Koro CE: The effects of antipsychotic therapy on serum lipids: a comprehensive review. Schizophr Res 70(1):1–17, 2004 15246458

Meyer-Massetti C, Cheng CM, Sharpe BA, et al: The FDA extended warning for intravenous haloperidol and torsades de pointes: how should institutions respond? J Hosp Med 5(4):E8–E16, 2010 20394022

Miller EA, Leslie DL, Rosenheck RA: Incidence of new-onset diabetes mellitus among patients receiving atypical neuroleptics in the treatment of mental illness: evidence from a privately insured population. J Nerv Ment Dis 193(6):387–395, 2005 15920379

Miller GM, Stripp R: A study of western pharmaceuticals contained within samples of Chinese herbal/patent medicines collected from New York City's Chinatown. Leg Med (Tokyo) 9(5):258–264, 2007 17652006

Miller JL, Ashford JW, Archer SM, et al: Comparison of intranasal administration of haloperidol with intravenous and intramuscular administration: a pilot pharmacokinetic study. Pharmacotherapy 28(7):875–882, 2008 18576902

Mills KC: Serotonin syndrome. A clinical update. Crit Care Clin 13(4):763–783, 1997 9330840

Minns AB, Clark RF: Toxicology and overdose of atypical antipsychotics. J Emerg Med 43(5):906–913, 2012 22555052

Mirassou MM: Rectal antidepressant medication in the treatment of depression. J Clin Psychiatry 59(1):29, 1998 9491063

Mitchell-Heggs P, Murphy K, Minty K, et al: Diazepam in the treatment of dyspnoea in the "Pink Puffer" syndrome. Q J Med 49(193):9–20, 1980 6776586

Mockenhaupt M, Messenheimer J, Tennis P, et al: Risk of Stevens-Johnson syndrome and toxic epidermal necrolysis in new users of antiepileptics. Neurology 64(7):1134–1138, 2005 15824335

Monti JM, Pandi-Perumal SR: Eszopiclone: its use in the treatment of insomnia. Neuropsychiatr Dis Treat 3(4):441–453, 2007 19300573

Mortensen PB: Neuroleptic treatment and other factors modifying cancer risk in schizophrenic patients. Acta Psychiatr Scand 75(6):585–590, 1987 2887088

Muir JF, DeFouilloy C, Broussier P, et al: Comparative study of the effects of zopiclone and placebo on respiratory function in patients with chronic obstructive respiratory insufficiency. Int Clin Psychopharmacol 5 (suppl 2):85–94, 1990 2201733

Mula M, Trimble MR, Yuen A, et al: Psychiatric adverse events during levetiracetam therapy. Neurology 61(5):704–706, 2003 12963770

Munar MY, Singh H: Drug dosing adjustments in patients with chronic kidney disease. Am Fam Physician 75(10):1487–1496, 2007 17555141

Murray R, Correll CU, Reynolds GP, et al: Atypical antipsychotics: recent research findings and applications to clinical practice: proceedings of a symposium presented at the 29th Annual European College of Neuropsychopharmacology Congress, 19 September 2016, Vienna, Austria. Ther Adv Psychopharmacol 7 (1 suppl):1–14, 2017 28344764

Najib J: Eszopiclone, a nonbenzodiazepine sedative-hypnotic agent for the treatment of transient and chronic insomnia. Clin Ther 28(4):491–516, 2006 16750462

Natural Medicines: Database, Therapeutic Research Center. 2017. Available at: https://naturalmedicines.therapeuticresearch.com. Accessed October 17, 2017.

Nemeroff CB: Safety of available agents used to treat bipolar disorder: focus on weight gain. J Clin Psychiatry 64(5):532–539, 2003 12755655

Neuvonen PJ, Tokola O: Bioavailability of rectally administered carbamazepine mixture. Br J Clin Pharmacol 24(6):839–841, 1987 3440107

Nezafati MH, Vojdanparast M, Nezafati P: Antidepressants and cardiovascular adverse events: a narrative review. ARYA Atheroscler 11(5):295–304, 2015 26715935

Nilsson MI, Widerlöv E, Meresaar U, et al: Effect of urinary pH on the disposition of methadone in man. Eur J Clin Pharmacol 22(4):337–342, 1982 6286317

Norman JL, Anderson SL: Novel class of medications, orexin receptor antagonists, in the treatment of insomnia—critical appraisal of suvorexant. Nat Sci Sleep 8:239–247, 2016 27471419

Norton J: The use of intravenous valproate in psychiatry. Can J Psychiatry 46(4):371–372, 2001 11387798

O'Brien CP: Benzodiazepine use, abuse, and dependence. J Clin Psychiatry 66 (suppl 2):28–33, 2005 15762817

Otsuka: Abilify Maintena. 2017. Available at: www.abilifymaintenahcp.com. Accessed October 18, 2017.

Owen JA, Crouse EL: Pharmacokinetics, pharmacodynamics, and principles of drug-drug interactions, in Clinical Manual of Psychopharmacology in the Medically Ill, 2nd Edition. Edited by Levenson JL, Ferrando SJ. Arlington, VA, American Psychiatric Publishing, 2017, pp 3–44

Papakostas GI: The efficacy, tolerability, and safety of contemporary antidepressants. J Clin Psychiatry 71 (suppl E1):e03, 2010 20371030

Park SH, Ishino R: Liver injury associated with antidepressants. Curr Drug Saf 8(3):207–223, 2013 23914755

Parkinson Study Group: Low-dose clozapine for the treatment of drug-induced psychosis in Parkinson's disease. N Engl J Med 340(10):757–763, 1999 10072410

Parsons RL: Drug absorption in gastrointestinal disease with particular reference to malabsorption syndromes. Clin Pharmacokinet 2(1):45–60, 1977 322910

Periclou A, Ventura D, Rao N, et al: Pharmacokinetic study of memantine in healthy and renally impaired subjects. Clin Pharmacol Ther 79(1):134–143, 2006 16413248

Perrott J, Murphy NG, Zed PJ: L-carnitine for acute valproic acid overdose: a systematic review of published cases. Ann Pharmacother 44(7–8):1287–1293, 2010 20587742

Pfizer: Zeldox (ziprasidone). FDA background on Zeldox; psychopharmacological drugs advisory committee. 2000. Available at: https://www.fda.gov/ohrms/dockets/ac/00/backgrd/3619b1b.pdf. Accessed October 18, 2017.

Pfizer: Pristiq (desvenlafaxine). 2016. Available at: http://www.pristiq.com. Accessed October 18, 2017.

Pfizer: Geodon (ziprasidone). 2017. Available at: http://www.geodon.com. Accessed October 18, 2017.

Pileggi DJ, Cook AM: Neuroleptic malignant syndrome: focus on treatment and rechallenge. Ann Pharmacother 50(11):973–981, 2016 27423483

Porter M, Chacko L: Antiepileptic drugs after first unprovoked seizure. Am Fam Physician 95(3):online, 2017 28145666

Pottegård A, Friis S, Andersen M, et al: Use of benzodiazepines or benzodiazepine related drugs and the risk of cancer: a population-based case-control study. Br J Clin Pharmacol 75(5):1356–1364, 2013 23043261

Pycha R, Miller C, Barnas C, et al: Intravenous flunitrazepam in the treatment of alcohol withdrawal delirium. Alcohol Clin Exp Res 17(4):753–757, 1993 8214408

Quilici S, Chancellor J, Löthgren M, et al: Meta-analysis of duloxetine vs. pregabalin and gabapentin in the treatment of diabetic peripheral neuropathic pain. BMC Neurol 9:6, 2009 19208243

Radomski JW, Dursun SM, Reveley MA, et al: An exploratory approach to the serotonin syndrome: an update of clinical phenomenology and revised diagnostic criteria. Med Hypotheses 55(3):218–224, 2000 10985912

Raja M: Clozapine safety, 35 years later. Curr Drug Saf 6(3):164–184, 2011 22122392

Ranløv PJ, Nielsen SP: Effect of zopiclone and diazepam on ventilatory response in normal human subjects. Sleep 10 (suppl 1):40–47, 1987 3125575

Rao A, Suliman A, Story G, et al: Meta-analysis of population-based studies comparing risk of cerebrovascular accident associated with first- and second-generation antipsychotic prescribing in dementia. Int J Methods Psychiatr Res 25(4):289–298, 2016 27121795

Rapport MD, Moffitt C: Attention deficit/hyperactivity disorder and methylphenidate. A review of height/weight, cardiovascular, and somatic complaint side effects. Clin Psychol Rev 22(8):1107–1131, 2002 12436807

Ravina B, Putt M, Siderowf A, et al: Donepezil for dementia in Parkinson's disease: a randomised, double blind, placebo controlled, crossover study. J Neurol Neurosurg Psychiatry 76(7):934–939, 2005 15965198

Ravindran AV, Balneaves LG, Faulkner G, et al; CANMAT Depression Work Group: Canadian Network for Mood and Anxiety Treatments (CANMAT) 2016 Clinical Guidelines for the

Management of Adults with Major Depressive Disorder: Section 5. Complementary and Alternative Medicine Treatments. Can J Psychiatry 61(9):576–587, 2016 27486153

Repetto MJ, Petitto JM: Psychopharmacology in HIV-infected patients. Psychosom Med 70(5):585–592, 2008 18519881

Reulbach U, Dütsch C, Biermann T, et al: Managing an effective treatment for neuroleptic malignant syndrome. Crit Care 11(1):R4, 2007 17222339

Rey E, Tréluyer JM, Pons G: Pharmacokinetic optimization of benzodiazepine therapy for acute seizures. Focus on delivery routes. Clin Pharmacokinet 36(6):409–424, 1999 10427466

Richard IH, Maughn A, Kurlan R: Do serotonin reuptake inhibitor antidepressants worsen Parkinson's disease? A retrospective case series. Mov Disord 14(1):155–157, 1999 9918360

Risch SC, Groom GP, Janowsky DS: The effects of psychotropic drugs on the cardiovascular system. J Clin Psychiatry 43(5 Pt 2):16–31, 1982 6122680

Robertson P Jr, Hellriegel ET: Clinical pharmacokinetic profile of modafinil. Clin Pharmacokinet 42(2):123–137, 2003 12537513

Robertson P Jr, Hellriegel ET, Arora S, et al: Effect of modafinil on the pharmacokinetics of ethinyl estradiol and triazolam in healthy volunteers. Clin Pharmacol Ther 71(1):46–56, 2002 11823757

Robinson RG, Jorge RE: Post-stroke depression: a review. Am J Psychiatry 173(3):221–231, 2016 26684921

Roose SP, Glassman AH, Giardina EG, et al: Nortriptyline in depressed patients with left ventricular impairment. JAMA 256(23):3253–3257, 1986 3783871

Roose SP, Dalack GW, Glassman AH, et al: Cardiovascular effects of bupropion in depressed patients with heart disease. Am J Psychiatry 148(4):512–516, 1991 1900980

Rosenberg MR, Green M: Neuroleptic malignant syndrome. Review of response to therapy. Arch Intern Med 149(9):1927–1931, 1989 2673115

Rosenstein DL, Nelson JC, Jacobs SC: Seizures associated with antidepressants: a review. J Clin Psychiatry 54(8):289–299, 1993 8253696

Roth T, Rippon GA, Arora S: Armodafinil improves wakefulness and long-term episodic memory in nCPAP-adherent patients with excessive sleepiness associated with obstructive sleep apnea. Sleep Breath 12(1):53–62, 2008 17874255

Rudolph JL, Salow MJ, Angelini MC, et al: The anticholinergic risk scale and anticholinergic adverse effects in older persons. Arch Intern Med 168(5):508–513, 2008 18332297

Rugino TA, Copley TC: Effects of modafinil in children with attention-deficit/hyperactivity disorder: an open-label study. J Am Acad Child Adolesc Psychiatry 40(2):230–235, 2001 11211372

Russell WJ: The impact of Alzheimer's disease medication on muscle relaxants. Anaesth Intensive Care 37(1):134–135, 2009 19160552

Sacchetti E, Trifirò G, Caputi A, et al: Risk of stroke with typical and atypical anti-psychotics: a retrospective cohort study including unexposed subjects. J Psychopharmacol 22(1):39–46, 2008 18187531

Sachdev PS: A rating scale for neuroleptic malignant syndrome. Psychiatry Res 135(3):249–256, 2005 15996751

Sanger DJ, Zivkovic B: Differential development of tolerance to the depressant effects of benzodiazepine and non-benzodiazepine agonists at the omega (BZ) modulatory sites of GABAA receptors. Neuropharmacology 31(7):693–700, 1992 1357576

Saper RB, Phillips RS, Sehgal A, et al: Lead, mercury, and arsenic in US- and Indian-manufactured Ayurvedic medicines sold via the Internet. JAMA 300(8):915–923, 2008 18728265

Sarris J, LaPorte E, Schweitzer I: Kava: a comprehensive review of efficacy, safety, and psychopharmacology. Aust N Z J Psychiatry 45(1):27–35, 2011 21073405

Schmid MM, Freudenmann RW, Keller F, et al: Non-fatal and fatal liver failure associated with valproic acid. Pharmacopsychiatry 46(2):63–68, 2013 22915484

Schmidt D, Elger CE: What is the evidence that oxcarbazepine and carbamazepine are distinctly different antiepileptic drugs? Epilepsy Behav 5(5):627–635, 2004 15380112

Schmitt L, Tonnoir B, Arbus C: Safety and efficacy of oral escitalopram as continuation treatment of intravenous citalopram in patients with major depressive disorder. Neuropsychobiology 54(4):201–207, 2006 17337913

Schrettl V, Felgenhauer N, Rabe C, et al: L-Arginine in the treatment of valproate overdose—five clinical cases. Clin Toxicol (Phila) 55(4):260–266, 2017 28152637

Silva MA, Key S, Han E, Malloy MJ: Acute pancreatitis associated with antipsychotic medication: evaluation of clinical features, treatment, and polypharmacy in a series of cases. J Clin Psychopharmacol 36(2):169–172, 2016 26859276

Singh NP, Despars JA, Stansbury DW, et al: Effects of buspirone on anxiety levels and exercise tolerance in patients with chronic airflow obstruction and mild anxiety. Chest 103(3):800–804, 1993 8449072

Sivertsen B, Salo P, Pentti J, et al: Use of sleep medications and risk of cancer: a matched case-control study. Sleep Med 16(12):1552–1555, 2015 26116466

Slim M, Medina-Caliz I, Gonzalez-Jimenez A, et al: Hepatic safety of atypical antipsychotics: current evidence and future directions. Drug Saf 39(10):925–943, 2016 27449495

Spina E, Hiemke C, De Leon J: Assessing drug-drug interactions through therapeutic drug monitoring when administering oral second-generation antipsychotics. Expert Opin Drug Metab Toxicol 12(4):407–422, 2016 26878495

Stancer HC, Kivi R: Lithium carbonate and oedema. Lancet 2(7731):985, 1971 4107943

Staner C, Joly F, Jacquot N, et al: Sublingual zolpidem in early onset of sleep compared to oral zolpidem: polysomnographic study in patients with primary insomnia. Curr Med Res Opin 26(6):1423–1431, 2010 20397964

Sternbach H: The serotonin syndrome. Am J Psychiatry 148(6):705–713, 1991 2035713

Stewart DE: Hepatic adverse reactions associated with nefazodone. Can J Psychiatry 47(4):375–377, 2002 12025437

Storey P, Trumble M: Rectal doxepin and carbamazepine therapy in patients with cancer. N Engl J Med 327(18):1318–1319, 1992 1406828

Strawn JR, Keck PE Jr, Caroff SN: Neuroleptic malignant syndrome. Am J Psychiatry 164(6):870–876, 2007 17541044

Sun H, Palcza J, Card D, et al: Effects of suvorexant, an orexin receptor antagonist, on respirations during sleep in patients with obstructive sleep apnea. J Clin Sleep Med 12(1):9–17, 2016 26194728

Sweetman AM, Lack LC, Catcheside PG, et al: Developing a successful treatment for co-morbid insomnia and sleep apnoea. Sleep Med Rev 33:28–38, 2017 27401786

Takeda: Rozerem (ramelteon). 2016. Available at: http://www.rozerem.com. Accessed October 18, 2017.

Tamim HM, Mahmud S, Hanley JA, et al: Antidepressants and risk of prostate cancer: a nested case-control study. Prostate Cancer Prostatic Dis 11(1):53–60, 2008 17684479

Taylor D: Antidepressant drugs and cardiovascular pathology: a clinical overview of effectiveness and safety. Acta Psychiatr Scand 118(6):434–442, 2008 18785947

Tenner S: Drug induced acute pancreatitis: does it exist? World J Gastroenterol 20(44):16529–16534, 2014 25469020

Teter CJ, Phan KL, Cameron OG, et al: Relative rectal bioavailability of fluoxetine in normal volunteers. J Clin Psychopharmacol 25(1):74–78, 2005 15643102

Tharwani HM, Yerramsetty P, Mannelli P, et al: Recent advances in poststroke depression. Curr Psychiatry Rep 9(3):225–231, 2007 17521519

Thompson A, Silverman B, Dzeng L, et al: Psychotropic medications and HIV. Clin Infect Dis 42(9):1305–1310, 2006 16586391

Toh S, Rodríguez LA, Hernández-Díaz S: Use of antidepressants and risk of lung cancer. Cancer Causes Control 18(10):1055–1064, 2007 17682831

Tracy TS, Kingston RL (eds): Herbal Products, 2nd Edition. Totowa, NJ, Humana Press, 2007

U.S. Food and Drug Administration: Abilify (Aripiprazole) tablets. Application No. 21–436, drug approval package, medical review(s). Food and Drug Administration Center for Drug Evaluation and Research, November 15, 2002. March 7, 2003. Available at: https://

www.accessdata.fda.gov/drugsatfda_docs/nda/2002/21-436_Abilify.cfm. Accessed October 18, 2017.

U.S. Food and Drug Administration: FDA Drug Safety Communication: FDA warns about serious risks and death when combining opioid pain or cough medicines with benzodiazepines; requires its strongest warning. U.S. Food and Drug Administration. 2016a. Available at: http://www.fda.gov/Drugs/DrugSafety/ucm518473.htm. Accessed October 17, 2017.

U.S. Food and Drug Administration: FDA Drug Safety Communication: Revised recommendations for Celexa (citalopram hydrobromide) related to potential risk of abnormal heart rhythms with high doses. Silver Spring, MD; Food and Drug Administration. 2016b. Available at: https://www.fda.gov/Drugs/DrugSafety/ucm297391.htm. Accessed October 17, 2017.

USPDI Editorial Board (ed): U.S. Pharmacopoeia Dispensing Information, Vol 1: Drug Information for the Health Care Professional, 27th Edition. Greenwood Village, CO, Thompson Micromedex, 2007

Valeant: Zelapar (selegiline oral disintegrating tablets). 2017. Available at: http://www.zelapar.com. Accessed October 18, 2017.

Van Amelsvoort T, Bakshi R, Devaux CB, et al: Hyponatremia associated with carbamazepine and oxcarbazepine therapy: a review. Epilepsia 35(1):181–188, 1994 8112243

Vanderkooy JD, Kennedy SH, Bagby RM: Antidepressant side effects in depression patients treated in a naturalistic setting: a study of bupropion, moclobemide, paroxetine, sertraline, and venlafaxine. Can J Psychiatry 47(2):174–180, 2002 11926080

van Gorp F, Whyte IM, Isbister GK: Clinical and ECG effects of escitalopram overdose. Ann Emerg Med 54(3):404–408, 2009 19556032

van Hoogdalem E, de Boer AG, Breimer DD: Pharmacokinetics of rectal drug administration, part I: general considerations and clinical applications of centrally acting drugs. Clin Pharmacokinet 21(1):11–26, 1991a 1717195

van Hoogdalem EJ, de Boer AG, Breimer DD: Pharmacokinetics of rectal drug administration, part II: clinical applications of peripherally acting drugs, and conclusions. Clin Pharmacokinet 21(2):110–128, 1991b 1884566

van Noord C, Straus SM, Sturkenboom MC, et al: Psychotropic drugs associated with corrected QT interval prolongation. J Clin Psychopharmacol 29(1):9–15, 2009 19142100

Varela Piñón M, Adán-Manes J: Selective serotonin reuptake inhibitor-induced hyponatremia: clinical implications and therapeutic alternatives. Clin Neuropharmacol 40(4):177–179, 2017 28622213

Velligan DI, Weiden PJ, Sajatovic M, et al; Expert Consensus Panel on Adherence Problems in Serious and Persistent Mental Illness: The expert consensus guideline series: adherence problems in patients with serious and persistent mental illness. J Clin Psychiatry 70 (suppl 4):1–46, quiz 47–48, 2009 19686636

Verrotti A, Scaparrotta A, Grosso S, et al: Anticonvulsant drugs and hematological disease. Neurol Sci 35(7):983–993, 2014 24619070

Vieweg WV: Mechanisms and risks of electrocardiographic QT interval prolongation when using antipsychotic drugs. J Clin Psychiatry 63 (suppl 9):18–24, 2002 12088172

Vieweg WVR, Hasnain M, Howland RH, et al: Citalopram, QTc interval prolongation, and torsade de pointes. How should we apply the recent FDA ruling? Am J Med 125(9):859–868, 2012 22748401

Wermeling DP, Record KA, Kelly TH, et al: Pharmacokinetics and pharmacodynamics of a new intranasal midazolam formulation in healthy volunteers. Anesth Analg 103(2):344–349, 2006 16861415

Werneke U, Jamshidi F, Taylor DM, et al: Conundrums in neurology: diagnosing serotonin syndrome—a meta-analysis of cases. BMC Neurol 16:97, 2016 27406219

Wernicke J, Lledó A, Raskin J, et al: An evaluation of the cardiovascular safety profile of duloxetine: findings from 42 placebo-controlled studies. Drug Saf 30(5):437–455, 2007 17472422

Whyte IM, Dawson AH, Buckley NA: Relative toxicity of venlafaxine and selective serotonin reuptake inhibitors in overdose compared to tricyclic antidepressants. QJM 96(5):369–374, 2003 12702786

Williams AM, Park SH: Seizure associated with clozapine: incidence, etiology, and management. CNS Drugs 29(2):101–111, 2015 25537107

Wooltorton E: Hua Fo tablets tainted with sildenafil-like compound. CMAJ 166(12):1568, 2002a 12074127

Wooltorton E: Risperidone (Risperdal): increased rate of cerebrovascular events in dementia trials. CMAJ 167(11):1269–1270, 2002b 12451085

Wroblewski BA, Leary JM, Phelan AM, et al: Methylphenidate and seizure frequency in brain injured patients with seizure disorders. J Clin Psychiatry 53(3):86–89, 1992 1548250

Wu CC, Pai TY, Hsiao FY, et al: The effect of different carbapenem antibiotics (ertapenem, imipenem/cilastatin, and meropenem) on serum valproic acid concentrations. Ther Drug Monit 38(5):587–592, 2016 27322166

Wu CS, Wang SC, Chang IS, Lin KM: The association between dementia and long-term use of benzodiazepine in the elderly: nested case-control study using claims data. Am J Geriatr Psychiatry 17(7):614–620, 2009 19546656

Wu CS, Lu ML, Liao YT, et al: Ovarian cancer and antidepressants. Psychooncology 24(5):579–584, 2015 25335924

Wu Chou AI, Wang YC, Lin CL, Kao CH: Female schizophrenia patients and risk of breast cancer: a population-based cohort study. Schizophr Res 188:165–171, 2017 28108225

Zaccara G, Franciotta D, Perucca E: Idiosyncratic adverse reactions to antiepileptic drugs. Epilepsia 48(7):1223–1244, 2007 17386054

Zhang L, Li H, Li S, Zou X: Reproductive and metabolic abnormalities in women taking valproate for bipolar disorder: a meta-analysis. Eur J Obstet Gynecol Reprod Biol 202:26–31, 2016 27160812

Zhang LS, Hu XY, Yao LY, et al: Prophylactic effects of duloxetine on post-stroke depression symptoms: an open single-blind trial. Eur Neurol 69(6):336–343, 2013 23549225

Zimbroff DL: Pharmacological control of acute agitation: focus on intramuscular preparations. CNS Drugs 22(3):199–212, 2008 18278976

Zin CS, Nissen LM, Smith MT, et al: An update on the pharmacological management of postherpetic neuralgia and painful diabetic neuropathy. CNS Drugs 22(5):417–442, 2008 18399710

Zivin K, Pfeiffer PN, Bohnert AS, et al: Evaluation of the FDA warning against prescribing citalopram at doses exceeding 40 mg. Am J Psychiatry 170(6):642–650, 2013 23640689

CHAPTER 37

Psychotherapy

Elspeth Guthrie, M.B., Ch.B., FRCPsych, M.Sc., M.D.

*The heartbeat of therapy is a process of learning how to go
on becoming a person together with others. That learning
never ends.*

R.F. Hobson (1985, p. xii)

The term *psychotherapy* has a very broad meaning. At its heart, however, the term implies the intent to help another person or persons through the medium of an interpersonal professional relationship. People usually seek or are referred for therapy because they are distressed or are struggling to cope with some major life problem or difficulty. Physical illness is scary, stressful, and at times unimaginably difficult to bear. What must it be like to be told that the tremor you have developed is the first sign of Parkinson's disease or that the cough that will not go away has been confirmed as lung cancer?

This chapter focuses on the role of psychological treatments in physical illness and is divided into two parts. In the first part, psychological approaches to helping people cope with physical illness are discussed, and in the second part, evidence for the effectiveness of psychological treatments in physical illness is reviewed. In this textbook there are separate chapters on psychological treatments and pharmacotherapy (see Chapter 36, "Psychopharmacology"). The two, however, are commonly used together to good effect, particularly in people with physical illness, and it is usually helpful when considering psychological treatment to also consider the potential benefits of pharmacological interventions. These delivery approaches will be discussed in more detail later in this chapter in relation to collaborative and stepped-care models (see section "Organization and Delivery of Psychological Treatments").

Psychological Approaches to Helping People Cope With Physical Illness

Rationale for Psychological Therapies in Physical Illness

Many people find it difficult to cope or adapt to physical illness, but given time and the right environment, most manage this process without the need to seek professional help. Approximately 10% of medically ill patients require specific psychiatric treatment (Royal College of Physicians and Royal College of Psychiatrists 2003). Although certain forms of physical illness (e.g., terminal cancer) carry huge emotional burdens, people's individual perceptions of their illness have a powerful influence on how they cope with the illness and how emotionally stressful they find it. At a very basic human level, physical illness can be understood as a threat to the self (Cassel 1982), and it can "attack" the very heart of who we are as people and human beings. For example, physical illness can interfere with our ability to work, parent, make love, socialize, and take part in sports, music, and other creative activities. It can threaten our body image, our physical independence, and our ability to care for ourselves. It can undermine and destabilize us—and, of course, in its most extreme form, threaten our very existence.

Minute Particulars of the Patient's Story of Illness

Whatever the modality of therapy, the starting point for most therapies involving patients with physical illness is a detailed account of the person's own illness story. Most people "need" to tell their story, retell it and reshape it, and finally, hopefully, make peace with it. William Blake wrote, "He who would do good to another must do it in the Minute Particulars: General Good is the plea of the scoundrel, hypocrite and flatterer, for Art and Science cannot exist but in minutely organized particulars" (*Jerusalem* III, 55:60–68; Erdman 1988).

It is through the exploration of the "Minute Particulars" of the person's illness that a real sharing and understanding of the person's suffering emerges. At its best, this process can foster a deep and positive therapeutic alliance with the client, which can provide a springboard for further work involving any therapeutic modality. In itself, it can bring relief from suffering, an understanding of the self and of the experience of illness, and a sense of mastery and empowerment.

Most people with physical illness explain changes in their mood, and particularly depression, in the context of their life story (Alderson et al. 2014). They may feel a sense of responsibility to keep their feelings from affecting their family or home life, and many still regard depression as a weakness that only occurs when people "give in" to their low mood (Alderson et al. 2014). People also report problems of a more general or personal nature, such as existential ideas about themselves, stigma related to depression, self-blame, and suicidal ideas (Alderson et al. 2012).

Necessary Adaptations

Participation in any form of meaningful psychotherapy requires an individual to be able to concentrate during the therapy and to recall and think about the therapy between sessions. In structured therapies, there is an explicit expectation that homework will be carried out between sessions. However, physical illness may prevent some people from participating in psychological treatments because they are too physically unwell. It is hard to concentrate in therapy if one is nauseated or exhausted or in pain. It may also be physically difficult for some people to attend psychotherapy sessions because of problems with mobility or transport. Sessions may have to be rescheduled or fitted around other medical commitments (e.g., chemotherapy, renal dialysis). The duration of sessions may have to be modified or breaks in therapy accommodated because of relapses in the person's illness or participation in challenging treatment regimens.

It is often appropriate for the therapist to involve other members of the patient's family in the therapeutic process, particularly if they have a role as a care provider. It may also be important for the therapist to liaise with other members of the health care team and to spend time with the patient discussing relationships with nursing, medical, and other professional staff.

Therapists who work in medical settings need to have an understanding of the illnesses the patients they see are suffering from and the kinds of investigations and treatment that patients are likely to experience. This will involve spending time in medical settings.

Three broad approaches will be described in this chapter: 1) basic supportive techniques and problem solving, 2) relational therapies, and 3) cognitive-behavioral therapies. As cognitive therapy continues to develop, and to incorporate many aspects of other treatment approaches into newer cognitive-behavioral therapy (CBT) treatments, the differences between therapies are becoming less distinct.

Supportive and Problem-Solving Approaches

Health care professionals play a key role in helping people adjust to illness and may prevent the development of long-term distress by a sensitive and judicious approach. This should involve establishing a trusting relationship with the patient based on warmth and a genuine desire to help. Fear and uncertainty can be reduced by providing individuals with clear information. This may need to be repeated on several occasions, and it is important to convey the right amount of information so that individuals are not overwhelmed. The information should be presented in an authoritative but jargon-free manner. There should be a continual process of checking out what the person knows and doesn't know and what they want to know. The health professional should be guided by the person's responses and tailor the information accordingly. The health professional should be optimistic but realistic and avoid false reassurance. Positive reassurance can be very helpful but must be based on and grow out of the physician's understanding of the patient's anxiety.

There should be a collaborative approach to treatment so that patients themselves can make most of the decisions about their treatment. However, sometimes patients want doctors to play a more active, authoritative role in decision making, as was found in women attending clinics for breast cancer (Wright et al. 2004). This emphasizes the need to find out what different people want and tailor responses accordingly.

If possible, patients should be given emotional space to voice their fears and uncertainties about their illness or reflect on loss and explore ways of coping. This is rarely possible in busy hospital clinics or ward settings, but it should be an ideal to which all health professionals aspire. Any opportunity to foster beliefs in the controllability of the disease process will help the patient feel more empowered and less vulnerable. Involvement of patients' families in the treatment process is crucial, as illness affects the whole family and not just the individual with the illness. The spiritual and cultural dimensions of peoples' lives are often overlooked by busy health professionals. Many religious organizations offer support and help for people at times of adversity, and other forms of cultural support may be available for certain groups of patients (e.g., gay men who are HIV positive).

Counseling

There are many different forms of counseling, ranging from the imparting of information (educational counseling) to quite intensive psychotherapeutic interventions. One of the most common forms of therapeutic counseling is *person-centered counseling*. This is nondirective counseling in which emphasis is placed on the development of a personal relationship in which an individual can talk openly and freely about his or her problems. The counselor employs specific skills, such as warmth, empathy, and attentive listening. Counseling involves skilled use of nonspecific psychotherapeutic techniques.

Counseling is widely employed in health service settings to help people adjust better to illness. There are relatively few controlled evaluations of the benefits of counseling in relation to physical illness. An exception is in the field of cancer, where there have been several evaluations by different research groups of the effects of counseling (Christensen 1983; Hersch et al. 2009; Maguire et al. 1980, 1983). A systematic review of psychosocial interventions for anxiety and depression in adult cancer patients concluded that interventions involving counseling can be currently recommended for improving patients' general functional ability or quality of life, degree of depression, and interpersonal relationships (Jacobsen and Jim 2008). However, the review noted the general poor methodological quality of many studies.

Hypnosis

Hypnosis has been used as a treatment for medical conditions for more than 300 years. It involves the induction of a state of mind in which a person's normal critical nature is bypassed, allowing for acceptance of suggestions. Hypnotherapy involves the induction of a hypnotic trance using progressive relaxation and other induction procedures to deepen the hypnotic state. This is followed by suggestions, imagery, and other individualized techniques directed toward control and improvement of bodily function or pain. Patients are given one-to-one treatment over several weeks and are also asked to practice skills on a daily basis by using an autohypnosis recording. This kind of treatment can also be delivered in a group format. The role of hypnosis in medicine has been reviewed by Stewart (2005). The best evidence for hypnotherapy in the field of consultation-liaison psychiatry comes from work in relation to irritable bowel syndrome (Schaefert et al. 2014) and fibromyalgia (Bernardy et al. 2011).

Problem-Solving Therapy

Problem-solving therapy improves individuals' abilities to cope with stressful life difficulties. It has three main steps: 1) symptoms and problems are identified, and the two are linked together; 2) the problems are defined and clarified; and 3) strategies are developed in a collaborative fashion with the patient to help solve the problems in a systematic way. The overall intention is to break problems down into very small components that then become easier to tackle and solve. Problem solving has been employed in a pure form to treat depression or other problems in primary care. It is a relatively brief intervention, with one of the earliest studies involving six sessions and a total contact time of less than 4 hours (Hawton and Kirk 1989).

Problem-solving therapy has been used to help patients with cancer (Nezu et al. 2003) and has also been incorporated into more complex treatment interventions involving stepped-care models for treating depression and collaborative care models for treating people with depression and chronic physical illness.

Supportive–Expressive Group Therapy and Support Groups

A variety of supportive group therapies have been investigated in medically ill patients, with most studies involving cancer patients. Early studies demonstrated emotional benefits and pain reduction, and some found apparent enhanced survival (e.g., Spiegel et al. 1989). The survival claims were controversial and were ultimately not replicated. More recent studies have not found evidence that supportive group therapies reduce distress or prolong survival (Classen et al. 2008; Ho et al. 2016).

The group approaches that have received the most attention are those employing *supportive–expressive group therapy,* which is an unstructured but quite intensive and existentially based treatment (Spiegel and Glafkides 1983). The rationale for the existential orientation presumes that living with a terminal illness amplifies existential concerns of death, meaning, freedom, and isolation. The treatment strategy is to facilitate discussion of issues that are uppermost in patients' minds rather than imposing the topics to be discussed.

Relational Therapies

A broad group of therapies have in common a model of human development and the mind in which the nature and quality of human interpersonal relationships play a key role in the maintenance of "emotional homeostasis." Close interpersonal relationships can either be a source of stress or act as a buffer against adversity to provide emotional support and foster resilience. Relational therapies are based on the premise that feelings, thoughts, and relationships are intimately tied up with each other. How we feel and think about others affects how we behave toward them, and this, in turn, affects how we feel about ourselves.

A variety of different theories and models of development, including psychodynamic, attachment, and interpersonal, link together previous relationship experiences, current relationship experiences, and emotions and coping. Individuals with a history of childhood adversity have an increased likelihood of both emotional and physical problems as adults. People with certain kinds of insecure attachment styles find physical illness more difficult to manage than those with secure attachment and may default on medical appointments or find it more difficult to establish trusting relationships with health professionals (Ciechanowski et al. 2004).

Physical illness is a threat to the self, and nearly all aspects of being physically ill impact the interpersonal domain. At a very deep level, some people construe their illness as a personal attack on themselves, asking, "Why me?" At other levels, physical illness can put an immense strain on families and their relationships. Severe or chronic physical illness often changes people and forces them to reappraise themselves and their relationships. Issues of loss—for example, fears of loss or dying, fears of becoming dependent and a burden on others, fears of having to cope alone—are extremely common in the physically ill and can be addressed by relational therapies (see also Chapter 3, "Psychological Responses to Illness").

Interpersonal Therapy

Interpersonal therapy (IPT) was originally developed as a time-limited treatment for depression (Klerman et al. 1984), based on the assumption that there is a relationship between the onset and recurrence of a depressive episode and a person's social and interpersonal relationships at the time.

There are three stages in IPT when it is used to treat depression. In the first phase, an interpersonal inventory is compiled of the patient's relationships, and the main interpersonal problem areas are identified, classified into four groups: grief, role transitions, role disputes, and interpersonal deficits. During the intermediate sessions of therapy, the therapist and client try to modify these problematic interactions using a variety of techniques, including role-play. In the final phase, the therapist works to consolidate the client's gains and addresses the termination of therapy, with a focus on strategies that can prevent the depression from recurring.

Several elements of IPT are highly relevant to the general medical setting and to patients who have emotional difficulties secondary to physical illness. In particular, grief (e.g., loss of a body part) and role transition (e.g., having to change from being an active and healthy person to someone who is confined to a wheelchair) are extremely common problem areas. IPT has been used to good effect to treat depression in HIV-positive patients (Markowitz et al. 1995), and it has also been adapted for the treatment of posttraumatic stress disorder, which is common in some medical settings. IPT has also been adapted for use in hypochondriasis, focusing on the interpersonal consequences of being preoccupied with physical illness (Stuart and Noyes 2005).

Psychodynamic Interpersonal Therapy ("Conversational Model" Therapy)

Psychodynamic interpersonal therapy (PIT) combines elements of psychodynamic and interpersonal therapies. It places greater emphasis on the patient–therapist relationship as a tool for resolving interpersonal issues than does IPT, and there is less emphasis on the interpretation of transference than in psychodynamic therapies. One of the central tenets of PIT is the importance of human experience and an individual's sense of self within a personal relationship. Human existence is regarded as being essentially relational, and man is regarded as a "creature of the between." This applies even to people who live a solitary existence.

The emphasis in the therapy is on getting to know someone, rather than merely knowing *about* them. In the words of Hobson (1985, p. xiii), "In an unrepeatable moment, I hope to respond to my unique client by sharing in an ongoing act of creation, expressing and shaping immediate experience in the making and remaking of a verbal and nonverbal language of feeling." This form of therapy, in addition to specific ingredients, targets the therapeutic bond between client and therapist and the expectations of the client. It places these two areas under the microscope, getting them right, before moving on to any other aspect of the treatment process.

The client and therapist begin by exploring the minute particulars of the client's physical symptom experience. The client is encouraged to explore and describe his or her physical symptoms in great depth, and the therapist assumes an attitude of intense listening, concern, and fascination. It is in the detail of the conversation that metaphors or feeling language emerges, as the client and therapist go deeper and deeper into the client's physical experience. Expressions such as "off balance," which used to describe neurological symptoms, come to also represent psychological and emotional states of mind. The process is collaborative, gradual, and nonthreatening. The conversation gradually moves from being about physical symptoms to what Hobson (1985) described as a "feeling language." This process of symbolic transformation leads to a change in the experience of the self and a move toward a greater understanding of the connection between physical and psychological, followed by psychological and emotional change.

Key features of the model include 1) the assumption that the patient's problems arise from or are exacerbated by disturbances of significant personal relationships; 2) a tentative, encouraging, supportive approach from the therapist, who seeks to develop a deeper understanding with the patient through negotiation, exploration of feelings, and use of metaphor; 3) the linkage of the patient's distress to specific interpersonal problems; and 4) the use of the therapeutic relationship to address problems and test out solutions in the "here and now."

PIT has efficacy comparable to that of cognitive therapy for the treatment of depression (Shapiro et al. 1994) and has been adapted for use in medically unexplained symptoms. PIT has been evaluated in several large randomized controlled trials (RCTs) (Creed et al. 2003; Guthrie et al. 1991; Hamilton et al. 2000; Sattel et al. 2012). It is cost effective, with the costs of therapy being recouped by reductions in health care use in the months posttherapy (Creed et al. 2003; Guthrie et al. 1999). It has also been used after self-harm and was found to result in a reduction in repetition in the subsequent 6 months following the index episode (Guthrie et al. 2001), and more recently for motor conversion disorder (Hubschmid et al. 2015).

Cognitive-Behavioral Therapy

The central tenet of CBT is that emotions, behavior, and cognitions are all interlinked. According to the cognitive model, distressing emotions such as anxiety or depression are linked to particular beliefs, assumptions, or thoughts. It is assumed that persistent distress is linked to underlying maladaptive beliefs, and that modification of these beliefs and cognitions will result in reductions in emotional distress.

In the general medical setting, the way a person thinks about his or her illness or bodily sensations is central to the cognitive model. If, for example, benign sensations are regarded as being symptomatic of disease, several consequences ensue. First, the patient will become emotionally distressed, which may cause further bodily sensations. Second, the patient will pay increased attention to these symptoms and may worry about them more. Third, the types of behaviors the patient employs to cope with the symptoms may exacerbate the symptoms rather than relieve them (e.g., rubbing one's chest if it is painful). Fourth, other people, including doctors, may respond to the patient in a way that intensifies, rather than reduces, the patient's concern with disease, attention to bodily sensations, and dysfunctional coping (Sharpe et al. 1992).

This model is applicable to patients with medically unexplained symptoms, but also to patients with medical disease (e.g., concerns about recurrence of a breast lump after previous diagnosis and treatment for breast cancer).

Sensky (2004) has described in detail how CBT has been adapted for use in people with physical illnesses. Crucial to the development of any treatment intervention is an understanding of the patient's model of his or her illness, and a useful model or framework for doing this has been developed by Moss-Morris et al. (2002) in relation to illness perception. This concept was originally developed by Leventhal et al. (1997). Within Leventhal and colleagues' model, illness representations are considered to be multidimensional, comprising five main components: identity, perceived consequences, timeline, perceived cause, and control/cure (Table 37–1).

A key principle in cognitive therapy is that the patient, rather than the therapist, is the expert in understanding the patient's problems. A detailed understanding of the patient's illness perceptions often leads to identification of maladaptive beliefs and underlying fears or anxieties, which can then be addressed.

CBT is tailored to the individual patient's beliefs and behavior, although certain cognitions are likely to be associated with particular presenting symptoms. For example, it is common for patients who experience chest pain to fear that they are going to have a heart attack, and they will become very anxious every time chest pain is experienced.

If someone believes that his chest pain is indicative of a heart attack and repeatedly seeks reassurance every time chest pain is experienced, that reassurance is characteristically short-lived, and the behavior becomes counterproductive. The therapist can address this kind of behavior in the therapy session, particularly if the client develops pain or seeks reassurance from the therapist during the session itself. The therapist can ask the patient to keep a diary between sessions, quantifying at various times the extent of his worry and/or reassurance on a 0–10 scale. Having identified that the behavior is unhelpful and only increases anxiety and worry, patient and therapist can then collaborate to devise ways of managing the problem behavior and beliefs more effectively.

This is done by devising behavioral and/or cognitive experiments aiming to produce more favorable outcomes. In the above example, a behavioral experiment might be for the patient to delay seeking reassurance about his chest pain for progressively longer periods, to demonstrate that he is able to tolerate the anxiety involved. A cognitive task might be to prepare a statement (and perhaps even to write it down on a "cue card") regarding the unhelpful outcomes of reassurance seeking that the patient can remind himself about when he experiences the urge to seek reassurance. Each of these tasks might be rehearsed in the therapy session, so that the patient has some confidence that the possible benefits of carrying out the tasks between sessions outweigh the perceived risks.

Other cognitive factors in the assessment of the physically ill have been described by Guthrie and Sensky (2008) and are summarized in Table 37–2.

CBT is a recognized treatment for many different psychiatric disorders (Butler et al. 2006). There is a substantial evidence base for CBT, both for the treatment of medically unexplained symptoms and for the treatment of depression in physical illness (Fekete et al. 2007). Both will be reviewed later in this chapter.

TABLE 37–1. Leventhal and colleagues' five components of illness representations

Identity: Label or name given to the condition and the symptoms that go with it.

Cause: Ideas about the perceived cause of the condition (may or may not be based on biomedical evidence).

Timeline: Predictive beliefs about how long the condition will last.

Consequences: Individual beliefs about the consequences of the condition and how these affect people physically and socially.

Curability/controllability: Beliefs about whether the condition can be cured or kept under control.

Source. Leventhal et al. 1997.

TABLE 37–2. Cognitive factors in the assessment of the physically ill

Illness model and illness perception: What is the patient's understanding of his/her illness, and how does this contribute to worry or distress, or to maladaptive behaviors and beliefs?

Personalized formulation of the patient's problem: How can the patient's physical symptoms, emotional response, behavior, and cognitions be linked together in an understandable and meaningful formulation?

Affective disturbance: Is the patient experiencing anxiety, fears, depression, or hopelessness?

Motivation: Prochaska's stages of change model (Prochaska et al. 1994):

Precontemplation—Is the patient avoiding thinking about the consequences of illness?

Contemplation—Is the patient beginning to face the fact that changes have to be made to adapt to the impact of the illness?

Preparation—Is the patient taking steps necessary for action?

Action—Is the patient making the required changes?

Maintenance—Are the changes/adaptations being maintained?

Coping: What are the patient's emotion-focused and problem-focused ways of coping? Which of these are helpful? Which are not helpful?

Life transitions: How is the individual managing the impact of illness on his or her life, and what can be learned from the way he/she has managed previous life transitions?

Influence of others: How are the patient's relationships with doctors and other professionals, family, and friends influenced by the patient's beliefs about his/her illness? Conversely, how do the patient's illness beliefs influence his or her relationships with others?

Resilience: What are the patient's areas of vulnerability in regard to his or her responses to stress? What are the patient's strengths?

Source. Adapted from Guthrie and Sensky 2008.

Mindfulness-Based Stress Reduction Interventions

Mindfulness-based stress reduction (MBSR) is a well-defined systematic, educational, patient-focused intervention that provides formal training in mindfulness meditation and its applications in everyday life, including self-management of physical and emotional pain. MBSR has grown rapidly in the medical setting, and MBSR programs are now offered in health care settings around the world. A useful review of its practice in the medical setting has been written by Ott et al. (2006). MBSR programs generally consist of 7–10 weekly group sessions. Each session lasts 1–1.5 hours, and in addition there is one silent retreat. Classes include both an educational component and an experiential component. During the groups, participants are taught meditation fundamentals and practice sitting meditation, awareness of sensations, body scan, and mindfulness movement, which they are expected to practice for 45 minutes on a daily basis.

Bringing attention to the senses is generally unthreatening and easy to experience. Patients are also asked to focus on their breathing during sitting meditation. They may become aware that they are not breathing fully, but rather are limiting inspiration to the upper part of the chest, losing the benefit of abdominal breathing. As patients continue to focus on breathing, the breath becomes a familiar focal point, and they are then able to move on and focus on other physical sensations. Even strong physical sensations such as pain can become less intense and less frightening through use of MBSR.

The body scan enables patients to develop a focused concentrated awareness of the body, moving attention methodically from the toes to the head. Patients become aware of subtle changes that are happening on a moment-to-moment basis, and unpleasant sensations become more tolerable. Mindfulness movement invites a compassionate, ongoing awareness of the body in motion (Ott et al. 2006).

Mindfulness-Based Cognitive Therapy

Mindfulness-based cognitive therapy (MBCT) has been adapted from mindfulness stress reduction approaches as a treatment for depression (Segal et al. 2002). It includes simple breathing meditations and yoga stretches to help participants become more aware of the present moment, including getting in touch with moment-to-moment changes in the mind and the body. MBCT also includes basic education about depression and several exercises from cognitive therapy that show the links between thinking and feeling and demonstrate how people can look after themselves when depression threatens to overwhelm them.

Numerous systematic reviews have examined mindfulness interventions for physical health problems, including stress from medical illness (Arias et al. 2006); cancer (Cramer et al. 2012b; Ledesma and Kumano 2009; Ott et al. 2006; J.E. Smith et al. 2005); chronic medical disease (Bohlmeijer et al. 2010); chronic pain (Chiesa and Serretti 2011); low back pain (Cramer et al. 2012a); fibromyalgia (Lauche et al. 2013); and multiple sclerosis (Simpson et al. 2014). Most reviews have reported promising results but note that further studies are needed before firm conclusions can be drawn. Acceptance-based therapies, which also employ mindfulness, have been developed (Ost 2014), and their beneficial effects for pain may be equivalent to those of CBT (Veehof et al. 2011).

Organization and Delivery of Psychological Treatments

Although psychological treatments can be offered as stand-alone treatments, they are increasingly delivered as part of a package of care or part of a stepped-care model. This delivery approach is widely used in the treatment of depressive disorders but is applicable to interventions for many other psychological conditions, including medically unexplained symptoms and depression in the context of chronic physical illness.

The stepped-care model involves five different intensities of treatment that are offered to the patient or client according to the severity or complexity of his or her problems. Most patients start at the bottom of this model and progress to the next step only if their symptoms do not improve:

- Step 1 involves watchful waiting, because many patients who present with symptoms will find that these resolve spontaneously without requiring any help.
- Step 2 usually involves some form of guided self-help and may include computerized CBT, psychoeducation, or help from volunteer organizations. Exercise may also be prescribed.
- Step 3 involves brief psychological therapy (e.g., CBT, counseling, interpersonal therapies) for six to eight sessions. Antidepressants may be prescribed if there is a previous history of moderate to severe depression.
- Step 4 involves depression case management, and the patient may be assigned a case manager or key worker. Medication and more intensive psychological treatments may be offered, with care coordinated by the case manager working with the patient's primary care physician.
- Step 5 is for patients who have not responded to the previous four steps. Step 5 may involve crisis intervention services, inpatient treatment, or even more intensive multicomponent treatment.

Collaborative care models have five essential elements:

1. Collaborative definition of problems, in which patient-defined problems are identified alongside medical problems diagnosed by health care professionals
2. Focus on specific problems and use of problem-solving techniques
3. Creation of a range of self-management training and support services
4. Provision of active follow-up in which patients are contacted at regular intervals to monitor health status and check and reinforce progress in implementing the care plan
5. Assignment of a case manager who has responsibility for delivering the care plan

Sometimes stepped-care programs are incorporated into collaborative care interventions, as in the Pathways Study (Katon et al. 2004), which tested a complex intervention to treat depression in patients with diabetes. The intervention involved an initial choice of two treatments, either an antidepressant or problem-solving therapy, followed by a stepped-care algorithm in which patients received different types and intensities of treatment according to their observed outcomes. In comparison with those receiving usual care, patients who received the complex intervention showed significant improvements in depression, but there was no impact on glycemic control. However, a later study by Katon et al. (2010) did show widespread positive effects from collaborative care on both physical and mental health outcomes, including diabetic control, in patients with diabetes and coronary heart disease. Coventry et al. (2015) likewise demonstrated positive effects from collaborative care in people with diabetes or cardiovascular disease in a U.K. population, and this approach has also shown benefit in depressed patients with cancer (Dwight-Johnson et al. 2005; Ell et al. 2008) and older patients with arthritis (Lin et al. 2003).

Evidence Base for Psychological Treatments for Specific Conditions

Patients With Medically Unexplained Symptoms or Somatic Symptom and Related Disorders

There is a substantial evidence base for the efficacy and effectiveness of psychological treatments for people with medically unexplained symptoms (or persistent physical symptoms). Most studies have involved patients with specific symptom-defined syndromes, such as chronic fatigue syndrome and irritable bowel syndrome. It remains unclear whether these conditions are discrete entities (Hamilton et al. 2009) or share a common underlying problem of bodily symptom distress (Fink et al. 2007). There is, however, substantial overlap among the conditions, and psychological approaches that are shown to be helpful for one condition are likely to benefit patients who present with different symptoms but similar concerns.

Psychosocial factors such as depression, anxiety, childhood adversity, stressful life events, and chronic difficulties are common in people who have medically unexplained symptoms that are persistent and severe and who seek treatment. Psychological morbidity is less prevalent in community subjects with medically unexplained symptoms who do not seek treatment. Most studies that have evaluated the efficacy or effectiveness of psychological interventions in patients with medically unexplained symptoms have been carried out on patients in secondary- or tertiary-care settings who have moderate to severe symptoms. There are far fewer primary care–based studies, and these tend to show less substantial treatment effects than studies conducted in secondary-care settings (Raine et al. 2002). A systematic review of the efficacy of treatment (pharmacological and nonpharmacological) for fibromyalgia concluded that there was little difference in treatment effects according to whether patients were treated in primary or secondary care (Garcia-Campayo et al. 2008).

Tables 37–3 and 37–4 summarize the findings of systematic or critical reviews of psychological treatment for two common functional somatic syndromes: chronic fatigue syndrome and irritable bowel syndrome. The strongest evidence for the efficacy of psychological interventions is in these two conditions, and they can be used as exemplars for other functional disorders. The majority of studies have focused on CBT interventions.

Fibromyalgia

Psychological treatment of fibromyalgia is reviewed in Chapter 25 ("Chronic Fatigue and Fibromyalgia Syndromes").

Chronic Fatigue Syndrome

As the number and quality of RCTs have increased over the years, the general effect sizes for CBT in CFS have fallen, with small to moderate effect sizes reported by the more recent reviews (Castell et al. 2011; Marques et al. 2015). In a study comparing treatments with and without cognitive elements, Malouff et al. (2008) found no evidence that including cognitive components led to greater effects. In fact, a trend was

TABLE 37–3. Systematic reviews, critical reviews, and meta-analyses of trials of psychological treatment in chronic fatigue syndrome (CFS)

Authors	Therapy	Type of review	Outcome
Whiting et al. 2001	Pharmacological and nonpharmacological	Systematic review (36 RCTs, 8 controlled trials)	Mixed results in terms of effectiveness; promising results shown for CBT and GET
Looper and Kirmayer 2002	CBT	Critical review (4 studies)	Positive outcomes in most studies
Rimes and Chalder 2005	Pharmacological and nonpharmacological	Systematic review	Most promising results shown for CBT and GET
Chambers et al. 2006	Pharmacological and nonpharmacological	Systematic review (70 studies)	Promising results shown for some behavioral interventions in reducing symptoms of CFS/ME and improving physical functioning
Malouff et al. 2008	CBT	Meta-analysis (13 RCTs)	Significant difference (Cohen's $d = 0.48$) in posttreatment fatigue favoring CBT over control conditions
Price et al. 2008	CBT	Meta-analysis (15 RCTs)	Posttreatment results favored CBT over usual care (SMD: –0.39; 95% CI: –0.60 to –0.19) and over other interventions (e.g., relaxation) (SMD: –0.43; 95% CI: –0.65 to –0.20); follow-up effects inconsistent
Castell et al. 2011	CBT and GET	Meta-analysis (16 RCTs CBT; 5 RCTs GET)	Equal efficacy for GET and CBT, but small effect sizes (Hedge's $g = 0.28$ for GET and 0.33 for CBT)
Marques et al. 2015	Behavioral interventions with graded physical activity component	Meta-analysis (16 RCTs)	Significant small to medium effect sizes (Hedge's $g = 0.25$ to 0.66) found for all outcomes posttreatment and at follow-up, except for physical activity ($g = 0.11$)

Note. CBT = cognitive-behavioral therapy; CI = confidence interval; ME = myalgic encephalomyelitis; RCT = randomized controlled trial; GET = graded exercise therapy; SMD = standardized mean difference.

TABLE 37–4. Systematic reviews, critical reviews, and meta-analyses of trials of psychological treatment in irritable bowel syndrome (IBS)

Authors	Therapy	Type of review	Outcome
Lackner et al. 2004	Psychological treatment	Systematic review and meta-analysis (17 RCTs)	Effectiveness of psychological treatments for IBS (NNT = 2)
Blanchard 2005	CBT	Critical review	Good evidence for efficacy of CBT interventions in the short term; long-term outcome rarely evaluated
Wilson et al. 2006	Hypnotherapy	Systematic review (6 controlled/RCT, 12 uncontrolled)	Suggestive evidence of significant benefit
Ford et al. 2009	Antidepressants and psychological therapies	Systematic review and meta-analysis (32 RCTs)	Effectiveness of antidepressants in treatment of IBS; less high-quality evidence for psychological therapies, although they may be of comparable efficacy
Ford et al. 2014	Antidepressants and psychological therapies	Systematic review and meta-analysis (48 RCTs; 32 RCTs involving psychological treatment)	Effectiveness of antidepressants and psychological therapies (CBT, hypnotherapy, multicomponent therapy, and dynamic therapy) in treatment of IBS

Note.   CBT = cognitive-behavioral therapy; NNT = number needed to treat; RCT = randomized controlled trial.

observed in favor of *not* including cognitive components. Graded exercise therapy, which can be delivered by either less-experienced or highly trained therapists, appears to have efficacy almost equivalent to that of CBT (see Chapter 25 for a more detailed discussion).

Irritable Bowel Syndrome

The most recent systematic review of treatment interventions for irritable bowel syndrome included an evaluation of the efficacy of antidepressants and psychological therapies (Ford et al. 2014). Thirty-two studies included in the review involved evaluations of psychological treatment. The reviewers calculated the relative risk (RR) of remaining symptomatic after treatment. The RR of symptoms not improving with psychological therapies was 0.68 (95% confidence interval [CI]: 0.61 to 0.76), and the benefits were small to moderate. CBT, hypnotherapy, multicomponent therapy, and psychodynamic interpersonal therapy were all beneficial. See Chapter 19, "Gastrointestinal Disorders," for a more detailed discussion.

Medically Unexplained Symptoms

There have been several reviews of psychological interventions for people with medically unexplained symptoms. The most recent reviews are those by Kleinstäuber et al. (2011) and van Dessel et al. (2014). The two groups came to similar conclusions that there was evidence of efficacy for improvement in physical symptoms, but these effects were of small to moderate size. The effects on depression were significant but small. As a specific treatment, CBT was the only intervention to have been studied adequately, and effect sizes were generally small, but with substantial differences in effects between studies.

Psychological Treatment of Depression in Physical Illness

A growing evidence base supports the treatment of depression in physical illness using either psychological interventions (alone or as part of a package of collaborative care) or some other form of complex intervention. Beltman et al. (2010) systematically reviewed CBT for the treatment of depression in patients with physical disease. Twenty-nine studies met inclusion criteria. The investigators found that CBT was superior to control conditions, with larger effect sizes found in studies restricted to participants with depressive disorder (standardized mean difference [SMD]: –0.83; 95% CI: –1.36 to –0.31; $P<0.001$) than in studies of participants with depressive symptoms (SMD: –0.16; 95% CI: –0.27 to –0.06; $P=0.001$). A subgroup analysis showed that CBT was not superior to other psychotherapies.

Many studies have been published in the last 5–10 years that provide support for the efficacy and effectiveness of psychological interventions for the treatment of depression in physical disease. Three of the most common chronic physical diseases will be taken as exemplars: diabetes, coronary heart disease, and chronic obstructive pulmonary disease (COPD). It must be remembered that chronic physical disease rarely occurs in isolation and that many people with a long-term physical illness have multiple comorbid conditions, although most research studies focus on one individual condition. Studies in the field of cancer are also discussed in the next section, because of the large numbers of trials in this area.

Diabetes

van der Feltz-Cornelis et al. (2010) carried out a systematic review and meta-analysis of 14 RCTs (involving a total of 1,724 patients) to determine the effectiveness of antidepressant therapies, including psychological treatments, in type 1 and type 2 diabetes mellitus. These researchers reported an effect size of –0.581 (95% CI: –0.770 to –0.391; $n=310$) for psychological treatments in reducing depressive symptoms, which was slightly higher than the effect size for combination treatment or for pharmacological treatment alone. There was no evidence, however, that treatments that improved depression had any impact on glycemic control. Baumeister et al. (2014) included seven trials in their meta-analysis of the effects of psychological treatment for depression. They concluded that psychological treatment resulted in moderate improvements in mood in the medium and long term, but only three studies were included in the longer-term analysis. Like van der Feltz-Cornelis et al. (2010), Baumeister et al. (2014) did not find evidence that psychological interventions had a positive effect on glycemic control.

Coronary Heart Disease

Dickens et al. (2013), in a systematic review, sought to determine which characteristics of psychological interventions led to improvement in depression among individuals with CHD. They identified 64 independent treatment comparisons. The overall treatment effects were small (SMD=0.18, $P<.001$), and no individual treatment component significantly improved depression. Problem solving (SMD=0.34), general education (SMD=0.19), skills training (SMD=0.25), CBT (SMD=0.23), and relaxation techniques (SMD=0.15) each had small effects in studies in which CHD patients were recruited irrespective of their depression status. In some studies, it was hypothesized that patients may benefit from psychological treatment approaches even if they are not depressed.

Chronic Obstructive Pulmonary Disease

Coventry et al. (2013) conducted a systematic review of psychological and/or lifestyle interventions for adults with COPD. In their review of 29 RCTs, which involved 30 independent comparisons of treatment ($N=2,063$), Coventry and colleagues found that the interventions were associated with small reductions in symptoms of depression (SMD: 0 to 0.28; 95% CI: –0.41 to –0.14) and anxiety (SMD: –0.23; 95% CI: –0.38 to –0.09). Multicomponent exercise training was the only intervention with significant treatment effects for depression (SMD: –0.47; 95% CI: –0.66 to –0.28) and for anxiety (SMD: –0.45; 95% CI: –0.71 to –0.18).

Two further reviews have reported small but positive effects for CBT interventions, but both commented on the poor quality of studies, with potential for bias (Farver-Vestergaard et al. 2015; S.M. Smith et al. 2014).

Summary

Findings from the reviews in the three chronic diseases discussed above were remarkably similar and suggest that psychological treatments have small but significant beneficial effects on depression in chronic physical illness. There is no evidence to support any specific form of psychological treatment, and it is not uncommon for therapies to be given in combination with either pharmacotherapy or other self-management strategies. There is little evidence that psychological treatments have significant impacts on the underlying disease states.

Psychological Therapies for Patients With Cancer

Psychosocial care is now recognized as an essential component of comprehensive cancer care. A wide range of therapies have been evaluated, including behavioral therapy, cognitive therapy, CBT, communication skills training, counseling, family therapy/counseling, guided imagery, mindfulness therapy, music therapy, problem-solving therapy, psychotherapy, stress management training, support groups, and supportive–expressive group therapy (Jacobsen and Jim 2008).

Many systematic reviews published over the past 30 years have evaluated the evidence supporting the benefits of psychosocial treatments for anxiety and depression in patients with cancer, as well as for other outcomes, including quality of life, emotional well-being, and survival.

Jacobsen and Jim (2008) carried out a "review of reviews" summarizing findings from 14 previous systematic reviews that had evaluated psychosocial interventions. These authors reported that nine of the reviews reached positive conclusions, with the best evidence for behavioral therapy and counseling/psychotherapy. However, they also identified a number of limitations and inconsistencies in the evidence base that have important clinical implications.

More recent systematic reviews of psychosocial therapies in the treatment of cancer are summarized in Table 37–5. Most, but not all, point to small but significant effects on mood or psychological well-being.

Internet-Based Psychological Treatments

In recent years, Internet-based psychological treatments have been developed for somatic symptom and related disorders, and the results have been encouraging. In contrast to face-to-face therapies, it is more difficult with Internet-based approaches to determine the representativeness of patient groups, but the advantage of Internet-based interventions is that they can reach a wider population and are relatively inexpensive to deliver. Relatively few studies have compared Internet-based approaches with face-to-face treatment; however, a systematic review by Andersson et al. (2014; 13 studies) found equivalent effects for the two approaches.

Cuijpers et al. (2008) conducted a systematic review of 12 studies of Internet-based therapies. Eleven involved comparison with a control condition, and one evaluated two different Internet-based therapies. The physical conditions were quite diverse, including headache, tinnitus, chronic pain, back pain, breast cancer, diabetes, and physical disability with accompanying loneliness ("people with physical disability who feel lonely"). The reviewers found that the effects of the interventions that targeted pain were comparable to those of face-to-face treatments, with less robust evidence for the other conditions.

Webb et al. (2010) reviewed the evidence for Internet-based interventions that are aimed to bring about positive changes in health behavior. The review, which included 85 studies and a total of 43,236 participants, found small but significant effects on health-related behavior ($d=0.16$; 95% CI: 0.09 to 0.23). The reviewers concluded that

TABLE 37–5. Systematic reviews and meta-analyses of psychosocial interventions for anxiety or depression in adults with cancer

Authors	Intervention	Number of RCTs	Total number of participants included	Main findings
Galway et al. 2012	Psychosocial interventions to improve quality of life and emotional well-being (recently diagnosed patients)	30	—	No significant effects on quality of life. General psychological distress improved in eight studies (SMD: –0.81; 95% CI: –1.44 to –0.18). Significant variation across participants and interventions suggests findings should be treated with caution.
Mustafa et al. 2013	Psychological interventions (metastatic breast cancer)	10	1,378 women	Most were group interventions. Overall effect favored intervention on 1-year survival (odds ratio: 1.46; 95% CI: 1.07 to 1.99). Positive effect on short-term outcomes for psychological symptoms. No evidence of long-term effects on survival.
Semple et al. 2013	Psychosocial interventions (head and neck cancer)	7	542 adults	No evidence that psychosocial interventions improve quality of life or depression in this group of patients. Conclusions limited by heterogeneity of studies and small evidence base.
Parahoo et al. 2013	Psychosocial interventions (prostate cancer)	19	3,204 men	Psychosocial interventions had small but significant positive effects on quality of life at end of treatment but not long term.
Jassim et al. 2015	Psychological interventions (nonmetastatic breast cancer)	28	3,940 women	Pooled SMD for depression was –1.01 (95% CI: –1.83 to –0.18). Significant effects also seen for anxiety (SMD: –0.48; 95% CI: –0.76 to –0.21). No significant effect on survival.

Note. CI=confidence interval; RCT=randomized controlled trial; SMD=standardized mean difference.

Source. Adapted from Jacobsen and Jim 2008.

Internet-based interventions that included more behavior change techniques had greater effects.

Internet-based therapies for chronic pain have been reviewed by Macea et al. (2010). The review authors included 11 studies and found small effects for the Internet-based approaches in comparison with mainly wait-list controls, on the order of 0.29 (95% CI: 0.15 to 0.42). Eccleston et al. (2014; 15 trials) and Buhrman et al. (2016; 22 trials) also reviewed this field and found similar results.

More recently, Ljótsson et al. (2010) evaluated Internet-based treatments for irritable bowel syndrome. In their first study, they found that Internet-delivered exposure-based treatment plus mindfulness was superior to a control condition (a discussion forum) and, in their second study (Ljótsson et al. 2011b), was superior to Internet-delivered stress management for irritable bowel syndrome. They have also reported that the positive treatment effects appear to be maintained in the long term (Ljótsson et al. 2011c) and that the intervention is cost-effective (Ljótsson et al. 2011a).

Conclusion

There is evidence that psychological therapies are beneficial for patients with physical health problems, although the treatment effects are generally small. Most interventions have involved CBT, but there is growing interest in third-wave cognitive-behavioral and psychodynamic therapies.

In head-to-head comparisons, there appears to be little difference between different therapeutic approaches, so we need better ways to target therapies at patients who are likely to benefit from psychological treatment, if effect sizes are to be increased. Psychological treatments are often delivered as components of either stepped-care or collaborative care models. Psychological therapies are often provided in conjunction with pharmacological treatments, particularly if there is poor initial response to psychological treatments alone.

Access to appropriate psychological treatment for patients with physical and psychological health problems remains a serious problem in many countries. Internet-based treatments may help with this problem, but it is still likely that face-to face psychological therapy will be required for people with chronic or complex problems. Improvement in access is unlikely to occur to a significant extent unless psychological therapies are better integrated into physical health care systems.

References

Alderson SL, Foy R, Glidewell L, et al: How patients understand depression associated with chronic physical disease—a systematic review. BMC Fam Pract 13:41, 2012 22640234

Alderson SL, Foy R, Glidewell L, House AO: Patients understanding of depression associated with chronic physical illness: a qualitative study. BMC Fam Pract 15:37, 2014 24555886

Andersson G, Cuijpers P, Carlbring P, et al: Guided Internet-based vs. face-to-face cognitive behavior therapy for psychiatric and somatic disorders: a systematic review and meta-analysis. World Psychiatry 13(3):288–295, 2014 25273302

Arias AJ, Steinberg K, Banga A, Trestman RL: Systematic review of the efficacy of meditation techniques as treatments for medical illness. J Altern Complement Med 12(8):817–832, 2006 17034289

Baumeister H, Hutter N, Bengel J: Psychological and pharmacological interventions for depression in patients with diabetes mellitus: an abridged Cochrane review. Diabet Med 31(7):773–786, 2014 24673571

Beltman MW, Voshaar RC, Speckens AE: Cognitive-behavioural therapy for depression in people with a somatic disease: meta-analysis of randomised controlled trials. Br J Psychiatry 197(1):11–19, 2010 20592427

Bernardy K, Füber N, Klose P, Häuser W: Efficacy of hypnosis/guided imagery in fibromyalgia syndrome—a systematic review and meta-analysis of controlled trials. BMC Musculoskelet Disord 12:133, 2011 21676255

Blanchard EB: A critical review of cognitive, behavioral, and cognitive-behavioral therapies for irritable bowel syndrome. J Cogn Psychother 19(2):101–123, 2005

Bohlmeijer E, Prenger R, Taal E, Cuijpers P: The effects of mindfulness-based stress reduction therapy on mental health of adults with a chronic medical disease: a meta-analysis. J Psychosom Res 68(6):539–544, 2010 20488270

Buhrman M, Gordh T, Andersson G: Internet interventions for chronic pain including headache. Internet Interventions 4(Pt 1):17–34, 2016

Butler AC, Chapman JE, Forman EM, Beck AT: The empirical status of cognitive-behavioral therapy: a review of meta-analyses. Clin Psychol Rev 26(1):17–31, 2006 16199119

Cassel EJ: The nature of suffering and the goals of medicine. N Engl J Med 306(11):639–645, 1982 7057823

Castell BD, Kazantzis N, Moss-Morris RE: Cognitive behavioral therapy and graded exercise for chronic fatigue syndrome: a meta-analysis. Clinical Psychology Science and Practice 18(4):311–324, 2011

Chambers D, Bagnall AM, Hempel S, Forbes C: Interventions for the treatment, management and rehabilitation of patients with chronic fatigue syndrome/myalgic encephalomyelitis: an updated systematic review. J R Soc Med 99(10):506–520, 2006 17021301

Chiesa A, Serretti A: Mindfulness-based interventions for chronic pain: a systematic review of the evidence. J Altern Complement Med 17(1):83–93, 2011 21265650

Christensen DN: Postmastectomy couple counseling: an outcome study of a structured treatment protocol. J Sex Marital Ther 9(4):266–275, 1983 6663643

Ciechanowski P, Russo J, Katon W, et al: Influence of patient attachment style on self-care and outcomes in diabetes. Psychosom Med 66(5):720–728, 2004 15385697

Classen CC, Kraemer HC, Blasey C, et al: Supportive-expressive group therapy for primary breast cancer patients: a randomized prospective multicenter trial. Psychooncology 17(5):438–447, 2008 17935144

Coventry PA, Bower P, Keyworth C, et al: The effect of complex interventions on depression and anxiety in chronic obstructive pulmonary disease: systematic review and meta-analysis. PLOS One 8(4):e60532, 2013 23585837

Coventry P, Lovell K, Dickens C, et al: Integrated primary care for patients with mental and physical multimorbidity: cluster randomised controlled trial of collaborative care for patients with depression comorbid with diabetes or cardiovascular disease. BMJ 350:h638, 2015 25687344

Cramer H, Haller H, Lauche R, Dobos G: Mindfulness-based stress reduction for low back pain. A systematic review. BMC Complement Altern Med 12:162, 2012a 23009599

Cramer H, Lauche R, Paul A, Dobos G: Mindfulness-based stress reduction for breast cancer—a systematic review and meta-analysis. Curr Oncol 19(5):e343–e352, 2012b 23144582

Creed F, Fernandes L, Guthrie E, et al; North of England IBS Research Group: The cost-effectiveness of psychotherapy and paroxetine for severe irritable bowel syndrome. Gastroenterology 124(2):303–317, 2003 12557136

Cuijpers P, van Straten A, Andersson G: Internet-administered cognitive behavior therapy for health problems: a systematic review. J Behav Med 31(2):169–177, 2008 18165893

Dickens C, Cherrington A, Adeyemi I, et al: Characteristics of psychological interventions that improve depression in people with coronary heart disease: a systematic review and meta-regression. Psychosom Med 75(2):211–221, 2013 23324874

Dwight-Johnson M, Ell K, Lee PJ: Can collaborative care address the needs of low-income Latinas with comorbid depression and cancer? Results from a randomized pilot study. Psychosomatics 46(3):224–232, 2005 15883143

Eccleston C, Fisher E, Craig L, et al: Psychological therapies (Internet-delivered) for the management of chronic pain in adults. Cochrane Database Syst Rev (2):CD010152, 2014 24574082

Ell K, Xie B, Quon B, et al: Randomized controlled trial of collaborative care management of depression among low-income patients with cancer. J Clin Oncol 26(27):4488–4496, 2008 18802161

Erdman DV (ed): The Complete Poetry and Prose of William Blake (Jerusalem Chapter III, Plate 55: verses 60–68). New York, Anchor Books, 1988

Farver-Vestergaard I, Jacobsen D, Zachariae R: Efficacy of psychosocial interventions on psychological and physical health outcomes in chronic obstructive pulmonary disease: a systematic review and meta-analysis. Psychother Psychosom 84(1):37–50, 2015 25547641

Fekete EM, Antoni MH, Schneiderman N: Psychosocial and behavioral interventions for chronic medical conditions. Curr Opin Psychiatry 20(2):152–157, 2007 17278914

Fink P, Toft T, Hansen MS, et al: Symptoms and syndromes of bodily distress: an exploratory study of 978 internal medical, neurological, and primary care patients. Psychosom Med 69(1):30–39, 2007 17244846

Ford AC, Talley NJ, Schoenfeld PS, et al: Efficacy of antidepressants and psychological therapies in irritable bowel syndrome: systematic review and meta-analysis. Gut 58(3):367–378, 2009 19001059

Ford AC, Quigley EMM, Lacy BE, et al: Effect of antidepressants and psychological therapies, including hypnotherapy, in irritable bowel syndrome: systematic review and meta-analysis. Am J Gastroenterol 109(9):1350–1365, quiz 1366, 2014 24935275

Galway K, Black A, Cantwell M, et al: Psychosocial interventions to improve quality of life and emotional wellbeing for recently diagnosed cancer patients. Cochrane Database Syst Rev (11):CD007064, 2012 23152241

Garcia-Campayo J, Magdalena J, Magallón R, et al: A meta-analysis of the efficacy of fibromyalgia treatment according to level of care. Arthritis Res Ther 10(4):R81, 2008 18627602

Guthrie E, Sensky T: The role of psychological treatments, in Handbook of Liaison Psychiatry. Edited by Lloyd GG, Guthrie E. Cambridge, UK, Cambridge University Press, 2008, pp 800–817

Guthrie E, Creed F, Dawson D, Tomenson B: A controlled trial of psychological treatment for the irritable bowel syndrome. Gastroenterology 100(2):450–457, 1991 1985041

Guthrie E, Moorey J, Margison F, et al: Cost-effectiveness of brief psychodynamic-interpersonal therapy in high utilizers of psychiatric services. Arch Gen Psychiatry 56(6):519–526, 1999 10359466

Guthrie E, Kapur N, Mackway-Jones K, et al: Randomised controlled trial of brief psychological intervention after deliberate self poisoning. BMJ 323(7305):135–138, 2001 11463679

Hamilton J, Guthrie E, Creed F, et al: A randomized controlled trial of psychotherapy in patients with chronic functional dyspepsia. Gastroenterology 119(3):661–669, 2000 10982759

Hamilton WT, Gallagher AM, Thomas JM, White PD: Risk markers for both chronic fatigue and irritable bowel syndromes: a prospective case-control study in primary care. Psychol Med 39(11):1913–1921, 2009 19366500

Hawton K, Kirk J: Problem-solving, in Cognitive Behaviour Therapy for Psychiatric Problems: A Practical Guide. Edited by Hawton K, Salkovskis P, Kirk J, et al. Oxford, UK, Oxford Medical Publications, 1989, pp 406–427

Hersch J, Juraskova I, Price M, Mullan B: Psychosocial interventions and quality of life in gynaecological cancer patients: a systematic review. Psychooncology 18(8):795–810, 2009 19090556

Ho RT, Fong TC, Lo PH, et al: Randomized controlled trial of supportive-expressive group therapy and body-mind-spirit intervention for Chinese non-metastatic breast cancer patients. Support Care Cancer 24(12):4929–4937, 2016 27470259

Hobson RF: Forms of Feeling. London, Tavistock, 1985

Hubschmid M, Aybek S, Maccaferri GE, et al: Efficacy of brief interdisciplinary psychotherapeutic intervention for motor conversion disorder and nonepileptic attacks. Gen Hosp Psychiatry 37(5):448–455, 2015 26099544

Jacobsen PB, Jim HS: Psychosocial interventions for anxiety and depression in adult cancer patients: achievements and challenges. CA Cancer J Clin 58(4):214–230, 2008 18558664

Jassim GA, Whitford DL, Hickey A, Carter B: Psychological interventions for women with non-metastatic breast cancer. Cochrane Database Syst Rev (5):CD008729, 2015 26017383

Katon WJ, Von Korff M, Lin EH, et al: The Pathways Study: a randomized trial of collaborative care in patients with diabetes and depression. Arch Gen Psychiatry 61(10):1042–1049, 2004 15466678

Katon WJ, Lin EHB, Von Korff M, et al: Collaborative care for patients with depression and chronic illnesses. N Engl J Med 363(27):2611–2620, 2010 21190455

Kleinstäuber M, Witthöft M, Hiller W: Efficacy of short-term psychotherapy for multiple medically unexplained physical symptoms: a meta-analysis. Clin Psychol Rev 31(1):146–160, 2011 20920834

Klerman G, Weissman M, Rounsaville B, et al: Interpersonal Psychotherapy of Depression. New York, Basic Books, 1984

Lackner JM, Mesmer C, Morley S, et al: Psychological treatments for irritable bowel syndrome: a systematic review and meta-analysis. J Consult Clin Psychol 72(6):1100–1113, 2004 15612856

Lauche R, Cramer H, Dobos G, et al: A systematic review and meta-analysis of mindfulness-based stress reduction for the fibromyalgia syndrome. J Psychosom Res 75(6):500–510, 2013 24290038

Ledesma D, Kumano H: Mindfulness-based stress reduction and cancer: a meta-analysis. Psychooncology 18(6):571–579, 2009 19023879

Leventhal H, Benyamini Y, Brownlee S: Illness representations: theoretical foundations, in Perceptions of Health and Illness: Current Research and Applications. Edited by Petrie KJ, Weinman J. Amsterdam, The Netherlands, Harwood Academic Publishers, 1997, pp 19–45

Lin EHB, Katon W, Von Korff M, et al; IMPACT Investigators: Effect of improving depression care on pain and functional outcomes among older adults with arthritis: a randomized controlled trial. JAMA 290(18):2428–2429, 2003 14612479

Ljótsson B, Falk L, Vesterlund AW, et al: Internet-delivered exposure and mindfulness based therapy for irritable bowel syndrome—a randomized controlled trial. Behav Res Ther 48(6):531–539, 2010 20362976

Ljótsson B, Andersson G, Andersson E, et al: Acceptability, effectiveness, and cost-effectiveness of Internet-based exposure treatment for irritable bowel syndrome in a clinical sample: a randomized controlled trial. BMC Gastroenterol 11:110, 2011a 21992655

Ljótsson B, Hedman E, Andersson E, et al: Internet-delivered exposure-based treatment vs. stress management for irritable bowel syndrome: a randomized trial. Am J Gastroenterol 106(8):1481–1491, 2011b 21537360

Ljótsson B, Hedman E, Lindfors P, et al: Long-term follow-up of Internet-delivered exposure and mindfulness based treatment for irritable bowel syndrome. Behav Res Ther 49(1):58–61, 2011c 21092934

Looper KJ, Kirmayer LJ: Behavioral medicine approaches to somatoform disorders. J Consult Clin Psychol 70(3):810–827, 2002 12090385

Macea DD, Gajos K, Daglia Calil YA, Fregni F: The efficacy of Web-based cognitive behavioral interventions for chronic pain: a systematic review and meta-analysis. J Pain 11(10):917–929, 2010 20650691

Maguire P, Tait A, Brooke M, et al: Effect of counselling on the psychiatric morbidity associated with mastectomy. BMJ 281(6253):1454–1456, 1980 7192170

Maguire P, Brooke M, Tait A, et al: The effect of counselling on physical disability and social recovery after mastectomy. Clin Oncol 9(4):319–324, 1983 6362943

Malouff JM, Thorsteinsson EB, Rooke SE, et al: Efficacy of cognitive behavioral therapy for chronic fatigue syndrome: a meta-analysis. Clin Psychol Rev 28(5):736–745, 2008 18060672

Markowitz JC, Klerman GL, Clougherty KF, et al: Individual psychotherapies for depressed HIV-positive patients. Am J Psychiatry 152(10):1504–1509, 1995 7573591

Marques MM, De Gucht V, Gouveia MJ, et al: Differential effects of behavioral interventions with a graded physical activity component in patients suffering from chronic fatigue (syndrome): an updated systematic review and meta-analysis. Clin Psychol Rev 40:123–137, 2015 26112761

Moss-Morris R, Weinman J, Petrie KJ, et al: The Revised Illness Perception Questionnaire (IPQ-R). Psychology & Health 17(1):1–16, 2002

Mustafa M, Carson-Stevens A, Gillespie D, Edwards AGK: Psychological interventions for women with metastatic breast cancer. Cochrane Database Syst Rev (6):CD004253, 2013 23737397

Nezu AM, Nezu CM, Felgoise SH, et al: Project Genesis: assessing the efficacy of problem-solving therapy for distressed adult cancer patients. J Consult Clin Psychol 71(6):1036–1048, 2003 14622079

Ost LG: The efficacy of Acceptance and Commitment Therapy: an updated systematic review and meta-analysis. Behav Res Ther 61:105–121, 2014 25193001

Ott MJ, Norris RL, Bauer-Wu SM: Mindfulness meditation for oncology patients: a discussion and critical review. Integr Cancer Ther 5(2):98–108, 2006 16685074

Parahoo K, McDonough S, McCaughan E, et al: Psychosocial interventions for men with prostate cancer. Cochrane Database Syst Rev (12):CD008529, 2013 24368598

Price JR, Mitchell E, Tidy E, Hunot V: Cognitive behaviour therapy for chronic fatigue syndrome in adults. Cochrane Database Syst Rev (3):CD001027, 2008 18646067

Prochaska JO, Norcross JC, DiClemente CC: Changing for Good: A Revolutionary Six-Stage Program for Overcoming Bad Habits and Moving Your Life Positively Forward. New York, William Morrow, 1994

Raine R, Haines A, Sensky T, et al: Systematic review of mental health interventions for patients with common somatic symptoms: can research evidence from secondary care be extrapolated to primary care? BMJ 325(7372):1082–1085, 2002 12424170

Rimes KA, Chalder T: Treatments for chronic fatigue syndrome. Occup Med (Lond) 55(1):32–39, 2005 15699088

Royal College of Physicians and Royal College of Psychiatrists: The Psychological Care of Medical Patients: A Practical Guide, 2nd Edition. London, Royal College of Physicians, 2003. Available at: http://www.rcpsych.ac.uk/files/pdfversion/cr108.pdf. Accessed February 5, 2010.

Sattel H, Lahmann C, Gündel H, et al: Brief psychodynamic interpersonal psychotherapy for patients with multisomatoform disorder: randomised controlled trial. Br J Psychiatry 200(1):60–67, 2012 22075651

Schaefert R, Klose P, Moser G, Häuser W: Efficacy, tolerability, and safety of hypnosis in adult irritable bowel syndrome: systematic review and meta-analysis. Psychosom Med 76(5):389–398, 2014 24901382

Segal Z, Teasdale J, Williams M: Mindfulness-Based Cognitive Therapy for Depression. New York, Guilford, 2002

Semple C, Parahoo K, Norman A, et al: Psychosocial interventions for patients with head and neck cancer. Cochrane Database Syst Rev (7):CD009441, 2013 23857592

Sensky T: Cognitive therapy with medical patients, in Cognitive-Behavior Therapy. Edited by Wright JH (Review of Psychiatry Series, Vol 23; Oldham JM and Riba MB, series eds). Washington, DC, American Psychiatric Publishing, 2004, pp 83–121

Shapiro DA, Barkham M, Rees A, et al: Effects of treatment duration and severity of depression on the effectiveness of cognitive-behavioral and psychodynamic-interpersonal psychotherapy. J Consult Clin Psychol 62(3):522–534, 1994 8063978

Sharpe M, Peveler R, Mayou R: The psychological treatment of patients with functional somatic symptoms: a practical guide. J Psychosom Res 36(6):515–529, 1992 1640390

Simpson R, Booth J, Lawrence M, et al: Mindfulness based interventions in multiple sclerosis—a systematic review. BMC Neurol 14:15, 2014 24438384

Smith JE, Richardson J, Hoffman C, Pilkington K: Mindfulness-Based Stress Reduction as supportive therapy in cancer care: systematic review. J Adv Nurse 52(3):315–327, 2005 [Erratum in: J Adv Nurs 53(5):618, 2006] 16194185

Smith SM, Sonego S, Ketcheson L, Larson JL: A review of the effectiveness of psychological interventions used for anxiety and depression in chronic obstructive pulmonary disease. BMJ Open Respir Res 1(1):e000042, 2014 25478188

Spiegel D, Glafkides MC: Effects of group confrontation with death and dying. Int J Group Psychother 33(4):433–447, 1983 6642804

Spiegel D, Bloom JR, Kraemer HC, Gottheil E: Effect of psychosocial treatment on survival of patients with metastatic breast cancer. Lancet 2(8668):888–891, 1989 2571815

Stewart JH: Hypnosis in contemporary medicine. Mayo Clin Proc 80(4):511–524, 2005 15819289

Stuart S, Noyes R Jr: Treating hypochondriasis with interpersonal psychotherapy. J Contemp Psychother 35(3):269–283, 2005

van Dessel N, den Boeft M, van der Wouden JC, et al: Non-pharmacological interventions for somatoform disorders and medically unexplained physical symptoms (MUPS) in adults. Cochrane Database Syst Rev (11):CD011142, 2014 25362239

van der Feltz-Cornelis CM, Nuyen J, Stoop C, et al: Effect of interventions for major depressive disorder and significant depressive symptoms in patients with diabetes mellitus: a systematic review and meta-analysis. Gen Hosp Psychiatry 32(4):380–395, 2010 20633742

Veehof MM, Oskam MJ, Schreurs KM, Bohlmeijer ET: Acceptance-based interventions for the treatment of chronic pain: a systematic review and meta-analysis. Pain 152(3):533–542, 2011 21251756

Webb TL, Joseph J, Yardley L, Michie S: Using the Internet to promote health behavior change: a systematic review and meta-analysis of the impact of theoretical basis, use of behavior changes techniques, and mode of delivery on efficacy. J Med Internet Res 12(1):e4, 2010 20164043

Whiting P, Bagnall AM, Sowden AJ, et al: Interventions for the treatment and management of chronic fatigue syndrome: a systematic review. JAMA 286(11):1360–1368, 2001 11560542

Wilson S, Maddison T, Roberts L, et al; Birmingham IBS Research Group: Systematic review: the effectiveness of hypnotherapy in the management of irritable bowel syndrome. Aliment Pharmacol Ther 24(5):769–780, 2006 16918880

Wright EB, Holcombe C, Salmon P: Doctors' communication of trust, care, and respect in breast cancer: qualitative study. BMJ 328(7444):864, 2004 15054034

CHAPTER 38

Electroconvulsive Therapy and Other Brain Stimulation Therapies

Keith G. Rasmussen, M.D.

Electroconvulsive therapy (ECT) is associated with low morbidity and mortality (Nuttall et al. 2004). Nonetheless, medical comorbidity in ECT patients is common, and the psychiatrist should be aware of a patient's medical status and familiar with strategies to prevent complications. The essence of the pre-ECT medical evaluation is a history and physical examination. Further testing or specialist consultation can be ordered as needed. Additionally, individual hospitals and clinics may have their own policies governing pre-procedural tests such as blood work or electrocardiograms (ECGs). As a general rule, stabilization of any suboptimally controlled medical conditions before commencing ECT is ideal, but it must be balanced with clinical urgency. For example, waiting a few days to stabilize a medical problem may be acceptable in a behaviorally well-modulated patient, but not in a mute, stuporous, catatonic patient. Good communication among the primary psychiatrist, other specialist consultants, and the anesthesiologist is essential. In many ECT clinics, the anesthesiologist of the day varies from treatment to treatment, so it falls on the psychiatrist to ensure that information obtained from previous treatments is passed on. Also, the patient's medical status prior to treatments may change during the course of treatments, so ongoing vigilance to assess new-onset medical issues is critical, and this too usually falls on the psychiatrist. Thus, it is unwise for a psychiatrist treating an ECT patient to assume an attitude that it is the anesthesiologist's or internist's responsibility to deal with medical problems—good care of these patients begins with the psychiatrist.

There are too many medical problems to discuss in detail here. In this chapter, the focus will be on common medical comorbidities in ECT patients and strategies for risk reduction. It is recommended, however, that any psychiatrist treating a patient with other medical issues not discussed in this chapter make an effort to obtain published literature and to consult with specialists pertinent to the medical issues at hand. This chapter will focus on pretreatment and intertreatment assessment of patients with medical problems. Intratreatment management of medical issues is the responsibility of anesthesiology staff and will be touched on only briefly. Finally, this chapter will focus on ECT. Readers interested in transcranial magnetic stimulation (TMS) are referred to an excellent practice guideline on that topic (Rossi et al. 2009).

Cardiovascular Disorders

Cardiac Physiology of ECT

After the electrical stimulus, there is a parasympathetically mediated short-lived bradycardia, occasionally with an asystole of several seconds. This is rapidly replaced by a sympathetically mediated tachycardia and a rise in blood pressure during and for a few minutes after the seizure. Myocardial workload and cardiac output increase significantly. Transient ECG abnormalities may occur during this time, including ST segment depression and T wave changes as well as temporary echocardiographic abnormalities, mainly abnormal wall motion. The parameters that are monitored routinely include blood pressure and ECG, and any untoward measurements can be treated promptly by the anesthesiologist (e.g., with blood pressure medication or antiarrhythmics) to prevent serious complications. These physiological changes might predispose cardiac patients to higher-than-usual risks during ECT, but the literature does not permit precise conclusions about such risks. Pre-ECT consultation with a cardiologist or an anesthesiologist familiar with the cardiac physiology of ECT should be undertaken in patients with known significant cardiac disease. No universally agreed-upon standards of pre-ECT cardiac testing, such as stress echocardiography or sestamibi scanning, have been developed. The need for such testing should be determined by the consulting cardiologist.

Congestive Heart Failure

Patients with congestive heart failure (CHF) are particularly sensitive to increased myocardial demand such as occurs in ECT. The keys to maximum safety with such patients are to stabilize ventricular pump function, optimally before proceeding, and to obtain expert anesthesiological management during the sessions. There have been six case series describing 58 patients with CHF given ECT, with two deaths, as described below.

Gerring and Shields (1982) provided detailed outcome data on four patients with CHF who were treated with ECT for depressive illness. A 60-year-old woman with mitral stenosis received ECT without complications. A 58-year-old woman, also with mitral stenosis in addition to CHF, experienced atrial fibrillation leading to severe decompensation of the CHF after the second treatment; on stabilization, she went on to receive another course of ECT without complications. A 71-year-old woman with a history of myocardial infarction (MI) in addition to CHF had a cardiopulmonary arrest 45 minutes after her fifth treatment and died. Finally, a 69-year-old woman showed transient ventricular and atrial dysrhythmias after several of her ECT treatments, which she otherwise tolerated well.

Zielinski et al. (1993) reported on 12 ECT patients with CHF. There were no deaths in this series. Ten of the patients had minor cardiac complications, consisting usually of transient dysrhythmias (atrial or ventricular) or ischemic changes on ECG. Goldberg and Badger (1993) treated two patients with CHF and implantable cardioverter defibrillators (ICDs). The first patient tolerated eight ECT treatments without consequences. The second, a 65-year-old man with dilated cardiomyopathy and a pre-ECT ejection fraction of 20%, underwent four treatments. After recovery from the first and third treatments, he had respiratory difficulties and bouts of hypotension that responded to ephedrine. After the fourth treatment, he developed a wide complex tachycardia without palpable pulse and was resuscitated. No further ECT was administered, but he had a hypotensive episode 5 days later that ultimately led to his death from progressive heart failure several days thereafter.

Petrides and Fink (1996), in a series of ECT patients with atrial fibrillation, reported that one 89-year-old woman with CHF converted to sinus rhythm after receiving a course of ECT. Also, a 76-year-old woman with CHF and atrial fibrillation received a course of seven ECT treatments, during which she fluctuated between atrial fibrillation and sinus rhythm. The CHF did not seem to worsen.

Stern et al. (1997) described three patients with CHF who received ECT without any cardiac complications. The authors used a nitroglycerin patch, sublingual nifedipine, and intravenous labetalol pre-ECT. In the largest and best-described series to date, Rivera et al. (2011) administered ECT to 35 patients with CHF, none of whom died. One patient experienced persistent tachycardia and was sent to the intensive care unit as a precaution, but was discharged after 1 day. Some transient benign dysrhythmias were noted in a few patients.

CHF should optimally be stabilized prior to commencing ECT. Cardiac medications should be administered in the morning before the treatments with a small amount of water, with enough time to ensure absorption. One practice guideline cautions against administration of diuretic agents the morning of ECT to avoid bladder rupture or incontinence during the seizure (American Psychiatric Association Committee on Electroconvulsive Therapy 2001). However, diuretics should be administered in the morning, if that is the usual time, to avoid any abrupt changes in the medical regimen. The full-bladder problem can be managed simply by having the patient void just before the treatment or, if necessary, by making transient use of a urinary catheter.

Whether to use an antimuscarinic agent in the patient with CHF must be decided on a case-by-case basis. The potential for such medication to increase myocardial workload through added tachycardia and hypertension has been established (Rasmussen et al. 1999). However, if a patient receives a subconvulsive electrical stimulus, especially if he or she is also receiving beta-blocking medication, there is a risk of unopposed parasympathetic stimulation and resultant prolonged asystole (Tang and Ungvari 2001).

The attending anesthesiologist may elect to use other cardioprotective agents when ECT is being administered to the patient with CHF. For example, a beta-blocker such as esmolol or labetalol may dampen the seizure-induced sympathetic stimulation. Other strategies include preload reduction (e.g., nitrates), peripheral vasodilators (e.g., hydralazine), and calcium channel blockade (e.g., verapamil or diltiazem).

Finally, intertreatment assessment in patients with CHF is especially important, as demonstrated by the case report of a patient who died several days after the last ECT treatment (Goldberg and Badger 1993). Daily rounds should include not only assessment of mood and cognitive status but also inquiries about symptoms of CHF (e.g., shortness of breath, orthopnea) and physical examination for signs of CHF (e.g., gallops, jugular venous distension, peripheral edema, pulmonary crackles). Any new or worsening findings should prompt careful evaluation and, if necessary, halting of ECT (even if temporarily) to stabilize the patient. As previously mentioned, patients with known CHF should be evaluated by an internist or a cardiologist prior to initiating treatment.

Coronary Artery Disease/Post–Myocardial Infarction

Easing the rise in myocardial oxygen demand during ECT is the goal in care of patients with coronary artery disease (CAD). In several case series (Gerring and Shields 1982; Magid et al. 2005; Petrides and Fink 1996; Rice et al. 1994; Zielinski et al. 1993), numerous patients with CAD—some with a remote history of MI—underwent ECT without major complications. In an echocardiographic/sestamibi study by Ruwitch et al. (1994) in patients with known CAD, ECT did not cause any clinical complications (e.g., angina, MI, clinically significant ventricular dysfunction).

After the prospective ECT patient with CAD has had the appropriate pretreatment evaluation and stabilization, some measures may further reduce cardiac risk. Many studies have shown that pretreatment with an antihypertensive agent (e.g., beta-blockers, calcium channel blockers, other vasodilators, nitrates) lowers the seizure-induced rise in heart rate or blood pressure (Abrams 2002, pp. 77–81). Whether this reliably translates into actual protection against cardiac complications is unknown. In fact, Castelli et al. (1995), O'Connor et al. (1996), and Zvara et al. (1997) found no evidence that use of beta-blockers during ECT reduced the incidence of myocardial ischemia, despite beneficial effects on blood pressure increases during the treatments. Thus, it remains uncertain whether beta-blocker pretreatment reduces morbidity associated with ECT. Given the well-documented salutary effects of such drugs in patients with ischemic heart disease, it seems reasonable to use them in selected cases before, during, or shortly after the treatment, depending on the patient's hemodynamic status, after carefully weighing the risks and potential benefits of such treatment.

Dysrhythmias, Pacemakers, and Implantable Defibrillators

The most common dysrhythmia in ECT patients is atrial fibrillation. There are several reports of patients in atrial fibrillation who safely received ECT (Petrides and Fink 1996). Occasionally, such patients will convert to sinus rhythm during ECT or convert back to atrial fibrillation if already converted before ECT to sinus rhythm. Atrial fibrillation newly identified before ECT should be assessed by a cardiologist for optimal management, including the decision of whether to choose rate control or cardioversion. Therapeutic anticoagulation should be maintained throughout the course of ECT if the patient is already anticoagulated. Close and meticulous monitoring of the patient's hemodynamic status, oxygenation, and ECG changes in response to treatment is critically important during ECT. ECG rhythm should be inspected before each treatment. The patient without a history of atrial fibrillation who develops this rhythm during ECT obviously should have a cardiac evaluation before treatment is resumed. In patients taking warfarin, therapeutic anticoagulation should be continued throughout ECT (Mehta et al. 2004).

Because cardiac patients are predisposed to a variety of atrial or ventricular dysrhythmias, it is important to ensure that electrolytes are normal. Electrolyte abnormalities and other metabolic perturbations (e.g., thyroid dysfunction) can cause arrhythmias, along with medications that can potentially prolong the QT interval, a group that includes many psychotropics, which are often prescribed for ECT patients (Rasmussen et al. 2006a).

A related issue concerns the prospective ECT patient with a cardiac pacemaker or an ICD. There have been numerous case reports of patients with pacemakers who have undergone successful and uncomplicated ECT (Dolenc et al. 2004), as well as a few reports of patients with ICDs (Dolenc et al. 2004; Lynch et al. 2008). Pre-ECT device assessment to ensure normal functioning is advisable. Some practitioners have used a magnet placed on the chest above the device to convert a demand-mode pacemaker to fixed mode during ECT to avoid spurious discharge of the device, which theoretically could occur as the result of muscle electrical activity; however, no evidence supports this practice. ICDs should be turned off prior to each ECT treatment while the patient is on an electrocardiographic monitor, the latter being continued until the ICD is turned back on. All patients with ICDs or pacemakers that have been reprogrammed prior to ECT should receive device assessment after the procedure.

Other Cardiac Disorders

Assuming that patients have no preexisting conditions or surgical complications, there is no specific reason to assume that patients who have had an aneurysm repair are at increased risk during ECT. The chief concern in patients with aneurysms is the potential risk of rupture or leakage caused by the rapid rise in blood pressure during ECT. If a patient is known to have an aortic aneurysm, the size should be evaluated (e.g., by ultrasound) prior to ECT. Consultation with a vascular surgeon would be prudent to evaluate the stability of the aneurysm and strategies for risk reduction. Pretreatment with antihypertensives before ECT anesthesia can optimize control of blood pressure and reduce arterial wall stress. Labetalol is ideal for this purpose because it has both alpha and beta blockade and thus can reduce peripheral vascular resistance and attenuate the rise in blood pressure during and shortly after the seizure. Repetitive imaging may be necessary during the course of ECT treatments if there is any concern with respect to the stability of the aneurysm. It is not known whether metallic implants in the brain (e.g., a metallic clip in an intracerebral aneurysm) can elevate the risk of complications during ECT. The same is true for other metallic devices in the brain, such as deep brain stimulators.

Hypertension is the most common cardiovascular disorder among ECT patients. Although it is intuitively obvious that good control of blood pressure is desirable prior to starting ECT, there must be no insistence on precise limits, because psychiatric patients often have difficult-to-control blood pressures. The anesthesiologist can always bring blood pressure down a bit with a beta blocker such as labetalol if needed. As patients improve with ECT, it is not uncommon for blood pressures to become easier to control as well.

Aortic stenosis is common, especially in elderly patients, and may require special attention by the anesthesiologist during ECT treatments to balance the risk of hyper- or hypotension, both of which may be problematic (Mueller et al. 2007). If a patient has had mechanical valve replacement and has received appropriate anticoagulation, the risk of ECT treatment should not be significantly increased (assuming that no other cardiac dysfunction, such as impaired ventricular function or dysrhythmia, is present). However, if a patient has a valvular abnormality that has not been optimally treated or is newly identified, then cardiac consultation should be obtained.

Heart transplant patients are rarely encountered in ECT practice. One should undertake ECT in a cardiac transplant patient only in close consultation with the patient's cardiologist.

Neurological Disorders

Neurophysiology of ECT

In contrast to cardiac physiology and testing, no known neurodiagnostic tests specifically predict neurological risk with ECT, and neuroprotective strategies are unavailable. Thus, brain imaging and electroencephalograms are not routinely indicated to assess ECT risk. If there is some other reason to perform a neurodiagnostic procedure, such as a newly found focal neurological sign, then that should be done prior to ECT as part of the diagnostic evaluation. ECT causes a brief rise in intracranial pressure, which theoretically implies risk of brain stem herniation in patients who already have increased intracranial pressure. However, such patients rarely are considered for ECT.

Neurodegenerative Disorders

In ECT practice, patients with Parkinson's, Alzheimer's, or Lewy body disease are commonly encountered. Much less frequently, patients with frontotemporal dementia are treated with ECT. Such patients are usually being treated for either depression or agitation (Acharya et al. 2015). There is no reason to believe that these conditions in themselves would increase the risk of medical complications during ECT. Although it would not be surprising if such patients were to experience greater-than-average acute cognitive impairment with ECT, it is not known whether the trajectory of their dementia would be worsened by a series of electrically induced seizures. The definitive study would be to randomly assign patients with well-characterized dementia syndromes who have psychopathology that normally would indicate ECT treatment to ECT or other interventions and follow up carefully with longitudinal assessments of cognition. Such a study has never been conducted and is not likely to be. Prudent advice for the ECT practitioner who treats patients with dementia is to use unilateral electrode placement and twice-weekly scheduling to minimize cognitive side effects. Nootropic agents such as donepezil or rivastigmine can be safely continued during ECT.

There is an interesting literature on the use of ECT in patients with Parkinson's disease (reviewed thoroughly by Borisovskaya et al. 2016). In brief, ECT may help the motor signs of parkinsonism as well as depressive or psychotic symptoms. Because relapse is high, maintenance ECT may help to sustain the initial benefits. Treatment-emergent dyskinesias are common and (after consultation with a neurologist) may call for careful reduction of levodopa doses during the index ECT. Given that cognitive side effects tend to be exaggerated in this population, unilateral electrode placement is recommended.

Other Neurological Disorders

Stroke

It is prudent for the ECT practitioner to avoid using ECT in patients with a recent stroke. However, occasionally such a patient is profoundly depressed, with marked decreases in psychomotor effort; has low or absent food intake; or is at high acute suicidal risk. In such cases, if ECT is judged to be necessary, risk-reduction strategies include continuing anticoagulation if it already is indicated (i.e., it should not be started just for ECT) and paying close attention to blood pressure to avoid high spikes and potentially dangerous declines. There is concern that intracerebral aneurysms may rupture during ECT because of the rapid increase in blood pressure during seizures. Most investigators reporting on ECT in patients with known aneurysms used antihypertensive drugs to dampen the ECT-related increase in blood pressure (Okamura et al. 2006; Sharma et al. 2005).

Epilepsy

Several case reports, a small case series, and one fairly large series suggested that epileptic patients can be given ECT effectively without worsening spontaneous seizure frequency (Lunde et al. 2006; Sienaert and Peuskens 2007). Before undertaking a course of ECT in a patient with epilepsy, consultation with the patient's neurologist is advised. Pretreatment brain imaging or electroencephalography is not needed unless such testing is indicated as part of the patient's neurological care.

The most common technical problem in ECT with epileptic patients is elicitation of therapeutic seizures in the context of concomitant treatment with anticonvulsant medications. Cautious lowering of the patient's anticonvulsant medication dosages might be needed; however, this action increases the risk of spontaneous seizures and should be undertaken only with the aid of a neurologist (Lunde et al. 2006).

Other Conditions

Some reports indicate that ECT can be safely used in patients with various types of intracranial masses (Kohler and Burock 2001; Patkar et al. 2000; Perry et al. 2007; Rasmussen and Flemming 2006; Rasmussen et al. 2007b). Presence of any central nervous system tumor may lead to an increased risk for neurological complications caused by ECT. In the absence of focal neurological signs, brain edema, mass effects, or papilledema, the risks likely are relatively small. In the presence of such findings, ECT should be considered only when no other reasonable option exists, and only after consultation with a neurosurgeon or neurologist to discuss strategies to reduce the increase in intracranial pressure that accompanies seizures.

ECT may be life-saving in some cases of refractory neuroleptic-induced malignant catatonia, which includes neuroleptic malignant syndrome.

Other Medical Conditions

The heart and brain bear most of the physiological effects of ECT. Fortunately, most of the other organ systems are not substantially affected, nor do their diseases generally cause much concern for greater risk of complications during ECT. Some additional considerations are discussed below.

Pregnancy

The most common adverse events in pregnant women during ECT are aspiration pneumonitis and induction of premature labor, uterine contractions, and vaginal bleeding, although ECT can be delivered safely during pregnancy (Calaway et al. 2016; Spodniaková et al. 2015). The period of greatest risk is the third trimester. Measures to prevent aspiration pneumonitis include tracheal intubation and alkalinizing intragastric pH with a nonparticulate antacid. Pretreatment obstetric assessment can identify high-risk pregnancies. Noninvasive monitoring of fetal heart tones before and after the seizure can document that no fetal distress occurred. Finally, probably the most important aspect of safe use of ECT in pregnant women is ready availability of obstetric intervention in case of untoward events.

Diabetes Mellitus

Single ECT treatments cause a brief rise (approximately 8%–10%) in blood sugar immediately after treatment in both diabetic and nondiabetic patients (Rasmussen and Ryan 2005; Rasmussen et al. 2006b). However, very little change occurs in blood sugar control over a course of treatments (Netzel et al. 2002). Diabetic patients should have blood glucose levels monitored closely during the ECT course, including fingerstick checks before treatment. Typically, patients with type 1 diabetes are administered half of their morning insulin dose and then promptly treated with ECT. They are then given breakfast and the remaining half of their insulin dose. Alternatively, the whole dose can be withheld, ECT can be delivered promptly early in the morning, and then posttreatment breakfast and the insulin dose can be given.

Chronic Pain

Chronic pain syndromes are quite common in psychiatric patients. When the pain symptom is clearly secondary to a melancholic or psychotic depression, the ECT clinician can be optimistic about resolution of the pain symptoms along with other psychiatric symptoms. When a chronic pain patient seems to have developed secondary depression, results are more mixed with ECT (Rasmussen 2003; Rasmussen and Rummans 2002). An intriguing finding is that phantom limb pain may abate with ECT even in the absence of apparent mood disturbance (Rasmussen and Rummans 2000).

Miscellaneous Considerations

Large case series attest to the safe use of ECT in patients with asthma (Mueller et al. 2006) or chronic obstructive pulmonary disease (Schak et al. 2008). Patients who are using inhalers should do so in the morning shortly before treatment. Mild sodium abnormalities have not been shown to be problematic for safe administration of ECT (Rasmussen et al. 2007a). Some anesthesiologists prefer to give an extra dose of steroid—a so-called stress dose—prior to ECT in patients who are already taking such medication. However, in a large series (Rasmussen et al. 2008), this practice was found to be unnecessary. Histamine-2 antagonists or antacids may decrease gastric acid secretion and the risk of aspiration pneumonitis in patients with gastroesophageal reflux disease, gastroparesis, or obesity (as well as pregnancy, as discussed earlier). Patients at severe risk of aspiration may require intubation. Urinary retention from antimuscarinic agents given during ECT is quite uncomfortable for patients and can predispose to urinary tract infections and even bladder rupture if not monitored. In those patients who do experience significant urinary retention after treatments, antimuscarinic agents can be withheld, while recognizing that the vagal effect of the electrical stimulus is not blocked and prolonged asystole can occur. Patients with severe osteoporosis or recent fractures require careful titration of muscle relaxant dosing; the adequacy of paralysis can be tested with a peripheral nerve stimulator. Extra care should be exercised when ventilating a patient with unstable cervical spine disease to avoid spinal cord injury. Given the brief increase in intraocular pressure lasting a few minutes after the seizures (Good et al. 2004), glaucoma patients should receive their medications in the mornings before treatment, an exception being anticholinesterase drugs, which may prolong the action of succinylcholine.

Other Brain Stimulation Therapies

Other brain stimulation therapies are increasingly being used in medically ill patients. U.S. Food and Drug Administration (FDA)–approved therapies include transcranial magnetic stimulation, vagal nerve stimulation, and deep brain stimulation. A variety of others are investigational for treatment of depression, including magnetic seizure therapy, transcranial direct current stimulation, transcranial low voltage pulsed electromagnetic fields, trigeminal nerve stimulation, and low field magnetic stimulation.

TMS is FDA approved for treatment-resistant depression. Its use is being actively investigated for other neuropsychiatric conditions (e.g., conversion disorder, chronic pain, cognitive impairment, migraine, Parkinson's disease, poststroke depression). (See Chapter 7, "Depression," for a review of the evidence supporting the efficacy of TMS for depression after stroke and in Parkinson's disease.) TMS, in common with brain magnetic resonance imaging, is contraindicated in patients with ferromagnetic implants, including electronic devices in or near the head (e.g., deep brain stimulators, carotid stents, aneurysm clips or coils, cerebrospinal fluid shunts, cochlear implants) and ferromagnetic fragments. The most common adverse effect of TMS is headache. There is a very small risk of inducing a single seizure with TMS. The estimated risk of seizure is approximately 1 in 30,000 treatments, but the risk may be higher in patients who have epilepsy or who are otherwise at increased risk for seizures. Caution has been advised in patients with cardiac pacemakers and implantable defibrillators, although there are no published case reports.

Vagal nerve stimulation (VNS) is FDA approved for treatment-resistant depression and epilepsy. VNS is contraindicated in patients who have cardiac conduction abnormalities or who have had a left vagotomy. VNS may aggravate sleep apnea and may affect programmable shunt valves. Patients with a VNS device cannot have short-wave diathermy, microwave diathermy, or therapeutic ultrasound diathermy, because the generated heating of the VNS components can cause tissue damage. Diagnostic ultrasound is not contraindicated. Common side effects of VNS include voice alteration/hoarseness, cough, dyspnea, and dysphagia. Bradycardia is very rare.

Deep brain stimulation (DBS) is FDA approved for use in treatment-resistant obsessive-compulsive disorder and for investigational use in depression. It is contraindicated in patients with increased bleeding risk, immunodeficiency, or cerebrovascular disease. DBS may be affected by—or may adversely affect—pacemakers and defibrillators. Diathermy, electrolysis, radiation therapy, and electrocautery should not be used directly over the implant site. Potential adverse effects include surgical and hardware complications, as well as mood disturbances and suicidality.

References

Abrams R: Electroconvulsive Therapy, 4th Edition. New York, Oxford University Press, 2002

Acharya D, Harper DG, Achtyes ED, et al: Safety and utility of acute electroconvulsive therapy for agitation and aggression in dementia. Int J Geriatr Psychiatry 30(3):265–273, 2015 24838521

American Psychiatric Association Committee on Electroconvulsive Therapy: The Practice of Electroconvulsive Therapy, 2nd Edition. Washington, DC, American Psychiatric Association, 2001

Borisovskaya A, Bryson WC, Buchholz J, et al: Electroconvulsive therapy for depression in Parkinson's disease: systematic review of evidence and recommendations. Neurodegener Dis Manag 6(2):161–176, 2016 27033556

Calaway K, Coshal S, Jones K, et al: A systematic review of the safety of electroconvulsive therapy use during the first trimester of pregnancy. J ECT 32(4):230–235, 2016 27327556

Castelli I, Steiner LA, Kaufmann MA, et al: Comparative effects of esmolol and labetalol to attenuate hyperdynamic states after electroconvulsive therapy. Anesth Analg 80(3):557–561, 1995 7864425

Dolenc TJ, Barnes RD, Hayes DL, Rasmussen KG: Electroconvulsive therapy in patients with cardiac pacemakers and implantable cardioverter defibrillators. Pacing Clin Electrophysiol 27(9):1257–1263, 2004 15461716

Gerring JP, Shields HM: The identification and management of patients with a high risk for cardiac arrhythmias during modified ECT. J Clin Psychiatry 43(4):140–143, 1982 7068545

Goldberg RJ, Badger JM: Major depressive disorder in patients with the implantable cardioverter defibrillator. Two cases treated with ECT. Psychosomatics 34(3):273–277, 1993 8493312

Good MS, Dolenc TJ, Rasmussen KG: Electroconvulsive therapy in a patient with glaucoma. J ECT 20(1):48–49, 2004 15087998

Kohler CG, Burock M: ECT for psychotic depression associated with a brain tumor (letter). Am J Psychiatry 158(12):2089, 2001 11729041

Lunde ME, Lee EK, Rasmussen KG: Electroconvulsive therapy in patients with epilepsy. Epilepsy Behav 9(2):355–359, 2006 16876485

Lynch AM, Pandurangi AK, Levenson JL: Electroconvulsive therapy in a candidate for heart transplant with an implantable cardiovertor defibrillator and cardiac contractility modulator. Psychosomatics 49(4):341–344, 2008 18621940

Magid M, Lapid MI, Sampson SM, et al: Use of electroconvulsive therapy in a patient 10 days after myocardial infarction. J ECT 21(3):182–185, 2005 16127311

Mehta V, Mueller PS, Gonzalez-Arriaza HL, et al: Safety of electroconvulsive therapy in patients receiving long-term warfarin therapy. Mayo Clin Proc 79(11):1396–1401, 2004 15544018

Mueller PS, Schak KM, Barnes RD, et al: Safety of electroconvulsive therapy in patients with asthma. Neth J Med 64(11):417–421, 2006 17179572

Mueller PS, Barnes RD, Nishimura R, et al: The safety of electroconvulsive therapy in patients with severe aortic stenosis. Mayo Clin Proc 82(11):1360–1363, 2007 17976355

Netzel PJ, Mueller PS, Rummans TA, et al: Safety, efficacy, and effects on glycemic control of electroconvulsive therapy in insulin-requiring type 2 diabetic patients. J ECT 18(1):16–21, 2002 11925516

Nuttall GA, Bowersox MR, Douglass SB, et al: Morbidity and mortality in the use of electroconvulsive therapy. J ECT 20(4):237–241, 2004 15591857

O'Connor CJ, Rothenberg DM, Soble JS, et al: The effect of esmolol pretreatment on the incidence of regional wall motion abnormalities during electroconvulsive therapy. Anesth Analg 82(1):143–147, 1996 8712391

Okamura T, Kudo K, Sata N, et al: Electroconvulsive therapy after coil embolization of cerebral aneurysm: a case report and literature review. J ECT 22(2):148–149, 2006 16801833

Patkar AA, Hill KP, Weinstein SP, et al: ECT in the presence of brain tumor and increased intracranial pressure: evaluation and reduction of risk. J ECT 16(2):189–197, 2000 10868329

Perry CL, Lindell EP, Rasmussen KG: ECT in patients with arachnoid cysts. J ECT 23(1):36–37, 2007 17435574

Petrides G, Fink M: Atrial fibrillation, anticoagulation, and electroconvulsive therapy. Convuls Ther 12(2):91–98, 1996 8744168

Rasmussen KG: The role of electroconvulsive therapy in chronic pain. Reviews in Analgesia 7(1):1–8, 2003

Rasmussen KG, Flemming KD: Electroconvulsive therapy in patients with cavernous hemangiomas. J ECT 22(4):272–273, 2006 17143161

Rasmussen KG, Rummans TA: Electroconvulsive therapy for phantom limb pain. Pain 85(1–2):297–299, 2000 10692632

Rasmussen KG, Rummans TA: Electroconvulsive therapy in the management of chronic pain. Curr Pain Headache Rep 6(1):17–22, 2002 11749873

Rasmussen KG, Ryan DA: The effect of electroconvulsive therapy treatments on blood sugar in nondiabetic patients. J ECT 21(4):232–234, 2005 16301883

Rasmussen KG, Jarvis MR, Zorumski CF, et al: Low-dose atropine in electroconvulsive therapy. J ECT 15(3):213–221, 1999 10492860

Rasmussen KG, Mueller M, Kellner CH, et al: Patterns of psychotropic medication use among patients with severe depression referred for electroconvulsive therapy: data from the Consortium for Research on Electroconvulsive Therapy. J ECT 22(2):116–123, 2006a 16801827

Rasmussen KG, Ryan DA, Mueller PS: Blood glucose before and after ECT treatments in type 2 diabetic patients. J ECT 22(2):124–126, 2006b 16801828

Rasmussen KG, Mohan A, Stevens SR: Serum sodium does not correlate with seizure length or seizure threshold in electroconvulsive therapy. J ECT 23(3):175–176, 2007a 17804992

Rasmussen KG, Perry CL, Sutor B, Moore KM: ECT in patients with intracranial masses. J Neuropsychiatry Clin Neurosci 19(2):191–193, 2007b 17431067

Rasmussen KG, Albin SM, Mueller PS, et al: Electroconvulsive therapy in patients taking steroid medication: should supplemental doses be given on the days of treatment? J ECT 24(2):128–130, 2008 18580555

Rice EH, Sombrotto LB, Markowitz JC, et al: Cardiovascular morbidity in high-risk patients during ECT. Am J Psychiatry 151(11):1637–1641, 1994 7943453

Rivera FA, Lapid MI, Sampson S, et al: Safety of electroconvulsive therapy in patients with a history of heart failure and decreased left ventricular systolic heart function. J ECT 27(3):207–213, 2011 21865957

Rossi S, Hallett M, Rossini PM, et al; Safety of TMS Consensus Group: Safety, ethical considerations, and application guidelines for the use of transcranial magnetic stimulation in clinical practice and research. Clin Neurophysiol 120(12):2008–2039, 2009 19833552

Ruwitch JF, Perez JE, Miller TR, et al: Myocardial ischemia induced by electroconvulsive therapy (abstract 2034). Circulation 90 (suppl 4, pt 2):I379, 1994

Schak KM, Mueller PS, Barnes RD, et al: The safety of ECT in patients with chronic obstructive pulmonary disease. Psychosomatics 49(3):208–211, 2008 18448774

Sharma A, Ramaswamy S, Bhatia SC: Electroconvulsive therapy after repair of cerebral aneurysm. J ECT 21(3):180–181, 2005 16127310

Sienaert P, Peuskens J: Anticonvulsants during electroconvulsive therapy: review and recommendations. J ECT 23(2):120–123, 2007 17548985

Spodniaková B, Halmo M, Nosáľová P: Electroconvulsive therapy in pregnancy—a review. J Obstet Gynaecol 35(7):659–662, 2015 25526509

Stern L, Hirschmann S, Grunhaus L: ECT in patients with major depressive disorder and low cardiac output. Convuls Ther 13(2):68–73, 1997 9253526

Tang W-K, Ungvari GS: Asystole during electroconvulsive therapy: a case report. Aust N Z J Psychiatry 35(3):382–385, 2001 11437814

Zielinski RJ, Roose SP, Devanand DP, et al: Cardiovascular complications of ECT in depressed patients with cardiac disease. Am J Psychiatry 150(6):904–909, 1993 8494067

Zvara DA, Brooker RF, McCall WV, et al: The effect of esmolol on ST-segment depression and arrhythmias after electroconvulsive therapy. Convuls Ther 13(3):165–174, 1997 9342132

CHAPTER 39

Palliative Care

Andrew Edelstein, M.D.

Yesne Alici, M.D.

William Breitbart, M.D.

Harvey Max Chochinov, M.D., Ph.D., FRCPC

One of the most challenging roles for the psychosomatic medicine psychiatrist is to help guide terminally ill patients physically, psychologically, and spiritually through the dying process. Patients with advanced cancer, AIDS, and other life-threatening medical illnesses are at increased risk for developing major psychiatric complications and have an enormous burden of both physical and psychological symptoms. Psychological symptoms such as depression, anxiety, and hopelessness are as frequent as, if not more frequent than, pain and other physical symptoms (Portenoy et al. 1994; Vogl et al. 1999). The psychiatrist, as a consultant to or member of a palliative care team, has a unique role in compassionate palliative care.

In 1999 the Academy of Psychosomatic Medicine published a position statement titled "Psychiatric Aspects of Excellent End-of-Life Care" (Shuster et al. 1999), which stressed the importance of psychiatric issues and the need for competent psychiatric care to be an integral component of palliative care. Major books have provided comprehensive reviews of the interface of psychiatry and palliative medicine (Breitbart and Alici 2014; Chochinov and Breitbart 2012), and an international journal with that focus has been in existence since 2003 (Breitbart 2003a).

The importance of the psychiatric, psychosocial, and spiritual aspects of palliative care has also been recognized in reports from the American Board of Internal Medicine (Subcommittee on Psychiatric Aspects of Life-Sustaining Technology 1996), the Institute of Medicine (Field and Cassel 1997; Foley and Helband 2001), the National Comprehensive Cancer Network (Levy et al. 2009), the U.S. Health Resources and Services Administration (O'Neill et al. 2003), and the National Consensus Project for Quality Palliative Care (2013). Several prominent national and international palliative

We would like to thank Ms. Shaunna Beckford for her editorial assistance in the preparation of this manuscript.

care organizations also exist, and more than 10 national and international palliative care scientific journals have been published (Stjernsward and Clark 2004).

In this chapter we summarize the most salient aspects of effective psychiatric care of individuals with advanced, life-threatening medical illnesses, including basic concepts of palliative care, as well as the assessment and management of common psychiatric disorders in this population. We describe the psychotherapies developed for use in palliative care settings and then discuss spirituality, grief and bereavement, and psychiatric contributions to the control of common physical symptoms.

Related topics are discussed elsewhere in this book, including advance directives and end-of-life decisions (see Chapter 2, "Legal and Ethical Issues," and Chapter 3, "Psychological Responses to Illness"), physician-assisted suicide (see Chapter 8, "Suicidality"), dialysis discontinuation (see Chapter 20, "Renal Disease"), and pain management (see Chapter 34, "Pain").

Palliative Care

Historical Perspectives

The term *palliation* is derived from the Latin root word *palliare*, which means "to cloak" or "to conceal." *Pallium* also refers to the cloth that covers or cloaks burial caskets. These root words suggest that the patient can be "cloaked" or "embraced" in the comforting arms of the caregiver, and treatment can be aimed at providing comfort irrespective of curative status.

The terms *palliative care* and *palliative medicine* are often used interchangeably. *Palliative medicine* refers to the medical discipline of palliative care. The nature and focus of palliative care have evolved, expanding beyond just comfort for the dying to include palliation and symptom control that begins with the onset of a life-threatening illness and proceeds past death to include bereavement interventions for family and others (Sepúlveda et al. 2002).

Modern palliative care is an outgrowth of the hospice movement, which began with Calvaires in Lyon, France, in the 1840s; continued with St. Joseph's Hospice in London, established in 1902; and culminated with St. Christopher's Hospice in London, established in 1967 by Cicely Saunders. By 1975, a large number of independent hospices had been established in the United Kingdom, Canada, and Australia. The first hospice in the United States was established in 1974 in Connecticut. Soon after, the U.S. government established limited Medicare coverage for hospice benefits. The first Canadian palliative care program was founded at Royal Victoria Hospital in Montreal. Hospital-based pain and palliative care consultation services were developed, such as the pain service established in 1978 by Kathleen Foley at the Memorial Sloan-Kettering Cancer Center (Canadian Palliative Care Association 1995). Modern palliative care thus evolved from the hospice movement into clinical care delivery systems that had components of home care and hospital-based services (Stjernsward and Clark 2004).

Evolving Definitions

At its inception, palliative care was circumscribed to terminally ill patients, or those deemed ineligible for traditional, life-prolonging treatment (Palliative Care Foundation 1981, p. 10). Over the span of decades, the role of palliation has transformed from an alternative to curative treatment to an important adjunct. Empirical data have shown that palliative intervention initiated close to initial diagnosis correlates with improved quality of life (Temel et al. 2010). In recognition of the expanded role of palliative care in the United States, the Department of Health and Human Services Centers for Medicare & Medicaid Services defined palliative care as

> Patient and family centered care that optimizes quality of life by anticipating, preventing, and treating suffering. Palliative care throughout the continuum of illness involves addressing physical, intellectual, emotional, social and spiritual needs and [facilitating] patient autonomy, access to information and choice. (73 Federal Register 32204, June 5, 2008)

This definition also emphasizes a multidisciplinary approach, in which mental health plays a pivotal, if not central, role.

Models of Care Delivery

Palliative care is not restricted to people who are dying, but rather can be applied to the control of symptoms in and the provision of support to those living with chronic life-threatening illnesses.

Model palliative care programs ideally include all of the following components: 1) a home care (e.g., hospice) program; 2) a hospital-based palliative care consultation service; 3) a day care program or ambulatory care clinic; 4) a palliative care inpatient unit (or dedicated palliative care beds in a hospital); 5) a bereavement program; 6) training and research programs; and 7) Internet-based services. An updated U.S. national expert consensus process led to publication of the third edition of the *Clinical Practice Guidelines for Quality Palliative Care* (National Consensus Project for Quality Palliative Care 2013).

Psychiatry at End of Life in the United States

What Is a "Good" Death?

A meaningful dying process is one throughout which the patient is physically, psychologically, spiritually, and emotionally supported by his or her family, friends, and caregivers. Weisman (1972) identified four criteria required for what he called an "appropriate death": 1) internal conflicts, such as fears about loss of control, should be reduced as much as possible; 2) the individual's personal sense of identity should be sustained; 3) critical relationships should be enhanced or at least maintained, and conflicts should be resolved, if possible; and 4) the person should be encouraged to set and attempt to reach meaningful goals, even though limited, such as attending a graduation, a wedding, or the birth of a child, as a way of providing a sense of continuity into the future. The World Health Organization (WHO) (2017) characterized a "good" death as one that is 1) free from avoidable distress and suffering for patient, family, and caregivers; 2) in general accord with the patient's and family's wishes; and 3) reasonably consistent with clinical, cultural, and ethical standards. Weisman's criteria and the WHO guidelines can serve as general principles for psychiatrists in caring for the dying.

What Is the Role of the Psychiatrist?

The traditional role of the psychiatrist is broadened in several ways in the care of the dying patient. The psychiatrist's primary role in the palliative care setting is the diagnosis and treatment of comorbid psychiatric disorders. Consultation-liaison psychiatrists can provide expert care and teaching about the management of depression, suicide, anxiety, delirium, fatigue, and pain in terminally ill patients (Chochinov and Breitbart 2012).

The role of the psychiatrist in the care of the dying extends beyond management of psychiatric symptoms and syndromes to encompass existential issues, family and caregiver support, bereavement, doctor–patient communication, and education and training. Psychiatrists can play an important role in addressing social, psychological, ethical, and spiritual issues that complicate the care of dying patients.

Psychiatrists also have a role in encouraging discussion of end-of-life ethical decisions regarding treatment provision or nonprovision (e.g., withholding of resuscitation, withdrawal of life support). The capacity of the patient to make rational judgments and/or the ability of the proxy to make appropriate decisions for the patient may require psychiatric evaluation. The decision to withdraw life support is highly emotional and may require psychiatric consultation (Subcommittee on Psychiatric Aspects of Life-Sustaining Technology 1996). Psychiatrists can assist in teaching providers how to deliver bad news and discuss do-not-resuscitate (DNR) orders and other treatment preferences, ideally with the patient, or with family members when the patient is incapacitated (Levin et al. 2008; Weissman 2004).

Psychiatric Disorders in the Palliative Care Setting

Patients with advanced disease are particularly vulnerable to psychiatric disorders and complications (Breitbart et al. 1995; Miovic and Block 2007). Unfortunately, medical specialists frequently fail to recognize emotional distress and common psychiatric disorders in terminally ill patients (Breitbart and Alici 2008; Miovic and Block 2007). In this section we review psychiatric disorders frequently encountered in palliative care settings, including anxiety disorders, depression, and delirium. The incidence, assessment, and treatment of psychiatric disorders in specific advanced diseases are discussed in earlier chapters in this volume.

Anxiety Disorders and Posttraumatic Stress Disorder

Prevalence

Estimates of the prevalence of anxiety disorders in palliative care settings have ranged from 15% to 28% (Kerrihard et al. 1999; Pidgeon et al. 2016). Mixed anxiety and depressive symptoms are more common than anxiety alone (Roth and Massie 2009). Anxiety prevalence increases with advancing disease and decline in the patient's physical status (Rabkin et al. 1997). Brandberg et al. (1995) reported that 28% of patients with advanced melanoma were anxious compared with 15% of control subjects. In the Canadian National Palliative Care Survey (Wilson et al. 2007), 24.4% of the patients receiving palliative care for cancer were found to have at least one

DSM-IV (American Psychiatric Association 1994) anxiety or depressive disorder. The prevalence of anxiety disorders in that survey was 13.9%. Younger patients and those with a lower performance status, smaller social networks, and less participation in organized religious services were more likely to have a psychiatric disorder. Compared with patients without a psychiatric disorder, those who met criteria for a DSM-IV anxiety and/or depressive disorder reported more severe distress in interviews assessing a range of common physical symptoms, social concerns, and existential issues (Wilson et al. 2007).

Assessment

Anxiety can occur in terminally ill patients as an adjustment disorder, a disease- or treatment-related condition, or an exacerbation of a preexisting anxiety disorder (Kerrihard et al. 1999; Massie 1989). Adjustment disorder with anxiety is often related to coping with the existential crisis and the uncertainty of the prognosis and the future (Holland 1989). When faced with terminal illness, patients with preexisting anxiety disorders are at risk for reactivation of symptoms. Generalized anxiety disorder or panic disorder is apt to recur, especially in the presence of dyspnea or pain. Patients with phobias will have an especially difficult time if the disease or treatment confronts them with their fears (e.g., claustrophobia, fear of needles, fear of isolation). Posttraumatic stress disorder (PTSD)[1] may be activated in dying patients as their circumstances remind them of prior traumatic experiences (e.g., intensive care unit stays). Patients with PTSD may present with high levels of anxiety, insomnia, frequent panic attacks, comorbid depressive symptoms, and avoidance of medical settings that trigger traumatic memories (Miovic and Block 2007).

Symptoms of anxiety in the terminally ill individual may arise from a medical complication of the illness or its treatment (Breitbart et al. 1995; Roth and Massie 2009). Hypoxia, sepsis, poorly controlled pain, medication side effects such as akathisia, and withdrawal states often present as anxiety (Miovic and Block 2007). In a patient who is dying, anxiety can represent impending cardiac or respiratory arrest, pulmonary embolism, sepsis, electrolyte imbalance, or dehydration. During the terminal phase of illness, when patients become less alert, there is a tendency to minimize the use of sedating medications. It is important to slowly taper benzodiazepines and opioids, which may have been sustained at high doses to provide extended relief of anxiety or pain, in order to prevent acute withdrawal. Withdrawal in terminally ill patients often manifests first as agitation or anxiety and becomes clinically evident days later than might be expected in younger, healthier patients because of impaired metabolism.

As disease progresses, patients' anxiety may include fears about the disease process, the clinical course, possible treatment outcomes, and death. Separation anxiety may intensify, as well as fear of the increasing financial consequences of treatment.

Despite the fact that anxiety in terminal illness commonly results from medical complications, it is important to consider psychological factors that may play a role, particularly in individuals who are alert and not confused (Holland 1989; Roth and

---

[1] In DSM-5, PTSD is now classified with the Trauma- and Stressor-Related Disorders, but for the purposes of this discussion it remains grouped with the Anxiety Disorders.

Massie 2009). Patients frequently fear the isolation and separation of death. Claustrophobic patients may fear the idea of being confined and buried in a coffin. These issues can be disconcerting to consultants, who may find themselves at a loss for words that might console the patient.

Treatment

The most effective management of anxiety is multimodal and usually involves a combination of psychotherapy and pharmacological management. The treatment of anxiety in terminal illness has been extensively reviewed (Breitbart et al. 1995; Levin and Alici 2010; Roth and Massie 2009) and is similar in most respects to its treatment in the medically ill in general (see Chapter 10, "Anxiety Disorders," Chapter 36, "Psychopharmacology," and Chapter 37, "Psychotherapy"). We note here selected aspects specific to the terminally ill.

Pharmacological treatment.   For patients who feel persistently anxious, the first-line antianxiety drugs are the benzodiazepines. For patients with severely compromised hepatic function, lorazepam, oxazepam, or temazepam is preferred, as these agents have no active metabolites (Roth and Massie 2009). To control anxiety, restlessness, and agitation in the final days of life, dying patients can be administered diazepam rectally when no other route is available, with dosages equivalent to those used in oral regimens. Clonazepam is available in an orally disintegrating formulation for patients with swallowing difficulties. See also the section "Alternative Routes of Administration" in Chapter 36. However, a Cochrane review of pharmacotherapy for anxiety in palliative care concluded that there was lack of high-quality evidence on the role of antianxiety medications in terminally ill patients (Salt et al. 2017). In anxious patients with severely compromised pulmonary function, benzodiazepines may suppress central respiratory mechanisms, making them unsafe. Low dosages of an antipsychotic or an antihistamine can be useful, but the anticholinergic effects of antihistamines make them problematic in debilitated patients prone to develop delirium. Anxiety symptoms in patients with delirium are better treated with antipsychotics than with benzodiazepines (Breitbart et al. 1996); however, none of the antipsychotics have been systematically studied in the treatment of anxiety among patients receiving palliative care (Levin and Alici 2010; Salt et al. 2017).

Sedating antidepressants such as trazodone or mirtazapine may help patients with persistent anxiety, insomnia, and anorexia. Selective serotonin reuptake inhibitors (SSRIs) are also effective in the management of anxiety disorders (Roth and Massie 2009). The utility of antidepressants and buspirone for anxiety disorders is often limited in the dying patient because they require weeks to achieve therapeutic effect.

Opioids are primarily indicated for pain but are also effective in relieving dyspnea and associated anxiety (Elia and Thomas 2008). Continuous intravenous infusions of morphine or other narcotic analgesics allow for careful titration and control of respiratory distress, anxiety, pain, and agitation (Portenoy and Foley 1989). Occasionally one must maintain the patient in a state of unresponsiveness to maximize comfort. When respiratory distress is not a major problem, it is preferable to use opioids solely for analgesia, and anxiolytics for concomitant anxiety.

Nonpharmacological treatment.   Nonpharmacological interventions for anxiety in palliative care settings include supportive psychotherapy, behavioral interventions, meaning-centered psychotherapy (MCP), and cognitive-behavioral therapy (CBT), used alone or in combination (see discussion later in this chapter and in Chapters 10 and 37). Brief supportive psychotherapy is often useful in dealing with both crises and existential issues confronted by the terminally ill (Roth and Massie 2009). Supportive–expressive group therapy has been shown to reduce distress and subsyndromal symptoms of PTSD in women with advanced breast cancer (Classen et al. 2001). Inclusion of the family in psychotherapeutic interventions should be considered, particularly as the patient with advanced illness becomes increasingly debilitated and less able to interact.

Relaxation, guided imagery, and hypnosis may help reduce anxiety and thereby increase the patient's sense of control. Many patients with advanced illness are still appropriate candidates for the use of behavioral techniques despite physical debilitation. A feasibility study of a brief cognitive-behavioral intervention demonstrated that it reduced anxiety and depression symptoms in a small population of hospice patients (Anderson et al. 2008). However, the utility of such interventions for terminally ill patients is limited by the degree of the patients' mental clarity (Breitbart et al. 1995). In some cases, techniques can be modified so as to include even mildly cognitively impaired patients. This involves the therapist taking a more active role by orienting the patient, creating a safe and secure environment, and evoking a conditioned response to his or her voice or presence. A typical behavioral intervention for anxiety in a terminally ill patient would include a relaxation exercise combined with some distraction or imagery technique. The patient is first taught to relax using passive breathing accompanied by either passive or active muscle relaxation. When in a relaxed state, the patient is taught a pleasant, distracting imagery exercise. Of course, relaxation techniques can be prescribed concurrently with anxiolytic medications in highly anxious terminal patients.

Depression

See also Chapter 7, "Depression," for additional information.

Epidemiology

Studies investigating psychiatric comorbidity in palliative care patients with advanced cancer suggest a major depressive disorder (MDD) prevalence of roughly 20% (Austin et al. 2011; Wilson et al. 2007), with variations based on population studied and screening tool used. For example, the Canadian National Palliative Care Survey found a prevalence rate of 20.7% for any depressive disorder among patients ($n=381$) receiving palliative care (Wilson et al. 2007), while studies in Australia using the Hospital Anxiety and Depression Scale (HADS) estimated that 45.8% of patients were "possibly depressed" (HADS score ≥ 8) and 22.7% were "probably depressed" (HADS score ≥ 11) (O'Connor et al. 2010). Family history of depression and history of previous depressive episodes further increase the patient's risk of developing a depressive episode (Miovic and Block 2007). Loss of meaning and low scores on measures of spiritual well-being have been associated with higher levels of depressive symptoms (Nelson et al. 2002). Depression is associated with poor treatment compliance, reduced quality of life, lower survival, and desire for hastened death among terminally ill patients (Breitbart et al. 2000; Chochinov et al. 1995; Lloyd-Williams et al. 2009; Potash and Breitbart 2002; van der Lee et al. 2005). Many studies have also found correlations among depression, pain, and functional status (Breitbart 1989; Potash and Breitbart 2002; Wilson et al. 2007). Gender can be an important mediator for all these factors. In one study conducted at a southeast London hospice, terminally ill men were nearly twice as likely as terminally ill women to be depressed (25.7% vs. 12.8%) (Hayes et al. 2012). The study authors attributed this difference to relative difficulty coping with physical dependence on others; in patients who were physically dependent, 37.8% of the men were depressed, compared with 2.4% of the women. Younger age and inadequate social support have also been identified as risk factors for depression in the terminally ill (Potash and Breitbart 2002).

Additional treatment factors include corticosteroids (Stiefel et al. 1989), chemotherapeutic agents, amphotericin, whole brain radiation, metabolic endocrine complications, and paraneoplastic syndromes, all of which can cause depressive symptoms (Potash and Breitbart 2002). The phenomenological similarities between depression and "sickness behavior syndrome" have led researchers to consider the role of proinflammatory cytokines in the development of depressive syndromes among patients with advanced disease (Jacobson et al. 2008).

Assessment

Depressed mood and sadness can be appropriate responses as the patient faces death. These emotions can be manifestations of anticipatory grief over the impending loss of one's life, health, loved ones, and autonomy (Block et al. 2000). Despite this, MDD is common in the palliative care setting, where it may be underdiagnosed and undertreated. Minimization of depressive symptoms as "normal reactions" and the difficulties of accurately diagnosing depression in the terminally ill both contribute to the underdiagnosis of depression, and undertreatment is due in part to the concern that severely medically ill patients will be unable to tolerate antidepressant side effects (Block et al. 2000). However, clinicians have become more vigilant in recognition and treatment of depression in the medically ill (Wilson et al. 2009). Strategies for accurately diagnosing depression in seriously medically ill patients are reviewed in Chapter 7. A detailed description of their application in palliative care settings can be found in Wilson et al. (2009).

The diagnosis of a major depressive syndrome in a terminally ill individual, as in medically ill patients in general, often relies more on the psychological or cognitive symptoms of MDD than on the neurovegetative ones. Relying on the psychological symptoms of depression for diagnostic specificity is not without problems. How is the clinician to interpret feelings of hopelessness in the dying patient when there is no hope for cure or recovery? Feelings of hopelessness, worthlessness, or suicidal ideation should be explored in detail. Although many dying patients lose hope for a cure, they are able to maintain hope for better symptom control. For many patients, hope is contingent on the ability to find continued meaning in their day-to-day existence. Hopelessness that is pervasive and accompanied by a sense of despair or despondency is more likely to represent a symptom of a depressive disorder. Such patients often state that they feel they are burdening their families unfairly, causing them great pain and inconvenience. MDD is even more likely in individuals who feel that their life has never had any worth or that their illness is punishment for evil things they have done. Even mild and passive forms of suicidal ideation are very often indicative of significant degrees of depression in terminally ill patients (Breitbart 1990).

Several screening instruments have been studied for detection of depression in palliative care settings, and a detailed description of these instruments can be found elsewhere (Wilson et al. 2009). Chochinov et al. (1997) studied brief screening instruments to measure depression in the terminally ill, including a single item assessing depressed mood ("Have you been depressed most of the time for the past 2 weeks?"), two items assessing depressed mood and loss of interest in activities, a visual analogue scale for depressed mood, and the Beck Depression Inventory. Semistructured diagnostic interviews served as the standard against which the screening performance of the four brief screening methods was assessed. The single-item question had a 100% concordance with diagnostic interviews, substantially outperforming the questionnaire and visual analogue measures, as well as marginally better specificity compared with the two-item screen (which generated occasional false positives). Although this specific study has not been replicated, more recent two-item screens based on the Palliative care Outcome Scale (POS) have been tested (Antunes et al. 2015). Combining two questions ("Is life worth living?" and "Do you feel good about yourself?") appeared to yield higher sensitivity compared with asking each question individually, showing an overall negative predictive value of 89.4%.

Treatment

Treatment of depression in the medically ill is reviewed in detail in Chapters 7, 36, and 37. Here we note specific aspects relevant to palliative care. A combination of pharmacotherapy, supportive psychotherapy, CBT, and psychoeducation is the mainstay of treatment for depression in palliative care settings (Miovic and Block 2007; Wilson et al. 2000). It is important to treat distressing physical symptoms (e.g., pain, dyspnea, nausea) concurrently while managing depression in patients with advanced disease (Potash and Breitbart 2002).

Pharmacological treatment.   Antidepressants are the mainstay of pharmacological management for gravely ill patients with symptoms that meet diagnostic criteria for MDD (Block et al. 2000; Wilson et al. 2000) and have established efficacy (Wilson et al. 2000, 2009). Factors such as prognosis and the time frame for treatment play an important role in determining the choice of pharmacotherapy for depression in the terminally ill. Unlike a depressed patient with only days or weeks to live, a depressed patient with several months of life expectancy can afford to wait the 2–4 weeks it may take to respond to a standard antidepressant. For terminally ill patients, antidepressants are usually initiated at approximately half the usual starting dosage because of patients' sensitivity to adverse effects. Recent meta-analyses suggest that antidepressants show their clearest benefit after 6 weeks of treatment, consistent with the current consensus favoring SSRIs; however, the significance of these findings is potentially clouded by high levels of publication bias favoring medication (Rayner et al. 2011; Ujeyl and Müller-Oerlinghausen 2012). In view of the time required for antidepressants to exert their effects, a depressed individual with less than 3 weeks to live may derive more benefit from a rapid-acting psychostimulant (Block et al. 2000; Homsi et al. 2001). Similarly, a distressed or agitated patient who is within hours or days of death may derive the most benefit from sedatives or from opioid infusions.

Psychostimulants are particularly helpful in the treatment of depression in the terminally ill because they have a rapid onset of action and energizing effects and typically do not cause anorexia, weight loss, or insomnia at therapeutic doses (M. Candy et al. 2008). In fact, at low doses, stimulants may actually increase appetite. Abuse is almost always an irrelevant concern in the terminally ill, and stimulants should not be withheld on the basis of a patient's previous history of substance abuse. Occasionally, treatment with an SSRI and a psychostimulant may be initiated concurrently so that depressed patients may receive the immediate benefits of the psychostimulant while waiting for the SSRI to work. At that point the psychostimulant may be withdrawn. Methylphenidate and dextroamphetamine are usually initiated at low dosages (2.5–5.0 mg in the morning and at noon). The benefits can be assessed during the first 1–2 days of treatment and the dose gradually titrated (usually to no greater than 30 mg/day total). An additional benefit of stimulants is that they reduce sedation secondary to opioids and provide adjuvant analgesic effects (Bruera et al. 1987). A review of 19 controlled trials of methylphenidate in medically ill older adults and patients in palliative care concluded that low-dose methylphenidate was well tolerated in the treatment of depression, fatigue, or apathy (Hardy 2009); however, evidence of treatment effectiveness is lacking (Sullivan et al. 2017). Modafinil and armodafinil produce increased alertness, wakefulness, and energy and might relieve depressive symptoms in palliative care settings.

Nonpharmacological treatment.   Depression in cancer patients with advanced disease is optimally managed with a combination of supportive psychotherapy, cognitive-behavioral techniques, psychoeducation, and antidepressants as discussed above. A recent meta-analysis of psychotherapeutic interventions, in the form of either individual or group counseling, demonstrated significant reductions in psychological distress and depressive symptoms in patients with advanced-stage cancer (Okuyama et al. 2017). However, this analysis spanned several decades of data, from the first published study of social support groups (Spiegel et al. 1981) to a more recent study of CBT (Greer et al. 2012), thus yielding considerable heterogeneity and limiting generalizability. Further research is needed to establish an evidence-based psychotherapeutic approach for treating depression in the palliative care setting, ideally expanded beyond English-speaking countries.

Suicidality, Demoralization, and Desire for Hastened Death

Suicide and suicidal ideation, particularly in the context of major medical illness, are important and serious consequences of unrecognized or inadequately treated clinical depression (see also Chapter 8, "Suicidality"). However, in the palliative care setting, it is also important to recognize a distinct clinical entity, desire for hastened death, which can be distressing for family members and providers as well as for the patient. Although clinical depression has been demonstrated to be a critically important factor in the desire for hastened death, diligent exploration of other factors that may lead terminally ill patients to wish or seek to hasten their own death remains a key obligation in the practice of palliative care.

Suicide in the Palliative Care Setting

A discussion of the legal and ethical implications of suicide in the terminally ill is beyond the scope of this chapter (see the section "Physician-Assisted Suicide" in Chapter 8). However, physicians are always obligated to treat distress, and it is important to identify and attempt to help vulnerable individuals before they take irreversible actions. A major challenge in the study of suicide in this population is the relative rarity of its occurrence or reporting. In two separate large-scale studies of patients in palliative care treatment (N=72,633 [Grzybowska and Finlay 1997] and N=17,964 [Ripamonti et al. 1999]), the respective suicide incidences were 0.027% and 0.029%.

Although terminally ill patients have the same risk factors for suicide that other medically ill populations have, certain risk factors are more prevalent in terminally ill patients and warrant special attention. In a "psychological autopsy" of five terminally ill patients who completed suicide, common themes included loss of control and autonomy (either anticipated or realized), fear of being a burden to others, uncontrolled pain, and profound hopelessness (Filiberti et al. 2001). It should be noted that these patients were part of a cohort of 17,594 patients who had similar diagnoses and degrees of distress but who did not commit suicide. These cases again highlight the low incidence of suicide in terminally ill patients—and, as a consequence, the low predictive value of any risk factor identified. Thus, the goal of the treating psychiatrist must extend beyond prevention of suicide to encompass identification and treatment of distress that can lead to it.

Broaching the topic of transition into purely palliative or comfort care should also be performed with care, and without the supposition that the patient will no longer receive treatment. In Scandinavia, the highest incidence of suicide was found in cancer patients who were offered no further treatment and no further contact with the health care system (Bolund 1985; Louhivuori and Hakama 1979). Palliative care offers hope in various forms: that patients can control aspects of their disease and symptoms and that they will continue to be connected to medical providers and others.

Suicidal Ideation

It is widely held that most terminally ill patients experience occasional thoughts of suicide as a means of escaping the threat of being overwhelmed by their illness ("If it gets too bad, I always have a way out") and will reveal such thoughts to a sensitive interviewer. However, some studies suggest that suicidal ideation is relatively infrequent and is limited to individuals who are significantly depressed (Brown et al. 1986). Studies examining the prevalence of suicidal ideation among patients with advanced cancer have reported estimates of 8.9% (Spencer et al. 2012) and 15.3% (Zhong et al. 2017). In these studies, clinical markers of suicidal ideation included low social and spiritual support, heightened physical distress, and a sense of helplessness and low self-efficacy. Patients who reported suicidal ideation had higher rates of comorbid PTSD (Spencer et al. 2012). Notably, patients who had accessed mental health services were more likely to report suicidal ideation (Spencer et al. 2012), a finding that may indicate nothing more than that these patients were more comfortable disclosing their thoughts to interviewers; however, it might also suggest that the mental health care interventions these patients received were ineffective in reducing their thoughts of suicide.

Desire for Hastened Death

Desire for hastened death may be thought of as a unifying construct underlying requests for assisted suicide or euthanasia as well as suicidal thoughts in general. Such desires often arise in the context of demoralization (discussed in greater detail below), in which the individual's identity and sense of future self are suppressed by a life-consuming illness or a disability (Kissane et al. 2001). This existential crisis of despair often leads to negative cognitions of personal failure, perceived helplessness, and being a burden on others, behaviorally manifesting in amotivation and social alienation, and ultimately leading to desire for hastened death. The prevalence of desire for hastened death varies based on intensity. For example, in studies in palliative care units, 45% of patients expressed "a fleeting desire to die," whereas only 9%–17% maintained a consistent desire for death (Breitbart et al. 2000; Chochinov et al. 1995). A study of Canadian palliative care programs found that 35% of patients experienced at least fleeting thoughts, with 12.2% expressing a moderate (stable but not all-consuming) to extreme (constant and pervasive) wish for death (Wilson et al. 2016). This latter group had a high prevalence of mental illness (52%), consistent with prior reports. Patients with a significant desire for hastened death but without a mental disorder still reported increased distress from physical, social, and existential difficulties. Thus, desire for hastened death should prompt clinicians to take inventory of the various somatic and psychosocial concerns affecting the patient, because it is often a red flag for other sources of distress.

Researchers have also explored the desire for hastened death among patients with a better illness prognosis to determine whether similar contributing factors play a role in this population (Rodin et al. 2007; Rosenfeld et al. 2006). In a sample of metastatic cancer patients with an expected prognosis of 6 months or longer, 5% of patients had a high desire for hastened death, a relatively lower rate compared with the 17% rate among patients with less than 1 month of survival expectancy. The desire for hastened death significantly correlated with high levels of depression and hopelessness in all the individuals in that sample (Rodin et al. 2007).

A recent cross-sectional study of 162 patients in palliative care in Australia explored factors that could potentially mediate the relationship between lower quality of life and desire for hastened death. Depression, loss of a sense of meaning/purpose, and low perceived control were deemed important mediators, while factors such as high levels of distress and reduced coping showed less significance (Robinson et al. 2017). Brief, easy-to-use validated measures are available, such as the six-item Schedule of Attitudes toward Hastened Death—abbreviated version (SAHD-A) (Kolva et al. 2017).

Demoralization

Kissane et al. (2001) described a syndrome of "demoralization" in the terminally ill that is distinct from depression and consists of a triad of hopelessness, loss of meaning, and existential distress expressed as a desire for death. It is associated with life-threatening medical illness, disability, bodily disfigurement, fear, loss of dignity, social isolation, and feelings of being a burden (Kissane et al. 2009). Because of the sense of impotence and hopelessness, those with the syndrome predictably progress to a desire to die or commit suicide. A brief five-item instrument, the Short Demoralization Scale (Galiana et al. 2017), is available for assessment of demoralization.

Interventions for Despair at the End of Life

Kissane et al. (2001) describe a multidisciplinary, multimodal treatment approach for demoralization consisting of 1) ensuring continuity of care and active symptom management; 2) ensuring dignity in the dying process; 3) using various types of psychotherapy to help sustain a sense of meaning, limit cognitive distortions, and maintain family relationships (i.e., meaning-based, cognitive-behavioral, interpersonal, and family psychotherapy interventions); 4) using life review and narrative and attention to spiritual issues; and 5) administering pharmacotherapy for comorbid anxiety, depression, and delirium.

Studies have demonstrated that desire for hastened death can often be ameliorated through treatment of depression with antidepressants (Breitbart et al. 2010a). If the treatment of depression reduces the wish for hastened death, it may also result in increased desire for life-sustaining medical therapies (Ganzini et al. 1994). When practical, decisions about withdrawal of treatment in severely depressed individuals—particularly those who feel hopeless—should be delayed until after treatment of their depression.

Psychiatric hospitalizations to prevent suicide offer limited and often undesirable treatment, from both patient and provider perspectives. Given that suicidality is often driven by loss of control and fear of being a burden to others, hospitalization on a locked unit could in fact make symptoms worse. Additionally, psychiatric facilities without medical psychiatry inpatient units are unequipped and unprepared to deal with the high medical comorbidity associated with terminal illness.

Novel psychotherapies have become important tools to address demoralization and existential despair. Specific therapeutic approaches are described in detail in the section "Psychotherapy Interventions in Palliative Care" later in this chapter.

Delirium

Delirium is discussed in detail in Chapter 4, "Delirium"; we focus here on aspects most relevant to palliative care. In the palliative care literature, delirium occurring in the last days of life is often referred to as "terminal delirium," "terminal restlessness," or "terminal agitation." Despite being the most common neuropsychiatric complication of advanced illness, delirium may be underdiagnosed and untreated in palliative care settings. Delirium is a harbinger of impending death among terminally ill patients, and also a significant source of distress for patients, families, and staff. Delirium can interfere dramatically with the recognition and control of other physical and psychological symptoms, such as pain. Palliative care clinicians should thus be familiar with the assessment and management of delirium, as well as the controversies regarding the goals of management in the terminally ill (Breitbart and Alici 2008; Breitbart et al. 2002).

Prevalence

Delirium is the most common and serious neuropsychiatric complication in patients with advanced illnesses such as cancer and AIDS, particularly in the last weeks of life, with prevalence rates ranging from 19% to 58% (de la Cruz et al. 2015; Hosie et al. 2016; Şenel et al. 2017).

The Experience of Delirium for Patients, Families, and Staff

Delirium causes significant distress in patients, families, and staff (Breitbart et al. 2002; Buss et al. 2007; Morita et al. 2004). In a study of terminally ill cancer patients, Breitbart et al. (2002) found that 54% of patients recalled their delirium experience after recovery from delirium. Factors predicting delirium recall included the degree of short-term memory impairment, delirium severity, and the presence of perceptual disturbances (the more severe, the less likely recall). The most significant factor predicting distress for patients was the presence of delusions. Patients with hypoactive delirium were just as distressed as patients with hyperactive delirium. Spousal distress was predicted by patients' Karnofsky Performance Status (the lower the Karnofsky score, the worse the spousal distress), and nurse distress was predicted by delirium severity and perceptual disturbances.

Assessment and Reversibility of Delirium in the Terminally Ill

Reversibility of delirium is often possible even in patients with advanced illness, but it may not be reversible in the last 24–48 hours of life, with the outcome probably attributable to irreversible processes such as multi-organ failure occurring in the final hours of life.

Instruments available for diagnosing and monitoring severity of delirium are described in detail in Chapter 4. Of those, the Delirium Rating Scale—Revised–98 (DRS-R-98), the Memorial Delirium Assessment Scale (MDAS), the Confusion Assessment Method (CAM), and the Delirium Observation Screening (DOS) Scale have been validated in palliative care settings (Breitbart et al. 1997; Jorgensen et al. 2017; Lawlor et al. 2000; Ryan et al. 2009). Lawlor et al. (2000) found that an MDAS cutoff score of 7 out of 30 yielded the highest sensitivity (98%) and specificity (76%) for a delirium diagnosis in patients with advanced cancer in a palliative care unit. In palliative care settings, the CAM had a sensitivity of 88% and a specificity of 100% when administered by well-trained clinicians (Ryan et al. 2009). In the home hospice setting, the DOS had a 92% concordance with the DRS-R-98, with a sensitivity of 97% and specificity of 89% (Jorgensen et al. 2017).

The standard approach to managing delirium, outlined in Chapter 4, remains relevant in the terminally ill, including a search for underlying causes, correction of those factors, and management of the symptoms of delirium (for review, see Grassi et al. 2015; for a practice guideline. see Bush et al. 2014). The ideal and often achievable outcome is a patient who is awake, alert, calm, cognitively intact, not psychotic, and communicating coherently with family and staff. In the terminally ill patient who develops delirium in the last days of life (terminal delirium), the management differs, presenting a number of dilemmas, and the desired clinical outcome may be significantly altered by the dying process.

Delirium can have multiple potential etiologies (see Table 4–4 in Chapter 4). Evaluation should focus on realistically reversible causes while avoiding investigations that would be burdensome for the patient. Physical examination should assess for evidence of infection, fecal impaction, and dehydration. Any medications that could contribute to delirium should be identified. Oximetry can rule out hypoxia; one blood draw can screen for metabolic disturbances (e.g., hypercalcemia) and hematological abnormalities (e.g., anemia, leukocytosis). Brain imaging and cerebrospinal fluid examination may be appropriate if they have the potential to identify lesions amenable to palliative treatment (e.g., radiosensitive central nervous system metastases).

Interventions

Pharmacological

Pharmacotherapy of delirium is reviewed in detail in Chapter 4. Detailed reviews of the use of antipsychotic medications in the treatment of delirium are available elsewhere (Breitbart and Alici 2012; Bush et al. 2014; Grassi et al. 2015). Although no medications have been approved by the U.S. Food and Drug Administration for treatment of delirium, treatment with antipsychotics or sedatives is often required to control the symptoms of delirium in palliative care settings. Low dosages of antipsychotics are usually sufficient for treating delirium in the terminally ill, but high dosages have sometimes been required (Breitbart and Alici 2008, 2012). Haloperidol continues to be the drug of first choice and may be given orally or parenterally (Breitbart and Alici 2008; Breitbart et al. 1996). Delivery of haloperidol by the subcutaneous route is utilized by many palliative care practitioners. The use of antipsychotics for delirium in palliative care remains the subject of active investigation (Agar et al. 2017; B. Candy et al. 2012; Hui et al. 2017).

Psychostimulants—alone or in combination with antipsychotics—have been suggested to be beneficial in treatment of the hypoactive subtype of delirium (Keen and Brown 2004). A systematic review supported the use of methylphenidate in hypoactive delirium, but the evidence was very limited (Elie et al. 2010).

Although antipsychotics are generally beneficial in reducing agitation, anxiety, and confusion in delirium, complete resolution of these symptoms is not always possible in the terminally ill. A significant group (at least 10%–20%) of terminally ill patients experience delirium that can only be controlled by sedation to the point of a significantly decreased level of consciousness (Fainsinger et al. 2000; Lo and Rubenfeld 2005; Rietjens et al. 2008). The goal of treatment in those cases is quiet sedation only with use of sedating agents such as benzodiazepines or propofol (Breitbart and Alici 2008). The alpha$_2$ agonist dexmedetomidine has shown promise, both for its sedating and for its analgesic properties (Hilliard et al. 2015; Prommer 2011), and the anesthetic ketamine has been shown to reduce opioid requirements and reverse opioid-induced neurotoxic symptoms in the palliative care setting (Winegarden et al. 2016).

Nonpharmacological

In addition to seeking out and potentially correcting underlying causes of delirium, environmental and supportive interventions are important, as described in Chapter 4. In fact, in the dying patient, these may be the only steps taken. The presence of family, frequent reorientation, correction of hearing and visual impairment, reversal of dehydration, and a quiet well-lit room with familiar objects all are helpful in reducing the severity and impact of delirium in seriously ill patients. However, these interventions are less applicable in the last days of life, and there is little likelihood that they would prevent terminal delirium.

Controversies in the Management of Terminal Delirium

Several aspects of the use of antipsychotics and other agents in the management of delirium in the dying patient remain controversial in some circles. Some view delirium as a natural part of the dying process that should not be altered and argue that pharmacological interventions are inappropriate. In particular, some who care for the dying view hallucinations and delusions in which dead relatives communicate with dying patients or welcome them to heaven as important elements in the transition from life to death. There are some patients who experience hallucinations during delirium that are pleasant and even comforting, and many clinicians question the appropriateness of intervening pharmacologically in such instances.

Another concern often raised is that these patients are so close to death that aggressive treatment is unnecessary. Parenteral antipsychotics or sedatives may be mistakenly avoided because of exaggerated fears that they might hasten death through hypotension or respiratory depression. There is the possibility that sedation may worsen confusion in delirium. Many clinicians are unnecessarily pessimistic about the possible results of antipsychotic treatment for delirium. They argue that since the underlying pathophysiological process, such as hepatic or renal failure, often continues unabated, no improvement can be expected in the patient's mental status.

Clinical experience in managing delirium in dying patients suggests that the use of antipsychotics in the management of agitation, paranoia, hallucinations, and altered sensorium is safe, effective, and often quite appropriate (Breitbart and Alici 2008; Breitbart et al. 2001). Management of delirium on a case-by-case basis seems wisest. The agitated, delirious dying patient should usually receive a trial of antipsychotics to help restore calm. A "wait and see" approach prior to using antipsychotics may be appropriate with some patients who have a lethargic, somnolent presentation of delirium or those who are having frankly pleasant or comforting hallucinations. Such an approach must be tempered by the knowledge that a lethargic delirium may very quickly and unexpectedly become an agitated delirium that can threaten the serenity and safety of the patient, family, and staff.

Finally, a very challenging clinical problem is management of terminal delirium that is unresponsive to antipsychotics and that can only be controlled by sedation to the point of significantly decreased consciousness. Before undertaking interventions such as midazolam or propofol infusions, in which the aim is a calm, comfortable, but sedated and unresponsive patient, the clinician should discuss with family members (and the patient if he or she has lucid moments) their preferences for the type of care that can best honor the patient's and family's values. Family members should be informed that the goal of sedation is to provide comfort and symptom control and not to hasten death. Terminal sedation intended to maximize the patient's comfort is not euthanasia. After the patient receives this degree of sedation, the family may experience a premature sense of loss, and they may feel their loved one is in some sort of limbo state, not yet dead but yet no longer alive in the vital sense. The distress and confusion that family members can experience during such a period can be ameliorated by including them in the decision making and emphasizing shared goals of care. Sedation in such patients is not always complete or irreversible; some patients have periods of wakefulness, despite sedation, and many clinicians will periodically lighten sedation to reassess the patient's condition.

Addressing Extra-Clinical Needs

Spirituality

Although chaplains and spiritual counselors have been instrumental in the palliative care movement since its inception, regulatory and medical bodies are now increasingly recognizing their importance. In the United States, the National Consensus Project (NCP) recommends that all palliative care and hospice programs have some form of spiritual care available (National Consensus Project for Quality Palliative Care 2013), and Medicare mandates such services through a Condition of Participation with hospices. As a result, psychiatrists should maintain some degree of competency but consult the experts when questions of spirituality arise. Although beyond the scope of this chapter, spirituality in palliative care is a growing area of research. Steinhauser et al. (2017) have provided a primer on the relevance and nomenclature of this field, and Balboni et al. (2017) delve into the topics of assessment and intervention.

Culture and Ethnicity

Ethnicity and culture strongly influence attitudes toward death and dying. A full discussion of specific cultural and ethnic differences in the face of life-threatening illness is beyond the scope of this chapter. In practice, however, cultural barriers can often generate psychiatric consultation when questions of decision-making capacity arise. Cultural barriers can lead to marginalization of minorities, who have been shown to underutilize palliative care services and receive aggressive end-of-life measures (Fang et al. 2016). As part of any psychiatric or palliative intervention, providers should be aware of cultural preferences for family-based medical decision making or means of communicating information.

Doctor–Patient Communication

Effective doctor–patient communication is an essential component in caring for a dying patient. Consulting psychiatrists can help improve communication skills in physicians and other providers caring for dying patients. Intensive training programs in doctor–patient communication that use a variety of teaching methods, including role-playing, videotaped feedback, experiential exercises, and didactics, have been demonstrated to have both short-term and long-term efficacy in improving communication skills among physicians (Barth and Lannen 2011; Epstein et al. 2017; Kissane et al. 2012; Moore et al. 2013).

Bereavement

One of the most controversial changes from DSM-IV to DSM-5 (American Psychiatric Association 2013) was removal of the so-called bereavement exclusion, which had previously excluded the diagnosis of MDD when symptoms followed the recent death of a loved one. While a discussion of the ongoing debate on this issue is beyond the scope of this chapter, psychiatrists working in the palliative care setting still have a unique opportunity to provide psychoeducation and referral. Given advances in treatment, it is important for families to be aware of resources that are available, and for providers to maintain a flexible stance in the face of ongoing research.

Although words such as *grief, mourning,* and *bereavement* are commonly used interchangeably, the following definitions may be helpful:

- *Bereavement* is the state of loss resulting from death.
- *Grief* is the emotional response associated with loss.
- *Uncomplicated grief* is the process of successfully integrating the loss of a loved one without significant detriment in self-care, social interaction, or overall well-being, with significant individual variation.
- *Mourning* is the process of adaptation to loss, including the cultural and social rituals prescribed as accompaniments.
- *Complicated grief,* as recently proposed, presumes a normative and adaptive grief response that has been interrupted or delayed (Shear et al. 2016).
- *Prolonged grief disorder* focuses on the intensity and length of grief itself as contributing to a pathological state (Prigerson et al. 2009).
- *Persistent complex bereavement disorder* is a clinical entity semantically synthesizing the above two terms. DSM-5 identifies it as a "condition for further study" involving intense emotional distress centered on preoccupation with the deceased and the circumstances of death (American Psychiatric Association 2013).
- *Integrated grief,* a term used in the context of attachment theory, refers to a stable state in which the individual maintains an emotional attachment to the lost loved one without impaired function (Shear et al. 2016).

Clinical Presentations of Grief

Since its inception, psychiatry has explored the distinction between normative and pathological grieving. In his seminal work *Mourning and Melancholy,* Freud described mourning as an intense, painful longing for a lost object, whether a person, a place, or even an ideal (Freud 1917 [1915]). He posited that this longing could be so intense that it came into conflict with reality, generating hallucinations and other phenomena to prolong the experienced existence of what has been lost. However, over time, "respect for reality gains the day" (Freud 1917 [1915], p. 244). Modern conceptualizations of grief have generally continued that view, describing a deep yearning, with multiaxial manifestations, including cognitive, emotional, somatic, and behavioral responses, all contingent on the individual.

In attachment theory, acute grief ideally transitions into *integrated grief,* in which the person maintains the emotional connection to the lost one but accepts reality and appropriately adapts to new routines and changes in life (Bowlby 1980). Individuals can still expect to intermittently experience a sense of loss, sadness, and deep nostalgia, in addition to joy and fond recollection, with memories triggered by anniversaries and meaningful dates. However, clinical data demonstrate that many people are unable to reach this state, instead experiencing high levels of persistent impairment and disabling distress, necessitating some clinical framework to identify and help them (Lichtenthal et al. 2004).

There are two prevailing theories about grief and mental dysfunction. *Prolonged grief* theory supports the idea that the grieving process itself can be pathological based on its intensity and prolongation (Maciejewski et al. 2016). *Complicated grief* theory states that the grieving process itself is not pathological per se but rather is a process of maintaining attachment that can be derailed. Complications include avoidant behaviors related to loss (including inappropriate substance use) and cognitive distortions that include catastrophic thinking, assignment of blame for loss, and frequent "if only" statements. In clinical practice, psychiatrists need not take a partisan approach, but instead can draw on both frameworks when providing psychoeducation to families, with the caveat that the issue still is being actively debated. However, it is important to note that complicated grief criteria appear to capture a larger number of people (30%) compared with prolonged grief (10%) (Maciejewski et al. 2016).

In regard to the expected time course of grief, DSM-IV criteria for MDD required that symptoms persist for at least 2 months after the death of a loved one before the diagnosis could be made; by contrast, the criteria for persistent complex bereavement disorder (listed under "conditions for further study" in DSM-5) require symptom persistence for at least 12 months after the death. Mental health professionals providing psychoeducation to patients or families should be mindful that neither time course has been empirically validated, although some naturalistic data suggest that intense grieving past 6 months is associated with diminished function, suicidal ideation, and mental disorder (Prigerson et al. 2009). The time course of grief is highly individualized, with some experiencing persistent, painful emotions; others experiencing fluctuations in intensity of emotions; and still others experiencing an admixture of positive and negative thoughts about the deceased.

Anticipatory Grief

Anticipatory grief generally draws a supportive family closer, but for some families, impaired coping is exhibited through protective avoidance, denial of the seriousness of the threat, anger, or withdrawal from involvement. Family dysfunction may be glaring or may develop gradually as individuals struggle to adapt. Although anticipatory grief was historically thought to reduce postmortem grief, intense anticipatory distress is now well recognized as a marker of risk for complicated grief. During the period of anticipatory grief, families that are capable of effective communication should be encouraged to openly share their feelings as they go about the care of their dying family member or friend. Saying goodbye should be a process that evolves over time, with opportunities for reminiscence, celebration of the life and contributions of the dying person, expressions of gratitude, and completion of any unfinished business. These tasks have the potential to generate creative and positive emotional experiences during what is otherwise a sad time for all.

Sometimes staff will have concerns about the emotional responses of bereaved family members. If there is uncertainty about the cultural appropriateness of responses, consultation with an informed cultural intermediary may be helpful.

Traumatic Grief

When death has been unexpected or its nature in some way shocking—traumatic, violent, stigmatized, or perceived as undignified—its integration and acceptance may be interfered with by the arousal and increased distress that memories can trigger. Intensive recollections, including flashbacks, nightmares, and recurrent intrusive memories, cause hyperarousal, disbelief, insomnia, irritability, and disturbed concentration that distort normal grieving (Prigerson and Jacobs 2001). The shock of the death can precipitate mistrust, anger, detachment, and an unwillingness to accept its reality. These reactions at a subthreshold level are on a continuum with the full features of acute stress disorder and PTSD, but subthreshold states have been observed to persist for years and contribute substantial morbidity. Palliative care deaths involving profound breakdown of bodily surfaces, gross disfigurement due to head and neck cancers, or other changes eliciting fear, disgust, or mortification may generate traumatic memories in the bereaved. The researchers who initially proposed the term *traumatic grief* have suggested returning to the original term, *complicated grief,* in order to avoid confusion between traumatic grief and PTSD (Zhang et al. 2006).

Psychiatric Disorders in Bereavement

The current consensus is that grief, whether normative, complicated, or prolonged, is an entity clinically distinct from MDD, generalized anxiety disorder, and PTSD, despite sharing many clinical manifestations (Golden and Dalgleish 2010). However, this conceptualization does not preclude the recognition that premorbid psychiatric disorders can manifest concurrently with grief. Frank psychiatric disorders that affect bereavement are more likely to be recognized and treated than subthreshold states. The recognition of psychiatric disorders in bereaved individuals calls for experienced clinical judgment that does not normalize the distress as understandable.

Rates of MDD in the bereaved have varied from 16% to 50%, peaking during the first 2 months (Clayton 1990; Zisook et al. 1991) and gradually decreasing to 15% across the next 2 years (Harlow et al. 1991; Zisook et al. 1994). The features of any major depressive episode following bereavement resemble MDD at other points of the life cycle (Kendler et al. 2008). There is a tendency toward chronicity, considerable social morbidity, and risk of inadequate treatment.

Anxiety disorders take the form of adjustment disorders, generalized anxiety disorder, phobias, and acute stress disorder and PTSD, and occur in up to 30% of bereaved individuals (Jacobs 1993).

Individuals predisposed to alcohol or other substance use disorders are at higher risk for relapse during grief, as are those with psychotic disorders. The latter should not be confused with the "normal" hallucinations that can occur in grief, typically limited to the voice, sight, and/or sense of the presence of the deceased.

Risk factors associated with greater risk of complicated grief include a death that is untimely within the life cycle (e.g., death of a child) or unexpected; a past history of psychiatric disorder or maladaptive coping; a cumulative experience of multiple losses; a problematic relationship with the deceased; and a dysfunctional family and support network.

Grief Therapies

The most basic model of grief therapy is a supportive–expressive intervention in which the person is invited to share his or her feelings about the loss with a health professional who will listen and seek to understand the other's distress in a comforting manner. The key therapeutic aspects of this encounter are the sharing of distress and, through the relational understanding that is acknowledged, some shifts in cognitive appraisals of the reality that has been forever altered. There are multiple possible formal interventions for bereaved people, but the first question is whether an intervention is actually warranted. Early intervention should be considered for persons at risk of maladaptive outcomes, and active treatment is required for those who later develop complicated bereavement. As a target of treatment, grief should be viewed beyond psychiatry's usual scope of individual pathology. Practitioners should look at the family and social system at large and should ideally have some training in family therapy.

"Complicated grief therapy," a manualized approach developed by Katherine Shear (Shear et al. 2005), is the most robustly studied and disseminated treatment for complex grief. This therapy incorporates the framework of attachment theory with elements of CBT, interpersonal therapy, and motivational interviewing. The ultimate goal is to resolve complications preventing integration of grief. Treatment is structured in a time-limited fashion, with individual sessions focused on core skills or themes, ranging from cognitive restructuring to a mediated conversation with the deceased. At least one designated social support is incorporated, and individuals are encouraged to develop a novel interest or pursuit. Repeat randomized clinical trials evaluating this therapy have shown benefit, with a response rate greater than 80%, a number needed to treat (NNT) of 3.6, and significant reductions in suicidal ideation (Shear et al. 2016). A citalopram treatment arm added to both the active psychotherapy and the control condition had no impact on overall results. The control condition included psychoeducation, grief monitoring, and encouragement to engage in activities. Further studies are needed to establish the applicability of this therapy to the community setting.

The spectrum of interventions spans individual-, group-, and family-oriented therapies and encompasses all schools of psychotherapy as well as appropriately indicated pharmacotherapy. A typical intervention entails six to eight sessions over several months. In this sense, grief therapy is focused and time limited, but multimodal therapies are common (Kissane and Zaider 2015). Table 39–1 lists commonly used forms of grief therapy (Kissane and Zaider 2015).

Pharmacotherapy is widely used to support the bereaved, but prescribing should be judicious. Benzodiazepines allay anxiety and assist sleep, but excessive use may interfere with adaptive mourning. Antidepressants are indicated when bereavement is complicated by MDD or panic disorder.

Caregiver Distress

Distress is highly prevalent among caregivers of patients in palliative care settings. Nearly one-quarter of hospice caregivers were found to be moderately to severely depressed, and nearly one-third of hospice caregivers reported moderate to severe symptoms of anxiety (Parker Oliver et al. 2017). However, the timely identification and treatment of these conditions remain inadequate. A comprehensive review of caregiver issues is beyond the scope of this chapter but can be found elsewhere (e.g., the February 2017 issue of the journal *Palliative and Supportive Care* is dedicated to the most recent studies on assessment and management of caregiver distress; see Applebaum 2017).

TABLE 39–1.   Models of grief therapy

Model	Potential focus for application	Clinical issues when indicated
Supportive–expressive therapy (guided grief work, crisis intervention)	Individual and/or group	Avoidance of emotional expression Inhibited or delayed grief Isolation and lack of support Established psychiatric disorders including depression
Interpersonal or psychodynamic therapy	Individual and/or group	Predominant relational issues Role transition difficulties
Cognitive-behavioral therapy	Individual and/or group	Chronic grief with "stuck" behaviors Traumatic grief Posttraumatic stress disorder
Family-focused grief therapy	Family	Family either at risk or clearly dysfunctional in its relating Adolescents or children at risk
Pharmacotherapy combined with any of the psychotherapeutic models	Individual	Depressive disorders Anxiety disorders Sleep disorders

Palliation of Selected Physical Symptoms

Although diagnosis and treatment of psychiatric disorders in patients with advanced illness are important, pain and other distressing physical symptoms must also be aggressively treated to optimize quality of life. Some key points are noted here, but for a comprehensive review of pharmacological and nonpharmacological interventions for common physical symptoms in the terminally ill, readers are referred to major palliative care texts (e.g., Cherny et al. 2017; Chochinov and Breitbart 2012).

Pain

Recent guidelines for managing cancer pain have been published by the National Comprehensive Cancer Network (NCCN Adult Cancer Pain Panel Members 2017; NCCN Palliative Care Panel Members 2017) (see also Chapter 34). After adequate medical treatment, mild to moderate levels of residual pain can be effectively managed with behavioral techniques that are quite similar to those used for anxiety, phobias, and anticipatory nausea and vomiting. Relaxation techniques, imagery, hypnosis, biofeedback, and multicomponent cognitive-behavioral interventions have been used to provide comfort and minimize pain in adults, children, and adolescents.

Anorexia and Weight Loss

Although physiological changes associated with terminal illness and its treatment account for most of the anorexia and cachexia in terminally ill individuals, psychological factors, including anxiety, depression, and conditioned food aversions, may also play a role (NCCN Palliative Care Panel Members 2017). Treatment of anorexia and weight loss begins with identification and correction of reversible causes (e.g., opioid-induced nausea, stomatitis from chemotherapy, thrush) (NCCN Palliative Care Panel Members 2017). For patients with months-to-weeks or weeks-to-days life expectancy, the NCCN Palliative Care Guidelines recommend considering the use of appetite stimulants (e.g., megestrol acetate, dexamethasone, olanzapine), especially if increased appetite is an important aspect of quality of life. Cannabinoid-based interventions (e.g., dronabinol, cannabis) have not yet been demonstrated to be effective for cancer-related anorexia (Davis 2016). Appetite-stimulating antidepressants (e.g., mirtazapine) should be considered when the cause is MDD, but depression should never be diagnosed solely on the basis of unexplained anorexia and weight loss.

Fatigue

Fatigue is extremely common in individuals with advanced cancer, AIDS, or organ failure. Although this symptom may arise from deconditioning, catabolism, malnutrition, infection, profound anemia, metabolic abnormalities, or adverse effects of treatment, in many cases a reversible cause cannot be identified. As with unexplained weight loss in advanced disease, there is a tendency to overdiagnose depression in terminally ill patients with extreme fatigue.

The literature in support of pharmacotherapy for fatigue in cancer patients is limited, but practice guidelines are available (NCCN Cancer-Related Fatigue Panel Members 2017). Antidepressants have been recommended to treat underlying depression when present (NCCN Cancer-Related Fatigue Panel Members 2017). Identifiable causes should receive targeted treatment when possible (e.g., erythropoietin for anemia). Some patients respond to corticosteroids, but the benefits tend to be fleeting, and prolonged use can cause proximal myopathy. A Cochrane review of pharmacological treatments of fatigue in palliative care concluded that modafinil and methylphenidate may be beneficial, although further research is needed. There was insufficient evidence to draw conclusions about corticosteroids, acetylsalicylic acid, armodafinil, amantadine, and L-carnitine (Mücke et al. 2015). Low doses of stimulants do not appear to cause appetite suppression or weight loss and may actually improve energy and appetite in fatigued terminally ill patients.

Nausea and Vomiting

Common causes of nausea and vomiting in patients with advanced cancer include radiation, medications, toxins, metabolic derangements, obstruction of the gastrointestinal tract, and chemotherapy (NCCN Antiemesis Panel Members 2017). Conditioned by the experience of profound nausea and vomiting secondary to highly emetic chemotherapy agents, some patients report being nauseated in anticipation of treatment. Anticipatory nausea and vomiting used to be very common but has become less so with current antiemetic therapy.

Antiemetic drugs are the mainstay of managing chemotherapy-induced nausea and vomiting in patients with advanced disease. Several antiemetics (e.g., metoclopramide, prochlorperazine, promethazine, haloperidol, olanzapine) have dopamine-blocking properties and thus can cause acute akathisia and dystonia. Extrapyramidal side effects are rarely a problem with newer antipsychotics (e.g., olanzapine) and newer antiemetics (e.g., serotonin 5-HT_3 antagonists such as ondansetron). Agents that target the cannabinoid system may be considered in treating refractory chemotherapy-induced nausea and vomiting. Dronabinol and nabilone are two cannabinoid agents approved for treating chemotherapy-induced nausea and vomiting that are refractory to standard antiemetic therapies, but there is insufficient evidence to support use of cannabinoids or cannabis as primary treatment (Davis 2016; Smith et al. 2015). For anxiety-related nausea, the addition of benzodiazepines can be considered.

Psychotherapy Interventions in Palliative Care

The potential benefits of psychotherapy for seriously medically ill patients are frequently underestimated by clinicians (Rodin 2009). This bias against psychotherapy tends to be even more pronounced in regard to patients who are months away from death. However, psychotherapeutic interventions have been demonstrated to be useful and effective for patients struggling with advanced, life-threatening medical illnesses (Kissane et al. 2009). Psychotherapy can be challenging in the palliative care setting. Several cultures, including the culture of medicine, create a taboo around death and illness, often fostering patterns of avoidance in both patient and provider. Providers are often confronted with themes of futility and despair that can become oppressive, particularly with their own a priori experience. However, with some flexibility, psychotherapy in this setting can be profoundly rewarding for both parties, particularly when these interventions engage with family systems. In this section we briefly describe different psychotherapeutic interventions and their relative applicability and efficacy for individuals near the end of life. Table 39–2 summarizes psychotherapies useful in palliative care. Psychotherapy in the medically ill is reviewed in detail in Chapter 37.

Therapeutic Stance

Supportive psychotherapy for the dying patient consists of active listening with supportive verbal interventions and occasional interpretation. Despite the seriousness of the patient's plight, it is not necessary for the therapist to appear overly solemn or emotionally restrained. The psychotherapist may be the only person among the patient's caregivers who is comfortable enough to converse lightheartedly and to allow the patient to talk about his or her life and experiences rather than focus solely on impending death. The dying patient who wishes to talk or ask questions about death should be encouraged to do so freely, with the therapist maintaining an interested, interactive stance.

Insight-Oriented and Cognitive-Behavioral Psychotherapy

Traditional insight-oriented psychotherapy has had limited application among dying patients, and there have been no clinical trials. Nevertheless, a psychodynamic formulation can be helpful in developing a deeper understanding of the patient's defenses and relationships and can usefully inform other psychotherapeutic interventions.

Several palliative psychotherapies have been derived from the principles of CBT. These therapies use a manualized approach, which allows for empirical testing and wide dissemination, and they often combine cognitive restructuring and exposure/response prevention components of traditional CBT with ancillary measures. For example, the ongoing TIRED study is assessing the efficacy of progressive behavioral activation through exercise combined with cognitive restructuring to address symptoms of fatigue in terminally ill cancer patients (Poort et al. 2017).

Existential Therapies

Existential therapies explore ways in which suffering can be experienced from a more positive and meaningful perspective, inspired by the work of Victor Frankl (1963).

Narrative Approaches

One form of existential therapy useful for demoralized patients is the *life narrative*. This treatment explores the meaning of the physical illness in the context of the patient's life trajectory. It is designed to create a new perspective of dealing with the illness, emphasize past strengths, increase self-esteem, and support effective past coping strategies. The therapist emphatically summarizes the patient's life history and response to the illness to convey a sense that the therapist understands the patient over time (Viederman 2000). Life narrative can bolster patients' psychological and physical well-being. Life narrative has traditionally been used for treating depressed patients whose depression is a response to physical illness. However, the written form of this approach can be too demanding for patients at the end stage of their illness.

TABLE 39–2.   Psychotherapy interventions in palliative care

	Core features addressed in palliative care setting	Form of intervention	Therapeutic frame
Meaning-centered psychotherapy	Meaningful existence through profound experiences, creative acts, active participation in life through, and finding context within, personal past/present/future	Combination of didactics and personal exploration; writing to promote self-reflection both in and outside of session	Seven to eight sessions; group and individual modalities
Dignity therapy	Illness-related concerns, conservation of dignity, maintenance of positive social interactions and support	Open account of life facilitated by therapist, recorded, transcribed, and self-edited for posterity	Time limited
Cognitive-behavioral therapy	Maladaptive behaviors and cognition; fatigue	Cognitive restructuring around "unhelpful" thoughts; behavioral activation; extinction of avoidant behaviors	Variable but time-limited exercises to reinforce therapeutic values (homework)
Acceptance and commitment therapy	"Psychological flexibility," maintenance of internal values in the face of distress, language as core of cognition	Mindfulness/meditation, perspective exercise (e.g., writing letter to self); teaching and fostering of "skills," identification and limiting of avoidance of distress	Using patient experiences to demonstrate principles; goal setting for each encounter
Insight-oriented therapy	Recognition and resolution of unconscious, internal conflicts	Interpretation of treater–patient relationship (transference); free association of thoughts; identification of "defenses"	Open-ended; often well-defined boundaries of treatment (although flexibility encouraged with terminal illness)

A similar method of intervention is the *life review,* which provides patients with the opportunity to identify and re-examine past experiences and achievements to find meaning, resolve old conflicts and make amends, or resolve unfinished business (Lichter et al. 1993). The process of life review can be achieved through written or taped autobiographies, by reminiscing, through storytelling about past experiences or discussion of the patient's career or life work, and by creating family trees (Lewis and Butler 1974). Examples of other life review activities include undertaking of pilgrimages, artistic expression (e.g., creating a collage or drawings, writing poetry), and journal writing (Pickrel 1989). Life review has traditionally been used in the elderly as a means of conflict resolution and to facilitate a dignified acceptance of death (Butler 1963). For dying patients, their stories have a special meaning. In negotiating one's way through serious illness and its treatment, the telling of one's own story takes on a renewed urgency. A recent systematic review and meta-analysis of eight clinical trials concluded that therapeutic life review is potentially beneficial for people near the end of life (Wang et al. 2017).

Meaning-Centered Psychotherapy

Breitbart and colleagues (Breitbart 2002, 2003b; Greenstein and Breitbart 2000) have applied Viktor Frankl's concepts of meaning-based psychotherapy (Logotherapy) to address spiritual suffering in dying patients (Frankl 1963). This form of MCP (Greenstein and Breitbart 2000) utilizes a mixture of didactics, discussion, and experiential exercises that focus on particular themes related to meaning and advanced cancer. It is designed to help individuals with advanced cancer sustain or enhance a sense of meaning, peace, and purpose in their lives even as they approach the end of life. In randomized controlled trials in patients with advanced cancer, meaning-centered group psychotherapy (MCGP) was superior to supportive group psychotherapy, with significant improvements in spiritual well-being and sense of meaning, and reductions in depression, hopelessness, physical symptom distress, and desire for hastened death (Breitbart et al. 2010b, 2015). Follow-up studies of MCGP have shown improvements in personal growth and environmental mastery, as measured using Ryff's Scales of Psychological Well-Being (van der Spek et al. 2017).

MCP has also been expanded to individuals with advanced cancer (Breitbart et al. 2012). This intervention takes a manualized approach to foster meaning in four domains—attitudinal (how patients are actively making choices in their life), experiential (how patients engage with art, humor, beauty, etc.), historical (how patients are contextualized in their past, their present, and after death), and creative (how patients affect the world by creating). Care is delivered in seven to eight sessions, with emphasis on a flexible frame to accommodate illness. An abbreviated form of MCP is being developed for use in palliative care patients, with treatment delivered in three sessions to accommodate significantly shortened life expectancies (Rosenfeld et al. 2017). A variant of MCP targeted toward cancer caregivers is also being developed (Applebaum et al. 2015).

Dignity-Conserving Care

Ensuring dignity in the dying process is a critical goal of palliative care and has significant overlap with concepts of purpose, spirituality, and existential meaning. Chochinov et al. (2002a, 2002b) examined how dying patients understand and define *dignity* in order to develop a model of dignity in the terminally ill (Figure 39–1). A semistructured interview was designed to explore how patients cope with their illness and their perceptions of dignity. Three major categories emerged: *illness-related concerns* (concerns related to the illness itself that threaten or impinge on the patient's sense of dignity), *dignity-conserving repertoire* (internally held qualities or personal approaches that patients use to maintain their sense of dignity), and *social dignity inventory* (social concerns or relationship dynamics that enhance or detract from a patient's sense of dignity). These broad categories and their carefully defined themes and subthemes form the foundation for an emerging model of dignity among the dying (Chochinov et al. 2006). The concept of dignity and the notion of dignity-conserving care offer a way of understanding how patients face advancing terminal illness and present an approach that clinicians can use to explicitly target the maintenance of dignity as a therapeutic objective.

Chochinov (2002) developed a short-term dignity-conserving care intervention for palliative care patients, called dignity therapy, which incorporates facets of the dignity model most likely to bolster dying patients' will to live, lessen their desire for death and their overall level of distress, and improve their quality of life. The dignity model establishes the importance of generativity as a significant dignity theme. The sessions are taped, transcribed, and edited, and the transcription is returned to the patient within 1–2 days. The creation of a tangible product that will live beyond the patient acknowledges the importance of generativity as a salient dignity issue. The immediacy of the returned transcript is intended to bolster the patient's sense of purpose, meaning, and worth, while giving the patient tangible evidence that his or her thoughts and words will continue to be valued. In most instances, these transcripts will be left for family or loved ones and form part of a personal legacy that the patient will have actively participated in creating and shaping.

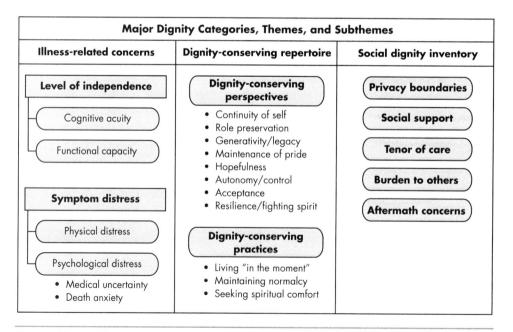

FIGURE 39–1.   Model of dignity for the terminally ill.

Conclusion

The consulting psychiatrist can play an important role in the care of patients with advanced, life-threatening medical illnesses. Palliative care for terminally ill patients must include not only control of pain and physical symptoms but also assessment and management of psychiatric and psychosocial complications. Psychiatrists working in the palliative care setting must be knowledgeable in how to adapt the assessment and management of major psychiatric complications, such as anxiety, depression, and delirium, and must be adept in dealing with issues of existential despair and spiritual suffering. Cultural issues, communication issues, ethical issues, and issues of bereavement are all areas requiring attention and awareness. As part of an interdisciplinary team, the psychiatrist can play an important role in the provision of comprehensive palliative care.

Web Resources

American Academy of Hospice and Palliative Medicine (AAHPM): http://www.aahpm.org
American Board of Hospice and Palliative Medicine (ABHPM): http://www.abhpm.org
American Board of Psychiatry and Neurology (ABPN) subspecialty certification in Hospice and Palliative Medicine: https://www.abpn.com/become-certified/taking-a-subspecialty-exam/hospice-and-palliative-medicine/
Center to Advance Palliative Care (CAPC): http://www.capc.org
National Consensus Project (NCP): http://www.nationalconsensusproject.org
National Hospice and Palliative Care Organization: http://www.nhpco.org/templates/1/homepage.cfm

References

Agar MR, Lawlor PG, Quinn S, et al: Efficacy of oral risperidone, haloperidol, or placebo for symptoms of delirium among patients in palliative care: a randomized clinical trial. JAMA Intern Med 177(1):34–42, 2017 27918778

American Psychiatric Association: Diagnostic and Statistical Manual of Mental Disorders, 4th Edition. Washington, DC, American Psychiatric Association, 1994

American Psychiatric Association: Diagnostic and Statistical Manual of Mental Disorders, 5th Edition. Arlington, VA, American Psychiatric Association, 2013

Anderson T, Watson M, Davidson R: The use of cognitive behavioural therapy techniques for anxiety and depression in hospice patients: a feasibility study. Palliat Med 22(7):814–821, 2008 18755828

Antunes B, Murtagh F, Bausewein C, et al; EURO IMPACT: Screening for depression in advanced disease: psychometric properties, sensitivity, and specificity of two items of the Palliative care Outcome Scale (POS). J Pain Symptom Manage 49(2):277–288, 2015 25131889

Applebaum AJ: Survival of the fittest...caregiver? Palliat Support Care 15(1):1–2, 2017 28112070

Applebaum AJ, Kulikowski JR, Breitbart W: Meaning-centered psychotherapy for cancer caregivers (MCP-C): rationale and overview. Palliat Support Care 13(6):1631–1641, 2015 26000705

Austin P, Wiley S, McEvoy PM, et al: Depression and anxiety in palliative care inpatients compared with those receiving palliative care at home. Palliat Support Care 9(4):393–400, 2011 22104415

Balboni TA, Fitchett G, Handzo G, et al: State of the Science of Spirituality and Palliative Care Research, part II: screening, assessment, and interventions. J Pain Symptom Manage 54(17):441–453, 2017 28734881

Barth J, Lannen P: Efficacy of communication skills training courses in oncology: a systematic review and meta-analysis. Ann Oncol 22(5):1030–1040, 2011 20974653

Block SD; ACP-ASIM End-of-Life Care Consensus Panel; American College of Physicians–American Society of Internal Medicine: Assessing and managing depression in the terminally ill patient. Ann Intern Med 132(3):209–218, 2000 10651602

Bolund C: Suicide and cancer, II: medical and care factors in suicide by cancer patients in Sweden, 1973–1976. Journal of Psychosocial Oncology 3(1):17–30, 1985

Bowlby J: Attachment and Loss, Vol 3: Loss: Sadness and Depression. London, Tavistock, 1980

Brandberg Y, Månsson-Brahme E, Ringborg U, et al: Psychological reactions in patients with malignant melanoma. Eur J Cancer 31A(2):157–162, 1995 7718319

Breitbart W: Psychiatric management of cancer pain. Cancer 63 (11 suppl):2336–2342, 1989 2655868

Breitbart W: Cancer pain and suicide, in Advances in Pain Research and Therapy, Vol 16. Edited by Foley K, Bonica JJ, Ventafridda V, et al. New York, Raven, 1990, pp 399–412

Breitbart W: Spirituality and meaning in supportive care: spirituality- and meaning-centered group psychotherapy interventions in advanced cancer. Support Care Cancer 10(4):272–280, 2002 12029426

Breitbart W: Palliative and Supportive Care: introducing a new international journal; the "care" journal of palliative medicine. Palliat Support Care 1(1):1–2, 2003a

Breitbart W: Reframing hope: meaning-centered care for patients near the end of life. Interview by Karen S. Heller. J Palliat Med 6(6):979–988, 2003b 14733692

Breitbart W, Alici Y: Agitation and delirium at the end of life: "We couldn't manage him." JAMA 300(24):2898–2910, 2008 19109118

Breitbart W, Alici Y: Evidence-based treatment of delirium in patients with cancer. J Clin Oncol 30(11):1206–1214, 2012 22412123

Breitbart W, Alici Y: Psychosocial Palliative Care. New York, Oxford University Press, 2014

Breitbart W, Bruera E, Chochinov H, et al: Neuropsychiatric syndromes and psychological symptoms in patients with advanced cancer. J Pain Symptom Manage 10(2):131–141, 1995 7730685

Breitbart W, Marotta R, Platt MM, et al: A double-blind trial of haloperidol, chlorpromazine, and lorazepam in the treatment of delirium in hospitalized AIDS patients. Am J Psychiatry 153(2):231–237, 1996 8561204

Breitbart W, Rosenfeld B, Roth A, et al: The Memorial Delirium Assessment Scale. J Pain Symptom Manage 13(3):128–137, 1997 9114631

Breitbart W, Rosenfeld B, Pessin H, et al: Depression, hopelessness, and desire for hastened death in terminally ill patients with cancer. JAMA 284(22):2907–2911, 2000 11147988

Breitbart W, Rosenfeld B, Kaim M, et al: A randomized, double-blind, placebo-controlled trial of psychostimulants for the treatment of fatigue in ambulatory patients with human immunodeficiency virus disease. Arch Intern Med 161(3):411–420, 2001 11176767

Breitbart W, Gibson C, Tremblay A: The delirium experience: delirium recall and delirium-related distress in hospitalized patients with cancer, their spouses/caregivers, and their nurses. Psychosomatics 43(3):183–194, 2002 12075033

Breitbart W, Rosenfeld B, Gibson C, et al: Impact of treatment for depression on desire for hastened death in patients with advanced AIDS. Psychosomatics 51(2):98–105, 2010a 20332284

Breitbart W, Rosenfeld B, Gibson C, et al: Meaning-centered group psychotherapy for patients with advanced cancer: a pilot randomized controlled trial. Psychooncology 19(1):21–28, 2010b 19274623

Breitbart W, Poppito S, Rosenfeld B, et al: Pilot randomized controlled trial of individual meaning-centered psychotherapy for patients with advanced cancer. J Clin Oncol 30(12):1304–1309, 2012 22370330

Breitbart W, Rosenfeld B, Pessin H, et al: Meaning-centered group psychotherapy: an effective intervention for improving psychological well-being in patients with advanced cancer. J Clin Oncol 33(7):749–754, 2015 25646186

Brown JH, Henteleff P, Barakat S, et al: Is it normal for terminally ill patients to desire death? Am J Psychiatry 143(2):208–211, 1986 3946656

Bruera E, Chadwick S, Brenneis C, et al: Methylphenidate associated with narcotics for the treatment of cancer pain. Cancer Treat Rep 71(1):67–70, 1987 3791269

Bush SH, Bruera E, Lawlor PG, et al: Clinical practice guidelines for delirium management: potential application in palliative care. J Pain Symptom Manage 48(2):249–258, 2014 24766743

Buss MK, Vanderwerker LC, Inouye SK, et al: Associations between caregiver-perceived delirium in patients with cancer and generalized anxiety in their caregivers. J Palliat Med 10(5):1083–1092, 2007 17985965

Butler RN: The life review: an interpretation of reminiscence in the aged. Psychiatry 26:65–76, 1963 14017386

Canadian Palliative Care Association: Palliative Care: Towards a Consensus in Standardized Principles of Practice. Ottawa, ON, Canadian Palliative Care Association, 1995

Candy B, Jackson KC, Jones L, et al: Drug therapy for delirium in terminally ill adult patients. Cochrane Database Syst Rev (11):CD004770, 2012 23152226

Candy M, Jones L, Williams R, et al: Psychostimulants for depression. Cochrane Database Syst Rev (2):CD006722, 2008 18425966

Cherny N, Fallon M, Kaasa S, et al: Oxford Textbook of Palliative Medicine, 5th Edition. Oxford, UK, Oxford University Press, 2017

Chochinov HM: Dignity-conserving care—a new model for palliative care: helping the patient feel valued. JAMA 287(17):2253–2260, 2002 11980525

Chochinov HM, Breitbart W (eds): Handbook of Psychiatry in Palliative Medicine, 2nd Edition. New York, Oxford University Press, 2012

Chochinov HM, Wilson KG, Enns M, et al: Desire for death in the terminally ill. Am J Psychiatry 152(8):1185–1191, 1995 7625468

Chochinov HM, Wilson KG, Enns M, et al: "Are you depressed?" Screening for depression in the terminally ill. Am J Psychiatry 154(5):674–676, 1997 9137124

Chochinov HM, Hack T, Hassard T, et al: Dignity in the terminally ill: a cross-sectional, cohort study. Lancet 360(9350):2026–2030, 2002a 12504398

Chochinov HM, Hack T, McClement S, et al: Dignity in the terminally ill: a developing empirical model. Soc Sci Med 54(3):433–443, 2002b 11824919

Chochinov HM, Krisjanson LJ, Hack TF, et al: Dignity in the terminally ill: revisited. J Palliat Med 9(3):666–672, 2006 16752972

Classen C, Butler LD, Koopman C, et al: Supportive-expressive group therapy and distress in patients with metastatic breast cancer: a randomized clinical intervention trial. Arch Gen Psychiatry 58(5):494–501, 2001 11343530

Clayton PJ: Bereavement and depression. J Clin Psychiatry 51 (suppl):34–38, discussion 39–40, 1990 2195011

Davis MP: Cannabinoids for symptom management and cancer therapy: the evidence. J Natl Compr Canc Netw 14(7):915–922, 2016 27407130

de la Cruz M, Ransing V, Yennu S, et al: The frequency, characteristics, and outcomes among cancer patients with delirium admitted to an acute palliative care unit. Oncologist 20(12):1425–1431, 2015 26417036

Elia G, Thomas J: The symptomatic relief of dyspnea. Curr Oncol Rep 10(4):319–325, 2008 18778558

Elie D, Gagnon P, Gagnon B, et al: [Using psychostimulants in end-of-life patients with hypoactive delirium and cognitive disorders: a literature review] [in French]. Can J Psychiatry 55(6):386–393, 2010 20540834

Epstein RM, Duberstein PR, Fenton JJ, et al: Effect of a patient-centered communication intervention on oncologist-patient communication, quality of life, and health care utilization in advanced cancer: the VOICE randomized clinical trial. JAMA Oncol 3(1):92–100, 2017 27612178

Fainsinger RL, Waller A, Bercovici M, et al: A multicentre international study of sedation for uncontrolled symptoms in terminally ill patients. Palliat Med 14(4):257–265, 2000 10974977

Fang ML, Sixsmith J, Sinclair S, et al: A knowledge synthesis of culturally and spiritually sensitive end-of-life care: findings from a scoping review. BMC Geriatr 16:107, 2016 27193395

Field MJ, Cassel CK (eds): Approaching Death: Improving Care at the End of Life. Committee on Care at the End of Life, Institute of Medicine. Washington, DC, National Academies Press, 1997

Filiberti A, Ripamonti C, Totis A, et al: Characteristics of terminal cancer patients who committed suicide during a home palliative care program. J Pain Symptom Manage 22(1):544–553, 2001 11516596

Foley KM, Helband H (eds): Improving Palliative Care for Cancer. National Cancer Policy Board, Institute of Medicine, and National Research Council. Washington, DC, National Academy Press, 2001

Frankl VF: Man's Search for Meaning. New York, Washington Square Press, 1963

Freud S: Mourning and melancholia (1917 [1915]), in Standard Edition of the Complete Psychological Works of Sigmund Freud, Vol 14. Translated and edited by Strachey J. London, Hogarth Press, 1957, pp 237–260

Galiana L, Rudilla D, Oliver A, et al: The Short Demoralization Scale (SDS): a new tool to appraise demoralization in palliative care patients. Palliat Support Care 9:1–8, 2017 28065203

Ganzini L, Lee MA, Heintz RT, et al: The effect of depression treatment on elderly patients' preferences for life-sustaining medical therapy. Am J Psychiatry 151(11):1631–1636, 1994 7943452

Golden AM, Dalgleish T: Is prolonged grief distinct from bereavement-related posttraumatic stress? Psychiatry Res 178(2):336–341, 2010 20493535

Grassi L, Caraceni A, Mitchell AJ, et al: Management of delirium in palliative care: a review. Curr Psychiatry Rep 17(3):550, 2015 25663153

Greenstein M, Breitbart W: Cancer and the experience of meaning: a group psychotherapy program for people with cancer. Am J Psychother 54(4):486–500, 2000 11109133

Greer JA, Pirl WF, Jackson VA, et al: Effect of early palliative care on chemotherapy use and end-of-life care in patients with metastatic non-small-cell lung cancer. J Clin Oncol 30(4):394–400, 2012 22203758

Grzybowska P, Finlay I: The incidence of suicide in palliative care patients. Palliat Med 11(4):313–316, 1997 9373583

Hardy SE: Methylphenidate for the treatment of depressive symptoms, including fatigue and apathy, in medically ill older adults and terminally ill adults. Am J Geriatr Pharmacother 7(1):34–59, 2009 19281939

Harlow SD, Goldberg EL, Comstock GW: A longitudinal study of the prevalence of depressive symptomatology in elderly widowed and married women. Arch Gen Psychiatry 48(12):1065–1068, 1991 1845223

Hayes RD, Lee W, Rayner L, et al: Gender differences in prevalence of depression among patients receiving palliative care: the role of dependency. Palliat Med 26(5):696–702, 2012 21775410

Hilliard N, Brown S, Mitchinson S: A case report of dexmedetomidine used to treat intractable pain and delirium in a tertiary palliative care unit. Palliat Med 29(3):278–281, 2015 25467740

Holland JC: Anxiety and cancer: the patient and the family. J Clin Psychiatry 50 (suppl):20–25, 1989 2681170

Homsi J, Nelson KA, Sarhill N, et al: A phase II study of methylphenidate for depression in advanced cancer. Am J Hosp Palliat Care 18(6):403–407, 2001 11712722

Hosie A, Lobb E, Agar M, et al: Measuring delirium point-prevalence in two Australian palliative care inpatient units. Int J Palliat Nurs 22(1):13–21, 2016 26804952

Hui D, Valentine A, Bruera E: Neuroleptics for delirium: more research is needed. JAMA Intern Med 177(7):1052–1053, 2017 28672351

Jacobs S: Pathological Grief. Washington, DC, American Psychiatric Press, 1993

Jacobson CM, Rosenfeld B, Pessin H, et al: Depression and IL-6 blood plasma concentrations in advanced cancer patients. Psychosomatics 49(1):64–66, 2008 18212178

Jorgensen SM, Carnahan RM, Weckmann MT: Validity of the Delirium Observation Screening Scale in Identifying Delirium in Home Hospice Patients. Am J Hosp Palliat Care 34(8):744–747, 2017 27413013

Keen JC, Brown D: Psychostimulants and delirium in patients receiving palliative care. Palliat Support Care 2(2):199–202, 2004 16594250

Kendler KS, Myers J, Zisook S: Does bereavement-related major depression differ from major depression associated with other stressful life events? Am J Psychiatry 165(11):1449–1455, 2008 18708488

Kerrihard T, Breitbart W, Dent R, et al: Anxiety in patients with cancer and human immunodeficiency virus. Semin Clin Neuropsychiatry 4(2):114–132, 1999 10378955

Kissane DW, Zaider TI: Bereavement, in The Oxford Textbook of Palliative Medicine, 5th Edition. Edited by Cherny N, Fallon M, Kassa S, et al. Oxford, UK, Oxford University Press, 2015, pp 1110–1133

Kissane D, Clarke DM, Street AF: Demoralization syndrome: a relevant psychiatric diagnosis for palliative care. J Palliat Care 17(1):12–21, 2001 11324179

Kissane D, Treece C, Breitbart W, et al: Dignity, meaning, and demoralization, in Handbook of Psychiatry in Palliative Medicine, 2nd Edition. Edited by Chochinov HM, Breitbart W. New York, Oxford University Press, 2009, pp 324–340

Kissane DW, Bylund CL, Banerjee SC, et al: Communication skills training for oncology professionals. J Clin Oncol 30(11):1242–1247, 2012 22412145

Kolva E, Rosenfeld B, Liu Y, et al: Using item response theory (IRT) to reduce patient burden when assessing desire for hastened death. Psychol Assess 29(3):349–353, 2017 27280743

Lawlor PG, Nekolaichuk C, Gagnon B, et al: Clinical utility, factor analysis, and further validation of the memorial delirium assessment scale in patients with advanced cancer: assessing delirium in advanced cancer. Cancer 88(12):2859–2867, 2000 10870073

Levin TT, Alici Y: Anxiety disorders, in Psycho-Oncology, 2nd Edition. Edited by Holland JC. New York, Oxford University Press, 2010, pp 324–330

Levin TT, Li Y, Weiner JS, et al: How do-not-resuscitate orders are utilized in cancer patients: timing relative to death and communication-training implications. Palliat Support Care 6(4):341–348, 2008 19006588

Levy MH, Back A, Benedetti C, et al: NCCN clinical practice guidelines in oncology: palliative care. J Natl Compr Canc Netw 7(4):436–473, 2009 19406043

Lewis MI, Butler RN: Life-review therapy. Putting memories to work in individual and group psychotherapy. Geriatrics 29(11):165–173, 1974 4417455

Lichtenthal WG, Cruess DG, Prigerson HG: A case for establishing complicated grief as a distinct mental disorder in DSM-V. Clin Psychol Rev 24(6):637–662, 2004 15385092

Lichter I, Mooney J, Boyd M: Biography as therapy. Palliat Med 7(2):133–137, 1993 8261183

Lloyd-Williams M, Shiels C, Taylor F, et al: Depression—an independent predictor of early death in patients with advanced cancer. J Affect Disord 113(1–2):127–132, 2009 18558439

Lo B, Rubenfeld G: Palliative sedation in dying patients: "we turn to it when everything else hasn't worked." JAMA 294(14):1810–1816, 2005 16219885

Louhivuori KA, Hakama M: Risk of suicide among cancer patients. Am J Epidemiol 109(1):59–65, 1979 433917

Maciejewski PK, Maercker A, Boelen PA, et al: "Prolonged grief disorder" and "persistent complex bereavement disorder," but not "complicated grief," are one and the same diagnostic entity: an analysis of data from the Yale Bereavement Study. World Psychiatry 15(3):266–275, 2016 27717273

Massie MJ: Anxiety, panic, phobias, in Handbook of Psychooncology: Psychological Care of the Patient With Cancer. Edited by Holland JC, Rowland JH. New York, Oxford University Press, 1989, pp 300–309

Miovic M, Block S: Psychiatric disorders in advanced cancer. Cancer 110(8):1665–1676, 2007 17847017

Moore PM, Rivera Mercado S, Grez Artigues M, et al: Communication skills training for health-care professionals working with people who have cancer. Cochrane Database Syst Rev (3):CD003751, 2013 23543521

Morita T, Hirai K, Sakaguchi Y, et al: Family perceived distress from delirium-related symptoms of terminally ill cancer patients. Psychosomatics 45(2):107–113, 2004 15016923

Mücke M, Mochamat, Cuhls H, et al: Pharmacological treatments for fatigue associated with palliative care. Cochrane Database Syst Rev (5):CD006788, 2015 26026155

National Consensus Project for Quality Palliative Care: Clinical Practice Guidelines for Quality Palliative Care, 3rd Edition. 2013. Available at: http://www.nationalconsensusproject.org. Accessed October 20, 2017.

NCCN Adult Cancer Pain Panel Members: National Comprehensive Cancer Network (v.2.2017) Adult Cancer Pain. NCCN Practice Guidelines in Oncology. 2017. Available at: https://www.nccn.org/professionals/physician_gls/pdf/pain.pdf. Accessed October 20, 2017.

NCCN Antiemesis Panel Members: National Comprehensive Cancer Network (v.2.2017) Antiemesis. NCCN Practice Guidelines in Oncology. 2017. Available at: http://www.nccn.org/professionals/physician_gls/PDF/antiemesis.pdf. Accessed October 20, 2017.

NCCN Cancer-Related Fatigue Panel Members: National Comprehensive Cancer Network (v.2.2017) Cancer-Related Fatigue. NCCN Practice Guidelines in Oncology. 2017. Available at: http://www.nccn.org/professionals/physician_gls/PDF/fatigue.pdf. Accessed October 20, 2017.

NCCN Palliative Care Panel Members: National Comprehensive Cancer Network (v.2.2017) Palliative Care. NCCN Practice Guidelines in Oncology. 2017. Available at: https://www.nccn.org/professionals/physician_gls/pdf/palliative.pdf. Accessed October 20, 2017.

Nelson CJ, Rosenfeld B, Breitbart W, et al: Spirituality, religion, and depression in the terminally ill. Psychosomatics 43(3):213–220, 2002 12075036

O'Connor M, White K, Kristjanson LJ, et al: The prevalence of anxiety and depression in palliative care patients with cancer in Western Australia and New South Wales. Med J Aust 193(5) (suppl):S44–S47, 2010 21542445

Okuyama T, Akechi T, Mackenzie L, et al: Psychotherapy for depression among advanced, incurable cancer patients: a systematic review and meta-analysis. Cancer Treat Rev 56:16–27, 2017 28453966

O'Neill JF, Selwyn PA, Schietinger H (eds): A Clinical Guide to Supportive and Palliative Care for HIV/AIDS. Washington, DC, U.S. Department of Health and Human Services, Health Resources and Services Administration, HIV/AIDS Bureau, 2003

Palliative Care Foundation: Palliative Care Services in Hospitals, Guidelines. Report of the Working Group on Special Services in Hospitals, Ottawa, Ontario. Toronto, ON, Canada, National Health and Welfare, Palliative Care Foundation, 1981

Parker Oliver D, Washington K, Smith J, et al: The prevalence and risks for depression and anxiety in hospice caregivers. J Palliat Med 20(4):366–371, 2017 27912042

Pickrel J: "Tell me your story": using life review in counseling the terminally ill. Death Studies 13(2):127–135, 1989

Pidgeon T, Johnson CE, Currow D, et al: A survey of patients' experience of pain and other symptoms while receiving care from palliative care services. BMJ Support Palliat Care 6(3):315–322, 2016 25743438

Poort H, Verhagen CA, Peters ME, et al: Study protocol of the TIRED study: a randomised controlled trial comparing either graded exercise therapy for severe fatigue or cognitive behaviour therapy with usual care in patients with incurable cancer. BMC Cancer 17(1):81, 2017 28129746

Portenoy R, Foley KM: Management of cancer pain, in Handbook of Psychooncology: Psychological Care of the Patient With Cancer. Edited by Holland JC, Rowland JH. New York, Oxford University Press, 1989, pp 369–382

Portenoy RK, Thaler HT, Kornblith AB, et al: The Memorial Symptom Assessment Scale: an instrument for the evaluation of symptom prevalence, characteristics and distress. Eur J Cancer 30A(9):1326–1336, 1994 7999421

Potash M, Breitbart W: Affective disorders in advanced cancer. Hematol Oncol Clin North Am 16(3):671–700, 2002 12170575

Prigerson H, Jacobs S: Traumatic grief as a distinct disorder: a rationale, consensus criteria, and a preliminary empirical test, in Handbook of Bereavement Research: Consequences, Coping, and Care. Edited by Stroebe M, Hansson R, Stroebe W, et al. Washington, DC, American Psychological Association, 2001, pp 613–637

Prigerson HG, Horowitz MJ, Jacobs SC, et al: Prolonged grief disorder: psychometric validation of criteria proposed for DSM-V and ICD-11. PLoS Med 6(8):e1000121, 2009 19652695

Prommer E: Review article: dexmedetomidine: does it have potential in palliative medicine? Am J Hosp Palliat Care 28(4):276–283, 2011 21131636

Rabkin JG, Goetz RR, Remien RH, et al: Stability of mood despite HIV illness progression in a group of homosexual men. Am J Psychiatry 154(2):231–238, 1997 9016273

Rayner L, Price A, Evans A, et al: Antidepressants for the treatment of depression in palliative care: systematic review and meta-analysis. Palliat Med 25(1):36–51, 2011 20935027

Rietjens JA, van Zuylen L, van Veluw H, et al: Palliative sedation in a specialized unit for acute palliative care in a cancer hospital: comparing patients dying with and without palliative sedation. J Pain Symptom Manage 36(3):228–234, 2008 18411017

Ripamonti C, Filiberti A, Totis A, et al: Suicide among patients with cancer cared for at home by palliative-care teams. Lancet 354(9193):1877–1878, 1999 10584730

Robinson S, Kissane DW, Brooker J, et al: The relationship between poor quality of life and desire to hasten death: a multiple mediation model examining the contributions of depression, demoralization, loss of control, and low self-worth. J Pain Symptom Manage 53(2):243–249, 2017 27744017

Rodin G: Individual psychotherapy for the patient with advanced disease, in Handbook of Psychiatry in Palliative Medicine, 2nd Edition. Edited by Chochinov HM, Breitbart W. New York, Oxford University Press, 2009, pp 443–453

Rodin G, Zimmermann C, Rydall A, et al: The desire for hastened death in patients with metastatic cancer. J Pain Symptom Manage 33(6):661–675, 2007 17531909

Rosenfeld B, Breitbart W, Gibson C, et al: Desire for hastened death among patients with advanced AIDS. Psychosomatics 47(6):504–512, 2006 17116952

Rosenfeld B, Saracino R, Tobias K, et al: Adapting meaning-centered psychotherapy for the palliative care setting: results of a pilot study. Palliat Med 31(2):140–146, 2017 27435603

Roth AJ, Massie MJ: Anxiety in palliative care, in Handbook of Psychiatry in Palliative Medicine, 2nd Edition. Edited by Chochinov HM, Breitbart W. New York, Oxford University Press, 2009, pp 69–80

Ryan K, Leonard M, Guerin S, et al: Validation of the confusion assessment method in the palliative care setting. Palliat Med 23(1):40–55, 2009 19010967

Salt S, Mulvaney CA, Preston NJ: Drug therapy for symptoms associated with anxiety in adult palliative care patients. Cochrane Database Syst Rev (5):CD004596, 2017 28521070

Şenel G, Uysal N, Oguz G, et al: Delirium frequency and risk factors among patients with cancer in palliative care unit. Am J Hosp Palliat Care 34(3):282–286, 2017 26722008

Sepúlveda C, Marlin A, Yoshida T, et al: Palliative care: the World Health Organization's global perspective. J Pain Symptom Manage 24(2):91–96, 2002 12231124

Shear K, Frank E, Houck PR, et al: Treatment of complicated grief: a randomized controlled trial. JAMA 293(21):2601–2608, 2005 15928281

Shear MK, Reynolds CF 3rd, Simon NM, et al: Optimizing treatment of complicated grief: a randomized clinical trial. JAMA Psychiatry 73(7):685–694, 2016 27276373

Shuster JL Jr, Breitbart W, Chochinov HM; Ad Hoc Committee on End-of-Life Care. The Academy of Psychosomatic Medicine: Psychiatric aspects of excellent end-of-life care. Psychosomatics 40(1):1–4, 1999 9989115

Smith LA, Azariah F, Lavender VT, et al: Cannabinoids for nausea and vomiting in adults with cancer receiving chemotherapy. Cochrane Database Syst Rev (11):CD009464, 2015 26561338

Spencer RJ, Ray A, Pirl WF, Prigerson HG: Clinical correlates of suicidal thoughts in patients with advanced cancer. Am J Geriatr Psychiatry 20(4):327–336, 2012 21989317

Spiegel D, Bloom JR, Yalom I: Group support for patients with metastatic cancer. A randomized outcome study. Arch Gen Psychiatry 38(5):527–533, 1981 7235853

Steinhauser KE, Fitchett G, Handzo G, et al: State of the Science of Spirituality and Palliative Care Research Part I: Definitions and Taxonomy, Measurement, and Outcomes. J Pain Symptom Manage 54(17):428–440, 2017 28733252

Stiefel FC, Breitbart WS, Holland JC: Corticosteroids in cancer: neuropsychiatric complications. Cancer Invest 7(5):479–491, 1989 2695230

Stjernsward J, Clark D: Palliative medicine: a global perspective, in Oxford Textbook of Palliative Medicine, 3rd Edition. Edited by Doyle D, Hanks GWC, Cherny N, et al. New York, Oxford University Press, 2004, pp 1197–1224

Subcommittee on Psychiatric Aspects of Life-Sustaining Technology: The role of the psychiatrist in end-of-life treatment decisions, in Caring for the Dying: Identification and Promotion of Physician Competency (Educational Resource Document). Philadelphia, PA, American Board of Internal Medicine, 1996, pp 61–67

Sullivan DR, Mongue-Tchokote S, Mori M, et al: Randomized, double-blind, placebo-controlled study of methylphenidate for the treatment of depression in SSRI-treated cancer patients receiving palliative care. Psychooncology 26(11):1763–1769, 2017 27429350

Temel JS, Greer JA, Muzikansky A, et al: Early palliative care for patients with metastatic non-small-cell lung cancer. N Engl J Med 363(8):733–742, 2010 20818875

Ujeyl M, Müller-Oerlinghausen B: [Antidepressants for treatment of depression in palliative patients: a systematic literature review] [in German]. Schmerz 26(5):523–536, 2012 22968366

van der Lee ML, van der Bom JG, Swarte NB, et al: Euthanasia and depression: a prospective cohort study among terminally ill cancer patients. J Clin Oncol 23(27):6607–6612, 2005 16116147

van der Spek N, Vos J, van Uden-Kraan CF, et al: Efficacy of meaning-centered group psychotherapy for cancer survivors: a randomized controlled trial. Psychol Med 47(11):1990–2001, 2017 28374663

Viederman M: The supportive relationship, the psychodynamic life narrative, and the dying patient, in Handbook of Psychiatry in Palliative Medicine. Edited by Chochinov HM, Breitbart W. New York, Oxford University Press, 2000, pp 215–223

Vogl D, Rosenfeld B, Breitbart W, et al: Symptom prevalence, characteristics and distress in AIDS outpatients. J Pain Symptom Manage 18(4):253–262, 1999 10534965

Wang CW, Chow AY, Chan CL: The effects of life review interventions on spiritual well-being, psychological distress, and quality of life in patients with terminal or advanced cancer: a systematic review and meta-analysis of randomized controlled trials. Palliat Med 31(10):883–894, 2017 28488923

Weisman AD: On Dying and Denying: A Psychiatric Study of Terminality. New York, Behavioral Publications, 1972

Weissman DE: Decision making at a time of crisis near the end of life. JAMA 292(14):1738–1743, 2004 15479939

Wilson KG, Chochinov HM, de Faye BJ, et al: Diagnosis and management of depression in palliative care, in Handbook of Psychiatry in Palliative Medicine. Edited by Chochinov HM, Breitbart W. New York, Oxford University Press, 2000, pp 25–49

Wilson KG, Chochinov HM, Skirko MG, et al: Depression and anxiety disorders in palliative cancer care. J Pain Symptom Manage 33(2):118–129, 2007 17280918

Wilson KG, Lander M, Chochinov HM: Diagnosis and management of depression in palliative care, in Handbook of Psychiatry in Palliative Medicine, 2nd Edition. Edited by Chochinov HM, Breitbart W. New York, Oxford University Press, 2009, pp 39–68

Wilson KG, Dalgleish TL, Chochinov HM, et al: Mental disorders and the desire for death in patients receiving palliative care for cancer. BMJ Support Palliat Care 6(2):170–177, 2016 24644212

Winegarden J, Carr DB, Bradshaw YS: Intravenous ketamine for rapid opioid dose reduction, reversal of opioid-induced neurotoxicity, and pain control in terminal care: case report and literature review. Pain Med 17(4):644–649, 2016 26234740

World Health Organization: Definition of palliative care. 2017. Available at: http://www.who.int/cancer/palliative/definition/en/. Accessed October 20, 2017.

Zhang B, El-Jawahri A, Prigerson HG: Update on bereavement research: evidence-based guidelines for the diagnosis and treatment of complicated bereavement. J Palliat Med 9(5):1188–1203, 2006 17040157

Zhong BL, Li SH, Lv SY, et al: Suicidal ideation among Chinese cancer inpatients of general hospitals: prevalence and correlates. Oncotarget 8(15):25141–25150, 2017 28212579

Zisook S, Shuchter SR, Lv SY, et al: Depression through the first year after the death of a spouse. Am J Psychiatry 148(10):1346–1352, 1991 1897615

Zisook S, Shuchter SR, Sledge PA, et al: The spectrum of depressive phenomena after spousal bereavement. J Clin Psychiatry 55 (suppl):29–36, 1994 8077167

Index

*Page numbers printed in **boldface** type refer to tables or figures.*

Glycopyrrolate
  anticholinergic effects of, **1215**
  for organophosphate poisoning, **1143,
    1160**
GnRH agonists. *See* Gonadotropin-releasing
  hormone agonists
Go/no-go task, 8
Gold, **701**
  for rheumatoid arthritis, 684
Gonadal disorders, 610–611
  polycystic ovary syndrome, 610
  premenstrual disorders and menopause,
    993, **994**
  testosterone deficiency, 610–611
Gonadotropin-releasing hormone (GnRH)
  agonists
  depression induced by, 198
  for endometriosis, 980
  for inappropriate sexual behavior, 421
  sexual effects of, **406, 412**
"Good death," 1299–1300
Graded exercise therapy (GET)
  in chronic fatigue syndrome, 722, 727,
    728–729, **1273**, 1275
  in fibromyalgia syndrome, 722, 727,
    728–729
  in somatic symptom disorder/illness
    anxiety disorder, 314
Graft-versus-host disease, 648
Granulomatosis with polyangiitis, 696, 700
Grapefruit juice–drug interactions, 491, 1211
Graves' disease, 602, 603
Grief, 1298, 1314–1317. *See also* Bereavement
  anticipatory, 1304, 1315
  clinical presentations of, 1314–1315
  complicated, 1314, 1315, 1316
    risk factors for, 1316
    after spontaneous abortion, 974, 975
    therapy for, 1317
  after death of child, 1018
    perinatal, 985
  definitions related to, 1314
  depression and, 193, 194, 1316
    in HIV disease, 753
    interpersonal therapy for, 1266
    in palliative care settings, 1304
  integrated, 1314
  pathological, 1314
  prolonged, 1314, 1315
  psychiatric disorders and, 1316
  related to child custody decisions, 988

  as response to medical illness, 9, 69, 71
    diabetes, 1037
    systemic lupus erythematosus, 692
  after spinal cord injury, 1073–1074, 1089
  suicidality and, 234
  therapies for, 1316–1317, **1318**
  time course of, 1315
  transplant surgery and, 866
  traumatic, 1315–1316
  uncomplicated, 1314
Group psychotherapy.
    See also Support groups
  for anxiety, 293, 294
  in bulimia nervosa, 363
  in cancer, 642, 649, 650, 1277, **1278,** 1303
  in chronic fatigue syndrome, 729
  in chronic obstructive pulmonary disease,
    515
  for depression, 207–208
    in diabetes, 596
    in end-stage renal disease, 574
    in HIV disease, 754
  for dissociative seizures, 935
  in heart disease, 484
  in hemophilia, 667
  for infertile patients, 969
  in inflammatory bowel disease, 541
  for migraine patients, 1114
  mindfulness-based stress reduction,
    1269–1270
  in palliative care settings
    grief therapy, 1317, **1318**
    meaning-centered psychotherapy,
      1322, 1323
  in psoriasis, 797
  in sickle cell disease, 667
  in somatic symptom disorder, 316
  supportive–expressive, 1265
    in cancer, 1277, 1303
  for transplant patients and families, 869
  in traumatic brain injury, 1087, 1088
  in urticaria, 799
Growth hormone (GH)
  acromegaly and, 608
  in anorexia nervosa, 362
  Creutzfeldt-Jakob disease and, 761
  deficiency of, after traumatic brain injury,
    1085
  gamma-hydroxybutyrate and, 455
GSH (glutathione), in acetaminophen
  overdose, 1146

Mallory-Weiss tears, 355
Malnutrition/nutritional deficiencies.
    See also Dietary factors
    acetaminophen toxicity and, 1147
    burning mouth syndrome and, 529
    catatonia and, 272
    chronic kidney disease and, 423, 575, 576
    cystic fibrosis and, 1029
    delirium and
        in cancer, 633
        in transplant patients, 883
    eating disorders and, 346, 347, 348, 349,
        350, 355, 357, 367, 790
        avoidant/restrictive food intake
            disorder, 343
        depression and, 347
        dermatological disorders and, 790
        differential diagnosis of, 351–353
        gastrointestinal disorders and, 355
        obsessive-compulsive disorder and, 348
    examination for, 12, **13**
    fatigue in terminally ill patients and, 1319
    fertility and, 968
    functional dysphagia and, 533
    HIV disease and, 752, 753
    inflammatory bowel disease and, 539
    iron deficiency anemia, 659–661, 674
    neuroleptic malignant syndrome and, 1202
    niacin deficiency, **256, 262,** 613
    pediatric feeding disorders and, 1021
        pica, 1024
        rumination disorder, 1025
    psychosis and, **256**
    substance use disorders and, 353, **437**
        alcohol, 443, 575
    thiamine deficiency, 135, 144, **256, 437**
        eating disorders and, 356
        Wernicke's encephalopathy and, 259,
            356, 443, 613, 922–923
    vitamin B$_6$ deficiency, 613
    vitamin B$_{12}$ deficiency, 661–663
    vitamin D deficiency, 919
    vitamin E deficiency, 613
Malpractice claims, 25, 28, 45–47
    factitious disorders and, 330
    four *D*s of, 46
    physicians' fear of, 46
Manganese
    hepatic encephalopathy and, 550
    "manganese madness," 1156
    toxicity of, 1153, 1155–1156

Mania. *See also* Bipolar disorder; Hypomania
    aggression and, 172
    "Bell's," 266
    bipolar disorder and, 260, 261
    cancer and, 633
    complementary medicines and
        S-adenosyl-L-methionine, **1228**
        ginseng, **1225**
        ma huang, **1226**
        St. John's wort, **1226**
    after deep brain stimulation for
        Parkinson's disease, 949
    delirious, 91, 260, 261, 266
    dementia and, 263
    drug-induced, 260, **262**
        antimicrobial agents, **768**
        antiretroviral agents, **769**
        corticosteroids, 264, 519, 633, 694, **697,**
            700, 701, **701**
        decongestants and related drugs, 1158
        fertility-enhancing drugs, 968
        hydroxychloroquine, **701**
        interferon, 549, **630**
        psychostimulants, 260
    endocrine disorders and, 263
        adrenal insufficiency, 607
        Cushing's syndrome, 606
        hyperthyroidism, 602
    epilepsy and, 263
    infectious diseases and, 263
        cryptococcal meningitis, 762
        dengue, 758
        HIV disease, 263, 264, 755
        leptospirosis, 746
        Lyme disease, 744
        measles, 759
        neurosyphilis, 134, 743
        postencephalitis syndromes, 760
        viral encephalitis, 757
    leukodystrophies and, 926
    multiple sclerosis and, 920
    neurodegenerative diseases and, 263
    perioperative, 824
    postpartum, 260
    poststroke, 261, 913
    rating scale for, 261
    sarcoidosis and, 517
    secondary, 249, 260–265
        clinical features of, 260
        course and prognosis for, 260
        diagnosis/assessment of, **254,** 260–261

Neuropathy *(continued)*
  thiamine deficiency and, 613
  toxin-induced
    arsenic, 1155
    inhalants, 1150
    insecticides, 1151, 1152
    lead, 1154
    thallium, 1155
  vitamin B$_{12}$ deficiency and, 662
  Wernicke-Korsakoff syndrome and, 923
Neuropsychiatric Inventory (NPI), 139
Neuropsychological testing, 15, 17, 19
  in aggression, 178
  in dementia, 139
  in diabetes, 601
  in factitious disorders, 324
  in hepatic encephalopathy, 551, 884
  in HIV-associated neurocognitive
      disorder, 751
  in Lyme disease, 745
  in malingering, 1168
  in multiple sclerosis, 919
  in rehabilitation settings, 1055
  after spinal cord injury, 1077
  in systemic lupus erythematosus, 694
  after traumatic brain injury, 1060, 1069,
      1077
Neurosarcoidosis, 516–517
Neurosurgical issues, 945–949
  assessment of fitness for surgery, 948–949
    epilepsy surgery, 948
    Parkinson's disease surgery, 948–949
  brain tumors, 945–946
  hydrocephalus, 946–947
  subarachnoid hemorrhage, 948
  subdural hematoma, 947
Neurosyphilis, 743. *See also* Syphilis
  autoenucleation and, 845
  dementia and, **124,** 128, 134, 927
  mania and, **262,** 263
  meningeal, 743
  meningovascular, 743
  parenchymatous, 743
  psychosis and, 253, **255**
  rheumatological disorders and, 700
Neurotic defenses, 64, **65**
Neuroticism
  eating disorders and, 353
  functional dyspepsia and, 538
  functional gastrointestinal disorders and,
      528

functional heartburn and, 531
hyperventilation and, 518
irritable bowel syndrome and, 544
posttraumatic stress disorder in cardiac
    disease and, 472
rheumatoid arthritis and, 688
Neurotransmitters.
    See also specific neurotransmitters
  in Alzheimer's disease, 130
  in delirium, 102
  in Parkinson's disease, 286, 1242
  in premenstrual dysphoric disorder, 993
  in traumatic brain injury, 1059, 1069, 1084
Neutrality of therapist, 7
Neutropenia
  benign ethnic, 671, 1207
  cancer and, 632
  drug-induced
    antipsychotics, 669, 1207
    carbamazepine, 673
    gabapentin, **670**
    lamotrigine, **670,** 1199
    valproate, 673, 1199
  mucormycosis and, 763
Nevirapine, **769**
NHANES (National Health and Nutrition
    Examination Survey), 468, 1031–1032
NIA (National Institute on Aging), 144
Niacin (nicotinic acid) deficiency, 135, **256,**
    262, 613
NICE. *See* National Institute for Health and
    Care Excellence guidelines
Nicergoline, 151
Nicotine, 449, 452–453.
    See also Smoking/tobacco use
  asking patient about use of, 438
  bariatric surgery and, 842
  drug interactions with, 452
  in e-cigarettes, 452
  insomnia and, 396
  restless legs syndrome and, 394
  withdrawal from, 452
    discharges against medical advice due
        to, 43
    head and neck cancers and, 646
    symptoms of, 168, 452
Nicotine replacement therapy (NRT), 76,
    452–453
  drug interactions with, 453
    bupropion, 877, 1192
  before transplant surgery, 877

Paliperidone
  adverse effects of
    breast cancer risk, 1245
    cardiac effects, 1205
    extrapyramidal symptoms, 1201
    hyperprolactinemia, 609, 1206
    hypotension, 1205
    sedation, 1202
    seizures, 1201
    weight gain, 1206
  alternative administration routes for, 1219
  in hepatic disease, 1231
  toxicity/overdose of, 1208
Palliative care, 1297–1325. *See also* Hospice care
  for anxiety disorders and posttraumatic
      stress disorder, 1300–1303
    assessment, 1301–1302
    nonpharmacological treatment,
        1302–1303
    pharmacological treatment, 1302
    prevalence, 1300–1301
  bereavement and, 1313–1317
    anticipatory grief, 1315
    clinical presentations of grief, 1314–1315
    definitions relevant to, 1314
    grief therapies, 1316–1317, **1318**
    psychiatric disorders and, 1316
    traumatic grief, 1315–1316
  caregiver distress and, 1317
  components of and practice guidelines for,
      1299
  culture, ethnicity and, 1313
  for delirium, 1309–1312
    assessment and reversibility in
        terminally ill, 1310–1311
    experience for patients, families, and
        staff, 1310
    management controversies, 1312
    nonpharmacological treatment, 1311
    pharmacological treatment, 1311
    prevalence, 1309
  for depression, 1303–1306
    assessment, 1304–1305
    epidemiology, 1303–1304
    nonpharmacological treatment, 1306
    pharmacological treatment, 1305–1306
  doctor–patient communication and, 1313
  in end-stage renal disease, 580
  evolving definitions of, 1298–1299
  "good death" and, 1299
    role of psychiatrist, 1300

  history of, 1298
  models of care delivery for, 1299
  psychotherapy in, 1320–1324, **1322**
    cognitive-behavioral therapy, 1321
    existential therapies, 1321–1324
      dignity-conserving care, 1323–1324,
          1324
      meaning-centered psychotherapy,
          1323
      narrative approaches, 1321, 1323
    insight-oriented psychotherapy,
        1321
    therapeutic stance for, 1321
  for specific symptoms, 1319–1320
    anorexia and weight loss, 1319
    fatigue, 1319–1320
    nausea and vomiting, 1320
    pain, 1319
  spiritual needs and, 1313
  for suicidality and despair, 1306–1309
    demoralization, 1308
    desire for hastened death, 1308
    interventions for despair at end of life,
        1309
Palliative care Outcome Scale (POS), 1305
Pancreas transplantation, 859
Pancreatic cancer, 55, 230, 553–554, 626,
    642–643
Pancreatitis
  drug-induced, **436,** 553, 1232
    anticonvulsants, 264, 553, 1198
    antidepressants, 553
    antipsychotics, 553, 1207
  pharmacokinetics in, 1182, 1233
  surgery in patients with alcohol use
      disorder and, 828
  trichotillomania and, 787
Pancytopenia
  factitious, **327**
  lamotrigine-induced, **670**
PANDAS (pediatric autoimmune
    neuropsychiatric disorder associated
    with streptococcal infection), 737,
    739–740, 939
Panic attacks, 283
  asthma and, 1030
  atypical chest pain and, 483
  brain tumors and, 946
  vs. chronic fatigue syndrome, 723
  conversion disorder and, 943
  coronary artery disease and, 479